Cons... Compatibility Chart

	Hydroxyzine	Meperidine	Metoclopramide	Midazolam	Morphine	Nalbu.	Penta.	Pento.	Perph.	Proc.	Prom.	Pron.	Ran.	Sco.	Secobarbital	Thiethylperazine
	C	C	C	C	C	C	C	C	C	C	C	C	C	C	I	
Phyllis																
Associat																
Saint Xa	C	C	C	C	C		C	I	C	C		C		C	I	C
School	C	C	C	C	C		C	I	C	C	C	C	C	C	I	
Chicago							I								I	
Jean K	I	I	I		I	I	I	I	I	I	I	I		I	I	I
A.R.N.P.	I	C	C	I	C		C	I	C	I	I	I	C	C	I	
Associa	C	C	C	C	C		C	I	C	C	C	C	C	C	I	
Univers	C	C	C		C	C	C	I	C	C	C	C		C	I	
Cent	C	C	C		C		C	I	C	C	C	C	C	C	I	
Colleg (Pha	C	C			C		I	I		C	C	C	C	C	I	
Omaha		I			I		I					I				
Barba		I			I		I					I				
Instru	■	C	C		C	C	C	I		C	C	C	I	C	I	
Schoo Sandu	C	■	C		I		C	I	C	C	C	C	C	C	I	
Marc	C	C	■		C		C		C	C	C	C	C	C	I	
Clinic	C		C	■	C	C		I	I	I	C	C	I	C		C
Clini Univ	C	I	C		■		C	I	C	C	C	C	C	C	I	
M	C					■		I		C		*	C	C	I	C
Dep Char	C	C	C		C		■	I	C	C	C	C	C	C	I	
	I	I			I	I	I	■	I	I	I	I		C	I	
Cor Ass		C	C		C		C	I	■		C		C	C	C	I
Niai C	C	C	C		C	C	C	I	C	■		C	C	C	C	I
San	C	C	C		C		C	I		C	■		C		C	I
	C	C	C		C	C	C	I	C	C	C	■	C	C	I	
Jud c.c		C	C	I	C	C	C		C	C		C	■		C		C
Cli	C	C	C		C	C	C	C	C	C	C	C	C	■		I
Un	I	I	I		I	I	I	I	I	I	I	I	I		I	■	I
Sa						C			I					C		I	

Parenteral compatibility occurs when two or more drugs are successfully mixed without liquefaction, deliquescence, or precipitation.

x   **Contents**

Individual drugs, 67

Appendixes

M I

A Harcourt

Editor-in-(
Editor-in-(
N. Darl
Senior de
Dana L
Project m
Designer:

Mosb
A Ha
1183(
St. L

ISSN
ISBN

(

ALPHA-ADRENERGIC BLOCKERS

Action: Acts by binding to α-adrenergic receptors, causing dilation of peripheral blood vessels. Lowers peripheral resistance, resulting in decreased blood pressure.

Uses: Used for pheochromocytoma, prevention of tissue necrosis and sloughing associated with extravasation of IV vasopressors.

Side effects/adverse reactions: The most common side effects are hypotension, tachycardia, nasal stuffiness, nausea, vomiting, and diarrhea.

Contraindications: Hypersensitive reactions may occur, and allergies should be identified before these products are given. Patients with myocardial infarction, coronary insufficiency, angina, or other evidence of coronary artery disease should not use these products.

Pharmacokinetics: Onset, peak, and duration vary among products.

Interactions: Vasoconstrictive and hypertensive effects of epinephrine are antagonized by α-adrenergic blockers.

Possible nursing diagnoses:
- Altered tissue perfusion *[uses]*
- Risk for injury *[adverse reactions]*
- Sleep pattern disturbance *[adverse reactions]*

NURSING CONSIDERATIONS

Assess:
- Electrolytes: K, Na, Cl, CO_2
- Weight daily, I&O
- B/P lying, standing before starting treatment, q4h thereafter
- Nausea, vomiting, diarrhea
- Skin turgor, dryness of mucous membranes for hydration status

Administer:
- Starting with low dose, gradually increasing to prevent side effects
- With food or milk for GI symptoms

Evaluate:
- Therapeutic response: decreased B/P, increased peripheral pulses

Teach patient/family:
- To avoid alcoholic beverages
- To report dizziness, palpitations, fainting
- To change position slowly or fainting may occur
- To take drug exactly as prescribed
- To avoid all OTC products (cough, cold, allergy) unless directed by prescriber

---

Generic names

phenoxybenzamine   phentolamine

ANESTHETICS—GENERAL/LOCAL

Action: Anesthetics (general) act on the CNS to produce tranquilization and sleep before invasive procedures. Anesthetics (local) inhibit conduction of nerve impulses from sensory nerves.

Uses: General anesthetics are used to premedicate for surgery, induction and maintenance in general anesthesia. For local anesthetics, refer to individual product listing for indications.

Side effects/adverse reactions: The most common side effects are dystonia, akathisia, flexion of arms, fine tremors, drowsiness, restlessness, and hypotension. Also common are chills, respiratory depression, and laryngospasm.

Contraindications: Persons with CVA, increased intracranial pressure, severe hypertension, cardiac decompensation should not use these products, since severe adverse reactions can occur.

Precautions: Anesthetics (general) should be used with caution in the elderly, cardiovascular disease (hypotension, bradydysrhythmias), renal disease, liver disease, Parkinson's disease, children <2 yr. The precaution for anesthetics (local) is pregnancy.

Pharmacokinetics: Onset, peak, and duration vary widely among products. Most products are metabolized in the liver and excreted in urine.

Interactions: MAOIs, tricyclics, phenothiazines may cause severe hypotension or hypertension when used with local anesthetics. CNS depressants will potentiate general and local anesthetics.

Possible nursing diagnoses:

General:
• Risk for injury *[adverse reactions]*
• Knowledge deficit *[teaching]*

Local:
• Pain *[uses]*
• Knowledge deficit *[teaching]*

NURSING CONSIDERATIONS

Assess:
• VS q10min during IV administration, q30min after IM dose

Administer:
• Anticholinergic preoperatively to decrease secretions
• Only with crash cart, resuscitative equipment nearby

Perform/provide:
• Quiet environment for recovery to decrease psychotic symptoms

Evaluate:
• Therapeutic response: maintenance of anesthesia, decreased pain

Generic names (Injectables only)

General anesthetics
droperidol
etomidate
fentanyl
fentanyl/droperidol
fentanyl transdermal
ketamine
methohexital
midazolam
procaine
thiopental

Local anesthetics
chloroprocaine
etidocaine
lidocaine
mepivacaine
propofol
ropivacaine
tetracaine

ANTACIDS

Action: Antacids are basic compounds that neutralize gastric acidity and decrease the rate of gastric emptying. Products are divided into those containing aluminum, magnesium, calcium, or a combination of these.

Uses: Hyperacidity is decreased by antacids in conditions such as peptic ulcer disease, reflux esophagitis, gastritis, and hiatal hernia.

Side effects/adverse reactions: The most common side effect caused by aluminum-containing antacids is constipation, which may lead to fecal impaction and bowel obstruction. Diarrhea occurs often when magnesium products are given. Alkalosis may occur when systemic products are used. Constipation occurs more frequently than laxation with calcium carbonate. The release of CO_2 from carbonate-containing antacids causes belching, abdominal distention, and flatulence. Sodium bicarbonate may act as a systemic antacid and produce systemic electrolyte disturbances and alkalosis. Calcium carbonate and sodium bicarbonate may cause rebound hyperacidity and milk-alkali syndrome. Alkaluria may occur when products are used on a long-term basis, particularly in persons with abnormal renal function.

Contraindications: Sensitivity to aluminum or magnesium products may cause hypersensitive reactions. Aluminum products should not be used by persons sensitive to aluminum; magnesium products should not be used by persons sensitive to magnesium. Check for sensitivity before administering.

Precautions: Magnesium products should be given cautiously to patients with renal insufficiency and during pregnancy and lactation. Sodium content of antacids may be significant; use with caution for patients with hypertension, CHF, or those on a low-sodium diet.

Pharmacokinetics: Duration is 20-40 min. If ingested 1 hr after meals, acidity is reduced for at least 3 hr.

Interactions: Drugs whose effects may be increased by some antacids: quinidine, amphetamines, pseudoephedrine, levodopa, valproic acid, dicumarol. Drugs whose effects may be decreased by some antacids: cimetadine, corticosteroids, ranitidine, iron salts, phenothiazines, phenytoin, digoxin, tetracyclines, ketoconazole, salicylates, isoniazid.

Possible nursing diagnoses:

• Pain *[uses]*

• Constipation *[adverse reactions]*

• Diarrhea *[adverse reactions]*

NURSING CONSIDERATIONS

Assess:

• Aggravating and alleviating factors of epigastric pain or hyperacidity; identify the location, duration, and characteristics of epigastric pain

• GI symptoms, including constipation, diarrhea, abdominal pain; if severe abdominal pain with fever occurs, these drugs should not be given

• Renal symptoms, including increasing urinary pH, electrolytes

Administer:

• All products with an 8-oz glass of water to ensure absorption in the stomach

• Another antacid if constipation occurs with aluminum products

Evaluate:

• The therapeutic effectiveness of the drug; absence of epigastric pain and decreased acidity should occur

Teach patient/family:

• Not to take other drugs within 1-2 hr of antacid administration, since antacids may impair absorption of other drugs

---

Generic names

aluminum hydroxide
bismuth subsalicylate
calcium carbonate
dihydroxyaluminum

magaldrate
magnesium oxide
sodium bicarbonate

ANTIANGINALS

Action: The antianginals are divided into the nitrates, calcium channel blockers, and β-adrenergic blockers. The nitrates dilate coronary arteries, causing decreased preload, and dilate systemic arteries, causing decreased afterload. Calcium channel blockers dilate coronary arteries, decrease SA/AV node conduction. β-Adrenergic blockers decrease heart rate so that myocardial O_2 use is decreased. Dipyridamole selectively dilates coronary arteries to increase coronary blood flow.

Uses: Antianginals are used in chronic stable angina pectoris, unstable angina, vasospastic angina. Some (i.e., calcium channel blockers and β-blockers) may be used for dysrhythmias and in hypertension.

Side effects/adverse reactions: The most common side effects are postural hypotension, headache, flushing, dizziness, nausea, edema, and drowsiness. Also common are rash, dysrhythmias, and fatigue.

Contraindications: Persons with known hypersensitivity, increased intracranial pressure, or cerebral hemorrhage should not use some of these products.

Precautions: Antianginals should be used with caution in postural hypotension, pregnancy, lactation, children, renal disease, and hepatic injury.

Pharmacokinetics: Onset, peak, and duration vary widely among coronary products. Most products are metabolized in the liver and excreted in urine.

Interactions: Please check individual monographs, since interactions vary widely among products.

Possible nursing diagnoses:
- Altered tissue perfusion: cardiopulmonary *[uses]*
- Pain *[uses]*
- Risk for injury *[uses]*
- Knowledge deficit *[teaching]*
- Decreased cardiac output *[adverse reactions]*

NURSING CONSIDERATIONS
Assess:
- Orthostatic B/P, pulse
- Pain: duration, time started, activity being performed, character
- Tolerance if taken over long period
- Headache, light-headedness, decreased B/P; may indicate a need for decreased dosage

Perform/provide:
- Storage protected from light, moisture; place in cool environment

Evaluate:
- Therapeutic response: decrease, prevention of anginal pain

Teach patient/family:
- To keep tabs in original container
- Not to use OTC products unless directed by prescriber
- To report bradycardia, dizziness, confusion, depression, fever
- To take pulse at home, advise when to notify prescriber
- To avoid alcohol, smoking, sodium intake
- To comply with weight control, dietary adjustments, modified exercise program
- To carry Medic Alert ID to identify drug that you are taking, allergies
- To make position changes slowly to prevent fainting

Generic names

Nitrates
amyl nitrite
erythrityl
isosorbide
nitroglycerin
pentaerythritol

β-*Adrenergic blockers*
atenolol
dipyridamole
metoprolol

nadolol
propranolol

Calcium channel blockers
amlodipine
bepridil
diltiazem
nicardipine
nifedipine
verapamil

ANTICHOLINERGICS

Action: Anticholinergics inhibit the muscarinic actions of acetylcholine at receptor sites in the autonomic nervous system; anticholinergics are also known as antimuscarinic drugs.

Uses: Anticholinergics are used for a variety of conditions: gastrointestinal anticholinergics are used to decrease motility (smooth muscle tone) in the GI, biliary, and urinary tracts and for their ability to decrease gastric secretions (propantheline, glycopyrrolate); decreasing involuntary movements in parkinsonism (benztropine, trihexyphenidyl); bradydysrhythmias (atropine); nausea and vomiting (scopolamine); and as cycloplegic mydriatics (atropine, hematropine, scopolamine, cyclopentolate, tropicamide).

Side effects/adverse reactions: The most common side effects are dry mouth, constipation, urinary retention, urinary hesitancy, headache, and dizziness. Also common is paralytic ileus.

Contraindications: Persons with narrow-angle glaucoma, myasthenia gravis, or GI/GU obstruction should not use some of these products.

Precautions: Anticholinergics should be used with caution in patients who are elderly, pregnant, or lactating or in those with prostatic hypertrophy, CHF, or hypertension; use with caution in presence of high environmental temp.

Pharmacokinetics: Onset, peak, and duration vary widely among products. Most products are metabolized in the liver and excreted in urine.

Interactions: Increased anticholinergic effects may occur when used with MAOIs and tricyclic antidepressants and amantadine. Anticholinergics may cause a decreased effect of phenothiazines and levodopa.

Possible nursing diagnoses:
- Decreased cardiac output [uses]
- Constipation [adverse reactions]
- Knowledge deficit [teaching]

NURSING CONSIDERATIONS
Assess:
- I&O ratio; retention commonly causes decreased urinary output
- Urinary hesitancy, retention; palpate bladder if retention occurs
- Constipation; increase fluids, bulk, exercise if this occurs
- For tolerance over long-term therapy, dose may need to be increased or changed
- Mental status: affect, mood, CNS depression, worsening of mental symptoms during early therapy

Administer:
- Parenteral dose with patient recumbent to prevent postural hypotension
- With or after meals to prevent GI upset; may give with fluids other than water
- Parenteral dose slowly; keep in bed for at least 1 hr after dose; monitor vital signs
- After checking dose carefully; even slight overdose can lead to toxicity

Perform/provide:
- Storage at room temp
- Hard candy, frequent drinks, sugarless gum to relieve dry mouth

Evaluate:
- Therapeutic response: decreased secretions, absence of nausea and vomiting

Teach patient/family:

• To avoid driving or other hazardous activities; drowsiness may occur
• To avoid OTC medication: cough, cold preparations with alcohol, antihistamines unless directed by prescriber

---

Generic names

atropine
belladonna alkaloids
benztropine
biperiden
clidinium
cyclopentolate (Appx C)
dicyclomine
glycopyrrolate
homatropine (Appx C)
hyoscyamine

mepenzolate
methantheline
methscopolamine
procyclidine
propantheline
scopolamine
scopolamine (transdermal)
trihexyphenidyl
tropicamide (Appx C)

ANTICOAGULANTS

Action: Anticoagulants interfere with blood clotting by preventing clot formation.

Uses: Anticoagulants are used for deep-vein thrombosis, pulmonary emboli, myocardial infarction, open-heart surgery, disseminated intravascular clotting syndrome, atrial fibrillation with embolization, transfusion, and dialysis.

Side effects/adverse reactions: The most serious adverse reactions are hemorrhage, agranulocytosis, leukopenia, eosinophilia, and thrombocytopenia, depending on the specific product. The most common side effects are diarrhea, rash, and fever.

Contraindications: Persons with hemophilia, leukemia with bleeding, peptic ulcer disease, thrombocytopenic purpura, blood dyscrasias, acute nephritis, and subacute bacterial endocarditis should not use these products.

Precautions: Anticoagulants should be used with caution in alcoholism, elderly, and pregnancy.

Pharmacokinetics: Onset, peak, and duration vary widely among products. Most products are metabolized in the liver and excreted in urine.

Interactions: Salicylates, steroids, and nonsteroidal antiinflammatories will potentiate the action of anticoagulants. Anticoagulants may cause serious effects; please check individual monographs.

Possible nursing diagnoses:
• Altered tissue perfusion *[uses]*
• Risk for injury *[side effects]*
• Knowledge deficit *[teaching]*

NURSING CONSIDERATIONS
Assess:
• Blood studies (Hct, platelets, occult blood in stools) q3mo
• Partial prothrombin time, which should be 1½-2 × control PPT qd, also APTT, ACT
• B/P, watch for increasing signs of hypertension
• Bleeding gums, petechiae, ecchymosis; black, tarry stools; hematuria
• Fever, skin rash, urticaria
• Needed dosage change q1-2wk

Administer:
• At same time each day to maintain steady blood levels
• Do not massage area or aspirate when giving SC injection; give in abdomen between pelvic bone, rotate sites; do not pull back on plunger, leave in for 10 sec; apply gentle pressure for 1 min
• Without changing needles
• Avoiding all IM injections that may cause bleeding

Perform/provide:
• Storage in tight container

Evaluate:
• Therapeutic response: decrease of deep-vein thrombosis

Teach patient/family:
• To avoid OTC preparations that may cause serious drug interactions unless directed by prescriber
• That drug may be held during active bleeding (menstruation), depending on condition
• To use soft-bristle toothbrush to avoid bleeding gums, avoid contact sports, use electric razor
• To carry a Medic Alert ID identifying drug taken
• To report any signs of bleeding: gums, under skin, urine, stools

---

Generic names

ardeparin (Appx A)	heparin
dalteparin	lepirudin
danaparoid	warfarin
enoxaparin	

ANTICONVULSANTS

Action: Anticonvulsants are divided into the barbiturates (p. 35), benzodiazepines (p. 37), hydantoins, succinimides, and miscellaneous products. Barbiturates and benzodiazepines are discussed in separate sections. Hydantoins act by inhibiting the spread of seizure activity in the motor cortex. Succinimides act by inhibiting spike and wave formation; they also decrease amplitude, frequency, duration, and spread of discharge in seizures.

Uses: Hydantoins are used in generalized tonic-clonic seizures, status epilepticus, and psychomotor seizures. Succinimides are used for absence (petit mal) seizures. Barbiturates are used in generalized tonic-clonic and cortical focal seizures.

Side effects/adverse reactions: Bone marrow depression is the most life-threatening adverse reaction associated with hydantoins or succinimides. The most common side effects are GI symptoms. Other common side effects for hydantoins are gingival hyperplasia and CNS effects such as nystagmus, ataxia, slurred speech, and mental confusion.

Contraindications: Hypersensitive reactions may occur, and allergies should be identified before these products are given.

Precautions: Persons with renal or hepatic disease should be watched closely.

Pharmacokinetics: Onset, peak, and duration vary widely among products. Most products are metabolized in the liver and excreted in urine, bile, and feces.

Interactions: Decreased effects of estrogens, oral contraceptives (hydantoins).

Possible nursing diagnoses:
- Risk for injury *[uses]*
- Noncompliance *[teaching]*
- Sleep pattern disturbance *[adverse reactions]*

NURSING CONSIDERATIONS
Assess:
- Renal function studies, including BUN, creatinine, serum uric acid, urine creatinine clearance before and during therapy
- Blood studies: RBC, Hct, Hgb, reticulocyte counts qwk for 4 wk then qmo
- Hepatic studies: AST (SGOT), ALT (SGPT), bilirubin, creatinine
- Mental status, including mood, sensorium, affect, behavorial changes; if mental status changes, notify prescriber
- Eye problems, including need for ophthalmic exam before, during, and after treatment (slit lamp, fundoscopy, tonometry)

• Allergic reactions, including red, raised rash; if this occurs, drug should be discontinued
• Blood dyscrasia, including fever, sore throat, bruising, rash, jaundice
• Toxicity, including bone marrow depression, nausea, vomiting, ataxia, diplopia, cardiovascular collapse, Stevens-Johnson syndrome

Administer:
• With food, milk to decrease GI symptoms

Perform/provide:
• Good oral hygiene is important for hydantoins

Evaluate:
• Therapeutic response, including decreased seizure activity; document on patient's chart

Teach patient/family:
• To carry ID card or Medic Alert bracelet stating drugs taken, condition, prescriber's name, phone number
• To avoid driving, other activities that require alertness

Generic names

Hydantoins
ethotoin
fosphenytoin
mephenytoin
phensuximide
phenytoin

Succinimides
ethosuximide
methsuximide
phensuximide

Miscellaneous
acetazolamide
carbamazepine

clonazepam
diazepam
felbamate
gabapentin
lamotrigine
magnesium sulfate
paraldehyde
paramethadione
phenacemide
phenobarbital
primidone
tiagabine (Appx A)
topiramate
trimethadione
valproate/valproic acid,
   divalproex sodium

ANTIDEPRESSANTS

Action: Antidepressants are divided into the tricyclics, MAOIs, and miscellaneous antidepressants. The tricyclics work by blocking reuptake of norepinephrine and serotonin into nerve endings and increasing action of norepinephrine and serotonin in nerve cells. MAOIs act by increasing concentrations of endogenous epinephrine, norepinephrine, serotonin, dopamine in storage sites in CNS by inhibition of MAO; increased concentration reduces depression.

Uses: Antidepressants are used for depression and in some cases enuresis in children.

Side effects/adverse reactions: The most serious adverse reactions are paralytic ileus, acute renal failure, hypertension, and hypertensive crisis, depending on the specific product. Common side effects are dizziness, drowsiness, diarrhea, dry mouth, retention, and orthostatic hypotension.

Contraindications: The contraindications to antidepressants are convulsive disorders, prostatic hypertrophy, severe renal, hepatic, cardiac disease depending on the type of medication.

Precautions: Antidepressants should be used cautiously in suicidal patients, severe depression, schizophrenia, hyperactivity, diabetes mellitus, pregnancy, and the elderly.

Pharmacokinetics: Onset, peak, and duration vary widely among products. Most products are metabolized in the liver and excreted in urine.

Interactions: Please check individual monographs, since interactions vary widely among products.

Possible nursing diagnoses:
- Ineffective individual coping [uses]
- Risk for injury [uses/adverse reactions]
- Knowledge deficit [teaching]

NURSING CONSIDERATIONS
Assess:
- B/P (lying, standing), pulse q4h; if systolic B/P drops 20 mm Hg, hold drug, notify prescriber; take vital signs q4h in patients with cardiovascular disease
- Blood studies: CBC, leukocytes, differential, cardiac enzymes if patient is receiving long-term therapy
- Hepatic studies: AST (SGOT), ALT (SGPT), bilirubin, creatinine
- Weight qwk; appetite may increase with drug
- EPS, primarily in elderly: rigidity, dystonia, akathisia
- Mental status: mood, sensorium, affect, suicidal tendencies, increase in psychiatric symptoms: depression, panic
- Urinary retention, constipation; constipation is more likely to occur in children, elderly
- Withdrawal symptoms: headache, nausea, vomiting, muscle pain, weakness; do not usually occur unless drug was discontinued abruptly
- Alcohol consumption; if alcohol is consumed, hold dose until morning
Administer:
- Increased fluids, bulk in diet if constipation, urinary retention occur
- With food or milk for GI symptoms
- Gum, hard candy, or frequent sips of water for dry mouth

Perform/provide:
• Storage in tight container at room temp; do not refreeze
• Assistance with ambulation during beginning therapy, since drowsiness, dizziness occur
• Safety measures including side rails primarily in elderly
• Checking to see PO medication swallowed

Evaluate:
• Therapeutic response: decreased depression

Teach patient/family:
• That therapeutic effects may take 2-3 wk
• To use caution in driving, other activities requiring alertness because of drowsiness, dizziness, blurred vision
• To avoid alcohol ingestion, other CNS depressants
• Not to discontinue medication quickly after long-term use; may cause nausea, headache, malaise
• To wear sunscreen or large hat, since photosensitivity may occur

---

Generic names

Tetracyclics	*Miscellaneous*	*SSRIs*
mirtazapine	bupropion	citalopram
	maprotiline	fluoxetine
Tricyclics	nefazodone	fluvoxamine
amitriptyline	trazodone	paroxetine
amoxapine	venlafaxine	sertraline
clomipramine		
desipramine	*MAOIs*	
doxepin	phenelzine	
imipramine	tranylcypromine	
nortriptyline		
protriptyline		
trimipramine		

ANTIDIABETICS

Action: Antidiabetics are divided into the insulins that decrease blood sugar, phosphate, and potassium and increase blood pyruvate and lactate; and oral antidiabetics that cause functioning β-cells in the pancreas to release insulin, improve the effect of endogenous and exogenous insulin.
Uses: Insulins are used for ketoacidosis and diabetes mellitus types I (IDDM) and II (NIDDM); oral antidiabetics are used for stable adult-onset diabetes mellitus type II (NIDDM).

Side effects/adverse reactions: The most common side effect of insulin and oral antidiabetics is hypoglycemia. Other adverse reactions to oral antidiabetics include blood dyscrasias, hepatotoxicity, and rarely, cholestatic jaundice. Adverse reactions to insulin products include allergic responses and more rarely, anaphylaxis.

Contraindications: Hypersensitive reactions may occur, and allergies should be identified before these products are given. Oral antidiabetics should not be used in juvenile or brittle diabetes, diabetic ketoacidosis, severe renal disease, or severe hepatic disease.

Precautions: Oral antidiabetics should be used with caution in the elderly, in cardiac disease, pregnancy, lactation, and in the presence of alcohol.

Pharmacokinetics: Onset, peak, and duration vary widely among products. Oral antidiabetics are metabolized in the liver, with metabolites excreted in urine, bile, and feces.

Interactions: Interactions vary widely among products. Check individual monograph for specific information.

Possible nursing diagnoses:
- Altered nutrition: more than body requirements *[uses]*

NURSING CONSIDERATIONS
Assess:
- Blood, urine glucose levels during treatment to determine diabetes control (oral products)
- Fasting blood glucose, 2 hr PP (60-100 mg/dl normal fasting level) (70-130 mg/dl normal 2-hr level)
- Hypoglycemic reaction that can occur during peak time

Administer:
- Insulin after warming to room temp by rotating in palms to prevent lipodystrophy from injecting cold insulin
- Human insulin to those allergic to beef or pork
- Oral antidiabetic 30 min before meals

Perform/provide:
- Rotation of injection sites when giving insulin; use abdomen, upper back, thighs, upper arm, buttocks; rotate sites within one of these regions; keep a record of sites

Evaluate:
- Therapeutic response, including decrease in polyuria, polydipsia, polyphagia, clear sensorium, absence of dizziness, stable gait

Teach patient/family:
- To avoid alcohol and salicylates except on advice of prescriber
- Symptoms of ketoacidosis: nausea, thirst, polyuria, dry mouth, decreased B/P; dry, flushed skin; acetone breath, drowsiness, Kussmaul respiration

• Symptoms of hypoglycemia: headache, tremors, fatigue, weakness; and that candy or sugar should be carried to treat hypoglycemia
• To test urine for glucose/ketones tid if this drug is replacing insulin
• To continue weight control, dietary restrictions, exercise, hygiene

Generic names

acetohexamide	insulin, zinc suspension
chlorpropamide	extended (Ultralente)
glipizide	insulin, zinc suspension,
glyburide	prompt (Semilente)
insulin lispro	metformin
insulin, regular	miglitol
insulin, regular concentrated	repaglinide
insulin, zinc suspension	tolbutamide
(Lente)	troglitazone

ANTIDIARRHEALS

Action: Antidiarrheals work by various actions, including direct action on intestinal muscles to decrease GI peristalsis; or by inhibiting prostaglandin synthesis responsible for GI hypermotility; by acting on mucosal receptors responsible for peristalsis; or by decreasing water content of stools.

Uses: Antidiarrheals are used for diarrhea of undetermined causes.

Side effects/adverse reactions: The most serious adverse reactions of some products are paralytic ileus, toxic megacolon, and angioneurotic edema. The most common side effects are constipation, nausea, dry mouth, and abdominal pain.

Contraindications: Persons with severe ulcerative colitis, pseudomembranous colitis with some products.

Precautions: Antidiarrheals should be used with caution in the elderly, pregnancy, lactation, children, dehydration.

Pharmacokinetics: Onset, peak, and duration vary widely among products. Most products are metabolized in the liver and excreted in urine.

Interactions: Please check individual monographs, since interactions vary widely among products.

Possible nursing diagnoses:
• Diarrhea *[uses]*
• Constipation *[adverse reactions]*
• Fluid volume deficit *[adverse reactions]*
• Knowledge deficit *[teaching]*

NURSING CONSIDERATIONS

Assess:

- Electrolytes (K, Na, Cl) if on long-term therapy
- Bowel pattern before; for rebound constipation after termination of medication
- Response after 48 hr; if no response, drug should be discontinued
- Dehydration in children

Administer:

- For 48 hr only

Evaluate:

- Therapeutic response: decreased diarrhea

Teach patient/family:

- To avoid OTC products
- Not to exceed recommended dose

Generic names

bismuth subsalicylate	loperamide
difenoxin	opium tincture
kaolin/pectin	

ANTIDYSRHYTHMICS

Action: Antidysrhythmics are divided into four classes and miscellaneous antidysrhythmics:

- Class I increases the duration of action potential and effective refractory period and reduces disparity in the refractory period between a normal and infarcted myocardium; further subclasses include Ia, Ib, Ic
- Class II decreases the rate of SA node discharge, increases recovery time, slows conduction through the AV node, and decreases heart rate, which decreases O_2 consumption in the myocardium
- Class III increases the duration of action potential and the effective refractory period
- Class IV inhibits calcium ion influx across the cell membrane during cardiac depolarization; decreases SA node discharge, decreases conduction velocity through the AV node
- Miscellaneous antidysrhythmics include those such as adenosine, which slows conduction through the AV node, and digoxin, which decreases conduction velocity and prolongs the effective refractory period in the AV node

Uses: These products are used for PVCs, tachycardia, hypertension, atrial fibrillation, angina pectoris.

Side effects/adverse reactions: Side effects and adverse reactions vary widely among products.

Contraindications: Contraindications vary widely among products.

Precautions: Precautions vary widely among products.

Pharmacokinetics: Onset, peak, and duration vary widely among products.

Interactions: Interactions vary widely among products; check individual monograph for specific information.

Possible nursing diagnoses:

• Decreased cardiac output *[uses]*
• Altered tissue perfusion: cardiopulmonary *[uses]*
• Diarrhea *[adverse reactions]*
• Impaired gas exchange *[adverse reactions]*

NURSING CONSIDERATIONS

Assess:

• ECG continuously to determine drug effectiveness, PVCs, or other dysrhythmias
• IV infusion rate to avoid causing nausea, vomiting
• For dehydration or hypovolemia
• B/P continuously for hypotension, hypertension
• I&O ratio
• Serum potassium
• Edema in feet and legs daily

Evaluate:

• Therapeutic response, including decrease in B/P in hypertension; decreased B/P, edema, moist rales in CHF

Teach patient/family:

• To comply with dosage schedule, even if patient is feeling better
• To report bradycardia, dizziness, confusion, depression, fever

Generic names

Class I	Class II
moricizine	acebutolol
	esmolol
Class Ia	propranolol
disopyramide	sotalol
procainamide	
quinidine	Class III
	amiodarone
Class Ib	bretylium
lidocaine	ibutilide
mexiletine	
phenytoin	Class IV
tocainide	verapamil
Class Ic	Miscellaneous
flecainide	adenosine
indecainide	atropine
propafenone	digoxin

ANTIFUNGALS (SYSTEMIC)

Action: Antifungals act by increasing cell membrane permeability in susceptible organisms by binding sterols and decreasing potassium, sodium, and nutrients in the cell.

Uses: Antifungals are used for infections of histoplasmosis, blastomycosis, coccidiomycosis, cryptococcosis, aspergillosis, phycomycosis, candidiasis, sporotrichosis causing severe meningitis, septicemia, and skin infections.

Side effects/adverse reactions: The most serious adverse reactions include renal tubular acidosis, permanent renal impairment, anuria, oliguria, hemorrhagic gastroenteritis, acute liver failure, and blood dyscrasias. Some common side effects include hypokalemia, nausea, vomiting, anorexia, headache, fever, and chills.

Contraindications: Persons with severe bone depression or hypersensitivity should not use these products.

Precautions: Antifungals should be used with caution in renal disease, pregnancy, and hepatic disease.

Pharmacokinetics: Onset, peak, and duration vary widely among products. Most products are metabolized in the liver and excreted in urine.

Interactions: Please check individual monographs, since interactions vary widely among products.

Possible nursing diagnoses:
• Risk for infection *[uses]*
• Risk for injury *[adverse reactions]*
• Knowledge deficit *[teaching]*

NURSING CONSIDERATIONS
Assess:
• VS q15-30min during first infusion; note changes in pulse, B/P
• I&O ratio; watch for decreasing urinary output, change in specific gravity; discontinue drug to prevent permanent damage to renal tubules
• Blood studies: CBC, K, Na, Ca, Mg q2wk
• Weight weekly; if weight increases over 2 lb/wk, edema is present; renal damage should be considered
• For renal toxicity: increasing BUN, if >40 mg/dl or if serum creatinine >3 mg/dl; drug may be discontinued or dosage reduced
• For hepatotoxicity: increasing AST, ALT, alk phosphatase, bilirubin
• For allergic reaction: dermatitis, rash; drug should be discontinued, antihistamines (mild reaction) or epinephrine (severe reaction) administered
• For hypokalemia: anorexia, drowsiness, weakness, decreased reflexes, dizziness, increased urinary output, increased thirst, paresthesias
• For ototoxicity: tinnitus (ringing, roaring in ears), vertigo, loss of hearing (rare)

Administer:
• IV using in-line filter (mean pore diameter >1 μm) using distal veins; check for extravasation, necrosis q8h
• Drug only after C&S confirms organism, drug needed to treat condition; make sure drug is used in life-threatening infections

Perform/provide:
• Protection from light during infusion, cover with foil
• Symptomatic treatment as ordered for adverse reactions: aspirin, antihistamines, antiemetics, antispasmodics
• Storage protected from moisture and light; diluted sol is stable for 24 hr

Evaluate:
• Therapeutic response: decreased fever, malaise, rash, negative C&S for infecting organism

Teach patient/family:
• That long-term therapy may be needed to clear infection (2 wk-3 mo depending on type of infection)

Generic names

amphotericin B
fluconazole
flucytosine
griseofulvin

itraconazole
ketoconazole
miconazole
nystatin

ANTIHISTAMINES

Action: Antihistamines compete with histamines for H_1-receptor sites. They antagonize in varying degrees most of the pharmacologic effects of histamines.

Uses: Products are used to control the symptoms of allergies, rhinitis, and pruritus.

Side effects/adverse reactions: Most products cause drowsiness; however, two of the newer products, astemizole and terfenadine, produce little, if any, drowsiness. Other common side effects are headache and thickening of bronchial secretions. Serious blood dyscrasias may occur, but are rare. Urinary retention, GI effects occur with many of these products.

Contraindications: Hypersensitivity to H_1-receptor antagonists occurs rarely. Patients with acute asthma and lower respiratory tract disease should not use these products, since thick secretions may result. Other contraindications include narrow-angle glaucoma, bladder neck obstruction, stenosing peptic ulcer, symptomatic prostatic hypertrophy, newborn, lactation.

Precautions: These products must be used cautiously in conjunction with intraocular pressure, since they increase intraocular pressure. Caution should also be used in patients with renal and cardiac disease, hypertension, seizure disorders, pregnancy, lactation, and in the elderly.

Pharmacokinetics: Onset varies from 20-60 min, with duration lasting 4-12 hr. In general, pharmacokinetics vary widely among products.

Interactions: Barbiturates, narcotics, hypnotics, tricyclic antidepressants, or alcohol can increase CNS depression when taken with antihistamines.

Possible nursing diagnoses:

• Ineffective airway clearance [uses]

NURSING CONSIDERATIONS
Assess:

• I&O ratio; be alert for urinary retention, frequency, dysuria; drug should be discontinued if these occur
• CBC during long-term therapy, since hemolytic anemia, although rare, may occur

• Blood dyscrasias: thrombocytopenia, agranulocytosis (rare)
• Respiratory status, including rate, rhythm, increase in bronchial secretions, wheezing, chest tightness
• Cardiac status, including palpitations, increased pulse, hypotension

Administer:
• With food or milk to decrease GI symptoms; absorption may be decreased slightly
• Whole (sustained release tabs)

Perform/provide:
• Hard candy, gum, frequent rinsing of mouth for dryness

Evaluate:
• Therapeutic response, including absence of allergy symptoms, itching

Teach patient/family:
• To notify prescriber if confusion, sedation, hypotension occur
• To avoid driving, other hazardous activity if drowsiness occurs
• To avoid concurrent use of alcohol, other CNS depressants
• To discontinue a few days before skin testing

Generic names

acrivastine/pseudoephedrine	cyproheptadine
astemizole	dexchlorpheniramine
azatadine	diphenhydramine
azelastine	fexofenadine
brompheniramine	loratadine
budesonide	promethazine
cetirizine	trimeprazine
chlorpheniramine	tripelennamine
clemastine	triprolidine

ANTIHYPERTENSIVES

Action: Antihypertensives are divided into angiotensin-converting enzyme (ACE) inhibitors, β-adrenergic blockers, calcium channel blockers, centrally acting adrenergics, diuretics, peripherally acting antiadrenergics, and vasodilators. β-Blockers, calcium channel blockers, and diuretics are discussed in separate sections. Angiotensin-converting enzyme inhibitors act by selectively suppressing renin-angiotensin I to angiotensin II; dilation of arterial and venous vessels occurs. Centrally acting adrenergics act by inhibiting the sympathetic vasomotor center in the CNS that reduces impulses in the sympathetic nervous system; blood pressure, pulse rate, and cardiac output decrease. Peripherally acting antiadrenergics inhibit sympathetic vasoconstriction by inhibiting release of norepinephrine and/or depleting norepinephrine stores in adrenergic nerve endings. Vasodilators act on arteriolar smooth muscle by producing direct relaxation or vasodilation; a reduction in blood pressure, with concomitant increases in heart rate and cardiac output, occurs.

Uses: Used for hypertension and for heart failure not responsive to conventional therapy. Some products are used in hypertensive crisis, angina, and for some cardiac dysrhythmias.

Side effects/adverse reactions: The most common side effects are marked hypotension, bradycardia, tachycardia, headache, nausea, and vomiting. Side effects and adverse reactions may vary widely between classes and specific products.

Contraindications: Hypersensitive reactions may occur, and allergies should be identified before these products are given. Antihypertensives should not be used in patients with heart block or in children.

Precautions: Antihypertensives should be used with caution in the elderly, in dialysis patients, and in the presence of hypovolemia, leukemia, and electrolyte imbalances.

Pharmacokinetics: Onset, peak, and duration vary widely among products. Most products are metabolized in the liver, with metabolites excreted in urine, bile, and feces.

Interactions: Interactions vary widely among products; check individual monograph for specific information.

Possible nursing diagnoses:
• Altered tissue perfusion *[uses]*
• Decreased cardiac output *[uses]*
• Diarrhea *[adverse reactions]*
• Impaired gas exchange *[adverse reactions]*

NURSING CONSIDERATIONS
Assess:
• Blood studies: neutrophil; decreased platelets occur with many of the products
• Renal studies: protein, BUN, creatinine; watch for increased levels that may indicate nephrotic syndrome; obtain baselines in renal and liver function studies before beginning treatment
• Edema in feet and legs daily
• Allergic reaction, including rash, fever, pruritus, urticaria: drug should be discontinued if antihistamines fail to help
• Symptoms of CHF: edema, dyspnea, wet rales, B/P
• Renal symptoms: polyuria, oliguria, frequency
Perform/provide:
• Supine or Trendelenburg position for severe hypotension

Evaluate:

• Therapeutic response, including decrease in B/P in hypotension; decreased B/P, edema, moist rales in CHF

Teach patient/family:

• To comply with dosage schedule, even if feeling better

• To rise slowly to sitting or standing position to minimize orthostatic hypotension

---

Generic names

Angiotensin-converting enzyme inhibitors
benazepril
enalapril
fosinopril
perindopril
quinapril
ramipril
spirapril
trandolapril

Angiotensin II receptor blocker
candesartan
irbesartan (Appx A)
losartan
telmisartan
valsartan

Centrally acting adrenergics
clonidine
guanabenz
guanfacine
methyldopa

Peripherally acting antiadrenergics
guanadrel
guanethidine
prazosin
reserpine
terazosin

Vasodilators
diazoxide
fenoldopam
esoprostenol
hydralazine
minoxidil
nitroprusside

Antiadrenergic combined α-/β-blocker
labetalol

ANTIINFECTIVES

Action: Antiinfectives are divided into several groups, which include but are not limited to penicillins, cephalosporins, aminoglycosides, sulfonamides, tetracyclines, monobactam, erythromycins, and quinolones. These drugs act by inhibiting the growth and replication of susceptible bacterial organisms.

Uses: Used for infections of susceptible organisms. These products are effective against bacterial, rickettsial, and spirochete infections.

Side effects/adverse reactions: The most common side effects are nausea, vomiting, and diarrhea. Adverse reactions include bone marrow depression and anaphylaxis.

24   Antiinfectives

Contraindications: Hypersensitivity reactions may occur, and allergies should be identified before these products are given. Cross-sensitivity can occur between products of different classes (penicillins or cephalosporins). Many persons allergic to penicillins are also allergic to cephalosporins.

Precautions: Antiinfectives should be used with caution in persons with renal and liver disease.

Pharmacokinetics: Onset, peak, and duration vary widely among products. Most products are metabolized in the liver, and metabolites are excreted in urine, bile, and feces.

Interactions: Interactions vary widely among products; check individual monograph for specific information.

Possible nursing diagnoses:
• Risk for infection *[uses]*
• Diarrhea *[adverse reactions]*

NURSING CONSIDERATIONS
Assess:
• Nephrotoxicity, including increased BUN, creatinine
• Blood studies: AST (SGOT), ALT (SGPT), CBC, Hct, bilirubin; test monthly if patient is on long-term therapy
• Bowel pattern qd; if severe diarrhea occurs, drug should be discontinued
• Urine output; if decreasing, notify prescriber; may indicate nephrotoxicity
• Allergic reaction, including rash, fever, pruritus, urticaria; drug should be discontinued
• Bleeding: ecchymosis, bleeding gums, hematuria, stool guaiac daily
• Overgrowth of infection: perineal itching, fever, malaise, redness, pain, swelling, drainage, rash, diarrhea, change in cough, sputum

Administer:
• For 10-14 days to ensure organism death, prevention of superinfection
• After C&S completed; drug may be taken as soon as culture is taken

Evaluate:
• Therapeutic response, including absence of fever, fatigue, malaise, draining wounds

Teach patient/family:
• To comply with dosage schedule, even if feeling better
• To report sore throat, bruising, bleeding, joint pain; may indicate blood dyscrasias (rare)

Generic names

Aminoglycosides
amikacin
azithromycin
clarithromycin
gentamicin
kanamycin
neomycin
netilmicin
streptomycin
tobramycin

Cephalosporins
cefaclor
cefadroxil
cefamandole
cefazolin
cefdinir
cefepime
cefixime
cefmetazole
cefonicid
cefoperazone
ceforanide
cefotaxime
cefprozil
ceftibuten
cefuroxime
cephalexin
cephalothin
cephapirin
cephradine
moxalactam

Fluoroquinolones
alatrofloxacin
ciprofloxacin
enoxacin
grepafloxacin
levofloxacin
lomefloxacin

nalidixic acid
norfloxacin
ofloxacin
sparfloxacin
trovafloxacin

Miscellaneous
meropenem

Penicillins
amoxicillin/clavulanate
ampicillin/sulbactam
azlocillin
bacampicillin
cloxacillin
dicloxacillin
imipenem/cilastatin
methicillin
mezlocillin
nafcillin
oxacillin
penicillin G benzathine
penicillin G potassium
penicillin G procaine
penicillin G sodium
penicillin V potassium
piperacillin
ticarcillin
ticarcillin/clavulanate

Sulfonamides
sulfasalazine
sulfisoxazole

Tetracyclines
demeclocycline
doxycycline
minocycline
oxytetracycline
tetracycline

ANTINEOPLASTICS

Action: Antineoplastics are divided into alkylating agents, antimetabolites, antibiotic agents, hormonal agents, and miscellaneous agents. Alkylating agents act by cross-linking strands of DNA. Antimetabolites act by inhibiting DNA synthesis. Antibiotic agents act by inhibiting RNA synthesis and by delaying or inhibiting mitosis. Hormones alter the effects of androgens, luteinizing hormone, follicle-stimulating hormone, and estrogen by changing the hormonal environment.

Uses: Uses vary widely among products and classes of drugs. They are used to treat leukemia, Hodgkin's disease, lymphomas, and other tumors throughout the body.

Side effects/adverse reactions: Most products cause thrombocytopenia, leukopenia, and anemia, and if these reactions occur, the drug may have to be stopped until the problem is corrected. Other side effects include nausea, vomiting, glossitis, and hair loss. Some products also cause hepatotoxicity, nephrotoxicity, and cardiotoxicity.

Contraindications: Hypersensitive reactions may occur, and allergies should be identified before these products are given. Also, persons with severe liver and kidney disease should not use these products unless the benefits outweigh the risks.

Precautions: Persons with bleeding, severe bone marrow depression, or renal or hepatic disease should be watched closely.

Pharmacokinetics: Onset, peak, and duration vary widely among products. Most products cross the placenta and are excreted in breast milk and in urine.

Interactions: Toxicity may occur when used with other antineoplastics or radiation.

Possible nursing diagnoses:
- Risk for infection *[adverse reactions]*
- Altered nutrition: less than body requirements *[adverse reactions]*
- Altered oral mucous membrane *[adverse reactions]*

NURSING CONSIDERATIONS
Assess:
- CBC, differential, platelet count weekly; withhold drug if WBC is <4000/mm^3 or platelet count is <75,000/mm^3; notify prescriber of results
- Renal function studies, including BUN, creatinine, serum uric acid, and urine creatinine clearance before and during therapy
- I&O ratio; report fall in urine output of 30 ml/hr
- Monitor temp q4h (may indicate beginning infection)
- Liver function tests before and during therapy (bilirubin, AST [SGOT], ALT [SGPT], LDH) as needed or monthly
- Bleeding, including hematuria, guaiac, bruising or petechiae, mucosa, or orifices q8h; obtain prescription for viscous Xylocaine (lidocaine)
- Yellowing of skin, sclera, dark urine, clay-colored stools, itchy skin, abdominal pain, fever, diarrhea
- Edema in feet, joint pain, stomach pain, shaking
- Inflammation of mucosa, breaks in skin

Administer:
• Checking IV site for irritation; phlebitis
• Epinephrine for hypersensitivity reaction
• Antibiotics for prophylaxis of infection

Perform/provide:
• Strict asepsis, protective isolation if WBC levels are low
• Comprehensive oral hygiene, using careful technique and soft-bristle brush

Evaluate:
• Therapeutic response, including decreased tumor size

Teach patient/family:
• To report signs of infection, including increased temp, sore throat, malaise
• To report signs of anemia, including fatigue, headache, faintness, shortness of breath, irritability
• To report bleeding and avoid use of razors or commercial mouthwash

---

Generic names

Alkylating agents
busulfan
carboplatin
carmustine
chlorambucil
cisplatin
cyclophosphamide
dacarbazine
lomustine
mechlorethamine
melphalan
streptozocin
thiotepa
uracil mustard

Antimetabolites
capecitabine
cytarabine
doxorubicin
etoposide
fludarabine
fluorouracil
mercaptopurine
thioguanine (6-TG)

Antibiotic agents
bleomycin
dactinomycin
daunorubicin
methotrexate
mitomycin
mitoxantrone
plicamycin

Hormonal agents
aminoglutethimide
estramustine
flutamide
goserelin
irinotecan
leuprolide
megestrol
mitotane
nilutamide
tamoxifen
testolactone
topotecan

Miscellaneous
altretamine
anastrozole
asparaginase
cladribine
gemcitabine
interferon alfa-2A
interferon alfa-2B
irinotecan
pentostatin
porfimer
procarbazine
rituximab
vinblastine
vincristine
vinorelbine

ANTIPARKINSON AGENTS

Action: Antiparkinson agents are divided into cholinergics and dopamine agonists. Cholinergics work by blocking or competing at central acetylcholine receptors; dopamine agonists work by decarboxylation to dopamine or by activation of dopamine receptors; monoamine oxidase type B inhibitors work by increasing dopamine activity by inhibiting MAO type B activity.

Uses: Antiparkinson agents are used alone or in combination for patients with Parkinson's disease.

Side effects/adverse reactions: Side effects and adverse reactions vary widely among products. The most common side effects include involuntary movements, headache, numbness, insomnia, nightmares, nausea, vomiting, dry mouth, and orthostatic hypotension.

Contraindications: Persons with hypersensitivity, narrow-angle glaucoma, and undiagnosed skin lesions should not use these products.

Precautions: Antiparkinson agents should be used with caution in pregnancy, lactation, children, renal, cardiac, hepatic disease, and affective disorder.

Pharmacokinetics: Onset, peak, and duration vary widely among products. Most products are metabolized in the liver and excreted in urine.

Interactions: Please check individual monographs, since interactions vary widely among products.

Possible nursing diagnoses:
• Risk for injury *[uses]*
• Risk for impaired physical mobility *[uses]*
• Knowledge deficit *[teaching]*

NURSING CONSIDERATIONS
Assess:
• B/P, respiration
• Mental status: affect, mood, behavioral changes, depression, complete suicide assessment
Administer:
• Drug up until NPO before surgery
• Adjust dosage depending on patient response
• With meals; limit protein taken with drug
• Only after MAOIs have been discontinued for 2 wk
Perform/provide:
• Assistance with ambulation, during beginning therapy
• Testing for diabetes mellitus, acromegaly if on long-term therapy

Evaluate:
• Therapeutic response: decrease in akathisia, increased mood
Teach patient/family:
• To change positions slowly to prevent orthostatic hypotension
• To report side effects: twitching, eye spasm; indicate overdose
• To use drug exactly as prescribed; if drug is discontinued abruptly, parkinsonian crisis may occur

---

Generic names

amantadine	levodopa
benztropine	pramipexole
biperiden	procyclidine
bromocriptine	selegiline
cabergoline	tolcapone
carbidopa-levodopa	trihexyphenidyl

ANTIPSYCHOTICS

Action: Antipsychotics/neuroleptics are divided into several subgroups: phenothiazines, thioxanthenes, butyrophenones, dibenzoxazepines, dibenzodiazepines, and indolones and other heterocyclic compounds. Although chemically different, these subgroups share many pharmacologic and clinical properties. All antipsychotics work to block postsynaptic dopamine receptors in the brain that are responsible for psychotic behavior, including hallucinations, delusions, and paranoia.

Uses: Antipsychotic behavior is decreased in conditions such as schizophrenia, paranoia, and mania. These agents are also effective for severe anxiety, intractable hiccups, nausea, vomiting, behavioral problems in children, and before surgery for relaxation.

Side effects/adverse reactions: The most common side effects include EPS such as pseudoparkinsonism, akathisia, dystonia, and tardive dyskinesia, which may be controlled by use of antiparkinsonian agents. Serious adverse reactions such as hypotension, agranulocytosis, cardiac arrest, and laryngospasm have occurred. Other common side effects include dry mouth and photosensitivity.

Contraindications: Persons with liver damage, severe hypertension or coronary disease, cerebral arteriosclerosis, blood dyscrasias, bone marrow depression, parkinsonism, severely depressed persons, narrow-angle glaucoma, children <12 yr, or persons withdrawing from alcohol or barbiturates should not use antipsychotics until these conditions are corrected.

Precautions: Caution must be used when antipsychotics are given to the elderly, since metabolism is slowed and adverse reactions can occur rapidly. Hepatic and renal disease may cause poor metabolism and excretion of the drug. Seizure threshold is decreased with these products; increases in the dose of anticonvulsants may be required. Persons with diabetes mellitus, prostatic hypertrophy, chronic respiratory disease, and peptic ulcer disease should be monitored closely.

Pharmacokinetics: Onset, peak, and duration vary widely with different products and routes. Products are metabolized by the liver, are excreted in urine as metabolites, are highly bound to plasma proteins, cross the placenta, and enter breast milk. Half-life can be extended over 3 days.

Interactions: Because other CNS depressants can cause oversedation, these combinations should be used carefully. Anticholinergics may decrease the therapeutic actions of phenothiazines and also cause increased anticholinergic effects.

Possible nursing diagnoses:
- Altered thought processes *[uses]*
- Sensory/perceptual alterations *[uses]*

NURSING CONSIDERATIONS
Assess:
- Bilirubin, CBC, liver function studies qmo, since these drugs are metabolized in the liver and excreted in urine
- I&O ratio: palpate bladder if low urinary output occurs, since urinary retention occurs with many of these products
- Affect, orientation, LOC, reflexes, gait, coordination, sleep pattern disturbances
- Dizziness, faintness, palpitations, tachycardia on rising
- B/P lying and standing; wide fluctuations between lying and standing B/P may require dosage or product change, since orthostatic hypotension is occurring
- EPS, including akathisia, tardive dyskinesia, pseudoparkinsonism

Administer:
- Antiparkinsonian agent if EPS occur
- Liquid concentrates mixed in glass of juice or cola, since taste is unpleasant; avoid contact with skin when preparing liquid concentrate or parenteral medications

Perform/provide:
- Supervised ambulation until stabilized on medication; do not involve in strenuous exercise program because fainting is possible; patient should not stand still for long periods
- Increased fluids to prevent constipation
- Sips of water, candy, gum for dry mouth

Evaluate:
• Therapeutic response: decrease in excitement, hallucinations, delusions, paranoia, reorganization of thought patterns, speech

Teach patient/family:
• To rise from sitting or lying position gradually, since fainting may occur
• To remain lying down for at least 30 min after IM injections
• To avoid hot tubs, hot showers, or tub baths, since hypotension may occur
• To wear a sunscreen or protective clothing to prevent burns
• To take extra precautions during hot weather to stay cool; heat stroke can occur
• To avoid driving, other activities requiring alertness until response to medication is known
• That drowsiness or impaired mental/motor activity is evident the first 2 wk, but tends to decrease over time

Generic names

Phenothiazines
chlorpromazine
fluphenazine
mesoridazine
perphenazine
prochlorperazine
promazine
thioridazine
thiothixene
trifluoperazine

Butyrophenone
haloperidol

Miscellaneous
loxapine
molindone
olanzapine
quetiapine (Appx A)
risperidone

ANTITUBERCULARS

Action: Antituberculars act by inhibiting RNA or DNA, or interfering with lipid and protein synthesis, thereby decreasing tubercle bacilli replication.
Uses: Antituberculars are used for pulmonary tuberculosis.
Side effects/adverse reactions: They vary widely among products. Most products can cause nausea, vomiting, anorexia, and rash. Serious adverse reactions include renal failure, nephrotoxicity, ototoxicity, and hepatic necrosis.
Contraindications: Persons with severe renal disease or hypersensitivity should not use these products.
Precautions: Antituberculars should be used with caution with pregnancy, lactation, and hepatic disease.
Pharmacokinetics: Onset, peak, and duration vary widely among products. Most products are metabolized in the liver and excreted in urine.

Interactions: Please check individual monographs, since interactions vary widely among products.

Possible nursing diagnoses:
• Risk for infection *[uses]*
• Risk for injury *[adverse reactions]*
• Knowledge deficit *[teaching]*
• Noncompliance *[teaching]*

NURSING CONSIDERATIONS
Assess:
• Signs of anemia: Hct, Hgb, fatigue
• Liver studies qwk: ALT (SGPT), AST (SGOT), bilirubin
• Renal status before, qmo: BUN, creatinine, output, specific gravity, urinalysis
• Hepatic status: decreased appetite, jaundice, dark urine, fatigue
Administer:
• For some of these agents on empty stomach, 1 hr ac (only for isoniazid and rifampin) or 2 hr pc
• Antiemetic if vomiting occurs
• After C&S is completed; qmo to detect resistance
Evaluate:
• Therapeutic response: decreased symptoms of TB, culture negative
Teach patient/family:
• That compliance with dosage schedule, duration is necessary
• That scheduled appointments must be kept; relapse may occur
• To avoid alcohol while taking drug
• To report flulike symptoms: excessive fatigue, anorexia, vomiting, sore throat; unusual bleeding, yellowish discoloration of skin/eyes

Generic names

capreomycin	kanamycin
cycloserine	pyrazinamide
ethambutol	rifabutin
ethionamide	rifampin
isoniazid	streptomycin

ANTITUSSIVES/EXPECTORANTS

Action: Antitussives act by suppressing the cough reflex by direct action on the cough center in the medulla. Expectorants act by liquefying and reducing the viscosity of thick, tenacious secretions.

Uses: Antitussives/expectorants are used to treat cough occurring in pneumonia, bronchitis, TB, cystic fibrosis, and emphysema; as an adjunct in atelectasis (expectorants); and nonproductive cough (antitussives).

Side effects/adverse reactions: The most common side effects are drowsiness, dizziness, and nausea.

Contraindications: Some products are contraindicated in hypothyroidism, iodine sensitivity, pregnancy, and lactation.

Precautions: Some products should be used cautiously in asthmatic, elderly, and debilitated patients.

Pharmacokinetics: Onset, peak, and duration vary widely among products. Some products are metabolized in the liver and excreted in urine.

Interactions: Please check individual monographs since interactions vary widely among products.

Possible nursing diagnoses:
- Ineffective breathing pattern *[uses]*
- Ineffective airway clearance *[uses]*
- Knowledge deficit *[teaching]*

NURSING CONSIDERATIONS

Assess:
- Cough: type, frequency, character (including sputum)

Administer:
- Decreased dose to elderly patients; their metabolism may be slowed

Perform/provide:
- Increased fluids to liquefy secretions
- Humidification of patient's room

Evaluate:
- Therapeutic response: absence of cough

Teach patient/family:
- To avoid driving, other hazardous activities until patient is stabilized on this medication
- To avoid smoking, smoke-filled rooms, perfumes, dust, environmental pollutants, cleaners that increase cough

---

Generic names

acetylcysteine
ammonium chloride
benzonatate
codeine
dextromethorphan

diphenhydramine
guaifenesin
hydrocodone
potassium iodide
terpin hydrate

ANTIVIRALS

Action: Antivirals act by interfering with DNA synthesis that is needed for viral replication.

Uses: Antivirals are used for mucocutaneous herpes simplex virus, herpes genitalis (HSV_1, HSV_2), advanced HIV infections, herpes simplex virus encephalitis, varicella-zoster encephalomyelitis.

Side effects/adverse reactions: Serious adverse reactions are fatal metabolic encephalopathy, blood dyscrasias, and acute renal failure. Common side effects are nausea, vomiting, anorexia, diarrhea, headache, vaginitis, and moniliasis.

Contraindications: Persons with hypersensitivity, herpes zoster in immunosuppressed individuals should not use these products.

Precautions: Antivirals should be used with caution in renal disease, liver disease, lactation, pregnancy, and dehydration.

Pharmacokinetics: Onset, peak, and duration vary widely among products. Most products are metabolized in the liver and excreted in urine.

Interactions: Please check individual monographs, since interactions vary widely among products.

Possible nursing diagnoses:

- Risk for infection *[uses]*
- Risk for injury *[adverse reactions]*
- Knowledge deficit *[teaching]*

NURSING CONSIDERATIONS
Assess:

- Signs of infection, anemia
- I&O ratio; report hematuria, oliguria, fatigue, weakness; may indicate nephrotoxicity; check for protein in urine during treatment
- Any patient with compromised renal system, since drug is excreted slowly in poor renal system function; toxicity may occur rapidly
- Liver studies: AST (SGOT), ALT (SGPT)
- Blood studies: WBC, RBC, Hct, Hgb, bleeding time; blood dyscrasias may occur; drug should be discontinued
- Renal studies: urinalysis, protein, BUN, creatinine, CrCl
- C&S before drug therapy; drug may be taken as soon as culture is taken; repeat C&S after treatment
- Bowel pattern before, during treatment; if severe abdominal pain with bleeding occurs, drug should be discontinued
- Skin eruptions: rash, urticaria, itching
- Allergies before treatment, reaction of each medication; record allergies on chart in bright red letters

Administer:
• Increased fluids to 3 L/day to decrease crystalluria when given IV

Perform/provide:
• Storage at room temp for up to 12 hr after reconstitution
• Adequate intake of fluids (2 L) to prevent deposit in kidneys

Evaluate:
• Therapeutic response: absence or control of infection

Teach patient/family:
• That drug does not cure infection, just controls symptoms
• To report sore throat, fever, fatigue; could indicate superinfection
• That drug must be taken in equal intervals around the clock to maintain blood levels for duration of therapy
• To notify prescriber of side effects of bruising, bleeding, fatigue, malaise; may indicate blood dyscrasias

---

Generic names

acyclovir	nelfinavir
amantadine	nevirapine
cidofovir	rimantadine
delavirdine	ritonavir
didanosine	saquinavir
famciclovir	stavudine
foscarnet	vidarabine
ganciclovir	zalcitabine
indinavir	zidovudine

BARBITURATES

Action: Barbiturates act by decreasing impulse transmission to the cerebral cortex.

Uses: All forms of epilepsy can be controlled, since the seizure threshold is increased. Uses also include febrile seizures in children, sedation, insomnia, hyperbilirubinemia, chronic cholestasis with some of these products. Ultra-short-acting barbiturates are used as anesthetics.

Side effects/adverse reactions: The most common side effects are drowsiness and nausea. Serious adverse reactions such as Stevens-Johnson syndrome and blood dyscrasias may occur with high doses and long-term treatment.

Contraindications: Hypersensitivity may occur, and allergies should be identified before administering. Barbiturates are identified as pregnancy category D and should not be used in pregnancy. Other contraindications include porphyria and marked impairment of liver function.

Precautions: Caution must be used when these products are given to the elderly or debilitated; usually smaller doses are needed, since metabolism is slowed. Persons with renal and hepatic disease may show delayed excretion. Barbiturates may produce excitability in children.

Pharmacokinetics: Onset of action can be slow, up to 1 hr, with a peak of 8 hr and a duration of 3-10 hr. These drugs are metabolized by the liver, excreted by the kidneys, cross the placenta, and enter breast milk.

Interactions: Increased CNS depressant effect may occur with alcohol, MAOIs, sedatives, or narcotics. These products should be used together cautiously. Oral anticoagulants, corticosteroids, griseofulvin, quinidine, oral contraceptives, and theophylline may show a decreased effect when used with barbiturates.

Possible nursing diagnoses:
• Sleep pattern disturbance [uses]
• Risk for injury [adverse reactions]

NURSING CONSIDERATIONS

Assess:
• Hepatic and renal studies: AST (SGOT), ALT (SGPT), bilirubin, creatinine, LDH, alkaline phosphatase, BUN if patient is on long-term therapy, since these products are metabolized and excreted by the liver and kidney
• Blood studies: CBC, hematocrit, hemoglobin, and prothrombin time if patient is on long-term therapy, since these products increase the possibility of bleeding and blood dyscrasias
• Barbiturate toxicity: hypotension, pulmonary constriction; cold, clammy skin; cyanosis of lips, insomnia, nausea, vomiting, hallucinations, delirium, weakness

Evaluate:
• Therapeutic response, including appropriate sedation or seizure control

Teach patient/family:
• That physical dependency may result when used for extended periods (45-90 days, depending on dose)
• To avoid driving, activities that require alertness, since drowsiness and dizziness may occur
• To abstain from alcohol or other psychotropic medications unless directed by prescriber
• Not to discontinue medication abruptly after long-term use; withdrawal symptoms will occur

---

Generic names

amobarbital	secobarbital
mephobarbital	talbutal
pentobarbital	thiopental
phenobarbital	

BENZODIAZEPINES

Action: Benzodiazepines potentiate the effects of γ-aminobutyric acid (GABA), including any other inhibitory transmitters in the CNS, resulting in decreased anxiety.

Uses: Anxiety is relieved in conditions such as phobic disorders. Benzodiazepines are also used for acute alcohol withdrawal to relieve the possibility of delirium tremens, and some products are used before surgery for relaxation.

Side effects/adverse reactions: The most common side effects are dizziness, drowsiness, blurred vision, and orthostatic hypotension. Most adverse effects are mediated through the CNS. There is a risk of physicial dependence and abuse.

Contraindications: Hypersensitivity, acute narrow-angle glaucoma, children <6 mo, liver disease (clonazepam), lactation (diazepam).

Precautions: Caution must be used when these products are given to the elderly or debilitated; usually smaller doses are needed, since metabolism is slowed. Persons with renal and hepatic disease may show delayed excretion. Clonazepam may increase incidence of seizures.

Pharmacokinetics: Onset of action is ½-1 hr, with a peak of 1-2 hr and a duration of 4-6 hr. These drugs are metabolized by the liver, excreted by the kidneys, cross the placenta, and enter breast milk.

Interactions: Increased CNS depressant effect may occur with other CNS depressants. These products should be used together cautiously. Alcohol should not be used; fatal reactions can occur. The serum concentration and toxicity of digoxin may be increased.

Possible nursing diagnoses:
* Anxiety [uses]
* Risk for injury [adverse reactions]

NURSING CONSIDERATIONS
Assess:
* B/P (lying, standing), pulse; if systolic B/P drops 20 mm Hg, hold drug, notify prescriber; orthostatic hypotension is severe
* Hepatic and renal studies: AST (SGOT), ALT (SGPT), bilirubin, creatinine, LDH, alkaline phosphatase
* Physical dependency, withdrawal symptoms, including headache, nausea, vomiting, muscle pain, weakness after long-term use

Administer:
* With food or milk for GI symptoms; may give crushed if patient is unable to swallow medication whole

Evaluate:

• Therapeutic response, including relaxation or decreased anxiety

Teach patient/family:

• That drug should not be used for everyday stress or long-term; not to take more than prescribed amount, since drug is habit forming

• To avoid driving and activities that require alertness, since drowsiness and dizziness occur

• To abstain from alcohol, other psychotropic medications unless directed by prescriber

• Not to discontinue medication abruptly after long-term use; withdrawal symptoms will occur

---

Generic names

alprazolam	lorazepam
chlordiazepoxide	midazolam
clonazepam	oxazepam
delavirdine (Appx A)	prazepam
diazepam	quazepam
flurazepam	temazepam
halazepam	triazolam

BETA-ADRENERGIC BLOCKERS

Action: β-Blockers are divided into selective and nonselective blockers. Nonselective blockers produce a fall in blood pressure without reflex tachycardia or reduction in heart rate through a mixture of β-blocking effects; elevated plasma renins are reduced. Selective β-blockers competitively block stimulation of β_1-receptors in cardiac smooth muscle; these drugs produce chronotropic and inotropic effects.

Uses: β-Blockers are used for hypertension, ventricular dysrhythmias, and prophylaxis of angina pectoris.

Side effects/adverse reactions: The most common side effects are orthostatic hypotension, bradycardia, diarrhea, nausea, vomiting. Serious adverse reactions include blood dyscrasias, bronchospasm, and CHF.

Contraindications: Hypersensitive reactions may occur, and allergies should be identified before these products are given. β-Adrenergic blockers should not be used in heart block, CHF, or cardiogenic shock.

Precautions: β-Blockers should be used with caution in the elderly or in renal and thyroid disease, COPD, CAD, diabetes mellitus, pregnancy, or asthma.

Pharmacokinetics: Onset, peak, and duration vary widely among products. Most products are metabolized in the liver, with metabolites excreted in urine, bile, and feces.

Interactions: Interactions vary widely among products; check individual monograph for specific information.

Possible nursing diagnoses:
- Altered tissue perfusion *[uses]*
- Decreased cardiac output *[uses]*
- Diarrhea *[adverse reactions]*
- Impaired gas exchange *[adverse reactions]*

NURSING CONSIDERATIONS

Assess:
- Renal studies, including protein, BUN, creatinine; watch for increased levels that may indicate nephrotic syndrome; obtain baselines in renal and liver function studies before beginning treatment
- I&O, weight daily
- B/P during beginning treatment and periodically thereafter; pulse q4h, note rate, rhythm, quality
- Apical/radial pulse before administration, notify prescriber of significant changes
- Edema in feet and legs daily

Administer:
- PO ac, hs; tablets may be crushed or swallowed whole
- Reduced dosage in renal dysfunction

Evaluate:
- Therapeutic response, including decrease in B/P in hypertension, decreased B/P, edema, moist rales in CHF

Teach patient/family:
- To comply with dosage schedule, even if feeling better
- To rise slowly to sitting or standing position to minimize orthostatic hypotension
- To report bradycardia, dizziness, confusion, depression, fever
- To take pulse at home; advise when to notify prescriber
- To comply with weight control, dietary adjustment, modified exercise program
- To wear support hose to minimize effects of orthostatic hypotension
- Not to discontinue drug abruptly; taper over 2 wk; may precipitate angina

Generic names

Selective β_1-receptor blockers
acebutolol
atenolol
esmolol
metoprolol

*Combined α_1-, β_1-, and β_2-
receptor blocker*
labetalol

*Nonselective β_1- and β_2-
blockers*
carteolol
nadolol
pindolol
propranolol
timolol

BRONCHODILATORS

Action: Bronchodilators are divided into anticholinergics, α/β-adrenergic agonists, β-adrenergic agonists, and phosphodiesterase inhibitors. Anticholinergics act by inhibiting interaction of acetylcholine at receptor sites on bronchial smooth muscle; α/β-adrenergic agonists by relaxing bronchial smooth muscle and increasing diameter of nasal passages; β-adrenergic agonists by action on β_2-receptors, which relaxes bronchial smooth muscle; phosphodiesterase inhibitors by blocking phosphodiesterase increase cAMP, which mediates smooth muscle relaxation in the respiratory system.

Uses: Bronchodilators are used for bronchial asthma, bronchospasm associated with bronchitis, emphysema, or other obstructive pulmonary diseases, Cheyne-Stokes respirations, prevention of exercise-induced asthma.

Side effects/adverse reactions: The most common side effects are tremors, anxiety, nausea, vomiting, and irritation in throat. The most serious adverse reactions include bronchospasm and dyspnea.

Contraindications: Persons with hypersensitivity, narrow-angle glaucoma, tachydysrhythmias, and severe cardiac disease should not use some of these products.

Precautions: Bronchodilators should be used with caution in lactation, pregnancy, hyperthyroidism, hypertension, prostatic hypertrophy, and seizure disorders.

Pharmacokinetics: Onset, peak, and duration vary widely among products. Most products are metabolized in the liver and excreted in urine.

Interactions: Please check individual monographs, since interactions vary widely among products.

Possible nursing diagnoses:
- Ineffective airway clearance *[uses]*
- Activity intolerance *[uses]*

- Risk for injury *[adverse reactions]*
- Knowledge deficit *[teaching]*

NURSING CONSIDERATIONS

Assess:
- Respiratory function: vital capacity, forced expiratory volume, ABGs, lung sounds, heart rate and rhythm

Administer:
- After shaking, exhale, place mouthpiece in mouth, inhale slowly, hold breath, remove, exhale slowly
- Gum, sips of water for dry mouth
- PO with meals to decrease gastric irritation

Perform/provide:
- Storage in light-resistant container, do not expose to temps over 86° F (30° C)

Evaluate:
- Therapeutic response: absence of dyspnea, wheezing

Teach patient/family:
- Not to use OTC medications; extra stimulation may occur
- Use of inhaler; review package insert with patient
- To avoid getting aerosol in eyes
- To wash inhaler in warm water qd and dry
- To avoid smoking, smoke-filled rooms, persons with respiratory infections

Generic names

albuterol	isoetharine
aminophylline	isoproterenol
atropine	metaproterenol
bitolterol	mibefradil
dyphylline	oxtriphylline
ephedrine	pirbuterol
epinephrine	terbutaline
ethylnorepinephrine	theophylline
ipratropium	

CALCIUM CHANNEL BLOCKERS

Action: These products act by inhibiting calcium ion influx across the cell membrane in cardiac and vascular smooth muscle. This action produces relaxation of coronary vascular smooth muscle, dilates coronary arteries, slows SA/AV node conduction, and dilates peripheral arteries.

Uses: These products are used for chronic stable angina pectoris, vasospastic angina, dysrhythmias, hypertension, and unstable angina.

Side effects/adverse reactions: The most common side effects are dysrhythmias and edema. Also common are headache, fatigue, drowsiness, and flushing.

Contraindications: Persons with 2nd or 3rd degree heart block, sick sinus syndrome, hypotension of <90 mm Hg systolic, Wolff-Parkinson-White syndrome, or cardiogenic shock should not use these products, since worsening of those conditions may occur.

Precautions: CHF may worsen, since edema may be increased. Hypotension may worsen, since B/P is decreased. Patients with renal and liver disease should use these products cautiously, since they are metabolized in the liver and excreted by the kidneys.

Pharmacokinetics: Onset, peak, and duration vary widely with route of administration. Drugs are metabolized by the liver and excreted in the urine primarily as metabolites.

Interactions: Increased levels of digoxin and theophylline may occur when used with these products. Increased effects of β-blockers and antihypertensives may occur with calcium channel blockers.

Possible nursing diagnoses:
• Altered tissue perfusion: cardiopulmonary *[uses]*
• Decreased cardiac output *[adverse reactions]*

NURSING CONSIDERATIONS
Assess:
• Cardiac system, including B/P, pulse, respirations, ECG intervals (PR, QRS, QT)
Administer:
• PO before meals and hs
Evaluate:
• Therapeutic response, including decreased anginal pain, decreased B/P, dysrhythmias
Teach patient/family:
• How to take pulse before taking drug; patient should record or graph pulses to identify changes
• To avoid hazardous activities until stabilized on this drug, since dizziness occurs frequently
• Need for compliance to all areas of medical regimen, including diet, exercise, stress reduction, drug therapy

Generic names

diltiazem	nifedipine
felodipine	verapamil
nicardipine	

CARDIAC GLYCOSIDES

Action: Products act by inhibiting sodium and potassium ATPase and then making more calcium available to activate contracted proteins. Cardiac contractility and cardiac output are increased.

Uses: These products are used for CHF, atrial fibrillation, atrial flutter, atrial tachycardia, and rapid digitalization in these disorders.

Side effects/adverse reactions: The most common side effects are cardiac disturbances, headache, hypotension, GI symptoms. Also common are blurred vision and yellow-green halos.

Contraindications: Hypersensitive reactions may occur, and allergies should be identified before these products are given. Also, persons with ventricular tachycardia, ventricular fibrillation, and carotid sinus syndrome should not use these products.

Precautions: Persons with acute MI and those who have or may develop serum potassium, calcium, or magnesium imbalances should use these products cautiously. Also, persons with AV block, severe respiratory disease, hypothyroidism, renal and liver disease, and the elderly should exercise caution when these drugs are prescribed.

Pharmacokinetics: Onset, peak, and duration vary widely with the route of administration. Digitoxin is inactivated by the liver, and inactive metabolites are excreted in urine. Digoxin is excreted in urine mainly as the parent drug and metabolites.

Interactions: Toxicity may occur when used with diuretics, succinylcholine, quinidine, and thioamines. Increased blood levels may occur with propantheline bromide, spironolactone, quinidine, verapamil, aminoglycosides (PO), amiodarone, anticholinergics, and quinine. Diuretics may increase toxicity.

Possible nursing diagnoses:

- Altered tissue perfusion: cardiopulmonary *[uses]*
- Decreased cardiac output *[adverse reactions]*

NURSING CONSIDERATIONS

Assess:

- Cardiac system, including B/P, pulse, respirations, and increased urine output

• Apical pulse for 1 min before giving drug; if pulse <60 bpm, take again in 1 hr; if still <60 bpm, notify prescriber
• Electrolytes, including K, Na, Cl, Mg; renal function studies, including BUN and creatinine; and blood studies, including AST (SGOT), ALT (SGPT), bilirubin
• I&O ratio, daily weights
• Monitor therapeutic drug levels

Administer:
• K supplements if ordered for K levels <3 mg/dl

Evaluate:
• Therapeutic response, including decreased weight, edema, pulse, respiration, and increased urine output

Teach patient/family:
• How to take pulse before taking drug; patient should record or graph pulse to identify changes
• To avoid hazardous activities until stabilized on this drug, since dizziness occurs frequently
• Need for compliance to all areas of medical regimen, including diet, exercise, stress reduction, drug therapy

---

Generic names

digitoxin   digoxin

CHOLINERGICS

Action: Cholinergics act by preventing destruction of acetylcholine, which increases concentration at sites where acetylcholine is released; this exaggerates the effects of acetylcholine and facilitates transmission of impulses across the myoneural junction. Cholinergics may also act by stimulating receptors for acetylcholine.

Uses: Cholinergics are used for myasthenia gravis, as antagonists of nondepolarizing neuromuscular blockade, postoperative bladder distention and urinary distention, postoperative ileus.

Side effects/adverse reactions: The most serious adverse reactions are respiratory depression, bronchospasm, constriction, laryngospasm, respiratory arrest, convulsions, and paralysis. The most common side effects are nausea, diarrhea, and vomiting.

Contraindications: Persons with obstruction of the intestine or renal system should not use these products.

Precautions: Caution should be used in patients with bradycardia, hypotension, seizure disorders, bronchial asthma, coronary occlusion, hyperthyroidism, lactation, and children.

Pharmacokinetics: Onset, peak, and duration vary widely among products. Most products are metabolized in the liver and excreted in urine.

Interactions: Please check individual monographs, since interactions vary widely among products.

Possible nursing diagnoses:
• Altered urinary elimination *[uses]*
• Ineffective breathing pattern *[uses]*
• Knowledge deficit *[teaching]*
• Noncompliance *[teaching]*

NURSING CONSIDERATIONS

Assess:
• VS, respiration q8h
• I&O ratio; check for urinary retention or incontinence
• Bradycardia, hypotension, bronchospasm, headache, dizziness, convulsions, respiratory depression; drug should be discontinued if toxicity occurs

Administer:
• Only with atropine sulfate available for cholinergic crisis
• Only after all other cholinergics have been discontinued
• Increased doses if tolerance occurs
• Larger doses after exercise or fatigue
• On empty stomach for better absorption

Perform/provide:
• Storage at room temp

Evaluate:
• Therapeutic response: increased muscle strength, hand grasp, improved muscle gait, absence of labored breathing (if severe)

Teach patient/family:
• That drug is not a cure; it only relieves symptoms (myasthenia gravis)
• To wear Medic Alert ID specifying myasthenia gravis, drugs taken

---

Generic names

bethanechol	physostigmine
edrophonium	pyridostigmine
neostigmine	

CHOLINERGIC BLOCKERS

Action: Cholinergic blockers inhibit or block acetylcholine at receptor sites in the autonomic nervous system.

Uses: Many products are used to decrease secretions before surgery, to reverse neuromuscular blockade, and to decrease motility of GI, biliary, urinary tracts. Other products are used for parkinsonian symptoms, including dystonia associated with neuroleptic drugs.

Side effects/adverse reactions: The most common side effects are dryness of the mouth and constipation, which can be prevented by frequent rinsing of the mouth and increasing water and bulk in the diet.

Contraindications: Hypersensitivity can occur, and allergies should be identified before administering these products. Persons with GI and GU obstruction should not use these products, since constipation and urinary retention may occur. They are also contraindicated in angle-closure glaucoma and myasthenia gravis.

Precautions: Caution must be used when these products are given to the elderly, since metabolism is slowed. Also, persons with tachycardia or prostatic hypertrophy should use these products with caution.

Pharmacokinetics: Onset, peak, and duration vary with route.

Interactions: Increase in anticholinergic effect occurs when used with narcotics, barbiturates, antihistamines, MAOIs, phenothiazines, amantadine.

Possible nursing diagnoses:
• Impaired physical mobility *[uses]*
• Pain *[uses]*

NURSING CONSIDERATIONS
Assess:
• I&O ratio; be alert for urinary retention, frequency, dysuria; drug should be discontinued if these occur
• Urinary hesitancy, retention; palpate bladder if retention occurs
• Constipation; increase fluids, bulk, exercise
• For tolerance over long-term therapy, dose may have to be increased or changed
• Mental status: affect, mood, CNS depression, worsening of mental symptoms during early therapy
Administer:
• With food or milk to decrease GI symptoms
• Parenteral dose with patient recumbent to prevent postural hypotension; give parenteral dose slowly, monitoring vital signs

Perform/provide:
• Hard candy, gum, frequent rinsing of mouth for dryness
Evaluate:
• Therapeutic response, including absence of cramps and EPS
Teach patient/family:
• To avoid driving, other hazardous activity if drowsiness occurs
• To avoid concurrent use of cough, cold preparations with alcohol, antihistamines unless directed by prescriber
• To use with caution in hot weather, since medication may increase susceptibility to heat stroke

---

Generic names

atropine	procyclidine
benztropine	scopolamine
biperiden	trihexyphenidyl
glycopyrrolate	

CORTICOSTEROIDS

Action: Corticosteroids are divided into glucocorticoids and mineralocorticoids. Glucocorticoids decrease inflammation by the suppression of migration of polymorphonuclear leukocytes, fibroblasts, increased capillary permeability, and lysosomal stabilization. They also have varied metabolic effects and modify the body's immune responses to many stimuli. Mineralocorticoids act by increasing resorption of sodium by increasing hydrogen and potassium excretion in the distal tubule.

Uses: Glucocorticoids are used to decrease inflammation and for immunosuppression. In addition, some products may be given for allergy, adrenal insufficiency, or cerebral edema. Mineralocorticoids are given for adrenal insufficiency or adrenogenital syndrome.

Side effects/adverse reactions: The most common side effects include change in behavior, including insomnia and euphoria; GI irritation, including peptic ulcer; metabolic reactions, including hypokalemia, hyperglycemia, and carbohydrate intolerance; and sodium and fluid retention. Most adverse reactions are dose dependent.

Contraindications: Hypersensitivity may occur and should be identified before administering. Since these products mask infection, they should not be used in systemic fungal infections or amebiasis. Mothers taking pharmacologic doses of corticosteroids should not nurse.

Precautions: Caution must be used when these products are prescribed for diabetic patients, since hyperglycemia may occur. Also, patients with glaucoma, seizure disorders, peptic ulcer, impaired renal function, CHF, hypertension, ulcerative colitis, or myasthenia gravis should be monitored closely if corticosteroids are given. Use with caution in children and the elderly and during pregnancy.

Pharmacokinetics: For oral preparations, the onset of action occurs between 1 and 2 hr, and duration can be up to 2 days, with a half-life of 2-4 days. Pharmacokinetics vary widely among products. These products cross the placenta and appear in breast milk.

Interactions: Decreased corticosteroid effect may occur with barbiturates, rifampin, phenytoin; corticosteroid dose may have to be increased. There is a possibility of GI bleeding when used with salicylates, indomethacin. Steroids may reduce salicylate levels. When using with digitalis glycosides, potassium-depleting diuretics, and amphotericin, serum potassium levels should be monitored.

Possible nursing diagnoses:
- Risk for infection *[adverse reactions]*
- Body image disturbance *[adverse reactions]*
- Risk for violence: self-directed (suicide) *[adverse reactions]*

NURSING CONSIDERATIONS
Assess:
- Potassium, blood sugar, urine glucose while on long-term therapy; hypokalemia and hyperglycemia are common
- Weight daily; notify prescriber of weekly gain >5 lb, since these products alter fluid and electrolyte balance
- I&O ratio; be alert for decreasing urinary output and increasing edema
- Plasma cortisol levels during long-term therapy (normal level is 138-635 nmol/L SI U when drawn at 8 AM)
- Infection, including increased temp, WBC, even after withdrawal of medication; drug masks symptoms of infection
- Adrenal insufficiency: nausea, anorexia, fatigue, dizziness, dyspnea, weakness, joint pain
- Potassium depletion, including paresthesias, fatigue, nausea, vomiting, depression, polyuria, dysrhythmias, weakness
- Mental status, including affect, mood, behavioral changes, aggression; if severe personality changes occur, including depression, drug may have to be tapered and then discontinued

Administer:
- With food or milk to decrease GI symptoms

Evaluate:
- Therapeutic response, including decreased inflammation

Teach patient/family:
• That ID as steroid user should be carried
• Not to discontinue this medication abruptly, or adrenal crisis can result
• Teach patient all aspects of drug use, including cushingoid symptoms
• That single daily or alternate-day doses should be taken in the morning before 9 AM (for replacement therapy)
• To take with meals or a snack

Generic names

Glucocorticoids
beclomethasone
betamethasone
cortisone
dexamethasone
flunisolide
hydrocortisone
hydrocortisone sodium phosphate
methylprednisolone

paramethasone
prednisolone
prednisone
rimexolone (Appx C)
triamcinolone

Mineralocorticoid
fludrocortisone

DIURETICS

Action: Diuretics are divided into subgroups: thiazides and thiazide-like diuretics, loop diuretics, carbonic anhydrase inhibitors, osmotic diuretics, and potassium-sparing diuretics. Each one of these subgroups has its own mechanism of action. Thiazides and thiazide-like diuretics increase excretion of water and sodium by inhibiting resorption in the early distal tubule. Loop diuretics inhibit resorption of sodium and chloride in the thick ascending limb of the loop of Henle. Carbonic anhydrase inhibitors increase sodium excretion by decreasing sodium-hydrogen ion exchange throughout the renal tubule. Carbonic anhydrase inhibitors also decrease secretion of aqueous humor in the eye and thus decrease intraocular pressure. Osmotic diuretics increase the osmotic pressure of glomerular filtrate, thus decreasing net absorption of sodium. The potassium-sparing diuretics interfere with sodium resorption at the distal tubule, thus decreasing potassium excretion.

Uses: Blood pressure is reduced in hypertension; edema is reduced in CHF; intraocular pressure is decreased in glaucoma.

Side effects/adverse reactions: Hypokalemia, hyperuricemia, and hyperglycemia occur most frequently with thiazide diuretics. Aplastic anemia, blood dyscrasias, volume depletion, and dehydration may occur when thiazide-like diuretics, loop diuretics, or carbonic anhydrase inhibitors are given. Side effects and adverse reactions vary widely for the miscellaneous products.

Contraindications: Persons with electrolyte imbalances (Na, Cl, K), dehydration, or anuria should not be given these products until the problem is corrected.

Precautions: Caution must be used when diuretics are given to the elderly, since electrolyte disturbances and dehydration can occur rapidly. Hepatic and renal disease may cause poor metabolism and excretion of the drug.

Pharmacokinetics: Onset, peak, and duration vary widely among the different subgroups of these drugs.

Interactions: Cholestyramine and colestipol will decrease the absorption of thiazide diuretics. Concurrent use of thiazides with diazoxide may increase hyperuricemia, hyperglycemia, and antihypertensive effects of thiazides. Ototoxicity may occur when loop diuretics are used with aminoglycosides. Thiazide and loop diuretics may increase therapeutic and toxic effects of lithium.

Possible nursing diagnoses:
• Fluid volume excess *[uses]*
• Decreased cardiac output *[adverse reactions]*

NURSING CONSIDERATIONS
Assess:
• Weight, I&O daily to determine fluid loss; check skin turgor for dehydration
• Electrolytes: K, Na, Cl; include BUN, blood sugar, CBC, serum creatinine, blood pH, ABGs, uric acid, Ca; electrolyte imbalances may occur quickly
• B/P lying, standing; postural hypotension may occur, since fluid loss occurs from intravascular spaces first
• Signs of metabolic alkalosis, including drowsiness and restlessness
• Signs of hypokalemia with some products, including postural hypotension, malaise, fatigue, tachycardia, leg cramps, weakness
Administer:
• In AM to avoid interference with sleep if using drug as a diuretic
• K replacement if K is less than 3 mg/dl
Evaluate:
• Therapeutic response: improvement in edema of feet, legs, sacral area daily if medication is being used in CHF; improvement in B/P if medication is being used as a diuretic; improvement in intraocular pressure if medication is being used to decrease aqueous humor in the eye
Teach patient/family:
• To take drug early in the day (diuretic) to prevent nocturia

Generic names

Thiazides
chlorothiazide
hydrochlorothiazide

Thiazide-like
chlorthalidone
indapamide
metolazone

Loop
bumetanide
ethacrynate/ethacrynic
furosemide
torsemide

Carbonic anhydrase inhibitors
acetazolamide
methazolamide

Potassium-sparing
amiloride
spironolactone
triamterene

Osmotic
mannitol
urea

HISTAMINE H$_2$ ANTAGONISTS

Action: Histamine H$_2$ antagonists act by inhibiting histamine at the H$_2$-receptor site in parietal cells, which inhibits gastric acid secretion.

Uses: Histamine H$_2$ antagonists are used for short-term treatment of duodenal and gastric ulcers and maintenance therapy for duodenal ulcer; gastroesophageal reflux disease.

Side effects/adverse reactions: The most serious adverse reactions are agranulocytosis, thrombocytopenia, neutropenia, aplastic anemia, exfoliative dermatitis. The most common side effects are confusion (not with ranitidine), headache, and diarrhea.

Contraindications: Persons with hypersensitivity should not use these products.

Precautions: Caution should be used in pregnancy, lactation, child <16 yr, organic brain syndrome, hepatic disease, renal disease.

Pharmacokinetics: Onset, peak, and duration vary widely among products. Most products are metabolized in the liver and excreted in urine.

Interactions: Antacids interfere with absorption of histamine H$_2$ antagonists. Check individual monographs for other interactions.

Possible nursing diagnoses:
- Pain *[uses]*
- Risk for injury *[bleeding]*
- Knowledge deficit *[teaching]*

NURSING CONSIDERATIONS
Assess:
- Gastric pH (>5 should be maintained)
- I&O ratio, BUN, creatinine

Administer:
- With meals for prolonged drug effect
- Antacids 1 hr before or 1 hr after cimetidine
- IV slowly; bradycardia may occur; give over 30 min

Perform/provide:
- Storage of diluted sol at room temp for up to 48 hr

Evaluate:
- Therapeutic response: decreased pain in abdomen

Teach patient/family:
- That gynecomastia, impotence may occur, but are reversible
- To avoid driving, other hazardous activities until patient is stabilized on this medication
- To avoid black pepper, caffeine, alcohol, harsh spices, extremes in temp of food
- To avoid OTC preparations: aspirin, cough, cold preparations
- That drug must be continued for prescribed time to be effective
- To report bruising, fatigue, malaise; blood dyscrasias may occur

---

Generic names

cimetidine   ranitidine
famotidine

IMMUNOSUPPRESSANTS

Action: Immunosuppressants act by inhibiting lymphocytes (T).

Uses: Most products are used for organ transplants to prevent rejection.

Side effects/adverse reactions: The most serious adverse reactions are albuminuria, hematuria, proteinuria, renal failure, and hepatotoxicity. The most common side effects are overgrowth of oral *Candida,* gum hyperplasia, tremors, and headache. The most serious adverse reactions for azathioprine are hematologic (leukopenia and thrombocytopenia) and GI (nausea and vomiting). There is a risk of secondary infection.

Contraindications: Products are contraindicated in hypersensitivity.

Precautions: Caution should be used in severe renal disease, severe hepatic disease, and pregnancy.

Pharmacokinetics: Onset, peak, and duration vary widely among products. Most products are metabolized in the liver and excreted in urine.

Interactions: Please check individual monographs, since interactions vary widely among products.

Possible nursing diagnoses:
- Risk for infection *[adverse reactions]*
- Risk for injury *[uses]*
- Knowledge deficit *[teaching]*

NURSING CONSIDERATIONS
Assess:
- Renal studies: BUN, creatinine at least qmo during treatment, 3 mo after treatment
- Liver function studies: alk phosphatase, AST (SGOT), ALT (SGPT), bilirubin
- Drug blood levels during treatment
- Hepatotoxicity: dark urine, jaundice, itching, light-colored stools; drug should be discontinued

Administer:
- For several days before transplant surgery
- With meals for GI upset or drug mixed with chocolate milk
- With oral antifungal for *Candida* infections

Evaluate:
- Therapeutic response: absence of rejection

Teach patient/family:
- To report fever, chills, sore throat, fatigue, since serious infections may occur
- To use contraceptive measures during treatment, for 12 wk after ending therapy

---

Generic names

azathioprine	muromonab-CD3
basiliximab	tacrolimus
cyclosporine	

LAXATIVES

Action: Laxatives are divided into bulk products, lubricants, osmotics, saline laxative stimulants, and stool softeners. Bulk laxatives work by absorbing water and expanding to increase moisture content and bulk in the stool. Lubricants increase water retention in the stool, causing reabsorption of water in the bowel. Stimulants act by increasing peristalsis by direct effect on the intestine. Saline draws water into the intestinal lumen.

Osmotics increase distention and promote peristalsis. Stool softeners reduce surface tension of liquids of the bowel.

Uses: Laxatives are used as a preparation for bowel and rectal exam, constipation, and stool softener.

Side effects/adverse reactions: The most common side effects are nausea, abdominal cramps, and diarrhea.

Contraindications: Persons with GI obstruction, perforation, gastric retention, toxic colitis, megacolon, abdominal pain, nausea, vomiting, or fecal impaction should not use these products.

Precautions: Caution should be used in rectal bleeding, large hemorrhoids, and anal excoriation.

Pharmacokinetics: Onset, peak, and duration vary among products.

Interactions: Please check individual monographs, since interactions vary widely among products.

Possible nursing diagnoses:

- Constipation [uses]
- Diarrhea [adverse reactions]
- Knowledge deficit [teaching]

NURSING CONSIDERATIONS

Assess:

- Blood, urine electrolytes if drug is used often by patient
- I&O ratio: to identify fluid loss
- Cause of constipation; identify whether fluids, bulk, or exercise is missing from lifestyle
- Cramping, rectal bleeding, nausea, vomiting; if these symptoms occur, drug should be discontinued

Administer:

- Alone only with water for better absorption; do not take within 1 hr of antacids, milk, or cimetidine

Evaluate:

- Therapeutic response: decrease in constipation

Teach patient/family:

- To swallow tabs whole; not to chew
- Not to use laxatives for long-term therapy; bowel tone will be lost
- That normal bowel movements do not always occur daily
- Not to use in presence of abdominal pain, nausea, vomiting
- To notify prescriber of abdominal pain, nausea, vomiting
- To notify prescriber if constipation is unrelieved or of symptoms of electrolyte imbalance: muscle cramps, pain, weakness, dizziness

Generic names

Bulk laxatives
calcium polycarbophil
methylcellulose
psyllium

Lubricants
mineral oil

Osmotic agents
glycerin
lactulose

Saline laxatives
magnesium salts
sodium biphosphate/phosphate

Stimulants
bisacodyl
cascara sagrada
phenolphthalein
senna

Stool softeners
docusate

NARCOTICS

Action: Narcotics act by depressing pain impulse transmission at the spinal cord level by interacting with opioid receptors. Products are divided into opiates and nonopiates.

Uses: Most products are used to control moderate to severe pain and are used before and after surgery.

Side effects/adverse reactions: GI symptoms, including nausea, vomiting, anorexia, constipation, and cramps are the most common side effects. Other common side effects include light-headedness, dizziness, sedation. Serious adverse reactions such as respiratory depression, respiratory arrest, circulatory depression, and increased intracranial pressure may result but are less common and usually dose dependent.

Contraindications: Hypersensitive reactions occur frequently. Check for sensitivity before administering. These drugs should not be used if narcotic addiction is suspected, and they are also contraindicated in acute bronchial asthma and upper airway obstruction.

Precautions: Caution must be used when these products are given to persons with an addictive personality, since the possibility of addiction is so great. Also, they may worsen intracranial pressure. Persons with severe heart disease, hepatic or renal disease, respiratory conditions, or seizure disorders should be monitored closely for worsening condition.

Pharmacokinetics: Onset of action is immediate by IV route and rapid by IM and PO routes. Peak occurs from 1-2 hr, depending on route, with a duration of 2-8 hr. These agents cross the placenta and appear in breast milk.

Interactions: Barbiturates, other narcotics, hypnotics, antipsychotics, or alcohol can increase CNS depression when taken with narcotics.

Possible nursing diagnoses:
• Pain *[uses]*
• Impaired gas exchange *[adverse reactions]*

NURSING CONSIDERATIONS
Assess:
• I&O ratio; be alert for urinary retention, frequency, dysuria; drug should be discontinued if these occur
• Respiratory dysfunction, including respiratory depression, rate, rhythm, character; notify prescriber if respirations are <12/min
• CNS changes: dizziness, drowsiness, hallucinations, euphoria, LOC, pupil reaction
• Allergic reactions: rash, urticaria
• Need for pain medication; use pain scoring

Administer:
• With antiemetic if nausea or vomiting occurs
• When pain is beginning to return; determine dosage interval by response

Perform/provide:
• Assistance with ambulation; patient should not be ambulating during drug peak

Evaluate:
• Therapeutic response, including decrease in pain

Teach patient/family:
• To report any symptoms of CNS changes, allergic reactions, or shortness of breath
• That physical dependency may result when used for extended periods
• That withdrawal symptoms may occur, including nausea, vomiting, cramps, fever, faintness, anorexia
• To avoid alcohol and other CNS depressants

Generic names

alfentanil
buprenorphine
butorphanol
codeine
dezocine
fentanyl
fentanyl transdermal
hydromorphone
levorphanol

meperidine
methadone
morphine
nalbuphine
oxycodone
oxymorphone
pentazocine
propoxyphene
remifentanil

NEUROMUSCULAR BLOCKING AGENTS

Action: Neuromuscular blocking agents are divided into depolarizing and nondepolarizing blockers. They act by inhibiting transmission of nerve impulses by binding with cholinergic receptor sites.

Uses: Neuromuscular blocking agents are used to facilitate endotracheal intubation and skeletal muscle relaxation during mechanical ventilation, surgery, or general anesthesia.

Side effects/adverse reactions: The most serious adverse reactions are prolonged apnea, bronchospasm, cyanosis, respiratory depression, and malignant hyperthermia. The most common side effects are bradycardia and decreased motility.

Contraindications: Persons who are hypersensitive should not be given this product.

Precautions: Caution should be used in pregnancy, thyroid disease, collagen disease, cardiac disease, lactation, children <2 yr, electrolyte imbalances, dehydration, neuromuscular disease (myasthenia gravis), and respiratory disease.

Pharmacokinetics: Onset, peak, and duration vary widely among products. Most products are metabolized in the liver and excreted in urine.

Interactions: Aminoglycosides potentiate neuromuscular blockade. See individual monographs.

Possible nursing diagnoses:
- Ineffective breathing pattern *[uses]*
- Risk for injury *[adverse reactions]*
- Knowledge deficit *[teaching]*

NURSING CONSIDERATIONS

Assess:
- For electrolyte imbalances (K, Mg); may lead to increased action of this drug
- Vital signs (B/P, pulse, respirations, airway) q15min until fully recovered; rate, depth, pattern of respirations, strength of hand grip
- I&O ratio; check for urinary retention, frequency, hesitancy
- Recovery: decreased paralysis of face, diaphragm, leg, arm, rest of body
- Allergic reactions: rash, fever, respiratory distress, pruritus; drug should be discontinued

Administer:
- Using nerve stimulator by anesthesiologist to determine neuromuscular blockade
- Anticholinesterase to reverse neuromuscular blockade

• IV undiluted over 1-2 min (only by qualified person, usually an anesthesiologist)

Perform/provide:

• Storage in light-resistant, cool area

• Reassurance if communication is difficult during recovery from neuromuscular blockade

Evaluate:

• Therapeutic response: paralysis of jaw, eyelid, head, neck, rest of body

---

Generic names

atracurium	pancuronium
cisatracurium	pipecuronium
doxacurium	succinylcholine
gallamine	tubocurarine
metocurine	vecuronium
mivacurium	

NONSTEROIDAL ANTIINFLAMMATORIES

Action: Nonsteroidals decrease prostaglandin synthesis by inhibiting an enzyme needed for biosynthesis.

Uses: Nonsteroidal antiinflammatories are used to treat mild to moderate pain, osteoarthritis, rheumatoid arthritis, and dysmenorrhea.

Side effects/adverse reactions: The most serious adverse reactions are nephrotoxicity (dysuria, hematuria, oliguria, azotemia), blood dyscrasias, and cholestatic hepatitis. The most common side effects are nausea, abdominal pain, anorexia, dizziness, and drowsiness.

Contraindications: Persons with hypersensitivity, asthma, severe renal disease, and severe hepatic disease should not use these products.

Precautions: Caution should be used in pregnancy, lactation, children, bleeding disorders, GI disorders, cardiac disorders, hypersensitivity to other antiinflammatory agents, and the elderly.

Pharmacokinetics: Onset, peak, and duration vary widely among products. Most products are metabolized in the liver and excreted in urine.

Interactions: Please check individual monographs, since interactions vary widely among products.

Possible nursing diagnoses:

• Chronic pain *[uses]*

• Impaired physical mobility *[uses]*

• Knowledge deficit *[teaching]*

• Noncompliance *[teaching]*

NURSING CONSIDERATIONS

Assess:

• Renal, liver, blood studies: BUN, creatinine, AST (SGOT), ALT (SGPT), Hgb, before treatment, periodically thereafter

• Audiometric, ophthalmic examination before, during, and after treatment

• For eye, ear problems: blurred vision, tinnitus; may indicate toxicity

Administer:

• With food to decrease GI symptoms; however, best to take on empty stomach to facilitate absorption

Perform/provide:

• Storage at room temp

Evaluate:

• Therapeutic response: decreased pain, stiffness in joints, decreased swelling in joints, ability to move more easily

Teach patient/family:

• To report blurred vision, ringing, roaring in ears; may indicate toxicity

• To avoid driving, other hazardous activities if dizziness, drowsiness occur, especially elderly

• To report change in urine pattern, increased weight, edema, increased pain in joints, fever, blood in urine; indicate nephrotoxicity

• That therapeutic effects may take up to 1 mo

Generic names

diclofenac	mefenamic acid
etodolac	nabumetone
fenoprofen	naproxen
flurbiprofen	oxyphenbutazone
ibuprofen	phenylbutazone
indomethacin	piroxicam
ketoprofen	sulindac
ketorolac	tolmetin
meclofenamate	

SALICYLATES

Action: Salicylates have analgesic, antipyretic, and antiinflammatory effects. The antiinflammatory and analgesic activities may be mediated through the inhibition of prostaglandin synthesis. Antipyretic action results from inhibition of the hypothalamic heat-regulating center.

Uses: The primary uses of salicylates are relief of mild to moderate pain and fever and in inflammatory conditions such as arthritis, thromboembolic disorders, and rheumatic fever.

Side effects/adverse reactions: The most common side effects are GI symptoms and rash. Serious blood dyscrasias and hepatotoxicity may result when used for long periods at high doses. Tinnitus or impaired hearing may indicate that blood salicylate levels are reaching or exceeding the upper limit of the therapeutic range.

Contraindications: Hypersensitivity to salicylates is common. Check for sensitivity before administering. Persons with bleeding disorders, GI bleeding, and vit K deficiency should not use these products, since salicylates increase prothrombin time. Children should not use these products, since salicylates have been associated with Reye's syndrome.

Precautions: Caution is needed when salicylates are given to patients with anemia, hepatic or renal disease, or Hodgkin's disease. Caution should also be exercised in pregnancy and lactation.

Pharmacokinetics: Onset of action occurs in 15-30 min, with a peak of 1-2 hr and a duration up to 6 hr. These drugs are metabolized by the liver and excreted by the kidneys.

Interactions: Increased effects of anticoagulants, insulin, methotrexate, heparin, valproic acid, and oral sulfonylureas may occur when used with salicylates. Aspirin may decrease serum concentrations of nonsteroidal antiinflammatory agents.

Possible nursing diagnoses:
- Pain *[uses]*
- Impaired physical mobility *[uses]*
- Activity intolerance *[uses]*
- Sensory/perceptual alterations: auditory *[adverse reactions]*
- Ineffective thermoregulation *[uses]*

NURSING CONSIDERATIONS
Assess:
- Hepatic and renal studies: AST (SGOT), ALT (SGPT), bilirubin, creatinine, LDH, alk phosphatase, BUN if patient is on long-term therapy, since these products are metabolized and excreted by the liver and kidney
- Blood studies: CBC, hematocrit, hemoglobin, and prothrombin time if patient is on long-term therapy, since these products increase the possibility of bleeding and blood dyscrasias
- Hepatotoxicity: dark urine, clay-colored stools; yellowing of skin, sclera; itching, abdominal pain, fever, diarrhea, which may occur with long-term use
- Ototoxicity: tinnitus; ringing, roaring in ears; audiometric testing is needed before and after long-term therapy

Administer:
- With food or milk to decrease gastric irritation; give 30 min before or 1 hr after meals with a full glass of water

Evaluate:
• Therapeutic response, including decreased pain, fever
Teach patient/family:
• That blood sugar levels should be monitored closely if patient is diabetic
• Not to exceed recommended dosage; acute poisoning may result
• That therapeutic response takes 2 wk in arthritis
• To avoid use of alcohol, since GI bleeding may result
• To notify prescriber of ringing in the ears or persistent GI pain
• To take with full glass of H_2O to reduce risk of lodging in esophagus

Generic names

aspirin	salsalate
choline salicylate	sodium thiosalicylate
magnesium salicylate	

THROMBOLYTICS

Action: Thrombolytics act by activating conversion of plasminogen to plasmin (fibrinolysin): plasmin is able to break down clots (fibrin).

Uses: Thrombolytics are used to treat deep-vein thrombosis, pulmonary embolism, arterial thrombosis, arterial embolism, arteriovenous cannula occlusion, lysis of coronary artery thrombi after MI, and acute, evolving transmural MI.

Side effects/adverse reactions: Serious adverse reactions include GI, GU, intracranial retroperitoneal bleeding, and anaphylaxis. The most common side effects are decreased Hct, urticaria, headache, and nausea.

Contraindications: Persons with hypersensitivity, active bleeding, intraspinal surgery, neoplasms of the CNS, ulcerative colitis/enteritis, severe hypertension, renal disease, hepatic disease, hypocoagulation, COPD, subacute bacterial endocarditis, rheumatic valvular disease, cerebral embolism/thrombosis/hemorrhage, intraarterial diagnostic procedure or surgery (10 days), and recent major surgery should not use these products.

Precautions: Caution should be used in arterial emboli from left side of heart and pregnancy.

Pharmacokinetics: Onset, peak, and duration vary widely among products. Most products are metabolized in the liver and excreted in urine.

Interactions: Please check individual monographs, since interactions vary widely among products.

Possible nursing diagnoses:
• Risk for injury *[uses]*

NURSING CONSIDERATIONS

Assess:

• VS, B/P, pulse, resp, neuro signs, temp at least q4h, temp >104° F (40° C) are indicators of internal bleeding; cardiac rhythm following intracoronary administration; systolic pressure increase of >25 mm Hg should be reported to prescriber

• For neurologic changes that may indicate intracranial bleeding

• Retroperitoneal bleeding: back pain, leg weakness, diminished pulses

• Allergy: fever, rash, itching, chill; mild reaction may be treated with antihistamines

• For bleeding during 1st hr of treatment: hematuria, hematemesis, bleeding from mucous membranes, epistaxis, ecchymosis

• Blood studies (Hct, platelets, PTT, PT, TT, APTT) before starting therapy; PT or APTT must be less than ×2 control before starting therapy; TT or PT q3-4h during treatment

Administer:

• As soon as thrombi identified; not useful for thrombi over 1 wk old

• Cryoprecipitate or fresh, frozen plasma if bleeding occurs

• Loading dose at beginning of therapy; may require increased loading doses

• Heparin after fibrinogen level is over 100 mg/dl. Heparin infusion to increase PTT to 1.5-2 × baseline for 3-7 days

• About 10% of patients have high streptococcal antibody titers requiring increased loading doses

• IV therapy using 0.8 μm filter

Perform/provide:

• Storage of reconstituted drug in refrigerator; discard after 24 hr

• Bed rest during entire course of treatment

• Avoidance of venous or arterial puncture, inj, rectal temp

• Treatment of fever with acetaminophen or aspirin

• Pressure for 30 sec to minor bleeding sites; inform prescriber if this does not attain hemostasis; apply pressure dressing

Evaluate:

• Therapeutic response: resolution of thrombosis, embolism

Generic names

alteplase
anistreplase

streptokinase
urokinase

THYROID HORMONES

Action: Acts by increasing metabolic rates, resulting in increased cardiac output, O_2 consumption, body temp, blood volume, growth, development at cellular level, respiratory rate, enzyme system activity.

Uses: Products are used for thyroid replacement.

Side effects/adverse reactions: The most common side effects include insomnia, tremors, tachycardia, palpitations, angina, dysrhythmias, weight loss, and changes in appetite. Serious adverse reactions include thyroid storm.

Contraindications: Persons with adrenal insufficiency, myocardial infarction, or thyrotoxicosis should not use these products.

Precautions: The elderly and patients with angina pectoris, hypertension, ischemia, cardiac disease, or diabetes mellitus or insipidus should be watched closely when using these products. Caution should be used in pregnancy (A) and lactation.

Pharmacokinetics: Pharmacokinetics vary widely among products; check specific monographs.

Interactions:
• Impaired absorption of thyroid products may occur when administered with cholestyramine (separate by 4-5 hr)
• Increased effects of anticoagulants, sympathomimetics, tricyclic antidepressants, catecholamines may occur
• Decreased effects of digitalis, glycosides, insulin, hypoglycemics may occur
• Decreased effects of thyroid products may occur with estrogens

Possible nursing diagnoses:
• Knowledge deficit [teaching]
• Noncompliance [teaching]
• Body image disturbance [adverse reactions]

NURSING CONSIDERATIONS

Assess:
• B/P, pulse before each dose
• I&O ratio
• Weight qd in same clothing, using same scale, at same time of day
• Height, growth rate if given to a child
• T_3, T_4, which are decreased; radioimmunoassay of TSH, which is increased; ratio uptake, which is decreased if patient is on too low a dosage of medication
• Increased nervousness, excitability, irritability; may indicate overdosage, usually after 1-3 wk of treatment

• Cardiac status: angina, palpitation, chest pain, change in VS
Administer:
• At same time each day to maintain drug level
• Only for hormone imbalances, not to be used for obesity, male infertility, menstrual conditions, lethargy
Perform/provide:
• Removal of medication 4 wk before RAIU test
Evaluate:
• Therapeutic response: absence of depression; increased weight loss; diuresis; pulse; appetite; absence of constipation; peripheral edema; cold intolerance; pale, cool, dry skin; brittle nails; alopecia; coarse hair; menorrhagia; night blindness; paresthesias; syncope; stupor; coma; rosy cheeks
Teach patient/family:
• That hair loss will occur in child and is temporary
• To report excitability, irritability, anxiety; indicates overdose
• Not to switch brands unless directed by prescriber
• That hypothyroid child will show almost immediate behavior/personality change
• That treatment drug is not to be taken to reduce weight
• To avoid OTC preparations with iodine; read labels
• To avoid iodine food, iodinized salt, soybeans, tofu, turnips, some seafood, some bread

---

Generic names

levothyroxine (T$_4$)	thyroglobulin
liothyronine (T$_3$)	thyroid USP
liotrix	thyrotropin (TSH)

VASODILATORS

Action: Vasodilators have various modes of action. Please check individual monograph for specific action.

Uses: Vasodilators are used to treat intermittent claudication, arteriosclerosis obliterans, vasospasm and muscular ischemia, ischemic cerebral vascular disease, hypertension, and angina.

Side effects/adverse reactions: The most common side effects are headache, nausea, hypotension or hypertension, and ECG changes.

Contraindications: Some drugs are contraindicated in acute MI, paroxysmal tachycardia, and thyrotoxicosis.

Precautions: Caution should be used in uncompensated heart disease or peptic ulcer disease.

Pharmacokinetics: Onset, peak, and duration vary widely among products. Most products are metabolized in the liver and excreted in urine.

Interactions: Please check individual monographs, since interactions vary widely among products.

Possible nursing diagnoses:
• Decreased cardiac output *[uses]*
• Altered tissue perfusion: cardiopulmonary *[uses]*
• Knowledge deficit *[teaching]*

NURSING CONSIDERATIONS

Assess:
• Bleeding time in individuals with bleeding disorders
• Cardiac status: B/P, pulse, rate, rhythm, character; watch for increasing pulse

Administer:
• With meals to reduce GI symptoms

Perform/provide:
• Storage in tight container at room temp

Evaluate:
• Therapeutic response: ability to walk without pain, increased temp in extremities, increased pulse volume

Teach patient/family:
• That medication is not cure; may need to be taken continuously
• That it is necessary to quit smoking to prevent excessive vasoconstriction
• That improvement may be sudden, but usually occurs gradually over several wk
• To report headache, weakness, increased pulse, as drug may have to be decreased or discontinued
• To avoid hazardous activities until stabilized on medication; dizziness may occur

---

Generic names

amyl nitrite	isoxsuprine
cyclandelate	minoxidil
dipyridamole	papaverine
hydralazine	tolazoline

VITAMINS

Action: Action varies widely among products and classes; check specific monographs.

Uses: Vitamins are used to correct and prevent vitamin deficiencies.

Side effects/adverse reactions: There are no side effects or adverse reactions with the water-soluble vitamins (C, B). However, fat-soluble vitamins (A, D, E, K) may accumulate in the body and cause adverse reactions (see specific monographs).

Contraindications: Hypersensitive reactions may occur, and allergies should be identified before these products are given.

Pharmacokinetics: Onset, peak, and duration vary widely among products; check individual monograph for specific information.

Possible nursing diagnoses:

• Altered nutrition: less than body requirements *[uses]*

NURSING CONSIDERATIONS
Administer:

• PO with food for better absorption

Perform/provide:

• Storage in tight, light-resistant container

Evaluate:

• Therapeutic response: no vitamin deficiency

Teach patient/family:

• Not to take more than prescribed amount

Generic names

Fat-soluble
menadione/menadiol
    sodium diphosphate
    (vitamin K₃)
phytonadione (vita-
    min K₁)
vitamin A
vitamin D
vitamin E

Water-soluble
ascorbic acid (C)
cyanocobalamin B₁₂/hydroxo-
    cobalamin (B₁₂a)
pyridoxine (B₆)
riboflavin (B₂)
thiamine (B₁)

Miscellaneous
    multivitamins

abciximab (℞)

(ab-six′i-mab)

ReoPro

Func. class.: Platelet aggregation inhibitor

Action: Decreases platelet aggregation by binding to receptors on platelet surfaces (glycoproteins)

Uses: Used with heparin and aspirin to prevent acute cardiac ischemia following percutaneous transluminal angioplasty (PTCA) in patients at high risk for reclosure of affected arteries

Dosage and routes:
• *Adult:* **IV** 250 μg (0.25 mg)/kg bolus 10-60 min prior to PTCA, followed by 10 μg/min **CONT INF** for 12 hr

Available forms: Inj 2 mg/ml

Side effects/adverse reactions:

CNS: Dizziness, abnormal thinking, hyperesthesia, confusion

CV: Hypotension, *atrial fibrillation/flutter,* bradycardia, vascular disorder, *supraventricular tachycardia,* weak pulse, AV block, peripheral edema

HEMA: Bleeding, *thrombocytopenia,* anemia, leukocytosis

RESP: Pleural effusion

Contraindications: Hypersensitivity to this drug or murine protein; GI, GU bleeding; CVA within 2 yr, bleeding disorders, intracranial neoplasm, intracranial arteriovenous malformations, intracranial aneurysm, platelet count >100,000/mm³, recent surgery, aneurysm, uncontrolled severe hypertension, vasculitis

Precautions: GI disease, pregnancy (C), lactation, children, patients >65 yr or <75 kg

Pharmacokinetics: Bound to platelet receptor sites for up to 10 days, half-life ½ hr

Interactions:
• Increased risk of bleeding: heparin, thrombolytics, dipyridamole, ticlopidine, oral anticoagulants, NSAIDs

🖊 Increased risk of bleeding: bromelain

NURSING CONSIDERATIONS
Assess:
⬥ For bleeding at all possible sites: (catheter, puncture sites, GI, GU, and retroperitoneal sites) during therapy; if bleeding occurs, stop the infusion; provide bed rest for 8 hr after infusion to prevent bleeding

• Hypersensitivity reactions: rash, pruritus, laryngeal edema, wheezing during treatment; if hypersensitivity reaction occurs, infusion should be stopped and appropriate action taken to treat the reaction; have epinephrine, antihistamines, corticosteroids in case of anaphylaxis

• Distal pulses of affected legs frequently while femoral artery sheath is in place and for several hours after sheath is removed

• ECG and vital signs during treatment

Administer:
• Visually inspect solution for opaque particles, do not use if these particles are present

• Discard any unused portion

Direct IV
• After withdrawing the amount of drug needed using a sterile, nonpyrogenic low protein binding 0.2-0.22 μm filter into a syringe; give by bolus dose 10-60 min before the start of PTCA

Continuous IV
• After withdrawing 4.5 ml of drug through a sterile, nonpyrogenic low protein binding 0.2-0.22 μm filter into a syringe; inject into 250 ml of

0.9% NaCl or D$_5$W; give at a rate of 17 ml/hr (10 µg/min) for 12 hr using an infusion pump and with an in-line filter as above

Perform/provide:
• Discontinuing heparin therapy at least 4 hr prior to removal of femoral artery sheath
• Pressure to the femoral artery using manual compression or a mechanical device for hemostasis; bed rest should be maintained for several hours after sheath removal
• Affected limb in straight position and complete bed rest with HOB at 30 degrees while the femoral artery sheath is in place

Teach patient/family:
• The reason for the medication and extent of treatment; hypersensitivity reaction including rash, bleeding, dyspnea
• The reason for bed rest, leg immobilization, and to avoid injury

---

acarbose (R)
(ay-car'bose)
Precose
Func. class.: Oral antidiabetic
Chem. class.: α-Glucosidase inhibitor

Action: Delays digestion of ingested carbohydrates, results in smaller rise in blood glucose after meals; does not increase insulin production

Uses: Non–insulin-dependent diabetes mellitus (NIDDM) Type II, alone or in combination with insulin or metformin

Dosage and routes:
• *Adult:* **PO** 25 mg tid initially, with first bite of meal; maintenance dose may be increased to 50 mg tid; may be increased to 100 mg tid if needed (only in patients >60 kg) with dosage adjustment at 4-9 wk intervals

Available forms: Tabs 50, 100 mg

Side effects/adverse reactions:
GI: Abdominal pain, diarrhea, flatulence

Contraindications: Hypersensitivity, diabetic ketoacidosis, cirrhosis, inflammatory bowel disease, colonic ulceration, partial intestinal obstruction, chronic intestinal disease, serum creatinine >2 mg/dl

Precautions: Pregnancy (B), renal disease, lactation, children, hepatic disease

Pharmacokinetics: Metabolized in GI tract, excreted as intact drug in urine, half-life 2 hr

Interactions:
• Effect of acarbose may be decreased: digestive enzymes, intestinal absorbents
• Increased hypoglycemia: sulfonylureas, insulin

Lab test interferences:
Decrease: Hct
Increase: AST

NURSING CONSIDERATIONS
Assess:
• Hypoglycemia, hyperglycemia; even though drug does not cause hypoglycemia, if patient is on sulfonylureas or insulin, hypoglycemia may be additive

Administer:
PO
• Tid with first bite of each meal

Perform/provide:
• Storage in tight container in cool environment

Evaluate:
• Therapeutic response: decreased signs/symptoms of diabetes mellitus (polyuria, polydipsia, polyphagia, clear sensorium, absence of dizziness, stable gait)

Teach patient/family:
• The symptoms of hypo/hyperglycemia, what to do about each

◆ = Nursing alert   ⫻ = Herb-drug interaction   ⊘ = Do not crush

• That medication must be taken as prescribed; explain consequences of discontinuing medication abruptly
• To avoid OTC medications unless approved by health-care provider
• That diabetes is lifelong illness; that this drug is not a cure
• To carry a Medic Alert ID for emergency purposes
• That diet and exercise regimen must be followed

---

acebutolol (℞)

(a-se-byoo'toe-lole)
Monitan*, Sectral

Func. class.: Antihypertensive, β_1-blocker, antidysrhythmic (II)

Action: Competitively blocks stimulation of β-adrenergic receptors within vascular smooth muscle; decreases rate of SA node discharge, increases recovery time, slows conduction of AV node resulting in decreased heart rate (negative chronotropic effect), which decreases O_2 consumption in myocardium; also decreases renin-aldosterone-angiotensin system at high doses, inhibits β_2-receptors in bronchial system (high doses)

Uses: Mild to moderate hypertension, sinus tachycardia, persistent atrial extrasystoles, tachydysrhythmias

Investigational uses: Prophylaxis of MI, treatment of angina pectoris, tremor, mitral valve prolapse, thyrotoxicosis, idiopathic hypertrophic subaortic stenosis

Dosage and routes:

Hypertension

• *Adult:* **PO** 400 mg qd or in 2 divided doses; may be increased to desired response; maintenance 200-1200 mg/qd in 2 divided doses

Ventricular dysrhythmia

• *Adult:* **PO** 200 mg bid, may increase gradually, usual range 600-1200 mg daily; should be tapered over 2 wk before discontinuing

Available forms: Caps 200, 400 mg; tabs 200, 400 mg*

Side effects/adverse reactions:

*CV: **Profound hypotension, bradycardia, CHF,** cold extremities, postural hypotension, **2nd- or 3rd-degree heart block***

CNS: Insomnia, fatigue, dizziness, mental changes, memory loss, hallucinations, depression, lethargy, drowsiness, strange dreams, catatonia*

GI: Nausea, diarrhea, vomiting, **mesenteric arterial thrombosis, ischemic colitis***

INTEG: Rash, fever, alopecia, dry skin

*HEMA: **Agranulocytosis, thrombocytopenia, purpura***

EENT: Sore throat, dry burning eyes

GU: Impotence, decreased libido, dysuria, nocturia

ENDO: Increased hypoglycemic response to insulin

*RESP: **Bronchospasm,** dyspnea, wheezing, cough*

MS: Joint pain, cramping

Contraindications: Hypersensitivity to β-blockers, cardiogenic shock, heart block (2nd-, 3rd-degree), sinus bradycardia, CHF, cardiac failure

Precautions: Major surgery, pregnancy (B), lactation, diabetes mellitus, renal disease, thyroid disease, COPD, asthma, well-compensated heart failure, aortic, mitral valve, hepatic disease

Pharmacokinetics:

PO: Onset 1-1½ hr, peak 2-4 hr, duration 10-12 hr, half-life 6-7 hr, excreted unchanged in urine, protein binding 5%-15%

Interactions:

• Increased hypotension, bradycar-

dia: reserpine, hydralazine, methyldopa, prazosin, anticholinergics
• Decreased antihypertensive effects: indomethacin
• Increased hypoglycemic effect: insulin
• Decreased bronchodilation: theophyllines, β_2 agonists
🖋 May increase acebutolol effect: buckthorn bark/berry, aloe, rhubarb root, senna leaf/fruits, cascara sagrada bark
🖋 Dysrhythmia: Ephedra
Lab test interferences:
Interference: Glucose/insulin tolerance tests
Increase: Uric acid, K, triglyceride, lipoproteins
NURSING CONSIDERATIONS
Assess:
• B/P during beginning treatment, periodically thereafter; pulse q4h; note rate, rhythm, quality
• Apical/radial pulse before administration; notify prescriber of any significant changes (pulse <50 bpm); signs of CHF (dyspnea, crackles, weight gain, jugular vein distension)
• Baselines in renal, liver function tests before therapy begins
• Edema in feet, legs daily: monitor I&O
• Skin turgor, dryness of mucous membranes for hydration status, especially elderly
Administer:
PO
• Drug ac, hs, tablet may be crushed or swallowed whole; give with food to prevent GI upset
• Reduced dosage in renal dysfunction
Perform/provide:
• Storage protected from light, moisture; place in cool environment
Evaluate:
• Therapeutic response: decreased

B/P after 1-2 wk; decreased dysrhythmias
Teach patient/family:
◆ Not to discontinue drug abruptly, taper over 2 wk; may cause precipitate angina if stopped abruptly; do not double dose; if a dose is missed, take as soon as remembered up to 4 hr before next dose
• Not to use OTC products containing α-adrenergic stimulants (such as nasal decongestants, OTC cold preparations) unless directed by prescriber
• To report bradycardia, dizziness, confusion, depression, fever
• To take pulse at home, advise when to notify prescriber
• To avoid alcohol, smoking, sodium intake
• To comply with weight control, dietary adjustments, modified exercise program
• To carry Medic Alert ID to identify drug, allergies
• To avoid hazardous activities if dizziness is present; that drug may cause sensitivity to cold
• To report symptoms of CHF: difficult breathing, especially on exertion or when lying down, night cough, swelling of extremities
• That if diabetic, monitor blood glucose; hyperglycemia, hypoglycemia occur
Treatment of overdose: Lavage, IV atropine for bradycardia, IV theophylline for bronchospasm, digitalis, O_2, diuretic for cardiac failure, IV glucose for hypoglycemia, IV diazepam (or phenytoin) for seizures

---

acetaminophen (OTC)

(a-seat-a-mee'noe-fen)
Abenol*, Acephen, Aceta, Actamin, Actimol, Aminofen, Apacet, APAP, Apo-Acetaminophen*, Aspirin Free Pain Relief, Atasol*, Banesin, Children's Feverall, Dapa, Datril, Exdol*, FemEtts, Genapap, Genebs, Halenol, Liquiprin, Mapap, Maranox, Meda, Panadol, Redutemp, Robigesic*, Rounax*, Snaplets-FR, Silapap, St. Joseph Aspirin-Free, Tapanol, Tempra, Tylenol, Uni-Ace, Valorin

Func. class.: Nonnarcotic analgesic, antipyretic

Chem. class.: Nonsalicylate, para-aminophenol derivative

Action: May block pain impulses peripherally that occur in response to inhibition of prostaglandin synthesis; does not possess antiinflammatory properties; antipyretic action results from inhibition of prostaglandins in the CNS (hypothalamic heat-regulating center)

Uses: Mild to moderate pain or fever

Dosage and routes:
• *Adult and child >12 yr:* **PO** 325-650 mg q4h prn, not to exceed 4 g/day; **RECT** 325-650 mg q4h prn, not to exceed 4 g/day
• *Child:* **PO** 10-15 mg/kg q4h
• *Child 6-12 yr:* **RECT** 325 mg q4-6h
• *Child 3-6 yr:* **RECT** 125 mg q4-6h
• *Child 1-3 yr:* **RECT** 80 mg q4h
• *Child 3-11 mo:* **RECT** 80 mg q6h
Available forms: Rect supp 120, 125, 325, 600, 650 mg; soft chew tabs 80, 160 mg; caps 500 mg; elix 120, 160, 325 mg/5 ml; liq 160 mg/5 ml, 500 mg/15 ml; sol 100 mg/1 ml, 120 mg/2.5 ml; granules 80 mg/ packet, 80 mg/cap; tabs 160, 325, 500, 650 mg

Side effects/adverse reactions:
SYST: **Anaphylaxis**
HEMA: **Leukopenia, neutropenia, hemolytic anemia (long-term use), thrombocytopenia, pancytopenia**
CNS: Stimulation, drowsiness
GI: Nausea, vomiting, abdominal pain, **hepatotoxicity**
INTEG: Rash, urticaria, **angioedema**
TOXICITY: **Cyanosis, anemia, neutropenia, jaundice, pancytopenia, CNS stimulation, delirium followed by vascular collapse, convulsions, coma, death**

Contraindications: Hypersensitivity, intolerance to tartrazine (yellow dye #4), alcohol, table sugar, saccharin

Precautions: Anemia, hepatic disease, renal disease, chronic alcoholism, pregnancy (B), elderly, lactation

Pharmacokinetics: Well absorbed PO, rectal absorption varies
PO: Onset 10-30 min, peak ½-2 hr, duration 3-4 hr
RECT: Onset slow, peak 1-2 hr, duration 3-4 hr; 85%-90% metabolized by liver, excreted by kidneys; metabolites may be toxic if overdose occurs; widely distributed, crosses placenta in low concentrations, excreted in breast milk, half-life 1-4 hr

Interactions:
• Increased effects of: chloramphenicol
• Decreased effects of acetaminophen: cholestyramine, oral contraceptives, anticholinergics, colestipol
• Increased effect of acetaminophen: diflunisal, caffeine
• Severe hypothermia: phenothiazines
• Increased chance of hepatotoxicity: alcohol

Side effects: *italics* = common; **bold italics** = life-threatening

Lab test interferences:
Interference: Chemstrip G, Dextrostix, Visidex II, 5-HIAA

NURSING CONSIDERATIONS
Assess:
• Liver function studies: AST, ALT, bilirubin, creatinine prior to therapy if long-term therapy is anticipated; may cause hepatic toxicity at doses >4 g/day with chronic use
• Renal function studies: BUN, urine creatinine, occult blood, albumin, if patient is on long-term therapy; presence of blood or albumin indicates nephritis
• Blood studies: CBC, pro-time if patient is on long-term therapy
• I&O ratio; decreasing output may indicate renal failure (long-term therapy)
• For fever and pain: type of pain, location, intensity, duration
• Mucosa, fingernail beds for cyanosis; inquire about dyspnea, vertigo, headache, weakness; symptoms indicate methemoglobinemia; notify prescriber immediately
• For chronic poisoning: rapid, weak pulse; dyspnea; cold, clammy extremities; report immediately to prescriber
• Hepatotoxicity: dark urine; clay-colored stools; yellowing of skin, sclera; itching, abdominal pain; fever; diarrhea if patient is on long-term therapy
• Allergic reactions: rash, urticaria; if these occur, drug may have to be discontinued

Administer:
PO
• To patient crushed or whole; chewable tablets may be chewed; give with full glass of water
• With food or milk to decrease gastric symptoms if needed
Perform/provide:
• Storage of suppositories <80° F (27° C)

Evaluate:
• Therapeutic response: absence of pain, fever

Teach patient/family:
Not to exceed recommended dosage; acute poisoning with liver damage may result
That acute toxicity includes symptoms of nausea, vomiting, abdominal pain; prescriber should be notified immediately
• To read label on other OTC drugs; many contain acetaminophen and may cause toxicity if taken concurrently
• To recognize signs of chronic overdose: bleeding, bruising, malaise, fever, sore throat
• That urine may become dark brown as a result of phenactin (metabolite of acetaminophen)
• To notify prescriber of pain or fever lasting over 3 days

Treatment of overdose: Drug level, gastric lavage, activated charcoal; administer oral acetylcysteine to prevent hepatic damage (see acetylcysteine monograph), monitor for bleeding

---

acetazolamide (℞)
(a-set-a-zole′a-mide)
acetazolamide, AK-Zol, apo-Acetazolam*, Dazamide, Diamox, Diamox Parenteral, Diamox Sequels, Storzolamide

Func. class.: Diuretic, carbonic anhydrase inhibitor, antiglaucoma agent, antiepileptic
Chem. class.: Sulfonamide derivative

Action: Inhibits carbonic anhydrase activity in proximal renal tubules to decrease reabsorption of water, sodium, potassium, bicarbonate; decreases carbonic anhydrase in CNS,

---

 = Nursing alert   = Herb-drug interaction   = Do not crush

increasing seizure threshold; able to decrease aqueous humor in eye, which lowers intraocular pressure

Uses: Open-angle glaucoma, narrow-angle glaucoma (preoperatively, if surgery delayed), epilepsy (petit mal, grand mal, mixed), edema in CHF, drug-induced edema, acute mountain sickness

Investigational uses: Prevention of uric acid/cystine renal stones, decrease CSF production in infants with hydrocephalus

Dosage and routes:

Closed-angle glaucoma
• *Adult:* **PO/IM/IV** 250 mg q4h or 250 mg bid, to be used for short-term therapy

Open-angle glaucoma
• *Adult:* **PO/IM/IV** 250 mg-1 g/day in divided doses for amounts over 250 mg or 500 mg SR bid

Edema in CHF
• *Adult:* **IM/IV** 250-375 mg/day in AM
  Child: **IM/IV** 5 mg/kg/day in AM

Seizures
• *Adult:* **PO/IM/IV** 4-30 mg/kg/day, in 1-4 divided doses usual range 375-1000 mg/day
• *Child:* **PO/IM/IV** 8-30 mg/kg/day in divided doses tid or qid, or 300-900 mg/m^2/day, not to exceed 1 g/day

Mountain sickness
• *Adult:* **PO** 250 mg q8-12h

Renal stones
• *Adult:* **PO** 250 mg hs

Infants with hydrocephalus
• *Infant:* **IV** 5 mg/kg/dose q6h, may be increased up to 100 mg/kg/day if tolerated

Available forms: Tabs 125, 250 mg; caps sust rel 500 mg; inj 500 mg

Side effects/adverse reactions:

GU: Frequency, polyuria, *uremia,* glucosuria, hematuria, dysuria, crystalluria, renal calculi

CNS: Drowsiness, paresthesia, anxiety, depression, headache, dizziness, confusion, stimulation, fatigue, *convulsions,* sedation, nervousness

GI: Nausea, vomiting, anorexia, constipation, diarrhea, melena, weight loss, *hepatic insufficiency,* taste alterations

EENT: Myopia, tinnitus

INTEG: Rash, pruritus, urticaria, fever, *Stevens-Johnson syndrome,* photosensitivity

ENDO: Hyperglycemia

HEMA: Aplastic anemia, hemolytic anemia, leukopenia, agranulocytosis, thrombocytopenia, purpura, pancytopenia

META: Hypokalemia, hyperchloremic acidosis

Contraindications: Hypersensitivity to sulfonamides, severe renal disease, severe hepatic disease, electrolyte imbalances (hyponatremia, hypokalemia), hyperchloremic acidosis, Addison's disease, long-term use in narrow-angle glaucoma, COPD

Precautions: Hypercalciuria, pregnancy (C), lactation

Pharmacokinetics:

PO: Onset 1-1½ hr, peak 1-4 hr, duration 6-12 hr

PO-SUS REL: Onset 2 hr, peak 3-6 hr, duration 18-24 hr

IV: Onset 2 min, peak 15 min, duration 4-5 hr, 65% absorbed if fasting (oral), 75% absorbed if given with food; half-life 2½-5½ hr; excreted unchanged by kidneys (80% within 24 hr), crosses placenta

Interactions:
• Increased action of amphetamines, procainamide, quinidine, tricyclics
• Increased excretion of barbiturates, ASA, lithium
• Increased toxicity: salicylates
• Hypokalemia: with other diuretics, corticosteroids, amphotericin B

Lab test interferences:

False positive: Urinary protein, 17 hydroxysteroid

Increase: Blood glucose levels, bilirubin, blood ammonia, calcium, chloride

Decrease: Urine citrate, K

NURSING CONSIDERATIONS
Assess:

• Weight daily, I&O daily to determine fluid loss; effect of drug may be decreased if used qd

• Rate, depth, rhythm of respiration, effect of exertion

• B/P lying, standing; postural hypotension may occur

• Electrolytes: K, Na, chloride; also BUN, blood sugar, CBC, serum creatinine, blood pH, ABGs, liver function tests

Administer:

• In AM to avoid interference with sleep if using drug as diuretic

• K replacement if K level is less than 3.0

PO

• With food if nausea occurs; absorption may be decreased slightly

🚫 Do not break, crush, or chew sus rel caps

IV

• After diluting 500 mg in >5 ml sterile H_2O for injection; direct IV—give at 100-500 mg/min; may be diluted further in LR, D_5W, $D_{10}W$, 0.45% NaCl, 0.9% NaCl, or Ringer's Sol and infused over 4-8 hr; use within 24 hr of dilution

Additive compatibilities: Cimetidine, ranitidine

Perform/provide:

• Storage in dark, cool area; use reconstituted solution within 24 hr

Evaluate:

• Therapeutic response: improvement in edema of feet, legs, sacral area daily if medication is being used

in CHF; or decrease in aqueous humor if medication is being used in glaucoma

Teach patient/family:

• To take exactly as prescribed; if dose is missed, take as soon as remembered; do not double dose

• To increase fluid intake by 2-3 L/day unless contraindicated; to rise slowly from lying or sitting position

• To notify prescriber if sore throat, unusual bleeding, bruising, paresthesias, tremors, flank pain, or skin rash occurs

• To use sunscreen to prevent photosensitivity

• To avoid hazardous activities if drowsiness occurs

Treatment of overdose: Lavage if taken orally; monitor electrolytes; administer dextrose in saline; monitor hydration, CV, renal status

---

acetohexamide (℞)
(a-set-oh-hex′a-mide)
acetohexamide, Dimelor*, Dymelor*
Func. class.: Antidiabetic
Chem. class.: Sulfonylurea (1st generation)

Action: Causes functioning β-cells in pancreas to release insulin, leading to drop in blood glucose levels; may improve binding between insulin and insulin receptors or increase number of insulin receptors with prolonged administration; may also reduce basal hepatic glucose secretion; not effective if patient lacks functioning β-cells

Uses: Stable adult-onset diabetes mellitus (type II), NIDDM

Dosage and routes:

• *Adult:* **PO** 250 mg-1.5 g/day; usually given before breakfast unless large dose is required; then dose is divided in two

Available forms: Tabs 250, 500 mg scored

Side effects/adverse reactions:

CNS: Headache, weakness, tinnitus, fatigue, dizziness, vertigo

GI: Nausea, vomiting, diarrhea, *hepatotoxicity, jaundice,* heartburn

HEMA: **Leukopenia, thrombocytopenia, agranulocytosis, aplastic anemia, hemolytic anemia,** increased AST, ALT, alk phosphatase

INTEG: Rash, allergic reactions, pruritus, urticaria, eczema, photosensitivity, erythema

ENDO: **Hypoglycemia,** hyponatremia

Contraindications: Hypersensitivity to sulfonylureas, type 1 diabetes, renal failure

Precautions: Pregnancy (C), elderly, cardiac disease, renal disease, hepatic disease, thyroid disease, severe hypoglycemic reactions

Pharmacokinetics:

PO: Completely absorbed by GI route, onset 1 hr, peak 2-4 hr, duration 12-24 hr, half-life 6-8 hr, metabolized in liver, excreted in urine (active metabolites, unchanged drug)

Interactions:

• Increased hypoglycemic effects: oral anticoagulants, salicylates, sulfonamides, nonsteroidal antiinflammatories, guanethidine, methyldopa, MAOIs, chloramphenicol, insulin, cimetidine

• Decreased action of acetohexamide: calcium channel blockers, corticosteroids, oral contraceptives, thiazide diuretics, thyroid preparations, estrogens, phenobarbital, phenothiazines, phenytoin, rifampin, sympathomimetics

• Decreased effect of both drugs: diazoxide

NURSING CONSIDERATIONS

Assess:

• Hypoglycemic/hyperglycemic reaction that can occur soon after meals

• Monitor glucose levels often; may need insulin therapy during severe stress, surgery

Administer:

PO

• Drug 30 min before meals; give in divided doses if GI upset occurs

Perform/provide:

• Storage in tight container in cool environment

Evaluate:

• Therapeutic response: decrease in polyuria, polydipsia, polyphagia, clear sensorium, absence of dizziness, stable gait

Teach patient/family:

• To check for symptoms of cholestatic jaundice: dark urine, pruritus, yellow sclera; if these occur, prescriber should be notified

• To use capillary blood glucose test or Chemstrip tid

• To recognize the symptoms of hypo/hyperglycemia, what to do about each

• That drug must be continued on daily basis; explain consequence of discontinuing drug abruptly

• To take drug in morning to prevent hypoglycemic reactions at night, to take as prescribed; if dose is missed, take when remembered

• To avoid OTC medications unless directed by prescriber

• That diabetes is lifelong illness; that this drug is not a cure

• That all food included in diet plan must be eaten to prevent hypoglycemia

• To carry Medic Alert ID for emergency purposes, carry a glucagon emergency kit

• That tabs may be crushed

Treatment of overdose: Glucose

25 g IV, via dextrose 50% sol, 50 ml or 1 mg glucagon

---

acetylcysteine (℞)

(a-se-teel-sis′tay-een)
Mucomyst*, Mucosal
Func. class.: Mucolytic; antidote—acetaminophen
Chem. class.: Amino acid L-cysteine

Action: Decreases viscosity of secretions by breaking disulfide links of mucoproteins; increases hepatic glutathione, which is necessary to inactivate toxic metabolites in acetaminophen overdose

Uses: Acetaminophen toxicity; bronchitis; pneumonia; cystic fibrosis; emphysema; atelectasis; tuberculosis; complications of thoracic, cardiovascular surgery; diagnosis in bronchial lab tests

Dosage and routes:
Mucolytic
• *Adult and child:* **INSTILL** 1-2 ml (10%-20% sol) q1-4h prn or 3-5 ml (20% sol) or 6-10 ml (10% sol) tid or qid
Acetaminophen toxicity
• *Adult and child:* **PO** 140 mg/kg, then 70 mg/kg q4h × 17 doses to total of 1330 mg/kg
Available forms: Sol 10%, 20%

Side effects/adverse reactions:
CNS: Dizziness, drowsiness, headache, fever, chills
GI: Nausea, stomatitis, constipation, vomiting, anorexia, *hepatotoxicity*
EENT: Rhinorrhea, tooth damage
CV: Hypotension
INTEG: Urticaria, rash, fever, clamminess
RESP: Bronchospasm, burning, *hemoptysis,* chest tightness

Contraindications: Hypersensitivity, increased intracranial pressure, status asthmaticus

Precautions: Hypothyroidism, Addison's disease, CNS depression, brain tumor, asthma, hepatic disease, renal disease, COPD, psychosis, alcoholism, convulsive disorders, lactation, pregnancy (B)

Pharmacokinetics:
INH/INSTILL: Onset 1 min, duration 5-10 min, metabolized by liver, excreted in urine

Interactions:
• Do not use with iron, copper, rubber
• Do not mix with antibiotics: tetracycline, chlortetracycline, oxytetracycline, erythromycin, lactobionate, amphotericin B, sodium ampicillin; iodized oil, chymotrypsin, trypsin, hydrogen peroxide

NURSING CONSIDERATIONS
Assess:
• Cough: type, frequency, character, including sputum
• Rate, rhythm of respirations, increased dyspnea; sputum; discontinue if bronchospasm occurs
• VS, cardiac status including checking for dysrhythmias, increased rate, palpitations
• ABGs for increased CO_2 retention in asthma patients
• Antidotal use: liver function tests, pro-time, BUN, glucose, electrolytes, acetaminophen levels; inform prescriber if dose is vomited or vomiting is persistent
• Nausea, vomiting, rash; notify prescriber if these occur

Administer:
PO
• Antidotal use: give within 24 hr; give with cola or soft drink to disguise taste; can be given with H_2O through tubes; use within 1 hr
INSTILL
• By syringe 2-3 doses of 1-2 ml of 20% or 2-4 ml of 10% solution

---

A

• Decreased dose to elderly patients; their metabolism may be slowed
• Only if suction machine is available
• Before meals ½-1 hr for better absorption, to decrease nausea
• 20% solutions diluted with NS or water for injection; may give 10% solution undiluted
• Only after patient clears airway by deep breathing, coughing
• Gum, hard candy, frequent rinsing of mouth for dryness of oral cavity
Perform/provide:
• Store in refrigerator; use within 96 hr of opening
• Assistance with inhaled dose: bronchodilator if bronchospasm occurs
• Mechanical suction if cough insufficient to remove excess bronchial secretions
Evaluate:
• Therapeutic response: absence of purulent secretions when coughing; absence of hepatic damage in acetaminophen toxicity
Teach patient/family:
• About mucolytic use
• To avoid driving, other hazardous activities until patient is stabilized on this medication
• To avoid alcohol, other CNS depressants; will enhance sedating properties of this drug
• That unpleasant odor will decrease after repeated use
• That discoloration of solution after bottle is opened does not impair its effectiveness
• To avoid smoking, smoke-filled rooms, perfume, dust, environmental pollutants, cleaners

acrivastine/pseudo-ephedrine (R)

(ac-ri-vas'teen)
Semprex-D
Func. class.: Antihistamine
Chem. class.: H_1-histamine antagonist

Action: Acts on blood vessels, GI, respiratory system by competing with histamine for H_1-receptor site; decreases allergic response by blocking pharmacologic effects of histamine; less sedation rate than with other antihistamines; causes increased heart rate, vasodilation, increased secretions
Uses: Rhinitis, allergy symptoms, chronic idiopathic urticaria
Dosage and routes:
• *Adult, child >12 yr:* **PO** 8 mg q4-6h
Available forms: Caps 8 mg/60 mg
Side effects/adverse reactions:
GU: Dysmenorrhea
RESP: Cough, pharyngitis
GI: *Nausea,* dry mouth
CNS: Headache, dizziness, nervousness, insomnia
Contraindications: Hypersensitivity to this drug or triprolidine, severe hypertension, cardiac disease
Precautions: Pregnancy (B), lactation, elderly, children, respiratory disease, hypertension, diabetes mellitus, ischemic heart disease, increased intraocular pressure, prostate hypertrophy
Pharmacokinetics: Metabolized by the liver; excreted in kidneys, feces; half-life 1½ hr, peak 1-1½ hr, duration 12 hr
Interactions:
• Increased CNS depression: alcohol, narcotics, sedatives, hypnotics
• Hypertensive crisis: MAO inhibitors

🍃 May increase CNS depression: kava kava

🍃 May increase anticholinergic effect: henbane leaf

Lab test interferences:

False negative: Skin allergy tests (discontinue antihistamine 3 days prior to testing)

NURSING CONSIDERATIONS

Assess:

• Respiratory status: rate, rhythm, increase in bronchial secretions, wheezing, chest tightness; provide fluids to 2 L/day to decrease thickness of secretions

Administer:

PO

• With food, fluid for GI symptoms

🚫 Do not break, crush, or chew caps

Perform/provide:

• Storage in tight, light-resistant container

Evaluate:

• Therapeutic response: absence of running or congested nose, rashes

Teach patient/family:

• All aspects of drug use; to avoid driving, other hazardous activity if drowsy; to avoid alcohol, other CNS depressants that may potentiate effect

• Not to exceed recommended dose

• To use hard candy, gum, or frequent rinsing of mouth for dryness

Treatment of overdose: Administer ipecac syrup or lavage, diazepam, vasopressors, barbiturates (short-acting)

activated charcoal (OTC)

Acta-Char Liquid-A, Actidose-Aqua, Aqueous-Charcodote*, Charac-50*, CharcoAid 2000, Charcocaps, Charcodote*, Charcotabs, Insta-Char, Insta-Char Aqueous Suspension, Liqui-Char, SuperChar

Func. class.: Antiflatulent; antidote

Action: Binds poisons, toxins, irritants; increases adsorption in GI tract; inactivates toxins and binds until excreted

Uses: Poisoning

Dosage and routes:

• Children should not get more than 1 dose of products with sorbitol

Poisoning

• *Adult and child:* **PO** 30-100 g or 1 g/kg, minimum dose 30 g/250 ml of water, may give 20-40 g q6h for 1-2 days in severe poisoning

Available forms: Powder 15, 25*, 30, 40, 120, 125, 240 g/container; oral susp 12.5 g/60 ml, 15 g/72 ml, 15 g/120 ml, 25 g/120 ml, 30 g/120 ml, 50 g/240 ml; Canada 15 g/120 ml, 25 g/125 ml, 50 g/225 ml, 50 g/250 ml

Side effects/adverse reactions:

GI: Nausea, black stools, vomiting, constipation, diarrhea

Contraindications: Hypersensitivity to this drug, unconsciousness, semiconsciousness, poisoning of cyanide, mineral acids, alkalies

Pharmacokinetics:

PO: Excreted in feces

Interactions:

• Decreased effectiveness of both drugs: ipecac, laxatives

• Do not mix with dairy products

NURSING CONSIDERATIONS

Assess:

• Respiration, pulse, B/P to determine charcoal effectiveness if taken for barbiturate/narcotic poisoning

Administer:

PO

• After inducing vomiting unless vomiting contraindicated (i.e., cyanide or alkalies)

• After mixing with water or fruit juice to form thick syrup; do not use dairy products to mix charcoal

• Repeat dose if vomiting occurs soon after dose; give with a laxative to promote elimination; alone, do not administer with ipecac

• After spacing at least 1 hr before or after other drugs, or absorption will be decreased

• Keeping container tightly closed to prevent absorption of gases

NG

• Through a nasogastric tube if patient unable to swallow

Evaluate:

• Therapeutic response: LOC-alert (poisoning)

Teach patient/family:

• That stools will be black

• How to prevent further poisonings

---

acyclovir (℞)

(ay-sye′kloe-ver)

Avirax*, Zovirax

Func. class.: Antiviral

Chem. class.: Acyclic purine nucleoside analog

Action: Interferes with DNA synthesis by conversion to acyclovir triphosphate, causing decreased viral replication, time of lesional healing

Uses: Mucocutaneous herpes simplex virus, herpes genitalis (HSV-1, HSV-2)

Investigational uses: Herpes zoster, cytomegalovirus, HSV after transplant, mononucleosis, varicella zoster, herpes simplex, varicella pneumonia

Dosage and routes:

• Lengthen dosing interval in renal disease CrCl <50 ml/min

Herpes simplex

• *Adult and child >12 yr:* IV INF 5 mg/kg over 1 hr q8h × 5 days

• *Child <12 yr:* IV INF 250 mg/m^2 or 30 mg/kg/day divided q8h over 1 hr q8h × 5 days

Genital herpes

• *Adult:* PO 200 mg q4h (5×/day while awake) for 5 days to 6 mo depending on whether initial, recurrent, or chronic

Herpes simplex encephalitis

• *Adult:* IV 10 mg/kg over 1 hr q8h × 10 days

• *Child >6 mo:* IV 500 mg/m^2 q8h × 10-14 days

Herpes zoster

• *Adult:* PO 800 mg × 7-10 days; IV 5 mg/kg q8h

Children with immunosuppression:

• *Child >2 yr:* 20 mg/kg qid × 5 days

Varicella-zoster

• *Adult:* PO 1000 mg q6h × 5 days or 600-800 mg q4h (5×/day while awake); IV 500 mg/m^2 q8h or 10 mg/kg q8h × 7d

• *Child:* PO 10-20 mg/kg (max 800 mg) qid × 5 days; IV 500 mg/m^2 q8h or 10 mg/kg q8h × 7d

Available forms: Caps 200 mg; inj 500 mg, oral susp, tabs 400, 800 mg

Side effects/adverse reactions:

CNS: Tremors, confusion, lethargy, hallucinations, ***convulsions,*** dizziness, *headache,* encephalopathic changes

GI: Nausea, vomiting, diarrhea, increased ALT, AST, abdominal pain, glossitis, colitis

GU: ***Oliguria, proteinuria, hematuria,*** vaginitis, moniliasis, ***glomer-***

ulonephritis, acute renal failure, changes in menses, polydipsia
EENT: Gingival hyperplasia
INTEG: Rash, urticaria, pruritus, pain or phlebitis at IV site, unusual sweating, alopecia
MS: Joint pain, leg pain, muscle cramps
Contraindications: Hypersensitivity
Precautions: Lactation, hepatic disease, renal disease, electrolyte imbalance, dehydration, pregnancy (B)
Pharmacokinetics:
IV: Peak 1 hr, half-life 20 min-3 hr (terminal); metabolized by liver, excreted by kidneys as unchanged drug (95%); crosses placenta; absorbed minimally (PO), distributed widely; crosses placenta, CSF concentrations are 50% plasma
PO: Onset unknown, peak 1½-2 hr, terminal half-life 3½ hr
Interactions:
• Increased neurotoxicity, nephrotoxicity: aminoglycosides, amphotericin, interferon, probenecid, methotrexate, zidovudine

NURSING CONSIDERATIONS
Assess:
• Signs of infection, anemia
• I&O ratio; report hematuria, oliguria, fatigue, weakness; may indicate nephrotoxicity; check for protein in urine during treatment
◆ Any patient with compromised renal system, since drug is excreted slowly in poor renal system function; toxicity may occur rapidly
• Liver studies: AST, ALT
• Blood studies: WBC, RBC, Hct, Hgb, bleeding time; blood dyscrasias may occur; drug should be discontinued
• Renal studies: urinalysis, protein, BUN, creatinine, CrCl
• C&S before drug therapy; drug may be taken as soon as culture is taken; repeat C&S after treatment; determine the presence of other sexually transmitted diseases
• Bowel pattern before, during treatment; if severe abdominal pain with bleeding occurs, drug should be discontinued
• Skin eruptions: rash, urticaria, itching
• Allergies before treatment, reaction of each medication; place allergies on chart in bright red letters
Administer:
PO
🚫 Do not break, crush, or chew caps
IV
• Increased fluids to 3 L/day to decrease crystalluria
• After reconstituting with 10 ml compatible solution/500 mg of drug, concentration of 50 mg/ml, shake, use within 12 hr (<7 mg/ml); give over at least 1 hr (constant rate) by infusion pump to prevent nephrotoxicity; do not reconstitute with sol containing benzyl alcohol in neonates
• Lower dose in acute or chronic renal failure
Additive compatibilities: Fluconazole
Solution compatibilities: D_5W, LR, or NaCl (D_5 0.9% NaCl, 0.9% NaCl) solutions
Y-site compatibilities: Allopurinol, amikacin, ampicillin, cefamandole, cefazolin, cefonicid, cefoperazone, cefotaxime, cefoxitin, ceftazidime, ceftizoxime, ceftriaxone, cefuroxime, cephapirin, chloramphenicol, cimetidine, clindamycin, dexamethasone sodium phosphate, dimenhydrinate, diphenhydramine, doxycycline, erythromycin, famotidine, filgrastim, fluconazole, gallium, gentamicin, granisetron, heparin, hydrocortisone sodium succinate, hydromorphone, imipenem/cilastatin,

---

◆ = Nursing alert   🌿 = Herb-drug interaction   🚫 = Do not crush

lorazepam, magnesium sulfate, melphalan, methylprednisolone sodium succinate, metoclopramide, metronidazole, multivitamin, nafcillin, oxacillin, paclitaxel, penicillin G potassium, pentobarbital, perphenazine, piperacillin, potassium chloride, propofol, ranitidine, sodium bicarbonate, tacrolimus, teniposide, theophylline, thiotepa, ticarcillin, tobramycin, trimethoprim-sulfamethoxazole, vancomycin, zidovudine

Perform/provide:

• Storage at room temperature for up to 12 hr after reconstitution; if refrigerated, sol may show a precipitate that clears at room temperature

• Adequate intake of fluids (2 L) to prevent deposit in kidneys

Evaluate:

• Therapeutic response: absence of itching, painful lesions; crusting and healed lesions

Teach patient/family:

• To take as prescribed; if dose is missed, take as soon as remembered up to 1 hr before next dose; do not double dose

• That drug may be taken orally before infection occurs; drug should be taken when itching or pain occurs, usually before eruptions

• That partners need to be told that patient has herpes; they can become infected; condoms must be worn to prevent reinfections

• That drug does not cure infection, just controls symptoms and does not prevent infection to others

◆ To report sore throat, fever, fatigue (may indicate superinfection)

• That drug must be taken in equal intervals around the clock to maintain blood levels for duration of therapy

• To notify prescriber of side effects of bruising, bleeding, fatigue,

malaise; may indicate blood dyscrasias

• To seek dental care during treatment to prevent gingival hyperplasia

Treatment of overdose: Discontinue drug, hemodialysis, resuscitate if needed

---

adenosine (℞)

(a-den'oh-seen)
Adenocard, Adenoscan
Func. class.: Antidysrhythmic
Chem. class.: Endogenous nucleoside

Action: Slows conduction through AV node, can interrupt reentry pathways through AV node, and can restore normal sinus rhythm in patients with paroxysmal supraventricular tachycardia (PSVT)

Uses: PSVT

Dosage and routes:

• *Adult:* **IV BOL** 6 mg; if conversion to normal sinus rhythm does not occur within 1-2 min, give 12 mg by rapid **IV BOL**; may repeat 12 mg dose again in 1-2 min

• *Infants/children:* 0.05 mg/kg, if not effective, increase dose by 0.05 mg/kg q2min to a max of 0.25 mg/kg or 12 mg

Available forms: Inj 3 mg/ml

Side effects/adverse reactions:

GI: Nausea, metallic taste, throat tightness, groin pressure

RESP: Dyspnea, chest pressure, hyperventilation

CNS: Lightheadedness, dizziness, arm tingling, numbness, apprehension, blurred vision, headache

CV: Chest pain, ***atrial tachydysrhythmias,*** sweating, palpitations, hypotension, *facial flushing*

Contraindications: Hypersensitivity, 2nd- or 3rd-degree heart block,

AV block, sick sinus syndrome, atrial flutter, atrial fibrillation

Precautions: Pregnancy (C), lactation, children, asthma, elderly

Pharmacokinetics: Cleared from plasma in <30 sec, half-life 10 sec

Interactions:

• Increased effects of adenosine: dipyridamole

• Decreased activity of adenosine: theophylline or other methylxanthines (caffeine)

• Higher degree of heart block: carbamazepine

🌿 May cause increased adenosine effect: buckthorn bark/berry, cascara sagrada bark, rhubarb root, senna leaf/fruits, aloe

Lab test interferences:

Increase: Liver function tests

NURSING CONSIDERATIONS
Assess:

• Cardiac status continually

• B/P continuously for fluctuations

• I&O ratio, electrolytes (K, Na, Cl)

• Cardiac status: B/P, pulse, respiration, ECG intervals (PR, QRS, QT)

• Respiratory status: rate, rhythm, lung fields for rales, watch for respiratory depression

• CNS effects: dizziness, confusion, psychosis, paresthesias, convulsions; drug should be discontinued

• Lung fields, bilateral rales may occur in CHF patient

• Increased respiration, increased pulse; drug should be discontinued

Administer:

IV bolus

• Undiluted; give 6 mg or less by rapid inj; if using an IV line, use port near insertion site, flush with normal saline (50 ml)

Perform/provide:

• Storage at room temperature; sol should be clear; discard unused drug

Evaluate:

• Therapeutic response: decreased anginal pain, decreased B/P, dysrhythmias, decreased heart rate

Treatment of overdose: Defibrillation, vasopressor for hypotension

---

albumin, normal serum 5%/25% (℞)

(al-byoo'min)

Albuminar 5%, Albuminar 25%, Albutein 5%, Albutein 25%, Buminate 5%, Buminate 25%, Plasbumin 5%, Plasbumin-25%

Func. class.: Blood derivative

Chem. class.: Placental human plasma

Action: Exerts oncotic pressure, which expands volume of circulating blood and maintains cardiac output

Uses: Restores plasma volume in burns, hyperbilirubinemia, shock, hypoproteinemia, prevention of cerebral edema, cardiopulmonary bypass procedures, ARDS

Dosage and routes:

Burns

• *Adult:* **IV** dose to maintain plasma albumin at 30-50 g/L, use 5% sol initially, then 25% sol after 24 hr

Shock

• *Adult:* **IV** 500 ml of 5% sol q30 min, as needed

• *Child:* 0.5-1 g/kg/dose

Hypoproteinemia

• *Adult:* **IV** 1000-2000 ml of 5% sol qd, not to exceed 5-10 ml/min or 25-100 g of 25% sol qd, not to exceed 3 ml/min, titrated to patient response

Hyperbilirubinemia/erythroblastosis fetalis

• *Infant:* **IV** 1 g of 25% sol/kg before transfusion

⬥ = Nursing alert　　🌿 = Herb-drug interaction　　🚫 = Do not crush

albuterol

and routes:

nt exercise-induced asthma
INH 2 puffs 15 min before
ng; **NEB/LPPB** 5 mg tid-

ospasm
and child >12 yr: **INH** 1-2
-6h; **PO** 2-4 mg tid-qid, not
ed 8 mg
2-6 yr: **PO** 0.1 mg/kg tid
mg tid); may increase to 0.2
tid (max 4 mg tid)
le forms: Aerosol 90 µg/
n; tabs 2, 4 mg; syr 2 mg/5
rel 8 mg; inh sol 0.5%

fects/adverse reactions:

remors, anxiety, insomnia,
e, dizziness, stimulation,
ness, hallucinations, flush-
tability

Dry nose, irritation of nose
oat

pitations, tachycardia, hy-
ion, angina, hypotension,
hmias

rtburn, nausea, vomiting
scle cramps

indications: Hypersensitiv-
mpathomimetics, tachydys-
as, severe cardiac disease

tions: Lactation, pregnancy
diac disorders, hyperthyroid-
abetes mellitus, hyperten-
ostatic hypertrophy, narrow-
aucoma, seizures, exercise-
l bronchospasm (aerosol) in
n <12 years

acokinetics: Well absorbed
ensively metabolized in the
d tissues, crosses placenta,
milk, blood-brain barrier
set ½ hr, peak 2½ hr, dura-
hr, half-life 2½ hr
Onset ½ hour; peak 2-3 hr;
12 hr
set 5-15 min, peak 1-1½ hr,
4-6 hr, half-life 4 hr

Interactions:

• Increased action of aerosol bronchodilators
• Increased action of albuterol: tricyclic antidepressants, MAOIs, other
adrenergics
• May inhibit action of albuterol:
other β-blockers

NURSING CONSIDERATIONS
Assess:

• Respiratory function: vital capacity, forced expiratory volume, ABGs,
lung sounds, heart rate and rhythm
(baseline)
• That patient has not received theophylline therapy before giving dose
• Patient's ability to self-medicate
• For evidence of allergic reactions

Administer:
Inhalation

• In geriatric patients, a spacing device is advised
• After shaking, exhale, place
mouthpiece in mouth, inhale slowly,
hold breath, remove, exhale slowly
• Gum, sips of water for dry mouth

PO

• With meals to decrease gastric irritation
• Syrup to children (no alcohol,
sugar)

Perform/provide:

• Storage in light resistant container,
do not expose to temperatures over
86° F (30° C)

Evaluate:

• Therapeutic response: absence of
dyspnea, wheezing after 1 hr, improved airway exchange, improved
ABGs

Teach patient/family:

• To use exactly as prescribed; take
missed dose when remembered, alter dosing schedule
• Not to use OTC medications; excess stimulation may occur
• Use of inhaler; review package
insert with patient; use demonstration, return demonstration

Available forms: Inj 50, 250 mg/ml (5%, 25%)

Side effects/adverse reactions:

GI: Nausea, vomiting, increased salivation

INTEG: Rash, urticaria

CNS: Fever, chills, flushing, headache

RESP: Altered respirations, *pulmonary edema*

CV: Fluid overload, hypotension, erratic pulse, tachycardia

Contraindications: Hypersensitivity, CHF, severe anemia, renal insufficiency

Precautions: Decreased salt intake, decreased cardiac reserve, lack of albumin deficiency, hepatic disease, renal disease, pregnancy (C)

Pharmacokinetics: In hyponutrition states, metabolized as protein/energy source

Lab test interferences:

False increase: Alk phosphatase

NURSING CONSIDERATIONS

Assess:

• Blood studies Hct, Hgb; if serum protein declines, dyspnea, hypoxemia can result

• Decreased B/P, erratic pulse, respiration

• I&O ratio: urinary output may decrease

◆CVP, pulmonary wedge pressure will increase if overload occurs

• Allergy: fever, rash, itching, chills, flushing, urticaria, nausea, vomiting, hypotension, requires discontinuation of infusion, use of new lot if therapy reinstituted

• CVP reading: distended neck veins indicate circulatory overload; shortness of breath, anxiety, insomnia, expiratory rales, frothy bloodtinged cough, cyanosis indicate pulmonary overload

Administer:

IV

• Slowly, to prevent fluid overload;

dilute with N
5% may be
may be give
give over 4 l

Solution con

Ringer's, D
dextrose/sali
tran₆ NaCl 0.
dextrose/LR

Y-site comp
lorazepam

Perform/pr

• Adequate l
ing administ

• Check typ
stored at roo
need to be re

Evaluate:

• Therapeutic
B/P, decrease
rum albumi
plasma prote

---

albutero

(al-byoo'ter-
Airet, albu
tamol*, No
til, Proven
Repetabs,
todisk*, Ve
tacaps, Vol
Func. class
agonist

Action: Caus
action on β_2 (
by increasing
relaxes smoo
bronchodilatic
ulation, as we
sis and gastric
acting than is

Uses: Preve
induced asthm
vention of pr

Investigation
mia in dialysi

Dosag

To prev

• *Adul*
exercis
qid

Bronc

• *Adul*
puffs q
to exce

• *Chil*
(max 2
mg/kg

Availa
actuatic
ml; ex

Side e

CNS: T
headac
restles
ing, in
EENT:
and th
CV: Pa
pertens
dysrhy
GI: He
MS: M

Contra
ity to s
rhythm

Precau
(C), ca
ism, d
sion, p
angle g
induce
childre

Pharm
PO, ex
liver a
breast
PO: O
tion 4-
PO-ER.
duratio
INH: O
duratio

Side effects: *italics* = common; *bold*   ◆ = N

- To avoid getting aerosol in eyes; blurring may result
- To wash inhaler in warm water qd and dry
- To avoid smoking, smoke-filled rooms, persons with respiratory infections

◆ That paradoxic bronchospasm may occur and to stop drug immediately

- To limit caffeine products such as chocolate, coffee, tea, and colas

Treatment of overdose: Administer a β_1-adrenergic blocker

---

aldesleukin (℞)

(al-dess-loo'ken)
Interleukin-2, IL-2, Proleukin
Func. class.: Miscellaneous antineoplastic
Chem. class.: Interleukin-2, human recombinant (cytokine)

Action: Enhancement of lymphocyte mitogenesis and stimulation of IL-2-dependent cell lines; enhancement of lymphocyte cytotoxicity; induction of killer cell activity; induction of interferon γ-production; results in activation of cellular immunity, cytokines, and inhibition of tumor growth

Uses: Metastatic renal cell carcinoma in adults, phase II for HIV in combination with zidovudine, melanoma

Investigational uses: Kaposi's sarcoma given with zidovudine, metastatic melanoma given with cyclophosphamide, non-Hodgkin's lymphoma given with lymphokine-activated killer cells, AIDS (phase I) given with zidovudine

Dosage and routes:
- *Adult:* **IV INF** 600,000 IU/kg (0.037 mg/kg) q8h over 15 min × 14 doses; off 9 days, repeat schedule for another 14 doses, for a max of 28 doses/course

Available forms: Powder for inj, lyophilized

Side effects/adverse reactions:

CV: Hypotension, sinus tachycardia, dysrhythmias, bradycardia, PVCs, PACs, myocardial ischemia, *myocardial infarction, cardiac arrest, capillary leak syndrome*

RESP: Pulmonary congestion, dyspnea, *pulmonary edema, respiratory failure,* tachypnea, pleural effusion, wheezing

GI: Nausea, vomiting, diarrhea, stomatitis, anorexia, GI bleeding, dyspepsia, constipation, *intestinal perforation*/ileus, jaundice, ascites

HEMA: Anemia, *thrombocytopenia, leukopenia, coagulation disorders, leukocytosis, eosinophilia*

CNS: Mental status changes, dizziness, sensory dysfunction, syncope, motor dysfunction, fever, chills, headache

GU: Oliguria/anuria, proteinuria, hematuria, dysuria, *renal failure*

INTEG: Pruritus, erythema, rash, dry skin, *exfoliative dermatitis,* purpura, petechiae, urticaria

MS: Arthralgia, myalgia

SYST: Infection

Contraindications: Hypersensitivity, abnormal thallium stress test or pulmonary function tests, organ allografts

Precautions: CNS metastases, bacterial infections, renal/hepatic/cardiac/pulmonary disease, pregnancy (C), lactation, children, anemia, thrombocytopenia

Pharmacokinetics: Renal elimination half-life 85 min

Interactions:
- Potentiate hypotension: antihypertensives
- Reduced antitumor effectiveness: corticosteroids

• Increased toxicity: aminoglycosides, indomethacin, cytotoxic chemotherapy, methotrexate, asparaginase, doxorubicin

Lab test interferences:

Increase: Bilirubin, BUN, serum creatinine, transaminase, alk phosphatase; hypomagnesemia, acidosis hypocalcemia, hypophosphatemia, hypokalemia, hyperuricemia, hypoalbuminemia, hypoproteinemia, hyponatremia, hyperkalemia, alkalosis

NURSING CONSIDERATIONS
Assess:

• CBC, differential, platelet count weekly; withhold drug if WBC is <4000/mm^3 or platelet count is <75,000/mm^3; notify prescriber of these results

◆▶Capillary leak syndrome including a drop in mean arterial pressure (2-12 hr after initiating therapy); hypotension and hypoperfusion will occur

• Renal function studies: BUN, serum uric acid, urine CrCl, electrolytes before, during therapy

• I&O ratio; report fall in urine output to <30 ml/hr

• Monitor temperature q4h; fever may indicate beginning infection

• Liver function tests before, during therapy: bilirubin, AST, ALT, alk phosphatase as needed or monthly

• ECG; watch for ST-T wave changes, low QRS and T, possible dysrhythmias (sinus tachycardia, PVCs)

• Baselines in pulmonary function; document FEV >2 L or ≥75% prior to therapy; check daily VS, pulse oximetry, dyspnea, rales, ABGs

• Stress thallium study prior to therapy; document normal ejection fraction, unimpaired wall motion

• Bleeding: hematuria, guaiac, bruising or petechiae, mucosa or orifices q8h

• Food preferences; list likes, dislikes

• Inflammation of mucosa, breaks in skin

• Buccal cavity q8h for dryness, sores, ulceration, white patches, oral pain, bleeding, dysphagia

• Alkalosis if severe vomiting is present

• Local irritation, pain, burning at injection site

• GI symptoms: frequency of stools, cramping

• Acidosis, signs of dehydration: rapid respirations, poor skin turgor, decreased urine output, dry skin, restlessness, weakness

• Cardiac status: B/P, pulse, character, rhythm, rate, ABGs, ECG

Administer:

IV

• Hydrocortisone, dexamethasone or sodium bicarbonate (1 mEq/1 ml) for extravasation, apply ice compresses

• Antiemetic 30-60 min before giving drug to prevent vomiting

• IV after diluting 22 million IU (1.3 mg)/1.2 ml sterile H_2O for inj at site of vial and swirl, do not shake; dilute dose with 50 ml D_5W and give over 15 min; use plastic bag; do not use an in-line filter, give through Y-tube or 3-way stopcock

• Dopamine 1-5 kg/min before onset of hypotension; decreased dose preserves kidney output

Y-site compatibilities: Amikacin, amphotericin B, calcium gluconate, diphenhydramine, dopamine, fluconazole, foscarnet, gentamicin, heparin, IV fat emulsion, magnesium sulfate, metoclopramide, morphine, ondansetron, piperacillin, potassium chloride, ranitidine, ticar-

---

◆▶ = Nursing alert   🥦 = Herb-drug interaction   🚫 = Do not crush cillin, tobramycin, TPN #145, trimethoprim/sulfamethoxazole

Perform/provide:

• Strict hand-washing technique, gloves, protective clothing

• Liquid diet: carbonated beverage, gelatin (Jell-O) may be added if patient is not nauseated or vomiting

• Rinsing of mouth tid-qid with water, club soda; brushing of teeth bid-tid with soft brush or cotton-tipped applicators for stomatitis; use unwaxed dental floss

• Storage in refrigerator of diluted drug; do not freeze; administer within 48 hr; bring to room temperature before infusing; discard unused portion

Evaluate:

• Therapeutic response: decreased tumor size, spread of malignancy

Teach patient/family:

• To use a nonhormonal contraceptive method during therapy

• To report any complaints, side effects to nurse or prescriber

• To avoid foods with citric acid, hot or rough texture

• To report any bleeding, white spots, ulcerations in mouth to prescriber; tell patient to examine mouth qd

• To avoid crowds and persons with infections when granulocyte count is low

---

alendronate (Rx)

(al-en-drone'ate)

Fosamax

Func. class.: Bone-resorption inhibitor

Chem. class.: Biphosphonate

Action: Absorbs calcium phosphate crystal in bone and may directly block dissolution of hydroxyapatite crystals of bone; inhibits bone resorption, apparently without inhibiting bone formation, mineralization

Uses: Osteoporosis in postmenopausal women, Paget's disease

Dosage and routes:

Osteoporosis in postmenopausal women

• *Adult and elderly:* **PO** 10 mg qd

Paget's disease

• *Adult and elderly:* **PO** 40 mg qd × 6 mo

Available forms: Tabs 10, 40 mg

Side effects/adverse reactions:

CNS: Headache

META: Anemia, hypokalemia, hypomagnesemia, hypophosphatemia

GI: Abdominal pain, anorexia, constipation, nausea, vomiting, esophageal ulceration

MS: Bone pain

CV: Hypertension

GU: UTI, fluid overload

Contraindications: Hypersensitivity to biphosphonates, hypocalcemia

Precautions: Children, lactation, pregnancy (C), CrCl <35 ml/min, esophageal disease, ulcers, gastritis

Pharmacokinetics: Rapidly cleared from circulation, taken up mainly by bones, eliminated primarily through kidneys

NURSING CONSIDERATIONS

Assess:

• Electrolytes: renal function studies, Ca, P, Mg, K

• For hypercalcemia: paresthesia, twitching, laryngospasm, Chvostek's, Trousseau's signs

Administer:

PO

• For 6 months to be effective in Paget's disease

Perform/provide:

• Storage in cool environment, out of direct sunlight

Evaluate:

• Therapeutic response: increased bone mass, absence of fractures

Teach patient/family:
• To remain upright for 30 min after dose
• To take in AM before food, other meds, take with 6-8 oz of water (no mineral water)

---

alfentanil (℞)

(al-fen'ta-nil)
Alfenta, Rapifen*
Func. class.: Narcotic analgesic
Chem. class.: Opiate, synthetic

Controlled Substance Schedule II
Action: Inhibits ascending pain pathways in limbic system, thalamus, midbrain, hypothalamus
Uses: In combination with other drugs in general anesthesia, as a primary anesthetic in general surgery, monitored anesthesia care (MAC)
Dosage and routes:
Anesthesia <30 min
Combination
• *Adult:* IV 8-50 µg/kg, may increase by 3-15 µg/kg
Anesthetic induction
• *Adult:* IV 3-5 µg/kg, then 0.5-1.5 µg/kg/min; total dose is 8-40 µg/kg
Anesthesia 30-60 min
Induction
• *Adult:* IV 20-50 µg/kg
Maintenance
• *Adult:* IV 5-15 µg/kg; may give up to 75 µg/kg total dose
Continuous anesthesia >45 min
Induction
• *Adult:* IV 50-75 µg/kg
Maintenance
• *Adult:* IV 0.5-3.0 µg/kg/min; rate should be decreased by 30%-50% after 1 hr maintenance inf; may be increased to 4 µg/kg/min or bol doses of 7 µg/kg
Induction of anesthesia >45 min
• *Adult:* IV 130-245 µg/kg, then 0.5-1.5 µg/kg/min

MAC
Induction
• *Adult:* IV duration ≤½ hr 3-8 µg/kg
Maintenance
• *Adult:* 3-5 µg/kg q5-20min to 1 µg/kg/min, total dose 3-40 µg/kg
Available forms: Inj 500 µg/ml
Side effects/adverse reactions:
CNS: Drowsiness, dizziness, confusion, headache, sedation, euphoria, delirium, agitation, anxiety
GI: Nausea, vomiting, anorexia, constipation, cramps, dry mouth
GU: Urinary retention, dysuria
INTEG: Rash, urticaria, bruising, flushing, diaphoresis, pruritus
EENT: Tinnitus, blurred vision, miosis, diplopia
CV: Palpitation, bradycardia, change in B/P, facial flushing, syncope, asystole
RESP: **Respiratory depression, apnea**
MS: Rigidity
Contraindications: Child <12 yr, hypersensitivity
Precautions: Pregnancy (C), lactation, increased intracranial pressure, acute MI, severe heart disease, renal disease, hepatic disease, asthma, respiratory conditions, convulsive disorders, elderly
Pharmacokinetics: Half-life 1-2 hr, 90% bound to plasma proteins, duration 30 min
Interactions:
• Respiratory depression, hypotension, profound sedation: alcohol, sedative/hypnotics, or other CNS depressants, antihistamines, phenothiazines, fluconazole
🖋 Increased CNS depression: kava kava
Lab test interferences:
Increase: Amylase
NURSING CONSIDERATIONS
Assess:
• I&O ratio, check for decreasing

◆ = Nursing alert   🖋 = Herb-drug interaction   🚫 = Do not crush

output; may indicate urinary retention, especially in elderly
• CNS changes: dizziness, drowsiness, hallucinations, euphoria, LOC, pupil reaction
• Allergic reactions: rash, urticaria
◆ Respiratory dysfunction: respiratory depression, character, rate, rhythm: notify prescriber if respirations are <12/min; CV status: bradycardia, syncope
• Use pain scoring to determine pain perception

Administer:

Direct IV
• Over 1½-3 min; use tuberculin syringe

Continuous IV
• By diluting 20 ml of drug in 230 ml of diluent (40 µg/ml); discontinue inf 15 min before surgery is completed

Solution compatibilities: LR, 0.9% NaCl, D_5W, D_5/0.9% NaCl

Syringe compatibilities: Atracurium

Y-site compatibilities: Etomidate propofol

Perform/provide:
• Storage in light-resistant area at room temperature

Evaluate:
• Therapeutic response: maintenance of anesthesia

Teach patient/family:
• Tell patient to call for assistance when ambulating or smoking; drowsiness, dizziness may occur
• Advise patient to make position changes slowly to prevent orthostatic hypotension

Treatment of overdose: Nalaxone HCl 0.2-0.8 mg IV, O_2, IV fluids, vasopressors

alglucerase (R)
(al-gloo'sir-ace)
Ceredase
Func. class.: Enzyme

Action: Catalyzes the breakdown of glucocerebroside, which accumulates in macrophages primarily in the liver, spleen, and bone marrow in Gaucher's disease

Uses: Long-term enzyme replacement for a confirmed diagnosis of type I Gaucher's disease

Dosage and routes:
• *Adult and child:* **IV** 60 U/kg diluted in up to 100 ml of 0.9% NaCl given over 1-2 hr; dose is repeated q2wk, but may be given qod or as infrequently as q4wk; dose should be adjusted downward at intervals of 3-6 mo

Available forms: Inj 10, 80 IU/ml

Side effects/adverse reactions:

CNS: Fever, malaise, chills

GI: Nausea, vomiting, diarrhea, abdominal discomfort

INTEG: Pain on injection, burning and swelling at site of injection

Contraindications: Hypersensitivity

Precautions: Pregnancy (C), lactation

Pharmacokinetics: Steady-state enzymatic activity occurs within 60 min after a single injection; elimination half-life 4-20 min

NURSING CONSIDERATIONS
Assess:
• GI status: transient nausea, vomiting, abdominal discomfort
• Hypersensitive reactions; rashes and local injection site reactions may occur
• For increased fluid retention in cardiac disease

Administer:

IV infusion
• Over 1-2 hr

• Dilute 60 U/kg in up to 100 ml of 0.9% NaCl

Perform/provide:
• Storage in refrigerator; do not freeze; do not shake, as this may inactivate the drug

Evaluate:
• Therapeutic response: reduction of splenomegaly and hepatomegaly; improvement of hematologic deficiencies; reduced cachexia and wasting in children

Teach patient/family:
• To use only as directed by prescriber
• To report unusual side effects and avoid all other medications unless prescribed

---

allopurinol (℞)

(al-oh-pure'i-nole)
allopurinol, Apo-Allopurinol*, Lopurin*, Purimol*, Zyloprim
Func. class.: Antigout drug
Chem. class.: Xanthene oxidase inhibitor

Action: Inhibits the enzyme xanthine oxidase, reducing uric acid synthesis

Uses: Chronic gout, hyperuricemia associated with malignancies, recurrent calcium oxalate calculi, Chagas' disease, cutaneous/visceral leishmaniasis

Dosage and routes:
Gout/hyperuricemia
• *Adult:* **PO** 200-600 mg qd depending on severity, not to exceed 800 mg/day
• *Child 6-10 yr:* 300 mg qd
• *Child <6 yr:* 150 mg qd
Impaired renal function
• *Adult:* **PO** 200 mg qd when CrCl is 20 to 10 ml/min
• *Adult:* **PO** 100 mg qd (CrCl <20 ml/min)

Recurrent calculi
• *Adult:* **PO** 200-300 mg qd
Uric acid nephropathy prevention
• *Adult and child >10 yr:* **PO** 600-800 mg qd × 2-3 days
Available forms: Tabs 100, 300 mg
Side effects/adverse reactions:
HEMA: Agranulocytosis, thrombocytopenia, aplastic anemia, pancytopenia, leukopenia, bone marrow suppression, eosinophilia
CNS: Headache, drowsiness, neuritis, paresthesia
GI: Nausea, vomiting, anorexia, malaise, metallic taste, cramps, peptic ulcer, diarrhea, stomatitis
MISC: Myopathy, arthralgia, hepatomegaly, *cholestatic jaundice, renal failure, exfoliative dermatitis*
EENT: Retinopathy, cataracts, epistaxis
INTEG: Fever, chills, dermatitis, pruritus, purpura, erythema, ecchymosis, alopecia
Contraindications: Hypersensitivity
Precautions: Pregnancy (B), lactation, renal disease, hepatic disease, children
Pharmacokinetics:
PO: Peak 2-4 hr; excreted in feces, urine; half-life 2-3 hr, terminal half-life 18-30 hr
Interactions:
• Increased action of oral anticoagulants, chlorpropamide, cyclophosphamide, hydantoin, theophylline, vidarabine, ACE inhibitors, mercaptopurine, azathioprine
• Decreased effects of probenecid
• Rash: ampicillin, amoxicillin
• Increased hypersensitivity: thiazide diuretics
• Decreased effects of allopurinol: aluminum salts
Lab test interferences:
Increase: AST/ALT, alk phosphatase

◆ = Nursing alert   ⚗ = Herb-drug interaction   🚫 = Do not crush

Decrease: Hct/Hgb, leukocytes, serum glucose

NURSING CONSIDERATIONS

Assess:
• Uric acid levels q2wk; uric acid levels should be 6 mg/dl or less
• CBC, AST, BUN, creatinine before starting treatment, monthly
• I&O ratio; increase fluids to prevent stone formation
• Nutritional status: discourage organ meat, sardines, salmon, legumes, gravies (high-purine foods), alcohol

Administer:

PO
• With meals, to prevent GI symptoms
• A few days before antineoplastic therapy

Evaluate:
• Therapeutic response: decreased pain in joints, decreased stone formation in kidney

Teach patient/family:
• That tabs may be crushed
• To take as prescribed; if dose is missed, take as soon as remembered; do not double dose
• To increase fluid intake to 3-4 L/day
• To report skin rash, stomatitis, malaise, fever, aching; drug should be discontinued
• To avoid hazardous activities if drowsiness or dizziness occurs
• To avoid alcohol, caffeine; will increase uric acid levels
• To avoid large doses of vitamin C; kidney stone formation may occur
• To maintain a diet enhancing urine alkalinity, e.g., milk

A

alpha₁-proteinase inhibitor, human (℞)

Prolastin

Func. class.: Enzyme inhibitor

Action: Prevents elastase destruction on alveolar tissue

Uses: Replacement in patients with α_1-antitrypsin deficiency

Dosage and routes:
• *Adult:* IV 60 mg/kg qwk, may give at a rate of 0.08 ml/kg/min or greater

Available forms: Inj 500 mg, 1000 mg vials

Side effects/adverse reactions:

HEMA: Leukocytosis, ***viral transmission possible***

CNS: Dizziness, light-headedness

MISC: Fever, delayed

Contraindications: Hypersensitivity to polyethylene glycol, emphysema associated with α_1-antitrypsin

Precautions: Irreversible destruction of lung tissue secondary to α_1-antitrypsin deficiency, pregnancy (C), lactation, children

Pharmacokinetics: Duration unknown

Interactions:
• Decreased effects: cigarette smoking

NURSING CONSIDERATIONS

Assess:
• Respiratory status: rate, lung sounds, rhythm prior to and weekly during treatment
• For fluid overload: hypertension, dyspnea, rales/crackles, jugular vein distention
• For fever, chills, dizziness, lightheadedness

Administer:

Direct IV
• After bringing to room temperature, reconstitute with sterile water for inj to a concentration of 20 mg/

---

ml; use instructions for vacuum transfer using filter needle; swirl to mix, do not shake; may be diluted in 0.9% NaCl, give at a rate of 0.08 mg/kg/min or greater

IV incompatibilities: Do not mix with other drugs or diluents

Teach patient/family:

• The purpose for medication and need for weekly treatment; tell patient to avoid smoking and report changes in breathing or sputum production

• That fever may be delayed for up to 12 hr after infection and resolves by 24 hr

• That periodic pulmonary function test may be required to determine progression of disease

---

alprazolam (R)

(al-pray'zoe-lam)
Apo-Alpraz*, Novo-Alprazol*, Nu-Alpraz*, Xanax
Func. class.: Antianxiety
Chem. class.: Benzodiazepine

Controlled Substance Schedule IV

Action: Depresses subcortical levels of CNS, including limbic system, reticular formation

Uses: Anxiety, panic disorders, anxiety with depressive symptoms

Investigational uses: Depression, social phobia, premenstrual syndrome

Dosage and routes:

Anxiety disorder
• *Adult:* PO 0.25-0.5 mg tid, not to exceed 4 mg/day in divided doses
• *Elderly:* PO 0.125-0.25 mg bid; increase by 0.125 as needed

Panic disorder
• *Adult:* PO 0.5 mg may increase q3-4d by 1 mg/day or less

Premenstrual syndrome
• *Adult:* PO 0.25 mg tid

Social phobia
• *Adult:* PO 2-8 mg/day

Available forms: Tabs 0.25, 0.5, 1, 2 mg

Side effects/adverse reactions:

CNS: Dizziness, drowsiness, confusion, headache, anxiety, tremors, stimulation, fatigue, depression, insomnia, hallucinations

GI: Constipation, dry mouth, nausea, vomiting, anorexia, diarrhea

INTEG: Rash, dermatitis, itching

CV: Orthostatic hypotension, ECG changes, tachycardia, hypotension

EENT: Blurred vision, tinnitus, mydriasis

Contraindications: Hypersensitivity to benzodiazepines, narrow-angle glaucoma, psychosis, pregnancy (D), lactation, child <18 yr

Precautions: Elderly, debilitated, hepatic disease, renal disease

Pharmacokinetics:

PO: Onset 30 min, peak 1-2 hr, duration 4-6 hr, therapeutic response 2-3 days; metabolized by liver, excreted by kidneys; crosses placenta, breast milk; half-life 12-15 hr

Interactions:

• Increased toxicity: benzodiazepines

• Increased CNS depression: anticonvulsants, alcohol, antihistamines, sedative/hypnotics

• Decreased action of alprazolam: disulfiram, cimetidine

• Decreased action of levodopa

⌀ Increased CNS depression: kava kava

Lab test interferences:

Increase: AST/ALT, serum bilirubin, neutropenia

False increase: 17-OHCS

Decrease: RAIU, HCT

NURSING CONSIDERATIONS

Assess:

• B/P lying, standing; pulse; if systolic B/P drops 20 mm Hg, hold drug, notify prescriber

---

• Blood studies: CBC during long-term therapy; blood dyscrasias have occurred rarely
• Hepatic studies: AST, ALT, bilirubin, creatinine, LDH, alk phosphatase
• I&O; may indicate renal dysfunction
• For indications of increasing tolerance and abuse
• Mental status: mood, sensorium, affect, sleeping pattern, drowsiness, dizziness, especially in elderly
◆Physical dependency, withdrawal symptoms: anxiety, panic attacks, agitation, convulsions, headache, nausea, vomiting, muscle pain, weakness; withdrawal seizures may occur after rapid decrease in dose or abrupt discontinuation
• Suicidal tendencies

Administer:
PO
• With food or milk for GI symptoms
• Crushed if patient is unable to swallow medication whole
• Sugarless gum, hard candy, frequent sips of water for dry mouth

Perform/provide:
• Assistance with ambulation during beginning therapy; drowsiness/dizziness occurs
• Safety measures, including side rails
• Check that PO medication has been swallowed

Evaluate:
• Therapeutic response: decreased anxiety, restlessness, sleeplessness

Teach patient/family:
• Not to double doses; take exactly as prescribed; if dose is missed, take within 1 hr as scheduled
• That drug may be taken with food
• Not to use for everyday stress or longer than 3 mo unless directed by prescriber; not to take more than

prescribed amount; may be habit forming
• To avoid OTC preparations unless approved by prescriber
• To avoid driving, activities that require alertness, since drowsiness may occur
• To avoid alcohol ingestion or other psychotropic medications unless directed by prescriber
• Not to discontinue medication abruptly after long-term use
• To rise slowly or fainting may occur, especially elderly
• That drowsiness may worsen at beginning of treatment
Treatment of overdose: Lavage, VS, supportive care

alprostadil (R)
(al-pros'ta-dil)
Caverject, Edex, Muse, PGEl, prostaglandin E₁, Prostin VR*, Prostin VR Pediatric
Func. class.: Hormone
Chem. class.: Prostaglandin E₁

Action: Relaxes smooth muscles of ductus arteriosus; results in increased O_2 content throughout body; causes erection by dilation of cavernosal arteries and relaxation of trabecular muscle, this leads to the trapping of blood
Uses: To maintain patent ductus arteriosus (temporary treatment), erectile dysfunction

Dosage and routes:
Patent ductus arteriosus
• *Infants:* **IV INF** 0.1 µg/kg/min, until desired response, then reduce to lowest effective amount, 0.4 µg/kg/min not likely to produce greater beneficial effects
Erectile dysfunction of vasculogenic or mixed etiology, psychogenic
• *Men:* **INTRACAVERNOSAL**

2.5 μg may increase by 2.5 μg; may then increase by 5-10 μg until adequate response occurs; **INTRA-URETHRAL:** administer as needed to achieve erection

Available forms: Inj 500 μg/ml; lyopholized powder for inj 6.15, 11.9, 23.2 μg; 5, 10, 20, 40 μg/ single dose vial; pellet 125, 250, 500, 1000 μg

Side effects/adverse reactions:

MS: Deformities of long bones in neonates treated for prolonged periods

MISC: Sepsis, hypokalemia, *peritonitis,* hypoglycemia, hyperkalemia

RESP: Apnea, bradypnea, wheezing, respiratory depression

HEMA: DIC (disseminated intravascular coagulation), *thrombocytopenia,* anemia, *bleeding*

CNS: Fever, *convulsions,* lethargy, hypothermia, stiffness, hyperirritability, *cerebral bleeding*

GI: Diarrhea, regurgitation, hyperbilirubinemia

GU: Oliguria, hematuria, *anuria*

CV: Bradycardia, tachycardia, hypotension, *CHF, ventricular fibrillation, shock,* flushing, *cardiac arrest,* edema

Local (Caverject): Penile pain, prolonged erection, penile fibrosis, penile rash, edema, hematoma, ecchymosis

Systems (Caverject): Headache, dizziness, flu symptoms, sinusitis, nasal congestion, hypertension, back pain, prostatic disorder

Contraindications: Hypersensitivity, respiratory distress syndrome (RDS)

Precautions: Bleeding disorders

Pharmacokinetics: Up to 80% metabolized in lungs, excreted in urine (metabolites)

Interactions:

• Do not mix in sol or syringe with other drugs; compatibility not known

NURSING CONSIDERATIONS
Assess:

• ABGs, arterial pH, arterial pressure, continuous ECG; if arterial pressure decreases, reduce or stop drug

 Apnea and bradycardia; if these occur, be prepared to support ventilation

• Increased pH, B/P, output, decreased ratio of PA to AP (restricted systemic blood flow)

Administer:

IV infusion

• Only with emergency equipment available and by trained clinicians (patent ductus arteriosus)

• After diluting with NS or D_5W injection to a concentration of 500 μg/ml, dilute further with 0.9% NaCl, D_5W; 500 μg of drug/250 ml of dilute = 2 μg/ml; 0.1 μg/kg/min run at 0.05 ml/kg/min, use infusion pump

Perform/provide:

• Arterial pressure measurement during infusion

• Refrigeration for drug; discard all mixed unused portion

Evaluate:

• Therapeutic response: increased PO_2 (cyanotic heart disease); erection

Teach patient/family:

• About the diagnosis, prognosis, treatment

• The method for self-injection (erectile disorder), amount to be used, disposal of needle; there is little control over erection; refrigerate; alternate sides of the penis with each inj; do not inj >3×/wk; allow 24 hr between doses; notify health-care provider of new penile pain, nodules, or signs of infection

Treatment of overdose: Discontinue drug, provide supportive measures

---

 = Nursing alert   = Herb-drug interaction   🚫 = Do not crush

alteplase (℞)

(al-ti-plaze′)

Activase, Activase rt-PA*, rt-Pa, tissue plasminogen activator, TPA

Func. class.: Thrombolytic enzyme

Chem. class.: Tissue plasminogen activator (TPA)

Action: Produces fibrin conversion of plasminogen to plasmin; able to bind to fibrin, convert plasminogen in thrombus to plasmin, which leads to local fibrinolysis, limited systemic proteolysis

Uses: Lysis of obstructing thrombi associated with acute MI, ischemic conditions requiring thrombolysis, i.e., PE, DVT, unclotting arteriovenous shunts, acute ischemic CVA

Investigational uses: Unstable angina

Dosage and routes:

• *Adult >65 kg:* **IV** a total of 100 mg; 6-10 mg given **IV BOL** over 1-2 min, 60 mg given over first hour, 20 mg given over second hour, 20 mg given over third hour; or 1.25 mg/kg given over 3 hr for smaller patients

Accelerated INF

• *Adult:* **IV BOL** 15 mg; then 0.75 mg/kg over ½ hr; 0.5 mg/kg over 1 hr

Available forms: Powder for inj 50 mg (29 million IU/vial), 100 mg (58 million IU/vial)

Side effects/adverse reactions:

*SYST: **GI, GU, intracranial, retroperitoneal bleeding,** surface bleeding*

*CV: **Sinus bradycardia, ventricular tachycardia, accelerated idioventricular rhythm***

INTEG: Urticaria, rash

Contraindications: Hypersensitivity, active internal bleeding, recent CVA, severe uncontrolled hypertension, intracranial/intraspinal surgery/trauma, aneurysm

Precautions: Pregnancy (C), lactation, children

Pharmacokinetics: Cleared by liver, 80% cleared within 10 min of drug termination

Interactions:

• Increased bleeding: heparin, acetylsalicylic acid, dipyridamole, NSAIDs

Lab test interferences:

Increase: PT, APTT, TT

NURSING CONSIDERATIONS

Assess:

• VS, B/P, pulse, respirations, neurologic signs, temperature at least q4h; temperature >104° F (40° C) indicates internal bleeding; monitor rhythm closely; ventricular dysrhythmias may occur with hyperfusion; monitor heart, breath sounds, neuro status, peripheral pulses

◆▶For bleeding during first hour of treatment and 24 hr after procedure: hematuria, hematemesis, bleeding from mucous membranes, epistaxis, ecchymosis; guaiac all body fluids, stools. Do not use 150 mg or more total dose; intracranial bleeding may occur

• Allergy: fever, rash, itching, chills; mild reaction may be treated with antihistamines

• Blood studies (Hct, platelets, PTT, PT, TT, APTT) before starting therapy; PT or APTT must be less than 2 × control before starting therapy TT or PT q3-4h during treatment

Administer:

Intermittent IV inf

• After reconstituting with provided diluent, add appropriate amount of sterile water for injection (no preservatives) 20 mg vial/20 ml or 50 mg vial/50 ml to make 1 mg/ml,

mix by slow inversion or dilute with NaCl, D_5W to a concentration of 0.5 mg/ml; 1.5 to <0.5 mg/ml may result in precipitation of drug; use 18 G needle; flush line with NaCl after administration
• Heparin therapy after thrombolytic therapy is discontinued, TT, ACT, or APTT less than 2 × control (about 3-4 hr)
• Reconstituted IV solution within 8 hr or discard
• Within 6 hr of coronary occlusion for best results
Additive compatibilities: Lidocaine, morphine, nitroglycerin
Y-site compatibilities: Lidocaine, metoprolol, propranolol
Perform/provide:
• Avoidance of invasive procedures, injection, rectal temperature
• Pressure for 30 sec to minor bleeding sites; 30 min to sites of atrial puncture, followed by pressure dressing; inform prescriber if this does not attain hemostasis; apply pressure dressing
• Storage of powder at room temperature or refrigerate; protect from excessive light
Evaluate:
• Therapeutic response: lysis of thrombi
Teach patient/family:
• The purpose and expected results of the treatment

altretamine (R)

(al-tret'a-meen)
Hexalen, hexamethylmelamine, Hexastat*
Func. class.: Misc. antineoplastic
Chem. class.: S-triazine derivative (formerly known as hexamethylmelamine)

Action: Products of metabolism form covalent adducts with tissue macromolecules including DNA, which may be responsible for cytotoxicity; activity is not cell cycle phase specific
Uses: Palliative treatment of recurrent, persistent ovarian cancer following first-line treatment with cisplatin or alkylating agent-based combination
Dosage and routes:
• *Adult:* **PO** 260 mg/m²/day for 14 or 21 days in a 28-day cycle; give in 4 divided doses after meals and at hs
Available forms: Caps 50 mg
Side effects/adverse reactions:
GI: Nausea, anorexia, vomiting, increased alk phosphatase, *hepatic toxicity*
CNS: Peripheral sensory neuropathy, fatigue, *seizures,* mood disorders, disorders of consciousness, ataxia, dizziness, vertigo
HEMA: Leukopenia, thrombocytopenia, anemia
GU: Increased BUN, serum creatinine
INTEG: Rash, pruritus, alopecia
Contraindications: Hypersensitivity, severe bone marrow depression, severe neurologic toxicity
Precautions: Pregnancy (D), lactation, children
Pharmacokinetics:
PO: Well absorbed orally, rapidly metabolized in liver, metabolites excreted in urine; peak ½-3 hr

Interactions:
• Possible increased toxicity of altretamine: cimetidine
• Severe orthostatic hypotension: MAOI

NURSING CONSIDERATIONS
Assess:
• CBC, differential, platelet count weekly, withhold drug if WBC is <2000 or platelet count is <75,000 or granulocyte count is <1000/mm^3; notify prescriber of results
• Renal function studies: BUN, serum uric acid, urine CrCl before, during therapy
• I&O ratio; report fall in urine output of 30 ml/hr
• Temperature q4h; may indicate beginning infection
• Liver function tests before, during therapy (bilirubin, AST, ALT, LDH) as needed or monthly

Administer:
PO
• Antacid before oral agent, give drug after meals, at hs
• Antiemetic 30-60 min before giving drug to prevent vomiting
• Antibiotics for prophylaxis of infection

Perform/provide:
• Strict medical asepsis, protective isolation if WBC levels are low

Evaluate:
• Therapeutic response: decreased tumor size, spread of malignancy

Teach patient/family:
• To report signs of infection: increased temperature, sore throat, flu symptoms
• To report signs of anemia: fatigue, headache, faintness, shortness of breath, irritability
• To report bleeding; avoid use of razors, commercial mouthwash
• To avoid use of aspirin products, ibuprofen
• That hair may be lost during therapy; a wig or hairpiece may make

patient feel better; new hair may be different in color, texture (rare)

---

aluminum acetate (OTC)

Bluboro Powder, Boropak Powder, Burow's Solution, Domeboro, Modified Burow's Solution, Pedi-boro Soak Paks

Func. class.: Astringent
Chem. class.: Aluminum product

Action: Maintains skin acidity, which is protective to skin surface
Uses: Skin irritation, inflammation, athlete's foot, insect bites, poison ivy, eczema, acne, rash, bruises, pruritus (anal)

Dosage and routes:
• *Adult and child:* **TOP** apply for 15-30 min q4-8h (1:10-40); gargle use 1:10 sol prn
Available forms: Solution, cream*

Side effects/adverse reactions:
INTEG. Irritation, increasing inflammation

Contraindications: Tight, occlusive dressing

Interactions:
• Inhibits action of topical collagenase ointment
• Decreased action of aluminum acetate: soap

NURSING CONSIDERATIONS
Assess:
• Area of body to receive topical application, irritation, rash, breaks, dryness

Administer:
Topical
• 1 pk/1 pt H$_2$O (1:10-40 H$_2$O) 2-4×/day

Perform/provide:
• Wet dressings using only loose-fitting dressing

Evaluate:
- Therapeutic response: decreased skin irritation

Teach patient/family:
- To discontinue use if irritation occurs
- To avoid using near eye area
- To retain otic preparation for 2-3 min

---

aluminum hydroxide (OTC)

AlternaGEL, Alu-Cap, Alugel*, aluminum hydroxide, Alu-Tab, Amphojel, Basaljel, Dialume

Func. class.: Antacid, hypophosphatemic

Chem. class.: Aluminum product

Action: Neutralizes gastric acidity, binds phosphates in GI tract; these phosphates are excreted

Uses: Antacid, hyperphosphatemia in chronic renal failure

Investigational uses: Stress ulcer, GI bleeding

Dosage and routes:
- *Adult:* SUSP 5-10 ml 1 hr pc, hs; PO 600 mg 1 hr pc, hs, chewed with milk or water

Hyperphosphatemia in renal failure
- *Adult:* SUSP 500 mg-2 g bid-qid

GI bleeding
- *Infant:* 2-5 ml/dose q1-2h
- *Child:* PO 5-15 ml/dose q1-2h

Available forms: Caps 475, 500 mg; tabs 300, 500 mg; chewable tabs 600 mg; susp (4%) 600 mg/5 ml; liq 320 mg/5 ml, 600 mg/5 ml

Side effects/adverse reactions:
GI: Constipation, anorexia, *obstruction,* fecal impaction
META: Hypophosphatemia, hypercalciuria

Contraindications: Hypersensitivity to this drug or aluminum products

Precautions: Elderly, fluid restriction, decreased GI motility, GI obstruction, dehydration, renal disease, sodium-restricted diets, pregnancy (C), lactation

Pharmacokinetics:
PO: Onset 20-40 min, excreted in feces

Interactions:
- Decreased effectiveness of tetracyclines, anticholinergics, phenothiazines, isoniazid, quinidine, phenytoin, digitalis, iron salts, warfarin, ketoconazole, ciprofloxacin; separate by at least 2 hr

NURSING CONSIDERATIONS
Assess:
- Phosphate levels, since drug is bound in GI system
- Hypophosphatemia: anorexia, weakness, fatigue, bone pain, hyporeflexia
- Constipation; increase bulk in diet if needed
- Urinary pH, Ca^{++}, electrolytes

Administer:
PO
- Laxatives or stool softeners if constipation occurs, especially elderly
- After shaking liquid
- With small amount of water or milk

NG
- By nasogastric tube if patient unable to swallow

Evaluate:
- Therapeutic response: absence of pain, decreased acidity

Teach patient/family:
- To increase fluids to 2 L/day unless contraindicated; measures to prevent constipation
- To avoid phosphate foods (most dairy products, eggs, fruits, carbonated beverages) during drug therapy
- Not to use for prolonged periods

---

in patients with low serum phosphate or if on a low-sodium diet
• To add cheese, corn, pasta, plums, prunes, lentils after drug is discontinued
• That stools may appear white or speckled
• To check with prescriber after 2 wk of self-prescribed antacid use

---

amantadine (℞)

(a-man'ta-deen)
amantadine HCl, Symadine, Symmetrel
Func. class.: Antiviral, antiparkinsonian agent
Chem. class.: Tricyclic amine

Action: Prevents uncoating of nucleic acid in viral cell, preventing penetration of virus to host; causes release of dopamine from neurons
Uses: Prophylaxis or treatment of influenza type A, extrapyramidal reactions, parkinsonism, respiratory tract infections
Investigational uses: Neuroleptic malignant syndrome, cocaine dependency, enuresis
Dosage and routes:
Influenza type A
• *Adult and child >12 yr:* **PO** 200 mg/day in single dose or divided bid
• *Child 9-12 yr:* **PO** 100 mg bid
• *Child 1-9 yr:* **PO** 4.4-8.8 mg/kg/day divided bid-tid, not to exceed 200 mg/day
Extrapyramidal reaction/parkinsonism
• *Adult:* **PO** 100 mg bid, up to 400 mg/day in EPS; give for 1 wk, then 100 mg as needed up to 400 mg in parkinsonism; CrCl 40-50 ml/min 100 mg/day; CrCl 30 ml/min 200 mg 2×/wk; CrCl 20 ml/min 100 mg 3×/wk; CrCl <10 ml/min 100 mg alternating with 200 mg q7days

Available forms: Caps 100 mg; syr 50 mg/5 ml
Side effects/adverse reactions:
CNS: Headache, dizziness, drowsiness, fatigue, *anxiety,* psychosis, *depression, hallucinations,* tremors, **convulsions,** confusion, *insomnia*
CV: Orthostatic hypotension, **CHF**
INTEG: Photosensitivity, dermatitis
EENT: Blurred vision
HEMA: **Leukopenia**
GI: Nausea, vomiting, constipation, dry mouth
GU: Frequency, retention
Contraindications: Hypersensitivity, lactation, child <1 yr, eczematic rash
Precautions: Epilepsy, CHF, orthostatic hypotension, psychiatric disorders, hepatic disease, renal disease, peripheral edema, elderly, pregnancy (C)
Pharmacokinetics:
PO: Onset 48 hr, half-life 24 hr, not metabolized, excreted in urine (90%) unchanged, crosses placenta, excreted in breast milk
Interactions:
• Increased anticholinergic response: atropine, other anticholinergics
• Increased CNS stimulation: CNS stimulants
• Decreased renal excretion of amantadine: triamterene, hydrochlorothiazide
🖋 Increased anticholinergic effect: belladonna leaf/root, henbane leaf
🖋 Increased action/side effects: pheasant's eye herb, scopolia root
NURSING CONSIDERATIONS
Assess:
• I&O ratio; report frequency, hesitancy
• CHF, confusion, mottling of skin
• Bowel pattern before, during treatment
• Skin eruptions, photosensitivity after administration of drug

• Respiratory status: rate, character, wheezing, tightness in chest
• Allergies before initiation of treatment, reaction of each medication
• Signs of infection

Administer:
• Before exposure to influenza; continue for 10 days after contact
• At least 4 hr before hs to prevent insomnia
• After meals for better absorption, to decrease GI symptoms
• In divided doses to prevent CNS disturbances: headache, dizziness, fatigue, drowsiness

Perform/provide:
• Storage in tight, dry container

Evaluate:
• Therapeutic response: absence of fever, malaise, cough, dyspnea in infection; tremors, shuffling gait in Parkinson's disease

Teach patient/family:
• To change body position slowly to prevent orthostatic hypotension
• About aspects of drug therapy: need to report dyspnea, weight gain, dizziness, poor concentration, dysuria, behavioral changes
• To avoid hazardous activities if dizziness, blurred vision occurs
• To take drug exactly as prescribed; parkinsonian crisis may occur if drug is discontinued abruptly; do not double dose; if a dose is missed, do not take within 4 hr of next dose; caps may be opened and mixed with food
• To avoid alcohol

Treatment of overdose: Withdraw drug, maintain airway, administer epinephrine, aminophylline, O₂, IV corticosteroids, physostigmine

amifostine (℞)

(a-mi-foss'teen)
Ethyl
Func. class.: Cytoprotective agent for cisplatin

Action: Binds and detoxifies damaging metabolites of cisplatin by converting this drug by alkaline phosphatase in tissue to an active free thiol compound

Uses: Used to reduce renal toxicity when cisplatin is given in ovarian cancer

Dosage and routes:
• *Adult:* **IV** 910 mg/m^2 qd, within ½ hr before chemotherapy
Available forms: Powder for inj 500 mg/vial with 500 mg mannitol

Side effects/adverse reactions:
CNS: Dizziness, somnolence
EENT: Sneezing
INTEG: Flushing
CV: Hypotension
GI: Nausea, vomiting, hiccoughs
MISC: Hypocalcemia, rash, chills

Contraindications: Hypersensitivity to mannitol, aminothiol; hypotension, dehydration, lactation

Precautions: Elderly, CV disease, pregnancy (UK), children

Pharmacokinetics: Metabolized to free thiol compound, half-life 8 min

Interactions:
• Increased hypotension: antihypertensives

NURSING CONSIDERATIONS
Assess:
• Fluid status before administration; administer antiemetic prior to administration to prevent severe nausea and vomiting; also, dexamethasone 20 mg IV and a serotonin antagonist such as ondansetron or granisetron
• Calcium levels before and during

◆ = Nursing alert ⦿ = Herb-drug interaction ⊘ = Do not crush treatment; calcium supplements may be given for low calcium levels

• B/P prior to and q5min during infusion; if severe hypotension occurs, give IV 0.9% NaCl to expand fluid volume, place in Trendelenburg position

Administer:

Intermittent IV inf

• Intermittent INF after reconstituting with 9.5 ml of sterile 0.9% NaCl, further dilute with 0.9% NaCl to a concentration of 5-40 mg/ml, give at a rate over 15 min within ½ hr of chemotherapy

Y-site compatibilities: Amikacin, aminophylline, ampicillin, ampicillin/sulbactam, aztreonam, bleomycin, bumetanide, buprenorphine, butorphanol, calcium gluconate, carboplatin, carmustine, cefazolin, cefonicid, cefotaxime, cefotetan, cefoxitin, ceftazidime, ceftizoxime, ceftriaxone, cefuroxime, cimetidine, ciprofloxacin, clindamycin, cyclophosphamide, cytarabine, dacarbazine, dactinomycin, daunorubicin, dexamethasone, diphenhydramine, dobutamine, dopamine, doxorubicin, doxycycline, droperidol, enalaprilat, etoposide, famotidine, floxuridine, fluconazole, fludarabine, fluorouracil, furosemide, gallium, gentamicin, granisetron, haloperidol, heparin, hydrocortisone, hydromorphone, idarubicin, ifosfamide, imipenem-cilastatin, leucovorin, lorazepam, magnesium sulfate, mannitol, mechlorethamine, meperidine, mesna, methotrexate, methylprednisolone, metoclopramide, metronidazole, mezlocillin, mitomycin, mitoxantrone, morphine, nalbuphine, netilmicin, ondansetron, piperacillin, plicamycin, potassium chloride, promethazine, ranitidine, sodium bicarbonate, streptozocin, teniposide, thiotepa, ticarcillin, ticarcillin/clavulanate, tobramycin, trimetho-prim-sulfamethoxazole, trimetrexate, vancomycin, vinblastine, vincristine, zidovudine

Additive incompatibilities: Do not mix with other drugs or solutions

Teach patient/family:

• The reason for the medication and expected results

• That side effects may cause severe nausea, vomiting, decreased B/P, chills, dizziness, somnolence, hiccoughs, sneezing

---

amikacin (℞)

(am-i-kay′sin)

amikacin sulfate, Amikin

Func. class.: Antibiotic

Chem. class.: Aminoglycoside

Action: Interferes with protein synthesis in bacterial cell by binding to ribosomal subunit, which causes misreading of genetic code; inaccurate peptide sequence forms in protein chain, causing bacterial death

Uses: Severe systemic infections of CNS, respiratory, GI, urinary tract, bone, skin, soft tissues caused by *P. aeruginosa, E. coli, Enterobacter, Acinetobacter, Providencia, Citrobacter, Staphylococcus, Serratia, Proteus, Klebsiella* pneumonia

Investigational uses: Mycobacterium avium complex (intrathecal or intraventricular)

Dosage and routes:

Severe systemic infections

• *Adult and child:* **IV INF** 15 mg/kg/day in 2-3 divided doses q8-12h in 100-200 ml D_5W over 30-60 min, not to exceed 1.5 g; decreased doses are needed in poor renal function as determined by blood levels, renal function studies; **IM** 15 mg/kg/day in divided doses q8-12h; qd or extended interval dosing as an alternative dosing regimen

---

• *Infant:* **IV INF** 10 mg/kg initially, then 7.5 mg/kg q12h in D$_5$W over 1-2 hr

Severe urinary tract infections
• *Adult:* **IM** 250 mg q12h

Adult with poor renal function:
5-7.5 mg/kg initially, then increased as determined by blood levels, renal function studies

Available forms: Inj 50, 250 mg/ml

Side effects/adverse reactions:

GU: Oliguria, hematuria, renal damage, azotemia, failure, nephrotoxicity

CNS: Confusion, depression, numbness, tremors, *convulsions,* muscle twitching, *neurotoxicity,* dizziness, vertigo, tinnitus

EENT: Ototoxicity, deafness, visual disturbances

HEMA: Agranulocytosis, thrombocytopenia, leukopenia, eosinophilia, anemia

GI: Nausea, vomiting, anorexia; increased ALT, AST, bilirubin; hepatomegaly, *hepatic necrosis,* splenomegaly

CV: Hypotension or hypertension, palpitations

INTEG: Rash, burning, urticaria, dermatitis, alopecia

Contraindications: Mild to moderate infections, hypersensitivity to aminoglycosides

Precautions: Neonates, mild renal disease, pregnancy (C), myasthenia gravis, lactation, hearing deficits, Parkinson's disease, elderly

Pharmacokinetics:

IM: Onset rapid, peak 1-2 hr

IV: Onset immediate, peak 1-2 hr; plasma half-life 2-3 hr, prolonged up to 7 hr in infants; not metabolized, excreted unchanged in urine, crosses placental barrier, poor penetration into CSF

Interactions:

• Increased ototoxicity, neurotoxicity, nephrotoxicity: other aminoglycosides, amphotericin B, polymyxin, vancomycin, ethacrynic acid, furosemide, mannitol, methoxyflurane, cisplatin, cephalosporins, penicillins

• Increased neuromuscular blockade, respiratory depression: anesthetics, nondepolarizing neuromuscular blockers, succinylcholine

NURSING CONSIDERATIONS

Assess:

• Weight before treatment; calculation of dosage is usually based on ideal body weight but may be calculated on actual body weight

• I&O ratio; urinalysis daily for proteinuria, cells, casts; report sudden change in urine output

• VS during infusion; watch for hypotension, change in pulse

• IV site for thrombophlebitis including pain, redness, swelling q30 min; change site if needed; apply warm compresses to discontinued site

• Serum peak, drawn at 30-60 min after IV infusion or 60 min after IM injection, trough level drawn just before next dose; peak 20-30 μg/ml, trough 4-8 μg/ml; adjust dosage per levels

• Urine pH if drug is used for UTI; urine should be kept alkaline

• Renal impairment by securing urine for CrCl testing, BUN, serum creatinine; lower dosage should be given in renal impairment (CrCl <80 ml/min)

◆ Deafness by audiometric testing, ringing, roaring in ears, vertigo; assess hearing before, during, after treatment

• Dehydration: high specific gravity, decrease in skin turgor, dry mucous membranes, dark urine

• Overgrowth of infection, including increased temperature, malaise, redness, pain, swelling, perineal itching, diarrhea, stomatitis, change in cough, sputum

• C&S before starting treatment to identify organism

• Vestibular dysfunction: nausea, vomiting, dizziness, headache; drug should be discontinued if severe

• Injection sites for redness, swelling, abscesses; use warm compresses at site

Administer:

IM

• Injection in large muscle mass; rotate injection sites

• Bicarbonate to alkalinize urine if ordered for UTI, as drug is most active in alkaline environment

Intermittent IV inf

• Dilute 500 mg of drug/100-200 ml of IV D_5W, D_5RL, D_5NaCl, or 0.9% NaCl and give over ½-1 hr; flush after administration with D_5W or 0.9% NaCl

• In evenly spaced doses to maintain blood level

Additive compatibilities: Amobarbital, ascorbic acid inj, bleomycin, calcium chloride, calcium gluconate, cefepime, cefoxitin, chloramphenicol, chlorpheniramine, cimetidine, ciprofloxacin, clindamycin, cloxacillin, colistimethate, dimenhydrinate, diphenhydramine, epinephrine, ergonovine, fluconazole, furosemide, hyaluronidase, hydrocortisone, lincomycin, metaraminol, metronidazole, metronidazole/sodium bicarbonate, norepinephrine, pentobarbital, phenobarbital, phytonadione, polymyxin B, prochlorperazine, promethazine, ranitidine, secobarbital, sodium bicarbonate, succinylcholine, vancomycin, verapamil

Syringe compatibilities: Clindamycin, doxapram

Y-site compatibilities: Acyclovir, amifostine, amiodarone, amsacrine, aztreonam, cefepime, cyclophosphamide, dexamethasone, diltiazem, enalaprilat, esmolol, filgrastim, fluconazole, fludarabine, foscarnet, furosemide, granisetron, idarubicin, IL-2, labetalol, lorazepam, magnesium sulfate, melphalan, midazolam, morphine, ondansetron, paclitaxel, perphenazine, sargramostim, teniposide, thiotepa, TPN #54, #61, #91, #203, #204, vinorelbine, warfarin, zidovudine

Perform/provide:

• Adequate fluids of 2-3 L/day, unless contraindicated, to prevent irritation of tubules

• Flush of IV line with NS or D_5W after infusion

• Supervised ambulation, other safety measures with vestibular dysfunction

Evaluate:

• Therapeutic response: absence of fever, draining wounds, negative C&S after treatment

Teach patient/family:

• To report headache, dizziness, symptoms for overgrowth of infection, renal impairment

➜To report loss of hearing, ringing, roaring in ears or feeling of fullness in head

Treatment of hypersensitivity: Hemodialysis, exchange transfusion in the newborn, monitor serum levels of drug, may give ticarcillin or carbenicillin

---

amiloride (℞)

(a-mill'oh-ride)

amiloride HCl, Midamor

Func. class.: Potassium-sparing diuretic

Chem. class.: Pyrazine

Action: Acts primarily on proximal distal tubule by inhibiting reabsorption of sodium, H_2O, and increasing potassium retention

Uses: Edema in CHF in combination with other diuretics, for hypertension, adjunct with other diuretics to maintain potassium

Investigational uses: Cystic fibrosis (INH), lithium-induced polyuria

Dosage and routes:
• *Adult:* PO 5 mg qd, may be increased to 10-20 mg qd if needed
Available forms: Tabs 5 mg

Side effects/adverse reactions:
GU: Polyuria, dysuria, frequency, impotence
ELECT: **Hyperkalemia**
RESP: Cough, dyspnea, shortness of breath
CNS: Headache, dizziness, fatigue, weakness, paresthesias, tremor, depression, anxiety
GI: Nausea, diarrhea, dry mouth, *vomiting, anorexia,* cramps, constipation, abdominal pain, jaundice, bleeding
EENT: Loss of hearing, tinnitus, blurred vision, nasal congestion, increased intraocular pressure
INTEG: Rash, pruritus, alopecia, urticaria
MS: Cramps, joint pain
CV: Orthostatic hypotension, dysrhythmias, angina
HEMA: Aplastic anemia, neutropenia

Contraindications: Anuria, hypersensitivity, hyperkalemia, impaired renal function

Precautions: Dehydration, pregnancy (B), diabetes, acidosis, lactation

Pharmacokinetics:
PO: Onset 2 hr, peak 6-10 hr, duration 24 hr; excreted in urine, feces, half-life 6-9 hr

Interactions:
• Enhanced action of antihypertensives

• Hyperkalemia: other potassium-sparing diuretics, potassium products, ACE inhibitors, salt substitutes
• Decreased effect of amiloride: NSAIDs

Lab test interferences:
Interference: GTT

NURSING CONSIDERATIONS
Assess:
• Weight, I&O daily to determine fluid loss; effect of drug may be decreased if used qd
• Rate, depth, rhythm of respiration, effect of exertion
• B/P lying, standing; postural hypotension may occur
• Electrolytes: K, Na, Cl; glucose (serum), BUN, CBC, serum creatinine, blood pH, ABGs
• Improvement in CVP q8h
• Signs of drowsiness, restlessness
• Rashes, temperature elevation qd
• Confusion, especially in elderly; take safety precautions if needed

Administer:
PO
• In AM to avoid interference with sleep if using drug as a diuretic
• With food; if nausea occurs, absorption may be decreased slightly

Evaluate:
• Therapeutic response: improvement in edema of feet, legs, sacral area daily if medication is being used in CHF

Teach patient/family:
• To take as prescribed; if dose is missed, take when remembered within 1 hr of next dose
• About adverse reactions: muscle cramps, weakness, nausea, dizziness, blurred vision
• To take with food or milk for GI symptoms
• To take early in day to prevent nocturia
• To avoid potassium-rich foods:

◆ = Nursing alert   ⊘ = Herb-drug interaction   ⊘ = Do not crush oranges, bananas; salt substitutes, dried fruits

Treatment of overdose: Lavage if taken orally, monitor electrolytes, administer sodium bicarbonate for $K^+ > 6.5$ mEq/L, monitor hydration, CV, renal status

---

amino acid injection (R)

(a-mee′noe)
FreAmine, HepatAmine
Func. class.: Nitrogen product

Action: Needed for anabolism to maintain structure, decrease catabolism, promote healing

Uses: Hepatic encephalopathy, cirrhosis, hepatitis, nutritional support in cancer

Dosage and routes:
• *Adult:* IV 80-120 g/day; 500 ml of amino acids/500 ml D_{50} given over 24 hr

Available forms: Inj; many strengths, types

Side effects/adverse reactions:
CNS: Dizziness, headache, confusion, *loss of consciousness*
CV: Hypertension, *CHF, pulmonary edema*
GI: Nausea, vomiting, liver fat deposits, abdominal pain
GU: Glycosuria, osmotic diuresis
ENDO: Hyperglycemia, rebound hypoglycemia, electrolyte imbalances, hyperosmolar syndrome, hyperosmolar hyperglycemic nonketotic syndrome, alkalosis, acidosis, hypophosphatemia, hyperammonemia, dehydration, hypocalcemia
INTEG: Chills, flushing, warm feeling, rash, urticaria, extravasation necrosis, phlebitis at injection site

Contraindications: Hypersensitivity, severe electrolyte imbalances, anuria, severe liver damage, maple syrup urine disease, PKU

Precautions: Renal disease, pregnancy (C), lactation, children, diabetes mellitus, CHF

NURSING CONSIDERATIONS
Assess:
• Electrolytes (K, Na, Ca, Cl, Mg), blood glucose, ammonia, phosphate, ketones
• Renal, liver function studies: BUN, creatinine, ALT (SGOT), AST (SGPT), bilirubin
• Injection site for extravasation: redness along vein, edema at site, necrosis, pain, hard tender area; site should be changed immediately
• Respiratory function q4h: auscultate lung fields bilaterally for crackles, respirations, quality, rate, rhythm
• Temperature q4h for increased fever, indicating infection; if infection suspected, infusion is discontinued, tubing bottle cultured

⬥For impending hepatic coma: asterixis, confusion, uremic fetor, lethargy
• Hyperammonemia: nausea, vomiting, malaise, tremors, anorexia, convulsions

Administer:
Continuous IV
• Up to 40% protein and dextrose (up to 12.5%) via peripheral vein; stronger solutions require central IV administration
• TPN only mixed with dextrose to promote protein synthesis
• Immediately after mixing under strict aseptic technique, use infusion pump, in-line filter (0.22 μm) unless mixed with fat emulsion and dextrose (3 in 1)

⬥ Using careful monitoring technique; do not speed up infusion; pulmonary edema, glucose overload will result

---

Additive compatibilities: Amikacin, aminophylline, aztreonam, calcium gluconate, cefamandole, cefazolin, cefepime, cefotaxime, cefoxitin, cefsulodin, ceftazidime, ceftriaxone, cefuroxime, cimetidine, clindamycin, cyanocobalamin, cyclophosphamide, cyclosporine, cytarabine, dopamine, epoetin, erythromycin, famotidine, folic acid, furosemide, heparin, insulin (regular), isoproterenol, lidocaine, meperidine, metaraminol, methicillin, methotrexate, methyldopate, methylprednisolone, metoclopramide, morphine, nafcillin, netilmicin, nizatidine, norepinephrine, ondansetron, oxacillin, penicillin G potassium, penicillin G sodium, phytonadione, polymyxin B, sodium bicarbonate, tacrolimus, tobramycin, vancomycin

Y-site compatibilities: Amoxicillin, ascorbic acid inj, atracurium, azlocillin, calcium gluconate, cefamandole, cefazolin, cefoperazone, cefotaxime, cefoxitin, ceftazidime, ceftriaxone, cephalothin, cephapirin, chloramphenicol, cimetidine, ciprofloxacin, clindamycin, clonazepam, dexamethasone, diazepam, digoxin, dobutamine, dopamine, doxycycline, epinephrine, erythromycin, fentanyl, flucloxacillin, fluconazole, folic acid, foscarnet, furosemide, gentamicin, haloperidol, heparin, hydrocortisone, idarubicin, IL-2, insulin (regular), isoproterenol, kanamycin, lidocaine, meperidine, methicillin, metronidazole, mezlocillin, miconazole, morphine, moxalactam, multivitamins, nafcillin, netilmicin, norepinephrine, oxacillin, penicillin G, penicillin G potassium, piperacillin, potassium chloride, ranitidine, salbutamol, sargramostim, thiotepa, ticarcillin, ticarcillin/clavulanate, tobramycin, urokinase, vancomycin, vecuronium, zidovudine

Perform/provide:
• Storage depends on type of solution; consult manufacturer
• Changing dressing and IV tubing to prevent infection q24-48h

Evaluate:
• Therapeutic response: weight gain, decrease in jaundice in liver disorders, increased LOC

Teach patient/family:
• The reason for use of TPN
• If chills, sweating are experienced, report at once
• About infusion pump and blood glucose monitoring

---

amino acid solution (Ⴗ)
Aminees, Aminosyn, Branch Amin, FreAmine III, NeprAmine, Novamine, ProcalAmine, Ren Amin, Travasol, Trophmine
Func. class.: Nitrogen product

Action: Needed for anabolism to maintain structure, decrease catabolism, promote healing

Uses: Nutritional support in cancer, trauma, intestinal obstruction, short bowel syndrome, severe malabsorption

Dosage and routes:
• *Adult:* **IV** 1-1.5 g/kg/day titrated to patient's needs
• *Child:* **IV** 2-3 g/kg/day titrated to patient's needs

Available forms: Inj, many types, strengths

Side effects/adverse reactions:
CNS: Dizziness, headache, confusion, *loss of consciousness*
CV: Hypertension, *CHF, pulmonary edema*
GI: Nausea, vomiting, liver fat deposits, abdominal pain, jaundice
GU: Glycosuria, osmotic diuresis

⬥ = Nursing alert   🌿 = Herb-drug interaction   🚫 = Do not crush

ENDO: Hyperglycemia, rebound hypoglycemia, electrolyte imbalances, hyperosmolar syndrome, hyperosmolar hyperglycemic nonketotic syndrome, alkalosis, acidosis, hypophosphatemia, hyperammonemia, dehydration, hypocalcemia

INTEG: Chills, flushing, warm feeling, rash, urticaria, extravasation necrosis, phlebitis at injection site

Contraindications: Hypersensitivity, severe electrolyte imbalances, anuria, severe liver damage, maple syrup urine disease, PKU

Precautions: Renal disease, pregnancy (C), lactation, children, diabetes mellitus, CHF

NURSING CONSIDERATIONS
Assess:

• Electrolytes (K, Na, Ca, Cl, Mg), blood glucose, ammonia, phosphate

• Renal, liver function studies: BUN, creatinine, ALT (SGOT), AST (SGPT), bilirubin

• Injection site for extravasation: redness along vein, edema at site, necrosis, pain, hard tender area; site should be changed immediately

• Monitor respiratory function q4h: auscultate lung fields bilaterally for crackles, respirations, quality, rate, rhythm

• Monitor temperature q4h for increased fever, indicating infection; if infection suspected, discontinue infusion, culture tubing, bottle

• Urine glucose q6h using Tes Tape, Clinistix, which are not affected by infusion substances; blood glucose is preferred testing method

• Hyperammonemia: nausea, vomiting, malaise, tremors, anorexia, convulsions

Administer:
Continuous IV

• Up to 40% protein and dextrose (up to 12.5%) via peripheral vein; stronger solutions require central IV administration, use infusion pump

• TPN only mixed with dextrose to promote protein synthesis

• Immediately after mixing in pharmacy under strict aseptic technique using laminar flow hood, use infusion pump, in-line filter (0.22 µm) unless mixed with fat emulsion and dextrose (3 in 1)

⬥ Using careful monitoring technique; do not speed up infusion; pulmonary edema, glucose overload will result

Y-site compatibilities: Cefamandole, cefazolin, cefoperazone, cefotaxime, cefoxitin, cephalothin, cephapirin, chloramphenicol, clindamycin, digoxin, dobutamine, dopamine, doxycycline, erythromycin lactobionate, fat emulsion, foscarnet, furosemide, gentamicin, isoproterenol, kanamycin, lidocaine, meperidine, methicillin, mezlocillin, miconazole, morphine, nafcillin, netilmicin, norepinephrine, oxacillin, penicillin G potassium, piperacillin, sargramostim, ticarcillin, tobramycin, urokinase, vancomycin

Perform/provide:

• Storage depends on type of solution; consult label

• Changing dressing and IV tubing to prevent infection q24-48h

Evaluate:

• Therapeutic response: weight gain, decrease in jaundice in liver disorders, increased serum albumin

Teach patient/family:

• The reason for use of TPN

• That any chills, sweating should be reported at once

• About infusion pump and blood glucose monitoring

---

aminoglutethimide (℞)

(a-meen-oh-gloo-teth'i-mide)

Cytadren

Func. class.: Antineoplastic , adrenal steroid inhibitor

Chem. class.: Hormone

Action: Acts by inhibiting DNA, RNA, protein synthesis; is derived from *Streptomyces verticillus;* replication is decreased by binding to DNA, which causes strand splitting; phase specific in G_2 and M phases; blocks biosynthesis of all steroid hormones (cortisol, androgens, progestins)

Uses: Suppression of adrenal function in Cushing's syndrome, metastatic breast cancer, adrenal cancer

Investigational uses: Advanced prostate cancer, metastatic postmenopausal breast cancer

Dosage and routes:

• *Adult:* **PO** 250 mg qid at 6 hr intervals, may increase by 250 mg/day q1-2wk, not to exceed 2 g/day

Available forms: Tabs 250 mg

Side effects/adverse reactions:

GI: Nausea, vomiting, anorexia, hepatotoxicity

INTEG: Rash, pruritus, hirsutism

CV: Hypotension, tachycardia

CNS: Drowsiness, morbilliform skin rash, dizziness, headache, lethargy

Contraindications: Hypersensitivity, hypothyroidism, pregnancy (D)

Precautions: Renal disease, hepatic disease, respiratory disease

Pharmacokinetics: Half-life 13 hr, metabolized in liver, excreted in urine, crosses placenta

Interactions:

• Accelerated metabolism: dexamethasone

NURSING CONSIDERATIONS

Assess:

• Renal function studies: BUN, serum uric acid, urine CrCl, electrolytes before, during therapy

• I&O ratio; report fall in urine output of 30 ml/hr

• Monitor temperature q4h; may indicate beginning infection

• Liver function tests before, during therapy (bilirubin, AST, ALT, LDH) as needed or monthly

• RBC, Hct, Hgb, since these may be decreased

• Food preferences; list likes, dislikes

• Inflammation of mucosa, breaks in skin

• Yellowing of skin, sclera, dark urine, clay-colored stools, itchy skin, abdominal pain, fever, diarrhea

• Symptoms indicating severe allergic reaction: rash, pruritus, urticaria, purpuric skin lesions, itching, flushing

Administer:

PO

• Antacid before oral agent; give last dose of the day after evening meal before bedtime

• Local or systemic drugs for infection if indicated

Perform/provide:

• Liquid diet, including cola, Jell-O; dry toast or crackers as ordered may be added if patient is not nauseated or vomiting

• Nutritious diet with iron and vitamin supplements as ordered

Evaluate:

• Therapeutic response: decrease in size of tumor or decrease in Cushing's syndrome

Teach patient/family:

• To report any complaints, side effects to nurse or prescriber

• That masculinization can occur, is reversible after discontinuing treatment

• To avoid self-administration of adjuvant corticosteroids

 = Nursing alert   = Herb-drug interaction   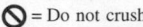 = Do not crush

• That drowsiness may occur and to avoid driving or operating heavy machinery

---

aminophylline (R)

(am-in-off'i-lin)

Amoline, Corophyllin*, Palaron*, Phyllocontin, Truphylline

Func. class.: Spasmolytic

Chem. class.: Xanthine, ethylenediamide

Action: Relaxes smooth muscle of respiratory system by blocking phosphodiesterase, which increases cyclic AMP; increased cyclic AMP alters intracellular calcium ion movements; produces bronchodilation, increased pulmonary blood flow, relaxation of respiratory tract

Uses: Bronchial asthma, bronchospasm, Cheyne-Stokes respirations

Investigational uses: Apnea in infancy for respiratory/myocardial stimulation, Cheyne-Stokes respirations as a respiratory stimulant

Dosage and routes:

• *Adult:* **PO** 500 mg, then 250-500 mg q6-8h; **CONT IV** 0.3-0.9 mg/kg/hr (maintenance); **RECT** 500 mg q6-8h

• *Child:* **PO** 7.5 mg/kg, then 3-6 mg/kg q6-8h; **IV** 7.5 mg/kg, then 3-6 mg/kg q6-8h injected over 5 min; do not exceed 25 mg/min; may give loading dose of 5.6 mg/kg over ½ hr; **CONT IV** 1 mg/kg/hr (maintenance); for children/infants use drug without preservative or alcohol

• *Neonate:* **IV/PO** 1 mg/kg initially for plasma increases of each 2 μg/ml, then 1 mg/kg q12h

Available forms: Inj IV, IM, rectal supp 250, 500 mg; rectal sol 300 mg/5 ml; elix 250 mg/5 ml; oral liq 105 mg/5 ml; tabs 100, 200 mg, tabs con rel 225 mg; tabs sus rel 300 mg

Side effects/adverse reactions:

CNS: Anxiety, restlessness, insomnia, *dizziness,* **convulsions,** headache, light-headedness, muscle twitching

CV: Palpitations, sinus tachycardia, hypotension, flushing, dysrhythmias, increased respiratory rate

GI: Nausea, vomiting, anorexia, diarrhea, bitter taste, dyspepsia, anal irritation (suppositories), epigastric pain

RESP: Tachypnea

INTEG: Flushing, urticaria, *rectal supp (irritation)*

GU: Urinary frequency

Contraindications: Hypersensitivity to xanthines, tachydysrhythmias

Precautions: Elderly, CHF, cor pulmonale, hepatic disease, active peptic ulcer disease, diabetes mellitus, hyperthyroidism, hypertension, children, pregnancy (C), lactation, glaucoma, prostatic hypertrophy

Pharmacokinetics: Well absorbed PO; extended rel well absorbed slowly, rectal supp is erratic, rectal sol is absorbed quickly; metabolized by liver (caffeine); excreted in urine; crosses placenta; appears in breast milk; half-life 3-12 hr; half-life increased in geriatric patients, hepatic disease, CHF

PO: Onset ¼ hr, peak 1-2 hr, duration 6-8 hr

PO-ER: Unknown, peak 4-7 hr, duration 8-12 hr

IV: Onset rapid, duration 6-8 hr

REC: Onset erratic, peak 1-2 hr, duration 6-8 hr

Interactions:

• Increased action of aminophylline: cimetidine, propranolol, erythromycin, troleandomycin

• Dysrhythmias: halothane

• May increase effects of anticoagulants

• Cardiotoxicity: β-blockers

- Increased elimination: smoking
- Increased toxicity: erythromycin, influenza vaccine, oral contraceptives, glucocorticoids, disulfiram
- Decreased effects of lithium
- Decreased effects of: rifampin, barbiturates, adrenergics, ketoconazole

Lab test interferences:
Increase: Plasma free fatty acids

NURSING CONSIDERATIONS
Assess:
- Theophylline blood levels (therapeutic level is 10-20 µg/ml); toxicity may occur with small increase above 20 µg/ml, especially elderly
- Monitor I&O; diuresis occurs; dehydration may result in elderly or children
- Whether theophylline was given recently (24 hr)
- Respiratory rate, rhythm, depth; auscultate lung fields bilaterally; notify prescriber of abnormalities
- Allergic reactions: rash, urticaria; if these occur, drug should be discontinued

Administer:
- Avoid IM injection; pain and tissue damage may occur

PO
- After meals to decrease GI symptoms; absorption may be affected with a full glass of water
- 🚫 Do not break, crush, or chew enteric-coated or ER tabs
- Only clear sol; flush IV line before dose

Rectal
- If patient is unable to take PO; retain rectal dose for ½ hr

IV
- After diluting in 5% dextrose to decrease burning sensation at injection site; only clear solutions
- May be diluted for IV INF in 100-200 ml in D_5W, $D_{10}W$, $D_{20}W$, 0.9% NaCl, 0.45% NaCl, LR

Additive compatibilities: Amobarbital, bretylium, calcium gluconate, chloramphenicol, cibenzoline, cimetidine, dexamethasone, diphenhydramine, dopamine, erythromycin lactobionate, esmolol, floxacillin, flumazenil, furosemide, heparin, hydrocortisone, lidocaine, mephentermine, meropenem, methicillin, methyldopa, metronidazole/sodium bicarbonate, nitroglycerin, pentobarbital, phenobarbital, potassium chloride, ranitidine, secobarbital, sodium bicarbonate, terbutaline

Syringe compatibilities: Heparin, metoclopramide, pentobarbital, thiopental

Y-site compatibilities: Allopurinol, amifostine, amrinone, aztreonam, ceftazidime, cimetidine, cladribine, enalaprilat, esmolol, famotidine, filgrastim, fluconazole, fludarabine, foscarnet, gallium, granisetron, heparin sodium with hydrocortisone sodium succinate, labetalol, melphalan, meropenem, morphine, netilmicin, paclitaxel, pancuronium, piperacillin/tazobactam, potassium chloride, propofol, ranitidine, sargramostim, tacrolimus, teniposide, thiotepa, tolazoline, vecuronium, vit B/C

Perform/provide:
- Storage of diluted solution for 24 hr if refrigerated

Evaluate:
- Therapeutic response: decreased dyspnea, respiratory stimulation in infancy, clear lung fields bilaterally

Teach patient/family:
- To take doses as prescribed, not to skip dose, not to double dose
- To check OTC medications, current prescription medications for ephedrine; will increase CNS stimulation; not to drink alcohol or caffeine products (tea, coffee, chocolate, colas)
- To avoid hazardous activities; dizziness may occur

• If GI upset occurs, to take drug with 8 oz water; avoid food, since absorption may be decreased

• To remain in bed 15-20 min after rectal suppository is inserted to avoid removal

◆ To notify prescriber of toxicity: insomnia, anxiety, nausea, vomiting, rapid pulse, convulsions

• To notify prescriber of change in smoking habit; a change in dose may be required

• To increase fluids to 2 L/day to decrease secretion viscosity

---

amiodarone (℞)

(a-mee-o'da-rone)
Cordarone

Func. class.: Antidysrhythmic (class III)

Chem. class.: Iodinated benzofuran derivative

Action: Prolongs duration of action potential and effective refractory period, noncompetitive α- and β-adrenergic inhibition; increases PR and QT intervals, decreases sinus rate

Uses: Severe ventricular tachycardia, supraventricular tachycardia, atrial fibrillation, ventricular fibrillation not controlled by first-line agents

Dosage and routes:

• *Adult:* **PO** loading dose 800-1600 mg/day 1-3 wk; then 600-800 mg/day 1 mo; maintenance 200-600 mg/day

• *Child:* **PO** loading dose 10-15 mg/kg/day in 1-2 divided doses for 4-14 days then 5 mg/kg/day

• *Adult:* **IV** loading dose (first rapid) 150 mg over the first 10 min then slow 360 mg over the next 6 hr; maintenance 540 mg given over the remaining 18 hr, decrease rate of the slow infusion to 0.5 mg/min

Available forms: Tabs 200 mg; inj 50 mg/ml

Side effects/adverse reactions:

CNS: Headache, dizziness, involuntary movement, tremors, peripheral neuropathy, malaise, fatigue, ataxia, paresthesias, insomnia

GI: Nausea, vomiting, diarrhea, abdominal pain, anorexia, constipation, *hepatotoxicity*

CV: Hypotension, bradycardia, *sinus arrest, CHF,* dysrhythmias, *SA node dysfunction*

INTEG: Rash, photosensitivity, blue-gray skin discoloration, alopecia, spontaneous ecchymosis

EENT: Blurred vision, halos, photophobia, *corneal microdeposits,* dry eyes

ENDO: Hyperthyroidism or hypothyroidism

MS: Weakness, pain in extremities

RESP: **Pulmonary fibrosis,** pulmonary inflammation

MISC: Flushing, abnormal taste or smell, edema, abnormal salivation, coagulation abnormalities

Precautions: Goiter, Hashimoto's thyroiditis, SN dysfunction, 2nd- or 3rd-degree AV block, electrolyte imbalances, pregnancy (C), bradycardia, lactation

Pharmacokinetics:

PO: Onset 1-3 wk, peak 2-10 hr; half-life 15-100 days; metabolized by liver, excreted by kidneys

Interactions:

• Bradycardia: β-blockers, calcium channel blockers, digitalis

• Increased levels of digitalis, quinidine, procainamide, flecainide, disopyramide, phenytoin, theophylline

• Increased anticoagulant effects: warfarin

• Bradycardia, arrest: lidocaine

🖋 May increase amiodarone effect:

---

aloe, buckthorn bark/berry, cascara sagrada bark, rhubarb root, senna leaf/fruits

Lab test interferences:
Increase: T_4

NURSING CONSIDERATIONS
Assess:
• I&O ratio; electrolytes (K, Na, Cl)
• Liver function studies: AST (SGOT), ALT (SGPT), bilirubin, alk phosphatase
• Chest x-ray, thyroid function tests
• ECG continuously to determine drug effectiveness, measure PR, QRS, QT intervals, check for PVCs, other dysrhythmias
• For dehydration or hypovolemia
• B/P continuously for hypotension, hypertension
• For rebound hypertension after 1-2 hr
• CNS symptoms: confusion, psychosis, numbness, depression, involuntary movements; if these occur, drug should be discontinued
• Hypothyroidism: lethargy, dizziness, constipation, enlarged thyroid gland, edema of extremities, cool, pale skin
• Hyperthyroidism: restlessness, tachycardia, eyelid puffiness, weight loss, frequent urination, menstrual irregularities, dyspnea; warm, moist skin
◆Pulmonary toxicity: dyspnea, fatigue, cough, fever, chest pain; drug should be discontinued
• Cardiac rate, respiration: rate, rhythm, character, chest pain

Administer:
PO
• Loading dose with food to decrease nausea

Intermittent IV inf
• 1000 mg/24 hr during loading/maintenance
• Initial loading: Add 3 ml (150 mg) 100 ml D_5W (1.5 mg/ml) give over 10 min

• Loading Inf: Add 18 ml (900 mg) 500 ml D_5W (1.8 mg/ml) give over next 6 hr
• Maintenance Inf: Give remainder of loading inf 540 mg over 18 hr (0.5 mg/min)

Continuous inf
• After 24 hr, give 1-6 mg/ml at 0.5 mg/ml, do not exceed 30 mg/min

Additive compatibilities: Dobutamine, lidocaine, potassium chloride, procainimide, verapamil

Y-site compatibilities: Amikacin, bretylium, clindamycin, dobutamine, dopamine, doxycycline, erythromycin, esmolol, gentamicin, insulin, isoproterenol, labetalol, lidocaine, metaraminol, metronidazole, midazolam, morphine, nitroglycerin, norepinephrine, penicillin G potassium, phentolamine, phenylephrine, potassium chloride, procainamide, tobramycin, vancomycin

Evaluate:
• Therapeutic response: decrease in ventricular tachycardia, supraventricular tachycardia or fibrillation

Teach patient/family:
• To take this drug as directed; avoid missed doses
• To use sunscreen or stay out of sun to prevent burns
• To report side effects immediately
• That skin discoloration is usually reversible
• That dark glasses may be needed for photophobia

Treatment of overdose: O_2, artificial ventilation, ECG, administer dopamine for circulatory depression, administer diazepam or thiopental for convulsions, isoproterenol

---

 = Nursing alert   = Herb-drug interaction   🚫 = Do not crush

amitriptyline (R)

(a-mee-trip'ti-leen)
Amitril, amitriptylline HCl, Apo-
Amitriptyline*, Elavil, Emi-
trip, Endep, Enovil, Levate*,
Meravil*, Novotriptyn*, Rolavil*
Func. class.: Antidepressant—
tricyclic
Chem. class.: Tertiary amine

Action: Blocks reuptake of norepinephrine, serotonin into nerve
endings, increasing action of
norepinephrine, serotonin in nerve
cells

Uses: Major depression

Investigational uses: Chronic pain
management, prevention of cluster/
migraine headaches

Dosage and routes:
Depression
• *Adult:* PO 50-100 mg hs, may in-
crease to 200 mg qd, not to exceed
300 mg/day; IM 20-30 mg qid, or
80-120 mg hs
• *Adolescent:* PO 30 mg/day in di-
vided doses, may be increased to
150 mg/day
• *Geriatric:* Generally avoided due
to anticholinergic side effects; if used
PO 10-25 mg at hs, increase by
10-25/wk as tolerated
Cluster/migraine headache
• *Adult:* PO 50-150 mg/day
Chronic pain
• *Adult:* PO 75-150 mg/day
Available forms: Tabs 10, 25, 50,
75, 100, 150 mg; inj 10 mg/ml

Side effects/adverse reactions:
*HEMA: **Agranulocytosis, thrombocytopenia, eosinophilia, leukopenia***
CNS: Dizziness, drowsiness, confusion, headache, anxiety, tremors,
stimulation, weakness, insomnia,
nightmares, EPS (elderly), increased
psychiatric symptoms, seizures

GI: Constipation, dry mouth, nausea, vomiting, ***paralytic ileus,*** increased appetite, cramps, epigastric
distress, jaundice, ***hepatitis,*** stomatitis
GU: Retention
INTEG: Rash, urticaria, sweating,
pruritus, photosensitivity
*CV: Orthostatic hypotension, **ECG
changes, tachycardia, hypertension,*** palpitations
EENT: Blurred vision, tinnitus, mydriasis, ophthalmoplegia

Contraindications: Hypersensitivity to tricyclic antidepressants, recovery phase of myocardial infarction, narrow-angle glaucoma

Precautions: Suicidal patients, convulsive disorders, prostatic hypertrophy, schizophrenia, psychosis, severe depression, increased intraocular pressure, narrow-angle glaucoma,
urinary retention, cardiac disease,
hepatic disease, renal disease, hyperthyroidism, electroshock therapy,
elective surgery, child <12 yr, pregnancy (C), lactation, elderly

Pharmacokinetics:
PO/IM: Onset 45 min, peak 2-12 hr,
therapeutic response 4-10 days; metabolized by liver; excreted in urine,
feces; crosses placenta, excreted in
breast milk, half-life 31-46 hr

Interactions:
• Decreased effects of guanethidine,
clonidine, indirect-acting sympathomimetics (ephedrine)
• Increased effects of direct-acting
sympathomimetics (epinephrine), alcohol, barbiturates, benzodiazepines,
CNS depressants
• Hyperpyretic crisis, convulsions,
hypertensive episode: MAOI (pargyline [Eutonyl])
✿ Increased CNS depression: kava
kava
✿ Increased anticholinergic effect:
belladonna leaf/root, henbane leaf

🖉 Increased action of amitriptyline: scopolia root

Lab test interferences:

Increase: Serum bilirubin, blood glucose, alk phosphatase

Decrease: VMA, 5-HIAA

False increase: Urinary catecholamines

NURSING CONSIDERATIONS
Assess:
• B/P lying, standing; pulse q4h; if systolic B/P drops 20 mm Hg, hold drug, notify prescriber; take vital signs q4h in patients with cardiovascular disease
• Blood studies: CBC, leukocytes, differential, cardiac enzymes if patient is receiving long-term therapy
• Blood level: ther 100-250 ng/ml; toxic >500 ng/ml
• Hepatic studies: AST (SGOT), ALT (SGPT), bilirubin
• Weight qwk; appetite may increase with drug
• ECG for flattening of T wave, bundle branch block, AV block, dysrhythmias in cardiac patients
• EPS primarily in elderly: rigidity, dystonia, akathisia
• Mental status: mood, sensorium, affect, suicidal tendencies; increase in psychiatric symptoms: depression, panic
• Urinary retention, constipation; constipation is most likely to occur in children and elderly
• Withdrawal symptoms: headache, nausea, vomiting, muscle pain, weakness; do not usually occur unless drug was discontinued abruptly
• Alcohol consumption; if alcohol is consumed, hold dose until morning

Administer:
PO
• Increased fluids, bulk in diet if constipation, urinary retention occur, especially elderly

• With food or milk for GI symptoms
• Crushed if patient is unable to swallow medication whole
• Dosage hs if oversedation occurs during day; may take entire dose hs; elderly may not tolerate once/day dosing
• Gum; hard, sugarless candy; or frequent sips of water for dry mouth

Perform/provide:
• Storage at room temperature; do not freeze
• Assistance with ambulation during beginning therapy, since drowsiness/dizziness occurs
• Safety measures, including side rails, primarily in elderly
• Checking to see PO medication swallowed

Evaluate:
• Therapeutic response: decrease in depression, absence of suicidal thoughts

Teach patient/family:
• To take medication as directed; do not double dose
• That therapeutic effects may take 2-3 wk
• To use caution in driving, other activities requiring alertness because of drowsiness, dizziness, blurred vision; to avoid rising quickly from sitting to standing, especially elderly
• To avoid alcohol ingestion, other CNS depressants
• Not to discontinue medication quickly after long-term use: may cause nausea, headache, malaise
• To wear sunscreen or large hat, since photosensitivity occurs

Treatment of overdose: ECG monitoring, induce emesis, lavage, activated charcoal, administer anticonvulsant

---

◆ = Nursing alert   🖉 = Herb-drug interaction   🚫 = Do not crush

amlodipine (R)

(am-loe'di-peen)
Norvasc
Func. class.: Antianginal, calcium channel blocker
Chem. class.: Dihydropyridine

Action: Inhibits calcium ion influx across cell membrane during cardiac depolarization; produces relaxation of coronary vascular smooth muscle, peripheral vascular smooth muscle; dilates coronary vascular arteries; increases myocardial oxygen delivery in patients with vasospastic angina

Uses: Chronic stable angina pectoris, hypertension, vasospastic angina

Dosage and routes:
Angina
• *Adult:* PO 5-10 mg qd
Hypertension
• *Adult:* PO 5 mg qd initially, may increase up to 10 mg/day
Available forms: Tabs 2.5, 5, 10 mg

Side effects/adverse reactions:
CV: Dysrhythmia, edema, bradycardia, hypotension, palpitations, syncope, AV block
GI: Nausea, vomiting, diarrhea, gastric upset, constipation, abdominal cramps, flatulence, anorexia
GU: Nocturia, polyuria
INTEG: Rash, pruritus, urticaria, hair loss
CNS: Headache, fatigue, dizziness, anxiety, depression, insomnia, paresthesia, somnolence, asthenia
OTHER: Flushing, nasal congestion, sweating, shortness of breath, sexual difficulties, muscle cramps, cough, weight gain, tinnitus, epistaxis

Contraindications: Sick sinus syndrome, 2nd- or 3rd-degree heart block, hypotension less than 90 mm Hg systolic, hypersensitivity

Precautions: CHF, hypotension, hepatic injury, pregnancy (C), lactation, children, renal disease, elderly

Pharmacokinetics:
PO: Onset not determined, peak 6-12 hr, half-life 30-50 hr; metabolized by liver, excreted in urine (90% as metabolites)

Interactions:
• Increased effects of digitalis, neuromuscular blocking agents, theophylline, prazosin, β-blockers, fentanyl

NURSING CONSIDERATIONS
Assess:
• Cardiac status: B/P, pulse, respiration, ECG
Administer:
PO
• Once a day
Evaluate:
• Therapeutic response: decreased anginal pain, decreased B/P
Teach patient/family:
○ Do not break, open, crush, or chew sust rel caps
• To take drug as prescribed, do not double or skip dose
• To avoid hazardous activities until stabilized on drug, dizziness is no longer a problem
• To avoid OTC drugs unless directed by prescriber
• To comply in all areas of medical regimen: diet, exercise, stress reduction, drug therapy
• To notify prescriber of irregular heartbeat, shortness of breath, swelling of feet and hands, pronounced dizziness, constipation, nausea, hypotension
Treatment of overdose: Defibrillation, β-agonists, IV calcium inotropic agents, diuretics, atropine for AV block, vasopressor for hypotension

amobarbital (℞)

(am-oh-bar'bi-tal)
amobarbital sodium, Amytal, Amytal Sodium, Amytal Sodium Pulvules, Novamobarb*

Func. class.: Sedative , hypnotic-barbiturate (intermediate acting)
Chem. class.: Amylobarbitone

Controlled Substance Schedule II (USA), Schedule G (Canada)

Action: Depresses activity in brain cells primarily in reticular activating system in brain stem; also selectively depresses neurons in posterior hypothalamus, limbic structures; able to decrease seizure activity by inhibition of impulses in CNS; depresses REM sleep

Uses: Sedation, preanesthetic sedation, insomnia, anticonvulsant, adjunct in psychiatry, hypnotic

Dosage and routes:
Preanesthetic sedation
• *Adult:* **PO/IM** 200 mg 1-2 hr preoperatively
• *Child:* **PO/IM** up to 100 mg
Sedation
• *Adult:* **PO** 30-50 mg bid or tid, may be 15-120 mg bid-qid
• *Child:* **PO** 2 mg/kg/day in 4 divided doses
Anticonvulsant/psychiatry
• *Adult:* **IV** 65-500 mg given over several min, not to exceed 100 mg/min; not to exceed 1 g
• *Child <6 yr:* **IV/IM** 3-5 mg/kg over several min
Insomnia
• *Adult:* **PO/IM** 65-200 mg hs, not to exceed 5 ml in one site
• *Child:* **IM** 3-5 mg/kg at hs, not to exceed 5 ml in one site
Available forms: Tabs 30, 50, 100 mg; caps 65, 200 mg; powder for inj 250, 500 mg/vial

Side effects/adverse reactions:
CNS: Lethargy, drowsiness, hangover, dizziness, stimulation in the elderly and children, light-headedness, physical dependence, CNS depression, mental depression, slurred speech
GI: Nausea, vomiting, diarrhea, constipation
INTEG: Rash, urticaria, pain, abscesses at injection site, *angioedema,* thrombophlebitis, *Stevens-Johnson syndrome*
CV: Hypotension, bradycardia
RESP: Depression, apnea, laryngospasm, bronchospasm
HEMA: Agranulocytosis, thrombocytopenia, megaloblastic anemia (long-term treatment)
Contraindications: Hypersensitivity to barbiturates, respiratory depression, addiction to barbiturates, severe liver impairment, porphyria, pregnancy (D), lactation
Precautions: Anemia, lactation, hepatic disease, renal disease, hypertension, elderly, acute/chronic pain
Pharmacokinetics:
PO: Onset 45-60 min, duration 6-8 hr
IV: Onset 5 min, duration 3-6 hr
Metabolized by liver, excreted by kidneys (inactive metabolites), crosses placenta, highly protein bound, excreted in breast milk, half-life 16-40 hr
Interactions:
• Increased CNS depression: alcohol, MAOIs, sedatives, narcotics, general anesthetics, antipsychotics
• Decreased effect of oral anticoagulants, corticosteroids, griseofulvin, quinidine, oral contraceptives, estrogens
• May increase or decrease phenytoin levels
• Increased half-life of doxycycline
 Increased CNS depression: kava kava, Indian snake root

Lab test interferences:
False increase: Sulfobromophthalein

NURSING CONSIDERATIONS
Assess:
• VS q30min after parenteral route for 2 hr
• Blood studies: Hct, Hgb, RBCs, serum folate, vit D (if on long-term therapy); pro-time in patients receiving anticoagulants
• Hepatic studies: AST (SGOT), ALT (SGPT), bilirubin; if increased, drug is usually discontinued
• Mental status: mood, sensorium, affect, memory (long, short), especially elderly
• Physical dependency: more frequent requests for medication, shakes, anxiety; elderly may be more sensitive due to decreased metabolism
◆ Barbiturate toxicity: hypotension; pulmonary constriction; cold, clammy skin; cyanosis of lips; CNS depression; nausea; vomiting; hallucinations; delirium; weakness; coma; pupillary constriction; mild symptoms may occur in 8-12 hr without drug
• Respiratory dysfunction: respiratory depression, character, rate, rhythm; hold drug if respirations are <10/min or if pupils are dilated
• Blood dyscrasias: fever, sore throat, bruising, rash, jaundice, epistaxis

Administer:
PO
• ½-1 hr before hs for expected sleeplessness
• On empty stomach for best absorption
• After removal of cigarettes, to prevent fires
• After trying conservative measures for insomnia

IM
• Deep injection in large muscle mass to prevent tissue sloughing, abscesses, no more than 5 ml/site
IV, direct
• After diluting each 125 mg/1.25 ml, give by direct IV at a rate of 100 mg or less/1 min (adult), or 60 mg/min child; titrate slowly to desired response with sterile water for injection to a concentration of 100 mg/ml; inject within 30 min of preparation; do not shake solution or use cloudy solution; use large vein; may cause thrombosis, extravasation
• IV only with resuscitative equipment available, administer at <100 mg/min (only by qualified personnel)
Additive compatibilities: Amikacin, aminophylline, sodium bicarbonate
Perform/provide:
• Assistance with ambulation after receiving dose
• Safety measures: side rails, nightlight, call bell within easy reach
• Checking to see PO medication swallowed
Evaluate:
• Therapeutic response: ability to sleep at night, decreased amount of early morning awakening if taking drug for insomnia, or decrease in number, severity of seizures if taking drug for seizure disorder
Teach patient/family:
• To take as directed; do not double dose
• That hangover is common
• That drug is indicated only for short-term treatment of insomnia and is probably ineffective after 2 wk
• That physical dependency may result when used for extended time (45-90 days, depending on dose)
• To avoid driving, other activities requiring alertness

---

* = Canada only   Side effects: *italics* = common; ***bold italics*** = life-threatening

- To avoid alcohol ingestion, CNS depressants; serious CNS depression may result
- Not to discontinue medication quickly after long-term use; drug should be tapered over 1 wk
- To tell all prescribers that a barbiturate is being taken
- That withdrawal insomnia may occur after short-term use; do not start using drug again; insomnia will improve in 1-3 nights; may experience increased dreaming
- That effects may take 2 nights for benefits to be noticed
- Alternative measures to improve sleep: reading, exercise several hours before hs, warm bath, warm milk, TV, self-hypnosis, deep breathing

Treatment of overdose: Lavage, activated charcoal, warming blanket, vital signs, hemodialysis, alkalinize urine; give IV volume expanders, IV fluids

---

amoxapine (℞)

(a-mox'a-peen)

amoxapine, Asendin

Func. class.: Antidepressant—tetracyclics

Chem. class.: Dibenzoxazepine derivative—secondary amine

Action: Blocks reuptake of norepinephrine, serotonin into nerve endings, increasing action of norepinephrine, serotonin in nerve cells

Uses: Depression

Dosage and routes:
- *Adult:* PO 50 mg tid, may increase to 100 mg tid on 3rd day of therapy; not to exceed 300 mg/day unless lower doses have been given for at least 2 wk, may be given daily dose hs, not to exceed 600 mg/day in hospitalized patients
- *Elderly:* PO 25 mg hs, may increase by 25 mg/wk, up to 150 mg/day in divided doses

Available forms: Tabs 10, 25, 50, 75, 100, 150 mg

Side effects/adverse reactions:

*HEMA: **Agranulocytosis, thrombocytopenia, eosinophilia, leukopenia***

CNS: Dizziness, drowsiness, confusion, headache, anxiety, tremors, stimulation, weakness, insomnia, nightmares, EPS (elderly), increased psychiatric symptoms, paresthesia, impairment of sexual functioning

GI: Dry mouth, constipation, nausea, vomiting, ***paralytic ileus,*** increased appetite, cramps, epigastric distress, jaundice, ***hepatitis,*** stomatitis

GU: Retention, ***acute renal failure***

INTEG: Rash, urticaria, sweating, pruritus, photosensitivity

*CV: Orthostatic hypotension, ECG changes, tachycardia, **hypertension,*** palpitations

EENT: Blurred vision, tinnitus, mydriasis, ophthalmoplegia

Contraindications: Hypersensitivity to tricyclic antidepressants, recovery phase of myocardial infarction, convulsive disorders, prostatic hypertrophy

Precautions: Suicidal patients, severe depression, increased intraocular pressure, narrow-angle glaucoma, urinary retention, cardiac disease, hepatic disease, hyperthyroidism, electroshock therapy, elective surgery, elderly, pregnancy (C)

Pharmacokinetics:

PO: Steady state 2-7 days; metabolized by liver, excreted by kidneys, crosses placenta, half-life 8 hr

Interactions:
- Decreased effects of guanethidine, clonidine, indirect-acting sympathomimetics (ephedrine)
- Increased effects of direct-acting sympathomimetics (epinephrine), al-

cohol, barbiturates, benzodiazepines, CNS depressants

• Hyperpyretic crisis, convulsions, hypertensive episode: MAOI (pargyline [Eutonyl])

⏮ Increased CNS depression: kava kava

⏮ May increase anticholinergic effects: belladonna leaf/root, henbane leaf

⏮ Increased action of amoxapine: scopolia root

Lab test interferences:
Increase: Serum bilirubin, blood glucose, alk phosphatase
False increase: Urinary catecholamines
Decrease: VMA, 5-HIAA

NURSING CONSIDERATIONS
Assess:

• B/P lying, standing; pulse q4h; if systolic B/P drops 20 mm Hg, hold drug, notify prescriber; take vital signs q4h in patients with cardiovascular disease

• Blood studies: CBC, leukocytes, differential, cardiac enzymes if patient is receiving long-term therapy

• Blood level: ther 20-100 ng/ml

• Hepatic studies: AST (SGOT), ALT (SGPT), bilirubin

• Weight qwk, appetite may increase with drug

• ECG for flattening of T wave, bundle branch block, AV block, dysrhythmias in cardiac patients

• EPS primarily in elderly: rigidity, dystonia, akathisia

• Mental status: mood, sensorium, affect, suicidal tendencies; increase in psychiatric symptoms: depression, panic; confusion (elderly)

• Urinary retention, constipation; constipation is more likely to occur in children, elderly

• Withdrawal symptoms: headache, nausea, vomiting, muscle pain, weakness; do not usually occur unless drug was discontinued abruptly

• Alcohol consumption; if alcohol is consumed, hold dose until morning

Administer:
PO

• Increased fluids, bulk in diet if constipation, urinary retention occur, especially in elderly

• Crushed if patient is unable to swallow medication whole, with food or milk for GI symptoms

• Dosage hs if oversedation occurs during day; may take entire dose hs; elderly may not tolerate once/day dosing

• Gum, hard candy, or frequent sips of water for dry mouth

Perform/provide:

• Storage at room temperature; do not freeze

• Assistance with ambulation during beginning therapy, since drowsiness/dizziness occurs

• Safety measures including side rails primarily for elderly

• Check to see PO medication swallowed

Evaluate:

• Therapeutic response: decreased depression, absence of suicidal thoughts

Teach patient/family:

• To take as directed, not to double dose

• That therapeutic effects may take 2-3 wk

• To use caution in driving or other activities requiring alertness because of drowsiness, dizziness, blurred vision

• To avoid alcohol ingestion, other CNS depressants

• Not to discontinue medication quickly after long-term use; may cause nausea, headache, malaise

• To wear sunscreen or large hat, since photosensitivity occurs

Treatment of overdose: ECG monitoring, induce emesis, lavage, acti-

vated charcoal, administer anticonvulsant

---

amoxicillin (R)

(a-mox-i-sill'in)
amoxicillin, Amoxil, Amoxil Pediatric Drops, Apo-moxi*,
Novamoxin*, Nu-Amoxi*, Polymox, Polymox Drops, Trimox
125, Trimox 250, Trimox 500,
Wymox
Func. class.: Broad-spectrum
antiinfective
Chem. class.: Aminopenicillin

Action: Interferes with cell wall replication of susceptible organisms;
the cell wall, rendered osmotically
unstable, swells and bursts from osmotic pressure
Uses: For gram-positive cocci (*S.
aureus, S. pyogenes, E. faecalis, S.
pneumoniae*), gram-negative cocci
(*N. gonorrhoeae, N. meningitidis*),
gram-positive bacilli (*C. diphtheriae, L. monocytogenes*), gram-
negative bacilli (*H. influenzae, E.
coli, P. mirabilis, Salmonella*); in
combination *H. pylori*
Investigational uses: Lyme disease, chlamydia trachomatis in pregnancy
Dosage and routes:
Systemic infections
• *Adult:* **PO** 750 mg-1.5 g qd in
divided doses q8h
• *Child:* **PO** 20-50 mg/kg/day in
divided doses q8h
Renal disease
• CrCl 10-50 ml/min dose q12h;
CrCl <10 ml/min dose q24h
Gonorrhea/urinary tract infections
• *Adult:* **PO** 3 g given with 1 g
probenecid as a single dose
Chlamydia trachomatis
• *Adult:* **PO** 500 mg/day × 1 wk

Bacterial endocarditis prophylaxis
• *Child:* **PO** 50 mg/kg/hr before and
25 mg/kg 6 hr after procedure
Available forms: Caps 250, 500, 875
mg; chew tabs 125, 250 mg; powder
for oral susp 50 mg/ml, 125, 250
mg/5 ml
Side effects/adverse reactions:
HEMA: Anemia, increased bleeding
time, *bone marrow depression,
granulocytopenia*
GI: Nausea, vomiting, diarrhea, increased AST (SGOT), ALT (SGPT),
abdominal pain, glossitis, colitis,
pseudomembranous colitis
CNS: Headache
*SYST: Anaphylaxis, respiratory dis-
tress, serum sickness*
INTEG: Urticaria, rash
Contraindications: Hypersensitivity to penicillins
Precautions: Pregnancy (B), lactation, hypersensitivity to cephalo-
sporins, neonates, renal disease
Pharmacokinetics:
PO: Peak 2 hr, duration 6-8 hr; half-
life 1-1⅓ hr, metabolized in liver,
excreted in urine, crosses placenta,
enters breast milk
Interactions:
• Increased amoxicillin concentrations: aspirin, probenecid, disulfiram
• Decreased effectiveness of oral
contraceptives
• Amoxicillin-induced skin rash: allopurinol
Lab test interferences:
False positive: Urine glucose, urine
protein
NURSING CONSIDERATIONS
Assess:
• I&O ratio; report hematuria, oliguria, since penicillin in high doses
is nephrotoxic
• Any patient with a compromised
renal system, since drug is excreted
slowly in poor renal system function; toxicity may occur rapidly

---

• Liver studies: AST (SGOT), ALT (SGPT)
• Blood studies: WBC, RBC, Hgb & Hct, bleeding time
• Renal studies: urinalysis, protein, blood, BUN, creatinine
• Culture, sensitivity before drug therapy; drug may be given as soon as culture is taken
• Bowel pattern before, during treatment
• Skin eruptions after administration of penicillin to 1 wk after discontinuing drug
• Respiratory status: rate, character, wheezing, tightness in the chest
• Allergies before initiation of treatment, reaction of each medication; place allergies on chart in bright red
Administer:
PO
• After C&S completed
• Shake suspension well before each dose
Perform/provide:
• Adrenaline, suction, tracheostomy set, endotracheal intubation equipment on unit
• Adequate intake of fluids (2 L) during diarrhea episodes
• Scratch test to assess allergy after securing order from prescriber; usually done when penicillin is only drug of choice
• Storage in tight container; after reconstituting, oral suspension refrigerated for 2 wk or stored at room temperature for 1 wk
Evaluate:
• Therapeutic response: absence of fever, draining wounds
Teach patient/family:
• That caps may be opened and contents taken with fluids
• To take as prescribed, not to double dose
• All aspects of drug therapy: need to complete entire course of medication to ensure organism death

(10-14 days); culture may be taken after completed course of medication
◆ To report sore throat, fever, fatigue, diarrhea (may indicate superimposed infection or agranulocytopenia)
• That drug must be taken in equal intervals around the clock to maintain blood levels; take on empty stomach with a full glass of water
• To wear or carry a Medic Alert ID if allergic to penicillins
Treatment of anaphylaxis: Withdraw drug, maintain airway, administer epinephrine, aminophylline, O_2, IV corticosteroids

---

amoxicillin/clavulanate potassium (Ŗ)

(a-mox-i-sill'in)
Augmentin, Clavulin*
Func. class.: Broad-spectrum antiinfective
Chem. class.: Aminopenicillin β-lactamase inhibitor

Action: Interferes with cell wall replication of susceptible organisms; the cell wall, rendered osmotically unstable, swells and bursts from osmotic pressure; combination increases spectrum of activity against β-lactamase resistant organisms
Uses: Sinus infections, pneumonia, otitis media, skin infection, UTI; effective for strains of *E. coli, P. mirabilis, H. influenzae, E. faeculis, S. pneumoniae,* and some β-lactamase-producing organisms
Dosage and routes:
• *Adult:* **PO** 250-500 mg q8h or 500-875 mg q12h depending on severity of infection
Renal disease
• CrCl 10-30 ml/min dose q12h; CrCl <10 ml/min dose q24h

- *Child:* **PO** 20-40 mg/kg/day in divided doses q8h or 25-45 mg/kg/day in divided doses q12h
Available forms: Tabs 250, 500, 875 mg/125 mg clavulanate; chew tabs 125, 200, 250, 400 mg; powder for oral susp 125, 200, 250, 400 mg/5 ml

Side effects/adverse reactions:
HEMA: Anemia, *bone marrow depression, granulocytopenia, leukopenia, eosinophilia,* thrombocytopenic purpura
GI: *Nausea, diarrhea, vomiting,* increased AST, ALT, abdominal pain, glossitis, colitis, black tongue, pseudomembranous colitis
GU: Oliguria, proteinuria, hematuria, *vaginitis, moniliasis, glomerulonephritis*
CNS: Headache, fever
META: Hyperkalemia, hypokalemia, alkalosis, hypernatremia
INTEG: Rash, urticaria
Contraindications: Hypersensitivity to penicillins
Precautions: Pregnancy (B), lactation, hypersensitivity to cephalosporins; neonates, renal disease
Pharmacokinetics:
PO: Peak 2 hr, duration 6-8 hr; half-life 1-1⅓ hr, metabolized in liver, excreted in urine, crosses placenta, excreted in breast milk
Interactions:
- Increased amoxicillin concentrations: aspirin, probenecid, disulfiram
- Decreased action of: oral contraceptives
- Amoxicillin-induced skin rash: allopurinol
Lab test interferences:
False positive: Urine glucose, urine protein

NURSING CONSIDERATIONS
Assess:
- I&O ratio; report hematuria, oli-guria, since penicillin in high doses is nephrotoxic
- Any patient with a compromised renal system, since drug is excreted slowly in poor renal system function; toxicity may occur
- Liver studies: AST (SGOT), ALT (SGPT)
- Blood studies: WBC, RBC, Hgb and Hct, bleeding time
- Renal studies: urinalysis, protein, blood, BUN, creatinine
- Culture, sensitivity before drug therapy; drug may be given as soon as culture is taken
- Bowel pattern before, during treatment
- Skin eruptions after administration of penicillin to 1 wk after discontinuing drug
- Respiratory status: rate, character, wheezing, tightness in chest
- Allergies before initiation of treatment, reaction of each medication; place allergies on chart in bright red
Administer:
PO
- After C&S completed
- Only as directed 2 (250 mg tab) not equivalent to 1 (500 mg tab) due to strength of clavulanate
- Shake suspension well before each dose
Perform/provide:
- Adrenaline, suction, tracheostomy set, endotracheal intubation equipment on unit
- Adequate intake of fluids (2 L) during diarrhea episodes
- Scratch test to assess allergy after securing order from prescriber; usually done when penicillin is only drug of choice
- Storage refrigerated for 2 wk or room temperature for 1 wk
Evaluate:
- Therapeutic response: absence of fever, draining wounds

Teach patient/family:
• To take as prescribed, not to double dose
• All aspects of drug therapy: need to complete entire course of medication to ensure organism death (10-14 days); culture may be taken after completed course of medication
⬦ To report sore throat, fever, fatigue (may indicate superinfection or agranulocytosis)
• That drug must be taken in equal intervals around the clock to maintain blood levels
• To wear or carry a Medic Alert ID if allergic to penicillins
• To notify nurse of diarrhea
Treatment of hypersensitivity: Withdraw drug, maintain airway, administer epinephrine, aminophylline, O_2, IV corticosteroids for anaphylaxis

---

amphetamine (℞)

(am-fet'a-meen)
amphetamine sulfate
Func. class.: Cerebral stimulant
Chem. class.: Amphetamine

Controlled Substance Schedule II
Action: Increases release of norepinephrine, dopamine in cerebral cortex to reticular activating system
Uses: Narcolepsy, exogenous obesity, attention deficit disorder
Dosage and routes:
Narcolepsy
• *Adult:* **PO** 5-60 mg qd in divided doses
• *Child >12 yr:* **PO** 10 mg qd increasing by 10 mg/day at weekly intervals
• *Child 6-12 yr:* **PO** 5 mg qd increasing by 5 mg/wk, max 60 mg/day

Attention deficit disorder
• *Child >6 yr:* **PO** 5 mg qd-bid increasing by 5 mg/day at weekly intervals
• *Child 3-6 yr:* **PO** 2.5 mg qd increasing by 2.5 mg/day at weekly intervals
Obesity
• *Adult:* **PO** 5-30 mg in divided doses 30-60 min before meals
Available forms: Tabs 5, 10 mg; long-acting capsules 5, 10 mg
Side effects/adverse reactions:
CNS: Hyperactivity, insomnia, restlessness, talkativeness, dizziness, headache, chills, stimulation, dysphoria, irritability, aggressiveness, tremor, dependence, addiction
GI: Nausea, vomiting, anorexia, dry mouth, diarrhea, constipation, weight loss, metallic taste, cramps
GU: Impotence, change in libido
CV: Palpitations, tachycardia, hypertension, dysrhythmias, decreased heart rate
INTEG: Urticaria
Contraindications: Pregnancy (X), hypersensitivity to sympathomimetic amines, hyperthyroidism, hypertension, glaucoma, severe arteriosclerosis, drug abuse, cardiovascular disease, anxiety, lactation
Precautions: Gilles de la Tourette's disorder, lactation, child <3 yr
Pharmacokinetics:
PO: Onset 30 min, peak 1-3 hr, duration 4-20 hr, metabolized by liver, excreted by kidneys, crosses placenta, breast milk, half-life 10-30 hr
Interactions:
• Hypertensive crisis: MAOIs or within 14 days of MAOIs or furazolidone
• Increased effect of amphetamine: acetazolamide, antacids, sodium bicarbonate urinary alkalinizers
• Decreased effect of amphetamine: barbiturates, tricyclics, urinary acidi-

---

fiers (ascorbic acid, ammonium chloride)

• Decreased effect of guanethidine

🔏 May decrease amphetamine effect: kava kava

NURSING CONSIDERATIONS
Assess:

• VS, B/P, since this drug may reverse antihypertensives; check patients with cardiac disease more often

• CBC, urinalysis, in diabetes: blood sugar, urine sugar; insulin changes may be required, since eating will decrease

• Height; growth rate in children may be decreased

• Mental status: mood, sensorium, affect, stimulation, insomnia; aggressiveness may occur

• Physical dependency; should not be used for extended time; dose should be discontinued gradually

◆ Withdrawal symptoms: headache, nausea, vomiting, muscle pain, weakness

• Drug tolerance will develop after long-term use

• Dosage should not be increased if tolerance develops

Administer:
PO

• At least 6 hr before hs to avoid sleeplessness

• For obesity only if patient is on weight-reduction program that includes dietary changes, exercise; patient will develop tolerance, and weight loss won't occur without additional methods; give 30-60 min before meals

• Gum, hard candy, frequent sips of water for dry mouth

Evaluate:

• Therapeutic response: decreased activity in attention deficit disorder; absence of sleeping during day in narcolepsy; decrease in weight

Teach patient/family:

• Not to double dose; if dose is missed, take up to 6 hr before hs

• To decrease caffeine consumption (coffee, tea, cola, chocolate), which may increase irritability, stimulation

• To avoid OTC preparations unless approved by prescriber

• To taper off drug over several weeks, or depression, increased sleeping, lethargy may occur

• To avoid alcohol ingestion

• To avoid hazardous activities until patient is stabilized on medication

• To get needed rest; patients will feel more tired at end of day

Treatment of overdose: Administer fluids, hemodialysis, peritoneal dialysis, antihypertensives for increased B/P; ammonium Cl for increased excretion

---

amphotericin B deoxycholate
(am-foe-ter′i-sin)
Fungizone
amphotericin B cholesteryl
Amphotec
amphotericin B lipid complex
Abelcet
amphotericin B liposome
AmBisome
Func. class: Antifungal
Chem. class.: Amphoteric polyene

Action: Increases cell membrane permeability in susceptible organisms by binding sterols; decreases potassium, sodium, and nutrients in cell

Uses: Histoplasmosis, blastomyco-

sis, coccidioidomycosis, cryptococcosis, aspergillosis, phycomycosis, candidiasis, sporotrichosis causing severe meningitis, septicemia, skin infections
Investigational uses: Candiduria (bladder irrigation)
Dosage and routes:
Deoxycholate
• *Adult:* IV Give test dose of 1 mg; then 0.25 mg/kg, increase qd slowly to 0.5 mg/kg, may give 1 mg/kg/day or 1.5 mg/kg qid
• *Child:* IV 0.25 mg/kg infused initially, increase by 0.25 mg/kg qod to max of 1 mg/kg/day
• *Adult/child:* **TOP** apply 2-4 × daily
• *Adult/child:* **PO** 1 ml qid
Cholesteryl sulfate
• *Adult/child:* IV 3-4 mg/kg/day, max 6 mg/kg/day
Lipid complex
• *Adult/child:* IV 5 mg/kg/day
Liposome
• *Adult/child:* IV Fungal infections 3-5 mg/kg q24h
Visceral Leishmaniasis 3-4 mg/kg q24h days 1-5, decrease dose
Available forms: Amphotericin deoxycholate inj 50 mg vial oral susp 100 mg/ml; *amphotericin B cholesteryl* powder for inj 50 mg, 100 mg; *amphotericin B lipid complex* susp for inj 100 mg/20 ml vial
Side effects/adverse reactions:
EENT: Tinnitus, deafness, diplopia, blurred vision
INTEG: Burning, irritation, pain, necrosis at injection site with extravasation, flushing, dermatitis, skin rash (topical route)
CNS: Headache, fever, chills, peripheral nerve pain, paresthesias, peripheral neuropathy, ***convulsions,*** dizziness
GU: Hypokalemia, azotemia, hyposthenuria, ***renal tubular acidosis,*** nephrocalcinosis, ***permanent renal impairment, anuria, oliguria***

GI: Nausea, vomiting, anorexia, diarrhea, cramps, ***hemorrhagic gastroenteritis, acute liver failure***
MS: ***Arthralgia, myalgia,*** generalized pain, weakness, weight loss
HEMA: Normochromic, normocytic anemia, ***thrombocytopenia, agranulocytosis, leukopenia, eosinophilia,*** hypokalemia, hyponatremia, hypomagnesemia
Contraindications: Hypersensitivity, severe bone marrow depression
Precautions: Renal disease, pregnancy (B), lactation
Pharmacokinetics:
IV: Peak 1-2 hr, initial half-life 24 hr, metabolized in liver, excreted in urine (metabolites), breast milk, highly bound to plasma proteins; penetrates poorly CSF, bronchial secretions, aqueous humor, muscle, bone
Interactions:
• Increased nephrotoxicity: other nephrotoxic antibiotics (aminoglycosides, cisplatin, vancomycin, cyclosporine, polymyxin B)
• Increased hypokalemia: corticosteroids, digitalis, skeletal muscle relaxants, thiazides
• Antagonism: miconazole
NURSING CONSIDERATIONS
Assess:
• VS q15-30min during first infusion; note changes in pulse, B/P
• I&O ratio; watch for decreasing urinary output, change in specific gravity; discontinue drug to prevent permanent damage to renal tubules
• Blood studies: CBC, K, Na, Ca, Mg q2wk, BUN, creatinine weekly
• Weight weekly; if weight increases over 2 lb/wk, edema is present; renal damage should be considered
◆ For renal toxicity: increasing BUN, serum creatinine; if BUN is >40 mg/dl or if serum creatinine >3 mg/dl, drug may be discontinued or dosage reduced

⬧ For hepatotoxicity: increasing AST (SGOT), ALT (SGPT), alk phosphatase, bilirubin
• For allergic reaction: dermatitis, rash; drug should be discontinued, antihistamines (mild reaction) or epinephrine (severe reaction) administered
• For hypokalemia: anorexia, drowsiness, weakness, decreased reflexes, dizziness, increased urinary output, increased thirst, paresthesias
• For ototoxicity: tinnitus (ringing, roaring in ears) vertigo, loss of hearing (rare)

Administer:
IV
• Drug only after C&S confirms organism, drug needed to treat condition; make sure drug is used in life-threatening infections
• After diluting 50 mg/10 ml sterile water (no preservatives) (5 mg-1 ml), shake, dilute with 500 ml of D₅W to concentration of 0.1 mg/ml
• Test dose of 1 mg/20 ml D₅W; give over 10-30 min

Intermittent IV inf
• IV using in-line filter (mean pore diameter >1 μm) using distal veins; check for extravasation, necrosis q8h; use an infusion pump; administer over 6 hr; rapid infusion may result in circulation collapse

Additive compatibilities: Fluconazole, heparin, hydrocortisone, sodium bicarbonate

Syringe compatibilities: Heparin

Y-site compatibilities: Aldesleukin, diltiazem, famotidine, tacrolimus, teniposide, thiotepa, zidovudine

Perform/provide:
• Acetaminophen and diphenhydramine 30 min prior to inf to reduce fever, chills, headache
• Storage, protected from moisture and light; diluted solution is stable for 24 hr at room temperature

Evaluate:
• Therapeutic response: decreased fever, malaise, rash, negative C&S for infecting organism

Teach patient/family:
• That long-term therapy may be needed to clear infection (2 wk-3 mo depending on type of infection)

---

ampicillin (℞)

(am-pi-sill'in)
Amcill, Ampicin*, Apo-Ampi*, D-Amp*, NovoAmpicillin*, Nu-Ampi*, Omnipen, Omnipen-N, Polycillin, Polycillin-N, Supen, Totacillin, Totacillin-N

Func. class.: Broad-spectrum antiinfective
Chem. class.: Aminopenicillin

Action: Interferes with cell wall replication of susceptible organisms; the cell wall, rendered osmotically unstable, swells, bursts from osmotic pressure

Uses: Effective for gram-positive cocci *(S. aureus, S. pyogenes, E. faecalis, S. pneumoniae),* gram-negative cocci *(N. gonorrhoeae, N. meningitidis),* gram-negative bacilli *(H. influenzae, P. mirabilis, Salmonella, Shigella, L. monocytogenes),* gram-positive bacilli

Dosage and routes:
Systemic infections
• *Adult:* PO 1-2 g qd in divided doses q6h; IV/IM 2-8 g qd in divided doses q4-6h

Renal disease
• CrCl 10-30 ml/min dose q6-12h; <10 ml/min dose q12h
• *Child:* PO 50-100 mg/kg/day in divided doses q6h; IV/IM 100-200 mg/kg/day in divided doses q6h

Meningitis
• *Adult:* IV 8-14 g/day in divided doses q3-4h

⬦ = Nursing alert　　🌿 = Herb-drug interaction　　🚫 = Do not crush

- *Child:* **IV** 200-300 mg/kg/day in divided doses q3-4h

Gonorrhea

- *Adult:* **PO** 3.5 g given with 1 g probenecid as a single dose

Available forms: Powder for inj 125, 250, 500 mg, 1, 2, 10 g; IV inj 500 mg, 1, 2 g; caps 250, 500 mg; powder for oral susp 100/1 ml, 125, 250, 500 mg/5 ml

Side effects/adverse reactions:

INTEG: Rash, urticaria

HEMA: Anemia, increased bleeding time, *bone marrow depression, granulocytopenia*

GI: Nausea, vomiting, diarrhea

GU: Oliguria, proteinuria, hematuria, *vaginitis, moniliasis, glomerulonephritis*

CNS: Lethargy, hallucinations, anxiety, depression, twitching, *coma, convulsions*

Contraindications: Hypersensitivity to penicillins

Precautions: Pregnancy (B), lactation; hypersensitivity to cephalosporins; neonates, renal disease

Pharmacokinetics:

PO: Peak 2 hr

IV: Peak 5 min

IM: Peak 1 hr

Half-life 50-110 min; metabolized in liver; excreted in urine, bile, breast milk; crosses placenta

Interactions:

- Possible increased bleeding: oral anticoagulants
- Increased ampicillin concentrations: aspirin, probenecid, disulfiram
- Decreased effectiveness of oral contraceptives
- Increased ampicillin-induced skin rash: allopurinol

Lab test interferences:

False positive: Urine glucose, urine protein

NURSING CONSIDERATIONS

Assess:

- I&O ratio; report hematuria, oliguria, since penicillin in high doses is nephrotoxic
- ◆ Any patient with compromised renal system, since drug is excreted slowly in poor renal system function; toxicity may occur
- Liver studies: AST (SGOT), ALT (SGPT)
- Blood studies: WBC, RBC, Hgb and Hct, bleeding time
- Renal studies: urinalysis, protein, blood, BUN, creatinine
- Culture, sensitivity before drug therapy; drug may be taken as soon as culture is taken
- Bowel pattern before, during treatment
- Skin eruptions after administration of penicillin to 1 wk after discontinuing drug
- Respiratory status: rate, character, wheezing, tightness in chest
- Allergies before initiation of treatment; reaction of each medication; place allergies on chart in bright red

Administer:

PO

- On empty stomach for best absorption (1-2 hr ac or 2-3 hr pc)
- Shake suspension well before each dose

IV

- After diluting with sterile H_2O 0.9-1.2 ml/125 mg drug, administer over 3-5 min (up to 500 mg), 10-15 min (>500 mg) by direct IV; may be diluted in 50 ml or more of D_5W, D_5 ½ NaCl to a concentration of 30 mg/ml or less; IV sol is stable for 1 hr; give at prescribed rate
- After C&S completed

Additive compatibilities: Cefotiam, clindamycin, erythromycin, floxacillin, furosemide

Syringe compatibilities: Chloramphenicol, colistimethate, diatrizoate, heparin, iohexol, iopamidol, iothalamate, ioxaglate, procaine

Y-site compatibilities: Acyclovir, allopurinol, amifostine, aztreonam, cyclophosphamide, enalaprilat, esmolol, famotidine, filgrastim, fludarabine, foscarnet, granisetron, heparin, insulin (regular), labetalol, magnesium sulfate, melphalan, meperidine, morphine, multivitamins, ofloxacin, perphenazine, phytonadione, potassium chloride, propofol, tacrolimus, teniposide, theophylline, thiotepa, tolazoline, vit B/C

Perform/provide:

• Adrenaline, suction, tracheostomy set, endotracheal intubation equipment on unit

• Adequate intake of fluids (2 L) during diarrhea episodes

• Scratch test to assess allergy after securing order from prescriber; usually done when penicillin is only drug of choice

• Storage in tight container; after reconstituting, oral suspension refrigerated for 2 wk or stored at room temperature for 1 wk

Evaluate:

• Therapeutic response: absence of temperature, draining wounds

Teach patient/family:

• That tabs may be crushed; caps may be opened and mixed with water

• To take oral ampicillin on empty stomach with full glass of water

• All aspects of drug therapy: need to complete entire course of medication to ensure organism death (10-14 days); culture may be taken after completed course of medication

◆ To report sore throat, fever, fatigue, diarrhea (may indicate superinfection); report rash or other signs of allergy

• That drug must be taken in equal intervals around the clock to maintain blood levels

• To wear or carry a Medic Alert ID if allergic to penicillins

Treatment of anaphylaxis: Withdraw drug, maintain airway, administer epinephrine, aminophylline, O_2, IV corticosteroids

ampicillin, sulbactam (℞)

Unasyn

Func. class.: Broad-spectrum antiinfective

Chem. class.: Aminopenicillin with β-lactamase inhibitor

Action: Interferes with cell wall replication of susceptible organisms; the cell wall, rendered osmotically unstable, swells, bursts from osmotic pressure; combination extends spectrum of activity by β-lactamase inhibition

Uses: Skin infections, pneumonia *(S. aureus, E. coli, Klebsiella, P. mirabilis, B. fragilis, H. influenzae, Enterobacter, A. calcoaceticus),* intraabdominal infections *(Enterobacter, Klebsiella, Bacteroides, E. coli),* gynecologic infections *(E. coli, Bacteroides),* meningitis, septicemia

Dosage and routes:

• *Adult:* **IV** 1 g ampicillin, 0.5 g sulbactam to 2 g ampicillin and 1 g sulbactam q6h, not to exceed 4 g/day sulbactam

Renal disease

• CrCl 15-29 ml/min dose q12h; CrCl 5-14 ml/min dose q24h

• *Child:* **PO** 100-200 mg/kg/day (ampicillin component) divided q6h

Available forms: Powder for inj 1.5 g (1 g ampicillin, 0.5 g sulbactam), 3.0 g (2 g ampicillin, 1 g sulbactam)

◆ = Nursing alert   ⫽ = Herb-drug interaction   ⊘ = Do not crush

Side effects/adverse reactions:
HEMA: Anemia, increased bleeding time, ***bone marrow depression, granulocytopenia***
GI: Nausea, vomiting, diarrhea, increased AST (SGOT), ALT (SGPT), abdominal pain, glossitis, colitis
GU: Oliguria, proteinuria, hematuria, *vaginitis, moniliasis, **glomerulonephritis***
CNS: Lethargy, hallucinations, anxiety, depression, twitching, ***coma, convulsions***
Contraindications: Hypersensitivity to penicillins
Precautions: Pregnancy (C), lactation, hypersensitivity to cephalosporins, neonates, renal disease
Pharmacokinetics:
IV: Peak 5 min; half-life 50-110 min; little metabolized in liver, 75% to 85% of both drugs excreted in urine, diffuses to breast milk, crosses placenta
Interactions:
• Increased ampicillin concentration: aspirin, probenecid, disulfiram
• Ampicillin-induced skin rash: allopurinol
Lab test interferences:
False positive: Urine glucose, urine protein
NURSING CONSIDERATIONS
Assess:
• Bowel pattern before, during treatment
• Respiratory status: rate, character, wheezing, tightness in chest
• I&O ratio; report hematuria, oliguria, since penicillin in high doses is nephrotoxic
◆ Any patient with compromised renal system, since drug is excreted slowly in poor renal system function; toxicity may occur rapidly
• Liver studies: AST (SGOT), ALT (SGPT)
• Blood studies: WBC, RBC, Hct, Hgb, bleeding time

• Renal studies: urinalysis, protein, blood, BUN, creatinine
• C&S before drug therapy; drug may be given as soon as culture is taken
• Skin eruptions after administration of ampicillin to 1 wk after discontinuing drug
• Allergies before initiation of treatment; reaction of each medication; report allergies on chart in bright red
Administer:
PO
• On empty stomach after C&S completed
IV
• After diluting 1.5 g/4 ml or more sterile H_2O for inj (375 mg/ml); allow to stand until foaming stops; dilute further in 50 ml or more of D_5W, NaCl, administer within 1 hr after reconstitution; give as an intermittent inf over 15-30 min
Additive compatibilities: Aztreonam
Y-site compatibilities: Amifostine, aztreonam, cefepime, enalaprilat, famotidine, filgrastim, fluconazole, fludarabine, gallium, granisetron, heparin, insulin (regular), meperidine, morphine, paclitaxel, tacrolimus, teniposide, theophylline, thiotepa
Perform/provide:
• Adrenaline, suction, tracheostomy set, endotracheal intubation equipment on unit for possible anaphylaxis
• Adequate intake of fluids (2 L) during diarrhea episodes
• Scratch test to assess allergy after securing order from prescriber; usually done when penicillin is only drug choice
• Storage in tight container, out of light
Evaluate:
• Therapeutic response: absence of

fever, draining wounds, negative C&S

Teach patient/family:

• To report sore throat, fever, fatigue, persistent diarrhea (may indicate superinfection)

• To wear or carry Medic Alert ID if allergic to penicillin products

Treatment of anaphylaxis: Withdraw drug, maintain airway, administer epinephrine, aminophylline, O_2, IV corticosteroids

---

amrinone (℞)

(am'ri-none)

Inocor

Func. class.: Cardiac inotropic agent

Chem. class.: Bipyrimidine derivative

Action: Positive inotropic agent with vasodilator properties; reduces preload and afterload by direct relaxation of vascular smooth muscle, increases cardiac output

Uses: Short-term management of CHF that has not responded to other medication; can be used with digitalis

Dosage and routes:

• *Adult and child:* **IV BOL** 0.75 mg/kg given over 2-3 min; start inf of 5-10 µg/kg/min; may give another bol 30 min after start of therapy, not to exceed 10 mg/kg total daily dose

Available forms: Inj 5 mg/ml

Side effects/adverse reactions:

HEMA: Thrombocytopenia

CV: Dysrhythmias, hypotension, headache, chest pain

GI: Nausea, vomiting, anorexia, abdominal pain, *hepatotoxicity, ascites,* jaundice, hiccups

INTEG: Allergic reactions, burning at injection site

RESP: Pleuritis, *pulmonary densities, hypoxemia*

Contraindications: Hypersensitivity to this drug or bisulfites, severe aortic disease, severe pulmonic valvular disease, acute MI

Precautions: Lactation, pregnancy (C), children, renal disease, hepatic disease, atrial flutter/fibrillation, elderly

Pharmacokinetics:

IV: Onset 2-5 min, peak 10 min, duration variable; half-life 4-6 hr, metabolized in liver, excreted in urine as drug and metabolites 60%-90%

Interactions:

• Excessive hypotension: antihypertensives

• Additive effect: cardiac glycosides

🖋 Possible increased action of amrinone: cascara sagrada bark, aloe, buckthorn bark/berry, ephedra, senna pod/leaf

NURSING CONSIDERATIONS

Assess:

• B/P and pulse q5min during infusion; if B/P drops 30 mm Hg, stop infusion and call prescriber

• Electrolytes: K, S, Cl, Ca; renal function studies: BUN, creatinine; blood studies: platelet count; monitor fluid status (CVP) in elderly

• ALT (SGOT), AST (SGPT), bilirubin daily

• I&O ratio and weight qd; diuresis should increase with continuing therapy

◆ If platelets are <150,000/mm^3, drug is usually discontinued and another drug started

• Extravasation; change site q48h

Administer:

IV

• Do not mix directly with glucose solutions; chemical reaction occurs over 24 hr; precipitate forms if am-

---

rinone and furosemide come in contact

• Into running dextrose infusion through Y-connector or directly into tubing; may give undiluted over 2-3 min or dilute with NS to 1-3 mg/ml, run at prescribed rate

• By infusion pump for doses other than bolus

• Potassium supplements if ordered for potassium levels <3.0

Syringe compatibilities: Propranolol, verapamil

Y-site compatibilities: Aminophylline, atropine, bretylium, calcium chloride, cimetidine, digoxin, dobutamine, dopamine, epinephrine, famotidine, hydrocortisone, isoproterenol, lidocaine, metaraminol, methylprednisolone, nitroglycerin, nitroprusside, norepinephrine, phenylephrine, potassium chloride, propofol, propranolol, verapamil

Evaluate:

• Therapeutic response: increased cardiac output, decreased PCWP, adequate CVP, decreased dyspnea, fatigue, edema, ECG

Treatment of overdose. Discontinue drug, support circulation

---

anagrelide (R)

(a-na'gre-lide)
Agrylin
Func. class.: Antiplatelet
Chem. class.: Imidazo-quinazolinone

Action: Reduces platelet count and prevents early platelet shape changes in response to aggregating agents thus inhibiting platelet aggregation

Uses: Essential thrombocythemia, polycythemia vera, chronic myelogenous leukemia

Dosage and routes:

• *Adult:* **PO** 0.5 mg qid or 1 mg bid,

may be adjusted after 1 wk, max 10 mg/day or 2.5 mg single dose

Available forms: Caps 0.5, 1.0 mg

Side effects/adverse reactions:

CV: Postural hypotension, tachycardia, palpitations, **CHF, MI, cardiomyopathy, cardiomegaly, complete heart block, atrial fibrillation,** arrhythmia

CNS: Headache, dizziness, seizures

INTEG: Rash

HEMA: **Anemia, thrombocytopenia, ecchymosis, lymphadenoma**

Contraindications: Hypersensitivity, hypotension

Precautions: Pregnancy (C), lactation

Pharmacokinetics:

PO: Peak 1 hr, duration >24 hr; metabolized in liver; excreted in feces/urine

NURSING CONSIDERATIONS

Assess:

• B/P pulse during treatment until stable; take B/P lying, standing; orthostatic hypotension is common

• Cardiac status: chest pain, what aggravates or ameliorates condition

Administer:

• On an empty stomach: 1 hr before meals or 2 hr after; give with 8 oz water for better absorption

Perform/provide:

• Storage at room temperature

Evaluate:

• Therapeutic response: increased platelet count

Teach patient/family:

• That medication is not a cure: may have to be taken continuously in evenly spaced doses only as directed

• That it is necessary to quit smoking to prevent excessive vasoconstriction

• To avoid hazardous activities until stabilized on medication; dizziness may occur

---

- To rise slowly from sitting or lying to prevent orthostatic hypotension
- Not to use alcohol or OTC medications unless approved by prescriber

---

anastrozole
(an-a-stroh′zole)
Arimidex
Func. class.: Antineoplastic
Chem. class.: Aromatase inhibitor

Action: Lowers serum estradiol concentrations; many breast cancers have strong estrogen receptors

Uses: Advanced breast carcinoma not responsive to other therapy in estrogen-receptor-positive patients (usually postmenopausal)

Dosage and routes:
- *Adult:* **PO** 1 mg qd

Available forms: Tabs 1 mg

Side effects/adverse reactions:
HEMA: Leukopenia
GI: Nausea, vomiting, altered taste (anorexia), diarrhea, constipation, abdominal pain, dry mouth
GU: Vaginal bleeding, pruritus vulvae, UTI
INTEG: Rash, alopecia
CV: Chest pain, hypertension, thrombophlebitis
CNS: Hot flashes, headache, lightheadedness, depression, dizziness, confusion, insomnia, anxiety
RESP: Cough, sinusitis
MS: Bone pain, myalgia

Contraindications: Hypersensitivity

Precautions: Leukopenia, thrombocytopenia, lactation, pregnancy (C), children, elderly, liver disease, renal disease

Pharmacokinetics:
PO: Peak 4-7 hr, half-life 50 hr, excreted in feces, urine

Lab test interferences:
Increase: GGT, AST, ALT, alk phosphatase, cholesterol, LDL

NURSING CONSIDERATIONS
Assess:
- CBC, differential, platelet count qwk; withhold drug if WBC is <3500/mm^3 or platelet count is <100,000/mm^3; notify prescriber
- Bleeding: hematuria, guaiac, bruising, petechiae, mucosa or orifices q8h
- Food preferences; list likes, dislikes
- Effects of alopecia on body image; discuss feelings about body changes
- Symptoms indicating severe allergic reactions: rash, pruritus, urticaria, purpuric skin lesions, itching, flushing

Administer:
PO
- Antacid before oral agent, give drug after evening meal, before bedtime
- Antiemetic 30-60 min before giving drug to prevent vomiting

Perform/provide:
- Liquid diet, if needed including cola, gelatin; dry toast or crackers may be added if patient is not nauseated or vomiting
- Increase fluid intake to 2-3 L/day to prevent dehydration
- Nutritious diet with iron, vitamin supplements as ordered
- Storage in light-resistant container at room temp

Evaluate:
- Therapeutic response: decreased tumor size, spread of malignancy

Teach patient/family:
- To report any complaints, side effects to prescriber
- That vaginal bleeding, pruritus, hot flashes are reversible after discontinuing treatment

---

◆ = Nursing alert   🌿 = Herb-drug interaction   🚫 = Do not crush

- To report vaginal bleeding immediately
- That tumor flare—increase in size of tumor, increased bone pain—may occur and will subside rapidly; may take analgesics for pain
- That hair may be lost during treatment; a wig or hairpiece may make patient feel better; new hair may be different in color, texture

---

anistreplase (℞)

(ah-nis′tre-place)
anisoylated plasminogen, APSAC, Eminase
Func. class.: Thrombolytic enzyme
Chem. class.: Anisoylated plasminogen streptokinase activator complex

---

Action: Promotes thrombolysis by promoting conversion of plasminogen to plasmin

Uses: Management of acute MI; although not yet approved, anistreplase will also be used for other conditions requiring thrombolysis, i.e., PE, DUT, unclotting arteriovenous shunts

Dosage and routes:
- *Adult:* IV INJ 30 U over 2-5 min as soon as possible after onset of symptoms

Available forms: Powder, lyophilized 30 U/vial

Side effects/adverse reactions:
HEMA: Decreased Hct; *GI, GU, intracranial, retroperitoneal,* surface bleeding; *thrombocytopenia*
INTEG: Rash, urticaria, phlebitis at inj site, itching, flushing
CNS: Headache, fever, sweating, agitation, dizziness, paresthesia, tremor, vertigo
GI: Nausea, vomiting
RESP: Altered respirations, dyspnea, *bronchospasm, lung edema*
MS: Low back pain, arthralgia
CV: Hypotension, dysrhythmias, conduction disorders
SYST: **Anaphylaxis (rare)**

Contraindications: Hypersensitivity, active internal bleeding, intraspinal or intracranial surgery, neoplasms of CNS, severe hypertension, cerebral embolism/thrombosis/hemorrhage, hypersensitivity to this drug or streptokinase

Precautions: Arterial emboli from left side of heart, pregnancy (C), ulcerative colitis/enteritis, renal disease, hepatic disease, hypocoagulation, COPD, subacute bacterial endocarditis, rheumatic valvular disease, intraarterial diagnostic procedure or surgery (10 days), recent major surgery, lactation

Pharmacokinetics: Half-life 105 min

Interactions:
- Increased bleeding potential: aspirin, indomethacin, phenylbutazone, anticoagulants
- Do not mix with any other sol or drug
- *⚕* Increased risk of bleeding: bromelain

Lab test interferences:
Increase: PT, APTT, TT
Decrease: Fibrinogen, plasminogen

NURSING CONSIDERATIONS
Assess:
- VS, B/P, pulse, respirations, neurologic signs, temperature at least q4h, temp >104° F (40° C) or indicators of internal bleeding, cardiac rhythm after intracoronary administration
- Allergy: fever, rash, itching, chills; mild reaction may be treated with antihistamines
- ◆Bleeding during first hr of treatment (hematuria, hematemesis, bleeding from mucous membranes,

epistaxis, ecchymosis), continue to monitor for 24 hr after treatment
• Blood studies (Hct, platelets, PTT, PT, TT, APTT) before starting therapy; PT or APTT must be less than 2 × control before starting therapy; TT or PT q3-4h during treatment

Administer:

IV, direct

• Reconstitute single-dose vial/5 ml sterile water for injection (not bacteriostatic water), and roll (not shake) to enhance reconstitution; give over 2-5 min by direct IV, give within ½ hr of reconstitution or discard, do not add other meds to vial or syringe; give within 6 hr of thrombi identification for best results
• Cryoprecipitate or fresh frozen plasma if bleeding occurs
• Heparin therapy after thrombolytic therapy is discontinued, TT or APTT less than 2 × control (about 3-4 hr)
• About 10% of patients have high streptococcal antibody titers, requiring increased loading doses

Perform/provide:

• Bed rest during entire course of treatment; handle patient as little as possible during therapy
• Storage of powder in refrigerator; use within 30 min after reconstitution
• Avoid invasive procedures: inj, rectal temperature
• Treat fever with acetaminophen
• Pressure of 30 sec to minor bleeding sites, 30 min to sites of arterial puncture followed by dressing; inform prescriber if hemostasis not attained; apply pressure dressing

Evaluate:

• Therapeutic response: absence of thrombi formation in MI, improved ventricular function

---

antihemophilic factor (AHF) (Rx)
(an-tee-hee-moe-fill'ik)
antihemophilic factor, Alphanate, Bioclate, Helixate, Humate-P, Koate H.P., Kogenate, Monoclate-P, Profilate HP, Recombinate
Func. class.: Hemostatic
Chem. class.: Factor VIII

Action: Necessary for clotting; activates factor X in conjunction with activated factor IX; transforms prothrombin to thrombin

Uses: Hemophilia A, patients with acquired circulating factor VIII inhibitors, factor VIII deficiency

Dosage and routes:

Massive hemorrhage
• *Adult and child:* IV 40-50 U/kg, then 20-25 U/kg q8-12h

Bleeding (frank, overt)
• *Adult and child:* IV 15-25 U/kg, then 8-15 U/kg q8-12h × 4 days

Hemorrhage near vital organs
• *Adult and child:* IV 15 U/kg, then 8 U/kg q8h × 2 days, then 4 U/kg q8h × 2 days

Minor hemorrhage
• *Adult and child:* IV 8-10 U/kg/ q24h × 2-3 days or 8 U/kg q12h × 2 days, then q24h × 2 days

Joint bleeding
• *Adult and child:* IV 5-10 U/kg q8-12h × 1-2 days

Available forms: Inj 250, 500, 1000, 1500 U/vial (number of units noted on label)

Side effects/adverse reactions:

GI: Nausea, vomiting, abdominal cramps, jaundice, *viral hepatitis*
INTEG: Rash, flushing, *urticaria*, stinging at injection site
CNS: Headache, *lethargy, chills, fever, flushing*

⬩ = Nursing alert   🌿 = Herb-drug interaction   🚫 = Do not crush

HEMA: ***Thrombosis, hemolysis, AIDS***

CV: Hypotension, tachycardia

RESP: ***Bronchospasm***

Contraindications: Hypersensitivity, monoclonal antibody-derived factor VIII

Precautions: Neonates/infants, hepatic disease; blood types A, B, AB; pregnancy (C), factor VIII inhibitor

Pharmacokinetics:

IV: Half-life 4 hr, terminal 15 hr

Interactions:

• Do not admix with other drugs

NURSING CONSIDERATIONS

Assess:

• Blood studies (coagulation factors assay by % normal: 5% prevents spontaneous hemorrhage, 30%-50% for surgery, 80%-100% for severe hemorrhage)

• I&O, urine color; notify prescriber if urine becomes orange, red

• Pulse: discontinue infusion if significant increase

• Hct, Coombs' test with blood types A, B, AB

• Test for factor VIII inhibitors before starting treatment, may require concomitant antiinhibitor coagulant complex therapy

• Allergy: fever, rash, itching, jaundice; give diphenhydramine HCl (Benadryl), continue therapy if reaction is mild

• Blood group of patient, donors (if applicable; most factor VIII not from specific blood group donors)

➡️ Bleeding: ankles, knees, elbows, other joints

Administer:

IV

• After rotating gently to mix

• Using plastic syringe to reconstitute, and administer; adheres to glass; use another needle as a vent when reconstituting

• After dilution with warm NS, D_5W, LR, give within 3 hr

IV infusion

• Give at ≤2 ml/min if concentration exceeds 34 U/ml or over 3 min if concentration is less than 34 U/ml

Perform/provide:

• Storage in refrigerator; do not freeze; after reconstitution, do not refrigerate; give within 3 hr

Evaluate:

• Therapeutic response: absence of bleeding

Teach patient/family:

• To report any signs of bleeding: gums, under skin, urine, stools, emesis; review methods to prevent bleeding

• To avoid salicylates (increase bleeding tendencies)

• To prepare, administer factor VIII concentrates at first sign of danger

• To advise health professionals of treatment for hemophilia

• The signs of viral hepatitis, AIDS

• That immunization for hepatitis B may be given first

• To report hives, urticaria, chest tightness, hypotension; may be monoclonal antibody-derived factor VIII

• To be checked q2-3mo for HIV screen

• To carry ID describing disease process

---

antithrombin III, human (℞)

(an'tee-throm'bin)

ATnativ, Kybernin, Thrombate III

Func. class.: Antithrombin

Chem. class.: Pooled human plasma

Action: Inactivates thrombin and the activated forms of factors IX, X, XI, XII, resulting in inhibition of coagulation

Uses: Hereditary antithrombin III deficiency in connection with surgical or obstetric procedures or for thromboembolism

Dosage and routes: Dosage is individualized; after first dose, antithrombin III level should increase to about 120% of normal; thereafter maintain at levels >80%; this is usually achieved by administering maintenance doses q24h

Available forms: Lyophilized powder, 50 ml infusion bottles containing 500 IU antithrombin III with 10 ml sterile water for injection; 1000 IU/0.2 ml sterile H_2O for inj

Side effects/adverse reactions:

SYST: Bleeding, surface bleeding, *anaphylaxis,* vasodilatory effects

Precautions: Pregnancy (C), lactation, children

Pharmacokinetics: Unknown

Interactions:

• Increased anticoagulant effect: heparin, aspirin

• Do not administer with other drugs in syringe or solutions

NURSING CONSIDERATIONS

Assess:

• VS, B/P, pulse, respirations, neurologic signs, temperature at least q4h, temperature 104° F (40° C) or indicators of internal bleeding, cardiac rhythm

◆ For neurologic changes that may indicate intracranial bleeding

◆ Retroperitoneal bleeding: back pain, leg weakness, diminished pulses

Administer:

• Heparin after fibrinogen level is over 100 mg/dl; heparin infusion to increase PTT to 1.5-2 × baseline for 3-7 days

IV

• After reconstituting 500 IU/10 ml of NS or D_5W; do not shake; rotate to dissolve; allow to warm to room temperature; use within 3 hr of reconstitution; give 50 IU or less/min; do not exceed 100 IU/min using 0.22 or 0.45 microfilter

Perform/provide:

• Bed rest during entire course of treatment

• Avoidance of venous or arterial puncture, inj, rectal temperature

• Treatment of fever with acetaminophen or aspirin

Evaluate:

• Therapeutic response: absence of thrombi formation

---

ardeparin (℞)

(are-de-pear′in)

Normiflo

Func. class.: Anticoagulant

Chem. class.: Low molecular weight heparin

Action: Prevents conversion of fibrinogen to fibrin and prothrombin to thrombin by enhancing inhibitory effects of antithrombin III

Uses: Prevention of deep vein thrombosis after knee replacement surgery

Dosage and routes:

• *Adult:* SC 50 antifactor XaU/kg q12h the evening of the day of knee replacement surgery or the following AM continued until patient is fully ambulatory or 2 wk, whichever is first

Available forms: Inj 5,000, 10,000 anti XaU/0.5 ml

Side effects/adverse reactions:

CNS: Intracranial bleeding, fever

SYST: Hypersensitivity, *hemorrhage, anaphylaxis* possible

HEMA: Thrombocytopenia, anemia

INTEG: Pruritus, superficial wound infection, ecchymosis, rash

Contraindications: Hypersensitivity to this drug, pork products, heparin, or other anticoagulants; hemo-

---

◆ = Nursing alert   ∥ = Herb-drug interaction   ⊘ = Do not crush

philia, leukemia with bleeding, thrombocytopenic purpura, cerebrovascular hemorrhage, cerebral aneurysm, severe hypertension, other severe cardiac disease

Precautions: Elderly, pregnancy (C), hepatic disease, severe renal disease, blood dyscrasias, subacute bacterial endocarditis, acute nephritis, lactation, child, recent childbirth, peptic ulcer disease, pericarditis, pericardial effusion, recent lumbar puncture, vasculitis, other diseases where bleeding is possible

Pharmacokinetics: Unknown

Interactions:
• Increased risk of bleeding: aspiration, oral anticoagulants, platelet inhibitors

🍴 May increase risk of bleeding: bromelain, cinchona bark

NURSING CONSIDERATIONS
Assess:
• For blood studies (Hct, occult blood in stools) during treatment since bleeding can occur

➡️For bleeding gums, petechiae, ecchymosis, black tarry stools, hematuria, epistaxis, decrease in Hct, B/P; may indicate bleeding, possible hemorrhage; notify prescriber immediately, drug should be discontinued
• For hypersensitivity: fever, skin rash, urticaria; notify prescriber immediately

Administer:
• Do not give IM or IV drug route; approved is SC only
• By SC only; have patient sit or lie down; SC inj may be around the navel in a U-shape, upper outer side of thigh or upper outer quadrangle of the buttocks; rotate inj sites
• Changing needles is not recommended

Evaluate:
• Therapeutic response: absence of deep-vein thrombosis

Teach patient/family:
• To avoid OTC preparations that may cause serious drug interactions unless directed by prescriber; may contain aspirin; other anticoagulants
• To use soft-bristle toothbrush to avoid bleeding gums, avoid contact sports, use electric razor, avoid IM injection
• To report any signs of bleeding: gums, under skin, urine, stools; unusual bruising

Treatment of overdose: Protamine sulfate 1% given IV

---

ascorbic acid (vit C) (OTC, ℞)
(a-skor'bic)
Apo-C*, ascorbic acid, Ascorbicap, Cebid, Cecon, Cemill, Cenolate, Cetane, Cevalin, Cevi-Bid, Ce-Vi-Sol, Flavorcee, Mega-C/A Plus, Ortho/CS, Sunkist Vitamin C, Vita-C
Func. class.: Vit C—water-soluble vitamin

Action: Needed for wound healing, collagen synthesis, antioxidant, carbohydrate metabolism

Uses: Vit C deficiency, scurvy, delayed wound and bone healing, chronic disease, urine acidification, before gastrectomy

Investigational uses: Acidification of urine, common cold prevention

Scurvy
• *Adult:* **PO/SC/IM/IV** 100 mg-500 mg qd, then 50 mg or more qd
• *Child:* **PO/SC/IM/IV** 100-300 mg qd, then 35 mg or more qd

Wound healing/chronic disease/fracture
• *Adult:* **SC/IM/IV/PO** 200-500 mg qd
• *Child:* **SC/IM/IV/PO** 100-200 mg added doses

Urine acidification
- *Adult:* 4-12 g qd in divided doses
- *Child:* 500 mg q6-8h

Available forms: Tabs 25, 50, 100, 250, 500, 1000, 1500 mg; tabs effervescent 1000 mg; tabs chewable 100, 250, 500 mg; tabs timed release 500, 750, 1000, 1500 mg; caps timed release 500 mg; crys 4 g/tsp; powd 4 g/tsp; liq 35 mg/0.6 ml; sol 100 mg/ml; syr 20 mg/ml, 500 mg/5 ml; inj SC, IM, IV 100, 250, 500 mg/ml

Side effects/adverse reactions:

CNS: Headache, insomnia, dizziness, fatigue, flushing

GI: Nausea, vomiting, diarrhea, anorexia, heartburn, cramps

GU: Polyuria, urine acidification, oxalate or urate renal stones

HEMA: Hemolytic anemia in patients with G6PD

Contraindications: None significant

Precautions: Gout, pregnancy (A); diabetes, renal calculi (large doses)

Pharmacokinetics:

PO, INJ: Metabolized in liver, unused amounts excreted in urine (unchanged) and metabolites, crosses placenta, breast milk

Interactions:
- Increased effects of salicylates, oral contraceptives
- Increased side effects of PAS, digitalis, sulfonamides
- Decreased effects of phenothiazines, disulfiram, amphetamines, heparin, coumadin (massive doses)

Lab test interferences:

False positive: Negatives in glucose tests

False negative: Occult blood

NURSING CONSIDERATIONS
Assess:
- I&O ratio
- Ascorbic acid levels throughout treatment if continued deficiency is suspected
- Nutritional status: citrus fruits, vegetables
- Injection sites for inflammation

Administer:
IV, direct
- Undiluted by direct IV 100 mg over at least 1 min

Intermittent IV inf
- Diluted with D_5W, D_5NaCl, NS, LR, Ringer's, sodium lactate and given over 15 min

Additive compatibilities: Amikacin, calcium chloride, calcium gluceptate, calcium gluconate, cephalothin, chloramphenicol, chlorpromazine, colistimethate, cyanocobalamin, diphenhydramine, heparin, kanamycin, methicillin, methyldopate, penicillin G potassium, polymyxin B, prednisolone, procaine, prochlorperazine, promethazine, verapamil

Syringe compatibilities: Metoclopramide

Y-site compatibilities: Warfarin

Evaluate:
- Therapeutic response: absence of anorexia, irritability, pallor, joint pain, hyperkeratosis, petechiae, poor wound healing

Teach patient/family:
- 🚫 Do not break, crush, or chew ext rel tab
- That caps may be opened and contents mixed with jelly
- The necessary foods in diet
- That if oral contraceptives are taken, increased levels of vit C are needed
- That smoking decreases vit C levels, not to exceed prescribed dose; increases will be excreted in urine, except time release

---

◆ = Nursing alert   ▮ = Herb-drug interaction   🚫 = Do not crush

asparaginase (℞)

(a-spare'a-gi-nase)
Elspar, Kidrolase*
Func. class.: Antineoplastic
Chem. class.: E. coli enzyme

Action: Indirectly inhibits protein synthesis in tumor cells; without amino acid, DNA, RNA synthesis is halted; asparagine, protein synthesis is halted; G_1 phase of cell cycle specific; a nonvesicant

Uses: Acute lymphocytic leukemia in combination with other antineoplastics

Investigational uses: Lymphosarcoma, other leukemias

Dosage and routes:

In combination

• *Adult:* **IV** 1000 IU/kg/day × 10 days given over 30 min; **IM** 6000 IU/m²/day

Sole induction

• *Adult:* **IV** 200 IU/kg/day × 28 days

Available forms: Inj 10,000 IU

Side effects/adverse reactions:

SYST: Anaphylaxis, hypersensitivity

HEMA: Thrombocytopenia, leukopenia, myelosuppression, anemia, decreased clotting factors

GI: Nausea, vomiting, anorexia, cramps, stomatitis, hepatotoxicity, pancreatitis

GU: Urinary retention, *renal failure,* glycosuria, polyuria, azotemia, uric acid neuropathy

INTEG: Rash, urticaria, chills, fever

ENDO: Hyperglycemia

RESP: Fibrosis, pulmonary infiltrate

CV: Chest pain

CNS: Neuritis, dizziness, headache, *coma,* depression, fatigue, confusion, hallucinations

Contraindications: Hypersensitivity, infants, pregnancy (D), lactation, pancreatitis

Precautions: Renal disease, hepatic disease

Pharmacokinetics: Half-life 4-9 hr, terminal 1.4-1.8 hr

Interactions:

• Decreased action of methotrexate
• Do not use with radiation
• Increased toxicity: vincristine, prednisone
• Synergism in combination with cytarabine, 6-azauridine

Lab test interferences:

Decrease: Thyroid function tests

NURSING CONSIDERATIONS

Assess:

• For signs and symptoms of pancreatitis (nausea, vomiting, severe abdominal pain), anaphylaxis (bronchospasm, dyspnea), cyanosis
• CBC, differential, platelet count weekly; withhold drug if WBC is <4000 or platelet count is <75,000; notify prescriber of these results
• Pulmonary function tests, chest x-ray studies before, during therapy; chest x-ray film should be obtained q2wk during treatment
• Renal function studies: BUN, serum uric acid, ammonia urine CrCl, electrolytes before, during therapy
• I&O ratio; report fall in urine output of 30 ml/hr
• Monitor temperature q4h; may indicate beginning infection
• Liver function tests before, during therapy (bilirubin, AST [SGOT], ALT [SGPT], LDH) as needed or monthly
• RBC, Hct, Hgb, since these may be decreased
• Serum, urine glucose levels
• Bleeding: hematuria, guaiac, bruising or petechiae, mucosa or orifices q8h
➤ Dyspnea, rales, nonproductive cough, chest pain, tachypnea, fatigue, increased pulse, pallor, leth-

argy, swelling around eyes or lips; anaphylaxis may occur

• Food preferences; list likes, dislikes

• Yellowing of skin and sclera, dark urine, clay-colored stools, itchy skin, abdominal pain, fever, diarrhea

• Local irritation, pain, burning, discoloration at injection site

• Symptoms indicating severe allergic reaction: rash, pruritus, urticaria, purpuric skin lesions, itching, flushing, dyspnea

• Frequency of stools, characteristics: cramping, acidosis; signs of dehydration: rapid respirations, poor skin turgor, decreased urine output, dry skin, restlessness, weakness

Administer:

IV, direct

• After intradermal skin testing and desensitization, give 0.1 ml (2 IU) intradermally after reconstituting with 5 ml sterile H_2O or 0.9% NaCl for injection; then add 0.1 ml of reconstituted drug to 9.9 ml diluent (20 IU/ml); observe for 1 hr, check for wheal

• Allopurinol or sodium bicarbonate to reduce uric acid levels, alkalinization of urine

Intermittent IV inf

• Using 21G, 23G, 25G needle; administer by slow IV infusion via Y-tube or 3-way stopcock of flowing D_5W or NS infusion over 30 min after diluting 10,000 IU/5 ml of sterile H_2O or 0.9% NaCl (no preservatives) (2000 IU/ml); use of filter may be necessary if fibers are present

Y-site compatibilities: Methotrexate, sodium bicarbonate

Perform/provide:

• Deep-breathing exercises with patient 3-4 × day; place in semi-Fowler's position

• Increase fluid intake to 2-3 L/day to prevent urate deposits, calculi formation

• Diet low in purines: absence of organ meats (kidney, liver), dried beans, peas to maintain alkaline urine

• Rinsing of mouth 3-4 × day with water, club soda

• Brushing of teeth 2-3 × day with soft brush or cotton-tipped applicators for stomatitis; use unwaxed dental floss

• Warm compresses at injection site for inflammation

• Nutritious diet with iron, vitamin supplements

• HOB raised to facilitate breathing

Evaluate:

• Therapeutic response: decreased exacerbations in ALL

Teach patient/family:

• To report any complaints or side effects to nurse or prescriber

• To report any changes in breathing or coughing

Treatment of anaphylaxis:

Administer epinephrine, diphenhydramine, IV corticosteroids

---

aspirin (OTC)

(as'pir-in)

acetylsalicylic acid, Acuprin, Apo-ASA*, Apo-Asen*, Arthrinol*, Arthrisin*, Artria S.R., A.S.A., Aspergum, Aspir-Low, Aspirin*, Aspirtab, Astrin*, Bayer, Easprin, Ecotrin, 8-Hour Bayer Timed Release, Empirin, Entrophen*, Norwich Extra-Strength, Novasen*, PMS-ASA*, Sloprin, St. Joseph Children's, Supasa*, Therapy Bayer, ZORprin

Func. class.: Nonnarcotic analgesic, nonsteroidal antiinflammatory, antipyretic, antiplatelet

Chem. class.: Salicylate

Action: Blocks pain impulses in CNS, inhibition of prostaglan-

 = Nursing alert   = Herb-drug interaction   = Do not crush

din synthesis; antipyretic action results from vasodilation of peripheral vessels; decreases platelet aggregation

Uses: Mild to moderate pain or fever including rheumatoid arthritis, osteoarthritis, thromboembolic disorders; transient ischemic attacks, rheumatic fever, postmyocardial infarction, prophylaxis of MI, ischemic stroke, angina

Investigational uses: Prevention of cataracts (long-term use)

Dosage and routes:
Arthritis
• *Adult:* PO 2.6-5.2 g/day in divided doses q4-6h
• *Child:* PO 90-130 mg/kg/day in divided doses q4-6h
Pain/fever
• *Adult:* PO/RECT 325-650 mg q4h prn, not to exceed 4 g/day
• *Child:* PO/RECT 40-100 mg/kg/ day in divided doses q4-6h prn
Kawasaki disease
• *Child:* PO 80-120 mg/kg/day in 4 divided doses, maintenance 3-8 mg/ kg/day as a single dose × 8 wk
Thromboembolic disorders
• *Adult:* PO 325-650 mg/day or bid
Transient ischemic attacks
• *Adult:* PO 650 mg qid or 325 mg qid
MI, stroke prophylaxis
• *Adult:* PO 81-650 mg/day
Available forms: Tabs 65, 81, 325, 500, 650, 975 mg; chewable tabs 81 mg; caps 325, 500 mg; tabs controlled-release 800 mg; tabs timerelease 650 mg; supp 60, 120, 125, 130, 195, 200, 300, 325, 600, 650 mg, 1.2 g; cream; gum 227.5 mg

Side effects/adverse reactions:
HEMA: ***Thrombocytopenia, agranulocytosis, leukopenia, neutropenia, hemolytic anemia,*** increased protime, APTT, bleeding time
CNS: Stimulation, drowsiness, dizziness, confusion, ***convulsion,*** headache, flushing, hallucinations, ***coma***
*GI: Nausea, vomiting, **GI bleeding,*** diarrhea, heartburn, anorexia, ***hepatitis***
INTEG: Rash, urticaria, bruising
EENT: Tinnitus, hearing loss
CV: Rapid pulse, pulmonary edema
RESP: Wheezing, hyperpnea
ENDO: Hypoglycemia, hyponatremia, hypokalemia
*SYST: **Reye's syndrome (children)***

Contraindications: Hypersensitivity to salicylates, tartrazine (FDC yellow dye #5), GI bleeding, bleeding disorders, children <12 yr, children with flulike symptoms, pregnancy (D), lactation, vit K deficiency, peptic ulcer

Precautions: Anemia, hepatic disease, renal disease, Hodgkin's disease, pre/postoperatively, gastritis, asthmatic patients with nasal polyps or aspirin sensitivity

Pharmacokinetics: Well absorbed PO; enteric and rectal products may be erratic
PO: Onset 15-30 min, peak 1-2 hr, duration 4-6 hr
REC: Onset slow, duration 4-6 hr; Metabolized by liver, inactive metabolites excreted by kidneys, crosses placenta, excreted in breast milk; half-life 1-3½ hr, up to 30 hr in large doses

Interactions:
• Decreased effects of aspirin: antacids, steroids, urinary alkalizers
• Increased bleeding: alcohol, heparin, valproic acid, plicamycin, cefamandole
• Increased effects of warfarin, insulin, methotrexate, thrombolytic agents, penicillins, phenytoin, valproic acid, oral hypoglycemics, sulfonamides
• Increased salicylate levels: urinary acidifiers

- Decreased effects of probenecid, spironolactone, sulfinpyrazone, sulfonylamides
- Toxic effects: PABA, furosemide, carbonic anhydrase inhibitors
- Decreased blood sugar levels: salicylates
- Gastric ulcer: steroids, antiinflammatories, nonsteroidal antiinflammatories
- Ototoxicity: vancomycin

Lab test interferences:

Increase: Coagulation studies, liver function studies, serum uric acid, amylase, CO_2, urinary protein

Decrease: Serum K, PBI, cholesterol

Interference: Urine catecholamines, pregnancy test, urine glucose tests (Clinistix, Tes-Tape)

NURSING CONSIDERATIONS
Assess:

- Liver function studies: AST (SGOT), ALT (SGPT), bilirubin, creatinine if patient is on long-term therapy
- Renal function studies: BUN, urine creatinine if patient is on long-term therapy
- Blood studies: CBC, Hct, Hgb, pro-time if patient is on long-term therapy
- I&O ratio; decreasing output may indicate renal failure (long-term therapy)
- ◆ Hepatotoxicity: dark urine, clay-colored stools, yellowing of skin, sclera, itching, abdominal pain, fever, diarrhea if patient is on long-term therapy
- Allergic reactions: rash, urticaria; if these occur, drug may have to be discontinued
- Renal dysfunction: decreased urine output
- Ototoxicity: tinnitus, ringing, roaring in ears; audiometric testing needed before, after long-term therapy
- Visual changes: blurring, halos; corneal, retinal damage
- Edema in feet, ankles, legs
- Drug history; many drug interactions
- Pain: location, duration, type, intensity, prior to dose and 1 hr after
- Musculoskeletal status: ROM prior to dose
- Fever; length of time and related symptoms

Administer:
PO

- To patient crushed or whole; chewable tablets may be chewed
  🚫 Do not crush enteric product
- With food or milk to decrease gastric symptoms; give 30 min before or 2 hr after meals

Evaluate:

- Therapeutic response: decreased pain, inflammation, fever

Teach patient/family:

- To report any symptoms of hepatotoxicity, renal toxicity, visual changes, ototoxicity, allergic reactions, bleeding (long-term therapy)
- To take with 8 oz H_2O and sit upright for ½ hr after dose
- Not to exceed recommended dosage; acute poisoning may result
- To read label on other OTC drugs; many contain aspirin
- That the therapeutic response takes 2 wk (arthritis)
- To report tinnitus, confusion, diarrhea, sweating, hyperventilation
- To avoid alcohol ingestion; GI bleeding may occur
- That patients who have allergies may develop allergic reactions
- To avoid buffered or effervescent products
- That medication is not to be given to children; Reye's syndrome may develop

---

◆ = Nursing alert   🖋 = Herb-drug interaction   🚫 = Do not crush

Treatment of overdose: Lavage, activated charcoal, monitor electrolytes, VS

---

astemizole (R)

(a-stem'ih-zole)
Hismanal
Func. class.: Antihistamine
Chem. class.: H_1-histamine antagonist

Action: Acts on blood vessels, GI, respiratory system by competing with histamine for H_1-receptor site; decreases allergic response by blocking pharmacologic effects of histamine

Uses: Rhinitis, allergy symptoms
Dosage and routes:
• *Adult and child >12 yr:* **PO** 10 mg qd; to reduce time to steady state may take 30 mg day 1, 20 mg day 2, followed by 10 mg daily
• *Child 6-12 yr:* **PO** 5 mg/day
Available forms: Tabs 10 mg
Side effects/adverse reactions:
GU: Frequency, dysuria, urinary retention, impotence
HEMA: **Hemolytic anemia, thrombocytopenia, leukopenia, agranulocytosis, pancytopenia**
RESP: Thickening of bronchial secretions, dry nose, throat
GI: Nausea, diarrhea, abdominal pain, vomiting, constipation
CNS: Headache, stimulation, drowsiness, sedation, fatigue, confusion, blurred vision, tinnitus, restlessness, tremors, paradoxical excitation in children or elderly
INTEG: Rash, eczema, photosensitivity, urticaria
CV: Hypotension, palpitations, bradycardia, tachycardia, *dysrhythmias* (rare)
Contraindications: Hypersensitivity, newborn or premature infants, lactation, severe hepatic disease

Precautions: Pregnancy (C), elderly, children, respiratory disease, narrow-angle glaucoma, prostatic hypertrophy, bladder neck obstruction, asthma, elderly
Pharmacokinetics:
PO: Peak 1-2 hr, 97% bound to plasma proteins; half-life is biphasic 3½ hr, 16-23 hr
Interactions:
• Increased CNS depression: alcohol, other CNS depressants, procarbazine
• Increased anticholinergic effects: MAOIs
• Decreased action of oral anticoagulants
• Serious CV reactions: ketoconazole, itraconazole, erythromycin
• Avoid use with antifungals, macrolide antibiotics
⚠ Increased CNS depression: kava kava
⚠ Increased anticholinergic effect: henbane leaf
Lab test interferences:
False negative: Skin allergy tests
NURSING CONSIDERATIONS
Assess:
• I&O ratio: be alert for urinary retention, frequency, dysuria, especially elderly; drug should be discontinued if these occur
• CBC during long-term therapy
• Respiratory status: rate, rhythm, increase in bronchial secretions, wheezing, chest tightness
Administer:
PO
• On empty stomach 1 hr before or 2 hr after meals
Perform/provide:
• Hard candy, gum, frequent rinsing of mouth for dryness
• Storage in tight, light-resistant container
Evaluate:
• Therapeutic response: absence of running or congested nose or rashes

Teach patient/family:
• All aspects of drug use; to notify prescriber if confusion, sedation, hypotension occur
• To avoid driving, other hazardous activity if drowsiness occurs
• To avoid alcohol, other CNS depressants
• Not to exceed recommended dose; dysrhythmias may occur

Treatment of overdose: Administer ipecac syrup or lavage, diazepam, vasopressors, barbiturates (short-acting)

---

atenolol (R)

(a-ten′oh-lole)
Apo-Atenol*, atenolol*, Novo-Atenol*, Tenormin

Func. class.: Antihypertensive, antianginal

Chem. class.: β-Blocker, β-1, β-2 blocker (high doses)

Action: Competitively blocks stimulation of β-adrenergic receptor within vascular smooth muscle; produces negative chronotropic activity, negative inotropic activity (decreases rate of SA node discharge, increases recovery time), slows conduction of AV node, decreases heart rate, decreases O_2 consumption in myocardium; also decreases renin-aldosterone-angiotensin system at high doses, inhibits β-2 receptors in bronchial system at higher doses

Uses: Mild to moderate hypertension, prophylaxis of angina pectoris, suspected or known myocardial infarction

Investigational uses: Dysrhythmia, mitral valve prolapse, pheochromocytoma, hypertrophic cardiomyopathy, vascular headaches, thyrotoxicosis, tremors, alcohol withdrawal

Dosage and routes:
• *Adult:* **IV** 5 mg, repeat in 10 min if initial dose is well tolerated, then start **PO** dose 10 min after last **IV** dose
• *Adult:* **PO** 50 mg qd, increasing q1-2wk to 100 mg qd; may increase to 200 mg qd for angina
• *Elderly:* **PO** 25 mg/day initially
Renal disease
• CrCl 15-35 ml/min, max 50 mg/day; CrCl <15 ml/min max dose 50 mg qod

Available forms: Tabs 25, 50, 100 mg; inj 5 mg/10 ml

Side effects/adverse reactions:
*CV: **Profound hypotension, bradycardia, CHF,** cold extremities, postural hypotension, 2nd- or 3rd-degree heart block*
CNS: Insomnia, fatigue, dizziness, mental changes, memory loss, hallucinations, depression, lethargy, drowsiness, strange dreams, catatonia
*GI: Nausea, diarrhea, vomiting, **mesenteric arterial thrombosis, ischemic colitis***
INTEG: Rash, fever, alopecia
*HEMA: **Agranulocytosis, thrombocytopenia, purpura***
EENT: Sore throat, dry burning eyes
GU: Impotence
ENDO: Increased hypoglycemic response to insulin
*RESP: **Bronchospasm,** dyspnea, wheezing*

Contraindications: Hypersensitivity to β-blockers, cardiogenic shock, 2nd- or 3rd-degree heart block, sinus bradycardia, cardiac failure

Precautions: Major surgery, pregnancy (C), lactation, diabetes mellitus, renal disease, thyroid disease, CHF, COPD, asthma, well-compensated heart failure

Pharmacokinetics:
PO: Peak 2-4 hr; half-life 6-7 hr,

excreted unchanged in urine, protein binding 5%-15%
Interactions:
• Increased hypotension, bradycardia: reserpine, hydralazine, methyldopa, prazosin, anticholinergics, digoxin
• Decreased antihypertensive effects: indomethacin
• Increased hypoglycemic effect: insulin
• Mutual inhibition: sympathomimetics (cough, cold preparations)
• Decreased bronchodilation: theophyllines, β₂-agonists
• Paradoxical hypertension: clonidine

Lab test Interferences:
Interference: Glucose/insulin tolerance tests

NURSING CONSIDERATIONS
Assess:
• I&O, weight daily
• B/P, pulse q4h; note rate, rhythm, quality
• Apical/radial pulse before administration; notify prescriber of any significant changes (<50 bpm)
• Baselines in renal, liver function tests before therapy begins
• Edema in feet, legs daily
• Skin turgor, dryness of mucous membranes for hydration status

Administer:
PO
• Drug ac, hs, tablet may be crushed or swallowed whole
• Reduced dosage in renal dysfunction

IV, direct
• Undiluted over 5 min

IV infusion
• Diluted in 10-50 ml of D₅W, D₅/NaCl, or NS and give as an infusion at prescribed rate

Y-site compatibilities: Meperidine, meropenem, morphine

Perform/provide:
• Storage protected from light, moisture; placed in cool environment

Evaluate:
• Therapeutic response: decreased B/P after 1-2 wk

Teach patient/family:
◆Not to discontinue drug abruptly
• Not to use OTC products unless directed by prescriber
• To report bradycardia, dizziness, confusion, depression, fever
• To take pulse at home; advise when to notify prescriber
• To limit alcohol, smoking, sodium intake
• To comply with weight control, dietary adjustments, modified exercise program
• To carry Medic Alert ID to identify drug that you are taking, allergies
• To avoid hazardous activities if dizziness is present
• That drug may mask symptoms of hypoglycemia in diabetic patients

Treatment of overdose: Lavage, IV atropine for bradycardia, IV theophylline for bronchospasm, digitalis, O₂, diuretic for cardiac failure, hemodialysis

---

atorvastatin (Ŗ)
(at-or'va-sta-tin)
Lipitor
Func. class.: Antilipidemic
Chem. class.: Synthetically derived fermentation product

Action: Inhibits HMG-CoA reductase enzyme, which reduces cholesterol synthesis
Uses: As an adjunct in primary hypercholesterolemia (types Ia, Ib)
Dosage and routes:
• *Adult:* **PO** 10 mg qd, usual range 10-80, dosage adjustments may be made in 2-4 wk intervals

---

Available forms: Tabs 10, 20, 40 mg

Side effects/adverse reactions:

INTEG: Rash, pruritus, alopecia

GI: Dyspepsia, flatus, *liver dysfunction,* pancreatitis

EENT: Lens opacities

MS: Myalgia

CNS: Headache

Contraindications: Hypersensitivity, pregnancy (X), lactation, active liver disease

Precautions: Past liver disease, alcoholism, severe acute infections, trauma, hypotension, uncontrolled seizure disorders, severe metabolic disorders, electrolyte imbalance

Pharmacokinetics: Metabolized in liver, highly protein bound, excreted primarily in urine, half-life 14 hr; protein binding 98%

Interactions:

• Increased effects of warfarin

• Increased myalgia, myositis: cyclosporine, gemfibrozil, niacin, erythromycin

• Increased serum level of digoxin

• Increased levels of oral contraceptives

• Decreased effects of atorvastatin: colestipol, antacids, bile acid sequestrants, propranolol

• Increased levels of atorvastatin: erythromycin, itraconazole

NURSING CONSIDERATIONS

Assess:

• Cholesterol levels periodically during treatment

• Liver function studies q1-2mo during the first 1½ yr of treatment; AST (SGOT), ALT (SGPT), liver function tests may be increased

• Renal studies in patients with compromised renal system: BUN, I&O ratio, creatinine

• Eyes with slit lamp before, 1 mo after treatment begins, annually; lens opacities may occur

Administer:

PO

• Total daily dose any time of day

Perform/provide:

• Storage in cool environment in tight container protected from light

Evaluate:

• Therapeutic response: decrease in cholesterol to desired level after 8 wk

Teach patient/family:

• That blood work and eye exam will be necessary during treatment

• To report blurred vision, severe GI symptoms, headache

• That previously prescribed regimen will continue: low-cholesterol diet, exercise program

---

atovaquone (R)

(a-toe′va-kwon)

Mepron

Func. class.: Antiprotozoal

Chem. class.: Aromatic diamide derivative, analog of ubiquinone

Action: Interferes with DNA/RNA synthesis in protozoa

Uses: *Pneumocystis carinii* infections in patients intolerant of trimethoprim/sulfamethoxazole

Dosage and routes:

• *Adult:* **PO** 750 mg/food tid for 21 days

Available forms: Tabs 250 mg, susp

Side effects/adverse reactions:

CV: Hypotension

HEMA: Anemia, leukopenia

INTEG: Pruritus, urticaria, *rash*, oral monilia

GI: Nausea, vomiting, diarrhea, anorexia, increased AST and ALT, acute pancreatitis, constipation, abdominal pain

CNS: Dizziness, headache, anxiety

META: Hyperkalemia, hyperglycemia, hyponatremia

 = Nursing alert   = Herb-drug interaction   ⊘ = Do not crush

Contraindications: Hypersensitivity or history of developing life-threatening allergic reactions to any component of the formulation,

Precautions: Blood dyscrasias, hepatic disease, diabetes mellitus, pregnancy (C), lactation, children, elderly

Pharmacokinetics: Excreted unchanged in feces (94%), highly protein bound (99%)

Interactions:

• Use caution when administering concurrently with other highly plasma protein-bound drugs with narrow therapeutic indices

• Decreased effect: rifampin, rifabutin

NURSING CONSIDERATIONS

Assess:

• Blood studies, blood glucose, CBC, platelets

• I&O ratio

• ECG for cardiac dysrhythmias, check B/P

• Liver studies: AST (SGOT), ALT (SGPT)

• Signs of infection, anemia

• Bowel pattern before, during treatment

• Respiratory status: rate, character, wheezing, dyspnea

• Dizziness, confusion, hallucination

• Allergies before treatment, reaction of each medication

Administer:

PO

• With food because of increased absorption of the drug and higher plasma concentrations

Evaluate:

• Therapeutic response: decreased temperature, ability to breathe

Teach patient/family:

◆ To report sore throat, fever, fatigue (may indicate superinfection)

• To take with food to increase plasma concentrations

atracurium (℞)

(a-tra-kyoor'ee-um)
Tracrium

Func. class.: Neuromuscular blocker (nondepolarizing)

Chem. class.: Biquaternary ammonium ester

Action: Inhibits transmission of nerve impulses by binding with cholinergic receptor sites, antagonizing action of acetylcholine

Uses: Facilitation of endotracheal intubation, skeletal muscle relaxation during mechanical ventilation, surgery, or general anesthesia

Dosage and routes:

• *Adult and child >2 yr:* **IV BOL** 0.3-0.5 mg/kg, then 0.08-0.10 mg/kg 20-45 min after first dose if needed for prolonged procedures

• *Child, 1 mo-2 yr:* **IV BOL** 0.3-0.4 mg/kg

Available forms: Inj 10 mg/ml

Side effects/adverse reactions:

CV: Bradycardia, tachycardia; increased, decreased B/P

*RESP: **Prolonged apnea, bronchospasm, cyanosis, respiratory depression***

EENT: Increased secretions

INTEG: Rash, flushing, pruritus, urticaria

MS: Inadequate or prolonged block

Contraindications: Hypersensitivity

Precautions: Pregnancy (C), cardiac disease, lactation, children <2 yr, electrolyte imbalances, dehydration, neuromuscular disease, respiratory disease

Pharmacokinetics:

IV: Onset 2 min, duration 20-60 min; half-life 2 min, terminal 29 min, excreted in urine, feces (metabolites), crosses placenta

---

Interactions:

• Increased neuromuscular blockade: aminoglycosides, clindamycin, enflurane, isoflurane, lincomycin, lithium, local anesthetics, narcotic analgesics, polymyxin antibiotics, procainamide, quinidine, thiazides, trimethaphan, verapamil

• Decreased neuromuscular blockade: edrophonium, neostigmine, phenytoin, pyridostigmine, theophylline

• Dysrhythmias: theophylline

NURSING CONSIDERATIONS

Assess:

• For electrolyte imbalances (K, Mg); may lead to increased action of this drug

• Vital signs (B/P, pulse, respirations, airway) until fully recovered; rate, depth, pattern of respirations, strength of hand grip

• I&O ratio; check for urinary retention, frequency, hesitancy

• Recovery: decreased paralysis of face, diaphragm, leg, arm, rest of body

• Allergic reactions: rash, fever, respiratory distress, pruritus; drug should be discontinued

Administer:

• Do not administer IM

IV

• Using nerve stimulator by anesthesiologist to determine neuromuscular blockade

• Anticholinesterase to reverse neuromuscular blockade

• IV undiluted by direct IV over 5 min, or diluted in 10-50 ml of D_5W, ½ NaCl or NS and give as an infusion at prescribed rate

• By slow IV over 1-2 min (only by qualified person)

Additive compatibilities: Bretylium, cimetidine, dobutamine, dopamine, esmolol, gentamicin, isoproterenol, lidocaine, morphine, potassium chloride, procainamide, vancomycin

Syringe compatibilities: Afantanil, fentanyl, midazolam, sufentanil

Y-site compatibilities: Cefazolin, cefuroxime, cimetidine, dobutamine, dopamine, epinephrine, esmolol, etomidate, fentanyl, gentamicin, heparin, hydrocortisone, isoproterenol, lorazepam, midazolam, morphine, nitroglycerine, ranitidine, sodium nitroprusside, trimethoprim/sulfamethoxazole, vancomycin

Perform/provide:

• Storage in light-resistant area

• Reassurance if communication is difficult during recovery from neuromuscular blockade

Evaluate:

• Therapeutic response: paralysis of jaw, eyelid, head, neck, rest of body

Treatment of overdose: Edrophonium or neostigmine, atropine, monitor VS; mechanical ventilation

---

atropine (Rx)

(a'troe-peen)

Atropair, Atro-Pen, Atropisol, Isopto-Atropine, I-Tropina, Minims Atopine*, Ocu-Tropine

Func. class.: Antidysrhythmic, anticholinergic parasympatholytic

Chem. class.: Belladonna alkaloid

Action: Blocks acetylcholine at parasympathetic neuroeffector sites; increases cardiac output, heart rate by blocking vagal stimulation in heart; dries secretions by blocking vagus

Uses: Bradycardia, bradydysrhythmia, anticholinesterase, insecticide poisoning, blocking cardiac vagal reflexes, decreasing secretions before surgery, antispasmodic with GU, biliary surgery, bronchodilator

---

◆ = Nursing alert   ⫸ = Herb-drug interaction   ⊘ = Do not crush

Dosage and routes:
Bradycardia/bradydysrhythmias
• *Adult:* **IV BOL** 0.5-1 mg given q3-5min, not to exceed 2 mg
• *Child:* **IV BOL** 0.01-0.03 mg/kg up to 0.4 mg or 0.3 mg/m²; may repeat q4-6h; min dose 0.1 mg to avoid paradoxical reaction
Insecticide poisoning
• *Adult and child:* **IM/IV** 2 mg qh until muscarinic symptoms disappear, may need 6 mg qh
Presurgery
• *Adult:* **SC/IM/IV** 0.4-0.6 mg before anesthesia
• *Child:* **SC** 0.1-0.4 mg 30 min before surgery
Available forms: Inj 0.05, 0.1, 0.3, 0.4, 0.5, 0.8, 1 mg/ml, 2 mg/0.7 ml, autoinjector tabs 0.4 mg; tabs sol 0.4, 0.6 mg
Side effects/adverse reactions:
GU: Retention, hesitancy, impotence, dysuria
CNS: Headache, dizziness, involuntary movement, confusion, psychosis, anxiety, **coma,** flushing, drowsiness, insomnia, weakness; delirium (elderly)
GI: Dry mouth, nausea, vomiting, abdominal pain, anorexia, constipation, *paralytic ileus,* abdominal distention, altered taste
CV: Hypotension, paradoxical bradycardia, angina, PVCs, hypertension, *tachycardia,* ectopic ventricular beats
INTEG: Rash, urticaria, contact dermatitis, dry skin, flushing
EENT: Blurred vision, photophobia, glaucoma, eye pain, pupil dilation, nasal congestion
MISC: Suppression of lactation, decreased sweating
Contraindications: Hypersensitivity to belladonna alkaloids, angle-closure glaucoma, GI obstructions, myasthenia gravis, thyrotoxicosis, ulcerative colitis, prostatic hypertrophy, tachycardia/tachydysrhythmias, asthma, acute hemorrhage, hepatic disease, myocardial ischemia

Precautions: Pregnancy (C), renal disease, lactation, CHF, tachydysrhythmias, hyperthyroidism, COPD, hepatic disease, child <6 yr, hypertension, elderly, intraabdominal infections, Down syndrome, spastic paralysis, gastric ulcer

Pharmacokinetics: Well absorbed PO, IM, SC; half-life 13-40 hr, excreted by kidneys unchanged (70%-90% in 24 hr); metabolized in liver, 40%-50% crosses placenta, excreted in breast milk
IV: Peak 2-4 min, duration 4-6 hr
IM/SC: Onset 15-50 min; peak 30 min, duration 4-6 hr
PO: Onset ½ hr; peak ½-1 hr; duration 4-6 hr

Interactions:
• Decreased effect of atropine; antacids
• Decreased effects of phenothiazines
• Increased anticholinergic effects of anticholinergics, tricylic antidepressants, amantadine, MAOIs, quinidine
🌿 Possible increased action of atropine: chronic use/abuse of cascara sagrada bark, buckthorn bark/berry, rhubarb root, senna leaf/fruits, aloe

NURSING CONSIDERATIONS
Assess:
• I&O ratio; check for urinary retention, daily output
• ECG for ectopic ventricular beats, PVC, tachycardia
• For bowel sounds; check for constipation
• Respiratory status: rate, rhythm, cyanosis, wheezing, dyspnea, engorged neck veins
• Increased intraocular pressure: eye

---

pain, nausea, vomiting, blurred vision, increased tearing
• Cardiac rate: rhythm, character, B/P continuously
• Allergic reaction: rash, urticaria

Administer:

PO
• Increased bulk, water in diet if constipation occurs
• ½ hr ac

IM
• Atropine flush may occur in children and is not harmful

IV
• Undiluted or diluted with 10 ml sterile H_2O, give at 0.6 mg/min, give through Y-tube or 3-way stopcock; do not add to IV sol; may cause paradoxical bradycardia lasting 2 min

Additive compatibilities: Dobutamine, furosemide, meropenem, netilmicin, sodium bicarbonate, verapamil

Syringe compatibilities: Benzquinamide, butorphanol, chlorpromazine, cimetidine, dimenhydrinate, diphenhydramine, droperidol, fentanyl, glycopyrrolate, heparin, hydromorphone, hydroxyzine, meperidine, metoclopramide, midazolam, milrinone, morphine, nalbuphine, pentazocine, perphenazine, prochlorperazine, promazine, promethazine, propiomazine, ranitidine, scopolamine, sufentanil

Y-site compatibilities: Amrinone, etomidate, famotidine, heparin, hydrocortisone, meropenem, nafcillin, potassium chloride, sufentanil, vit B/C

Perform/provide:
• Sugarless hard candy, gum, frequent rinsing of mouth for dryness

Evaluate:
• Therapeutic response: decreased dysrhythmias, increased heart rate, secretions; GI, GU spasms; bronchodilation

Teach patient/family:
• To report blurred vision, chest pain, allergic reactions
• Not to perform strenuous activity in high temperatures; heat stroke may result
• To take as prescribed; not to skip doses
• Not to operate machinery if drowsiness occurs
• Not to take OTC products without approval of prescriber

Treatment of overdose: O_2, artificial ventilation, ECG; administer dopamine for circulatory depression; administer diazepam or thiopental for convulsions; assess need for antidysrhythmics

---

auranofin (℞)

(au-rane'oh-fin)
Ridaura
Func. class.: Antiinflammatory
Chem. class.: Active gold compound (29%)

Action: Antiinflammatory action unknown; may decrease phagocytosis, lysosomal activity, or prostaglandin synthesis; decreases concentration of rheumatoid factor, immunoglobulins

Uses: Rheumatoid arthritis

Investigational uses: SLE, psoriatic arthritis, pemphigus

Dosage and routes:
• *Adult:* **PO** 6 mg qd or 3 mg bid; may increase to 9 mg/day after 3 mo

Available forms: Caps 3 mg

Side effects/adverse reactions:

HEMA: **Thrombocytopenia, agranulocytosis, aplastic anemia, leukopenia, eosinophilia, neutropenia**

INTEG: Rash, pruritus, dermatitis, **exfoliative dermatitis**, urticaria, alopecia, photosensitivity

CNS: Dizziness, confusion, halluci-

◆ = Nursing alert   ∥ = Herb-drug interaction   ⊘ = Do not crush

nations, *seizures,* EEG abnormalities

GI: Diarrhea, abdominal cramping, stomatitis, nausea, vomiting, enterocolitis, anorexia, flatulence, metallic taste, dyspepsia, jaundice, increased AST, ALT, glossitis, gingivitis, melena, constipation

GU: **Proteinuria, hematuria,** increased BUN, creatinine, vaginitis

MISC: Iritis, corneal ulcers, gold deposits in ocular tissues

RESP: **Interstitial pneumonitis, fibrosis,** cough, dyspnea

Contraindications: Hypersensitivity to gold, necrotizing enterocolitis, bone marrow aplasia, child <6 yr, lactation, pulmonary fibrosis, exfoliative dermatitis, blood dyscrasias, recent radiation therapy, renal/hepatic disease, marked hypertension, uncontrolled CHF

Precautions: Elderly, CHF, diabetes mellitus, allergic conditions, ulcerative colitis, renal disease, liver disease, pregnancy (C)

Pharmacokinetics:
PO: Absorbed by GI tract, peak 2 hr, steady state 8-16 wk, excreted in urine, feces

Interactions:
• Do not use with penicillamine or antimalarials
• May increase levels of phenytoin

Lab test interferences:
False positive: TB test

NURSING CONSIDERATIONS
Assess:
• Respiratory status: dyspnea, wheezing; if respiratory problems occur, drug should be discontinued
• I&O ratio
• Urine: hematuria, proteinuria; increased BUN, creatinine; may require decrease in dosage
• Platelet counts qmo; drug should be discontinued if <100,000/mm^3
• Hepatic test: ALT (SGOT), AST (SGPT), alk phosphatase

• Diarrhea stools; if severe, drug should be discontinued
• Allergy: rash, dermatitis, pruritus; drug should be discontinued if any of these occur
⬥ Gold toxicity: decreased Hgb, WBC <4000/mm^3, granulocytes <1500/mm^3, platelets <100,000/mm^3, severe diarrhea, stomatitis, hematuria, rash, itching, proteinuria

Administer:
PO
• Bid or may give as single dose qAM with food or drink

Evaluate:
• Therapeutic response: ability to move joints with less pain

Teach patient/family:
• That drug must be taken as prescribed to be useful, to obtain lab work monthly
🚫 Not to break, crush, or chew caps
• That diarrhea is common, but if blood appears in stools or urine, notify prescriber at once; that patient should check for bruising, petechiae, bleeding gums
• To report abnormal skin conditions, stomatitis, fatigue, jaundice; may indicate blood dyscrasias
• To avoid exposure to sunlight or ultraviolet light; to use sunscreen to prevent burns
• That therapeutic effect may take 3-4 mo
• To use diluted hydrogen peroxide for mild stomatitis, avoid hot spicy foods, food with high acidic content; use soft toothbrush, rinse more frequently, floss daily
• That contraception should be used during treatment

aurothioglucose/gold sodium thiomalate (℞)

(aur-oh-thye-oh-gloo′kose)
Solganal/Myochrysine
Func. class.: Antiinflammatory
Chem. class.: Active gold compound (50%)

Action: Antiinflammatory action unknown; may decrease phagocytosis, lysosomal activity, prostaglandin synthesis

Uses: Rheumatoid arthritis, psoriatic arthritis

Dosage and routes:
• *Adult:* **IM** 10 mg, then 25 mg qwk × 2-3 wk, then 50 mg/wk until total of 1 g is administered, then 25-50 mg q3-4wk if there is improvement without toxicity (aurothioglucose) total of 800 mg-1 g
• *Adult:* **IM** 10 mg, then 25 mg after 1 wk, then 50 mg qwk for total of 14-20 doses, then 50 mg q2wk × 4, then 50 mg q3wk × 4, then 50 mg qmo for maintenance (gold sodium thiomalate)
• *Child 6-12 yr:* **IM** 1 mg/kg/wk × 20 wk, or ¼ of adult dose (aurothioglucose)
• *Child:* **IM** 1 mg/kg/wk × 20 wk, then q3-4wk if improvement without toxicity (gold sodium thiomalate) not to exceed 2.5 mg

Available forms: Inj 50 mg/ml, 25 mg/ml

Side effects/adverse reactions:
EENT: Iritis, corneal ulcers
HEMA: **Thrombocytopenia, agranulocytosis, aplastic anemia, leukopenia, eosinophilia, neutropenia**
INTEG: Rash, pruritus, dermatitis, urticaria, alopecia, photosensitivity, **exfoliative dermatitis, angioedema**
GI: Stomatitis, nausea, vomiting, metallic taste, jaundice, **hepatitis,** diarrhea, cramping, flatulence
GU: Proteinuria, hematuria, **nephrosis, tubular necrosis**
RESP: Interstitial pneumonitis, pharyngitis, **pulmonary fibrosis**
CNS: Dizziness, EEG abnormalities, **encephalitis,** confusion, hallucinations
CV: Bradycardia, rapid pulse
SYST: **Anaphylaxis**

Contraindications: Hypersensitivity to gold, systemic lupus erythematosus, uncontrolled diabetes mellitus, marked hypertension, recent radiation therapy, CHF, lactation, renal disease, liver disease,

Precautions: Decreased tolerance in elderly, children, blood dyscrasias, pregnancy (C)

Pharmacokinetics:
IM: Peak 4-6 hr; half-life 3-27 days; excreted in urine, feces; half-life increases up to 168 days with 11th dose

Interactions:
• Increased blood dyscrasias: antimalarials, cytotoxic agents, immunosuppressants, phenylbutazone, penicillamine

Lab test interferences:
False positive: TB test

NURSING CONSIDERATIONS
Assess:
• Respiratory status: dyspnea, wheezing; if respiratory problems occur, drug should be discontinued
• I&O ratio
• For pregnancy before administration; do not give in pregnancy
• Urine: hematuria, proteinuria; increased BUN, creatinine; may require decrease in dosage
• Platelet counts qmo; drug should be discontinued if <100,000/mm³
• Hepatic test: ALT, AST, alk phosphatase
• Diarrhea stools; if severe, drug should be discontinued

◆ = Nursing alert   ∥ = Herb-drug interaction   ⊘ = Do not crush

• Allergy: rash, dermatitis, pruritus; drug should be discontinued if any of these occur

◆ Gold toxicity: decreased Hgb, WBC <4000/mm³, granulocytes <1500/mm³, platelets <100,000/mm³, severe diarrhea, stomatitis, hematuria, rash, itching, proteinuria

Administer:
• Never give IV

IM
• Bid or may give as single dose qAM
• Deep IM, never IV
• Slowly, keep patient recumbent for 10 min after injection, monitor for transient reaction

Evaluate:
• Therapeutic response: ability to move joints with less pain

Teach patient/family:
• That drug must be taken as prescribed to be useful
• To obtain lab work monthly
• That diarrhea is common, but if blood appears in stools or urine, notify prescriber at once; that patient should check for bruising, petechiae, bleeding gums
• To report skin conditions, stomatitis, fatigue, jaundice, which may indicate blood dyscrasias; report fever, chills, which may indicate infection
• That therapeutic effect may take 3-4 mo
• To use dilute hydrogen peroxide for mild stomatitis; avoid hot, spicy foods and food with high acidic content; use soft toothbrush, rinse more frequently
• That contraception should be used during treatment
• To use sunscreen to prevent burns

azatadine (℞)

(a-za′ta-deen)
Optimine
Func. class.: Antihistamine
Chem. class.: Piperidine H_1-receptor antagonist

Action: Acts on blood vessels, GI, respiratory system by competing with histamine for H_1-receptor site; decreases allergic response by blocking histamine

Uses: Allergy symptoms, rhinitis, chronic urticaria

Investigational uses: Cluster headaches; anorexia nervosa (as appetite stimulant)

Dosage and routes:
• *Adult:* PO 1-2 mg bid, not to exceed 4 mg/day
• *Geriatric:* PO 1 mg qd-bid
Available forms: Tabs 1 mg

Side effects/adverse reactions:
CNS: Dizziness, drowsiness, poor coordination, fatigue, anxiety, euphoria, confusion, paresthesia, neuritis, sweating, chills
CV: Hypotension, palpitations, tachycardia
RESP: Increased thick secretions, wheezing, chest tightness
*HEMA: **Thrombocytopenia, agranulocytosis, hemolytic anemia***
GI: Constipation, dry mouth, nausea, vomiting, anorexia, diarrhea
INTEG: Rash, urticaria, photosensitivity
GU: Retention, dysuria, frequency, impotence
EENT: Blurred vision, dilated pupils, tinnitus, nasal stuffiness, dry nose, throat, mouth

Contraindications: Hypersensitivity to H_1-receptor antagonist, acute asthma attack, lower respiratory tract disease, child <12 yr

Precautions: Increased intraocular

pressure, renal disease, cardiac disease, bronchial asthma, seizure disorder, stenosed peptic ulcers, hyperthyroidism, prostatic hypertrophy, bladder neck obstruction, pregnancy (B), lactation, elderly
Pharmacokinetics:
PO: Peak 4 hr; metabolized in liver, excreted by kidneys, crosses placenta, crosses blood-brain barrier, minimally bound to plasma proteins, half-life 9-12 hr
Interactions:
• Increased CNS depression: barbiturates, narcotics, hypnotics, tricyclic antidepressants, alcohol
• Decreased effect of oral anticoagulants, heparin
• Increased effect of azatadine: MAOIs
🍃 Increased CNS depression: kava kava
🍃 Increased anticholinergic effect: henbane leaf
Lab test interferences:
False negative: Skin allergy tests
NURSING CONSIDERATIONS
Assess:
• I&O ratio; be alert for urinary retention, frequency, dysuria, especially elderly; drug should be discontinued if these occur
• CBC during long-term therapy
• Blood dyscrasias: thrombocytopenia, agranulocytosis; these occur rarely
• Respiratory status: rate, rhythm, increase or thickening in bronchial secretions, wheezing, chest tightness
Administer:
PO
• With meals if GI symptoms occur; absorption may slightly decrease
Perform/provide:
• Hard candy, gum, frequent rinsing of mouth for dryness
• Storage in tight container at room temperature

Evaluate:
• Therapeutic response: absence of running or congested nose; rash
Teach patient/family:
• All aspects of drug use; to notify prescriber if confusion, sedation, or hypotension occurs
• To avoid driving or other hazardous activities if drowsiness occurs
• To avoid concurrent use of alcohol, other CNS depressants
Treatment of overdose: Administer ipecac syrup or lavage, diazepam, vasopressors, barbiturates (short-acting)

---

azathioprine (℞)

(ay-za-thye'oh-preen)
Imuran
Func. class.: Immunosuppressant
Chem. class.: Purine analog

Action: Produces immunosuppression by inhibiting purine synthesis in cells
Uses: Renal transplants to prevent graft rejection, refractory rheumatoid arthritis, refractory ITP, glomerulonephritis, nephrotic syndrome, bone marrow transplant
Investigational uses: Myasthenia gravis, chronic ulcerative colitis, Crohn's disease, Behçet's disease
Dosage and routes:
Prevention of rejection
• *Adult and child:* **PO, IV** 3-5 mg/kg/day, then maintenance (PO) of at least 1-2 mg/kg/day
Refractory rheumatoid arthritis
• *Adult:* **PO** 1/mg/kg/day, may increase dose after 2 mo by 0.5 mg/kg/day, not to exceed 2.5 mg/kg/day
Renal disease
• CrCl 10-50 ml/min 75% of dose; CrCl <10 ml/min 50% of dose

◆ = Nursing alert   🍃 = Herb-drug interaction   🚫 = Do not crush

Available forms: Tabs 50 mg; inj 100 mg

Side effects/adverse reactions:

GI: Nausea, vomiting, stomatitis, esophagitis, ***pancreatitis, hepatotoxicity, jaundice***

HEMA: ***Leukopenia, thrombocytopenia, anemia, pancytopenia***

INTEG: Rash

MS: Arthralgia, muscle wasting

Contraindications: Hypersensitivity, pregnancy (D), lactation

Precautions: Severe renal disease, severe hepatic disease, elderly

Pharmacokinetics: Metabolized in liver, excreted in urine (active metabolite), crosses placenta

Interactions:

• Increased action of azathioprine: allopurinol

• Do not admix with other drugs

NURSING CONSIDERATIONS

Assess:

• Blood studies: Hgb, WBC, platelets during treatment monthly; if leukocytes are < 3000/mm^3, drug should be discontinued

• Liver function studies: alk phosphatase, AST (SGOT), ALT (SGPT), bilirubin

◆ Hepatotoxicity: dark urine, jaundice, itching, light-colored stools; drug should be discontinued

Administer:

• All medications PO if possible, avoiding IM injections, since bleeding may occur

PO

• With meals to reduce GI upset

IV

• After diluting 100 mg/10 ml of sterile H$_2$O for inj; rotate to dissolve; may further dilute with 50 ml or more saline or glucose in saline

• For several days before transplant surgery

Solution compatibilities: D$_5$W, NaCl 0.9%, NaCl 0.45%

Evaluate:

• Therapeutic response: absence of graft rejection, immunosuppression in autoimmune disorders

Teach patient/family:

• That therapeutic response may take 3-4 mo in rheumatoid arthritis

• To report fever, rash, severe diarrhea, chills, sore throat, fatigue, since serious infections may occur

• To use contraceptive measures during treatment, for 12 wk after ending therapy; to avoid vaccinations

• To avoid crowds to reduce risk of infection

---

azelastine (Ŗ)

(ay´ze-lass-teen)

Astelin

Func. class.: Leukotriene synthesis inhibitor

Chem. class.: Phthalazinone derivative

Action: Inhibits synthesis and release of leukotrienes; antagonizes action of acetylcholine, histamine, serotonin

Uses: Seasonal allergic rhinitis

Dosages and routes:

• *Adult and child ≥12 yr:* **Nasal** 2 sprays/nostril bid

Available forms: Spray 137 μg/actuation

Side effects/adverse reactions:

CNS: Sedation (more common with increased doses), increased drowsiness

MISC: Weight increases, myalgia

Contraindications: Hypersensitivity, acute asthma attacks, lower respiratory tract disease

Precautions: Pregnancy (B), increased intraocular pressure, bronchial asthma

Pharmacokinetics: Peak 4-5 hr, half-life 25-42 hr; metabolized in liver, excreted in urine

---

Interactions:
• Additive CNS depressant effects: alcohol, other CNS depressants

NURSING CONSIDERATIONS
Administer:
• By nasal spray: remove cap/safety clip from spray pump
• Prime pump if using for 1st time by pushing 4 times quickly, away from face, blow nose, then place tip of pump into one nostril, while holding other nostril closed, tilt head forward and spray into nostril; repeat in other nostril; put cover/safety clip back on

Perform/provide:
• Storage in tight container at room temperature

Evaluate:
• Therapeutic response: absence of running or congested nose

Teach patient/family:
• To avoid driving, other hazardous activities if drowsiness occurs

---

azithromycin (℞)

(ay-zi-thro-my´sin)
Zithromax
Func. class.: Antiinfective
Chem. class.: Macrolide (azalide)

Action: Binds to 50S ribosomal subunits of susceptible bacteria and suppresses protein synthesis; much greater spectrum of activity than erythromycin

Uses: Mild to moderate infections of the upper respiratory tract, lower respiratory tract; uncomplicated skin and skin structure infections caused by *M. catarrhalis, S. pneumoniae, S. pyogenes, S. aureus, S. agalactiae, M. pneumoniae, H. influenzae, Clostridium, L. pneumophila;* nongonococcal urethritis or cervicitis due to *C. trachomatis*; in children: acute otitis media (*H. influenzae, M. catarrhalis, S. pneumoniae*) PO; community-acquired pneumonia; *(C. pneumoniae, H. influenzae, M. pneumoniae, S. pneumoniae)* PO; pharyngitis/tonsillitis *(S. pyogenes);* prophylaxis of disseminated *M. avium* complex (MAC)

Dosage and routes:
• *Adult:* PO 500 mg on day 1, then 250 mg qd on days 2-5 for a total dose of 1.5 g; may give a one-time dose of 1 g for chlamydial infections; 1200 mg qwk for MAC prophylaxis IV 500 mg qd ≥2 days, then 500 mg qd to complete 7-10 day therapy for community-acquired pneumonia
• *Adult:* IV 500 mg qd × 2 days, then 250 mg qd to complete 7 day therapy for pelvic inflammatory disease (PID)
• *Child ≥2 yr:* 12 mg/kg qd for 5 days
• *Child <6 mo:* 10 mg/kg on day 1, then 5 mg/kg qd

Available forms: Caps 250; tabs 250, 600 mg; powder for inj 500 mg; powder for oral susp 100 mg/5 ml, 200 mg/5 ml, 1 g/packet, 300 mg/15 ml, 600 mg/15 ml, 900 mg/22.5 ml

Side effects/adverse reactions:
INTEG: Rash, urticaria, pruritus, photosensitivity
CV: Palpitations, chest pain
CNS: Dizziness, headache, vertigo, somnolence
GI: Nausea, vomiting, diarrhea, hepatotoxicity, abdominal pain, stomatitis, heartburn, dyspepsia, flatulence, melena, *cholestatic jaundice*
GU: Vaginitis, moniliasis, nephritis

Contraindications: Hypersensitivity to azithromycin or erythromycin

Precautions: Pregnancy (B), lactation; hepatic, renal, cardiac disease; elderly, <6 mo for otitis media, <2 yr for pharyngitis, tonsillitis

Pharmacokinetics: Peak 2-4 hr, duration 24 hr, half-life 11-57 hr, ex-

---

⬦ = Nursing alert   🥄 = Herb-drug interaction   🚫 = Do not crush creted in bile, feces, urine primarily as unchanged drug

Interactions:
• Increased effects of oral anticoagulants, digoxin, theophylline, methylprednisolone, cyclosporine, bromocriptine, disopyramide, triazolam, carbamazepine, phenytoin
• Decreased action of clindamycin
• Toxicity: carbamazepine, terfenadine, astemizole
• Dysrhythmias: astemizole, terfenadine, cisapride
• Decreased absorption of azithromycin: food, aluminium, magnesium antacids

Lab test interferences:
False increase: 17-OHCS/17-KS, AST (SGOT), ALT (SGPT)
Decrease: Folate assay

NURSING CONSIDERATIONS
Assess:
• I&O ratio; report hematuria, oliguria in renal disease
• Liver studies: AST (SGOT), ALT (SGPT); CBC with differential
• Renal studies: urinalysis, protein, blood
• C&S before drug therapy; drug may be taken as soon as culture is taken; C&S may be repeated after treatment
• Bowel pattern before, during treatment
• Skin eruptions, itching
• Respiratory status: rate, character, wheezing, tightness in chest; discontinue drug if these occur
• Allergies before treatment, reaction of each medication

Administer:
• Adequate intake of fluids (2 L) if diarrhea occurs
• On an empty stomach, 1 hr ac, or 2-3 hr pc

Perform/provide:
• Storage at room temperature

Evaluate:
• Therapeutic response: C&S negative for infection; decreased signs of infection

Teach patient/family:
• To take with 8 oz H_2O; not to take with food; take 1 hr before or 2 hr after meals; do not take with fruit juices
• To report sore throat, fever, fatigue (may indicate superinfection)
• Not to take aluminum/magnesium-containing antacids simultaneously with this drug
• To notify nurse of diarrhea stools, dark urine, pale stools, yellow discoloration of eyes or skin, severe abdominal pain
• To take at evenly spaced intervals; complete dosage regimen

Treatment of hypersensitivity: Withdraw drug, maintain airway, administer epinephrine, aminophylline, O_2, IV corticosteroids

---

azlocillin (℞)
(az-loc-sill'in)
Azlin
Func. class.: Broad-spectrum antibiotic
Chem. class.: Extended-spectrum penicillin

Action: Interferes with cell wall replication of susceptible organisms; the cell wall, rendered osmotically unstable, swells, bursts from osmotic pressure; a β-lactam antibiotic

Uses: Lower respiratory infections, skin, bone, bacterial septicemia, urinary tract infections, yaws; effective for gram-positive bacilli *(C. perfringens, C. tetani),* gram-negative bacilli *(Bacteroides, P. aeruginosa, E. coli, H. influenzae, P. mirabilis)*

Dosage and routes:
- *Adult:* **IV** 100-350 mg/kg/day in 4-6 divided doses, max 24 g

Cystic fibrosis
- *Child:* **IV** 75 mg/kg q4h, max total dose 24 g

Available forms: Powder for inj 2, 3, 4 g

Side effects/adverse reactions:

HEMA: Anemia, increased bleeding time, **bone marrow depression, granulocytopenia**

GI: Nausea, vomiting, diarrhea, increased AST, ALT, abdominal pain, glossitis, colitis

GU: Oliguria, proteinuria, hematuria, *vaginitis, moniliasis, **glomerulonephritis***

CNS: Lethargy, hallucinations, anxiety, depression, twitching, **coma, convulsions**

META: Hypokalemia, alkalosis, hypernatremia

Contraindications: Hypersensitivity to penicillins

Precautions: Pregnancy (B), lactation, hypersensitivity to cephalosporins; neonates

Pharmacokinetics: Half-life 55-70 min, metabolized in liver; excreted in urine, bile, breast milk (small amount); crosses placenta

Interactions:
- Decreased antimicrobial effectiveness of azlocillin: tetracyclines, erythromycins
- Increased azlocillin concentrations: aspirin, probenecid
- Incompatible in sol with aminoglycosides, amphotericin B, chloramphenicol, lincomycin, oxytetracycline, polymyxin B, promethazine, tetracycline, vit B/C

Lab test interferences:

False positive: Urine glucose, urine protein

Decrease: Uric acid

NURSING CONSIDERATIONS
Assess:
- I&O ratio; report hematuria, oliguria, since penicillin in high doses is nephrotoxic
- Any patient with compromised renal system, since drug is excreted slowly in poor renal system function; toxicity may occur rapidly
- Liver studies: AST (SGOT), ALT (SGPT)
- Blood studies: WBC, RBC, Hgb, Hct, bleeding time
- Renal studies: urinalysis, protein, blood
- Culture, sensitivity before drug therapy; drug may be given as soon as culture is taken
- Bowel pattern before, during treatment
- Skin eruptions after administration of penicillin to 1 wk after discontinuing drug
- Respiratory status: rate, character, wheezing, tightness in chest
- Allergies before initiation of treatment; reaction of each medication; place allergies on chart in bright red

Administer:
IV
- After reconstituting 1 g/10 ml of D₅W, NS, or sterile water, shake
- After further dilution in 50-100 ml of compatible solution, give over 30 min; change IV site q48h
- After C&S completed
- Slowly (direct IV) over 5 min to prevent chest discomfort

Perform/provide:
- Adrenaline, suction, tracheostomy set, endotracheal intubation equipment on unit
- Adequate intake of fluids (2 L) during diarrhea episodes
- Scratch test to assess allergy after securing order from prescriber; usually done when penicillin is only drug of choice

---

 = Nursing alert   = Herb-drug interaction   = Do not crush

• Storage in cool environment; solution is stable for 24 hr at room temperature

Evaluate:
• Therapeutic response: absence of fever, draining wounds

Teach patient/family:
• That culture may be taken after completed course of medication
• To report sore throat, fever, fatigue (may indicate superinfection)
• To wear or carry a Medic Alert ID if allergic to penicillins
• To notify nurse of diarrhea

Treatment of anaphylaxis: Withdraw drug, maintain airway, administer epinephrine, aminophylline, O₂, IV corticosteroids

---

aztreonam (℞)

(az-tree'oh nam)

Azactam

Func. class.: Miscellaneous antibiotic

Chem. class.: Monobactam

Action: Inhibits organisms by inhibiting bacterial cell wall synthesis, which causes death of organism (bactericidal)

Uses: Urinary tract infection; septicemia; skin, muscle, bone infection; and other infections caused by gram-negative organisms

Dosage and routes:
Urinary tract infections
• *Adult:* IV/IM 500 mg-1 g q8-12h
Systemic infections
• *Adult:* IV/IM 1-2 g q8-12h
• *Child:* IV/IM 90-120 mg/kg/day divided q6-8h
Severe systemic infections
• *Adult:* IV/IM 2 g q6-8h; do not exceed 8 g/day
Continue treatment for 48 hr after negative culture or until patient is asymptomatic

Available forms: Powder for inj 500 mg, 1, 2 g; inj

Side effects/adverse reactions:
HEMA: Anemia, increased bleeding time, ***bone marrow depression, granulocytopenia***
GI: Nausea, vomiting, diarrhea, increased AST (SGOT), ALT (SGPT), abdominal pain, glossitis, colitis
CNS: Lethargy, hallucinations, anxiety, depression, twitching, ***coma, convulsions,*** malaise
EENT: Tinnitus, diplopia, nasal congestion
GU: Vaginal candidiasis, vaginitis, breast tenderness

Contraindications: Hypersensitivity to this drug, penicillins, cephalosporins

Precautions: Pregnancy (B), lactation, children, impaired renal, hepatic function, elderly

Pharmacokinetics:
IV: Peak immediate, trough 8 hr
IM: Peak 1 hr
Half-life: 1.7 hr; half-life prolonged in renal disease; protein binding 56%; metabolized by liver; excreted in urine 60%-70%; small amounts appear in breast milk, placenta

Interactions:
• Incompatible with nafcillin, metronidazole, cephradine

NURSING CONSIDERATIONS
Assess:
• Signs of bruising, bleeding, anemia
• Bowel pattern before, during treatment
• Respiratory status: rate, character, wheezing, tightness in chest
• I&O ratio; report hematuria, oliguria, since this drug in high doses is nephrotoxic
◆ Any patient with compromised renal system, since drug is excreted slowly in poor renal system function; toxicity may occur rapidly

---

- Liver studies: AST (SGOT), ALT (SGPT)
- Blood studies: WBC, RBC, Hgb, Hct, bleeding time
- Renal studies: urinalysis, protein, blood, serum creatinine, BUN
- Skin eruptions after administration of drug to 1 wk after discontinuing drug
- Allergies before initiation of treatment, reaction of medication; highlight allergies on chart

Administer:

IM

- Dilute each g with at least 3 ml of 0.9% NaCl; give into large muscle
- Drug after C&S completed

IV, direct

- After diluting with 6-10 ml sterile H_2O/15 ml drug; give over 3-5 min

IV inf

- After diluting with 3 ml or more sterile H_2O/1 g drug; then dilute with 50-100 ml of D_5W, 0.9% NaCl solution; give over ½-1 hr, by Y-tube or 3-way stopcock; flush tubing before and after administration

Additive compatibilities: Ampicillin/sulbactam, cefazolin, ciprofloxacin, clindamycin, gentamicin, tobramycin

Syringe compatibilities: Clindamycin

Y-site compatibilities: Allopurinol, amifostine, amikacin, aminophylline, ampicillin, ampicillin/sulbactam, bleomycin, bumetanide, buprenorphine, butorphanol, calcium gluconate, carboplatin, carmustine, cefazolin, cefepime, cefonicid, cefoperazone, cefotaxime, cefotetan, cefoxitin ceftazidime, ceftizoxime, ceftriaxone, cefuroxime, cimetidine, ciprofloxacin, cisplatin, clindamycin, cyclophosphamide, cytarabine, dacarbazine, dactinomycin, dexamethasone, diltiazem, diphenhydramine, dobutamine, dopamine, doxorubicin, doxycycline, droperidol, enalaprilat, etoposide, famotidine, filgrastim, floxuridine, fluconazole, fludarabine, fluorouracil, foscarnet, furosemide, gallium, gentamicin, granisetron, haloperidol, heparin, hydrocortisone, hydromorphone, hydroxyzine, idarubicin, ifosfamide, imipenem-cilastatin, insulin (regular), leucovorin, magnesium sulfate, mannitol, mechlorethamine, melphalan, meperidine, mesna, methotrexate, methylprednisolone, metoclopramide, mezlocillin, minocycline, morphine, nalbuphine, netilmicin, ondansetron, piperacillin, piperacillin/tazobactam, plicamycin, potassium chloride, promethazine, propofol, ranitidine, sargramostim, sodium bicarbonate, teniposide, theophylline, thiotepa, ticarcillin, ticarcillin/clavulanate, tobramycin, trimethoprim-sulfamethoxazole, vinblastine, vincristine, vinorelbine, zidovudine

Perform/provide:

- Adequate fluid intake (2 L) during diarrhea episodes
- Storage in refrigerator

Evaluate:

- Therapeutic response: absence of fever, purulent drainage, redness, inflammation

Teach patient/family:

- That culture may be taken after completed course of medication
- To report sore throat, fever, fatigue (may indicate superinfection)

---

bacampicillin (℞)

(ba-kam-pi-sill'in)

Penglobe*, Spectrobid*

Func. class.: Broad-spectrum antiinfective

Chem. class.: Aminopenicillin

Action: Interferes with cell wall replication of susceptible organisms; the cell wall, rendered osmotically

---

unstable, swells, bursts from osmotic pressure; drug is hydrolyzed to ampicillin during absorption

Uses: Respiratory tract, skin, urinary tract infections; effective for gram-positive cocci *(E. faecalis, S. pneumoniae),* gram-negative cocci *(N. gonorrhoeae),* gram-negative bacilli *(E. coli, H. influenzae, P. mirabilis)*

Dosage and routes:
• *Adult:* **PO** 400-800 mg q12h
• *Child:* **PO** 25-50 mg/kg/day in divided doses q12h

Available forms: Tabs 400 mg; powder for oral susp 125 mg/5 ml (equivalent to 87.5 mg ampicillin)

Side effects/adverse reactions:

HEMA: Anemia, increased bleeding time, **bone marrow depression, granulocytopenia**

GI: Nausea, vomiting, diarrhea, increased AST (SGOT), ALT (SGPT), abdominal pain, glossitis, pseudomembranous colitis

GU: Oliguria, proteinuria, hematuria, *vaginitis, moniliasis,* **glomerulonephritis**

CNS: Lethargy, hallucinations, anxiety, depression, twitching, **coma, convulsions**

Contraindications: Hypersensitivity to penicillins

Precautions: Pregnancy (B), lactation, hypersensitivity to cephalosporins, neonates, renal disease

Pharmacokinetics:

PO: Peak 30-60 min, duration 5-6 hr, half-life ½-1 hr, metabolized in liver, excreted in urine

Interactions:
• Increased bacampicillin concentrations: aspirin, probenecid, disulfiram
• Decreased action of: oral contraceptives

Lab test interferences:

False positive: Urine glucose, urine protein

Decrease: Uric acid

NURSING CONSIDERATIONS

Assess:
• I&O ratio; report hematuria, oliguria, since penicillin in high doses is nephrotoxic

➡ Any patient with compromised renal system, since drug is excreted slowly in poor renal system function; toxicity may occur
• Liver studies: AST (SGOT), ALT (SGPT)
• Blood studies: WBC, RBC, Hgb, Hct, bleeding time
• Renal studies: urinalysis, protein, blood, BUN, creatinine
• Culture, sensitivity before drug therapy; drug may be given as soon as culture is taken
• Bowel pattern before, during treatment
• Skin eruptions after administration of penicillin to 1 wk after discontinuing drug
• Respiratory status: rate, character, wheezing, tightness in chest
• Allergies before initiation of treatment; reaction of each medication

Administer:

PO
• After C&S completed
• Oral susp 1 hr before or 2 hr after meals; shake well before each dose

Perform/provide:
• Adrenaline, suction, tracheostomy set, endotracheal intubation equipment on unit
• Adequate intake of fluids (2 L) during diarrhea episodes
• Scratch test to assess allergy after securing order from prescriber; usually done when penicillin is only drug of choice
• Storage in dry tight container, oral suspension refrigerated for 2 wk or at room temperature for 1 wk

Evaluate:
• Therapeutic response: absence of fever, draining wounds

Teach patient/family:

• All aspects of drug therapy: culture may be taken after completed course of medication; patient must complete course of therapy

• To report sore throat, fever, fatigue (may indicate superinfection)

• To wear or carry a Medic Alert ID if allergic to penicillins

• To notify nurse of diarrhea

• That drug should be taken on an empty stomach, with a full glass of water

Treatment of hypersensitivity:

Withdraw drug, maintain airway, administer epinephrine, aminophylline, O_2, IV corticosteroids

---

bacitracin (Rx)

(bass-i-tray'sin)
Baci-IM, Bacitracin Sterile, Bacitracin U.S.P.
Func. class.: Antiinfective, misc.
Chem. class.: Bacillus subtilis derivative (polypeptide)

Action: Inhibits bacterial cell wall synthesis, interfering with osmotic pressure within cell

Uses:

Staphylococcal pneumonia, empyema, pseudomembranous colitis

Dosage and routes:

• *Infant >2.5 kg:* **IM** 1,000 U/kg/day in divided doses q8-12h

• *Infant ≤2.5 kg:* **IM** 900 U/kg/day in divided doses q8-12h

• *Adult:* **PO** 20,000-25,000 U q6h × 7-10 days; **IM** 10,000-25,000 U q6h × 7-10 days

• *Child:* **PO** 800-1200 U/kg/day divided q8h

Available forms: Inj IM 10,000, 50,000 U

Side effects/adverse reactions:

CV: Hypotension
INTEG: Rash, pain at injection site
GI: Nausea, vomiting, diarrhea
*GU: **Proteinuria, casts, azotemia***

Contraindications: Hypersensitivity, severe renal disease (IM use)

Precautions: Pregnancy (C), lactation, renal disease

Pharmacokinetics: Peak 1-2 hr, duration > 12 hr, metabolized in liver, excreted in urine

Interactions:

• Increased nephrotoxicity, neurotoxicity: aminoglycosides, polymyxin

• Increased neuromuscular blockade: nondepolarizing skeletal muscle relaxants, anesthetics

NURSING CONSIDERATIONS
Assess:

• I&O ratio; report oliguria, change in urinary output; high doses are nephrotoxic

• Any patient with compromised renal system; drug is excreted slowly in poor renal system function; toxicity may occur rapidly

• Renal studies: urinalysis, protein, blood, BUN, creatinine, urine pH (keep at 6.0)

• C&S before drug therapy; drug may be taken as soon as culture is taken; repeat C&S after treatment

• Bowel pattern before, during treatment; if severe diarrhea occurs, drug should be discontinued

• Skin eruptions, itching; rash, urticaria, erythema

• Respiratory status: rate, character, wheezing, tightness in chest, dyspnea on exertion

• Allergies before treatment, reaction of each medication; report allergies on chart in bright red; notify all people giving drugs

Administer:

IM

• After reconstituting with NS

• IM in deep muscle mass; rotate injection site; do not give IV/SC

◆ = Nursing alert   ⫙ = Herb-drug interaction   ⊘ = Do not crush

B

Perform/provide:
• Storage in refrigerator; protect from direct sunlight
• Adrenalin, suction, tracheostomy set, endotracheal intubation equipment on unit
• Adequate intake of fluids (2 L) during diarrhea episodes

Evaluate:
• Therapeutic response: absence of fever, cough, dyspnea, malaise

Teach patient/family:
• To report sore throat, fever, fatigue (may indicate superinfection); reduced frequency of urination

---

baclofen (℞)
(bak′loe-fen)
Alpha-Baclofen*, baclofen*, Lioresal, Lioresal DS, Lioresal Intrathecal
Func. class.: Skeletal muscle relaxant, central acting
Chem. class.: GABA chlorophenyl derivative

Action: Inhibits synaptic responses in CNS by decreasing GABA, which decreases neurotransmitter function; decreases frequency, severity of muscle spasms

Uses: Spinal cord injury, spasticity in multiple sclerosis

Dosage and routes:
• *Adult:* **PO** 5 mg tid × 3 days, then 10 mg tid × 3 days, then 15 mg tid × 3 days, then 20 mg tid × 3 days, then titrated to response, not to exceed 80 mg/day
• *Child >2 yr:* **PO** 10-15 mg/kg/day divided q8h titrate to max 40 mg/day
• *Child ≥8 yr:* as above, max 60 mg/day
• **INTRATHECAL:** Use implantable intrathecal INF pump; use screening trial of 3 separate BOL doses if needed (50 µg/ml, 75 µg/1.5 ml, 100 µg/2 ml). Initial: double screening dose that produced result and give over 24 hr: increase by 10%-30% q24h only. Maintenance: 1200-1500 µg/day

Available forms: Tabs 10, 20 mg; intrathecal inj 10 mg/20 ml (500 µg/ml), 10 mg/5 ml (2000 µg/ml)

Side effects/adverse reactions:
CNS: Dizziness, weakness, fatigue, drowsiness, headache, disorientation, insomnia, paresthesias, tremors
EENT: Nasal congestion, blurred vision, mydriasis, tinnitus
CV: Hypotension, chest pain, palpitations, edema
GI: Nausea, constipation, vomiting, increased AST (SGOT), alk phosphatase, abdominal pain, dry mouth, anorexia
GU: Urinary frequency
INTEG: Rash, pruritus

Contraindications: Hypersensitivity

Precautions: Peptic ulcer disease, renal disease, hepatic disease, stroke, seizure disorder, diabetes mellitus, pregnancy (C), lactation, elderly

Pharmacokinetics:
PO: Peak 2-3 hr, duration >8 hr, half-life 2½-4 hr, partially metabolized in liver, excreted in urine (unchanged)
INTRATHECAL: CSF levels with plasma levels 100 times oral route

Interactions:
• Increased CNS depression: alcohol, tricyclic antidepressants, narcotics, barbiturates, sedatives, hypnotics
⚕ May increase CNS depression: kava kava

Lab test interferences:
Increase: AST, alk phosphatase, blood glucose

NURSING CONSIDERATIONS
Assess:
• B/P, weight, blood sugar, and hepatic function periodically

◆ For increased seizure activity in epilepsy patient; this drug decreases seizure threshold

• I&O ratio; check for urinary retention, frequency, hesitancy
• ECG in epileptic patients; poor seizure control has occurred in patients taking this drug
• Allergic reactions: rash, fever, respiratory distress
• Severe weakness, numbness in extremities
• Tolerance: increased need for medication, more frequent requests for medication, increased pain
• CNS depression: dizziness, drowsiness, psychiatric symptoms
• Dosage, as individual titration is required

Administer:
PO
• With meals for GI symptoms
• Gum, frequent sips of water for dry mouth
IT
Additive compatibilities: Morphine
Perform/provide:
• Storage in tight container at room temperature
• Assistance with ambulation if dizziness or drowsiness occurs

Evaluate:
• Therapeutic response: decreased pain, spasticity

Teach patient/family:
• Not to discontinue medication quickly; hallucinations, spasticity, tachycardia will occur; drug should be tapered off over 1-2 wk
• Not to take with alcohol, other CNS depressants
• To avoid hazardous activities if drowsiness or dizziness occurs
• To avoid using OTC medication:

cough preparations, antihistamines, unless directed by prescriber
• To increase fluid intake >2 L/day; to take with food
Treatment of overdose: Induce emesis of conscious patient, lavage, dialysis

---

beclomethasone (℞)
(be-kloe-meth′a-sone)
Beclo disk*, Becloforte Inhaler*, Beclovent Rotocaps*, Vancenase Nasal Inhaler, Vanceril
Func. class.: Corticosteroid, synthetic
Chem. class.: Glucocorticoid

Action: Prevents inflammation by depression of migration of polymorphonuclear leukocytes, fibroblasts, reversal of increased capillary permeability and lysosomal stabilization; does not suppress hypothalamus and pituitary function
Uses: Chronic asthma, rhinitis
Dosage and routes:
• *Adult:* **INH** 2-4 puffs tid-qid, not to exceed 20 inhalations/day
• *Child: 6-12 yr:* **INH** 1-2 puffs tid-qid, not to exceed 10 inhalations/day
Available forms: Aerosol 42 μg/actuation
Side effects/adverse reactions:
RESP: **Bronchospasm**
GI: Dry mouth
EENT: Hoarseness, candidal infections of oral cavity, sore throat
Contraindications: Hypersensitivity, status asthmaticus (primary treatment), nonasthmatic bronchial disease; bacterial, fungal, viral infections of mouth, throat, lungs; children <3 yr
Precautions: Nasal disease/surgery, pregnancy (C), lactation
Pharmacokinetics:
INH: Onset 10 min, excreted in fe-

◆ = Nursing alert   🖋 = Herb-drug interaction   ⊘ = Do not crush

ces (metabolites), half-life 3-15 hr, crosses placenta, metabolized in lungs, liver, GI system

NURSING CONSIDERATIONS

Assess:

• Adrenal function periodically for HPA axis suppression

Administer:

• INH with water to decrease possibility of fungal infections

• Titrated dose, use lowest effective dose

Perform/provide:

• Gum, rinsing of mouth for dry mouth

Evaluate:

• Therapeutic response: decreased dyspnea, wheezing, dry rales on auscultation

Teach patient/family:

• To carry or wear ID as steroid user

• To notify prescriber if therapeutic response decreases; dosage adjustment may be needed

• Proper administration technique

• To wash inhaler with warm water and dry after each use

• All aspects of drug usage, including cushingoid symptoms

• The symptoms of adrenal insufficiency: nausea, anorexia, fatigue, dizziness, dyspnea, weakness, joint pain, depression

• To keep drug out of children's reach

---

belladonna alkaloids (℞)

(bell-a-don′a)

Bellafoline

Func. class.: Gastrointestinal anticholinergic

Chem. class.: Belladonna alkaloid

Action: Inhibits muscarinic actions of acetylcholine at postganglionic parasympathetic neuron effector sites

Uses: Treatment of peptic ulcer disease, irritable bowel syndrome in combination with other drugs; for other GI disorders

Dosage and routes:

• *Adult:* **PO** 0.25-0.5 mg tid; **SC** 0.125-0.5 mg qd or bid

• *Child >6 yr:* **PO** 0.125-0.25 mg tid

Available forms: Tabs 0.25 mg; inj 0.5 mg/ml

Side effects/adverse reactions:

CNS: Confusion, stimulation in elderly, headache, insomnia, dizziness, drowsiness, anxiety, weakness, hallucination

*GI: Dry mouth, constipation, **paralytic ileus,*** heartburn, nausea, vomiting, dysphagia, absence of taste

GU: Hesitancy, retention, impotence

CV: Palpitations, tachycardia

EENT: Blurred vision, photophobia, mydriasis, cycloplegia, increased ocular tension

INTEG: Urticaria, rash, pruritus, anhidrosis, fever, allergic reactions, flushing

Contraindications: Hypersensitivity to anticholinergics, narrow-angle glaucoma, GI obstruction, myasthenia gravis, paralytic ileus, GI atony, toxic megacolon

Precautions: Hyperthyroidism, coronary artery disease, dysrhythmias, CHF, ulcerative colitis, hypertension, hiatal hernia, hepatic disease, renal disease, pregnancy (C), lactation, urinary obstruction, elderly

Pharmacokinetics:

PO: Duration 4-6 hr; metabolized by liver, excreted in urine, half-life 13-38 hr

Interactions:

• Increased anticholinergic effect: amantadine, tricyclic antidepressants, MAOIs

---

- Increased effect of nitrofurantoin
- Decreased effect of phenothiazines, levodopa

NURSING CONSIDERATIONS
Assess:

- VS, cardiac status: checking for dysrhythmias, increased rate, palpitations, flushing
- I&O ratio; check for urinary retention or hesitancy
- GI complaints: pain, bleeding (frank or occult), nausea, vomiting, anorexia, constipation

Administer:
PO

- ½-1 hr ac for better absorption
- Decreased dose to elderly patients; their metabolism may be slowed
- Gum, hard candy, frequent rinsing of mouth for dryness of oral cavity

Perform/provide:

- Storage in tight container protected from light
- Increased fluids, bulk, exercise to decrease constipation

Evaluate:

- Therapeutic response: absence of epigastric pain, bleeding, nausea, vomiting

Teach patient/family:

- To avoid driving, other hazardous activities until stabilized on medication
- To avoid alcohol, other CNS depressants; will enhance sedating properties of this drug
- To avoid hot environments; heat stroke may occur; drug suppresses perspiration
- To use sunglasses when outside to prevent photophobia

---

benazepril (℞)

(ben-aze'uh-pril)
Lotensin
Func. class.: Antihypertensive
Chem. class.: Angiotensin-converting enzyme (ACE) inhibitor

Action: Selectively suppresses renin-angiotensin-aldosterone system; inhibits ACE, preventing conversion of angiotensin I to angiotensin II; results in dilation of arterial, venous vessels

Uses: Hypertension, alone or in combination with thiazide diuretics

Dosage and routes:

- *Adult:* **PO** 10 mg qd initially, then 20-40 mg/day divided bid or qd.
- *Renal impairment:* 5 mg qd with CrCl <30 ml/min, increase as needed to maximum of 40 mg/day
- *Geriatric:* **PO** 5-10 mg/day initially

Available forms: Tabs 5, 10, 20, 40 mg

Side effects/adverse reactions:

CV: Hypotension, postural hypotension, syncope, palpitations, angina
GU: Increased BUN, creatinine, decreased libido, impotence, urinary tract infection
HEMA: Neutropenia, agranulocytosis
INTEG: Angioedema, rash, flushing, sweating
RESP: Cough, asthma, bronchitis, dyspnea, sinusitis
META: Hyperkalemia, hyponatremia
GI: Nausea, constipation, vomiting, gastritis, melena
CNS: Anxiety, hypertonia, insomnia, paresthesia, headache, dizziness, fatigue
MS: Arthralgia, arthritis, myalgia

Contraindications: Hypersensitiv-

 = Nursing alert   ✦ = Herb-drug interaction   🚫 = Do not crush ity to ACE inhibitors, pregnancy (D), lactation, children

Precautions: Impaired renal, liver function, dialysis patients, hypovolemia, blood dyscrasias, CHF, COPD, asthma, elderly, bilateral renal artery stenosis

Pharmacokinetics:

PO: Peak ½-1 hr, serum protein binding 97%, half-life 10-11 hr, metabolized by liver (metabolites), excreted in urine

Interactions:

• Increased hypotension: diuretics, other antihypertensives, ganglionic blockers, adrenergic blockers

• Increased toxicity: vasodilators, hydralazine, prazosin, potassium-sparing diuretics, sympathomimetics, potassium supplements

• Decreased absorption: antacids

• Decreased antihypertensive effect: indomethacin

• Increased serum levels of digoxin, lithium

• Increased hypersensitivity: allopurinol

Lab test interferences:

False positive: Urine acetone

NURSING CONSIDERATIONS

Assess:

• Blood studies: neutrophils, decreased platelets

• B/P, orthostatic hypotension, syncope

• Renal studies: protein, BUN, creatinine; increased levels may indicate nephrotic syndrome; monitor urine for protein

• Baselines in renal, liver function tests before therapy begins

• Potassium levels, although hyperkalemia rarely occurs

• Edema in feet, legs daily

• Allergic reactions: rash, fever, pruritus, urticaria; drug should be discontinued if antihistamines fail to help

• Renal symptoms: polyuria, oliguria, frequency, dysuria

Perform/provide:

• Storage in tight container at 86° F (30° C) or less

• Supine or Trendelenburg position for severe hypotension

Evaluate:

• Therapeutic response: decrease in B/P

Teach patient/family:

• Not to discontinue drug abruptly

• Not to use OTC products (cough, cold, allergy) unless directed by prescriber; do not use salt substitutes containing potassium without consulting prescriber

• The importance of complying with dosage schedule, even if feeling better

• To rise slowly to sitting or standing position to minimize orthostatic hypotension

• To notify prescriber of mouth sores, sore throat, fever, swelling of hands or feet, irregular heartbeat, chest pain

• To report excessive perspiration, dehydration, vomiting, diarrhea; may lead to fall in B/P

• That drug may cause dizziness, fainting, light-headedness; may occur during first few days of therapy

• That drug may cause skin rash or impaired perspiration

• How to take B/P, and normal readings for age group

Treatment of overdose: 0.9% NaCl IV INF, hemodialysis

benztropine (Ⓡ)

(benz'troe-peen)
Apo-Benztropin*, benztropine
mesylate, Cogentin
Func. class.: Cholinergic blocker
Chem. class.: Tertiary amine

Action: Blockade of central acetylcholine receptors

Uses: Parkinson symptoms, EPS associated with neuroleptic drugs

Dosage and routes:

Drug-induced EPS

• *Adult:* **IM/IV** 1-4 mg qd-bid; give **PO** dose as soon as possible; **PO** 1-2 mg bid/tid, increase by 0.5 mg q5-6 days

• *Child:* **IM/IV** 0.02-0.05 mg/kg/dose 1-2 ×/day

• *Geriatric:* **PO** 0.5 mg qd-bid, increase by 0.5 mg q5-6d

Parkinson symptoms

• *Adult:* **PO** 0.5-1 mg qd, increase 0.5 mg q5-6d titrated to patient response

Acute dystonic reactions

• *Adult:* **IM/IV** 1-2 mg, may increase to 1-2 mg bid (PO)

Available forms: Tabs 0.5, 1, 2 mg; inj 1 mg/ml

Side effects/adverse reactions:

MS: Muscular weakness, cramping

INTEG: Rash, urticaria, dermatoses

MISC: Increased temperature, flushing, decreased sweating, hyperthermia, heat stroke, numbness of fingers

CNS: Anxiety, restlessness, irritability, delusions, hallucinations, headache, sedation, depression, incoherence, dizziness, memory loss; confusion, delirium (elderly)

EENT: Blurred vision, photophobia, dilated pupils, difficulty swallowing, dry eyes, mydriasis, increased intraocular tension, angle-closure glaucoma

CV: Palpitations, tachycardia, hypotension, bradycardia

GI: Dryness of mouth, constipation, nausea, vomiting, abdominal distress, *paralytic ileus,* epigastric distress

GU: Hesitancy, retention, dysuria

Contraindications: Hypersensitivity, narrow-angle glaucoma, myasthenia gravis, GI/GU obstruction, child <3 yr, peptic ulcer, megacolon, prostate hypertrophy

Precautions: Pregnancy (C), elderly, lactation, tachycardia, liver, kidney disease, drug abuse history, dysrhythmias, hypotension, hypertension, psychiatric patients, children

Pharmacokinetics:

IM/IV: Onset 15 min, duration 6-10 hr

PO: Onset 1 hr, duration 6-10 hr

Interactions:

• Increased anticholinergic effect: antihistamines, phenothiazines, amantadine

• Decreased effect of levodopa

• Increased schizophrenic symptoms: haloperidol

NURSING CONSIDERATIONS

Assess:

• I&O ratio; commonly causes decreased urinary output

• Parkinsonism, EPS: shuffling gait, muscle rigidity, involuntary movements

• Urinary hesitancy, retention; palpate bladder if retention occurs

• Constipation; increase fluids, bulk, exercise if this occurs

• For tolerance over long-term therapy; dose may have to be increased or changed

• Mental status: affect, mood, CNS depression, worsening of mental symptoms during early therapy

• Use caution in hot weather; drug

◆ = Nursing alert   ✒ = Herb-drug interaction   ⊘ = Do not crush

may increase susceptibility to stroke by decreasing sweating

• For benztropine "buzz" or "high," patients may imitate EPS

Administer:

PO

• With or after meals to prevent GI upset; may give with fluids other than water

• At hs to avoid daytime drowsiness in patient with parkinsonism

IV

• Undiluted IV (1 mg = 1 ml) dose at ≤1 mg/>1 min; keep in bed for at least 1 hr after dose

Syringe compatibilities: Chlorpromazine, fluphenazine, metoclopramide, perphenazine, thiothixene

Y-site compatibilities: Fluconazole, tacrolimus

Perform/provide:

• Storage at room temperature

• Hard candy, frequent drinks, gum to relieve dry mouth

Evaluate:

• Therapeutic response: absence of involuntary movements

Teach patient/family:

• That tabs may be crushed and mixed with food

• Not to discontinue this drug abruptly; to taper off over 1 wk

• To avoid driving, other hazardous activities; drowsiness may occur

• To avoid OTC medication: cough, cold preparations with alcohol, antihistamines unless directed by prescriber

---

bepridil (℞)

(be'pri-dil)

Bepadin, Vascor

Func. class.: Calcium channel blocker, antianginal

Action: Inhibits calcium ion influx across cell membrane during cardiac depolarization; produces relaxation of coronary vascular smooth muscle, dilates coronary arteries, decreases SA/AV node conduction, dilates peripheral arteries

Uses: Chronic stable angina, used alone or in combination with propranolol

Dosage and routes:

Angina

• *Adult:* **PO** 200 mg qd, after 10 days may increase dose if needed, max dose 400 mg/day

Available forms: Tabs, film-coated, 200, 300, 400 mg

Side effects/adverse reactions:

CV: Dysrhythmia, edema, CHF, bradycardia, hypotension, palpitations, AV block, *torsades de pointes*

GI: Nausea, vomiting, diarrhea, gastric upset, constipation, increased liver function studies

GU: Nocturia, polyuria

CNS: Headache, fatigue, drowsiness, dizziness, anxiety, depression, weakness, insomnia, confusion, light-headedness, nervousness

HEMA: Agranulocytosis

Contraindications: Sick sinus syndrome, 2nd- or 3rd-degree heart block, Wolff-Parkinson-White syndrome, hypotension less than 90 mm Hg systolic, cardiogenic shock, history of serious ventricular dysrhythmias

Precautions: CHF, hypotension, hepatic injury, pregnancy (C), lactation, children, renal disease, idiopathic hypertropic subaortic stenosis (IHSS), concomitant β-blocker therapy

Pharmacokinetics: Peak 2-3 hr, 99% plasma protein bound, half-life 42 hr; completely metabolized in the liver and excreted in urine and feces

Interactions:

• Increased effects: β-blockers

• Decreased effects of lithium, rifampin

• Increased levels of digoxin

 Increased antianginal effect: cat's claw, chicory

Lab test interferences:

Increase: Liver function tests, aminotransferase, CPK, LDH

NURSING CONSIDERATIONS

Assess:

• Cardiac status: B/P, pulse, respiration, ECG intervals (PR, QRS, QT), dysrhythmias

Administer:

PO

• Before meals, hs

Evaluate:

• Therapeutic response: decreased anginal pain

Teach patient/family:

• How to take pulse before taking drug; record or graph should be kept; use demonstration, return demonstration

• To avoid hazardous activities until stabilized on drug, dizziness no longer a problem

• To limit caffeine consumption

🚫 Not to break, crush, or chew tabs

• To avoid OTC drugs unless directed by a prescriber

• The importance of compliance with all areas of medical regimen: diet, exercise, stress reduction, drug therapy

Treatment of overdose: Defibrillation, atropine for AV block, vasopressor for hypotension

---

betamethasone/ betamethasone sodium phosphate/ betamethasone disodium phosphate/ betamethasone acetate/betamethasone sodium phosphate (℞)

(bay-ta-meth′a-sone)

Alphatrex*, Betacort*, Betaderm*, Betatrex, Beta-Val Betnelan*, Betamethasone Dipropionate, Celestone/Alphatrex, Celestone Phosphate, Cel-U-Jec, Diprolene AF/Betamethasone Sodium Phosphate, Diprosone, Maxivate, Selestoject, Teladar/Diprolene

Func. class.: Corticosteroid, synthetic

Chem. class.: Glucocorticoid, long-acting

Action: Decreases inflammation by suppressing migration of polymorphonuclear leukocytes, fibroblasts, reversal of increased capillary permeability and lysosomal stabilization

Uses: Immunosuppression, severe inflammation, prevention of neonatal respiratory distress syndrome (by administration to mother)

Dosage and routes:

• *Adult:* **PO** 0.6-7.2 mg qd; **IM/IV** 0.6-7.2 mg qd in joint or soft tissue (sodium phosphate)

• *Child:* **PO** 17.5 µg/kg/day in 3 divided doses; **IM** 17.5 µg/kg/day in 3 divided doses every 3rd day or 5.8-8.75 µg/kg/day as a single dose (adrenal insufficiency)

• *Child:* **PO** 62.5-250 µg/kg/day in 3 divided doses; **IM** 20.8-125 µg/kg/day of the base q12-24h (other uses)

Available forms: Tabs 0.6 mg; syr 0.6 mg/5 ml; inj 3, 4 mg/ml

Side effects/adverse reactions:

INTEG: Acne, poor wound healing, ecchymosis, bruising, petechiae

CNS: Depression, flushing, sweating, headache, ecchymosis, bruising, mood changes

*CV: Hypertension, **circulatory collapse, thrombophlebitis, embolism,** tachycardia, **necrotizing angiitis, CHF***

*HEMA: **Thrombocytopenia***

MS: Fractures, osteoporosis, weakness

*GI: Diarrhea, nausea, abdominal distention, **GI hemorrhage,** increased appetite, pancreatitis*

EENT: Fungal infections, increased intraocular pressure, blurred vision

Contraindications: Psychosis, hypersensitivity, idiopathic thrombocytopenia, acute glomerulonephritis, amebiasis, fungal infections, nonasthmatic bronchial disease, child <2 yr, AIDS, TB

Precautions: Pregnancy (C), lactation, diabetes mellitus, glaucoma, osteoporosis, seizure disorders, ulcerative colitis, CHF, myasthenia gravis, renal disease, esophagitis, peptic ulcer

Pharmacokinetics:

PO: Onset 1-2 hr, peak 1 hr, duration 3 days

IM/IV: Onset 10 min, peak 4-8 hr, duration 1-1½ days

Metabolized in liver, excreted in urine as steroids, crosses placenta

Interactions:

• Decreased action of betamethasone: cholestyramine, colestipol, barbiturates, rifampin, ephedrine, phenytoin, theophylline

• Decreased effects of anticoagulants, anticonvulsants, antidiabetics, ambenonium, neostigmine, isoniazid, toxoids, vaccines, anticholinesterases, salicylates, somatrem

• Increased side effects: alcohol, salicylates, indomethacin, amphotericin B, digitalis, cyclosporine, diuretics

• Increased action of betamethasone: salicylates, estrogens, indomethacin, oral contraceptives, ketoconazole, macrolide antibiotics

💋 Potassium deficiency: chronic use/abuse of cascara sagrada bark, buckthorn bark/berry, rhubarb root, senna leaf/fruits, aloe

💋 Increased action/side effects: squill, lily of the valley herb, pheasant's eye herb

Lab test interferences:

Increase: Cholesterol, sodium, blood glucose, uric acid, calcium, urine glucose

Decrease: Calcium, potassium, T_4, T_3, thyroid ^{131}I uptake test, urine 17-OHCS, 17-KS, PBI

False negative: Skin allergy tests

NURSING CONSIDERATIONS

Assess:

• Potassium, blood sugar, urine glucose while on long-term therapy; hypokalemia and hyperglycemia

• Weight daily; notify prescriber of weekly gain >5 lb

• B/P q4h, pulse; notify prescriber if chest pain occurs

• I&O ratio; be alert for decreasing urinary output and increasing edema

• Plasma cortisol levels during long-term therapy (normal level: 138-635 nmol/L SI units when drawn at 8 AM)

Administer:

PO

• With food or milk to decrease GI symptoms

IM

• Injection deeply in large muscle mass, rotate sites, avoid deltoid, use 21G needle

• In one dose in AM to prevent adrenal suppression, avoid SC administration; may damage tissue

IV

• Only sodium phosphate product; give >1 min; may be given by IV INF in compatible sol
• After shaking suspension (parenteral)
• Titrated dose; use lowest effective dose

Y-site compatibilities: Heparin, hydrocortisone, potassium chloride, vit B/C

Perform/provide:

• Assistance with ambulation in patient with bone tissue disease to prevent fractures

Evaluate:

• Therapeutic response: ease of respirations, decreased inflammation
• Infection: increased temperature, WBC even after withdrawal of medication; drug masks infection symptoms
• Potassium depletion: paresthesias, fatigue, nausea, vomiting, depression, polyuria, dysrhythmias, weakness
• Edema, hypertension, cardiac symptoms
• Mental status: affect, mood, behavioral changes, aggression

Teach patient/family:

• That ID as steroid user should be carried
• To notify prescriber if therapeutic response decreases; dosage adjustment may be needed
◆ Not to discontinue abruptly; adrenal crisis can result
• To avoid OTC products: salicylates, alcohol in cough products, cold preparations unless directed by prescriber
• All aspects of drug usage including cushingoid symptoms
• The symptoms of adrenal insufficiency: nausea, anorexia, fatigue, dizziness, dyspnea, weakness, joint pain

bethanechol (℞)

(be-than′e-kole)
bethanechol chloride, Duvoid, Urebeth, Urecholine

Func. class.: Cholinergic stimulant

Chem. class.: Synthetic choline ester

Action: Stimulates muscarinic ACh receptors directly; mimics effects of parasympathetic nervous system stimulation; stimulates gastric motility, stimulates micturition

Uses: Urinary retention (postoperative, postpartum), neurogenic atony of bladder with retention

Dosage and routes:

• *Adult:* **PO** 10-50 mg bid-qid; **SC** 2.5-10 mg tid-qid prn
• *Child:* **PO** 0.6 mg/kg/day divided in 3-4 doses/day

Test dose

• *Adult:* **SC** 2.5 mg repeated 15-30 min intervals × 4 doses to determine effective dose

Available forms: Tabs 5, 10, 25, 50 mg; inj 5 mg/ml

Side effects/adverse reactions:

INTEG: Rash, urticaria, flushing, increased sweating
CNS: Dizziness
GI: Nausea, bloody diarrhea, belching, vomiting, cramps, fecal incontinence
CV: Hypotension, bradycardia, orthostatic hypotension, reflex tachycardia, *cardiac arrest, circulatory collapse*
GU: Urgency
RESP: *Acute asthma, dyspnea*
EENT: Miosis, increased salivation, lacrimation, blurred vision

Contraindications: Hypersensitivity, severe bradycardia, asthma, severe hypotension, hyperthyroidism, peptic ulcer, parkinsonism, seizure

---

◆ = Nursing alert   ✐ = Herb-drug interaction   🚫 = Do not crush disorders, CAD, COPD, coronary occlusion, mechanical obstruction, peritonitis, recent urinary or GI surgery

Precautions: Hypertension, pregnancy (C), lactation, child <8 yr

Pharmacokinetics:

PO: Onset 30-90 min, duration 1-6 hr

SC: Onset 5-15 min, duration 2 hr, excreted by kidneys

Interactions:

• Increased action of bethanechol: other cholinergics, donezepril

• Hypotension: ganglionic blockers

• Decreased action of bethanechol: procainamide, quinidine

Lab test interferences:

Increase: AST, lipase/amylase, bilirubin, BSP

NURSING CONSIDERATIONS

Assess:

• B/P, pulse; observe after parenteral dose for 1 hr

• I&O ratio; check for urinary retention or incontinence

• Bradycardia, hypotension, bronchospasm, headache, dizziness, convulsions, respiratory depression; drug should be discontinued if toxicity occurs

Administer:

• To avoid nausea and vomiting, take on an empty stomach

SC

• Parenteral dose by SC route; use of IM, IV may result in cardiac arrest

◆Only with atropine sulfate available for cholinergic crisis

• Only after all other cholinergics have been discontinued

• Increased doses if tolerance occurs

Perform/provide:

• Storage at room temperature

• Bedpan/urinal if given for urinary retention

• Use of rectal tube if ordered, to increase passage of gas when used for abdominal distention

Evaluate:

• Therapeutic response: absence of urinary retention, abdominal distention

Teach patient/family:

• To take drug exactly as prescribed; 1 hr ac or 2 hr pc

• To make position changes slowly; orthostatic hypotension may occur

Treatment of overdose: Administer atropine 0.6-1.2 mg IV or IM (adult)

---

bicalutamide (℞)

(bye-kal-u'ta-mide)

Casodex

Func. class.: Antineoplastic hormone

Chem. class.: Nonsteroidal antiandrogen

Action: Binds to cytosol androgen in target tissue, which competitively inhibits the action to androgens

Uses: Prostate cancer in combination with luteinizing hormone releasing hormone (LHRH) analog

Dosage and routes:

• *Adult:* PO 50 mg qd with LHRH

Available forms: Tabs 50 mg

Side effects/adverse reactions:

GI: Diarrhea, constipation, nausea, vomiting, increased liver enzyme test

CV: Hot flashes, hypertension

CNS: Dizziness, paresthesia, insomnia

INTEG: Rash, sweating

GU: Nocturia, hematuria, UTI, impotence, gynecomastia, urinary incontinence

MISC: Infection, anemia, dyspnea, bone pain, headache, asthenia, back pain, flu syndrome

Contraindications: Hypersensitivity, pregnancy (X)

Precautions: Renal, hepatic disease, elderly, lactation

Pharmacokinetics: Well absorbed, metabolized by liver, excreted in urine, feces

Interactions:
• May displace anticoagulants from their binding sites

Lab test interferences:
Increase: AST, ALT, bilirubin, BUN, creatinine
Decrease: Hgb, WBC

NURSING CONSIDERATIONS
Assess:
• For diarrhea, constipation, nausea, vomiting
• For hot flashes, gynecomastia (assure patient that these are common side effects)
• Prostate specific antigen (PSA), liver function studies

Administer:
PO
• At same time each day, either AM or PM, with/without food
• With LHRH treatment

Evaluate:
• Therapeutic response: decreased tumor size, decreased spread of malignancy

Teach patient/family:
• To recognize, report signs of anemia, hepatoxicity, renal toxicity

---

biperiden (℞)
(bye-per´i-den)
Akineton
Func. class.: Cholinergic blocker

Action: Centrally acting competitive anticholinergic

Uses: Parkinson symptoms, EPS secondary to neuroleptic drug therapy

Dosage and routes:
Extrapyramidal symptoms
• *Adult:* **PO** 2 mg qd-tid; **IM/IV** 2 mg q30min, if needed, not to exceed 8 mg/24 hr
• *Child:* **IM** 40 µg/kg or 1.2 mg/m^2, may repeat q30min (max 4 doses/24 hr)

Parkinson symptoms
• *Adult:* **PO** 2 mg tid-qid; max 16 mg/24 hr

Available forms: Tabs 2 mg; inj 5 mg/ml (lactate)

Side effects/adverse reactions:
CNS: Confusion, anxiety, restlessness, irritability, delusions, hallucinations, headache, sedation, depression, incoherence, dizziness, euphoria, tremors, memory loss
EENT: Blurred vision, photophobia, dilated pupils, difficulty swallowing, mydriasis, increased intraocular tension, angle-closure glaucoma
CV: Palpitations, tachycardia, postural hypotension, bradycardia
GI: Dryness of mouth, constipation, nausea, vomiting, abdominal distress, *paralytic ileus*
GU: Hesitancy, retention, dysuria
INTEG: Rash, urticaria, dermatoses
MISC: Increased temperature, flushing, decreased sweating, hyperthermia, heat stroke, numbness of fingers, weakness, cramping

Contraindications: Hypersensitivity, narrow-angle glaucoma, myasthenia gravis, GI/GU obstruction, megacolon, stenosing peptic ulcers, prostatic hypertrophy

Precautions: Pregnancy (C), elderly, lactation, tachycardia, dysrhythmias, liver or kidney disease, drug abuse, hypotension, hypertension, psychiatric patients, children

Pharmacokinetics:
IM/IV: Onset 15 min, duration 6-10 hr
PO: Onset 1 hr, duration 6-10 hr

Interactions:
• Increased levels of digoxin, levodopa

◆ = Nursing alert   = Herb-drug interaction   🚫 = Do not crush

• Increased schizophrenic symptoms: haloperidol
• Increased anticholinergic effect: antihistamines, phenothiazines, amantadine
• Incompatibilities are unknown
NURSING CONSIDERATIONS
Assess:
• I&O ratio; retention commonly causes decreased urinary output
• Parkinsonism, EPS: shuffling gait, muscle rigidity, involuntary movements
• Patient response if anticholinergics are given
• Urinary hesitancy, retention; palpate bladder if retention occurs
• Constipation; increase fluids, bulk, exercise if this occurs
• For tolerance over long-term therapy; dose may have to be increased or changed
• Mental status: affect, mood, CNS depression, worsening of mental symptoms during early therapy
Administer:
PO
• With or after meals to prevent GI upset; may give with fluids other than water
• At hs to avoid daytime drowsiness in patients with parkinsonism
IM/IV
• With patient recumbent to prevent postural hypotension, give undiluted 2 mg or less≻1 min
Perform/provide:
• Storage at room temperature
• Hard candy, frequent drinks, gum to relieve dry mouth
Evaluate:
• Therapeutic response: absence of involuntary movements
Teach patient/family:
• To use caution in hot weather; drug may increase susceptibility to heat stroke, decreases sweating
• Not to discontinue this drug abruptly; to taper off over 1 wk

• To avoid driving, other hazardous activities; drowsiness may occur
• To avoid OTC medication: cough, cold preparations with alcohol, antihistamines unless directed by prescriber

---

bisacodyl

(bis-a-koe'dill)
Bisacolax*, Bisc-Evac, Bisco-Lax, Carter's Little Pills, Dacodyl, Deficol, Dulcagen, Dulcolax, Fleet Bisacodyl Laxit*, Therelax
Func. class.: Laxative, stimulant
Chem. class.: Diphenylmethane

Action: Acts directly on intestine by increasing motor activity; thought to irritate colonic intramural plexus
Uses: Short-term treatment of constipation, bowel or rectal preparation for surgery, examination
Dosage and routes:
• *Adult ≥12 yr:* PO 5-15 mg in PM or AM; may use up to 30 mg for bowel or rectal preparation; RECT 10 mg
• *Child >3 yr:* PO 5-10 mg as a single dose
• *Child >2 yr-11 yr:* RECT 10 mg as a single dose
• *Child <2 yr:* RECT 5 mg as a single dose
Available forms: Enteric coated tabs 5 mg; rect supp 5, 10 mg; rect sol: 10 mg/37 ml
Side effects/adverse reactions:
CNS: Muscle weakness
GI: Nausea, vomiting, anorexia, cramps, diarrhea, rectal burning (suppositories)
META: Protein-losing enteropathy, alkalosis, hypokalemia, ***tetany,*** electrolyte, fluid imbalances
Contraindications: Hypersensitivity, rectal fissures, abdominal pain,

---

nausea, vomiting, appendicitis, acute surgical abdomen, ulcerated hemorrhoids, acute hepatitis, fecal impaction, intestinal/biliary tract obstruction

Precautions: Pregnancy (C), lactation

Pharmacokinetics:

PO: Onset 6-10 min; acts within 6-12 hr

REC: Onset 15-16 min

Metabolized by liver; excreted in urine, bile, feces, breast milk

Interactions:

• Gastric irritation: antacids, milk, H_2-blockers

 Increased action/side effects: lily of the valley, pheasant's eye, squill

NURSING CONSIDERATIONS

Assess:

• Blood, urine electrolytes if drug is used often by patient

• I&O ratio to identify fluid loss

• Cause of constipation; identify whether fluids, bulk, or exercise missing from lifestyle

• Cramping, rectal bleeding, nausea, vomiting; if these symptoms occur, drug should be discontinued

Administer:

PO

• Alone only with water for better absorption; do not take within 1 hr of other drugs or within 1 hr of antacids, milk, or cimetidine

• In AM or PM

Evaluate:

• Therapeutic response: decrease in constipation

Teach patient/family:

Ⓝ To swallow tabs whole; do not break, crush, or chew tabs

• Not to use laxatives for long-term therapy; bowel tone will be lost

• That normal bowel movements do not always occur daily

• Not to use in presence of abdominal pain, nausea, vomiting

• To notify prescriber if constipation is unrelieved or if symptoms of electrolyte imbalance occur: muscle cramps, pain, weakness, dizziness

---

bismuth subsalicylate (OTC)

(bis′muth sub-sal-iss′uh-late)

Bismatrol, Bismed, Pepto-Bismol, Pepto-Bismol Maximum Strength, Pink Bismuth, PMS-Bismuth Subsalicylate

Func. class.: Antidiarrheal

Chem. class.: Salicylate

Action: Inhibits prostaglandin synthesis responsible for GI hypermotility; stimulates absorption of fluid and electrolytes

Uses: Diarrhea (cause undetermined), prevention of diarrhea when traveling; may be included to treat *H. pylori*

Dosage and routes:

• *Adult:* **PO** 30 ml or 2 tabs q30-60min, not to exceed 8 doses per day for >2 days

• *Child 10-14 yr:* **PO** 15 ml

• *Child 6-9 yr:* **PO** 10 ml

• *Child 3-6 yr:* **PO** 5 ml

Available forms: Chewable tabs 262 mg; susp 262 mg/15 ml

Side effects/adverse reactions:

HEMA: Increased bleeding time

GI: Increased fecal impaction (high doses), dark stools

CNS: Confusion, twitching

EENT: Hearing loss, tinnitus, metallic taste, blue gums, black tongue (chew tabs)

Contraindications: Child <3 yr, history of GI bleeding, renal disease

Precautions: Anticoagulant therapy, immobility

Pharmacokinetics:

PO: Onset 1 hr, peak 2 hr, duration 4 hr

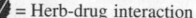 ◆ = Nursing alert   ◢ = Herb-drug interaction   Ⓝ = Do not crush

Interactions:

- Increased side effects: alcohol, aminosalicyclic acid, carbonic anhydrase inhibitors
- Increased action of bismuth: ammonium chloride
- Decreased action of bismuth: antacids, corticosteroids
- Decreased action of uricosurics, indomethacin, antidiabetics, tetracyclines
- Increased action of: anticoagulants, aspirin, warfarin
- 🍃 Increased absorption of bismuth: sarsaparilla root

Lab test interferences:

Interference: Radiographic studies of GI system

NURSING CONSIDERATIONS

Assess:

- Skin turgor
- Electrolytes (K, Na, Cl) if diarrhea is severe or continues long term
- Bowel pattern before drug therapy, after treatment

Administer:

PO

- Increased fluids to rehydrate the patient

Evaluate:

- Therapeutic response: decreased diarrhea or absence of diarrhea when traveling

Teach patient/family:

- To chew or dissolve in mouth; do not swallow whole; shake liquid before using
- To avoid other salicylates unless directed by prescriber; not to give to children, possibility of Reye's syndrome
- That stools may turn black; tongue may darken; impaction may occur in debilitated patients
- To stop use if symptoms do not improve within 2 days or become worse, or if diarrhea is accompanied by high fever

---

bisoprolol (℞)

(bis-oh'pro-lole)

Zebeta

Func. class.: Antihypertensive

Chem. class.: β_1-blocker

Action: Preferentially and competitively blocks stimulation of β_1-adrenergic receptors within cardiac muscle (decreases rate of SA node discharge, increases recovery time), slows conduction of AV node, decreases heart rate, which decreases O_2 consumption in myocardium; decreases renin-aldosterone-angiotensin system; inhibits β_2-receptors in bronchial and vascular smooth muscle at high doses

Uses: Mild to moderate hypertension

Investigational uses: Angina pectoris, supraventricular tachycardia

Dosage and routes:

- *Adult:* **PO** 2.5-5 mg qd; may increase if necessary to 20 mg qd; may need to reduce dose in presence of renal or hepatic impairment

Available forms: Tabs 5, 10 mg

Side effects/adverse reactions:

MS: Joint pain, arthralgia

MISC: Facial swelling, weight gain, decreased exercise tolerance

*CV: **Ventricular dysrhythmias, profound hypotension, bradycardia, CHF,** cold extremities, postural hypotension, **2nd- or 3rd-degree heart block***

CNS: Vertigo, headache, insomnia, fatigue, dizziness, mental changes, memory loss, hallucinations, depression, lethargy, drowsiness, strange dreams, catatonia, peripheral neuropathy

GI: Nausea, diarrhea, vomiting, ***mesenteric arterial thrombosis,*** isch-

---

emic colitis, flatulence, gastritis, gastric pain

INTEG: Rash, fever, alopecia, pruritus, sweating

HEMA: **Agranulocytosis, thrombocytopenia,** purpura, eosinophilia

EENT: Sore throat; dry, burning eyes

GU: Impotence, decreased libido

ENDO: Increased hypoglycemic response to insulin

RESP: **Bronchospasm,** dyspnea, wheezing, cough, nasal stuffiness

Contraindications: Hypersensitivity to β-blockers, cardiogenic shock, heart block (2nd, 3rd degree), sinus bradycardia, CHF, cardiac failure

Precautions: Major surgery, pregnancy (C), lactation, children, diabetes mellitus, renal or hepatic disease, thyroid disease, COPD, asthma, well-compensated heart failure, aortic or mitral valve disease, peripheral vascular disease, myasthenia gravis

Pharmacokinetics:

PO: Peak 2-4 hr; half-life 9-12 hr, 50% excreted unchanged in urine, protein binding 30%; metabolized in liver to inactive metabolites

Interactions:

• Increased hypotension, bradycardia: reserpine, hydralazine, methyldopa, quinidine, prazosin

• Decreased antihypertensive effects: indomethacin, nonsteroidal antiinflammatories, barbiturates, cholestyramine, colestipol, penicillins, salicylates

• Increased hypoglycemic effect: insulin

• Decreased bronchodilation: theophylline

• Decreased hypoglycemic effect of sulfonylureas

Lab test interferences:

Increase: AST and ALT

Interference: Glucose/insulin tolerance tests

NURSING CONSIDERATIONS
Assess:

• B/P during beginning treatment, periodically thereafter; pulse q4h: note rate, rhythm, quality

• Apical/radial pulse before administration; notify prescriber of any significant changes (pulse <50 bpm)

• Baselines in renal, liver function tests before therapy begins

• Edema in feet, legs daily

• Skin turgor, dryness of mucous membranes for hydration status, especially elderly

Administer:

PO

• Drug ac, hs, tablet may be crushed or swallowed whole

• Reduced dosage in renal and hepatic dysfunction

Perform/provide:

• Storage protected from light, moisture; placed in cool environment

Evaluate:

• Therapeutic response: decreased B/P after 1-2 wk

Teach patient/family:

• Not to discontinue drug abruptly, may cause precipitate angina

• Not to use OTC products containing α-adrenergic stimulants (such as nasal decongestants, OTC cold preparations) unless directed by prescriber

• To report bradycardia, dizziness, confusion, depression, fever

• To take pulse at home; advise when to notify prescriber

• To avoid alcohol, smoking, sodium intake

• To comply with weight control, dietary adjustments, modified exercise program

• To carry Medic Alert ID to identify drug taking, allergies

• To avoid hazardous activities if dizziness is present

To report symptoms of CHF: difficult breathing, especially on exertion or when lying down, night cough, swelling of extremities

Treatment of overdose: Lavage, IV atropine for bradycardia, IV theophylline for bronchospasm; digitalis, O_2, diuretic for cardiac failure; hemodialysis, IV glucose for hypoglycemia; IV diazepam (or phenytoin) for seizures

---

bitolterol (℞)

(bye-tole'ter-ole)
Tornalate
Func. class.: Bronchodilator, adrenergic β_2-agonist
Chem. class.: Acid ester of colterol

Action: Causes bronchodilation by action on β_2-receptors with increased synthesis of cAMP; relaxes bronchial smooth muscle; inhibits mast cell degranulation; stimulates cilia to remove secretions with very little effect on heart rate

Uses: Asthma, bronchospasm

Dosage and routes:

Inhaler

• *Adult and child >12 yr:* **INH** 2 puffs, wait 1-3 min before 3rd puff if needed, not to exceed 3 **INH** q6h or 2 **INH** q4h

Nebulization

• *Adult and child >12 yr:* **INH** 0.5 ml (1 mg) tid by intermittent flow or 1.25 mg tid by continuous flow

Available forms: Aerosol 0.37 mg/actuation, 0.02% neb sol

Side effects/adverse reactions:

CNS: Tremors, anxiety, insomnia, headache, dizziness, stimulation, restlessness, hallucinations

EENT: Dry nose, irritation of nose and throat

CV: Palpitations, tachycardia, hypertension, angina, hypotension

GI: Heartburn, nausea, vomiting, anorexia

MS: Muscle cramps

*RESP: **Bronchospasm,*** dyspnea

Contraindications: Hypersensitivity to sympathomimetics

Precautions: Lactation, pregnancy (C), cardiac disorders, hyperthyroidism, diabetes mellitus

Pharmacokinetics:

INH: Onset 3 min, peak ½-1 hr, duration 5-8 hr

Interactions:

• Increased action of aerosol bronchodilators

• Increased action of bitolterol: tricyclic antidepressants, MAOIs

• May inhibit action when used with other β-blockers

NURSING CONSIDERATIONS

Assess:

• Respiratory function: vital capacity, forced expiratory volume, ABGs

Administer:

Inhalation

• After shaking, exhale, place mouthpiece in mouth, inhale slowly, hold breath, remove, exhale slowly

• Gum, sips of water for dry mouth

Perform/provide:

• Storage in light-resistant container, do not expose to temperatures over 86° F (30° C)

Evaluate:

• Therapeutic response: absence of dyspnea, wheezing over 1 hr

Teach patient/family:

• Not to use OTC medications; excess stimulation may occur

• To use inhaler; review package insert with patient, provide demonstration, return demonstration

• To avoid getting aerosol in eyes

• To wash inhaler in warm water and dry qd

• All aspects of drug; to avoid smoking, smoke-filled rooms, persons with respiratory infections

---

Treatment for overdose: Administer a β_2-adrenergic blocker

---

bleomycin (R̟)

(blee-oh-mye′sin)
Blenoxane
Func. class.: Antineoplastic, antibiotic
Chem. class.: Glycopeptide

Action: Inhibits synthesis of DNA, RNA, protein; derived from *Streptomyces verticillus;* replication is decreased by binding to DNA, which causes strand splitting; phase specific in the G_2 and M phases; a nonvesicant

Uses: Cancer of head, neck, penis, cervix, vulva of squamous cell origin, Hodgkin's disease, lymphosarcoma, reticulum cell sarcoma, testicular carcinoma, malignant pleural effusion

Dosage and routes:
• *Adult and child:* SC/IV/IM 0.25-0.5 U/kg 1-2 times/wk or 10-20 U/m², then 1 U/day or 5 U/wk; may also be given by **CONT INF;** do not exceed total dose, 400 U in lifetime

Malignant pleural effusion
• *Adult:* 60 U as a single bolus intrapleural inj; 0.9% NaCl given through a thoracostomy tube following drainage of excess pleural fluid and complete lung expansion, remove after 4 hr

Available forms: Powder for inj, 15, 30 units

Side effects/adverse reactions:
SYST: Anaphylaxis
GI: Nausea, vomiting, anorexia, stomatitis, weight loss
INTEG: Rash, hyperkeratosis, nail changes, alopecia, fever and chills
RESP: Fibrosis, pneumonitis, wheezing, pulmonary toxicity
CNS: Fever, chills

IDIOSYNCRATIC REACTION: Hypotension, confusion, fever, chills, wheezing

Contraindications: Hypersensitivity

Precautions: Renal, hepatic, respiratory disease, pregnancy (D)

Pharmacokinetics: Half-life 2 hr; when CrCl >35 ml/min, half-life is increased in lower clearance; metabolized in liver, 50% excreted in urine (unchanged)

Interactions:
• Increased toxicity: other antineoplastics, radiation therapy
• Decreased serum digoxin levels: digoxin

NURSING CONSIDERATIONS
Assess:
• IM test dose
• Pulmonary function tests: chest x-ray film before and during therapy; should be obtained q2wk during treatment
• Temperature q4h; fever may indicate beginning infection
• Serum creatinine
• Dyspnea, rales, unproductive cough, chest pain, tachypnea, fatigue, increased pulse, pallor, lethargy
• Effects of alopecia and skin color on body image; discuss feelings about body changes
• Buccal cavity q8h for dryness, sores, ulceration, white patches, oral pain, bleeding, dysphagia
• Local irritation, pain, burning, discoloration at injection site
◆ Symptoms indicating severe allergic reaction: rash, pruritus, urticaria, purpuric skin lesions, itching, flushing

Administer:
• Antiemetic 30-60 min before giving drug to prevent vomiting, continue antiemetics 6-10 hr after treatment
• Topical or systemic analgesics for

◆ = Nursing alert   𝄞 = Herb-drug interaction   ⊘ = Do not crush pain of stomatitis as ordered; antihistamines and antipyretics for fever and chills

IM/SC

• After reconstituting 5 U/1-5 ml sterile H_2O, D_5W, 0.9% NaCl, or bacteriostatic water for inj; do not use products containing benzyl alcohol when giving to neonates

Direct IV

• After reconstituting 15 U or less/5 ml or more of D_5W or 0.9% NaCl; after further diluting with 50-100 ml D_5W or 0.9% NaCl, give 15 U or less/10 min through Y-tube or 3-way stopcock

• Two test doses 2-5 U before initial dose; monitor for anaphylaxis

Intrapleural

• 60 U/50-100 ml of 0.9% NaCl

Additive compatibilities: Amikacin, cephapirin, dexamethasone, diphenhydramine, fluorouracil, gentamicin, heparin, hydrocortisone, phenytoin, streptomycin, tobramycin, vinblastine, vincristine

Solution compatibilities: 0.9% NaCl

Syringe compatibilities: Cisplatin, cyclophosphamide, doxorubicin, droperidol, fluorouracil, furosemide, heparin, leucovorin, methotrexate, metoclopramide, mitomycin, vinblastine, vincristine

Y-site compatibilities: Allopurinol, amifostine, aztreonam, cefepime, cisplatin, cyclophosphamide, doxorubicin, droperidol, filgrastim, fludarabine, fluorouracil, granisetron, heparin, leucovorin, melphalan, methotrexate, metoclopramide, mitomycin, ondansetron, paclitaxel, piperacillin/tazobactam, sargramostim, teniposide, thiotepa, vinblastine, vincristine, vinorelbine

Perform/provide:

• Storage for 2 wk after reconstituting at room temperature; discard unused portions

• Deep-breathing exercises with patient tid-qid; place in semi-Fowler's position

• Liquid diet: carbonated beverage; gelatin may be added if patient is not nauseated or vomiting

• Rinsing of mouth tid-qid with water, club soda; brushing of teeth with baking soda bid-tid with soft brush or cotton-tipped applicators for stomatitis; use unwaxed dental floss

• HOB raised to facilitate breathing

Evaluate:

• Therapeutic response: decrease in size of tumor

Teach patient/family:

• To report any complaints, side effects to nurse or prescriber

• To report any changes in breathing, coughing, fever

• That hair may be lost during treatment, and wig or hairpiece may make patient feel better; that new hair may be different in color, texture

• To avoid foods with citric acid, hot or rough texture

• To report any bleeding, white spots, ulcerations in mouth; to examine mouth qd and report symptoms

---

bretylium (R)

(bre-til'ee-um)

Bretylate*, bretylium tosylate, Bretylol

Func. class.: Antidysrhythmic (Class III)

Chem class.: Quaternary ammonium compound

Action: After a transient release of norepinephrine, inhibits further release by postganglionic nerve endings; prolongs duration of action potential and effective refractory period

Uses: Serious ventricular tachycardia, cardioversion, ventricular fibrillation; for short-term use only

Dosage and routes:
Severe ventricular fibrillation
• *Adult:* IV BOL 5 mg/kg, over 15-30 sec; increase to 10 mg/kg repeated q15min, up to 30 mg/kg; IV INF 1-2 mg/min or give 5-10 mg/kg over 10 min q6h (maintenance)
Ventricular tachycardia
• *Adult:* IV INF 500 mg diluted in 50 ml D_5W or NS, infuse over 10-30 min, may repeat in 1 hr, maintain with 1-2 mg/min or 5-10 mg/kg over 10-30 min q6h; IM 5-10 mg/kg undiluted; repeat in 1-2 hr if needed; maintain with same dose q6-8h
• *Child:* 2-5 mg/kg/dose
Renal disease
• CrCl 10-50 ml/min 25%-50% dose; CrCl <10 ml/min avoid use
Available forms: Inj 50 mg/ml; 1, 2, 4 mg/ml prefilled syringes
Side effects/adverse reactions:
CNS: Syncope, dizziness, confusion, psychosis, anxiety
GI: Nausea, vomiting
CV: Hypotension, postural hypotension, bradycardia, angina, PVCs, substernal pressure, transient hypertension, precipitation of angina
RESP: Respiratory depression
Contraindications: Hypersensitivity, digitalis toxicity, aortic stenosis, pulmonary hypertension, children
Precautions: Renal disease, pregnancy (C), lactation, children
Pharmacokinetics: Well absorbed by IM/IV routes
IV: Onset 5 min, duration 6-24 hr
IM: Onset ½-2 hr, duration 6-24 hr
Half-life 4-17 hr, excreted unchanged by kidneys (70%-80% in 24 hr), not metabolized
Interactions:
• Increased or decreased effects of bretylium: quinidine, procainamide, propranolol, other antidysrhythmics
• Hypotension: antihypertensives
• Toxicity: digitalis
🌿 Increased action of bretylium:

chronic use/abuse of cascara sagrada bark, aloe, buckthorn bark/berry, rhubarb root, senna leaf/fruits
Lab test interferences:
Decrease: Urinary epinephrine, urinary norepinephrine, urinary VMA epinephrine

NURSING CONSIDERATIONS
Assess:
• ECG continuously to determine drug effectiveness, PVCs, other dysrhythmias
• IV INF rate to avoid causing nausea, vomiting
• For dehydration or hypovolemia
• B/P continuously for hypotension, hypertension; orthostatic hypotension; keep supine until hypotension subsides
• I&O ratio
• If systolic B/P <75 mm Hg, notify prescriber
• For rebound hypertension after 1-2 hr
• Cardiac status: rate, rhythm, character, continuously
Administer:
IM
• Inj, rotate sites, inject <5 ml in any one site to prevent tissue necrosis, may repeat 1-2 hr
IV, direct
• Undiluted over 15-30 sec (ventricular fibrillation); may repeat in 15-30 min, not to exceed 30 mg/kg/24 hr
Intermittent IV inf
• Dilute 500 mg of drug/50 ml or more D_5W, 0.9% NaCl, D_5/0.45%, D_5/0.9% NaCl, D_5/LR, give over 15-30 min
Continuous IV inf
• Dilute further; give at 1-2 mg diluted sol/min via infusion pump
• Reduced dosage slowly with ECG monitoring, discontinue over 3-5 days, maintain on oral dysrhythmic
Additive compatibilities: Aminophylline, atracurium, calcium chlo-

ride, calcium gluconate, digoxin, dopamine, esmolol, insulin (regular), lidocaine, potassium chloride, quinadine, verapamil

Y-site compatibilities: Amiodarone, amrinone, diltiazem, dobutamine, famotidine, isoproterenol, ranitidine

Perform/provide:

• Place patient in supine position unless otherwise ordered; assist with ambulation

• Have suction equipment available

Evaluate:

• Therapeutic response: absence of ventricular tachycardia, fibrillation

Teach patient/family:

• To make position changes slowly; orthostatic hypotension may occur

Treatment of overdose: O_2, artificial ventilation, ECG; administer dopamine for circulatory depression; administer diazepam or thiopental for convulsions

---

bromocriptine (℞)

(broe-moe-krip'teen)
Parlodel
Func. class.: Dopamine receptor agonist, ovulation stimulant
Chem. class.: Ergot alkaloid derivative

Action: Inhibits prolactin release by activating postsynaptic dopamine receptors; activation of striatal dopamine receptors may be reason for improvement in Parkinson's disease

Uses: Female infertility, Parkinson's disease, prevention of postpartum lactation, amenorrhea caused by hyperprolactinemia, acromegaly

Dosage and routes:
Hyperprolactinemic indications/female infertility
• *Adult:* PO 1.25-2.5 mg with meals; may increase by 2.5 mg q3-7d, usual 5-7.5 mg

Acromegaly
• *Adult:* PO 1.25-2.5 mg × 3 days hs; may increase by 1.25-2.5 mg q3-7d; usual range 20-30 mg/day, max 100 mg/day

Postpartum lactation
• *Adult:* PO 2.5 mg qd-tid with meal × 14 or 21 days

Parkinson's disease
• *Adult:* PO 1.25 mg bid with meals, may increase q2-4wk by 2.5 mg/day, not to exceed 100 mg qd

Available forms: Caps 5 mg; tabs 2.5 mg

Side effects/adverse reactions:
EENT: Blurred vision, diplopia, burning eyes, nasal congestion

CNS: Headache, depression, restlessness, anxiety, nervousness, confusion, ***convulsions,*** hallucinations, dizziness, fatigue, drowsiness, abnormal involuntary movements, psychosis

GU: Frequency, retention, incontinence, diuresis

GI: Nausea, vomiting, anorexia, cramps, constipation, diarrhea, dry mouth, GI hemorrhage

INTEG: Rash on face, arms, alopecia

CV: Orthostatic hypotension, decreased B/P, palpitation, extra systole, ***shock,*** dysrhythmias, bradycardia

Contraindications: Hypersensitivity to ergot, severe ischemic disease, pregnancy (D), severe peripheral vascular disease

Precautions: Lactation, hepatic disease, renal disease, children, pituitary tumors

Pharmacokinetics:
PO: Peak 1-3 hr, duration 4-8 hr, 90%-96% protein bound, half-life 3 hr, metabolized by liver (inactive metabolites), 85%-98% of dose excreted in feces

---

Side effects: *italics* = common; ***bold italics*** = life-threatening

Interactions:
• Decreased action of bromocriptine: phenothiazines, imipramine, haloperidol, droperidol, amitriptyline
• Increased action of antihypertensives
🌿 Decreased effect of bromocriptine: chaste tree fruit

Lab test interferences:
Increase: Growth hormone, AST (SGOT), ALT (SGPT), CPK, BUN, uric acid, alk phosphatase, GGTP

NURSING CONSIDERATIONS
Assess:
• B/P; establish baseline, compare with other reading; this drug decreases B/P

Administer:
PO
• With meal to prevent GI symptoms
• At hs so dizziness, orthostatic hypotension do not occur

Perform/provide:
• Storage at room temperature in tight container

Evaluate:
• Therapeutic response (Parkinson's disease): decreased dyskinesia, decreased slow movements, decreased drooling

Teach patient/family:
• That tabs may be crushed and mixed with food
• To change position slowly to prevent orthostatic hypotension
• To use contraceptives during treatment with this drug; pregnancy may occur; to use methods other than oral contraceptives
• That therapeutic effect for Parkinson's disease may take 2 mo: galactorrhea, amenorrhea
• To avoid hazardous activity if dizziness occurs

---

brompheniramine (℞)
(brome-fen-ir′a-meen)
Bromphen, brompheniramine, Chlorphed, Codimal-A, Conjec-B, Cophene-B, Dehist, Dimetane, Dimetane Extentabs, Dimetapp Allergy Liqui-Gels, Histaject Modified, Nasahist-B, ND Stat Revised, Oraminic II, Veltane

Func. class.: Antihistamine
Chem. class.: Alkylamine, H$_1$-receptor antagonist

Action: Acts on blood vessels, GI, respiratory system by competing with histamine for H$_1$-receptor site; decreases allergic response by blocking histamine

Uses: Allergy symptoms, rhinitis

Dosage and routes:
• *Adult:* PO 4-8 mg tid-qid, not to exceed 36 mg/day; time rel 8-12 mg bid-tid, not to exceed 36 mg/day; **IM/IV/SC** 10 mg q6-12h, not to exceed 40 mg/day
• *Child >6 yr:* PO 2 mg tid-qid, not to exceed 12 mg/day; **IM/IV/SC** 0.125 mg/kg
• *Child <6 yr:* Only as directed by prescriber

Available forms: Tabs 4, 8, 12 mg; tabs, time rel 8, 12 mg; elix 2 mg/5 ml; inj 10, 100 mg/ml

Side effects/adverse reactions:
CNS: Dizziness, drowsiness, poor coordination, fatigue, anxiety, euphoria, confusion, paresthesia, neuritis
CV: Hypotension, palpitations, tachycardia
RESP: Increased thick secretions, wheezing, chest tightness
HEMA: Thrombocytopenia, agranulocytosis, hemolytic anemia
GI: Dry mouth, nausea, vomiting, anorexia, constipation, diarrhea

---

INTEG: Photosensitivity

GU: Retention, dysuria, frequency, impotence

EENT: Blurred vision, dilated pupils, tinnitus, nasal stuffiness, dry nose, throat, mouth

Contraindications: Hypersensitivity to H_1-receptor antagonists, acute asthma attack, lower respiratory tract disease, child <6 yr

Precautions: Increased intraocular pressure, renal disease, cardiac disease, hypertension, bronchial asthma, seizure disorder, stenosed peptic ulcers, hyperthyroidism, prostatic hypertrophy, bladder neck obstruction, pregnancy (C), lactation

Pharmacokinetics:
PO: Peak 2-5 hr, duration to 48 hr; metabolized in liver, excreted by kidneys, excreted in breast milk, half-life 12-34 hr

Interactions:
• Increased CNS depression: barbiturates, narcotics, hypnotics, tricyclic antidepressants, alcohol
• Decreased effect of oral anticoagulants, heparin
• Increased drying effect: MAOIs
• Incompatible with aminophylline, insulins, pentobarbital
🚱 Increased CNS depression: kava kava
🚱 Increased anticholinergic effect: henbane leaf

Lab test interferences:
False negative: Skin allergy tests

NURSING CONSIDERATIONS
Assess:
• I&O ratio; be alert for urinary retention, frequency, dysuria; drug should be discontinued if these occur
• CBC during long-term therapy
• Blood dyscrasias: thrombocytopenia, agranulocytosis (rare)
• Respiratory status: rate, rhythm, increase in bronchial secretions, wheezing, chest tightness

Administer:
PO
• With meals if GI symptoms occur; absorption may slightly decrease
IV, direct
• Undiluted or diluted with 10 ml 0.9% NaCl, given over 1 min or more
IV inf
• Dilute in D_5W, 0.9% NaCl given at prescribed rate

Perform/provide:
• Hard candy, gum, frequent rinsing of mouth for dryness
• Storage in tight container at room temperature

Evaluate:
• Therapeutic response: absence of running or congested nose or rashes

Teach patient/family:
🚫 Not to break, crush, or chew sustained release forms
• All aspects of drug use; to notify prescriber if confusion/sedation/hypotension occurs
• To avoid driving, other hazardous activities if drowsiness occurs
• To avoid use of alcohol, other CNS depressants while taking drug

Treatment of overdose: Administer ipecac syrup or lavage, diazepam, vasopressors, barbiturates (short-acting)

---

buclizine (℞)
(byoo′kli-zeen)
Bucladin-S, Softabs
Func. class.: Antiemetic, antihistamine, anticholinergic
Chem. class.: H_1-receptor antagonist (piperazine)

Action: Acts centrally by blocking chemoreceptor trigger zone, which in turn acts on vomiting center

Uses: Motion sickness, dizziness, nausea, vomiting

Dosage and routes:
• *Adult:* **PO** 25-50 mg prn ½ hr before travel; may be repeated q4-6h prn
Available forms: Tabs 50 mg
Side effects/adverse reactions:
CNS: Drowsiness, dizziness, fatigue, restlessness, headache, insomnia
GI: Nausea, anorexia, bitterness, constipation
EENT: Dry mouth, blurred vision
Contraindications: Hypersensitivity to cyclizines, shock
Precautions: Children, narrow-angle glaucoma, lactation, prostatic hypertrophy, elderly, pregnancy (C)
Pharmacokinetics:
PO: Duration 4-6 hr; other pharmacokinetics not known
Interactions:
🌿 Increased anticholinergic effect: henbane leaf
🌿 Increased CNS depression: kava kava

NURSING CONSIDERATIONS
Assess:
• VS, B/P
• Signs of toxicity of other drugs or masking of symptoms of disease: brain tumor, intestinal obstruction
• Drowsiness, dizziness
Administer:
PO
• Tablets may be swallowed whole, chewed, or allowed to dissolve
Evaluate:
• Therapeutic response: absence of dizziness, nausea, vomiting
Teach patient/family:
• To avoid hazardous activities, activities requiring alertness; dizziness may occur; instruct patient to request assistance with ambulation
• To avoid alcohol, depressants

budesonide (℞)
(byoo-des′oh-nide)
Pulmicort, Rhinocort, Turbuhaler
Func. class.: Glucocorticoid
Chem. class.: Nonhalogenated

Action: Prevents inflammation by depression of migration of polymorphonuclear leukocytes, fibroblasts, reversal of increased capillary permeability and lysosomal stabilization; does not suppress hypothalamus and pituitary function
Uses: Rhinitis, asthma
Dosage and routes:
• *Adult and child >12 yr:* **INH** 400-600 µg/day; **NASAL:** 200-400 µg/day
Available forms: Nasal aerosol 50 µg; dry powder for INH 200 µg/metered dose
Side effects/adverse reactions:
RESP: Nasal irritation, pharyngitis, cough, nasal bleeding
GI: Dry mouth, dyspepsia
INTEG: Itching, dermatitis
Contraindications: Hypersensitivity, status asthmaticus
Precautions: Pregnancy (C), lactation, child, TB, fungal, bacterial, systemic viral infections, ocular herpes simplex, nasal septal ulcers
Pharmacokinetics: Unknown
Interactions:
• Increased effects: terbutaline
NURSING CONSIDERATIONS
Assess:
• Respiratory status: rate, rhythm, increase in bronchial secretions, wheezing, chest tightness; provide fluids to 2 L/day to decrease thickness of secretions; check for oral candidiasis
Administer:
Inhalation
• Use scissors to open pouch

◆ = Nursing alert   🌿 = Herb-drug interaction   ⊘ = Do not crush

Perform/provide:
• Storage at 59°-86° F (15°-30° C); keep away from heat, open flame

Evaluate:
• Therapeutic response: absence of asthma, rhinitis

Teach patient/family:
• All aspects of drug use; to notify prescriber of pharyngitis, nasal bleeding
• Not to exceed recommended dose; adrenal suppression may occur

---

bumetanide (℞)
(byoo met′a-nide)
Bumex
Func. class.: Loop diuretic
Chem. class.: Sulfonamide derivative

Action: Acts on ascending loop of Henle by inhibiting reabsorption of chloride, sodium

Uses: Edema in CHF, liver disease, renal disease (nephrotic syndrome), pulmonary edema, ascites (nephrotic syndrome), hypertension, anasarca

Investigational uses: May be used alone or as adjunct with antihypertensives such as spironolactone, triamterene

Dosage and routes:
• *Adult:* **PO** 0.5-2.0 mg qd; may give 2nd or 3rd dose at 4-5 hr intervals, not to exceed 10 mg/day; may be given on alternate days or intermittently; **IV/IM** 0.5-1.0 mg; may give 2nd or 3rd dose at 2-3 hr intervals, not to exceed 10 mg/day
• *Child:* **PO/IM/IV** 0.02-0.1 mg/kg q12h, max 10 mg/day

Available forms: Tabs 0.5, 1, 2 mg; inj 0.25 mg/ml

Side effects/adverse reactions:
*GU: Polyuria, **renal failure,** glycosuria
*ELECT: Hypokalemia, hypochlo-*remic alkalosis, hypomagnesemia, hyperuricemia, hypocalcemia, hyponatremia

CNS: Headache, fatigue, weakness, vertigo

GI: Nausea, diarrhea, dry mouth, vomiting, anorexia, cramps, upset stomach, abdominal pain, ***acute pancreatitis, jaundice***

EENT: Loss of hearing, ear pain, tinnitus, blurred vision

INTEG: Rash, pruritus, purpura, ***Stevens-Johnson syndrome,*** sweating, photosensitivity

MS: Muscular cramps, arthritis, stiffness, tenderness

ENDO: Hyperglycemia

*HEMA: **Thrombocytopenia***

*CV: **Chest pain,*** hypotension, ***circulatory collapse,*** ECG changes, dehydration

Contraindications: Hypersensitivity to sulfonamides, anuria, hepatic coma

Precautions: Dehydration, ascites, severe renal disease, pregnancy (C), hepatic cirrhosis, lactation

Pharmacokinetics:
PO: Onset ½-1 hr, duration 4 hr
IM: Onset 40 min, duration 4 hr
IV: Onset 5 min, duration 2-3 hr, excreted by kidneys, crosses placenta, excreted in breast milk

Interactions:
• Decreased diuretic effect: indomethacin, NSAIDs, probenecid
• Ototoxicity: cisplatin, aminoglycosides, vancomycin
• Increased effect: antihypertensives
• Increased toxicity: lithium, nondepolarizing skeletal muscle relaxants, digitalis
• May increase anticoagulant activity
• Decreased effects of antidiabetics

NURSING CONSIDERATIONS
Assess:
• Hearing with high IV doses

- Weight, I&O daily to determine fluid loss; effect of drug may be decreased if used qd
- Rate, depth, rhythm of respiration, effect of exertion
- B/P lying, standing; postural hypotension may occur
- Electrolytes: K, Na, Cl; include BUN, blood sugar, CBC, serum creatinine, blood pH, ABGs, uric acid, Ca, Mg
- Glucose in urine if patient is diabetic
- Improvement in edema of feet, legs, sacral area daily if medication is being used in CHF
- Improvement in CVP q8h
- Signs of metabolic alkalosis: drowsiness, restlessness
- Signs of hypokalemia: postural hypotension, malaise, fatigue, tachycardia, leg cramps, weakness
- Rashes, temperature elevation qd
- Confusion, especially in elderly; take safety precautions if needed
- For digitalis toxicity in patients taking digitalis products

Administer:
- In AM to avoid interference with sleep if using drug as a diuretic
- Potassium replacement if potassium is less than 3.0

PO
- With food if nausea occurs; absorption may be decreased slightly

IV, direct
- Direct IV undiluted over at least 1 min through Y-tube or 3-way stopcock or heplock

Intermittent IV
- Dilute in LR, D_5W, 0.9% NaCl (rarely given by this method)

Additive compatibilities: Floxacillin, furosemide

Syringe compatibilities: Doxapram

Y-site compatibilities: Allopurinol, amifostine, aztreonam, cefepime, cladribine, diltiazem, filgrastim, granisetron, lorazepam, melphalan, me-

peridine, morphine, piperacillin/tazobactam, propofol, teniposide, thiotepa, vinorelbine

Evaluate:
- Therapeutic response: decreased edema, B/P

Teach patient/family:
- To increase fluid intake to 2-3 L/day unless contraindicated, to take K supplement, to rise slowly from lying or sitting position
- To recognize adverse reactions: muscle cramps, weakness, nausea, dizziness
- To take with food or milk for GI symptoms
- To take early in day to prevent nocturia
- To use sunscreen to prevent photosensitivity

Treatment of overdose: Lavage if taken orally; monitor electrolytes; administer dextrose in saline; monitor hydration, CV, renal status

---

buprenorphine (℞)

(byoo-pre-nor'feen)
Buprenex
Func. class.: Opioid analgesic
Chem. class.: Thebaine derivative

Controlled Substance Schedule V
Action: Depresses pain impulse transmission at the spinal cord level by interacting with opioid receptors
Uses: Moderate to severe pain
Dosage and routes:
- *Adult:* **IM/IV** 0.3-0.6 mg q6h prn, reduce dosage in elderly
- *Child 2-12 yr:* **IM/IV** 2-6 µg/kg q4-6h
- *Geriatric:* **PO** 0.15 mg q6h prn
Available forms: Inj 0.3 mg/ml (1 ml vials)
Side effects/adverse reactions:
CNS: Drowsiness, dizziness, confusion, headache, sedation, euphoria

◆ = Nursing alert   🖊 = Herb-drug interaction   🚫 = Do not crush

GI: Nausea, vomiting, anorexia, constipation, cramps

GU: Increased urinary output, dysuria

INTEG: Rash, urticaria, bruising, flushing, diaphoresis, pruritus

EENT: Tinnitus, blurred vision, miosis, diplopia

CV: Palpitations, bradycardia, change in B/P

*RESP: **Respiratory depression***

Contraindications: Hypersensitivity, addiction (narcotic)

Precautions: Addictive personality, pregnancy (C), lactation, increased intracranial pressure, MI (acute), severe heart disease, respiratory depression, hepatic disease, renal disease

Pharmacokinetics:

IM: Onset 10-30 min, peak ½ hr, duration 3-4 hr

IV: Onset 1 min, peak 5 min, duration 2-5 hr

Metabolized by liver; excreted by kidneys; crosses placenta; excreted in breast milk; half-life 2½-3½ hr; 96% bound to plasma proteins

Interactions:

• Effects may be increased with other CNS depressants: alcohol, narcotics, sedative/hypnotics, antipsychotics, skeletal muscle relaxants

🍃 Increased CNS depression: kava kava

NURSING CONSIDERATIONS

Assess:

• I&O ratio; check for decreasing output; may indicate urinary retention

• CNS changes, dizziness, drowsiness, hallucinations, euphoria, LOC, pupil reaction

• Allergic reactions: rash, urticaria

• Respiratory dysfunction: respiratory depression, character, rate, rhythm; notify prescriber if respirations are <12/min

• Need for pain medication, tolerance

Administer:

IV, direct

• Undiluted over 3-5 min, titrate to patient response

• With antiemetic if nausea, vomiting occur

• When pain is beginning to return; determine dosage interval by patient response

Additive compatibilities: Atropine, bupivacaine, diphenhydramine, droperidol, glycopyrrolate, haloperidol, hydroxyzine, promethazine, scopolamine

Syringe compatibilities: Midazolam

Y-site compatibilities: Allopurinol, amifostine, aztreonam, cefepime, cladribine, filgrastim, granisetron, melphalan, piperacillin/tazobactam, propofol, teniposide, thiotepa, vinorelbine

Perform/provide:

• Assistance with ambulation if needed

Evaluate:

• Therapeutic response: decrease in pain, absence of grimacing

Teach patient/family:

• To report any symptoms of CNS changes, allergic reactions

• That tolerance may result when used for extended periods

Treatment of overdose: Naloxone HCl (Narcan) 0.2-0.8 mg IV, O₂, IV fluids, vasopressors

---

bupropion (℞)

(byoo-proe′pee-on)

Wellbutrin, Wellbutrin SR, Zyban

Func. class.: Misc. antidepressant, smoking deterrent

Action: Inhibits reuptake of dopamine, serotonin, norepinephrine

Uses: Depression, smoking cessation

Dosage and routes:
Depression
• *Adult:* **PO** 100 mg bid initially, then increase after 3 days to 100 mg tid if needed; may increase after 1 mo to 150 mg tid
• *Geriatric:* **PO** 50-100 mg/day, may increase by 50-100 mg q3-4 day
Smoking cessation
• *Adult:* **PO** 150 mg bid, begin with 150 mg qd × 3 days, then 300 mg/day; continue for 7-12 wk
Available forms: Tabs 75, 100 mg; tab sust rel 100, 150 mg

Side effects/adverse reactions:
CNS: Headache, agitation, confusion, seizures, akathisia, delusions, insomnia, sedation, tremors
CV: Dysrhythmias, hypertension, palpitations, tachycardia, hypotension
GI: Nausea, vomiting, dry mouth, increased appetite, constipation
GU: Impotence, frequency, retention
INTEG: Rash, pruritus, sweating
EENT: Blurred vision, auditory disturbance

Contraindications: Hypersensitivity, seizure disorder, eating disorders

Precautions: Renal and hepatic disease, recent MI, cranial trauma, pregnancy (B), lactation, children

Pharmacokinetics: Onset 2-4 wk, half-life 8-24 hr; metabolized by liver, steady state 1½-5 wk

Interactions:
• Increased adverse reactions: levodopa, MAOIs, phenothiazines, tricyclic antidepressants, benzodiazepines, alcohol
 Increased CNS depression: kava kava
 May increase anticholinergic effect: belladonna leaf/root

NURSING CONSIDERATIONS
Assess:
• Blood studies: CBC, leukocytes, differential, cardiac enzymes if patient is on long-term therapy
• Liver function tests before, during therapy: bilirubin, AST (SGOT), ALT (SGPT)
• ECG: watch for flattening of T wave, bundle branch block, AV block, dysrhythmias in cardiac patients
• Mental status: mood, sensorium, affect, suicidal tendencies, increase in psychiatric symptoms
• EPS primarily in elderly: akathisia
• Withdrawal symptoms: headache, nausea, vomiting, muscle pain, weakness if drug is discontinued abruptly
• Alcohol consumption: if alcohol is consumed, hold dose until morning

Administer:
PO
• Increased fluids, bulk in diet if constipation occurs
• With food or milk for GI symptoms
• Gum, hard candy, or frequent sips of water for dry mouth

Perform/provide:
• Assistance with ambulation during beginning therapy, since sedation occurs
• Safety measures, including side rails, primarily in elderly
• Checking to see PO medication is swallowed

Evaluate:
• Therapeutic response: decreased depression, ability to function in daily activities, ability to sleep throughout the night

Teach patient/family:
• That therapeutic effects may take 2-4 wk
• To use caution in driving, other

activities requiring alertness; sedation, blurred vision may occur
• To avoid alcohol ingestion, other CNS depressants
• Not to discontinue medication quickly after long-term use; may cause nausea, headache, malaise
Treatment of overdose: ECG monitoring; induce emesis, lavage, activated charcoal; administer anticonvulsant

---

buspirone (Ŗ)

(byoo-spye'rone)

BuSpar

Func. class.: Antianxiety agent

Chem. class.: Azaspirodecanedione

Action: Acts by inhibiting the action of serotonin (5-HT)
Uses: Management and short-term relief of anxiety disorders
Dosage and routes:
• *Adult:* PO 5 mg tid; may increase by 5 mg/day q2-3d, not to exceed 60 mg/day
Available forms: Tabs 5, 10, 15 mg
Side effects/adverse reactions:
CNS: Dizziness, headache, depression, stimulation, insomnia, nervousness, light-headedness, numbness, paresthesia, incoordination, tremors, excitement, involuntary movements, confusion, akathisia
GI: Nausea, dry mouth, diarrhea, constipation, flatulence, increased appetite, rectal bleeding
CV: Tachycardia, palpitations, hypotension, hypertension, ***CVA, CHF, MI***
EENT: Sore throat, tinnitus, blurred vision, nasal congestion; red, itching eyes; change in taste, smell
GU: Frequency, hesitancy, menstrual irregularity, change in libido

MS: Pain, weakness, muscle cramps, spasms
RESP: Hyperventilation, chest congestion, shortness of breath
INTEG: Rash, edema, pruritus, alopecia, dry skin
MISC: Sweating, fatigue, weight gain, fever
Contraindications: Hypersensitivity, child <18 yr
Precautions: Pregnancy (B), lactation, elderly, impaired hepatic/renal function
Pharmacokinetics: Half-life 2-3 hr, metabolized by liver, excreted in feces, rapidly absorbed
Interactions:
• Increased B/P: MAOIs; do not use together
• Increased effects: psychotropic drugs, alcohol (avoid use)
• Increased ALT: trazodone
🖋 Increased CNS depression: kava kava
NURSING CONSIDERATIONS
Assess:
• B/P (lying, standing), pulse; if systolic B/P drops 20 mm Hg, hold drug, notify prescriber
• Blood studies: CBC during long-term therapy; blood dyscrasias have occurred rarely
• Hepatic studies: AST (SGOT), ALT (SGPT), bilirubin, creatinine, LDH, alk phosphatase
• I&O; may indicate renal dysfunction
• Mental status: mood, sensorium, affect, sleeping pattern, drowsiness, dizziness
• Suicidal tendencies
Administer:
PO
• With food or milk for GI symptoms
• Crushed if patient unable to swallow medication whole
• Sugarless gum, hard candy, frequent sips of water for dry mouth

Perform/provide:

• Assistance with ambulation during beginning therapy; drowsiness, dizziness occur

• Safety measures, including side rails, if drowsiness occurs

• Check to see PO medication swallowed

Evaluate:

• Therapeutic response: decreased anxiety, restlessness, sleeplessness

Teach patient/family:

• That drug may be taken with food

• To avoid OTC preparations unless approved by prescriber

• To avoid alcohol, activities requiring alertness, since drowsiness may occur

• To avoid alcohol ingestion, other psychotropic medications, unless directed by prescriber

• Not to discontinue medication abruptly after long-term use

• To rise slowly or fainting may occur, especially elderly

• That drowsiness may worsen at beginning of treatment

• That 1-2 wk of therapy may be required before therapeutic effects occur

Treatment of overdose: Gastric lavage, VS, supportive care

---

busulfan (℞)

(byoo-sul'fan)

Myleran

Func. class.: Antineoplastic alkylating agent

Chem. class.: Nitrosurea

Action: Changes essential cellular ions to covalent bonding with resultant alkylation; this interferes with normal biologic function of DNA; activity is not phase specific; action is due to myelosuppression

Uses: Chronic myelocytic leukemia

Dosage and routes:

• *Adult:* **PO** 4-12 mg/day initially until WBC levels fall to 10,000/mm^3, then drug is stopped until WBC levels raise over 50,000/mm^3, then 1-3 mg/day

• *Child:* **PO** 0.06-0.12 mg/kg or 1.8-4.6 mg/m^2 day; dose is titrated to maintain WBC levels at 20,000/mm^3

Available forms: Tabs 2 mg

Side effects/adverse reactions:

HEMA: **Thrombocytopenia, leukopenia, pancytopenia, severe bone marrow depression**

GI: Nausea, vomiting, *diarrhea, weight loss*

GU: Impotence, sterility, amenorrhea, gynecomastia, **renal toxicity,** hyperuremia, adrenal insufficiency-like syndrome

INTEG: Dermatitis, hyperpigmentation, alopecia

RESP: **Irreversible pulmonary fibrosis,** pneumonitis

OTHER: **Chromosomal aberrations**

Contraindications: Radiation, chemotherapy, lactation, pregnancy (3rd trimester) (D), blastic phase of chronic myelocytic leukemia, hypersensitivity

Precautions: Childbearing age men and women, leukopenia, thrombocytopenia, anemia, hepatotoxicity, renal toxicity

Pharmacokinetics: Well absorbed orally; excreted in urine; crosses placenta; excreted in breast milk

Interactions:

• Increased toxicity: other antineoplastics or radiation

NURSING CONSIDERATIONS

Assess:

• CBC, differential, platelet count weekly; withhold drug if WBC is <4000/mm^3 or platelet count is <75,000/mm^3; notify prescriber of results

---

◆ = Nursing alert   ▮ = Herb-drug interaction   🚫 = Do not crush

• Pulmonary function tests, chest x-ray films before, during therapy; chest film should be obtained q2wk during treatment
• Renal function studies: BUN, serum uric acid, urine CrCl before, during therapy
• I&O ratio; report fall in urine output <30 ml/hr
• Monitor for cold, fever, sore throat (may indicate beginning infection)
• For decreased hyperuricemia
• Bleeding: hematuria, guaiac, bruising or petechiae, mucosa or orifices q8h, no rectal temps
• Dyspnea, rales, nonproductive cough, chest pain, tachypnea
• Food preferences; list likes, dislikes
• Edema in feet, joint, stomach pain, shaking
• Inflammation of mucosa, breaks in skin; use viscous xylocaine for oral pain

Administer:

PO

• Antacid before oral agent, give drug after evening meal, before bedtime, antiemetic 30-60 min before giving drug to prevent vomiting
• Allopurinol or sodium bicarbonate to maintain uric acid levels, alkalinization of urine

Perform/provide:

• Comprehensive oral hygiene
• Strict medical asepsis, protective isolation if WBC levels are low
• Deep breathing exercises with patient tid-qid; place in semi-Fowler's position for pulmonary reactions
• Increase fluid intake to 2-3 L/day to prevent urate deposits, calculi formation
• Diet low in purines: organ meats (kidney, liver), dried beans, peas to maintain alkaline urine
• Storage in tight container

Evaluate:
• Therapeutic response: decreased exacerbations of chronic myelocytic leukemia

Teach patient/family:
• About protective isolation precautions
• To avoid use of products containing aspirin or ibuprofen, razors, commercial mouthwash
• To report signs of anemia (fatigue, headache, irritability, faintness, shortness of breath)
• To report symptoms of bleeding (hematuria, tarry stools)
• That impotence or amenorrhea can occur, are reversible after discontinuing treatment
• To report any changes in breathing or coughing even several months after treatment

---

butorphanol (R)

(byoo-tor′fa-nole)
Stadol, Stadol NS
Func. class.: Narcotic analgesics
Chem. class.: Opiate

Controlled Substance Schedule V
Action: Depresses pain impulse transmission at the spinal cord level by interacting with opioid receptors
Uses: Moderate to severe pain
Investigational uses: Migraine headache, pain
Dosage and routes:
• *Adult:* **IM** 1-4 mg q3-4h prn; **IV** 0.5-2 mg q3-4h prn; **INTRANASAL,** 1 spray in one nostril; may give another dose 1-1½ hr later; repeat if needed q3-4h
Renal disease
• CrCl 10-50 ml/min 75% dose; CrCl <10 ml/min 50% dose
Available forms: Inj 1, 2, 10 mg/ml
Side effects/adverse reactions:
CNS: Drowsiness, dizziness, confu-

sion, headache, sedation, euphoria, weakness, hallucinations
GI: Nausea, vomiting, anorexia, constipation, cramps
GU: Increased urinary output, dysuria, urinary retention
INTEG: Rash, urticaria, bruising, flushing, diaphoresis, pruritus
EENT: Tinnitus, blurred vision, miosis, diplopia
CV: Palpitations, bradycardia, change in B/P
RESP: **Respiratory depression,** pulmonary hypertension
Contraindications: Hypersensitivity, addiction (narcotic), CHF, myocardial infarction
Precautions: Addictive personality, pregnancy (B), lactation, increased intracranial pressure, respiratory depression, hepatic disease, renal disease, child <18 yr
Pharmacokinetics:
IM: Onset 10-30 min, peak ½ hr, duration 3-4 hr
IV: Onset 1 min, peak 5 min, duration 2-4 hr
INTRANASAL: Onset within 15 min, peak 1-2 hr, duration 4-5 hr
Metabolized by liver; excreted by kidneys; crosses placenta; excreted in breast milk; half-life 2½-3½ hr
Interactions:
• Effects may be increased with other CNS depressants: alcohol, narcotics, sedative/hypnotics, antipsychotics, skeletal muscle relaxants
⚕ Increased CNS depression: kava kava
Lab test interferences:
Increase: Amylase
NURSING CONSIDERATIONS
Assess:
• I&O ratio; check for decreasing output; may indicate urinary retention
◆ For withdrawal symptoms in narcotic-dependent patients: pulmo-

nary embolus, vascular occlusion, abscesses, ulcerations
• CNS changes: dizziness, drowsiness, hallucinations, euphoria, LOC, pupil reaction
• Allergic reactions: rash, urticaria
• Respiratory dysfunction: respiratory depression, character, rate, rhythm; notify prescriber if respirations are <10/min
• Need for pain medication, physical dependence
Administer:
• With antiemetic if nausea, vomiting occur
• When pain is beginning to return; determine dosage interval by patient response
IM
• Deeply in large muscle mass
IV
• Undiluted at a rate of <2 mg/>3-5 min, titrate to patient response
Syringe compatibilities: Atropine, chlorpromazine, cimetidine, diphenhydramine, droperidol, fentanyl, hydroxyzine, meperidine, methotrimerprazine, metoclopramide, midazolam, morphine, pentazocine, perphenazine, prochlorperazine, promethazine, scopolamine, thiethylperazine
Y-site compatibilities: Allopurinol, amifostine, aztreonam, cefepime, cladribine, enalaprilat, esmolol, filgrastim, fludarabine, granisetron, labetalol, melphalan, paclitaxel, piperacillin/tazobactam, propofol, sargramostim, tenoposide, thiotepa, vinorelbine
Perform/provide:
• Storage in light-resistant area at room temperature
• Assistance with ambulation
• Safety measures: side rails, nightlight, call bell within easy reach, especially elderly

◆ = Nursing alert   ⚕ = Herb-drug interaction   ⊘ = Do not crush

Evaluate:

• Therapeutic response: decrease in pain

Teach patient/family:

• To report any symptoms of CNS changes, allergic reactions

• That physical dependency may result when used for extended periods

• That withdrawal symptoms may occur: nausea, vomiting, cramps, fever, faintness, anorexia

Treatment of overdose: Naloxone HCl (Narcan) 0.2-0.8 mg IV, O_2, IV fluids, vasopressors

---

cabergoline (℞)

(ka-bear'joe-leen)

Dostinex

Func. class.: Dopamine receptor/agonist

Action: Inhibits prolactin release by activating postsynaptic dopamine receptors

Uses: Reduced prolactin/secretion in postpartum lactation

Investigational uses: Parkinson's disease, normalization of androgen levels and improved menstrual cycles in polycystic ovarian syndrome

Dosage and routes:

Hyperprolactinemic indications

• *Adult:* **PO** 0.25 mg 2×/wk, may increase by 0.25 mg 2×/wk at 4 wk intervals, max 1 mg 2×/wk; maintenance therapy may be needed for 6 mo

Available forms: Tabs 0.5 mg

Side effects/adverse reactions:

EENT: Blurred vision

CNS: Headache, depression, nervousness, dizziness, fatigue

GU: Breast pain, dysmenorrhea

GI: Nausea, vomiting, anorexia, abdominal pain, dyspepsia, constipation

INTEG: Acne, flushing

CV: Orthostatic hypotension, decreased B/P

MISC: Asthenia, malaise, flulike symptoms

Contraindications: Hypersensitivity to uncontrolled hypertension

Precautions: Lactation, hepatic disease, renal disease, children, pituitary tumors, pregnancy (B), eclampsia, pre-eclampsia, PIH, CV disease

Pharmacokinetics:

PO: Peak 2-3 hr, duration 24 hr, half-life 2.7-14 days, metabolized by liver, excreted in feces, urine

Interactions:

• Do not use with droperidol, metoclopramide, butyrophenones, thioxanthines, dopamine antagonists

🍂 Decreased action of cabergoline: chaste tree fruit

NURSING CONSIDERATIONS

Assess:

• B/P; establish baseline, compare with other reading; this drug decreases B/P

Administer:

• At hs so dizziness, orthostatic hypotension do not occur

Perform/provide:

• Storage at room temperature in tight container

Evaluate:

• Therapeutic response: prevention of postpartum lactation

Teach patient/family:

• To change position slowly to prevent orthostatic hypotension

• To avoid hazardous activity if dizziness occurs

---

calcifediol (℞)

(kal-si-fe-dye′ole)
Calderol
Func. class.: Vit D analog, 25-Hydroxyvitamin D$_3$
Chem. class.: Sterol

Action: Increases intestinal absorption of calcium for bones; increases renal tubular absorption of phosphate; increases mobilization of calcium from bones, bone resorption

Uses: Metabolic bone disease with chronic renal failure, osteopenia, osteomalacia, hypocalcemia

Dosage and routes:
• *Adult:* **PO** 300-350 μg qwk divided into qd or qod doses; may increase q4wk
• *Supplement Elderly:* **PO** 20 μg qd
Available forms: Caps 20, 50 μg

Side effects/adverse reactions:
EENT: Tinnitus, conjunctivitis, photophobia, rhinorrhea
CNS: Drowsiness, headache, vertigo, fever, lethargy
GI: Nausea, diarrhea, vomiting, jaundice, anorexia, dry mouth, constipation, cramps, metallic taste
MS: Myalgia, arthralgia, decreased bone development
GU: Polyuria, hypercalciuria, hyperphosphatemia, hematuria
CV: Dysrhythmias

Contraindications: Hypersensitivity, hyperphosphatemia, hypercalcemia, vit D toxicity

Precautions: Pregnancy (C), renal calculi, lactation, CV disease, elderly

Pharmacokinetics:
PO: Peak 4 hr, duration 15-20 days; half-life 12-22 days

Interactions:
• Decreased absorption of calcifediol: cholestyramine, colestipol HCl, mineral oil, fat-soluble vitamins
• Hypercalcemia: thiazide diuretics
• Cardiac dysrhythmias: cardiac glycosides
• Decreased effect of this drug: corticosteroids

Lab test interferences:
False increase: Cholesterol

NURSING CONSIDERATIONS
Assess:
• BUN, urinary calcium, AST, ALT, cholesterol, creatinine, uric acid, chloride, magnesium, electrolytes, urine pH, phosphate; may increase; calcium should be kept at 9-10 mg/dl, vit D 50-135 IU/dl, phosphate 70 mg/dl
• Alk phosphatase; may be decreased
• For increased blood level, since toxic reactions may occur rapidly
• For dry mouth, metallic taste, polyuria, bone pain, muscle weakness, headache, fatigue, tinnitus, change in LOC, irregular pulse, dysrhythmias, increased respirations, anorexia, nausea, vomiting, cramps, diarrhea, constipation; may indicate hypercalcemia
• Renal status: decreased urinary output (oliguria, anuria), edema in extremities, weight gain 5 lb, periorbital edema
• Nutritional status, diet for sources of vit D (milk, some seafood), calcium (dairy products, dark green vegetables), phosphates (dairy products)

Administer:
PO
🚫 Do not break, crush, or chew caps
• May be increased q4wk depending on blood level

Perform/provide:
• Storage in tight, light-resistant containers at room temperature
• Restriction of sodium, potassium if required; ensure adequate calcium intake

 = Nursing alert   = Herb-drug interaction   = Do not crush

- Restriction of fluids if required for chronic renal failure

Evaluate:
- Therapeutic response: calcium levels 9-10 mg/dl, decreasing symptoms of bone disease

Teach patient/family:
- The symptoms of hypercalcemia
- About foods rich in calcium

---

calcitonin (human) (℞)
(kal-si-toe′nin)
Cibacalcin
Func. class.: Parathyroid agents (calcium regulator)
Chem. class.: Polypeptide hormone

Action: Decreases bone resorption, blood calcium levels; increases deposits of calcium in bones
Uses: Paget's disease
Dosage and routes:
Paget's disease
- *Adult:* SC 0.5 mg/day initially; may require 0.5 mg bid × 6 mo, then decrease until symptoms reappear
Available forms: Inj (SC) 500 mg vial
Side effects/adverse reactions:
INTEG: Rash, flushing, pruritus of earlobes, edema of feet
CNS: Headache, tetany, chills, weakness, dizziness
GU: Diuresis
GI: Nausea, diarrhea, vomiting, anorexia, abdominal pain, salty taste, epigastric pain
MS: Swelling, tingling of hands
CV: Chest pressure
RESP: Dyspnea
Contraindications: Hypersensitivity
Precautions: Renal disease, children, lactation, osteogenic sarcoma, pregnancy (C)

Pharmacokinetics:
IM/SC: Onset 15 min, peak 4 hr, duration 8-24 hr; metabolized by kidneys, excreted as inactive metabolites

NURSING CONSIDERATIONS
Assess:
- GI symptoms, polyuria, flushing, head swelling, tingling, headache; may indicate hypercalcemia
- Nutritional status; diet for sources of vit D (milk, some seafood), calcium (dairy products, dark green vegetables), phosphates
- BUN, creatinine, uric acid, chloride, electrolytes, urine pH, urinary calcium, magnesium, phosphate, urinalysis (calcium should be kept at 9-10 mg/dl, vit D 50-135 IU/dl), alk phosphatase baseline, q3-6mo
- Increased drug level, since toxic reactions occur rapidly; have calcium chloride on hand if calcium level drops too low; check for tetany
- Urine for sediment

Administer:
SC
- By SC route only; rotate injection sites; use within 6 hr of reconstitution; give hs to minimize nausea, vomiting

Perform/provide:
- Store at <77° F (25° C); protect from light

Evaluate:
- Therapeutic response: calcium levels 9-10 mg/dl, decreasing symptoms of Paget's disease

Teach patient/family:
- The method of injection if patient will be responsible for self-medication

---

Side effects: *italics* = common; ***bold italics*** = life-threatening

calcitonin (salmon) (℞)

(kal-si-toe′nin)
Calcimar, Miacalcin, Osteocalcin, Salmonine

Func. class.: Parathyroid agents (calcium regulator)
Chem. class.: Polypeptide hormone

Action: Decreases bone resorption, blood calcium levels; increases deposits of calcium in bones

Uses: Hypercalcemia, postmenopausal osteoporosis, Paget's disease

Dosage and routes:
Postmenopausal osteoporosis
• *Adult:* SC/IM 100 IU/day; NASAL 200 IU qd alternating nostrils qd, activate pump before 1st dose
Paget's disease
• *Adult:* SC/IM 100 IU qd, maintenance 50-100 IU qd or qod
Hypercalcemia
• *Adult:* SC/IM 4 IU/kg q12h, increase to 8 IU/kg q12h if response is unsatisfactory

Available forms: Inj 200 IU/ml; nasal spray 200 IU/activation (0.09 ml/dose)

Side effects/adverse reactions:
INTEG: Rash, pruritus of earlobes, edema of feet
CNS: Headache, flushing, *tetany,* chills, weakness, dizziness
GU: Diuresis
GI: Nausea, diarrhea, vomiting, anorexia, abdominal pain, salty taste
MS: Swelling, tingling of hands

Contraindications: Hypersensitivity, children, lactation

Precautions: Renal disease, pernicious anemia, Zollinger-Ellison syndrome, pregnancy (C)

Pharmacokinetics:
IM/SC: Onset 15 min, peak 4 hr, duration 8-24 hr; metabolized by kidneys, excreted as inactive metabolites

NURSING CONSIDERATIONS
Assess:
• BUN, creatinine, uric acid, chloride, electrolytes, urine pH, urinary calcium, magnesium, phosphatase, urinalysis, calcitonin antibody formation (calcium should be kept at 9-10 mg/dl, vit D 50-135 IU/dl), alk phosphatase
• Urine for sediment and casts
• History of allergies
• GI symptoms, polyuria, flushing, head swelling, tingling, headache; may indicate hypercalcemia
• Nutritional status; diet for sources of vit D (milk, some seafood), calcium (dairy products, dark green vegetables), phosphates
• Systemic allergic reaction to drug: skin test before first dose

Administer:
• After test dose of 10 IU/ml, 0.1 ml intradermally; watch 15 min; give only with epinephrine and emergency meds available
• IM injection in deep muscle mass slowly; rotate sites

Perform/provide:
• Storage in light-resistant area; refrigerate; nasal prep can be stored at room temp for 2 wk
• Restriction of sodium, potassium if required

Evaluate:
• Therapeutic response: calcium 9-10 mg/dl, decreasing symptoms of bone disease

Teach patient/family:
• To administer drug SC if patient will be responsible for self-medication
• To report difficulty swallowing or change in side effects immediately to prescriber

calcitriol (℞)

(kal-sih-try'ole)
Calcijex, Rocaltrol Vitamin D₃,
(1,25-dihydroxycholecalciferol)
Func. class.: Parathyroid agents
(calcium regulator)
Chem. class.: Vit D hormone

Action: Increases intestinal absorption of calcium, provides calcium for bones, increases renal tubular resorption of phosphate

Uses: Hypocalcemia in chronic renal disease, hypoparathyroidism, pseudohypoparathyroidism

Dosage and routes:

Hypocalcemia
• *Adult:* **PO** 0.25 μg qd, may increase by 0.25 μg/day q4-8wk, maintenance 0.25 μg qod-1 μg qd

Hypoparathyroidism/pseudohypoparathyroidism
• *Adult and child >1 yr:* **PO** 0.25 μg qd, may be increased q2-4wk; maintenance 0.25-2 μg qd

Available forms: Caps 0.25, 0.5 μg; inj 1 μg, 2 μg/ml

Side effects/adverse reactions:

CNS: Drowsiness, headache, vertigo, fever, lethargy

GI: Nausea, diarrhea, vomiting, jaundice, anorexia, dry mouth, constipation, cramps, metallic taste

MS: Myalgia, arthralgia, decreased bone development

GU: Polyuria, hypercalciuria, hyperphosphatemia, hematuria

Contraindications: Hypersensitivity, hyperphosphatemia, hypercalcemia, vit D toxicity

Precautions: Pregnancy (C), renal calculi, lactation, CV disease

Pharmacokinetics:

PO: Peak 4 hr, duration 15-20 days, half-life 3-6 hr

Interactions:
• Decreased absorption of calcitriol: cholestyramine, mineral oil
• Hypercalcemia: thiazide diuretics, calcium supplement
• Cardiac dysrhythmias: cardiac glycosides, verapamil
• Decreased effect of calcifediol: barbiturates, phenytoin, corticosteroids

Lab test interferences:
False increase: Cholesterol

NURSING CONSIDERATIONS

Assess:
• BUN, urinary calcium, AST (SGOT), ALT (SGPT), cholesterol, creatinine, albumin, uric acid, chloride, magnesium, electrolytes, urine pH, phosphate; may increase calcium, should be kept at 9-10 mg/dl, vit D 50-135 IU/dl, phosphate 70 mg/dl
• Alk phosphatase; may be decreased
• For increased drug level, since toxic reactions may occur rapidly
• For dry mouth, metallic taste, polyuria, bone pain, muscle weakness, headache, fatigue, change in LOC, dysrhythmias, increased respirations, anorexia, nausea, vomiting, cramps, diarrhea, constipation; may indicate hypercalcemia
• Renal status: decreased urinary output (oliguria, anuria), edema in extremities, weight gain 5-7 lb, periorbital edema
• Nutritional status, diet for sources of vit D (milk, some seafood); calcium (dairy products, dark green vegetables), phosphates (dairy products) must be avoided

Perform/provide:
• Storage protected from light, heat, moisture
• Restriction of sodium, potassium if required
• Restriction of fluids if required for chronic renal failure

Evaluate:

• Therapeutic response: calcium 9-10 mg/dl, decreasing symptoms of hypocalcemia, hypoparathyroidism

Teach patient/family:

• The symptoms of hypercalcemia
• About foods rich in calcium
• To avoid products with sodium: cured meats, dairy products, cold cuts, olives, beets, pickles, soups, meat tenderizers in chronic renal failure
• To avoid products with potassium: oranges, bananas, dried fruit, peas, dark green leafy vegetables, milk, melons, beans in chronic renal failure
• To avoid OTC products containing calcium, potassium, or sodium in chronic renal failure
• To avoid all preparations containing vit D
• To monitor weight weekly
🚫 Not to break, crush, or chew caps

---

calcium carbonate
(PO-OTC, IV-℞)

Alka-Mints, Amitone, Apo-Cal*, BioCal, Calcarb, Calci-Chew, Calci-Mix, Calcilac, Calcite*, Calglycine*, Cal-Plus, Calsan*, Caltrate 600, Caltrate Jr., Chooz, Dicarbosil, Equilet, Gencalc, Liquid-Cal, Liquid-Cal-600, Maalox Antacid Caplets, Mallamint, Mylanta Lozenges*, Nephro-Calci, Nu-Cal*, Os-Cal 500, Oysco 500, Oystercal 500, Oyst-Cal 500, Rolaids Calcium Rich, Titralac, Tums, Tums E-X Extra Strength

Func. class.: Antacid, calcium supplement

Chem. class.: Calcium product

Action: Neutralizes gastric acidity
Uses: Antacid, calcium supplement; not suitable for chronic therapy

Dosage and routes:

• *Adult:* **PO** 1 g 4-6 ×/day, chewed with water; **SUSP** 1 g 1 hr pc, hs
Available forms: Chewable tabs 350, 420, 500, 750 mg; tabs 650 mg; gum 500 mg; susp 1 g/5 ml

Side effects/adverse reactions:

GI: Constipation, anorexia, ***obstruction,*** nausea, vomiting, flatulence, diarrhea, rebound hyperacidity, eructation

CV: ***Hemorrhage, rebound hypertension***

META: Hypercalcemia, metabolic alkalosis

GU: Renal dysfunction, renal stones, ***renal failure***

Contraindications: Hypersensitivity, hypercalcemia, hyperparathyroidism, bone tumors

Precautions: Elderly, fluid restriction, decreased GI motility, GI obstruction, dehydration, renal disease, pregnancy (C), lactation

Pharmacokinetics:

PO: Onset 3 min, excreted in feces

Interactions:

• Increased plasma levels of quinidine, amphetamines
• Decreased levels of salicylates, calcium channel blockers, ketoconazole, tetracyclines, iron salts
• Hypercalcemia: thiazide diuretics
🌿 Increased action/side effects: lily of the valley herb, pheasant's eye herb, squill

NURSING CONSIDERATIONS
Assess:

• Ca^+ (serum, urine), Ca^+ should be 8.5-10.5 mg/dl, urine Ca^+ should be 150 mg/day, monitor weekly
◆ Milk-alkali syndrome: nausea, vomiting, disorientation, headache
• Constipation; increase bulk in the diet if needed
• Hypercalcemia: headache, nausea, vomiting, confusion

◆ = Nursing alert   🌿 = Herb-drug interaction   🚫 = Do not crush

Administer:
PO
- As antacid 1 hr pc and hs
- As supplement 1½ hr pc and hs
- Only with regular tablets or capsules; do not give with enteric-coated tablets
- Laxatives or stool softeners if constipation occurs

Evaluate:
- Therapeutic response: absence of pain, decreased acidity

Teach patient/family:
- To increase fluids to 2 L unless contraindicated, to add bulk to diet for constipation
- Not to switch antacids unless directed by prescriber
- That therapeutic dose recommendations are figured as elemental calcium

---

calcium chloride/ calcium gluceptate/ calcium gluconate/ calcium lactate (℞)

Func. class.: Electrolyte replacement—calcium product

Action: Cation needed for maintenance of nervous, muscular, skeletal, enzyme reactions, normal cardiac contractility, coagulation of blood; affects secretory activity of endocrine, exocrine glands

Uses: Prevention and treatment of hypocalcemia, hypermagnesemia, hypoparathyroidism, neonatal tetany, cardiac toxicity caused by hyperkalemia, lead colic, hyperphosphatemia, vit D deficiency

Dosage and routes:
Calcium chloride
- *Adult:* IV 500 mg-1 g q1-3d as indicated by serum calcium levels, give at <1 ml/min; IV 200-800 mg injected in ventricle of heart

- *Child:* IV 25 mg/kg over several min

Calcium gluceptate
- *Adult:* IV 5-20 ml; IM 2-5 ml
- *Newborn:* 0.5 ml/100 ml of blood transfused

Calcium gluconate
- *Adult:* PO 0.5-2 g bid-qid; IV 0.5-2 g at 0.5 ml/min (10% solution)
- *Child:* PO/IV 500 mg/kg/day in divided doses

Calcium lactate
- *Adult:* PO 325 mg-1.3 g tid with meals
- *Child:* PO 500 mg/kg/day in divided doses

Available forms: Many; check product listings

Side effects/adverse reactions:
INTEG: Pain, burning at IV site, severe venous thrombosis, necrosis, extravasation
HYPERCALCEMIA: Drowsiness, lethargy, muscle weakness, headache, constipation, *coma,* anorexia, nausea, vomiting, polyuria, thirst
CV: Shortened QT, heart block, hypotension, bradycardia, dysrhythmias, *cardiac arrest*
GI: Vomiting, nausea, constipation

Contraindications: Hypercalcemia, digitalis toxicity, ventricular fibrillation, renal calculi

Precautions: Pregnancy (C), lactation, children, renal disease, respiratory disease, cor pulmonale, digitalized patient, respiratory failure

Interactions:
- Increased dysrhythmias: digitalis glycosides
- *Calcium chloride*
  Increased action/side effects: lily of the valley herb, pheasant's eye herb, squill

Lab test interferences:
Increase: 11-OCHS
False decrease: Magnesium
Decrease: 17-OHCS

NURSING CONSIDERATIONS
Assess:
• ECG for decreased QT and T wave inversion: hypercalcemia, drug should be reduced or discontinued, consider cardiac monitoring
• Calcium levels during treatment (8.5-11.5 g/dl is normal level)
• Cardiac status: rate, rhythm, CVP, (PWP, PAWP if being monitored directly)

Administer:
PO
• With or following meals to enhance absorption
IM
• IM injection may cause severe burning, necrosis, tissue sloughing; warm sol to body temp before administering only gluconate/gluceptate
IV
• Undiluted or diluted with equal amounts of NS for inj to a 5% sol, give 0.5-1 ml/min
• Through small-bore needle into large vein; if extravasation occurs, necrosis will result (IV)

• *Calcium chloride*
Additive compatibilities: Amikacin, ascorbic acid, bretylium, cephapirin, chloramphenicol, dopamine, hydrocortisone, isoproterenol, lidocaine, methicillin, norepinephrine, penicillin G potassium, penicillin G sodium, pentobarbital, phenobarbital, sodium bicarbonate, verapamil, vit B/C
Syringe compatibilities: Milrinone
Y-site compatibilities: Amrinone, dobutamine, epinephrine, esmolol, morphine, paclitaxel

• *Calcium gluceptate*
Additive compatibilities: Ascorbic acid injection, isoproterenol, lidocaine, norepinephrine, phytonadione, sodium bicarbonate

• *Calcium gluconate*
Additive compatibilities: Amikacin, aminophylline, ascorbic acid injection, bretylium, cephapirin, chloramphenicol, corticotropin, dimenhydrinate, erythromycin, furosemide, heparin, hydrocortisone, lidocaine, magnesium sulfate, methicillin, norepinephrine, penicillin G potassium, penicillin G sodium, phenobarbital, potassium chloride, tobramycin, vancomycin, verapamil, vit B/C
Syringe compatibilities: Aldesleukin, allopurinol, amifostine, aztreonam, cefazolin, cefepime, ciprofloxacin, cladribine, dobutamine, enalaprilat, epinephrine, famotidine, filgrastim, granisetron, heparin/hydrocortisone, labetalol, melphalan, midazolam, netilmicin, piperacillin/tazobactam, potassium chloride, prochlorperazine, propofol, sargramostim, tacrolimus, teniposide, thiotepa, tolazoline, vinorelbine, vit B/C

Perform/provide:
• Seizure precautions: padded side rails, decreased stimuli, (noise, light); place airway suction equipment, padded mouth gag if Ca levels are low
• Store at room temperature

Evaluate:
• Therapeutic response: decreased twitching, paresthesias, muscle spasms, absence of tremors, convulsions, dysrhythmias, dyspnea, laryngospasm, negative Chvostek's sign, negative Trousseau's sign

Teach patient/family:
• To remain recumbent ½ hr after IV dose
• To add food high in vit D content
• To add calcium-rich foods to diet: dairy products, shellfish, dark green leafy vegetables; decrease oxalate-rich and zinc-rich foods: nuts, legumes, chocolate, spinach, soy
• To prevent injuries, avoid immobilization

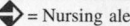 = Nursing alert   = Herb-drug interaction   = Do not crush

calcium polycarbophil (OTC)
(pol-i-kar'boe-fil)
Fiber Norm, Mitrolan
Func. class.: Laxative
Chem. class.: Bulk-forming

Action: Attracts water, expands in intestine to increase peristalsis; also absorbs excess water in stool; decreases diarrhea
Uses: Constipation, irritable bowel syndrome (diarrhea), acute, nonspecific diarrhea
Dosage and routes:
• *Adult:* PO 1 g qd-qid prn, not to exceed 6 g/24 hr
• *Child 6-12 yr:* PO 500 mg bid prn, not to exceed 3 g/24 hr
• *Child 3-6 yr:* PO 500 mg bid prn, not to exceed 1.5 g/24 hr
Available forms: Chew tabs 500, 625, 1250 mg
Side effects/adverse reactions:
GI: Obstruction, abdominal distention, flatus
Contraindications: Hypersensitivity, GI obstruction
Precautions: Pregnancy (C), lactation
Pharmacokinetics:
PO: Onset 12-24 min, peak 1-3 days
Interactions:
 Increased action/side effects: lily of the valley herb, pheasant's eye herb, squill
NURSING CONSIDERATIONS
Assess:
• Blood, urine electrolytes if used often
• I&O ratio to identify fluid loss
• Cause of constipation; identify whether fluids, bulk, or exercise is missing from lifestyle
• Cramping, rectal bleeding, nausea, vomiting; if these symptoms occur, drug should be discontinued

Administer:
PO
• Alone for better absorption; do not take within 1 hr of other drugs
• In morning or evening (oral dose)
Evaluate:
• Therapeutic response: decreased constipation
Teach patient/family:
• Not to use laxatives for long-term therapy; bowel tone will be lost
• That normal bowel movements do not always occur daily
• Not to use in presence of abdominal pain, nausea, vomiting
• To notify prescriber if constipation unrelieved or if symptoms of electrolyte imbalance occur: muscle cramps, pain, weakness, dizziness
• To chew thoroughly and follow with water

capreomycin (R)
(kap-ree-oh-mye'sin)
Capastat Sulfate
Func. class.: Antitubercular
Chem. class.: S. capreolus polypeptide antibiotic

Action: Inhibits RNA synthesis, decreases tubercle bacilli replication
Uses: Pulmonary TB as adjunct
Dosage and routes:
• *Adult:* IM 1 g qd × 2-4 mo, then 1 g 2-3 ×/wk × 18-24 mo, not to exceed 20 mg/kg/day; must be given with another antitubercular medication
• *Child:* 15 mg/kg/day (max 1 g)
Available forms: Powder for inj 1 g/10 ml vial
Side effects/adverse reactions:
INTEG: Pain, irritation, sterile abscess at injection site, rash, urticaria
CNS: Vertigo, fever, headache
EENT: Tinnitus, *deafness, ototoxicity*

*GU: **Proteinuria**,* decreased CrCl, increased BUN, serum Cr, ***tubular necrosis,*** hypokalemia, alkalosis, ***hematuria, albuminuria, nephrotoxicity***

*HEMA: **Eosinophilia, leukocytosis, leukopenia***

Contraindications: Hypersensitivity

Precautions: Renal disease, hearing impairment, allergy history, hepatic disease, pregnancy (C), lactation

Pharmacokinetics:

IM: Peak 1-2 hr, half-life 4-6 hr; excreted in urine unchanged

Interactions:

• Increased renal toxicity: aminoglycosides, polymyxin, colistin, vancomycin

• Increased neuroblocking action: phenothiazine, tubocurarine, neostigmine

NURSING CONSIDERATIONS
Assess:

• Liver studies qwk: ALT, AST, bilirubin; potassium

• Renal status: before; qwk: BUN, creatinine, output, specific gravity, urinalysis

• Blood levels of drug

• Audiometric testing before, during, after treatment

• Ototoxicity: tinnitus, vertigo, change in hearing

• Hepatic status: decreased appetite, jaundice, dark urine, fatigue

Administer:

IM

• After reconstituting with 2 ml NS or sterile water for injection, wait 2-3 min before giving; IM in large muscle mass; rotate sites

• With other antituberculars

• Reduced dosage in renal impairment; if BUN >20 mg/dl, drug should be decreased or discontinued

Evaluate:

• Therapeutic response: decreased dyspnea, fatigue

Teach patient/family:

• That compliance with dosage schedule, duration is necessary

• To notify health-care provider of side effects, adverse reactions: hearing loss, change in urine or urinary habits

---

captopril (℞)

(kap′toe-pril)
Capoten
Func. class.: Antihypertensive
Chem. class.: Angiotensin-converting enzyme inhibitor (ACE)

Action: Selectively suppresses renin-angiotensin-aldosterone system; inhibits ACE; preventing conversion of angiotensin I to angiotensin II; results in dilation of arterial, venous vessels

Uses: Hypertension, CHF, left ventricular dysfunction after MI, diabetic nephropathy

Dosage and routes:

Malignant hypertension

• *Adult:* **PO** 25 mg increasing q2h until desired response, not to exceed 450 mg/day

Hypertension

• *Initial dose:* 25 mg bid-tid; may increase to 50 mg bid-tid at 1-2 wk intervals; usual range: 25-150 mg bid-tid; max 450 mg

• *Child:* **PO** 0.3-0.5 mg/kg/dose, titrate up to 6 mg/kg/day in 2-4 divided doses

CHF

• *Adult:* **PO** 12.5 mg bid-tid; may increase to 50 mg bid-tid; after 14 days, may increase to 150 mg tid if needed

LVD after MI

• *Adult:* **PO** 50 mg tid, may begin treatment 3 days after MI; give 6.25

◆ = Nursing alert   🌢 = Herb-drug interaction   🚫 = Do not crush mg as a single dose, then 12.5 mg tid, increase to 25 mg tid for several days, then to 50 mg tid

Diabetic nephropathy
• *Adult:* **PO** 25 mg tid

Available forms: Tabs 12.5, 25, 50, 100 mg

Side effects/adverse reactions:

CV: Hypotension, postural hypotension

GU: Impotence, dysuria, nocturia, proteinuria, *nephrotic syndrome, acute reversible renal failure,* polyuria, oliguria, frequency

HEMA: **Neutropenia**

INT: Rash, *angioedema*

RESP: **Bronchospasm,** dyspnea, *cough*

META: Hyperkalemia

GI: Loss of taste

CNS: Fever, chills

Contraindications: Hypersensitivity, lactation, heart block, children, K-sparing diuretics, bilateral renal artery stenosis

Precautions: Dialysis patients, hypovolemia, leukemia, scleroderma, lupus erythematosus, blood dyscrasias, CHF, diabetes mellitus, renal disease, thyroid disease, COPD, asthma, pregnancy (C)

Pharmacokinetics:

PO: Peak 1 hr; duration 2-6 hr; half-life 6-7 hr; metabolized by liver (metabolites), excreted in urine; crosses placenta; excreted in breast milk

Interactions:

• Increased hypotension: diuretics, other antihypertensives, ganglionic blockers, adrenergic blockers

• Do not use with potassium-sparing diuretics, sympathomimetics, potassium supplements

Lab test interferences:

False positive: Urine acetone

NURSING CONSIDERATIONS

Assess:

• Blood studies: neutrophils, decreased platelets

• B/P

• Renal studies: protein, BUN, creatinine; watch for increased levels that may indicate nephrotic syndrome

• Baselines in renal, liver function tests before therapy begins

• Dipstick of urine for protein qd in first morning specimen; if protein is increased, a 24-hr urinary protein should be collected

• Edema in feet, legs daily

• Allergic reaction: rash, fever, pruritus, urticaria; drug should be discontinued if antihistamines fail to help

• Symptoms of CHF: edema, dyspnea, wet rales, B/P

• Renal symptoms: polyuria, oliguria, frequency

Administer:

• 1 hr ac or 1½ hr pc

Perform/provide:

• Storage in tight container at 86° F (30° C) or less

• Supine or Trendelenburg position for severe hypotension

Evaluate:

• Therapeutic response: decrease in B/P in hypertension, edema, moist rales (CHF)

Teach patient/family:

• That tabs may be crushed and mixed with food

• To administer 1 hr before meals

• Not to discontinue drug abruptly

• Not to use OTC (cough, cold, or allergy) products unless directed by prescriber

• To avoid sunlight or wear sunscreen if in sunlight; photosensitivity may occur

• To comply with dosage schedule, even if feeling better

• To rise slowly to sitting or standing position to minimize orthostatic hypotension

• To notify prescriber of mouth sores, sore throat, fever, swelling of

hands or feet, irregular heartbeat, chest pain, signs of angioedema
• That excessive perspiration, dehydration, vomiting; diarrhea may lead to fall in blood pressure; consult prescriber if these occur
• That dizziness, fainting, light-headedness may occur during first few days of therapy
• That skin rash or impaired perspiration may occur
• How to take B/P

Treatment of overdose: 0.9% NaCl IV/INF; hemodialysis

---

carbamazepine (℞)

(kar-ba-maz′e-peen)
Apo-Carbamazepine*, Atretol, Carbatrol, Epitol, Novo Carbamaz*, Tegretol, Tegretol CR*, Tegretol-XR
Func. class.: Anticonvulsant
Chem. class.: Iminostilbene derivative

Action: Inhibits nerve impulses by limiting influx of sodium ions across cell membrane in motor cortex
Uses: Tonic-clonic, complex-partial, mixed seizures; trigeminal neuralgia, diabetic neuropathy
Investigational uses: Diabetes insipidus, bipolar disorder, neurogenic pain, schizophrenia, psychotic behavior with dementia
Dosage and routes:
Seizures
• *Adult and child >12 yr:* **PO** 200 mg bid, may be increased by 200 mg/day in divided doses q6-8h; maintenance 800-1200 mg/day maximum 1200 mg/day; adjustment is needed to minimum dose to control seizures; ext rel give bid
• *Child <12 yr:* **PO** 10-20 mg/kg/day in 3-4 divided doses

Trigeminal neuralgia
• *Adult:* **PO** 100 mg bid with meals; may increase 100 mg q12h until pain subsides, not to exceed 1.2 g/day; maintenance is 200-400 mg bid
Available forms: Tabs, chewable 100 mg; tabs 200 mg; ext-rel tabs 100, 200, 400 mg; oral susp 100 mg/5 ml
Side effects/adverse reactions:
HEMA: ***Thrombocytopenia, agranulocytosis, leukocytosis, neutropenia, aplastic anemia, eosinophilia,*** increased pro-time
ENDO: SIADH (elderly)
CNS: Drowsiness, dizziness, confusion, fatigue, *paralysis,* headache, hallucinations, worsening of seizures
GI: Nausea, constipation, diarrhea, anorexia, vomiting, abdominal pain, stomatitis, glossitis, increased liver enzymes, ***hepatitis***
INTEG: Rash, ***Stevens-Johnson syndrome,*** urticaria
EENT: Tinnitus, dry mouth, blurred vision, diplopia, nystagmus, conjunctivitis
CV: ***Hypertension, CHF,*** hypotension, aggravation of cardiac artery disease
RESP: Pulmonary hypersensitivity (fever, dyspnea, pneumonitis)
GU: Frequency, retention, albuminuria, glycosuria, impotence, increased BUN
Contraindications: Hypersensitivity to carbamazepine or tricyclic antidepressants, bone marrow depression, concomitant use of MAOIs
Precautions: Glaucoma, hepatic disease, renal disease, cardiac disease, psychosis, pregnancy (C), lactation, child <6 yr
Pharmacokinetics:
PO: Onset slow, peak 4-8 hr; metabolized by liver; excreted in urine, feces; crosses placenta, blood-brain barrier; excreted in breast milk; half-life 14-16 hr

---

Interactions:
• Toxicity: troleandomycin, erythromycin, cimetidine, diltiazem, isoniazid, propoxyphene, lithium, verapamil, clarithromycin
• Decreased effects of phenobarbital, phenytoin, primidone, warfarin, oral contraceptives, theophylline, thyroid hormones, benzodiazepines
• Increased effects of vasopressin, lypressin, desmopressin, lithium
• Fatal reaction: MAOIs
Lab test interferences:
Decrease: Thyroid function tests
NURSING CONSIDERATIONS
Assess:
• Renal studies: urinalysis, BUN, urine creatinine q3mo
• Blood studies: RBC, Hct, Hgb, reticulocyte counts qwk for 4 wk then qmo; if myelosuppression occurs, drug should be discontinued
• Hepatic studies: ALT, AST, bilirubin
• Drug levels during initial treatment or when changing dose; should remain at 3-9 µg/ml; anorexia may indicate increased blood levels
• Description of seizures
• Mental status: mood, sensorium, affect, behavioral changes; if mental status changes, notify prescriber
• Eye problems: need for ophthalmic examinations before, during, after treatment (slit lamp, fundoscopy, tonometry)
• Allergic reaction: purpura, red, raised rash; if these occur, drug should be discontinued
• Blood dyscrasias: fever, sore throat, bruising, rash, jaundice
◆ Toxicity: bone marrow depression, nausea, vomiting, ataxia, diplopia, cardiovascular collapse, Stevens-Johnson syndrome

Administer:
PO
• With food, milk to decrease GI symptoms
• Chewable tablets; tell patient to chew tablet, not swallow it whole
Perform/provide:
• Storage at room temperature
• Hard candy, frequent rinsing of mouth, gum for dry mouth
• Assistance with ambulation during early part of treatment; dizziness occurs
Evaluate:
• Therapeutic response: decreased seizure activity, document on patient's chart
Teach patient/family:
• To carry Medic Alert ID stating patient's name, drugs taken, condition, prescriber's name, phone number
• To avoid driving, other activities that require alertness
• To avoid alcohol ingestion; convulsions may result
• Not to discontinue medication quickly after long-term use
• That urine may turn pink to brown
Treatment of overdose: Lavage, VS

carbidopa-levodopa (R̶)
(kar-bi-doe′pa) (lee-voe doe′pa)
carbidopa/levodopa
Sinemet, Sinemet CR
Func. class.: Antiparkinson agent
Chem. class.: Catecholamine

Action: Decarboxylation of levodopa to periphery is inhibited by carbidopa; more levodopa is made available for transport to brain and conversion to dopamine in the brain
Uses: Parkinson's disease, parkinsonism resulting from carbon

monoxide, chronic manganese intoxication, cerebral arteriosclerosis, restless leg syndrome

Dosage and routes:
• *Adult:* **PO** 3-6 tabs of 25 mg carbidopa/250 mg levodopa qd in divided doses, not to exceed 8 tabs/day; **SUST REL** 1 tablet bid at intervals of not less than 6 hr usual: 2-8 tabs/day at intervals of 4-8 hr

Available forms: Tabs 10/100, 25/100, 25 mg carbidopa/250 mg levodopa sust rel tab: 50 mg/200 mg carbidopa/levodopa

Side effects/adverse reactions:
HEMA: **Hemolytic anemia, leukopenia, agranulocytosis**
CNS: Involuntary choreiform movements, hand tremors, fatigue, headache, anxiety, twitching, numbness, weakness, confusion, agitation, insomnia, nightmares, psychosis, hallucination, hypomania, severe depression, dizziness
GI: Nausea, vomiting, anorexia, abdominal distress, dry mouth, flatulence, dysphagia, bitter taste, diarrhea, constipation
INTEG: Rash, sweating, alopecia
CV: Orthostatic hypotension, tachycardia, hypertension, palpitation
EENT: Blurred vision, diplopia, dilated pupils
MISC: Urinary retention, incontinence, weight change, dark urine

Contraindications: Hypersensitivity, narrow-angle glaucoma, undiagnosed skin lesions

Precautions: Renal disease, cardiac disease, hepatic disease, respiratory disease, MI with dysrhythmias, convulsions, peptic ulcer, pregnancy (C), lactation

Pharmacokinetics:
PO: Peak 1-3 hr, exceted in urine (metabolites)

Interactions:
• Hypertensive crisis: MAOIs, furazolidone

• Decreased effects of levodopa: anticholinergics, hydantoins, methionine, papaverine, pyridoxine, tricyclics, benzodiazepines
• Increased effects of levodopa: antacids, metoclopramide
• Drug/food: increased pyridoxine will decrease levodopa effect

💉 Decreased action, increased EPS: Indian snakeroot

Lab test interferences:
False positive: Urine ketones
False negative: Urine glucose
False increase: Uric acid, urine protein
Decrease: VMA, BUN, creatinine

NURSING CONSIDERATIONS
Assess:
• B/P, respiration; orthostatic B/P
• Mental status: affect, mood, behavioral changes, depression, complete suicide assessment

Administer:
PO
• Drug until NPO before surgery
• Adjust dosage to response
• With meals; limit protein taken with drug
• Only after MAOIs have been discontinued for 2 wk; if previously on levodopa, discontinue for at least 8 hr before change to carbidopa-levodopa

Perform/provide:
• Assistance with ambulation during beginning therapy
• Testing for diabetes mellitus, acromegaly if on long-term therapy

Evaluate:
• Therapeutic response: decrease in akathisia, improved mood

Teach patient/family:
🚫 Not to crush or chew cont rel tabs; may be broken in half
• To change positions slowly to prevent orthostatic hypotension
• To report side effects: twitching, eye spasms; indicate overdose

---

◆ = Nursing alert   💉 = Herb-drug interaction   🚫 = Do not crush

- To use drug exactly as prescribed; if discontinued abruptly, parkinsonian crisis may occur; prescriber may recommend drug-free holidays
- That urine, sweat may darken
- To use physical activities to maintain mobility, lessen spasms
- That improvement may not occur for 3-4 mo

---

carboplatin (R)
(kar-boe-pla′-tin)
Paraplatin, Paraplatin-AQ*
Func. class.: Antineoplastic alkylating agent
Chem. class.: Platinum coordination compound

Action: Produces interstrand DNA cross-links and to a lesser extent DNA protein cross-links; activity is not cell cycle phase specific

Uses: Palliative treatment of ovarian carcinoma recurrent after treatment with other antineoplastic agents

Dosage and routes (single agent):
- *Adult:* IV INF 360 mg/m^2 given over >15 min on day 1 q4wk; do not repeat single intermittent courses until neutrophil count is >2,000/mm^3 and platelet count is >100,000/mm^3

Available forms: Inj 50, 150, 450 mg/vial

Side effects/adverse reactions:

EENT: Tinnitus, hearing loss, *vestibular toxicity*

HEMA: **Thrombocytopenia, leukopenia, pancytopenia, neutropenia,** anemia, bleeding

CV: Cardiac abnormalities

GI: Severe nausea, vomiting, diarrhea, weight loss

GU: **Renal tubular damage,** renal insufficiency, impotence, sterility, amenorrhea, gynecomastia

INTEG: Alopecia, dermatitis, rash, erythema, pruritus, urticaria

CNS: **Convulsions, central neurotoxicity,** peripheral neuropathy

RESP: Mucositis

META: Hypomagnesemia, hypocalcemia, hypokalemia, hyponatremia, hyperuremia

Contraindications: Hypersensitivity to this drug, platinum products, mannitol; severe bone marrow depression, significant bleeding, pregnancy (D)

Precautions: Radiation therapy within 1 mo, chemotherapy within 1 mo, lactation, liver disease

Pharmacokinetics: Initial half-life 1-2 hr, postdistribution half-life 2 ½-6 hr, not bound to plasma proteins, excreted by the kidneys

Interactions:
- Increased nephrotoxicity or ototoxicity: aminoglycosides

NURSING CONSIDERATIONS
Assess:
- CBC, differential, platelet count weekly; withhold drug if WBC count is <4000/mm^3 or platelet count is <100,000/mm^3; notify prescriber of results
- Renal function studies: BUN, creatinine, serum uric acid, urine CrCL before and during therapy
- I&O ratio; report fall in urine output to <30 ml/hr
- Monitor temperature q4h (may indicate beginning of infection)
- Liver function tests before and during therapy (bilirubin, AST [SGOT], ALT [SGPT], LDH) as needed or monthly
- Bleeding; hematuria, stool guaiac, bruising or petechiae, mucosa or orifices q8h
- Dyspnea, rales, unproductive cough, chest pain, tachypnea
- Food preferences; list likes, dislikes

• Effects of alopecia on body image; discuss feelings about body changes
• Yellowing of skin, sclera, dark urine, clay-colored stools, itchy skin, abdominal pain, fever, diarrhea
• Edema in feet, joint pain, stomach pain, shaking
• Inflammation of mucosa, breaks in skin

Administer:
• Antiemetic 30-60 min before giving drug and prn for vomiting
• Allopurinol or sodium bicarbonate to maintain uric acid levels, alkalinization of urine

IV
• After diluting 10 mg/ml of sterile water for inj, D_5W, NS (10 mg/ml); then further dilute with the same sol 1-4 mg/ml; give over 15 min or more (INT INF)
• IV INF over 5-6 hr; do not use needles or IV administration sets containing aluminum; may cause precipitate
• Diuretic (furosemide 40 mg IV) after infusion

Additive compatibilities: Cisplatin, etoposide, floxuridine, ifosfamide, ifosfamide/etoposide

Solution compatibilities: D_5/0.2% NaCl, D_5/0.45% NaCl, D_5/0.9% NaCl, 0.9% NaCl, D_5W, sterile water for inj

Y-site compatibilities: Allopurinol, amifostine, aztreonam, cefepime, cladribine, filgrastim, fludarabine, granisetron, melphalan, ondansetron, paclitaxel, piperacillin/tazobactam, propofol, sargramostim, teniposide, thiotepa, vinorelbine

Perform/provide:
• Storage protected from light at room temperature; reconstituted sol stable for 8 hr at room temp
• Deep-breathing exercises with patient tid-qid; place in semi-Fowler's position

• Increase fluid intake to 2-3 L/day to prevent urate deposits and calculi formation and to speed elimination of drug
• Diet low in purines: organ meats (kidney, liver), dried beans, peas to maintain alkaline urine

Evaluate:
• Therapeutic response: decreasing size of tumor, spread of malignancy

Teach patient/family:
• To report any complaints or side effects to nurse or prescriber
• That impotence or amenorrhea can occur; reversible after treatment is discontinued
• To report any changes in breathing or coughing
• That hair may be lost during treatment; a wig or hairpiece may make patient feel better; new hair may be different in color, texture

---

carboprost (Ŗ)

(kar'boe-prost)
Hemabate, Prostin/15M*
Func. class.: Oxytocic
Chem. class.: Prostaglandin

Action: Stimulates uterine contractions, causing complete abortion in approximately 16 hr

Uses: Abortion at 13-20 wk gestation

Dosage and routes:
• *Adult:* **IM** 250 μg, then 250 μg q1½- 3½ h, may increase to 500 μg if no response, not to exceed 12 mg total dose

Available forms: Inj 250 μg/ml carboprost, 83 μg/ml tromethamine

Side effects/adverse reactions:
CNS: Fever, chills, headache
GI: Nausea, vomiting, diarrhea

Contraindications: Hypersensitivity, severe hepatic disease, severe renal disease, PID, respiratory disease, cardiac disease

---

◆ = Nursing alert   ∅ = Herb-drug interaction   ⊘ = Do not crush

Precautions: Asthma, anemia, jaundice, diabetes mellitus, convulsive disorders, past uterine surgery, pregnancy (C)

Pharmacokinetics: Onset 15 min, peak 2 hr; metabolized in lungs, liver; excreted in urine (metabolites)

Interactions:

🕭 Hypertension: Ephedra

NURSING CONSIDERATIONS

Assess:

• B/P, pulse; watch for change that may indicate hemorrhage

• Respiratory rate, rhythm, depth; notify prescriber of abnormalities

• For length, duration of contraction; notify prescriber of contractions lasting over 1 min or absence of contractions

• For incomplete abortion, pregnancy must be terminated by another method; drug is teratogenic

Administer:

IM

• In deep muscle mass; rotate injection sites if additional doses are given

Perform/provide:

• Emotional support before and after the abortion

Evaluate:

• Therapeutic response: expulsion of fetus

Teach patient/family:

• To report increased blood loss, abdominal cramps, increased temperature, foul smelling lochia

• Some methods of comfort control and pain control

---

carisoprodol (℞)

(kar-eye-soe-proe′dole)
carisoprodol, Soma, Vanadom

Func. class.: Skeletal muscle relaxant, central acting

Chem. class.: Meprobamate congener

Action: Depresses CNS by blocking interneuronal activity in descending reticular formation, spinal cord, producing sedation

Uses: Relieving pain, stiffness in musculoskeletal disorders

Dosage and routes:

• *Adult and child >12 yr·* **PO** 350 mg tid, hs

Available forms: Tabs 350 mg

Side effects/adverse reactions:

CNS: Dizziness, weakness, drowsiness, headache, tremor, depression, insomnia, ataxia, irritability

EENT: Diplopia, temporary loss of vision

CV: Postural hypotension, tachycardia

GI: Nausea, vomiting, hiccups, epigastric discomfort

INTEG: Rash, pruritus, fever, facial flushing

Contraindications: Hypersensitivity, child <12 yr, intermittent porphyria

Precautions: Renal disease, hepatic disease, addictive personality, pregnancy (C), elderly, lactation

Pharmacokinetics:

PO: Onset ½ hr, duration 4-6 hr; metabolized by liver; excreted in urine; crosses placenta; excreted in breast milk (large amounts); half-life 8 hr

Interactions:

• Increased CNS depression: alcohol, tricyclic antidepressants, narcotics, barbiturates, sedatives, hypnotics

---

🖊 May increase CNS depression: kava kava

NURSING CONSIDERATIONS
Assess:
• Blood studies: CBC, WBC, differential; blood dyscrasias may occur
• Liver function studies: AST, ALT, alk phosphatase; hepatitis may occur
• ECG in epileptic patients; poor seizure control has occurred with patients taking this drug
• Idiosyncratic reaction, anaphylaxis within a few min or hr of 1st to 4th dose
• Allergic reactions: rash, fever, respiratory distress
• Severe weakness, numbness in extremities
• Psychologic dependency: increased need for medication, more frequent requests for medication, increased pain
• CNS depression: dizziness, drowsiness, psychiatric symptoms

Administer:
PO
• With meals for GI symptoms

Perform/provide:
• Storage in tight container at room temperature
• Assistance with ambulation if dizziness, drowsiness occurs, especially elderly

Evaluate:
• Therapeutic response: decreased pain, spasticity

Teach patient/family:
• Not to discontinue medication quickly; insomnia, nausea, headache, spasticity, tachycardia will occur; drug should be tapered off over 1-2 wk
• Not to take with alcohol, other CNS depressants
• To avoid hazardous activities if drowsiness, dizziness occur
• To avoid using OTC medication:

cough preparations, antihistamines, unless directed by prescriber

Treatment of overdose: Induce emesis of conscious patient, lavage, dialysis

---

carmustine (℞)
(kar-mus′teen)
BiCNU, BCNU, Gliadel
Func. class.: Antineoplastic alkylating agent
Chem. class.: Nitrosourea

Action: Alkylates DNA, RNA; is able to inhibit enzymes that allow synthesis of amino acids in proteins; activity is not cell cycle phase specific

Uses: Brain tumors such as glioblastoma, medulloblastoma, astrocytoma; multiple myeloma, Hodgkin's disease, other lymphomas; GI, breast, bronchogenic, renal carcinomas

Dosage and routes:
• *Adult:* **IV** 75-100 mg/m^2 over 1-2 hr × 2 days or 200 mg/m^2 × 1 dose q6-8wk; if leukocytes fall below 2000 or platelets below 75,000, only 50% of dose should be given
• *Adult:* **INTRACAVITARY** wafer: 8 inserted into resection cavity
Available forms: Powder for inj 100 mg; wafer 7.7 mg

Side effects/adverse reactions:
HEMA: **Thrombocytopenia, leukopenia, myelosuppression, anemia**
GI: Nausea, vomiting, anorexia, stomatitis, **hepatotoxicity**
GU: Azotemia, **renal failure**
INTEG: Burning, hyperpigmentation at injection site
RESP: **Fibrosis, pulmonary infiltrate**

Contraindications: Hypersensitivity, leukopenia, thrombocytopenia
Precautions: Pregnancy (D), lactation

Pharmacokinetics: Degraded within 15 min; crosses blood-brain barrier; 70% excreted in urine within 96 hr; 10% excreted as CO_2; fate of 20% is unknown

Interactions:

• Increased toxicity: other antineoplastics, radiation
• Enhanced action: vit A, caffeine
• Increased toxicity: cimetidine, other antineoplastics, radiation

NURSING CONSIDERATIONS
Assess:

• CBC, differential, platelet count weekly; withhold drug if WBC is <4000 or platelet count is <75,000; notify prescriber of results
• Liver function tests: AST, ALT, bilirubin
• Pulmonary function tests, chest x-ray films before, during therapy; chest film should be obtained q2wk during treatment
• Renal function studies: BUN, serum uric acid, urine CrCl before, during therapy
• I&O ratio; report fall in urine output of 30 ml/hr
• Monitor for cold, cough, fever (may indicate beginning infection)
• Bleeding: hematuria, guaiac, bruising, petechiae, mucosa, orifices q8h
• Dyspnea, rales, unproductive cough, chest pain, tachypnea
• Food preferences; list likes, dislikes
• Inflammation of mucosa, breaks in skin

Administer:

• Antiemetic 30-60 min before giving drug to prevent vomiting
• Antibiotics for prophylaxis of infection

IV

• After diluting 100 mg drug/3 ml ethyl alcohol (provided); then further dilute 27 ml sterile H_2O for inj; then dilute with 100-500 ml 0.9% NaCl or D_5W, give over 1 hr or more, reduce rate if discomfort is felt

Y-site compatibilities: Amifostine, aztreonam, cefepime, filgrastim, fludarabine, granisetron, melphalan, ondansetron, piperacillin/tazobactam, sargramostim, teniposide, thiotepa, vinorelbine

Perform/provide:

• Storage in refrigerator
• Strict medical asepsis, protective isolation if WBC levels are low
• Special skin care
• Deep-breathing exercises with patient tid-qid; place in semi-Fowler's position
• Increase fluid intake to 2-3 L/day to prevent urate deposits, calculi formation
• Rinsing of mouth tid-qid with water or club soda; brushing of teeth bid-tid with soft brush or cotton-tipped applicators for stomatitis; use unwaxed dental floss, use viscous lidocaine (Xylocaine)
• Warm compresses at injection site for inflammation; reduce flow rate if patient complains of burning at infusion site

Evaluate:

• Therapeutic response: decreasing size of tumor, spread of malignancy

Teach patient/family:

• Protective isolation precautions
• To report any changes in breathing or coughing
• To avoid foods with citric acid, hot or rough texture
• To report any bleeding, white spots, ulceration in mouth to prescriber; tell patient to examine mouth qd
• To avoid use of aspirin, ibuprofen, razors, commercial mouthwash
• To report signs of anemia (fatigue, irritability, shortness of breath, faintness)
• To report signs of infection (sore throat, fever)

---

carteolol (℞)

(kar-tee'oh-lole)

Cartrol, Ocupress

Func. class.: Antihypertensive

Chem. class.: Nonselective β-blocker

Action: Produces fall in B/P without reflex tachycardia or significant reduction in heart rate through mixture of α-blocking, β-blocking effects and intrinsic sympathomimetic activity; elevated plasma renins are reduced

Uses: Mild to moderate hypertension, ophthalmic, intraocular, open-angle glaucoma

Dosage and routes:
• *Adult:* **PO** 2.5 mg qd initially, may gradually increase to desired response, max 10 mg/day; **OPHTH** 1 gtt bid

Renal disease
• CrCl 20-60 ml/min give dose q48h; CrCl <20 ml/min give dose q72h

Available forms: Tabs 2.5, 5 mg; ophth sol 1%

Side effects/adverse reactions:

CV: Orthostatic hypotension, *bradycardia, CHF, chest pain, ventricular dysrhythmias, AV block, peripheral vascular insufficiency,* palpitations

CNS: Dizziness, mental changes, drowsiness, fatigue, headache, catatonia, depression, anxiety, nightmares, paresthesia, lethargy, insomnia, decreased concentration

GI: Nausea, vomiting, diarrhea, dry mouth, flatulence, constipation, anorexia

INTEG: Rash, alopecia, urticaria, pruritus, fever

HEMA: Agranulocytosis, thrombocytopenic purpura (rare)

EENT: Tinnitus, visual changes, sore throat, double vision, dry burning eyes

GU: Impotence, dysuria, ejaculatory failure, urinary retention

RESP: **Bronchospasm,** dyspnea, wheezing, nasal stuffiness, pharyngitis

MS: Joint pain, arthralgia, muscle cramps, pain

OTHER: Facial swelling, decreased exercise tolerance, weight change, Raynaud's disease

Contraindications: Hypersensitivity to β-blockers, cardiogenic shock, heart block (2nd or 3rd degree), sinus bradycardia, bronchial asthma

Precautions: Major surgery, pregnancy (C), lactation, CHF, diabetes mellitus, renal disease, thyroid disease, COPD, well-compensated heart failure, nonallergic bronchospasm

Pharmacokinetics:

PO: Onset 1-2 hr, peak 2-4 hr, duration 8-12 hr, half-life 6-8 hr; metabolized by liver (metabolites inactive); excreted in urine, bile; crosses placenta; excreted in breast milk

Interactions:
• Increased hypotension: diuretics, other antihypertensives, halothane, nitroglycerin, prazosin
• Decreased β-blocker effects: sympathomimetics, nonsteroidal antiinflammatory agents, salicylates
• Increased hypoglycemic effect: insulin
• Increased effects of lidocaine
• Decreased bronchodilating effects of theophylline, β-agonists

Lab test interferences:

False increase: Urinary catecholamines

Interference: Glucose, insulin tolerance tests

NURSING CONSIDERATIONS

Assess:
• I&O, weight daily

 = Nursing alert   = Herb-drug interaction   = Do not crush

- B/P, pulse q4h; note rate, rhythm, quality
- Apical/radial pulse before administration; notify prescriber of any significant changes
- Baselines in renal, liver function tests before therapy begins
- Edema in feet, legs daily
- Skin turgor, dryness of mucous membranes for hydration status

Administer:

PO

- Drug ac, hs; tablet may be crushed or swallowed whole
- Reduced dosage in renal dysfunction

Perform/provide:

- Storage in dry area at room temperature; do not freeze

Evaluate:

- Therapeutic response: decreased B/P after 1-2 wk

Teach patient/family:

- Not to discontinue drug abruptly; taper over 2 wk, or may precipitate angina
- Not to use OTC products containing α-adrenergic stimulants (nasal decongestants, OTC cold preparations) unless directed by prescriber
- To report bradycardia, dizziness, confusion, depression, fever
- To take pulse at home, advise when to notify prescriber
- To avoid alcohol, smoking, sodium intake
- To comply with weight control, dietary adjustments, modified exercise program
- To carry Medic Alert ID to identify drug being taken, allergies
- To avoid hazardous activities if dizziness is present
- To report symptoms of CHF: difficult breathing, especially on exertion or when lying down, night cough, swelling of extremities
- To take medication hs to minimize orthostatic hypotension

- The method of instillation if using ophthalmic

Treatment of overdose: Lavage, IV atropine for bradycardia, IV theophylline for bronchospasm, digitalis, O_2, diuretic for cardiac failure; administer vasopressor (norepinephrine) for hypotension, isoproterenol for heart block

---

carvedilol (R)

(kar-ved′i-lole)
Coreg
Func. class.: α/β-adrenergic blocker

Action: A mixture of nonselective α/β-adrenergic blocking activity; decreases cardiac output, exercise-induced tachycardia, reflex orthostatic tachycardia; causes vasodilation, reduction in peripheral vascular resistance

Uses: Essential hypertension alone or in combination with other antihypertensives, CHF

Investigational uses: Angina pectoris, idiopathic cardiomyopathy

Dosage and routes:

Essential hypertension

- *Adult:* **PO** 6.25 mg bid × 7-14 days; if tolerated well, then increase to 12.5 mg bid × 7-14 days; if tolerated well, may be increased (if needed) to 25 mg bid; not to exceed 50 mg qd

Congestive heart failure

- *Adult:* **PO** 3.125 mg bid × 2 wk; if tolerated well, give 6.25 mg bid × 2 wk, then double q2wk to max dose

Angina pectoris

- *Adult:* **PO** 25-50 mg bid

Idiopathic cardiomyopathy

- *Adult:* **PO** 6.25-25 mg bid

Available forms: Tabs 3.125, 6.25, 12.5, 25 mg

Side effects/adverse reactions:
CNS: Dizziness, somnolence, insomnia, ataxia, hyperesthesia, paresthesia, vertigo, depression
GI: Diarrhea, abdominal pain
CV: Bradycardia, postural hypotension, dependent edema, peripheral edema, *AV block,* extrasystoles, hypertension, hypotension, palpitations, peripheral ischemia
RESP: Rhinitis, pharyngitis, dyspnea
MISC: Fatigue, injury, back pain, UTI, viral infection, hypertriglyceridemia, *thrombocytopenia*

Contraindications: Hypersensitivity, bronchial asthma, class IV decompensated cardiac failure, 2nd- or 3rd-degree heart block, cardiogenic shock, severe bradycardia

Precautions: Cardiac failure, hepatic injury, peripheral vascular disease, anesthesia, major surgery, diabetes mellitus, thyrotoxicosis, elderly, pregnancy (C), lactation, children, emphysema, chronic bronchitis, renal disease

Pharmacokinetics: Readily and extensively absorbed PO, >98% bound to plasma proteins, extensively metabolized by liver, excreted through bile into feces, terminal half-life 5-9 hr with increases in elderly, hepatic disease

Interactions:
• Increased hypoglycemia: antidiabetic agents
• Increased heart rate, B/P: clonidine
• Increased concentrations of digoxin
• Increased levels of carvedilol: cimetidine
• Decreased levels of carvedilol: rifampin

NURSING CONSIDERATIONS
Assess:
⬥ Renal studies, including protein, BUN, creatinine; watch for increased levels that may indicate nephrotic syndrome; obtain baselines in renal, liver function studies before beginning treatment
• I&O, weight daily
• B/P during beginning treatment, periodically thereafter; pulse q4h, note rate, rhythm, quality
• Apical/radial pulse before administration; notify prescriber of significant changes
• Edema in feet, legs daily

Administer:
PO
• Drug ac, hs; tablets may be crushed or swallowed whole
• Reduced dosage in renal dysfunction; give with food to decrease orthostatic hypotension

Evaluate:
• Therapeutic response: decreased B/P in hypertension

Teach patient/family:
• To comply with dosage schedule, even if feeling better
• To rise slowly to sitting or standing position to minimize orthostatic hypotension
• To report bradycardia, dizziness, confusion, depression, fever
• To take pulse at home; advise when to notify prescriber
• Not to discontinue drug abruptly

---

cascara sagrada/ cascara sagrada aromatic fluid extract/ cascara sagrada fluid extract (OTC)
(kas-kar'a)
Func. class.: Laxative
Chem. class.: Anthraquinone

Action: Direct chemical irritation in colon; increases propulsion of stool
Uses: Constipation; bowel or rectal

⬥ = Nursing alert   / = Herb-drug interaction   Ⓝ = Do not crush preparation for surgery or examination

Dosage and routes:
• *Adult:* **PO** 325 mg hs; **FLUID** 1 ml qd; **AROMATIC FLUID** 5 ml qd
• *Child 2-12 yr:* **PO/FLUID/AROMATIC FLUID** ½ adult dose
• *Child <2 yr:* **PO/FLUID/AROMATIC FLUID** ¼ adult dose
Available forms: Powder; tabs 325 mg; oral sol

Side effects/adverse reactions:
GI: Nausea, vomiting, anorexia, cramps, diarrhea
META: Hypocalcemia, enteropathy, alkalosis, hypokalemia, ***tetany***

Contraindications: Hypersensitivity, GI bleeding, obstruction, CHF, lactation, abdominal pain, nausea/vomiting, appendicitis, acute surgical abdomen, alcoholics (aromatic form)

Precautions: Pregnancy (C)

Pharmacokinetics:
PO: Peak 6-12 hr; metabolized by liver; excreted by kidneys, in feces

Interactions:
• Decreased absorption of these drugs: antibiotics, digitalis, nitrofurantoin, salicylates, tetracyclines, oral anticoagulants
🚫 Increased action/side effects: lily of the valley herb, pheasant's eye herb, squill

NURSING CONSIDERATIONS
Assess:
• Blood, urine electrolytes if drug is used often by patient
• I&O ratio to identify fluid loss
• Cause of constipation; identify whether fluids, bulk, or exercise missing from lifestyle
• Cramping, rectal bleeding, nausea, vomiting; if these symptoms occur, drug should be discontinued

Administer:
• Alone for better absorption; do not take within 1 hr of other drugs or within 1 hr of antacids, milk
• In morning or evening (oral dose)

Evaluate:
• Therapeutic response: decrease in constipation

Teach patient/family:
🚫 To swallow tabs whole; do not break, crush, or chew
• Not to use laxatives for long-term therapy; bowel tone will be lost
• That normal bowel movements do not always occur daily
• Not to use in presence of abdominal pain, nausea, vomiting
• To notify prescriber if constipation unrelieved or of symptoms of electrolyte imbalance: muscle cramps, pain, weakness, dizziness

cefaclor

cefadroxil
cefazolin

cefepime
cefixime

cefmandole
cefmetazole
cefonicid

cefoperazone
cefotaxime

cefotetan
cefoxitin

cefpodoxime

cefprozil

ceftazidime
ceftibuten
ceftizoxime
ceftriaxone

cefuroxime

cephalexin
cephalothin
cephapirin
cephradine

CEPHALOSPORINS—1ST GENERATION

cefadroxil (Rx)
(sef-a-drox'ill)
cefadroxil, Duricef, Ultracef

cefazolin (Rx)
(sef-a'zoe-lin)
Ancef, cefazolin, Gen-Cefazolin*, Kefzol, Zolicef

cephalexin (Rx)
(sef-a-lex'in)
Apo-Cephalex*, Cefanex, C-Lexin, cephalexin, Keflex, Keftab, Novo-Lexin*, Nu-Cephalex*

cephalothin (Rx)
(sef-a-loe'thin)
cephalothin, Keflin

cephapirin (Rx)
(sef-a-pye'rin)
Cefadyl, cephapirin

cephradine (Rx)
(sef'ra-deen)
cephradine, Velosef

Func. class.: Antiinfective
Chem. class.: Cephalosporin (1st generation)

Action: Inhibits bacterial cell wall synthesis, rendering cell wall osmotically unstable, leading to cell death by binding to cell wall membrane

Uses:

cefadroxil: gram-negative bacilli: *E. coli, P. mirabilis, Klebsiella* (UTI only); gram-positive organisms: *S. pneumoniae, S. pyogenes, S. aureus;* upper, lower respiratory tract, urinary tract, skin infections, otitis media; tonsillitis; and UTIs

cefazolin: gram-negative bacilli: *H. influenzae, E. coli, P. mirabilis, Klebsiella;* gram-positive organisms: *S. pneumoniae, S. pyogenes, S. aureus;* upper, lower respiratory tract, urinary tract, skin infections, bone, joint, biliary, genital infections, endocarditis, surgical prophylaxis, septicemia

cephalexin: gram-negative bacilli: *H. influenzae, E. coli, P. mirabilis, Klebsiella;* gram-positive organisms: *S. pneumoniae, S. pyogenes, S. aureus;* upper, lower respiratory tract, urinary tract, skin, bone infections, otitis media

cephalothin: gram-negative bacilli: *H. influenzae, E. coli, P. mirabilis, Klebsiella, Salmonella, Shigella;* gram-positive organisms: *S. pneumoniae, S. pyogenes, S. aureus;* upper, lower respiratory tract, skin infections, bone infections, endocarditis, septicemia, bacterial peritonitis

cephapirin: gram-negative bacilli: *H. influenzae, E. coli, P. mirabilis, Klebsiella;* gram-positive organisms: *S. pneumoniae, S. viridans, S. aureus;* lower respiratory tract, skin infections, endocarditis, bacterial peritonitis

cephradine: gram-negative bacilli: *H. influenzae, E. coli, P. mirabilis, Klebsiella;* gram-positive organisms: *S. pneumoniae, S. pyogenes, S. aureus;* serious respiratory tract, skin infections, urinary tract infections, otitis media

Dosage and routes:
cefadroxil
• *Adult:* **PO** 1-2 g qd or q12h in divided doses, give a loading dose of 1 g initially, reduce dose in renal disease (CrCl <50 ml/min)
• *Child:* **PO** 30/kg/day in divided doses

Available forms: Caps 500 mg; tabs 1 g; oral susp 125, 250, 500 mg/5 ml
cefazolin
Life-threatening infections
• *Adult:* **IM/IV** 1-2 g q6h
• *Child >1 mo:* **IM/IV** 100 mg/kg in 3-4 divided doses

Mild/moderate infections
• *Adult:* **IM/IV** 250 mg-1 g q8h
• *Child >1 mo:* **IM/IV** 25-50 mg/kg in 3-4 equal doses
Renal dose: CrCl 35-54 ml/min: 250-1000 mg q12h; CrCl 10-34 ml/min: 125-500 mg q12h; CrCl <10 ml/min: 125-500 mg q24h
Available forms: Inj 500 mg, 1, 5, 10, 20 g
cephalexin
Renal dose: CrCl <40 ml/min give q8-12h; CrCl 5-10 ml/min give q12h; CrCl <5 ml/min give q24h
Moderate infections
• *Adult:* **PO** 250-500 mg q6h
• *Child:* **PO** 25-50 mg/kg/day in 4 equal doses
Moderate skin infections
• *Adult:* **PO** 500 mg q12h
Severe infections
• *Adult:* **PO** 500 mg-1 g q6h
• *Child:* **PO** 50-100 mg/kg/day in 4 equal doses
Available forms: Caps 250, 500 mg; tabs 250, 500 mg, 1 g; oral susp 125, 250 mg/5ml
cephalothin
Renal dose: CrCl 26-50 ml/min 1.5 g q6h; CrCl 10-25 ml/min 1 g q6h; CrCl <10 ml/min 500 mg q6h
Moderate infections
• *Adult:* **IM/IV** 500 mg-1 g q4-6h
• *Child:* **IM/IV** 14-27 mg/kg q4h or 20-40 mg/kg q6h
Uncomplicated gonorrhea
• *Adult:* **IM** 2 g as a single dose
Severe infections
• *Adult:* **IM/IV** 1-2 g q4h
• *Child:* **IM/IV** 80-160 mg/kg/day in divided doses q4h
Available forms: Powder for inj 1, 2, 20 g
cephapirin
• *Adult:* **IM/IV** 500 mg-1 g q4-6h
• *Child:* **IM/IV** 40-80 mg/kg/day in divided doses q6h or 10-20 mg/kg q6h

Renal dose: CrCl <10 ml/min give q12h

Available forms: Powder for inj 500 mg, 1, 2, 20 g; IV only 1, 2, 4 g

cephradine
- *Adult:* **PO** 250 mg-1 g q6-12h
- *Child > 1 yr:* **PO** 6-12 mg/kg q6h

Renal dose: CrCl > 20 ml/min 500 mg q6h; CrCl 5-20 ml/min 250 mg q6h

Available forms: Caps 250, 500 mg; oral susp 125, 250 mg/5ml

Side effects/adverse reactions:

CNS: Headache, dizziness, weakness, paresthesia, fever, chills

GI: Nausea, vomiting, *diarrhea, anorexia,* pain, glossitis, bleeding; increased AST (SGOT), ALT (SGPT), bilirubin, LDH, alk phosphatase; abdominal pain, *pseudomembranous colitis*

GU: Proteinuria, vaginitis, pruritus, candidiasis, increased BUN, *nephrotoxicity, renal failure*

HEMA: Leukopenia, thrombocytopenia, agranulocytosis, anemia, *neutropenia, lymphocytosis, eosinophilia, pancytopenia, hemolytic anemia*

INTEG: Rash, urticaria, dermatitis, *anaphylaxis*

RESP: Dyspnea

Contraindications: Hypersensitivity to cephalosporins, infants <1 mo

Precautions: Hypersensitivity to penicillins, pregnancy (B), lactation, renal disease

Pharmacokinetics:

cefadroxil: Peak 1-1½ hr, half-life 1-2 hr; 20% bound by plasma proteins; crosses placenta; excreted in breast milk

cefazolin
IM: Peak ½-2 hr, half-life 1½-2¼ hr
IV: Peak 10 min; eliminated unchanged in urine; 70% to 86% protein bound

cephalexin: Peak 1 hr, duration 6-8 hr, half-life 30-72 min; 5%-15% bound by plasma proteins; 90%-100% eliminated unchanged in urine; crosses placenta; excreted in breast milk

cephalothin
IV: Peak 15 min
IM: Peak 30 min
Half-life ½-1 hr, 65%-80% bound by plasma proteins, 50%-75% eliminated unchanged in urine in 8 hr; crosses placenta, excreted in breast milk, deacetylated in kidneys, liver

cephapirin
IV: Peak 5 min
IM: Peak 30 min
Half-life 21-47 min; 44%-50% bound by plasma proteins; 40%-70% eliminated unchanged in urine; crosses placenta; excreted in breast milk; metabolized in liver

cephradine: Peak 1 hr, half-life 0.75-1.5 hr; 20% bound by plasma proteins; 80%-90% eliminated unchanged in urine; crosses placenta; excreted in breast milk

Interactions:
- Increased toxicity: aminoglycosides, furosemide, probenecid, ethacrynic acid
- Decreased action of: oral contraceptives

Lab test interferences:

False increase: Creatinine (serum urine), urinary 17-KS

False positive: Urinary protein, direct Coombs' test, urine glucose

Interference: Cross-matching

NURSING CONSIDERATIONS
Assess:
- Sensitivity to penicillin and other cephalosporins
- Nephrotoxicity: increased BUN, creatinine
- I&O daily
- Blood studies: AST (SGOT), ALT (SGPT), CBC, Hct, bilirubin,

LDH, alk phosphatase, Coombs' test monthly if patient is on long-term therapy
• Electrolytes: K, Na, Cl monthly if patient is on long-term therapy
• Bowel pattern qd; if severe diarrhea occurs, drug should be discontinued; may indicate pseudomembranous colitis
• Urine output: if decreasing, notify prescriber; may indicate nephrotoxicity
• Allergic reactions: rash, urticaria, pruritus, chills, fever, joint pain; angioedema; may occur few days after therapy begins
• Bleeding: ecchymosis, bleeding gums, hematuria, stool guaiac daily
• Overgrowth of infection: perineal itching, fever, malaise, redness, pain, swelling, drainage, rash, diarrhea, change in cough, sputum

Administer:
cefadroxil
• For 10-14 days to ensure organism death, prevent superinfection
• With food if needed for GI symptoms
• Shake susp, refrigerate, discard after 2 wk
• After C&S completed
cefazolin
• IV; check for irritation, extravasation often; dilute in 10 ml sterile H₂O for inj and run over 3-5 min; may be further diluted with 50-100 ml of NS, D₅W sol and run over ½-1 hr by Y-tube or 3-way stopcock
• For 10-14 days to ensure organism death, prevent superinfection
• After C&S completed

Additive compatibilities: Aztreonam, clindamycin, famotidine, fluconazole, metronidazole, verapamil

Syringe compatibilities: Heparin, vit B

Y-site compatibilities: Acyclovir, allopurinol, amifostine, atracurium, aztreonam, calcium gluconate, cy-

clophosphamide, diltiazem, enalaprilat, esmolol, famotidine, filgrastim, fluconazole, fludarabine, foscarnet, heparin, insulin (regular), labetalol, lidocaine, magnesium sulfate, melphalan, meperidine, midazolam, morphine, multivitamins, ondansetron, perphenazine, pancuronium, sargramostim, tacrolimus, teniposide, theophylline, thiotepa, vecuronium, vit B/C
cephalexin
• Shaking susp, refrigerate, discard after 2 wk
• For 10-14 days to ensure organism death, prevent superinfection
• With food if needed for GI symptoms
• After C&S
cephalothin
• Clear solution; do not give cloudy sol
• IV after diluting 1 g or less/10 ml or more of sterile H₂O for inj; give over 3-5 min; may be further diluted with 50 ml D₅W, NS by Y-tube or 3-way stopcock; run over 15-30 min; discontinue primary IV during administration; may also be given by continuous infusion
• Store 96 hr refrigerated, 24 hr room temp
• IM after reconstituting with 4 ml sterile H₂O for inj/1 g vial
• For 10-14 days to ensure organism death, prevent superinfection
• After C&S
• Insert IM in deep muscle mass, massage

Additive compatibilities: Ascorbic acid, chloramphenicol, clindamycin, fluorouracil, hydrocortisone, isoproterenol, magnesium sulfate, metaraminol, methicillin, methotrexate, potassium chloride, prednisolone, procaine, sodium bicarbonate, vit B/C

Syringe compatibilities: Cimetidine

Y-site compatibilities: Cyclophosphamide, famotidine, heparin, hydromorphone, magnesium sulfate, meperidine, morphine, multivitamins, perphenazine, potassium chloride, vit B/C

cephapirin
• IV after diluting 1 g or less/10 ml or more NS, D_5W, or bacteriostatic H_2O for inj; give 1 g or less/5 min or more; may be further diluted in 50-100 ml of D_5W, NS; run over 15 min; discontinue primary IV during administration; may also be given by continuous infusion, store refrigerated 96 hr, room temp 24 hr
• For 10-14 days to ensure organism death, prevent superinfection
• After C&S

Additive compatibilities: Bleomycin, calcium chloride, calcium gluconate, chloramphenicol, diphenhydramine, ergonovine, heparin, hydrocortisone, metaraminol, oxacillin, penicillin G potassium, pentobarbital, phenobarbital, phytonadione, potassium chloride, sodium bicarbonate, succinylcholine, verapamil, warfarin, vit B

Y-site compatibilities: Acyclovir, cyclophosphamide, famotidine, heparin, hydrocortisone, hydromorphone, magnesium sulfate, meperidine, morphine, multivitamins, perphenazine, potassium chloride, vit B/C

cephradine
• Shake suspension well before each dose
• For 10-14 days to ensure organism death, prevent superinfection
• With food if needed for GI symptoms
• After C&S

Evaluate:
• Therapeutic response: decreased symptoms of infection, negative C&S

Teach patient/family:
• If diabetic, to use Clinistix or Ketodiastix to check blood glucose level
• Not to drink alcohol or use meds with alcohol: reaction may occur
• To use yogurt or buttermilk to maintain intestinal flora, decrease diarrhea
• To take all medication prescribed for length of time ordered
• To report sore throat, bruising, bleeding, joint pain (may indicate blood dyscrasias [rare])

Treatment of anaphylaxis: Epinephrine, antihistamines; resuscitate if needed

CEPHALOSPORINS—2ND GENERATION

cefaclor (℞)
(sef'a-klor)
Ceclor

cefamandole (℞)
(sef-a-man'dole)
Mandol

cefmetazole (℞)
(sef-met'a-zole)
Zefazone

cefonicid (℞)
(se-fon'i-sid)
Monocid

cefotetan (℞)
(sef'oh-tee-tan)
Cefotan

cefoxitin (℞)
(se-fox'i-tin)
Mefoxin

cefprozil (℞)
(sef-proe'zill)
Cefzil

cefuroxime (℞)
(sef yoor-ox'eem)
Ceftin, Kefurox, Zinacef

loracarbef (℞)
(lor-a-kar'beff)
Lorabid

Func. class.: Antiinfective
Chem. class.: Cephalosporin
(2nd generation)

Action: Inhibits bacterial cell wall synthesis, rendering cell wall osmotically unstable, leading to cell death by binding to cell wall membrane

Uses:
cefaclor: Gram-negative bacilli: *H. influenzae, E. coli, P. mirabilis, Klebsiella;* gram-positive organisms: *S. pneumoniae, S. pyogenes, S. aureus;* upper and lower respiratory tract, urinary tract, skin, bone, joint infections, otitis media

cefamandole: Gram-negative bacilli: *H. influenzae, E. coli, P. mirabilis, Klebsiella;* gram-positive organisms: *S. pneumoniae, S. pyogenes, S. aureus;* upper, lower respiratory tract, urinary tract, skin infections, peritonitis, septicemia, surgical prophylaxis

cefmetazole: Gram-negative bacilli: *H. influenzae, E. coli, Proteus, Klebsiella, B. fragilis;* gram-positive organisms: *S. pneumoniae, S. pyogenes, S. aureus;* anaerobes, including *Clostridium;* infections of lower respiratory tract, urinary tract, skin, bone, intraabdominal infections

cefonicid: Gram-negative bacilli: *H. influenzae, E. coli, P. mirabilis, Klebsiella;* gram-positive organisms: *S. pneumoniae, S. pyogenes, S. aureus,* lower respiratory tract, urinary tract, skin infections, otitis media, peritonitis, septicemia

cefotetan: Gram-negative organisms: *H. influenzae, E. coli, E. aerogenes, P. mirabilis, Klebsiella, Citrobacter, Enterobacter, Salmonella, Shigella, Acinetobacter, B. fragilis, Neisseria, Serratia;* gram-positive organisms: *S. pneumoniae, S. pyogenes, S. aureus;* upper, lower, serious respiratory tract, urinary tract, skin, bone, joint, gynecologic, gonococcal, intraabdominal infections

cefoxitin: Gram-negative bacilli: *H. influenzae, E. coli, Proteus, Klebsiella, B. fragilis, N. gonorrhoeae, E. corrodens;* gram-positive organisms: *S. pneumoniae, S. pyogenes, S. aureus;* anaerobes including *Clostridium,* lower respiratory tract, urinary tract, skin bone, gynecologic, gonococcal infections, septicemia, peritonitis

cefprozil: Pharyngitis/tonsillitis, otitis media, secondary bacterial infection of acute bronchitis, and acute bacterial exacerbation of chronic bronchitis and uncomplicated skin and skin structure infections; acute sinusitis

cefuroxime: Gram-negative bacilli: *H. influenzae, E. coli, Neisseria, P. mirabilis, Klebsiella;* gram-positive organisms: *S. pneumoniae, S. pyogenes, S. aureus;* serious lower respiratory tract, urinary tract, skin, bone, joint, gonococcal infections, septicemia, meningitis

loracarbef: Gram-negative bacilli: *H. influenzae, E. coli, P. mirabilis, Klebsiella;* gram-positive organisms: *S. pneumoniae, S. pyogenes, S. aureus;* upper and lower respiratory tract, urinary tract, skin infections, otitis media; pharyngitis, tonsillitis

Dosage and routes:

cefaclor

• *Adult:* **PO** 250-500 mg q8h, not to exceed 4 g/day or 375-500 mg (ext rel) q12h × 7-10 days

• *Child >1 mo:* **PO** 20-40 mg/kg qd in divided doses q8h, or total daily dose may be divided and given q12h, not to exceed 1 g/day

Acute bacterial exacerbations of chronic bronchitis or acute bronchitis

• *Adult:* 500 mg/12 hr × 1 wk (ext rel)

Pharyngitis/tonsillitis

• *Adult:* 375 mg/12 hr × 10 days (ext rel)

Available forms: Caps 250, 500 mg; oral susp 125, 187, 250, 375 mg/5 ml; tabs, ext rel 375, 500 mg

cefamandole

• *Adult:* **IM/IV** 500 mg-1 g q4-8h; may give up to 2 g q4h for severe infections

• *Child >1 mo:* **IM/IV** 8.3-16.7 mg/kg q4h, not to exceed adult dose

• Dosage reduction indicated in renal impairment (CrCl <50 ml/min)

Available forms: Inj 1, 2, 10 g

cefmetazole

Renal dose: CrCl <50 ml/min 1-2 g q12h; CrCl 10-29 ml/min 1-2 g q24h; CrCl <10 ml/min 1-2 g q48h

• *Adult:* **IV** 2 g divided q6-12h × 5-14 days

Available forms: Powder for inj 1, 2 g/vial

cefonicid

Life-threatening infections

• *Adult:* **IM/IV BOL** or **INF** 0.5-2 g/24 hr; divide in two doses if giving 2 g

• Dosage reduction indicated in renal impairment

Available forms: Inj 500 mg, 1, 10 g

cefotetan

Renal dose: CrCl 10-30 ml/min give q24h; CrCl <10 ml/min give q48h

• *Adult:* **IV/IM** 1-2 g q12h × 5-10 days

Perioperative prophylaxis

• *Adult:* **IV** 1-2 g ½-1 hr before surgery

Available forms: Inj 1, 2, 10 g

cefoxitin

Renal dose: CrCl <50 ml/min give q8-12h; CrCl 10-29 ml/min give q24h; CrCl <10 ml/min give q24-48h

• *Adult:* **IM/IV** 1-2 g q6-8h

• Dosage reduction indicated in renal impairment (CrCl <50 ml/min) Uncomplicated gonorrhea 2 g IM as single dose with 1 g **PO** probenecid at same time

Severe infections

• *Adult:* **IM/IV** 2 g q4h

• *Child ≥3 mo:* **IM/IV** 80-160 mg/kg/day divided q4-6h; max 12 g/day

Available forms: Powder for inj 1, 2, 10 g

cefprozil

Renal dose: CrCl <30 ml/min 50% of dose

Upper respiratory infections

• *Adult:* **PO** 500 mg q24h × 10 days

Otitis media
• *Child 6 mo-12 yr:* **PO** 15 mg/kg q12h × 10 days

Lower respiratory infections
• *Adult:* **PO** 500 mg q12h × 10 days

Skin/skin structure infections
• *Adult:* **PO** 250-500 mg q12h × 10 days

Available forms: Tabs 250, 500 mg; susp 125, 250 mg/5 ml

cefuroxime
• *Adult and child:* **PO** 250 mg q12h; may increase to 500 mg q12h in serious infections
• *Adult:* **IM/IV** 750 mg-1.5 g q8h for 5-10 days

Urinary tract infections
• *Adult:* **PO** 125 mg q12h; may increase to 250 mg q12h if needed

Otitis media
• *Child <2 yr:* **PO** 125 mg bid
• *Child >2 yr:* **PO** 250 mg bid

Surgical prophylaxis
• *Adult:* **IV** 1.5 g ½-1 hr preop

Severe infections
• *Adult:* **IM/IV** 1.5 g q6h; may give up to 3 g q8h for bacterial meningitis
• *Child >3 mo:* **IM/IV** 50-100 mg/kg/day; may give up to 200-240 mg/kg/day **IV** in divided doses for bacterial meningitis (not recommended)
• Dosage reduction indicated in severe renal impairment (CrCl <20 ml/min)

Uncomplicated gonorrhea
• *Adult:* 1.5 g **IM** as single dose with oral probenecid in 2 separate sites

Available forms: Tabs 125, 250, 500 mg; inj 150, 750 mg, 1.5, 7.5 g; inj 750 mg; 1.5 g powder

loracarbef
Renal dose: CrCl 10-49 ml/min 50% of dose; CrCl <10 ml/min q3-5 days
• *Adult and child >13:* **PO** 200-400 mg q12h
• *Child to 12 yr:* **PO** 15-30 mg/kg/day in 2 divided doses q12h

Available forms: Caps 200, 400 mg; 100, 200 mg/5 ml oral susp

Side effects/adverse reactions:
CNS: Dizziness, headache, fatigue, paresthesia, fever, chills, confusion
GI: Diarrhea, nausea, vomiting, anorexia, dysgeusia, glossitis, bleeding; increased AST (SGOT), ALT (SGPT), bilirubin, LDH, alk phosphatase; abdominal pain, loose stools, flatulence, heartburn, stomach cramps, colitis, jaundice
INTEG: Rash, urticaria, dermatitis, *Stevens-Johnson syndrome*
GU: Vaginitis, pruritus, candidiasis, increased BUN, *nephrotoxicity, renal failure,* pyuria, dysuria, reversible interstitial nephritis
HEMA: Leukopenia, thrombocytopenia, agranulocytosis, anemia, *neutropenia, lymphocytosis, eosinophilia, pancytopenia, hemolytic anemia, leukocytosis, granulocytopenia*
RESP: Dyspnea
SYST: Anaphylaxis, serum sickness
Contraindications: Hypersensitivity to cephalosporins or related antibiotics, seizures
Precautions: Pregnancy (B), lactation, children, renal disease
Pharmacokinetics:
cefaclor: Peak ½-1 hr, half-life 36-54 min; 25% bound by plasma proteins; 60%-85% eliminated unchanged in urine in 8 hr; crosses placenta; excreted in breast milk (low concentrations)
cefamandole: Peak 1-1½ hr, half-life ½-1 hr; 60%-75% bound by plasma proteins; crosses placenta; excreted in breast milk; poor penetration into CSF
cefmetazole
IM: Peak 30-45 min; 68% bound by plasma proteins, excreted by kidneys; half-life 1-3 hr
cefonicid
IV: Onset 5 min

IM: Peak 1 hr

Half-life 4½ hr; excreted in breast milk (small amounts); 98% protein bound; poor penetration in CSF

cefotetan

IV/IM: Peak 1½-3 hr; half-life 3-5 hr, 70%-90% bound by plasma proteins, 50%-80% eliminated unchanged in urine, crosses placenta, excreted in breast milk

cefoxitin

IV: Peak 3 min

IM: Peak 15-60 min

Half-life 1 hr, 55%-75% bound by plasma proteins, 90%-100% eliminated unchanged in urine; crosses placenta, blood-brain barrier; eliminated in breast milk, not metabolized

cefprozil

PO: Peak 6-10 hr; plasma protein binding 99%; elimination half-life 25 hr; extensively metabolized to an active metabolite

cefuroxime: 65% excreted unchanged in urine, half-life 1-2 hr in normal renal function

loracarbef

PO: Peak 1 hr, half-life 1 hr; excreted in urine as unchanged drug

Interactions:

• Increased effect/toxicity: aminoglycosides, furosemide, probenecid, ethacrynic acid, vancomycin

• May decrease effects of: oral contraceptives

• Disulfiram-like reaction: alcohol

• Increased anticoagulant effect: heparin, warfarin

Lab test interferences:

False increase: Creatinine (serum urine), urinary 17-KS

False positive: Urinary protein, direct Coombs' test, urine glucose testing (Clinitest)

Interference: Cross-matching

NURSING CONSIDERATIONS

Assess:

◆ Nephrotoxicity: increased BUN, creatinine

• I&O ratio

• Blood studies: AST (SGOT), ALT (SGPT), CBC, Hct, bilirubin, LDH, alk phosphatase, Coombs' test qmo if patient is on long-term therapy

• Electrolytes: K, Na, Cl qmo if patient is on long-term therapy

• Bowel pattern qd; if severe diarrhea occurs, drug should be discontinued; may indicate pseudomembranous colitis

• Urine output; if decreasing, notify prescriber (may indicate nephrotoxicity)

• Allergic reactions: rash, flushing, urticaria, pruritus

• Bleeding: ecchymosis, bleeding gums, hematuria, stool guaiac daily

• Overgrowth of infection: perineal itching, fever, malaise, redness, pain, swelling, drainage, rash, diarrhea, change in cough, sputum

Administer:

cefaclor

• Shake susp, refrigerate, discard after 2 wk

• For 10-14 days to ensure organism death, prevent superinfection

• With food if needed for GI symptoms

• After C&S completed

🚫 Do not break, crush, or chew ext rel tabs

cefamandole

• IV; check often for irritation, extravasation; dilute 1 g or less of drug/10 ml or more normal saline or sterile H_2O for inj; run over 3-5 min; may be further diluted with 100 ml of compatible sol and run over 15-30 min via Y-tube or 3-way stopcock; may also be diluted in 1 L compatible sol, run over prescribed rate

---

◆ = Nursing alert   🌿 = Herb-drug interaction   🚫 = Do not crush

- For 10-14 days to ensure organism death, prevent superinfection
- After C&S completed

Additive compatibilities: Clindamycin, floxacillin, furosemide, metronidazole, verapamil

Syringe compatibilities: Heparin

Y-site compatibilities: Acyclovir, cyclophosphamide, hydromorphone, magnesium sulfate, meperidine, morphine, perphenazine

cefmetazole

- For 10-14 days to ensure organism death, prevent superinfection
- After C&S completed

Additive compatibilities: Clindamycin, famotidine, KCl

- IV after diluting 3.7 or 10 ml sterile H_2O for inj, 2 g/7 or 15 ml, shake, let stand until clear, run over 3-5 min; may be further diluted in 50-100 ml of D_5W, NS, LR to 1-20 mg/ml and run over ½-1 hr by Y-tube or 3-way stopcock

cefonicid

- IV direct dilute 0.5 g/2 ml or 1 g/2.5 ml sterile H_2O for inj and give by Y-tube or 3-way stopcock over 3-5 min
- IV INT INF may be further diluted in 50-100 ml D_5W, NS and given over 30 min; slight yellowing of sol does not affect potency
- IV; check for irritation, extravasation often

Additive compatibilities: Clindamycin

Y-site compatibilities: Acyclovir, amifostine, aztreonam, teniposide, thiotepa

cefotetan

- IV direct after diluting 1 g/10 ml sterile H_2O for inj and give over 3-5 min; may be diluted further with 50-100 ml of normal saline or D_5W, shake; run over ½-1 hr by Y-tube or 3-way stopcock; discontinue primary inf during administration

- May be stored 96 hr refrigerated or 24 hr room temp

Y-site compatibilities: Allopurinol, amifostine, aztreonam, diltiazem, famotidine, filgrastim, fluconazole, fludarabine, heparin, insulin (regular), melphalan, meperidine, morphine, paclitaxel, sargramostim, tacrolimus, teniposide, theophylline, thiotepa

cefoxitin

- IV after diluting 1 g or less/10 ml or more D_5W, NS and give over 3-5 min; may be diluted further with 50-100 ml of normal saline or D_5W; run over ½-1 hr by Y-tube or 3-way stopcock; discontinue primary inf during administration; by cont inf at prescribed rate; may store 96 hr refrigerated or 24 hr room temp
- For 10-14 days to ensure organism death, prevent superinfection
- After C&S completed

Additive compatibilities: Amikacin, cimetidine, clindamycin, gentamicin, kanamycin, multivitamins, sodium bicarbonate, tobramycin, verapamil, vit B/C

Syringe compatibilities: Heparin, insulin

Y-site compatibilities: Acyclovir, amifostine, aztreonam, cyclophosphamide, diltiazem, famotidine, fluconazole, foscarnet, hydromorphone, magnesium sulfate, meperidine, morphine, ondansetron, perphenazine, teniposide, thiotepa

cefprozil

- For 10-14 days to ensure organism death, prevent superinfection
- After C&S
- Refrigerate/shake susp prior to use

cefuroxime

- For 10-14 days to ensure organism death, prevent superinfection
- With food if needed for GI symptoms
- After C&S

Additive compatibilities: Clindamycin, floxacillin, furosemide, metronidazole, netilmicin

Y-site compatibilities: Acyclovir, allopurinol, amifostine, atracurium, aztreonam, cyclophosphamide, diltiazem, famotidine, fludarabine, foscarnet, hydromorphone, melphalan, meperidine, morphine, ondansetron, pancuronium, perphenazine, sargramostim, tacrolimus, teniposide, thiotepa, vecuronium

loracarbef

• Oral susp should be shaken before giving; store for 2 wk at room temp, discard after 2 wk

• 1 hr before or 2 hr after a meal

• After C&S is completed

• For 7 days to ensure organism death, prevent superinfection

Evaluate:

• Therapeutic response: negative C&S

Teach patient/family:

• If diabetic, to use blood glucose testing

• Not to drink alcohol or take meds with alcohol or reaction may occur

• To complete full course of drug therapy, to report persistent diarrhea

• To take on an empty stomach 1 hr before or 2 hr after a meal

🚫 Not to break, crush, or chew caps

• To notify prescriber if breastfeeding or of any side effects

Treatment of overdose: Epinephrine, antihistamines; resuscitate if needed (anaphylaxis)

CEPHALOSPORINS—3RD GENERATION

cefepime (℞)
(sef'e-peem)
Maxipime

cefixime (℞)
(sef-icks'ime)
Suprax

cefoperazone (℞)
(sef-oh-per'a-zone)
Cefobid

cefotaxime (℞)
(sef-oh-taks'eem)
Claforan

cefpodoxime (℞)
(sef-poe-docks'eem)
Vantin

ceftazidime (℞)
(sef'tay-zi-deem)
Ceptaz, Fortaz, Magnacef*, Pentacef, Tazicef, Tazidime

ceftibuten (℞)
(sef-ti-byoo'tin)
Cedax

ceftizoxime (℞)
(sef-ti-zox'eem)
Cefizox

ceftriaxone (℞)
(sef-try-ax'one)
Rocephin

moxalactam (℞)
(mox'a-lak-tam)
Moxam

Func. class.: Broad-spectrum antibiotic

Chem. class.: Cephalosporin (3rd generation)

Action: Inhibits bacterial cell wall synthesis, rendering cell wall osmotically unstable, leading to cell death

Uses:

cefepime: Gram-negative bacilli: *E. coli, Proteus, Klebsiella;* gram-positive organisms: *S. pneumoniae, S. pyogenes, S. aureus;* lower respiratory tract, urinary tract, skin, bone infections

cefixime: Uncomplicated UTI *(E. coli, P. mirabilis),* pharyngitis and tonsillitis *(S. pyogenes),* otitis media *(H. influenzae),* M. catarrhalis, acute bronchitis, and acute and exacerbations of chronic bronchitis *(S. pneumoniae, H. influenzae)*

cefoperazone: Gram-negative bacilli: *H. influenzae, E. coli, P. mirabilis, Klebsiella, Enterobacter, Serratia, Citrobacter, Providencia, P. aeruginosa;* lower respiratory tract, urinary tract, skin, bone infections, bacterial septicemia, peritonitis, PID

cefotaxime: Gram-negative organisms: *H. influenzae, E. coli, N. gonorrhoeae, N. meningitidis, P. mirabilis, Klebsiella, Citrobacter, Serratia, Salmonella, Shigella;* grampositive organisms: *S. pneumoniae, S. pyogenes, S. aureus,* lower serious respiratory tract, urinary tract, skin, bone, gonococcal infections; bacteremia, septicemia, meningitis

cefpodoxime: Gram-negative bacilli: *N. gonorrhoeae, H. influenzae, E. coli, P. mirabilis, Klebsiella;* gram-positive organisms: *S. pneumoniae, S. pyogenes, S. aureus;* upper and lower respiratory tract, urinary tract, skin infections; otitis media, sexually transmitted diseases

ceftazidime: Gram-negative organisms: *H. influenzae, E. coli, E. aerogenes, P. aeruginosa, P. mirabilis, Klebsiella, Citrobacter, Enterobacter, Salmonella, Shigella, Acinetobacter, B. fragilis, Neisseria, Serratia;* gram-positive organisms: *S. pneumoniae, S. pyogenes, S. aureus;* upper, lower, serious respiratory tract, urinary tract, skin, gynecologic, bone, joint, intraabdominal infections; septicemia, meningitis

ceftibuten: Pharyngitis/tonsillitis,

otitis media, secondary bacterial infection of acute bronchitis

ceftizoxime: Gram-negative organisms: *H. influenzae, E. coli, E. aerogenes, P. mirabilis, Klebsiella, Enterobacter;* gram-positive organisms: *S. pneumoniae, S. pyogenes, S. aureus;* lower serious respiratory tract, urinary tract, skin, intraabdominal infections, septicemia, meningitis, bone and joint infections, PID caused by *N. gonorrhoeae*

ceftriaxone: Gram-negative organisms: *H. influenzae, E. coli, E. aerogenes, P. mirabilis, Klebsiella, Citrobacter, Enterobacter, Salmonella, Shigella, Acinetobacter, B. fragilis, Neisseria, Serratia;* gram-positive organisms: *S. pneumoniae, S. pyogenes, S. aureus;* serious lower respiratory tract, urinary tract, skin, gonococcal, intraabdominal infections, septicemia, meningitis, bone, joint infections

moxalactam: Gram-negative organisms: *H. influenzae, E. coli, P. mirabilis, Klebsiella, Citrobacter, Salmonella, Shigella, Serratia;* gram-positive organisms: *S. pneumoniae, S. pyogenes, S. aureus;* serious lower respiratory tract, urinary tract, skin, bone infections; septicemia, meningitis, intraabdominal infections

Dosage and routes:

cefepime
Urinary tract infections (mild to moderate)
• *Adult:* IV/IM 0.5-1 g q12h × 7-10 days
Urinary tract infections (severe)
• *Adult:* IV 2 g q12h × 10 days
Pneumonia (moderate to severe)
• *Adult:* IV 1-2 g q12h × 10 days
Dosage reduction indicated in renal impairment (CrCl <50 ml/min)
Uncomplicated gonorrhea
• IM 2 g as a single dose with 1 g PO probenecid at the same time

Available forms: Powder for inj 500 mg, 1, 2 g

cefixime

Renal dose: CrCl 21-60 ml/min give 75% of dose; CrCl <20 ml/min give 50% of dose

• *Adult:* **PO** 400 mg qd as a single dose or 200 mg q12h

• *Child >50 kg or >12 yr:* **PO** use adult dosage

• *Child <50 kg or <12 yr:* **PO** 8 mg/kg/day as a single dose or 4 mg/kg q12h

Available forms: Tabs 200, 400 mg; powder for oral susp 100 mg/5 ml

cefoperazone

Hepatic dose: give 50% of dose

Mild/moderate infections

• *Adult:* **IM/IV** 1-2 g q12h

Severe infections

• *Adult:* **IM/IV** 6-12 g/day divided in 2-4 equal doses

Available forms: Inj 1, 2 g

cefotaxime

• *Adult:* **IM/IV** 1-2 g q12h as a single dose

• *Child 1 mo-12 yr:* **IM/IV** 50-180 mg/kg/day divided q6h

Severe infections

• *Adult:* **IM/IV** 2 g q4h, not to exceed 12 g/day

• *Child 1 mo-12 yr:* **IM/IV** 50 mg/kg q6h

Uncomplicated gonorrhea

• *Adult:* **IM** 1 g

Dosage reduction indicated for severe renal impairment (CrCl <30 ml/min)

Available forms: Powder for inj 1, 2, 10 g; frozen inj 20, 40 mg/ml

cefpodoxime

• Reduce dose in renal disease

• *Adult >13 yr: Pneumonia:* 200 mg q12h for 14 days; *uncomplicated gonorrhea:* 200 mg single dose; *skin and skin structure:* 400 mg q12h for 7-14 days; *pharyngitis and tonsillitis:* 100 mg q12h for 10 days; *uncomplicated UTI:* 100 mg q12h for 7 days; dosing interval increased in presence of severe renal impairment

• *Child 5 mo-12 yr: acute otitis media:* 5 mg/kg q12h for 10 days; *pharyngitis/tonsillitis:* 5 mg/kg q12h (max 100 mg/dose or 200 mg/day) × 5-10 days

Available forms: Tabs 100, 200 mg/ granules for susp 50, 100 mg/5 ml

ceftazidime

Renal dose: CrCl <50 ml/min give q12h; CrCl 10-30 ml/min give q24h; CrCl <10 ml/min give q48h

• *Adult:* **IV/IM** 1-2 g q8-12h × 5-10 days

• *Child:* **IV** 30-50 mg/kg q8h not to exceed 6 g/day

• *Neonate:* **IV** 30-50 mg/kg q12h

Available forms: Inj 500 mg, 1, 2, 6 g

ceftibuten

Renal dose: CrCl <50 ml/min give 200 mg q24h; CrCl 5-20 ml/min give 100 mg q24h

• *Adult:* **PO** 400 mg qd × 10 days

• *Child 6 mo-12 yr:* **PO** 9 mg/kg qd × 10 days

Available forms: Caps 400 mg; 90, 180 mg/5 ml

ceftizoxime

Renal dose: CrCl <80 ml/min give 500-1500 mg q8h; CrCl 10-49 ml/min give 250-1000 mg q12h

• *Adult:* **IM/IV** 1-2 g q8-12h, may give up to 4 g q8h in life-threatening infections

• *Child <6 mo:* **IM/IV** 50 mg/kg q6-8h

PID

• *Adult:* **IV** 2 g q8h, may increase to 4 g q8h in severe infections

Available forms: Powder for inj 500 mg, 1, 2, 10 g; premixed 1 g, 2 g/50 ml

ceftriaxone

• *Adult:* **IM/IV** 1-2 g qd, max 2 g q12h

• *Child:* **IM/IV** 50-75 mg/kg/day in equal doses q12h

Uncomplicated gonorrhea
• *Adult:* 250 mg **IM** as single dose
• Reduce dosage in severe renal impairment (CrCl <10 ml/min)

Meningitis
• *Adult and child:* **IM/IV** 100 mg/kg/day in equal doses q12h, max 4 g/day

Surgical prophylaxis
• *Adult:* **IV** 1 g ½-2 hr preop

Available forms: Inj 500 mg, 1, 2, 10 g

moxalactam

Mild infections
• *Adult:* **IM/IV** 250-500 mg q8-12h

Severe infections
• *Adult:* **IM/IV** 2-6 g q8h
• *Child:* **IM/IV** 50 mg/kg q6-8h
• Dosage reduction indicated even for mild renal impairment (CrCl <80 ml/min)

Available forms: Powder for inj 1, 2, 10 g

Side effects/adverse reactions:

CNS: Headache, dizziness, weakness, paresthesia, fever, chills, seizures

GI: Nausea, vomiting, diarrhea, anorexia, pain, glossitis, ***bleeding;*** increased AST (SGOT), ALT (SGPT), bilirubin, LDH, alk phosphatase; abdominal pain, *pseudomembranous colitis*

*GU: **Proteinuria,*** vaginitis, pruritus, candidiasis, increased BUN, ***nephrotoxicity, renal failure***

*HEMA: **Leukopenia, thrombocytopenia, agranulocytosis,*** anemia, ***neutropenia, lymphocytosis, eosinophilia, pancytopenia, hemolytic anemia***

INTEG: Rash, urticaria, dermatitis

RESP: Dyspnea

*SYST: **Anaphylaxis,*** serum sickness

Contraindications: Hypersensitivity to cephalosporins, infants <1 mo

Precautions: Hypersensitivity to penicillins, pregnancy (B), lactation, renal disease, children

Pharmacokinetics:

cefepime
Peak 79 min, half-life 2 hr, 20% bound by plasma proteins, 90% excreted unchanged in urine; crosses placenta, blood-brain barrier; excreted in breast milk; not metabolized

cefixime
PO: Peak 1-2 hr, half-life 3-4 hr, 65% bound by plasma proteins, 50% eliminated unchanged in urine; crosses placenta; excreted in breast milk

cefoperazone
IV: Onset 5 min, peak 5-20 min, duration 6-8 hr
IM: Peak 1-2 hr, duration 6-8 hr
Half-life 2 hr; 70%-75% is eliminated unchanged in bile; 20%-30% unchanged in urine; excreted in breast milk (small amounts)

cefotaxime
IV: Onset 5 min
IM: Onset 30 min
Half-life 1 hr; 35%-65% is bound by plasma proteins; 40%-65% is eliminated unchanged in urine in 24 hr; 25% metabolized to active metabolites; excreted in breast milk (small amounts)

cefpodoxime
Half-life 2-3 hr; 25% bound by plasma proteins; 30% eliminated unchanged in urine in 8 hr; crosses placenta; excreted in breast milk

ceftazidime
IV/IM: Peak 1 hr, half-life ½-1 hr, 90% bound by plasma proteins, 80% eliminated unchanged in urine, crosses placenta, excreted in breast milk

ceftibuten
PO: Peak 6-10 hr; plasma protein binding 99%; elimination half-life

25 hr; extensively metabolized to an active metabolite

ceftizoxime

IV: Onset 5 min
IM: Peak 1 hr

Half-life 5-8 hr; 90% bound by plasma proteins; 36%-60% eliminated unchanged in urine; crosses placenta; excreted in breast milk

ceftriaxone

IV: Onset 5 min
IM: Peak 1 hr

Half-life 5-8 hr, 90% bound by plasma proteins; 35%-60% eliminated unchanged in urine; crosses placenta; excreted in breast milk

moxalactam

IV: Peak 5 min
IM: Peak ½-2 hr

Half-life 1½-2½ hr, 25% bound by plasma proteins; 60%-97% eliminated unchanged in urine in 24 hr; crosses placenta, blood-brain barrier; excreted in breast milk; not metabolized

Interactions:

• Increased toxicity: aminoglycosides, furosemide, probenecid, ethacrynic acid
• May decrease action of oral contraceptives

Lab test interferences:

False increase: Urinary 17-KS
False positive: Urinary protein, direct Coombs' test, urine glucose
Interference: Cross-matching

NURSING CONSIDERATIONS
Assess:

• Sensitivity to penicillin, other cephalosporins
• Nephrotoxicity: increased BUN, creatinine
• Blood studies: AST (SGOT), ALT (SGPT), CBC, Hct, bilirubin, LDH, alk phosphatase, Coombs' test monthly if patient is on long-term therapy
• Electrolytes: K, Na, Cl monthly if patient is on long-term therapy

• Bowel pattern qd; if severe diarrhea occurs, drug should be discontinued; may indicate pseudomembranous colitis
• IV site for extravasation, phlebitis; change site q72h
⬥ Urine output: if decreasing, notify prescriber; may indicate nephrotoxicity
• Allergic reactions: rash, urticaria, pruritus, chills, fever, joint pain, angioedema; may occur few days after therapy begins
• Bleeding: ecchymosis, bleeding gums, hematuria, stool guaiac
• Overgrowth of infection: perineal itching, fever, malaise, redness, pain, swelling, drainage, rash, diarrhea, change in cough, sputum

Administer:

cefepime

• IV after diluting in 50-100 ml or more D_5, NS and give over 30 min
• For 7-10 days to ensure organism death, prevent superinfection

Solution compatibilities: 0.9% NaCl, D_5, 0.5%, 10% lidocaine, bacteriostatic water for inj with parabens/benzyl alcohol

cefixime

• For 10-14 days to ensure organism death, prevent superinfection

cefoperazone

• IV after diluting 1 g/ml sterile H_2O for inj, or 0.9% NaCl; shake, give over 3-5 min; each g may be further diluted with 20-40 ml D_5W, NS given over 30 min or as a cont inf over 6-24 hr to a concentration no greater than 25 mg/ml
• IM for concentration >250 mg/ml, dilute in sterile water, then lidocaine, inject deeply
• For 10-14 days to ensure organism death, prevent superinfection

Additive compatibilities: Cimetidine, clindamycin, furosemide
Syringe compatibilities: Heparin
Y-site compatibilities: Acyclovir,

allopurinol, aztreonam, cyclophosphamide, enalaprilat, esmolol, famotidine, foscarnet, fludarabine, hydromorphone, magnesium sulfate, melphalan, morphine, teniposide, thiotepa

cefotaxime

• IV after diluting 1g/10 ml D₅W, NS, sterile H₂O for inj and give over 3-5 min by Y-tube or 3-way stopcock; may be diluted further with 50-100 ml of normal saline or D₅W; run over ½-1 hr; discontinue primary inf during administration; or may be diluted in larger vol of sol and given as a cont inf over 6-24 hr
• For 10-14 days to ensure organism death, prevent superinfection

Additive compatibilities: Clindamycin, metronidazole, verapamil

Syringe compatibilities: Heparin, ofloxacin

Y-site compatibilities: Acyclovir, amifostine, aztreonam, cyclophosphamide, diltiazem, famotidine, fludarabine, hydromorphone, lorazepam, magnesium sulfate, melphalan, meperidine, midazolam, morphine, ondansetron, perphenazine, sargramostim, teniposide, thiotepa, tolazoline, vinorelbine

cefpodoxime

• For 10-14 days to ensure organism death, prevent superinfection
• With food to enhance absorption

Y-site compatibilities: Famotidine, fluconazole, fludarabine, insulin (regular), meperidine, morphine, sargramostim

ceftazidime

• IV after diluting 1 g/10 ml sterile H₂O for inj, shake, invert needle, push plunger, insert needle through stopper and keep in sol, expel bubbles and give over 3-5 min; may be diluted further with 50-100 ml of normal saline or D₅W; run over ½-1 hr, give through Y-tube or 3-way stopcock, discontinue primary inf

during administration; store for 96 hr refrigerated, 24 hr room temp
• For 5-10 days to ensure organism death, prevent superinfection

Additive compatibilities: Ciprofloxacin, clindamycin, fluconazole, metronidazole, ofloxacin

Y-site compatibilities: Acyclovir, allopurinol, amifostine, aztreonam, ciprofloxacin, diltiazem, enalaprilat, esmolol, famotidine, filgrastim, fludarabine, foscarnet, granisetron, heparin, hydromorphone, labetalol, meperidine, melphalan, morphine, ondansetron, paclitaxel, ranitidine, tacrolimus, teniposide, theophylline, thiotepa, vinorelbine, zidovudine

ceftibuten

• For 10 days to ensure organism death, prevent superinfection

ceftizoxime

• IV after diluting 1 g/10 ml sterile water, shake and give over 3-5 min; may be diluted further with 50-100 ml NS or D₅W give through Y-tube or 3-way stopcock; run over ½-1 hr
• For 10-14 days to ensure organism death, prevent superinfection

Additive compatibilities: Clindamycin

Y-site compatibilities: Acyclovir, allopurinol, aztreonam, enalaprilat, esmolol, famotidine, fludarabine, foscarnet, hydromorphone, labetalol, melphalan, meperidine, morphine, ondansetron, sargramostim, teniposide, vinorelbine

ceftriaxone

• For 10-14 days to ensure organism death, prevent superinfection
• IV after diluting 250 mg/2.4 ml D₅W, H₂O for inj, 0.9% NaCl; may be further diluted with 50-100 ml NS, D₅W, D₁₀W, shake; run over ½-1 hr

Additive compatibilities: Amino acids or sodium bicarbonate

Y-site compatibilities: Acyclovir,

allopurinol, aztreonam, diltiazem, fludarabine, foscarnet, heparin, melphalan, meperidine, methotrexate, morphine, paclitaxel, sargramostim, tacrolimus, teniposide, theophylline, vinorelbine, zidovudine

moxalactam

• For 10-14 days to ensure organism death, prevent superinfection

• IV after diluting 1 g/10 ml sterile H_2O, D_5, 0.9% NaCl; give through Y-tube over 3-5 min; may be further diluted 1 g/20 ml in D_5, 0.9% NaCl, give over ½ hr; may be added to 500-1000 ml, give over 6-24 hr

• Vit K for bleeding (10 mg/wk)

Additive compatibilities: Metronidazole, ranitidine, verapamil

Syringe compatibilities: Heparin

Y-site compatibilities: Cyclophosphamide, hydromorphone, magnesium sulfate, meperidine, morphine, perphenazine

Evaluate:

• Therapeutic response: decreased symptoms of infection; negative C&S

Teach patient/family:

• If diabetic, to check blood glucose

• To report sore throat, bruising, bleeding, joint pain; may indicate blood dyscrasias (rare)

• To report persistent diarrhea

Treatment of anaphylaxis: Epinephrine, antihistamines; resuscitate if needed

---

cerivistatin (℞)

(ser-iv'i-sta-tin)

Baycol

Func. class.: Cholesterol-lowering agent

Chem. class.: HMG-CoA reductase inhibitor

Action: Inhibits HMG-CoA reductase enzyme, which reduces cholesterol synthesis

Uses: As an adjunct in primary hypercholesterolemia (types IIa, IIb), mixed hyperlipidemia

Dosage and routes:

(Patient should first be placed on a cholesterol-lowering diet)

• *Adult:* **PO** 0.3 mg qd PM, may be given with a bile-acid-binding resin

Available forms: Tabs 0.2, 0.3 mg

Side effects/adverse reactions:

*GI: Flatus, nausea, constipation, diarrhea, dyspepsia, abdominal pain, heartburn, **liver dysfunction***

*MS: Muscle cramps, myalgia, **myositis, rhabdomyolysis***

CNS: Dizziness, headache, tremor

INTEG: Rash, pruritus

EENT: Blurred vision, dysgeusia, lens opacities

Contraindications: Hypersensitivity, pregnancy (X), lactation, active liver disease

Precautions: Past liver disease, alcoholism, severe acute infections, trauma, hypotension, uncontrolled seizure disorders, severe metabolic disorders, electrolyte imbalances, visual disorder, children

Pharmacokinetics:

PO: Unknown

Interactions:

• Increased effects: bile acid sequestrants, warfarin

• Increased myalgia, myositis: cyclosporine, gemfibrozil, niacin

Lab test interferences:

Increase: CPK, liver function tests

NURSING CONSIDERATIONS

Assess:

• Cholesterol levels periodically during treatment

• Liver function studies q1-2mo during the first 1½ yr of treatment; AST (SGOT), ALT (SGPT), liver function tests may increase

• Renal function in patients with compromised renal system: BUN, creatinine, I&O ratio

---

◆ = Nursing alert　　🖊 = Herb-drug interaction　　🚫 = Do not crush

• Eyes with slit lamp before, 1 mo after treatment begins, annually; lens opacities may occur

Administer:
• In evening with meal; if dose is increased, take with breakfast and evening meal

Perform/provide:
• Storage in cool environment in airtight, light-resistant container

Evaluate:
• Therapeutic response: cholesterol at desired level after 8 wk

Teach patient/family:
• That treatment will take several years
• That blood work and eye exam will be necessary during treatment
• To report blurred vision, severe GI symptoms, dizziness, headache
• That previously prescribed regimen will continue: low-cholesterol diet, exercise program

---

cetirizine (℞)

(se-teer'i-zeen)

Zyrtec

Func. class.: Antihistamine

Chem. class.: H_1-histamine antagonist

Action: Acts on blood vessels, GI, respiratory system by competing with histamine for H_1-receptor site; decreases allergic response by blocking pharmacologic effects of histamine

Uses: Rhinitis, allergy symptoms

Dosage and routes:
• *Adult and child >12 yr:* **PO** 5-10 mg qd
• *Child 6-11 yr:* **PO** 5-10 mg qd
• *Geriatric:* **PO** 5 mg qd, may increase to 10 mg/day

Available forms: Tabs 5, 10 mg; syrup 5 mg/5 ml

Side effects/adverse reactions:
GU: Frequency, dysuria, urinary retention, impotence

HEMA: **Hemolytic anemia, thrombocytopenia, leukopenia, agranulocytosis, pancytopenia**

RESP: Thickening of bronchial secretions, dry nose, throat

GI: Nausea, diarrhea, abdominal pain, vomiting, constipation

CNS: Headache, stimulation, drowsiness, sedation, fatigue, confusion, blurred vision, tinnitus, restlessness, tremors, paradoxical excitation in children or elderly

INTEG: Rash, eczema, photosensitivity, urticaria

CV: Hypotension, palpitations, bradycardia, tachycardia, ***dysrhythmias*** (rare)

Contraindications: Hypersensitivity, newborn or premature infants, lactation, severe hepatic disease

Precautions: Pregnancy (C), elderly, children, respiratory disease, narrow-angle glaucoma, prostatic hypertrophy, bladder neck obstruction, asthma, elderly

Pharmacokinetics:
PO: Peak 1-2 hr

Interactions:
• Increased CNS depression: alcohol, other CNS depressants, procarbazine
• Increased anticholinergic effects: MAOIs
• Decreased action of oral anticoagulants
• Serious CV reactions: ketoconazole, itraconazole, erythromycin
• Avoid use with antifungals, macrolide antibiotics
⚕ Increased CNS depression: kava kava

Lab test interferences:
False negative: Skin allergy tests

NURSING CONSIDERATIONS

Assess:
• I&O ratio: be alert for urinary re-

tention, frequency, dysuria, especially elderly; drug should be discontinued if these occur
• CBC during long-term therapy
• Respiratory status: rate, rhythm, increase in bronchial secretions, wheezing, chest tightness

Administer:
• On empty stomach 1 hr before or 2 hr after meals

Perform/provide:
• Hard candy, gum, frequent rinsing of mouth for dryness
• Storage in tight, light-resistant container

Evaluate:
• Therapeutic response: absence of running or congested nose or rashes

Teach patient/family:
• All aspects of drug use; to notify prescriber if confusion, sedation, hypotension occur
• To avoid driving, other hazardous activity if drowsiness occurs
• To avoid alcohol, other CNS depressants
• Not to exceed recommended dose; dysrhythmias may occur

Treatment for overdose: Administer ipecac syrup or lavage, diazepam, vasopressors, barbiturates (short-acting)

---

chenodiol (℞)
(kee-noe-dye'ole)
Chenix
Func. class.: Antilithic
Chem. class.: Chenodeoxycholic acid

Action: Suppresses synthesis of cholesterol, cholic acid, replacing cholic acid with drug metabolite, which leads to degradation of gallstones
Uses: Dissolving gallstones instead of surgery; drug has no effect on radiopaque, calcified gallstones or bile pigment stones

Dosage and routes:
• *Adult:* **PO** 250 mg bid × 2 wk, then increased by 250 mg/day, not to exceed 16 mg/kg/day × 24 mo
Available forms: Tabs 250 mg

Side effects/adverse reactions:
HEMA: **Leukopenia**
GI: Diarrhea, fecal urgency, heartburn, nausea, cramps; increased ALT, AST, LDH; vomiting, dysphagia, absence of taste, *hepatotoxicity,* flatulence, dyspepsia

Contraindications: Hypersensitivity, hepatic disease, bile duct obstruction, biliary GI fistula, pregnancy (X)

Precautions: Lactation, children, atherosclerosis, elderly

Pharmacokinetics: Metabolized by liver; excreted in feces (metabolite/unchanged drug); crosses placenta

Interactions:
• Decreased action of chenodiol: cholestyramine, colestipol, aluminum antacids, estrogens, clofibrate

NURSING CONSIDERATIONS
Assess:
• Vital signs, cardiac status: checking for dysrhythmias, increased rate, palpitations
• I&O ratio; check for urinary retention or hesitancy, especially elderly
• Oral cholecystogram or ultrasonogram q6-9mo
• GI complaints: nausea, vomiting, anorexia, diarrhea; if diarrhea is severe, dosage may have to be decreased

Administer:
• With meals for better absorption
• Antidiarrheals if diarrhea occurs

Perform/provide:
• Storage at room temperature
• Increased fluids, bulk, exercise to patient's lifestyle to decrease constipation

---

C

Evaluate:
• Therapeutic response: absence of pain (epigastric), gallstones on diagnostic testing
Teach patient/family:
• That stone dissolution may take 6-24 mo; therapy is discontinued in 18 mo if gallstones are still intact
• To notify prescriber if pregnancy is suspected; birth defects may occur

---

chloral hydrate (℞)

(klor-al hye'drate)
Aquachloral, chloral hydrate, Novochlorhydrate*, PMS-chloral hydrate*
Func. class.: Sedative/hypnotic
Chem. class.: Chloral derivative

Controlled Substance Schedule IV (USA), Schedule F (Canada)
Action: Reduction product trichloroethanol produces mild cerebral depression, which causes sleep
Uses: Sedation, insomnia
Dosage and routes:
Sedation
• *Adult:* **PO/RECT** 250 mg tid pc
• *Child:* **PO** 25-50 mg/kg tid, not to exceed 500 mg tid
Insomnia
• *Adult:* **PO/RECT** 500 mg-1 g ½ hr before hs
Procedure sedation
• *Child:* **PO/RECT** 25-50 mg/kg, not to exceed 100 mg/kg or 2 g
Renal disease
• CrCl <50 ml/min avoid use
Available forms: Caps 250, 500 mg; syr 250, 500 mg/5 ml; supp 325, 500, 650 mg
Side effects/adverse reactions:
*HEMA: **Eosinophilia, leukopenia***
*CNS: **Drowsiness,** dizziness, stimulation, nightmares, ataxia, hangover* (rare), light-headedness, headache, paranoia
GI: Nausea, vomiting, flatulence, diarrhea, unpleasant taste, ***gastric necrosis***
INTEG: Rash, urticaria, ***angioedema,*** fever, purpura, eczema
CV: Hypotension, ***dysrhythmias***
*RESP: **Depression***
Contraindications: Hypersensitivity to this drug or triclofos, severe renal disease, severe hepatic disease, GI disorders (oral forms), gastritis
Precautions: Severe cardiac disease, depression, suicidal individuals, asthma, intermittent porphyria, pregnancy (C), lactation, elderly
Pharmacokinetics:
PO: Onset 30 min-1 hr, duration 4-8 hr
REC: Onset slow, duration 4-6 hr; metabolized by liver; excreted by kidneys (inactive metabolite) and feces; crosses placenta; excreted in breast milk; metabolite is highly protein bound
Interactions:
• Increased action: oral anticoagulants, furosemide
• Increased action of both drugs: alcohol, CNS depressants
🍴 Increased CNS depression: kava kava
Lab test interferences:
Interference: Urine catecholamines, urinary 17-OHCS
False positive: Urine glucose (copper sulfate test)
NURSING CONSIDERATIONS
Assess:
• Blood studies: Hct, Hgb, RBCs, serum folate (if on long-term therapy), pro-time in patients receiving anticoagulants
• Mental status: mood, sensorium, affect, memory (long, short)

• Physical dependency: more frequent requests for medication, shakes, anxiety, pinpoint pupils
• Respiratory dysfunction: respiratory depression, character, rate, rhythm; hold drug if respirations <10/min or if pupils dilated (rare)
• Blood dyscrasias: fever, sore throat, bruising, rash, jaundice, epistaxis (rare)
• History of substance abuse, cardiac disease, gastritis
Administer:
• After trying conservative measures for insomnia
• ½-1 hr before hs for sleeplessness
🚫 On empty stomach with full glass of water or juice for best absorption and to decrease corrosion (do not break, crush, or chew); after meals to decrease GI symptoms if using for sedation
Perform/provide:
• Assistance with ambulation after receiving dose, especially elderly
• Safety measure: side rails, nightlight, call bell within easy reach
• Checking to see PO medication swallowed
• Storage in dark container, suppositories in refrigerator
Evaluate:
• Therapeutic response: ability to sleep at night, decreased amount of early morning awakening if taking drug for insomnia
Teach patient/family:
• To avoid driving, other activities requiring alertness
• To avoid alcohol ingestion, CNS depressants; serious CNS depression may result
• Not to discontinue medication quickly after long-term use; drug should be tapered over 1-2 wk
• That effects may take 2 nights for benefits to be noticed
🚫 Not to break, crush, or chew caps

• Alternative measures to improve sleep (reading, exercise several hours before hs, warm bath, warm milk, TV, self-hypnosis, deep breathing)
Treatment of overdose: Lavage, activated charcoal; monitor electrolytes, vital signs

---

chlorambucil (℞)

(klor-am'byoo-sil)
Leukeran
Func. class.: Antineoplastic alkylating agent
Chem. class.: Nitrogen mustard

Action: Alkylates DNA, RNA; inhibits enzymes that allow synthesis of amino acids in proteins; activity is not cell cycle phase specific
Uses: Chronic lymphocytic leukemia, Hodgkin's disease, other lymphomas, macroglobulinemia, nephrotic syndrome, breast carcinoma, choreocarcinoma, ovarian carcinoma
Dosage and routes:
• *Adult:* **PO** 0.1-0.2 mg/kg/day for 3-6 wk initially, then 2-6 mg/day; maintenance 0.2 mg/kg for 2-4 wk; course may be repeated at 2-4 wk intervals
• *Child:* **PO** 0.1-0.2 mg/kg/day in divided doses or 4.5 mg/m²/day as 1 dose or in divided doses
Available forms: Tabs 2 mg
Side effects/adverse reactions:
CNS: Convulsions in children
HEMA: Thrombocytopenia, leukopenia, pancytopenia (prolonged use), *permanent bone marrow depression*
GI: Nausea, vomiting, diarrhea, weight loss, hepatoxicity, jaundice
GU: Hyperuremia
INTEG: Alopecia (rare), dermatitis, rash
RESP: Fibrosis, pneumonitis
Contraindications: Radiation therapy within 1 mo, chemotherapy

---

within 1 mo, thrombocytopenia, smallpox vaccination, pregnancy (1st trimester) (D), lactation

Precautions: *Pneumococcus* vaccination

Pharmacokinetics: Well absorbed orally; metabolized in liver; excreted in urine; half-life 2 hr

Interactions:

• Increased toxicity: other antineoplastics, radiation

NURSING CONSIDERATIONS
Assess:

• Bleeding: hematuria, guaiac, bruising or petechiae, mucosa or orifices q8h

• Food preferences; list likes, dislikes

• Yellowing of skin, sclera, dark urine, clay-colored stools, itchy skin, abdominal pain, fever, diarrhea

• Dyspnea, rales, unproductive cough, chest pain, tachypnea

• Effects of alopecia on body image; discuss feelings about body changes (rare)

• CBC, differential, platelet count weekly, withhold drug if WBC is <4000 or platelet count is <75,000; notify prescriber of results

• Pulmonary function tests, chest x-ray films before, during therapy; chest film should be obtained q2wk during treatment

• Renal function studies: BUN, serum uric acid, urine CrCl before, during therapy

• I&O ratio; report fall in urine output of <30 ml/hr

• Monitor temperature q4h (may indicate beginning infection)

• Liver function tests before, during therapy (bilirubin, AST, ALT, LDH) as needed or monthly

Administer:

PO

• Antacid before oral agent; give drug 2 hr after evening meal, before bedtime

• Antiemetic 30-60 min before giving drug to prevent vomiting

• Allopurinol or sodium bicarbonate to maintain uric acid levels, alkalinization of urine

• Antibiotics for prophylaxis of infection

Perform/provide:

• Storage in tight container

• Strict medical asepsis, protective isolation if WBC levels are low

• Increase fluid intake to 2-3 L/day to prevent urate deposits, calculi formation

• Diet low in purines: organ meats (kidney, liver), dried beans, peas to maintain alkaline urine

Evaluate:

• Therapeutic response: decreased size of tumor, spread of malignancy

Teach patient/family:

• To report signs of infection: increased temperature, sore throat, flu symptoms

• To report signs of anemia: fatigue, headache, faintness, shortness of breath, irritability

• To report bleeding; avoid use of razors, commercial mouthwash

• To avoid use of aspirin products, ibuprofen

• About protective isolation precautions

• To report any changes in breathing or coughing

• That hair may be lost during treatment; a wig or hairpiece may make patient feel better; new hair may be different in color, texture (rare)

---

chloramphenicol (R)

(klor-am-fen'i-kole)

Ak-Chlor, Chloracol, chloramphenicol, Chlorofair, Chloromycetin, Chloroptic, Econochlor, Fenicol*, I-Chlor, Novochlorocap*

Func. class.: Antiinfective, misc
Chem. class.: Dichloroacetic acid derivative

Action: Binds to 50S ribosomal subunit, which interferes with or inhibits protein synthesis

Uses: Infections caused by *H. influenzae, S. typhi, Rickettsia, Neisseria,* mycoplasma

Dosage and routes:
• *Adult and child:* **PO/IV** 50-75 mg/kg/day in divided doses q6h, 100 mg/kg/day (for meningitis only) max 4 g/day
• *Premature infants and neonates:* **IV/PO** 25 mg/kg/day in divided doses q12-24h
Available forms: Inj 1 g; caps 250 mg

Side effects/adverse reactions:
HEMA: Anemia, thrombocytopenia, aplastic anemia, granulocytopenia, leukopenia (rare)
EENT: Optic neuritis, blindness
GI: Nausea, vomiting, diarrhea, abdominal pain, xerostomia, glossitis, colitis, pruritus ani
INTEG: Itching, urticaria, contact dermatitis, rash
CV: Gray syndrome in newborns: failure to feed, pallor, cyanosis, abdominal distention, irregular respiration, vasomotor collapse
CNS: Headache, *depression,* confusion

Contraindications: Hypersensitivity, severe renal disease, severe hepatic disease, minor infections

Precautions: Hepatic disease, renal disease, infants, children, bone marrow depression (drug-induced), pregnancy (C), lactation

Pharmacokinetics:
PO/IV: Peak 1-2 hr, duration 8 hr, half-life 1½-4 hr; conjugated in liver; excreted in urine (up to 15% as free drug, up to 80% in neonates), breast milk, feces; crosses placenta

Interactions:
• Increased action of phenytoin, tolbutamide, chlorpropamide, phenobarbital
• Increased prothrombin time: anticoagulants
• Decreased action of iron, vit B_{12}, folic acid, penicillins
• Avoid use with myelosuppressive drugs

NURSING CONSIDERATIONS
Assess:
• Signs of infection, anemia
◆ Any patient with compromised renal system; drug is excreted slowly in poor renal system function; toxicity may occur rapidly
• Liver studies: AST (SGOT), ALT (SGPT)
• Blood studies: WBC, RBC, Hct, Hgb, platelets, serum iron, reticulocytes; drug should be discontinued if bone marrow is depressed
• Renal studies: urinalysis, protein, blood, BUN, creatinine
• C&S before drug therapy; may be given as soon as culture is taken
• Drug level in impaired hepatic, renal systems; peak 15-20 mg/ml 3 hr after dose, trough 5-10 mg/ml prior to next dose
• Bowel pattern before, during treatment
• Skin eruptions, itching, dermatitis after administration
• Respiratory status: rate, character, wheezing, tightness in chest
• Allergies before treatment, reac-

tion of each medication; place allergies on chart, bright red letters; notify all people giving drugs

• Neonates for beginning Gray syndrome: cyanosis, abdominal distention, irregular respiration, failure to feed; drug should be discontinued immediately

Administer:

• Oral form on empty stomach with full glass of water

• IM route not recommended

IV

• After diluting 1 g/10 ml of sterile H_2O for inj or D_5W (10% sol); give >1 min; may be further diluted in 50-100 ml of D_5W; give through Y-tube, 3-way stopcock, or additive inf set; run over ½-1 hr

Additive compatibilities: Amikacin, aminophylline, ascorbic acid, calcium chloride or gluconate, cephalothin, cephapirin, colistimethate, corticotropin, cyanocobalamin, dimenhydrinate, dopamine, ephedrine, heparin, hydrocortisone, kanamycin, lidocaine, magnesium sulfate, metaraminol, methicillin, methyldopate, methylprednisolone, metronidazole, nafcillin, oxacillin, oxytocin, penicillin G potassium, penicillin G sodium, pentobarbital, phenylephrine, phytonadione, plasma protein fraction, potassium chloride, promazine, ranitidine, sodium bicarbonate, thiopental, verapamil, vit B/C

Syringe compatibilities: Ampicillin, cloxacillin, heparin, methicillin, penicillin G sodium

Y-site compatibilities: Acyclovir, cyclophosphamide, enalaprilat, esmolol, foscarnet, hydromorphone, labetalol, magnesium sulfate, meperidine, morphine, perphenazine, tacrolimus

Perform/provide:

• Storage of capsules in tight container at room temperature, reconstituted sol at room temp 30 days

• Adrenalin, suction, tracheostomy set, endotracheal intubation equipment on unit

• Adequate intake of fluids (2 L) during diarrhea episodes

Evaluate:

• Therapeutic response: decreased symptoms of infection

Teach patient/family:

• All aspects of drug therapy: the need to complete entire course to ensure organism death (10-14 days); culture may be taken after complete course of medication

🚫 Not to break, crush, or chew caps

• To report sore throat, fever, fatigue, unusual bleeding, bruising; could indicate bone marrow depression (may occur weeks or months after termination of drug)

• That drug must be taken in equal intervals around clock to maintain blood levels

Treatment of hypersensitivity: Withdraw drug, maintain airway, administer epinephrine, aminophylline, O_2, IV corticosteroids

---

chlordiazepoxide (℞)

(klor-dye-az-e-pox′ide)
Apo-Chlordiazepoxide*, chlordiazepoxide HCl*, Libritabs, Librium, Novopoxide*, Solium*

Func. class.: Antianxiety
Chem. class.: Benzodiazepine

Controlled Substance Schedule IV
Action: Potentiates the actions of GABA, especially in the limbic system, reticular formation
Uses: Short-term management of anxiety, acute alcohol withdrawal, preoperatively for relaxation

---

Dosage and routes:
Mild anxiety
• *Adult:* **PO** 5-10 mg tid-qid
• *Child* >6 yr: 5 mg bid-qid, not to exceed 10 mg bid-tid
Severe anxiety
• *Adult:* **PO** 20-25 mg tid-qid
Preoperatively
• *Adult:* **PO** 5-10 mg tid-qid on day before surgery; **IM** 50-100 mg 1 hr before surgery
Alcohol withdrawal
• *Adult:* **PO/IM/IV** 50-100 mg, not to exceed 300 mg/day
Available forms: Caps 5, 10, 25 mg; tabs 5, 10, 25 mg; powder for inj 100 mg ampule

Side effects/adverse reactions:
CNS: Dizziness, drowsiness, confusion, headache, anxiety, tremors, stimulation, fatigue, depression, insomnia, hallucinations
GI: Constipation, dry mouth, nausea, vomiting, anorexia, diarrhea
INTEG: Rash, dermatitis, itching
CV: Orthostatic hypotension, **ECG changes, tachycardia,** hypotension
EENT: Blurred vision, tinnitus, mydriasis

Contraindications: Hypersensitivity to benzodiazepines, narrow-angle glaucoma, psychosis, pregnancy (D), lactation, child <18 yr

Precautions: Elderly, debilitated, hepatic disease, renal disease

Pharmacokinetics:
PO: Onset 30 min, peak ½ hr, duration 4-6 hr; metabolized by liver, excreted by kidneys; crosses placenta, excreted in breast milk; half-life 5-30 hr (increased in elderly)

Interactions:
• Decreased effects of chlordiazepoxide: oral contraceptives, rifampin, valproic acid
• Increased effects of chlordiazepoxide: CNS depressants, alcohol, cimetidine, disulfiram, oral contraceptives

📁 Increased CNS depression: kava kava

Lab test interferences:
Increase: AST/ALT, serum bilirubin
False increase: 17-OHCS
Decrease: RAIU

NURSING CONSIDERATIONS
Assess:
• B/P (lying, standing), pulse; if systolic B/P drops 20 mm Hg, hold drug, notify prescriber
• Blood studies: CBC during long-term therapy; blood dyscrasias have occurred rarely
• Hepatic studies: AST (SGOT), ALT (SGPT), bilirubin, creatinine, LDH, alk phosphatase
• I&O; may indicate renal dysfunction
• For ataxia, oversedation in elderly, debilitated patients
• Mental status: mood, sensorium, affect, sleeping pattern, drowsiness, dizziness
• Physical dependency, withdrawal symptoms: headache, nausea, vomiting, muscle pain, weakness after long-term use
• Suicidal tendencies, paradoxic reactions such as excitement, stimulation, acute rage

Administer:
• With food or milk for GI symptoms
• Crushed if patient is unable to swallow medication whole
• Sugarless gum, hard candy, frequent sips of water for dry mouth
IV
• 5 ml NS/100 mg powder; agitate ampule gently; give through Y-tube or 3-way stopcock; give 100 mg or less ≥1 min; do not use IM diluent for IV use

Solution compatibilities: D_5W, 0.9% NaCl

Y-site compatibilities: Heparin, hy-

◆ = Nursing alert   📁 = Herb-drug interaction   🚫 = Do not crush drocortisone, potassium chloride, vit B/C

Perform/provide:
• Assistance with ambulation during beginning therapy, since drowsiness/dizziness occurs
• Safety measures, including side rails
• Check to see PO medication has been swallowed

Evaluate:
• Therapeutic response: decreased anxiety, restlessness, sleeplessness

Teach patient/family:
• That drug may be taken with food
• Not to use drug for everyday stress or use longer than 4 mo, unless directed by prescriber
• Not to take more than prescribed amount; may be habit forming
• To avoid OTC preparations unless approved by prescriber
• To avoid driving, activities that require alertness; drowsiness may occur
• To avoid alcohol ingestion, other psychotropic medications, unless directed by prescriber
• Not to discontinue medication abruptly after long-term use; may precipitate convulsions
• To rise slowly or fainting may occur, especially elderly
• That drowsiness may worsen at beginning of treatment

Treatment of overdose: Lavage, VS, supportive care, give flumazenil

---

chloroprocaine (℞)

(klor'-oh-pro-kane)
Nesacaine, Nesacaine-MPF
Func. class.: Local anesthetic
Chem. class.: Ester

Action: Competes with calcium for sites in nerve membrane that control sodium transport across cell membrane; decreases rise of depolarization phase of action potential

Uses: Epidural anesthesia, peripheral nerve block, caudal anesthesia, infiltration block

Dosage and routes:
• Varies by route of anesthesia
Available forms: Inj 1%, 2%, 3%

Side effects/adverse reactions:
CNS: Anxiety, restlessness, ***convulsions, loss of consciousness,*** drowsiness, disorientation, tremors, shivering
CV: ***Myocardial depression, cardiac arrest, dysrhythmias,*** bradycardia, hypotension, hypertension, fetal bradycardia
GI: Nausea, vomiting
EENT: Blurred vision, tinnitus, pupil constriction
INTEG: Rash, urticaria, allergic reactions, edema, burning, skin discoloration at injection site, tissue necrosis
RESP: ***Status asthmaticus, respiratory arrest, anaphylaxis***

Contraindications: Hypersensitivity, child <12 yr, elderly, severe liver disease

Precautions: Elderly, severe drug allergies, pregnancy (C), lactation

Pharmacokinetics: Duration ½-1 hr; metabolized by liver; excreted in urine (metabolites)

Interactions:
• Dysrhythmias: epinephrine, halothane, enflurane
• Hypertension: MAOIs, tricyclic antidepressants, phenothiazines

NURSING CONSIDERATIONS

Assess:
• B/P, pulse, respiration during treatment
• Fetal heart tones if used during labor
• Allergic reactions: rash, urticaria, itching

• Cardiac status: ECG for dysrhythmias, pulse, B/P during anesthesia

Administer:

• Only with crash cart, resuscitative equipment nearby
• Only drugs without preservatives for epidural or caudal anesthesia

Perform/provide:

• Use of new solution; discard unused portions

Evaluate:

• Therapeutic response: anesthesia necessary for procedure

Treatment of overdose: Airway, O_2, vasopressor, IV fluids, anticonvulsants for seizures

---

chloroquine (℞)

(klor'oh-kwin)

Aralen HCl, chloroquine phosphate

Func. class.: Antimalarial

Chem. class.: Synthetic 4-aminoquinoline derivative

Action: Inhibits parasite replications, transcription of DNA to RNA by forming complexes with DNA of parasite

Uses: Malaria of *Plasmodium vivax, P. malariae, P. ovale, P. falciparum* (some strains), amebiasis

Dosage and routes:

Malaria suppression

• *Adult and child:* PO 5 mg base/kg/wk on same day of week, not to exceed 300 mg base; treatment should begin 1-2 wk before exposure and for 8 wk after; if treatment begins after exposure, 600 mg base for adult and 10 mg base/kg for children in 2 divided doses 6 hr apart

Extraintestinal amebiasis

• *Adult:* IM 160-200 mg base qd × 10-12 days or PO (HCl) 600 mg base qd × 2 days, then 300 mg base qd × 2-3 wk (phosphate)

• *Child:* **IM/PO** 10 mg/kg qd (HCl) × 2-3 wk, not to exceed 300 mg/day

Available forms: Tabs 250 mg (150 mg base), 500 mg (300 mg base) phosphate; inj 50 mg (140 mg base)/ml HCl

Side effects/adverse reactions:

CV: Hypotension, ***heart block, asystole with syncope,*** ECG changes

INTEG: Pruritus, pigmentary changes, skin eruptions, lichen planus-like eruptions, eczema, ***exfoliative dermatitis***

CNS: Headache, stimulation, fatigue, ***convulsion,*** psychosis

EENT: Blurred vision, corneal changes, retinal changes, difficulty focusing, tinnitus, vertigo, deafness, photophobia, corneal edema

GI: Nausea, vomiting, anorexia, diarrhea, cramps

*HEMA: **Thrombocytopenia, agranulocytosis, hemolytic anemia, leukopenia***

Contraindications: Hypersensitivity, retinal field changes, porphyria

Precautions: Pregnancy (C), children, blood dyscrasias, severe GI disease, neurologic disease, alcoholism, hepatic disease, G6PD deficiency, psoriasis, eczema, lactation, porphyria

Pharmacokinetics:

PO: Peak 1-6 hr, half-life 3-5 days; metabolized in liver; excreted in urine, feces, breast milk; crosses placenta

Interactions:

• Decreased action of chloroquine: magnesium, aluminum compounds, kaolin
• Reduced oral clearance and metabolism of chloroquine: cimetidine

NURSING CONSIDERATIONS

Assess:

• Ophthalmic test if long-term treatment or dosage >150 mg/day
• Liver studies qwk: AST (SGOT), ALT (SGPT), bilirubin

◆ = Nursing alert   ∥ = Herb-drug interaction   🚫 = Do not crush

• Blood studies: CBC, since blood dyscrasias occur
• ECG during therapy
• Watch for depression of T waves, widening of QRS complex
• Allergic reactions: pruritus, rash, urticaria
• Blood dyscrasias: malaise, fever, bruising, bleeding (rare)
• For ototoxicity (tinnitus, vertigo, change in hearing); audiometric testing should be done before, after treatment
➤ For toxicity: blurring vision; difficulty focusing; headache; dizziness; decreased knee, ankle reflexes; drug should be discontinued immediately

Administer:
• IM after aspirating to avoid injection into blood system, which may cause hypotension, asystole, heart block; rotate injection sites
IV
• Before or after meals at same time each day to maintain drug level

Additive compatibilities: Promethazine

Perform/provide:
• Storage in tight, light-resistant container at room temp; keep injection in cool environment

Evaluate:
• Therapeutic response: decreased symptoms of infection

Teach patient/family:
• To use sunglasses in bright sunlight to decrease photophobia
• That urine may turn rust or brown color
• To report hearing, visual problems, fever, fatigue, bruising, bleeding, which may indicate blood dyscrasias

Treatment of overdose: Induce vomiting, gastric lavage, administer barbiturate (ultrashort-acting), vasopressor; tracheostomy may be necessary

chlorothiazide (℞)
(klor-oh-thye′a-zide)
Diuril
Func. class.: Diuretic
Chem. class.: Thiazide; sulfonamide derivative

Action: Acts on distal tubule and thick ascending limb of the loop of Henle by increasing excretion of water, sodium, chloride, potassium, magnesium

Uses: Edema, hypertension, diuresis

Dosage and routes:
Edema, hypertension
• *Adult:* PO/IV 500 mg-2 g qd in 2 divided doses
Diuresis
• *Adult:* IV 250 mg q6-12h
• *Child >6 mo:* PO 20 mg/kg/day in 2 divided doses
• *Child <6 mo:* PO up to 40 mg/kg/day in 2 doses
Available forms: Tabs 250, 500 mg; inj 500 mg

Side effects/adverse reactions:
CNS: Paresthesia, anxiety, depression, headache, *dizziness, fatigue, weakness,* insomnia
CV: Irregular pulse, orthostatic hypotension, palpitations, volume depletion
EENT: Blurred vision
ELECT: *Hypokalemia,* hypercalcemia, hyponatremia, hypochloremia, hypophosphatemia, hypomagnesemia
GI: Nausea, vomiting, anorexia, constipation, diarrhea, cramps, pancreatitis, GI irritation, *hepatitis*
GU: Frequency, polyuria, *uremia,* glucosuria, hematuria
*HEMA: **Aplastic anemia, hemolytic anemia, leukopenia, agranulocytosis, thrombocytopenia, neutropenia***

INTEG: Rash, urticaria, purpura, photosensitivity, fever, alopecia
META: Hyperglycemia, *hyperuricemia,* increased creatinine, BUN
Contraindications: Hypersensitivity to thiazides or sulfonamides, hepatic coma, anuria, renal decompensation, pregnancy (B), lactation
Precautions: Hypokalemia, renal disease, hepatic disease, gout, COPD, lupus erythematosus, diabetes mellitus, elderly, hyperlipidemia
Pharmacokinetics: Not well absorbed PO
PO: Onset 2 hr, peak 4 hr, duration 6-12 hr; crosses placenta, excreted in breast milk, excreted unchanged by kidneys; half-life 2 hr
Interactions:
• Increased toxicity: lithium, nondepolarizing skeletal muscle relaxants, digitalis, allopurinol
• Increased hypotension: other antihypertensives, alcohol
• Decreased effects of: antidiabetics, sulfonylureas, anticoagulants
• Decreased absorption of thiazides: cholestyramine, colestipol
• Decreased hypotensive response: indomethacin, other NSAIDs
• Hypokalemia: ticarcillin, glucocorticoids, amphotericin, mezlocillin, piperacillin
• Hyperglycemia, hypotension: diazoxide
🥀 Potassium deficiency: chronic use/abuse cascara sagrada bark, aloe, buckthorn bark/berry, licorice root, senna pod/leaf
Lab test interferences:
False negative: Phentolamine and tyramine tests
Interference: Urine steroid tests
Increase: BSP retention, Ca, amylase, parathyroid test
Decrease: PBI, PSP

NURSING CONSIDERATIONS
Assess:
• Weight, I&O daily to determine fluid loss; effect of drug may be decreased if used qd
• Rate, depth, rhythm of respirations; effect of exertion
• B/P lying, standing; postural hypotension may occur, especially in elderly
• Electrolytes: K, Na, Cl; include BUN, blood glucose, CBC, serum creatinine, blood pH, ABGs, uric acid, Ca, Mg
• Glucose in urine if patient is diabetic
• Improvement in CVP q8h
• Signs of metabolic alkalosis: drowsiness, restlessness
• Rashes, temp elevation qd
• Confusion, especially in elderly; take safety precautions if needed
Administer:
• In AM to avoid interference with sleep if using drug as a diuretic
• K replacement if K less than 3 mg/dl
• With food if nausea occurs; absorption may be decreased slightly; tablets may be crushed
• After shaking suspension
IV
• After diluting 0.5 g/18 ml or more of sterile water for inj; may be diluted further with 0.9% NaCl, D_5W, check for extravasation; give over 5 min (0.5 g/5 m)
Additive compatibilities: Cimetidine, lidocaine, nafcillin, ranitidine, sodium bicarbonate
Evaluate:
• Therapeutic response: improvement in edema of feet, legs, sacral area daily if medication is being used for CHF
Teach patient/family:
• To rise slowly from lying or sit-

◆ = Nursing alert   🥀 = Herb-drug interaction   🚫 = Do not crush ting position; orthostatic hypotension may occur

• To notify prescriber of muscle weakness, cramps, nausea, dizziness

• That drug may be taken with food or milk; to take at same time each day; not to double dose; dehydration may occur

• That blood sugar may be increased in diabetics

• To take early in day to avoid nocturia

• To use sunscreen (not with PABA); use protective clothing to prevent photosensitivity

• To weigh weekly and notify prescriber of change of >3 lb

• To eat diet high in K

• Not to take OTC medications without consulting prescriber

Treatment of overdose: Lavage if taken orally; monitor electrolytes; administer dextrose in saline; monitor hydration, CV, renal status

---

chlorpheniramine
(OTC, ℞)

(klor-fen-hir'a-meen)

Aller-Chlor, Chlo-Amine, Chlorate, Chlor-100, Chlor-Niramine, chlorpheniramine maleate, Chlor-Pro, Chlor-Span, Chlortab, Chlor-Trimeton, Chlor-Tripolon*, Gen-Allerate, Novo-Pheniram*, Pedia Care Allergy Formula, Pfeiffer's Allergy, Phenetron, Telachlor, Teldrin, Trimegen

Func. class.: Antihistamine
Chem. class.: Alkylamine, H_1-receptor antagonist

Action: Acts on blood vessels, GI system, respiratory system, by competing with histamine for H_1-receptor site; decreases allergic response by blocking histamine

Uses: Allergy symptoms, rhinitis

Dosage and routes:

• *Adult:* **PO** 2-4 mg tid-qid, not to exceed 36 mg/day; **TIME-REL** 8-12 mg bid-tid, not to exceed 24 mg/day; **IM/IV/SC** 5-40 mg/day

• *Child 6-12 yr:* **PO** 2 mg q4-6h, not to exceed 12 mg/day; **SUS REL** 8 mg hs or qd, **SUS REL** not recommended for child <6 yr

• *Child 2-5 yr:* **PO** 1 mg q4-6h, not to exceed 4 mg/day

Available forms: Tabs, chewable 2 mg; tabs 4, 8, 12 mg; tabs, time-rel 8, 12 mg; caps, time-rel 8, 12 mg; syr 1, 2 mg/5 ml; inj 10, 100 mg/ml

Side effects/adverse reactions:

CNS: Dizziness, drowsiness, poor coordination, fatigue, anxiety, euphoria, confusion, paresthesia, neuritis

RESP: Increased thick secretions, wheezing, chest tightness

*HEMA. **Thrombocytopenia, agranulocytosis, hemolytic anemia***

GI: Dry mouth, nausea, anorexia, diarrhea

INTEG: Photosensitivity

GU: Retention, dysuria, frequency

EENT: Blurred vision, dilated pupils, tinnitus, nasal stuffiness, dry nose, throat, mouth

Contraindications: Hypersensitivity to H_1-receptor antagonists, acute asthma attack, lower respiratory tract disease

Precautions: Increased intraocular pressure, renal disease, cardiac disease, hypertension, bronchial asthma, seizure disorder, stenosed peptic ulcers, hyperthyroidism, prostatic hypertrophy, bladder neck obstruction, pregnancy (B), lactation, elderly

Pharmacokinetics:

PO: Onset 20-60 min, duration 8-12 hr; detoxified in liver; excreted by

---

kidneys (metabolites/free drug); half-life 20-24 hr

Interactions:
• Increased CNS depression: barbiturates, narcotics, hypnotics, tricyclic antidepressants, alcohol
• Decreased effect of oral anticoagulants, heparin
• Increased effect of chlorpheniramine: MAOIs

 Increased CNS depression: kava kava

 Increased anticholinergic effect: henbane leaf

Lab test interferences:
False negative: Skin allergy tests

NURSING CONSIDERATIONS
Assess:
• I&O ratio; be alert for urinary retention, frequency, dysuria; drug should be discontinued
• CBC during long-term therapy
• Blood dyscrasias: thrombocytopenia, agranulocytosis (rare)
• Respiratory status: rate, rhythm, increase in bronchial secretions, wheezing, chest tightness

Administer:
• With meals for GI symptoms; absorption may slightly decrease

IV
• Undiluted at ≥10 mg/1 min

Additive compatibilities: Amikacin

Perform/provide:
• Hard candy, gum, frequent rinsing of mouth for dryness
• Storage in tight container at room temp

Evaluate:
• Therapeutic response: absence of running, congested nose, rashes

Teach patient/family:
 Not to break, crush, or chew sustained-release forms
• All aspects of drug use; to notify prescriber of confusion/sedation/hypotension, difficulty voiding

• That this drug decreases anticoagulant (oral) effect
• To avoid driving, other hazardous activity if drowsiness occurs, especially elderly
• To avoid concurrent use of alcohol, other CNS depressants

Treatment of overdose: Administer ipecac syrup or lavage, diazepam, vasopressors, barbiturates (short-acting)

---

chlorpromazine (R)
(klor-proe'ma-zeen)
Chlorpromanyl*, chlorpromazine HCl, Largactil*, Novo-Chlorpromazine*, Thorazine, Thor-Prom
Func. class.: Antipsychotic/neuroleptic/antiemetic
Chem. class.: Phenothiazine-aliphatic

Action: Depresses cerebral cortex, hypothalamus, limbic system, which control activity aggression; blocks neurotransmission produced by dopamine at synapse; exhibits a strong α-adrenergic, anticholinergic blocking action; mechanism for antipsychotic effects is unclear

Uses: Psychotic disorders, mania, schizophrenia, anxiety, intractable hiccups, nausea, vomiting; preoperatively for relaxation; acute intermittent porphyria, behavioral problems in children, nonpsychotic, demented patients

Dosage and routes:
Psychiatry
• *Adult:* **PO** 10-50 mg q1-4h initially, then increase up to 2 g/day if necessary
• *Adult:* **IM** 10-50 mg q1-4h
• *Geriatric:* Use lowest effective dose

 = Nursing alert   = Herb-drug interaction   = Do not crush

- *Child:* **PO** 0.25 mg/lb q4-6h or 0.5 mg/kg
- *Child:* **IM** 0.25 mg/lb q6-8h or 0.5 mg/kg
- *Child:* **RECT** 0.5 mg/lb q6-8h or 1 mg/kg

Nausea and vomiting
- *Adult:* **PO** 10-25 mg q4-6h prn; **IM** 25-50 mg q3h prn; **RECT** 50-100 mg q6-8h prn, not to exceed 400 mg/day; **IV** 25-50 mg qd-qid
- *Child:* **PO** 0.25 mg/lb q4-6h prn; **IM** 0.25 mg/lb q6-8h prn not to exceed 40 mg/day (<5 yr) or 75 mg/day (5-12 yr); **RECT** 0.5 mg/lb: q6-8h prn; **IV** 0.55 mg/kg q6-8h

Intractable hiccups
- *Adult:* **PO** 25-50 mg tid-qid; **IM** 25-50 mg (only if PO dose does not work); **IV** 25-50 mg in 500-1000 ml **NS** (only for severe hiccups)

Available forms: Tabs 10, 25, 50, 100, 200 mg; time-rel caps 30, 75, 150, 200, 300 mg; syr 10 mg/5ml; conc 30, 100 mg/ml; supp 25, 100 mg; inj 25 mg/ml

Side effects/adverse reactions:
CV: Orthostatic hypotension, hypertension, ***cardiac arrest***, ECG changes, *tachycardia*
EENT: Blurred vision, glaucoma, dry eyes
GI: Dry mouth, nausea, vomiting, anorexia, constipation, diarrhea, jaundice, weight gain
GU: Urinary retention, enuresis, impotence, amenorrhea, gynecomastia, breast engorgement
HEMA: Anemia, ***leukopenia, leukocytosis, agranulocytosis***
INTEG: Rash, photosensitivity, dermatitis
RESP: ***Laryngospasm,*** dyspnea, ***respiratory depression***
CNS: EPS: pseudoparkinsonism, akathisia, dystonia, tardive dyskinesia, seizures, *headache,* ***neuroleptic malignant syndrome*** *(rare)*

Contraindications: Hypersensitivity, circulatory collapse, liver damage, cerebral arteriosclerosis, coronary disease, severe hypertension/hypotension, blood dyscrasias, coma, child <2 yr, brain damage, bone marrow depression, alcohol and barbiturate withdrawal

Precautions: Pregnancy (C), lactation, seizure disorders, hypertension, hepatic disease, cardiac disease, elderly

Pharmacokinetics:
PO: Absorption variable, widely distributed; onset erratic 30-60 min, duration 4-6 hr
IM: Well absorbed; peak 15-20 min, duration 4 to 8 hr
IV: Onset 5 min, peak 10 min, duration unknown
PO-ER: Onset 30-60 min, peak unknown, duration 10-12 hr
REC: Onset erratic, duration 3 hr; metabolized by liver, excreted in urine (metabolites), crosses placenta, enters breast milk; 95% bound to plasma proteins; elimination half-life 10-30 hr

Interactions:
- Oversedation: other CNS depressants, alcohol, barbiturate anesthetics, antihistamines, sedatives/hypnotics, antidepressants
- Toxicity: epinephrine
- Decreased absorption: aluminum hydroxide, magnesium hydroxide antacids
- Decreased antiparkinson activity: levodopa, bromocriptine
- Decreased serum chlorpromazine: lithium
- Increased effects of both drugs: β-adrenergic blockers, alcohol
- Increased anticholinergic effects: anticholinergics
- Agranulocystosis: antithyroid agents

Increased CNS depression: kava kava

 Increased anticholinergic effect: henbane leaf

Lab test interferences:

Increase: Liver function tests, cardiac enzymes, cholesterol, blood glucose, prolactin, bilirubin, PBI, cholinesterase, ^{131}I, alk phosphatase, leukocytes, granulocytes, platelets

Decrease: Hormones (blood and urine)

False positive: Pregnancy tests, PKU

False negative: Urinary steroids, 17-OHCS

NURSING CONSIDERATIONS

Assess:

• Mental status: orientation, mood, behavior, presence of hallucinations and type before initial administration and monthly

• Any potentially reversible causes of behavior problems in the elderly before and during therapy

• Swallowing of PO medication; check for hoarding or giving of medication to other patients

• I&O ratio; palpate bladder if low urinary output occurs, especially in elderly

• Bilirubin, CBC, liver function studies monthly

• Urinalysis recommended before, during prolonged therapy

• Affect, orientation, LOC, reflexes, gait, coordination, sleep pattern disturbances

• B/P sitting, standing, lying; take pulse and respirations q4h during initial treatment; establish baseline before starting treatment; report drops of 30 mm Hg; obtain baseline ECG, Q-wave and T-wave changes

• Dizziness, faintness, palpitations, tachycardia on rising

 For neuroleptic malignant syndrome: hyperpyrexia, muscle rigidity, increased CPK, altered mental status, for acute dystonia (check chewing, swallowing, eyes, pin rolling)

• EPS including akathisia (inability to sit still, no pattern to movements), tardive dyskinesia (bizarre movements of the jaw, mouth, tongue, extremities), pseudoparkinsonism (rigidity, tremors, pill rolling, shuffling gait)

• Skin turgor daily

• Constipation, urinary retention daily; increase bulk, H_2O in diet

Administer:

• IM, inject in deep muscle mass, do not give SC

• Rectal after placing in refrigerator for ½ hr if too soft to insert

PO

• With full glass of water, milk; or with food to decrease GI upset

• Drug in liquid form mixed in glass of juice or cola if hoarding is suspected

• Periodically attempt dosage reduction in behavioral problems

IV

• After diluting 1 mg/1 ml with NS, give 1 mg or less/2 min or more; may be further diluted in 500-1000 ml of NS

• Antiparkinsonian agent for EPS

Additive compatibilities: Ascorbic acid, ethacrynate, netilmicin, theophylline, vit B/C

Syringe compatibilities: Atropine, benztropine, butorphanol, diphenhydramine, doxapram, droperidol, fentanyl, glycopyrrolate, hydromorphone, hydroxyzine, meperidine, metoclopramide, midazolam, morphine, pentazocine, perphenazine, prochlorperazine, promazine, promethazine, scopolamine

Y-site compatibilities: Amsacrine, cisplatin, cladribine, cyclophosphamide, cytarabine, doxorubicin, famotidine, filgrastim, fluconazole, granisetron, heparin, hydrocortisone, ondansetron, potassium chloride,

---

 = Nursing alert   = Herb-drug interaction   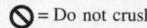 = Do not crush propofol, teniposide, thiotepa, vinorelbine, vit B/C

Perform/provide:
• Decreased stimuli by dimming lights, avoiding loud noises
• Supervised ambulation until stabilized on medication; do not involve in strenuous exercise program because fainting is possible; patient should not stand still for long periods
• Increased fluids to prevent constipation
• Sips of water, candy, gum for dry mouth
• Storage in tight, light-resistant container, oral sol in amber bottle

Evaluate:
• Therapeutic response: decrease in emotional excitement, hallucinations, delusions, paranoia, reorganization of patterns of thought, speech, increase in target behaviors

Teach patient/family:
• To use good oral hygiene; frequent rinsing of mouth, sugarless gum for dry mouth
• To avoid hazardous activities until drug response is determined
🚫 Not to break, crush, or chew time-rel caps
• That orthostatic hypotension occurs often and to rise from sitting or lying position gradually
• To remain lying down after IM injection for at least 30 min
• To avoid hot tubs, hot showers, tub baths, since hypotension may occur
• To avoid abrupt withdrawal of this drug, or EPS may result; drug should be withdrawn slowly
• To avoid OTC preparations (cough, hay fever, cold) unless approved by prescriber, since serious drug interactions may occur; avoid use with alcohol, CNS depressants; increased drowsiness may occur

• To use a sunscreen and sunglasses to prevent burns
• About EPS and necessity of meticulous oral hygiene, since oral candidiasis may occur
• To take antacids 2 hr before or after this drug
• To report sore throat, malaise, fever, bleeding, mouth sores; CBC should be drawn and drug discontinued
• That in hot weather, heat stroke may occur; take extra precautions to stay cool
• Contraceptive measures
• That urine may turn pink or red

Treatment of overdose: Lavage if orally ingested; provide airway; *do not induce vomiting or use epinephrine*

---

chlorthalidone (℞)

(klor-thal'i-done)
Apo-Chlorthalidone*, chlor–thalidone, Hygroton, Hylidone, Novothalidone*, Thalitone, Uridon*

Func. class.: Diuretic
Chem. class.: Thiazide-like phthalimidine derivative

Action: Acts on distal tubule and thick ascending limb of the loop of Henle by increasing excretion of water, sodium, chloride, potassium, magnesium, bicarbonate

Uses: Edema, hypertension, diuresis, CHF, nephrotic syndrome

Dosage and routes:
• *Adult:* PO 25-200 mg/day or 100 mg every other day
• *Geriatric:* PO 12.5 mg qd, initially
• *Child:* PO 2 mg/kg 3 ×/wk

Available forms: Tabs 15, 25, 50, 100 mg

Side effects/adverse reactions:
GU: Frequency, polyuria, ***uremia,*** glucosuria, impotence
CNS: Paresthesia, headache, *dizziness, fatigue, weakness*
GI: Nausea, vomiting, anorexia, constipation, diarrhea, cramps, pancreatitis, GI irritation, ***hepatitis***
EENT: Blurred vision
INTEG: Rash, urticaria, purpura, photosensitivity, fever
META: Hyperglycemia, hyperuremia, increased creatinine, BUN, gout
HEMA: ***Aplastic anemia, hemolytic anemia, leukopenia, agranulocytosis, thrombocytopenia, neutropenia***
CV: Irregular pulse, orthostatic hypotension, palpitations, volume depletion
ELECT: Hypokalemia, hypomagnesemia, hypercalcemia, hyponatremia, hypochloremia
Contraindications: Hypersensitivity to thiazides or sulfonamides, anuria, renal decompensation, lactation
Precautions: Hypokalemia, renal disease, pregnancy (B), lactation, hepatic disease, gout, diabetes mellitus, elderly, hyperlipidemia
Pharmacokinetics:
PO: Onset 2 hr, peak 6 hr, duration 24-72 hr; excreted unchanged by kidneys; crosses placenta; enters breast milk; half-life 40 hr
Interactions:
• Increased toxicity of: lithium, nondepolarizing skeletal muscle relaxants, allopurinol
• Decreased effects of antidiabetics, anticoagulants, antigout agents
• Decreased absorption of thiazides: cholestyramine, colestipol
• Decreased hypotensive response: indomethacin, NSAIDs
• Hyperglycemia, hypotension: diazoxide

• Hypokalemia: glucocorticoids, amphotericin B
 Potassium deficiency: chronic use/abuse of aloe, buckthorn bark/berry, cascara sagrada bark, licorice root, senna pod/leaf
Lab test interferences:
Increase: BSP retention, Ca, cholesterol, triglycerides, amylase
Decrease: PBI, PSP, parathyroid test
NURSING CONSIDERATIONS
Assess:
• Weight, I&O daily to determine fluid loss; effect of drug may be decreased if used qd
• Rate, depth, rhythm of respiration, effect of exertion
• B/P lying, standing; postural hypotension may occur
• Electrolytes: K, Mg, Na, Cl; include BUN, blood sugar, CBC, serum creatinine, blood pH, ABGs, uric acid, Ca
• Glucose in urine if patient is diabetic
• Signs of metabolic alkalosis: drowsiness, restlessness
• Signs of hypokalemia: postural hypotension, malaise, fatigue, tachycardia, leg cramps, weakness
• Rashes, temp elevation qd
• Confusion, especially in elderly; take safety precautions if needed
Administer:
• In AM to avoid interference with sleep if using drug as a diuretic
• K replacement if K less than 3 mg/dl
• With food if nausea occurs; absorption may be decreased slightly
Evaluate:
• Therapeutic response: improvement in edema of feet, legs, sacral area daily if medication used in CHF
Teach patient/family:
• To increase fluid intake to 2-3 L/day unless contraindicated, to rise slowly from lying or sitting position

---

◆ = Nursing alert　　　 = Herb-drug interaction　　　⊘ = Do not crush

C

• To notify prescriber of muscle weakness, cramps, nausea, dizziness

• That drug may be taken with food or milk

• That blood sugar may be increased in diabetics

• To use sunscreen to protect against photosensitivity

• To take early in day to avoid nocturia

Treatment of overdose: Lavage if taken orally, monitor electrolytes, administer dextrose in NS, monitor hydration, CV, renal status

---

chlorzoxazone (R)

(klor-zox′a-zone)
chlorzoxazone, Paraflex, Parafon Forte DSC, Remular-S
Func. class.: Skeletal muscle relaxant
Chem. class.: Benzoxazole derivative

Action: Inhibits multisynaptic reflex arcs

Uses: Relieving pain, spasm in musculoskeletal conditions

Dosage and routes:
• *Adult:* PO 250-750 mg tid-qid
• *Child:* PO 20 mg/kg/day in divided doses bid-tid
Available forms: Tabs 250 mg

Side effects/adverse reactions:
GU: Urine discoloration
HEMA: **Granulocytopenia, anemia**
CNS: Dizziness, drowsiness, headache, insomnia, stimulation, malaise
GI: Nausea, vomiting, anorexia, diarrhea, constipation, **hepatotoxicity, jaundice**
INTEG: Rash, pruritus, petechiae, ecchymoses, **angioedema**
SYST: **Anaphylaxis**

Contraindications: Hypersensitivity, impaired hepatic function
Precautions: Pregnancy (C), lactation, hepatic disease, elderly
Pharmacokinetics:
PO: Onset 1 hr, peak 3-4 hr, duration 6 hr, half-life 1 hr; metabolized in liver; excreted in urine (metabolites)
Interactions:
• Increased CNS depression: alcohol, tricyclic antidepressants, narcotics, barbiturates, sedatives, hypnotics
🌿 May increase CNS depression: kava kava

NURSING CONSIDERATIONS
Assess:
• Blood studies: CBC, WBC, differential for blood dyscrasias
• Liver function studies: AST, ALT, alk phosphatase; hepatitis may occur; hold dose and notify prescriber of signs of hepatotoxicity
• EEG in epileptic patients; poor seizure control has occurred
• Allergic reactions: rash, fever, respiratory distress
• Severe weakness, numbness in extremities
• Psychologic dependency: increased need for medication, more frequent requests for medication, increased pain
• CNS depression: dizziness, drowsiness, psychiatric symptoms
Administer:
• With meals for GI symptoms
Perform/provide:
• Storage in tight container at room temperature
• Assistance with ambulation if dizziness or drowsiness occurs, especially elderly
Evaluate:
• Therapeutic response: decreased pain, spasticity
Teach patient/family:
• Not to discontinue quickly; insomnia, nausea, headache, spastic-

ity, tachycardia will occur; drug should be tapered over 1-2 wk

• Not to take with alcohol, other CNS depressants; take with food

• To avoid hazardous activities if drowsiness, dizziness occurs

• To avoid using OTC medication: cough preparations, antihistamines, unless directed by prescriber

• That urine may be orange or purple

Treatment of overdose: Gastric lavage or induce emesis, then administer activated charcoal; use other supportive treatment as necessary; monitor cardiac function

---

cholestyramine (℞)

(koe-less-tir′a-meen)
Cholybar, Questran, Questran Light
Func. class.: Antilipemic
Chem. class.: Bile acid sequestrant

Action: Absorbs, combines with bile acids to form insoluble complex that is excreted through feces; loss of bile acids lowers cholesterol levels

Uses: Primary hypercholesterolemia, pruritus associated with biliary obstruction, diarrhea caused by excess bile acid, xanthomas

Dosage and routes:

• *Adult:* PO 4 g ac, and hs, not to exceed 32 g/day

• *Child:* PO 240 mg/kg/day in 3 divided doses with food or drink

Available forms: Pwd 9 g/4 g cholestyramine

Side effects/adverse reactions:

CNS: Headache, dizziness, drowsiness, vertigo, tinnitus

MS: Muscle, joint pain

GI: Constipation, abdominal pain, nausea, fecal impaction, hemorrhoids, flatulence, vomiting, steatorrhea, peptic ulcer

INTEG: Rash, irritation of perianal area, tongue, skin

HEMA: Decreased vit A, D, K, red cell folate content; **hyperchloremic acidosis, bleeding,** decreased protime

Contraindications: Hypersensitivity, biliary obstruction

Precautions: Pregnancy (C), lactation, children

Pharmacokinetics:

PO: Excreted in feces, maximum effect in 2 wk

Interactions:

• Decreased absorption of phenylbutazone, warfarin, thiazides, digitalis, penicillin G, tetracyclines, cephalexin, phenobarbital, folic acid, corticosteroids, iron, thyroid, clindamycin, trimethoprim, chenodiol, fat-soluble vitamins

Lab test interferences:

Increase: Liver function studies, Cl, PO_4

NURSING CONSIDERATIONS

Assess:

• Cardiac glycoside level, if both drugs are being administered

• For signs of vit A, D, K deficiency

• Fasting LDL, HDL, total cholesterol, triglyceride levels, electrolytes if on extended therapy

• Bowel pattern daily; increase bulk, H_2O in diet for constipation

Administer:

• Drug ac, hs; give all other medications 1 hr before cholestyramine or 4 hr after cholestyramine to avoid poor absorption

• Drug mixed with applesauce or stirred into beverage (2-6 oz), do not take dry, let stand for 2 min; avoid inhaling powder

• Supplemental doses of vit A, D, K, if levels are low

Evaluate:

• Therapeutic response: decreased cholesterol level (hyperlipidemia); diarrhea, pruritus (excess bile acids)

Teach patient/family:

◆The symptoms of hypoprothrombinemia: bleeding mucous membranes, dark tarry stools, hematuria, petechiae; report immediately
• The importance of compliance; toxicity may result if doses missed
• That risk factors should be decreased: high-fat diet, smoking, alcohol consumption, absence of exercise
• Not to discontinue suddenly

---

choline salicylate (Ŗ)

(koe'leen sa-liss'ih-late)
Arthropan
Func. class.: Nonnarcotic analgesic
Chem. class.: Salicylate

Action: Blocks pain impulses in CNS that occur in response to inhibition of prostaglandin synthesis; antipyretic action results from inhibition of hypothalamic heat-regulating center to produce vasodilation to allow heat dissipation

Uses: Mild to moderate pain or fever including arthritis, juvenile rheumatoid arthritis

Dosage and routes:
• *Adult and child >12 yr:* **PO** 870-1740 mg qid; max 6 ×/day
Pain/fever
• *Adult:* **PO** 870 mg q3-4h prn
Available forms: Liq 870 mg/5 ml

Side effects/adverse reactions:
HEMA: ***Thrombocytopenia, agranulocytosis, leukopenia, neutropenia, hemolytic anemia,*** increased protime
CNS: Stimulation, drowsiness, dizziness, confusion, ***convulsion,*** headache, flushing, hallucinations, ***coma***
GI: Nausea, vomiting, GI bleeding, diarrhea, heartburn, anorexia, ***hepatitis***

INTEG: Rash, urticaria, bruising
EENT: Tinnitus, hearing loss
CV: Rapid pulse, pulmonary edema
RESP: Wheezing, hyperpnea
ENDO: Hypoglycemia, hyponatremia, hypokalemia

Contraindications: Hypersensitivity to salicylates, GI bleeding, bleeding disorders, children <3 yr, vit K deficiency, children with flulike symptoms

Precautions: Anemia, hepatic disease, renal disease, Hodgkin's disease, pregnancy (C), lactation

Pharmacokinetics:
PO: Onset 15-30 min; metabolized by liver; crosses placenta; excreted in breast milk, by kidneys, half-life 2-3 hr, large doses 15-30 hr

Interactions:
• Decreased effects of choline: antacids, steroids, urinary alkalizers
• Increased blood loss: alcohol, heparin
• Increased effects of anticoagulants, insulin, methotrexate, penicillins, phenytoin
• Decreased effects of probenecid, spironolactone, sulfinpyrazone, sulfonylamides
• Toxic effects: PABA, furosemide, carbonic anhydrase inhibitors
• Decreased blood sugar levels: salicylates
• GI bleeding: steroids, antiinflammatories

Drug/food
• Foods that acidify the urine, increase salicylate level

Lab test interferences:
Increase: Coagulation studies, liver function studies, serum uric acid, amylase, CO_2, urinary protein
Decrease: Serum K, PBI, cholesterol
Interference: Urine catecholamines, pregnancy test

NURSING CONSIDERATIONS
Assess:

- Liver function studies: AST, ALT, bilirubin, creatinine (long-term therapy)
- Renal function studies: BUN, urine creatinine (long-term therapy)
- Blood studies: CBC, Hct, Hgb, pro-time (long-term therapy)
- I&O ratio; decreasing output may indicate renal failure (long-term therapy)

◆ Hepatotoxicity: dark urine; clay-colored stools; yellowing of skin, sclera; itching; abdominal pain; fever; diarrhea (long-term therapy)

- Allergic reactions: rash, urticaria; drug may have to be discontinued
- Renal dysfunction: decreased urine output
- Ototoxicity: tinnitus, ringing, roaring in ears; audiometric testing needed before, after long-term therapy
- Visual changes: blurring, halos, corneal, retinal damage
- Edema in feet, ankles, legs
- Drug history; many interactions

Administer:

- Mixed with fruit juice, carbonated beverage, water

Evaluate:

- Therapeutic response: decreased pain, fever, stiffness of joints

Teach patient/family:

- To report any symptoms of hepatotoxicity, renal toxicity, visual changes, ototoxicity, allergic reactions, bleeding (long-term therapy)
- Not to exceed recommended dosage; acute poisoning may result
- To read label on other OTC drugs; many contain aspirin
- That therapeutic response takes 2 wk (arthritis)
- To avoid alcohol ingestion; GI bleeding may occur
- That if anticoagulants are given with this drug, this drug should be decreased 2 wk before surgery

Treatment of overdose: Lavage, activated charcoal, monitor electrolytes, VS

---

chorionic gonadotropin, human (℞)

(go-nad'oh-troe-pin)
APL, Chorex-5, Chorex-10, Choron 10, Gonic, Pregnyl, Profasi

Func. class.: Human chorionic gonadotropin

Chem. class.: Polypeptide hormone

Action: Stimulates production of gonadal steroids, androgens; stimulates corpus luteum to produce progesterone

Uses: Infertility, anovulation, hypogonadism, nonobstructive cryptorchidism

Dosage and routes:
Dosage regimens vary widely

Infertility/anovulation
- *Adult:* IM 10,000 U 1 day after last dose of menotropins

Hypogonadism
- *Adult:* IM 500-1000 U 3 × wk × 3 wk, then 2 × wk × 3 wk, or 4000 U 3 × wk × 6-9 mo, then 2000 U 3 × wk × 3 mo

Cryptorchidism
- *Child (boy 4-9 yr):* IM 5000 U qod × 4 doses

Available forms: Powder for inj 500, 1000, 2000 U/ml

Side effects/adverse reactions:
CNS: Headache, depression, fatigue, anxiety, irritability
GU: Gynecomastia, early puberty, edema, *ectopic pregnancy*
INTEG: Pain at injection site

Contraindications: Hypersensitiv-

◆ = Nursing alert   ⫻ = Herb-drug interaction   🚫 = Do not crush

ity, pituitary hypertrophy/tumor, early puberty, prostatic cancer, pregnancy (X)

Precautions: Asthma, migraine headache, convulsive disorders, cardiac disease, renal disease, lactation, children <4 yr

Pharmacokinetics:
IM: Peak 6 hr, half-life 11-24 hr, excreted by kidneys

NURSING CONSIDERATIONS
Assess:
• Weight weekly; notify prescriber if weekly weight gain is >5 lb
• B/P before, during treatment
• Be alert for decreasing urinary output, increasing edema
• Edema, hypertension

Administer:
• Only after clomiphene citrate has been tried on anovulatory patient
• After reconstitution with diluent enclosed in package

Perform/provide:
• Refrigeration for up to 2 mo

Evaluate:
• Therapeutic response: ovulation, fertility

Teach patient/family:
• To report facial, axillary, pubic hair, change in voice, penile enlargement, acne in male, abdominal pain, distention; vaginal bleeding in women
• To report symptoms of ectopic pregnancy: dizziness, pain on one side or in shoulder, pallor, weak and thready pulse, hemorrhage; shock may proceed rapidly

---

chymopapain (R)
(kye'moe-pa-pane)
Chymodiactin
Func. class.: Enzyme
Chem. class.: Proteolytic

Action: Hydrolyzes noncollagenous polypeptides that maintain structure of chondromucoprotein; activity decreases pressure on disk

Uses: Herniated lumbar intervertebral disk

Dosage and routes:
• *Adult:* **INJ** 2-4 mKat U/disk injected intradiskally, not to exceed 10 mKat U in a multiple herniation

Available forms: Powder for inj 4, 10 mKat U/vial

Side effects/adverse reactions:
CNS: **Paraplegia, cerebral hemorrhage,** headache, dizziness, paresthesia, numbness of extremities
INTEG: Rash, urticaria, itching
GI: Nausea, paralytic ileus
MS: *Back pain, stiffness, spasm, acute transverse myelitis,* weakness, leg pain
SYST: **Anaphylaxis**
GU: Urinary retention

Contraindications: Hypersensitivity to this drug, papaya, meat tenderizer; severe spondylolisthesis; severe progressing paralysis; spinal cord tumor; cauda equina lesion, previous use

Precautions: Pregnancy (C), lactation, children

Pharmacokinetics: Onset 30 min, duration 24 hr

Interactions:
• Dysrhythmias: halothane anesthetics plus epinephrine

NURSING CONSIDERATIONS
Assess:
• RBCs, ESR before treatment
• Respiratory rate, rhythm, depth; notify prescriber of abnormalities
• Anaphylaxis for several days after injection
• Neuro status after surgery; elimination status for paralytic ileus
• For allergies: iodine, papaya, meat tenderizer; if allergies are identified, drug should not be used

Administer:
• Only with epinephrine available for anaphylaxis

- Only in lumbar spine by prescriber
- After diluting with sterile water for inj, use within 1 hr
- After completing allergy test (ChymoFAST)

Evaluate:
- Therapeutic response: absence of back pain, increased mobility

Teach patient/family:
- To report allergic reactions up to 2 wk after inj
- To be aware of possible infection: redness, swelling, pain

---

cidofovir (Ŗ)

(si-doh-foh'veer)
Vistide
Func. class.: Antiviral
Chem. class.: Nucleotide analog

Action: Suppresses cytomegalovirus (CMV) replication by selective inhibition of viral DNA synthesis

Uses: CMV retinitis in patients with AIDS

Dosage and routes:
- Dilute in 100 ml 0.9% saline sol before administration; probenecid must be given **PO** 2 g 3 hr prior to the cidofovir infusion and 1 g at 2 and 8 hr after ending the cidofovir infusion; give 1 L of 0.9% saline sol **IV** with each **INF** of cidofovir, give saline **INF** over 1-2 hr period immediately prior to cidofovir; patient should be given a 2nd L if the patient can tolerate the fluid load (2nd L given at time of cidofovir or immediately afterward and should be given over a 1-3 hr period)

Renal dose
- CrCl <50 ml/min reduce dose

Induction
- *Adult:* **IV INF** 5 mg/kg given over 1 hr at a constant rate qwk × 2 consecutive wk

Maintenance
- *Adult:* **IV INF** 5 mg/kg given over 1 hr q2wk

Available forms: Inj 75 mg/ml

Side effects/adverse reactions:

*CNS: Fever, chills, **coma,** confusion, abnormal thought, dizziness, bizarre dreams, headache, psychosis, tremors, somnolence, paresthesia, amnesia, anxiety, insomnia, seizures*

CV: Dysrhythmias, hypertension/hypotension

EENT: Retinal detachment in CMV retinitis

*GI: Abnormal LFTs, nausea, vomiting, anorexia, diarrhea, abdominal pain, **hemorrhage***

*GU: **Hematuria,** increased creatinine, BUN*

*HEMA: **Granulocytopenia, thrombocytopenia, irreversible neutropenia, anemia, eosinophilia***

INTEG: Rash, alopecia, pruritus, acne, urticaria, pain at inj site, phlebitis

RESP: Dyspnea

Contraindications: Hypersensitivity to this drug or probenecid, sulfa drugs

Precautions: Preexisting cytopenias, renal function impairment, pregnancy (C), lactation, children <6 mo, elderly, platelet count <25,000/mm^3

Pharmacokinetics: Unknown

Interactions:
- Nephrotoxicity: amphotericin B, foscarnet, aminoglycosides

NURSING CONSIDERATIONS

Assess:
- Culture before treatment is initiated; cultures of blood, urine, and throat may all be taken; CMV is not confirmed by this method; the diagnosis is made by an ophth exam
- Kidney, liver function, increased hemopoietic studies and BUN; serum creatinine, AST (SGOT), ALT

◆ = Nursing alert   ∥ = Herb-drug interaction   ⊘ = Do not crush

(SGPT), creatinine, AST (SGOT), ALT (SGPT), creatinine clearance, A-G ratio, baseline and drip treatment, blood counts should be done q2wk; watch for decreasing granulocytes, Hgb; if low, therapy may have to be discontinued and restarted after hematologic recovery; blood transfusions may be required

• For GI symptoms: severe nausea, vomiting, diarrhea; severe symptoms may necessitate discontinuing drug

• Electrolytes and minerals: calcium, phosphorous, magnesium, sodium, potassium; watch closely for tetany during first administration

• For symptoms of blood dyscrasias (anemia, granulocytopenia); bruising, fatigue, bleeding, poor healing

• Allergic reactions: flushing, rash, urticaria, pruritus

• For leukopenia, neutropenia, thrombocytopenia: WBCs, platelets q2d during 2×/day dosing and qwk thereafter; check for leukopenias, with qd WBC count in patients with prior leukopenia, with other nucleoside analogs, or for whom leukopenia counts are <1000 cells/mm³ at start of treatment

• Monitor serum creatinine or creatinine clearance at least q2wk

Administer:

IV

• Mix under strict aseptic conditions using gloves, gown, and mask, and using precautions for antineoplastic

• After diluting in 100 ml NS

• Slowly; do not give by bolus IV, SC inj

• Use diluted sol within 12 hr, do not refrigerate or freeze; do not use sol with particulate matter or discoloration

Evaluate:

• Therapeutic response: Decreased symptoms of CMV

Teach patient/family:

• To notify prescriber if sore throat, swollen lymph nodes, malaise, fever occur; may indicate other infections

• To report perioral tingling, numbness in extremities, and paresthesias

• That serious drug interactions may occur if OTC products are ingested; check first with prescriber

• That drug is not a cure, but will control symptoms

• That regular ophth exams must be continued

• That major toxicities may necessitate discontinuing drug

• To use contraception during treatment and that infertility may occur; men should use barrier contraception for 90 days after treatment

Treatment of overdose: Discontinue drug; use hemodialysis, and increase hydration

---

cimetidine (OTC, R)

(sye-met′i-deen)

Apo-Cimetidine*, Cimetidine, Novocimetine*, Peptol*, Tagamet

Func. class.: H₂-histamine receptor antagonist

Chem. class.: Imidazole derivative

Action: Inhibits histamine at H₂-receptor site in the gastric parietal cells, which inhibits gastric acid secretion

Uses: Short-term treatment of duodenal and gastric ulcers and maintenance; management of GERD and Zollinger-Ellison syndrome

Investigational uses: Prevention of aspiration pneumonitis, stress ulcers, upper GI bleeding, herpes infection, hirsutism

---

Dosage and routes:
Treatment of active ulcers
• *Adult:* **PO** 300 mg qid with meals, hs × 8 wk or 400 mg bid, 800 mg hs; after 8 wk give hs dose only; **IV BOL** 300 mg/20 ml 0.9% NaCl over 1-2 min q6h; **IV INF** 300 mg/50 ml D_5W over 15-20 min; **IM** 300 mg q6h, not to exceed 2400 mg/day
• *Child:* 20-40 mg/kg/day
Prophylaxis of duodenal ulcer
• *Adult and child >16 yr:* 400 mg hs
GERD
• *Adult:* **PO** 800-1600 mg/day in divided doses
Hypersecretory conditions (Zollinger-Ellison syndrome)
• *Adult:* **PO/IM/IV** 300-600 mg q6h; may increase to 12 g/day if needed
Upper GI bleeding prophylaxis
• *Adult:* **IV** 50 mg/hr; lowered in renal disease
Aspiration pneumonitis prophylaxis
• *Adult:* **IM/IV** 300 mg **IM** 1 hr before anesthesia, then 300 mg **IV** q4h until patient is alert
Renal disease
• CrCl 20-40 ml/min 300 mg q8h; CrCl <20 ml/min 300 mg q12h
Available forms: Tabs 100, 200, 300, 400, 800 mg; liq 300 mg/5 ml; inj 300 mg/2 ml, 300 mg/50 ml 0.9% NaCl

Side effects/adverse reactions:
CNS: Confusion, headache, depression, dizziness, anxiety, weakness, psychosis, tremors, *convulsions*
CV: Bradycardia, tachycardia
GI: Diarrhea, abdominal cramps, *paralytic ileus, jaundice*
GU: Gynecomastia, galactorrhea, impotence, increase in BUN, creatinine
HEMA: Agranulocytosis, thrombocytopenia, neutropenia, aplastic anemia, increase in pro-time
INTEG: Urticaria, rash, alopecia, sweating, flushing, *exfoliative dermatitis*

Contraindications: Hypersensitivity
Precautions: Pregnancy (B), lactation, child <16 yr, organic brain syndrome, hepatic disease, renal disease, elderly
Pharmacokinetics: Well absorbed (PO, IM)
IM/IV: Onset 10 min, peak ½ hr, duration 4-5 hr
PO: Peak 1-1½ hr, half-life 1½-2 hr; 30%-40% metabolized by liver, excreted in urine unchanged, crosses placenta, enters breast milk
Interactions:
• Increased toxicity: oral anticoagulants, benzodiazepines, metoprolol, propranolol, phenytoin, quinidine, theophylline, tricyclic antidepressants, lidocaine, procainamide, carmustine, flecainide, narcotic analgesics, succinylcholine, warfarin
• Decreased absorption of cimetidine: antacids, anticholinergics, metoclopramide
• Decreased effectiveness: smoking
• Decreased absorption: ketoconazole, iron salts, tetracyclines, indomethacin
• Decreased absorption of tocainide
Lab test interferences:
Increase: Alk phosphatase, AST, creatinine
False positive: Gastric bleeding test, hemoccult

NURSING CONSIDERATIONS
Assess:
• Gastric pH (5 or more should be maintained), also epigastric pain and duration, intensity; aggravating, ameliorating factors
• I&O ratio, BUN, creatinine, CBC with differential monthly
Administer:
• With meals for prolonged drug ef-

fect; antacids 1 hr before or 1 hr after cimetidine

IV

• After diluting 300 mg/20 ml of NS for inj; give ≥2 min; may be diluted 300 mg/50 ml of D_5W; run over 15-20 min; or total daily dose (900 mg) diluted in 100-1000 ml D_5W given over 24 hr

Additive compatibilities: Acetazolamide, amikacin, aminophylline, atracurium, cefoperazone, cefoxitin, chlorothiazide, clindamycin, colistimethate, dexamethasone, digoxin, epinephrine, erythromycin, ethacrynate, floxacillin, flumazenil, furosemide, gentamicin, insulin (regular), isoproterenol, lidocaine, lincomycin, meropenem, metaraminol, methylprednisolone, norepinephrine, nitroprusside, penicillin G potassium, phytonadione, polymyxin B, potassium chloride, protamine, quinidine, tacrolimus, vancomycin, verapamil, vit B/C

Syringe compatibilities: Atropine, butorphanol, cephalothin, diazepam, diphenhydramine, doxapram, droperidol, fentanyl, glycopyrrolate, heparin, hydromorphone, hydroxyzine, lorazepam, meperidine, midazolam, morphine, nafcillin, nalbuphine, penicillin G sodium, pentazocine, perphenazine, prochlorperazine, promazine, promethazine, scopolamine

Y-site compatibilities: Acyclovir, amifostine, aminophylline, amrinone, atracurium, aztreonam, cisplatin, cladribine, cyclophosphamide, cytarabine, diltiazem, doxorubicin, enalaprilat, esmolol, filgrastim, fluconazole, fludarabine, foscarnet, gallium, granisetron, haloperidol, heparin, hetastarch, idarubicin, labetalol, melphalan, meropenem, methotrexate, midazolam, ondansetron, paclitaxel, pancuronium, piperacillin/tazobactam, propofol, sargramostim, tacrolimus, teniposide, theophylline, thiotepa, tolazoline, vecuronium, vinorelbine, zidovudine

Perform/provide:

• Storage of diluted sol at room temp up to 48 hr

Evaluate:

• Therapeutic response: decreased pain in abdomen; healing of ulcers, absence of gastroesophageal reflux, gastric pH 5

Teach patient/family:

• That gynecomastia, impotence may occur, are reversible

• To avoid driving, other hazardous activities until patient is stabilized on this medication; drowsiness or dizziness may occur

• To avoid black pepper, caffeine, alcohol, harsh spices, extremes in temp of food

• To avoid OTC preparations: aspirin, cough, cold preparations; condition may worsen

• That smoking decreases the effectiveness of the drug

• That drug must be continued for prescribed time to be effective and taken exactly as prescribed; doses not to be doubled

• To report bruising, fatigue, malaise; blood dyscrasias may occur

• To report to prescriber diarrhea, black tarry stools, sore throat, rash

ciprofloxacin (℞)

(sip-ro-floks′a-sin)

Ciloxan, Cipro, Cipro IV

Func. class.: Broad-spectrum antibiotic

Chem. class.: Fluoroquinolone antibacterial

Action: Interferes with conversion of intermediate DNA fragments into high-molecular-weight DNA in bacteria; DNA gyrase inhibitor

Uses: Infection caused by susceptible *E. coli, E. cloacae, P. mirabilis, K. pneumoniae, P. vulgaris, C. freundii, S. marcescens, P. aeruginosa, S. aureus, Enterobacter, Campylobacter jejuni, Salmonella;* chronic bacterial prostatitis, acute sinusitis

Dosage and routes:

Uncomplicated urinary tract infections

• *Adult:* **PO** 250 mg q12h; **IV** 200 mg q12h

Complicated/severe urinary tract infections

• *Adult:* **PO** 500 mg q12h; **IV** 400 mg q12h

Respiratory, bone, skin, joint infections

• *Adult:* **PO** 500-750 mg q12h; **IV** 400 mg q12h

Renal disease

• CrCl <50 ml/min **PO** 250-500 mg q12h; CrCl 5-29 ml/min **PO** 250-500 mg q18h; **IV** 200-400 mg q18-24h

Corneal ulcers, conjunctivitis

• *Adult:* **OPHTH** 1-2 drops q15-30 min until infection is controlled, then 1-2 drops 4-6 times daily

Available forms: Tabs 250, 500, 750 mg; inj 200 mg/100 ml D$_5$, 400 mg/200 ml D$_5$; 200, 400 mg vial; ophth sol 0.3% (base)

Side effects/adverse reactions:

CNS: Headache, dizziness, fatigue, insomnia, depression, *restlessness,* seizures, confusion

GI: Nausea, diarrhea, increased ALT (SGOT), AST (SGOT), flatulence, heartburn, *vomiting,* oral candidiasis, dysphagia

INTEG: Rash, pruritus, urticaria, photosensitivity, flushing, fever, chills

MS: Tremor, arthralgia, tendon rupture

Contraindications: Hypersensitivity to quinolones

Precautions: Pregnancy (C), lactation, children, renal disease, epilepsy

Pharmacokinetics:

PO: Peak 1 hr, half-life 3-4 hr; excreted in urine as active drug, metabolites

Interactions:

• Decreased absorption of ciproflaxin: magnesium antacids, aluminum hydroxide, zinc, iron, sucralfate, calcium, enteral feeding, didanosine

• Increased serum levels of ciprofloxacin: probenecid

• Increased toxicity: caffeine, theophylline, cyclosporine

• Increased warfarin, cyclosporine effect

NURSING CONSIDERATIONS

Assess:

• CNS symptoms: headache, dizziness, fatigue, insomnia, depression

• Kidney, liver function studies: BUN, creatinine, AST (SGOT), ALT (SGPT)

• I&O ratio, urine pH <5.5 is ideal

• Allergic reactions: fever, flushing, rash, urticaria, pruritus

Administer:

• 2 hr before or 2 hr after antacids, zinc, iron, calcium

IV

• Over 1 hr as an INF, comes in premixed plastic INF container or diluted 20 or 40 ml vial to a final conc of 0.5-2 mg/ml of NS or D$_5$W; give through Y-tube or 3-way stopcock

• After clean-catch urine for C&S

Additive compatibilities: Amikacin, aztreonam, ceftazidime, cyclosporine, gentamicin, metronidazole, netilmicin, piperacillin, potassium acetate, potassium chloride, potassium phosphates, prednisolone, promethazine, propofol, ranitidine, Ringer's, sodium chloride, tobramycin, vit B/C

Y-site compatibilities: Amifostine,

◆ = Nursing alert   ⫸ = Herb-drug interaction   ⃠ = Do not crush amino acids, aztreonam, calcium gluconate, ceftazidime, digoxin, diltiazem, diphenhydramine, dobutamine, dopamine, gallium, gentamicin, granisetron, hydroxyzine, lidocaine, lorazepam, metoclopramide, midazolam, midodrine, piperacillin, potassium acetate, potassium chloride, potassium phosphates, prednisolone, promethazine, propofol, ranitidine, Ringer's, sodium chloride, tacrolimus, teniposide, thiotepa, tobramycin, verapamil

Perform/provide:
• Limited intake of alkaline foods, drugs: milk, dairy products, alkaline antacids, sodium bicarbonate

Evaluate:
• Therapeutic response: decreased pain, frequency, urgency, C&S; absence of infection

Teach patient/family:
• Not to take any products containing magnesium or calcium (such as antacids), iron, or aluminum with this drug or within 2 hr of drug
• That photosensitivity may occur; patient should avoid sunlight or use sunscreen to prevent burns
• That fluids must be increased to 3 L/day to avoid crystallization in kidneys
• If dizziness occurs, to ambulate, perform activities with assistance
• To complete full course of drug therapy
• To contact prescriber if adverse reaction occurs or if inflammation or pain in tendon occurs

---

cisapride (℞)

(siss'a-pride)
Prepulsid*, Propulsid
Func. class.: Cholinergic

Action: Enhances response to acetylcholine at the myenteric plexus

Uses: Treatment of heartburn

Dosage and routes:
• *Adult:* **PO** 10 mg qid at least 15 min ac and hs; may increase to 20 mg; elderly may need higher dosage
• *Child:* 0.15-0.3 mg/kg/dose 3-4 ×/day

Available forms: Tabs 10, 20 mg; susp 1 mg/ml

Side effects/adverse reactions:
*CV: **Prolonged QT**, palpitation*, tachycardia, ***ventricular tachycardia, torsades de pointes***
RESP: Rhinitis, sinusitis, coughing
CNS: Headache, sleeplessness, anxiety, nervousness, pain, fever
GI: Diarrhea, constipation, nausea, anorexia, abdominal pain, flatulence, dyspepsia
GU: UTI, frequency
INTEG: Pruritus, rash

Contraindications: Hypersensitivity; GI hemorrhage, obstruction, perforation, premature neonates, infants <6 mo

Precautions: Pregnancy (C), lactation, children, elderly, electrolyte disturbances, congenital prolonged QT syndrome, history of cardiac dysrhythmias, cardiac disease, renal disease, GI perforation or obstruction

Pharmacokinetics:
PO: Rapidly absorbed; onset ½-1 hr, peak 1-1½ hr; extensively metabolized by liver, excreted in urine (metabolite); 98% bound to plasma proteins; terminal half life 6-12 hr

Interactions:
• Inhibition of metabolism of cisapride: erythromycin, ketoconazole, itraconazole, clarithromycin, miconazole, troleandomycin, antidysrhythmic (class IA/III), antidepressants, antipsychotics, astemizole, bepridil, protease inhibitors, sparfloxacin, terodiline; do not use together
• Decreased action of cisapride: anticholinergics

• Increased peak plasma levels: cimetidine, H_2-antagonists
• Increased coagulation time: anticoagulants

NURSING CONSIDERATIONS
Assess:

• GI complaints: nausea, vomiting, anorexia, constipation
Administer:

• ½-1 hr before meals for better absorption
Evaluate:

• Therapeutic response: absence of heartburn
Teach patient/family:

• To avoid alcohol, other CNS depressants that will enhance sedating properties of this drug
• To increase fluids, bulk in diet for constipation
• That all health-care providers are aware of all meds taken by patient
• To inform health-care provider of heart palpitations
Treatment of overdose: Gastric lavage or activated charcoal, general support

---

cisatracurium

(sis-a-tra-kyoor'ee-um)
Nimbex
Func. class.: Neuromuscular blocker (nondepolarizing)

Action: Inhibits transmission of nerve impulses by binding with cholinergic receptor sites, antagonizing action of acetylcholine

Uses: Facilitation of endotracheal intubation, skeletal muscle relaxation during mechanical ventilation, surgery, or general anesthesia

Dosage and routes:
• *Adult:* IV 0.15-0.2 mg/kg depending on desired time to intubate and length of surgery; use peripheral nerve stimulation to evaluate dosage
• *Child 2-12 yr:* IV 0.1 mg/kg over 5-10 sec with halothane or opioid anesthesia

Available forms: Inj 2 mg/ml, 10 mg/ml

Side effects/adverse reactions:

CV: Bradycardia, tachycardia; increased, decreased B/P
RESP: **Prolonged apnea, bronchospasm, cyanosis, respiratory depression**
EENT: Increased secretions
INTEG: Rash, flushing, pruritus, urticaria

Contraindications: Hypersensitivity

Precautions: Pregnancy (B), cardiac disease, lactation, children <2 yr, electrolyte imbalances, dehydration, neuromuscular disease, respiratory disease

Pharmacokinetics: Onset 1-3 min, peak 2-5 min

Interactions:

• Increased neuromuscular blockade: aminoglycosides, clindamycin, lincomycin, quinidine, local anesthetics, polymyxin antibiotics, lithium, narcotic analgesics, thiazides, enflurane, isoflurane, bacitracin, tetracyclines
• Dysrhythmias: theophylline

NURSING CONSIDERATIONS
Assess:

• For electrolyte imbalances (K, Mg); may lead to increased action of this drug
• Vital signs (B/P, pulse, respirations, airway) until fully recovered; rate, depth, pattern of respirations; strength of hand grip
• I&O ratio; check for urinary retention, frequency, hesitancy
• Recovery: decreased paralysis of face, diaphragm, leg, arm, rest of body
• Allergic reactions: rash, fever, respiratory distress, pruritus; drug should be discontinued

Administer:
• Using nerve stimulator by anesthesiologist to determine neuromuscular blockade
• Anticholinesterase to reverse neuromuscular blockade
• By slow IV only by qualified person, do not administer IM

Perform/provide:
• Storage in light-resistant area
• Reassurance if communication is difficult during recovery from neuromuscular blockade

Evaluate:
• Therapeutic response: paralysis of jaw, eyelid, head, neck, rest of body

Treatment of overdose: Edrophonium or neostigmine, atropine, monitor VS; mechanical ventilation

---

cisplatin (℞)

(sis'pla-tin)

Platinol-AQ

Func. class.: Antineoplastic alkylating agent

Chem. class.: Inorganic heavy metal

Action: Alkylates DNA, RNA; inhibits enzymes that allow synthesis of amino acids in proteins; activity is not cell cycle phase specific

Uses: Advanced bladder cancer, adjunctive in metastatic testicular cancer, adjunctive in metastatic ovarian cancer, head, neck cancer, esophagus, prostate, lung and cervical cancer, lymphoma

Dosage and routes:

Testicular cancer
• **Adult:** IV 20 mg/m^2 qd × 5 days, repeat q3wk for 3 cycles or more, depending on response

Bladder cancer
• **Adult:** IV 50-70 mg/m^2 q3-4wk

Ovarian cancer
• **Adult:** IV 100 mg/m^2 q4wk or 50 mg/m^2 q3wk with doxorubicin therapy; mix with 2 L NaCl and 37.5 g mannitol over 6 hr

Available forms: Inj 10, 50, 100 mg; 1 mg/ml

Side effects/adverse reactions:

EENT: Tinnitus, hearing loss, vestibular toxicity

HEMA: ***Thrombocytopenia, leukopenia, pancytopenia***

CV: Cardiac abnormalities

GI: Severe nausea, vomiting, diarrhea, weight loss

GU: ***Renal tubular damage,*** renal insufficiency, impotence, sterility, amenorrhea, gynecomastia, hyperuremia

INTEG: Alopecia, dermatitis

CNS: ***Convulsions,*** peripheral neuropathy

RESP: ***Fibrosis***

META: Hypomagnesemia, hypocalcemia, hypokalemia, hypophosphatemia

SYST: ***Hypersensitivity reaction***

Contraindications: Radiation therapy or chemotherapy within 1 mo, thrombocytopenia, smallpox vaccination, pregnancy (D)

Precautions: Pneumococcus vaccination, lactation

Pharmacokinetics: Well absorbed orally, metabolized in liver, excreted in urine; half-life 2 hr

Interactions:
• Increased nephrotoxicity: aminoglycosides
• Decreased effects of phenytoin

NURSING CONSIDERATIONS

Assess:
• CBC, differential, platelet count weekly; withhold drug if WBC is <4000 or platelet count is <75,000; notify prescriber of results
• Renal function studies: BUN, creatinine, serum uric acid, urine CrCl before, electrolytes during therapy
• I&O ratio; report fall in urine output of <30 ml/hr

• Monitor temp q4h (may indicate beginning infection)
• Liver function tests before, during therapy (bilirubin, AST [SGOT], ALT [SGPT], LDH) as needed or monthly
• Bleeding: hematuria, guaiac, bruising or petechiae, mucosa or orifices q8h; obtain prescription for viscous lidocaine (Xylocaine)
• Dyspnea, rales, nonproductive cough, chest pain, tachypnea
• Food preferences; list likes, dislikes
• Effects of alopecia on body image; discuss feelings about body changes
• Yellowing of skin, sclera; dark urine; clay-colored stools; itchy skin; abdominal pain; fever; diarrhea
• Edema in feet, joint pain, stomach pain, shaking
• Inflammation of mucosa, breaks in skin

Administer:

IV

• After diluting 10 mg/10 ml or 50 mg/50 ml sterile H_2O for inj; withdraw prescribed dose, dilute ½ dose with 1000 ml D_5 0.2 NaCl or D_5 0.45 NaCl with 37.5 g mannitol; IV INF is given over 3-4 hr; use a 0.45 µm filter; total dose 2 L over 6-8 hr; check site for irritation, phlebitis; do not use equipment containing aluminum
• Hydrate patient with 1-2 L fluids over 8-12 hr before treatment
• Epinephrine for hypersensitivity reaction
• Antiemetic 30-60 min before giving drug and prn
• Allopurinol or sodium bicarbonate to maintain uric acid levels, alkalinization of urine
• Antibiotics for prophylaxis of infection
• Diuretic (furosemide 40 mg IV) or mannitol after infusion

Additive compatibilities: Carboplatin, cyclophosphamide with etoposide, etoposide, etoposide with floxuridine, floxuridine, floxuridine with leucovorin, hydroxyzine, ifosfamide, ifosfamide with etoposide, leucovorin, magnesium sulfate, mannitol, ondansetron

Solution compatibilities: D_5/0.225% NaCl, D_5/0.45% NaCl, D_5/0.9% NaCl, D_5/0.45% NaCl with mannitol 1.875%, D_5/0.33% NaCl with KCl 20 mEq and mannitol 1.875%, 0.9% NaCl, 0.45% NaCl, 0.3% NaCl, 0.225% NaCl

Syringe compatibilities: Bleomycin, cyclophosphamide, doxapram, doxorubicin, droperidol, fluorouracil, furosemide, heparin, leucovorin, methotrexate, metoclopramide, mitomycin, vinblastine, vincristine

Y-site compatibilities: Allopurinol, aztreonam, bleomycin, chlorpromazine, cimetidine, cladribine, cyclophosphamide, dexamethasone, diphenhydramine, doxorubicin, droperidol, famotidine, filgrastim, fludarabine, fluorouracil, furosemide, ganciclovir, granisetron, heparin, hydromorphone, leucovorin, lorazepam, melphalan, methotrexate, methylprednisolone, metoclopramide, mitomycin, morphine, ondansetron, paclitaxel, prochlorperazine, promethazine, propofol, ranitidine, sargramostim, teniposide, vinblastine, vincristine, vinorelbine

Perform/provide:

• Strict medical asepsis, protective isolation if WBC levels are low
• Comprehensive oral hygiene
• Storage protected from light in refrigerator (dry powder)
• Deep breathing exercises with patient tid-qid; place in semi-Fowler's position
• Increase fluid intake to 2-3 L/day to prevent urate deposits, calculi formation; elimination of drug

◆ = Nursing alert   ▨ = Herb-drug interaction   ⊘ = Do not crush

- Monitor temp q4h; fever may indicate beginning infection
- Liver function tests before, during therapy: bilirubin, AST, ALT, alk phosphatase as needed or monthly
- Local irritation, pain, burning at injection site

⬥ Symptoms indicating severe allergic reaction: rash, pruritus, urticaria, purpuric skin lesions, itching, flushing

- GI symptoms: frequency of stools, cramping

Administer:

IV

- Antiemetic 30-60 min before giving drug to prevent vomiting
- Use gloves, gown to mix IV sol
- Use bacteriostatic (0.9% NaCl, 0.9% benzyl alcohol preserved) to prepare 7-day inf; pass both cladribine and diluent through sterile 0.22 μm hydrophilic syr filter as each sol is introduced into inf reservoir; add dose of cladribine to inf reservoir using filter, then bacteriostatic 0.9% NaCl to bring sol total to 100 ml; after preparation, clamp line, disconnect filter, discard; aspirate air bubbles (reservoir) using syr, dry filter or sterile vat filter assembly; reclamp line, discard filter and syr; infuse continuously × 7 days
- Add dose for single daily dose to inf bag (500 ml 0.9% NaCl); infuse continuously over 24 hr; repeat daily dose × 7 days

Y-site compatibilities: Aminophylline, bumetanide, buprenorphine, butorphanol, calcium gluconate, carboplatin, chlorpromazine, cimetidine, cisplatin, cyclophosphamide, cytarabine, dexamethasone, diphenhydramine, dobutamine, dopamine, doxorubicin, droperidol, enalaprilat, etoposide, famotidine, furosemide, gallium, granisetron, halo-peridol, heparin, hydrocortisone, hydrocortisone sodium phosphate, hydromorphone, imipenem, hydroxyzine, idarubicin, lorazepam, mesna, leucovorin, mesna, methyl, meperidine, clopramide, melone, meto-phine, nalbuphine, mor-paclitaxel, potassi, mor-chlorperazine, pron, nsetron, dine, sodium bicar, pro-side, vincristine niti-

Perform/provide:

- Hydrocortisone, sodi fate to infiltration area, press after stopping inf
- Strict hand-washing te gloves, protective covering
- Liquid diet: carbonated bev gelatin may be added if pat. not nauseated or vomiting
- Storage in refrigerator; pro from light; reconstituted or dilu sol may be stored at room temp longer than 8 hr; discard single-us vials of unused sol

Evaluate:

- Therapeutic response: decrease in symptoms of hairy cell leukemia

Teach patient/family:

- To report any complaints, side effects to nurse or prescriber
- To avoid crowds, sources of infection when granulocyte count low

---

clarithromycin (℞)

(klare-ith′row-my-sin)
Biaxin

Func. class.: Antibacterial
Chem. class.: Macrolide antibiotic

Action: Binds to 50S ribosomal subunits of susceptible bacteria and suppresses protein synthesis
Uses: Mild to moderate infections of the upper respiratory tract, lower

---

⬥ = Nursing alert   ✏ = Herb-drug interaction   🚫 = Do not crush respiratory tract, uncomplicated skin and skin structure infections caused by *S. pneumoniae, M. pneumoniae, L. pneumophilia, M. catarrhalis, N. gonorrhoeae, C. diphtheriae, L. monocytogenes, H. influenzae, S. pyogenes, S. aureus, M. avium* (MAC), complex infection in AIDS patients, *M. intracellulare, H. pylori* in combination with omeprazole

Dosage and routes:
• *Adult:* **PO** 250-500 mg bid for 7-14 days; 500 mg bid continues for *M. avium* (MAC)
• *Child:* **PO** 15 mg/kg/day (max 1000 mg) divided q12h × 10 days
H. pylori *infection*
• *Adult:* **PO** 500 mg qd plus omeprazole 2 × 20 mg q AM (day 1-14), then omeprazole 20 mg q AM (days 15-28)
Available forms: Tabs 250, 500 mg; granules for oral susp 125 mg/5 ml, 250 mg/5 ml

Side effects/adverse reactions:
INTEG: Rash, urticaria, pruritus
*GI: Nausea, vomiting, diarrhea, **hepatotoxicity**, abdominal pain,* stomatitis, heartburn, anorexia, *abnormal taste*
GU: Vaginitis, moniliasis
MISC: Headache

Contraindications: Hypersensitivity to this drug or macrolide antibiotics

Precautions: Pregnancy (C), lactation, hepatic, renal disease, elderly

Pharmacokinetics: Peak 2 hr, duration 12 hr, half-life 4-6 hr; metabolized by liver; excreted in bile, feces

Interactions:
• Dysrhythmias: terfenadine, astemizole, cisapride, pimozide
• Increased clarithromycin levels: fluconazole, delavirdine
• Increased CNS effects: triazolam
• Increased effects of oral anticoagulants, digoxin, theophylline, carbamazepine, tacrolimus, cyclosporine, bromocriptine, disopyramide, hexobarbital, lorvastatin, phenytoin, pimozide, valproate
• Decreased action: clindamycin, rifampin
• Increased or decreased action: zidovudine

Lab test interferences:
False increase: 17-OHCS/17-KS, AST, ALT, BUN, creatinine, LDH, total bilirubin
Decrease: Folate assay, WBC

NURSING CONSIDERATIONS
Assess:
• I&O ratio; report hematuria, oliguria in renal disease
• Liver studies: AST, ALT
• Renal studies: urinalysis, protein, hematuria
• C&S before drug therapy; drug may be given as soon as culture is taken; C&S may be repeated after treatment
• Bowel pattern before, during treatment
• Skin eruptions, itching
• Respiratory status: rate, character, wheezing, tightness in chest; discontinue drug
• Allergies before treatment, reaction of each medication

Administer:
• Adequate intake of fluids (2 L) during diarrhea episodes
• q12h to maintain serum level

Perform/provide:
• Storage at room temp

Evaluate:
• Therapeutic response: C&S negative for infection

Teach patient/family:
• To take with full glass H_2O; may give with food to decrease GI symptoms
• To report sore throat, fever, fatigue; may indicate superinfection

• To notify nurse of diarrhea stools, dark urine, pale stools, yellow discoloration of eyes or skin, severe abdominal pain

• To take at evenly spaced intervals; complete dosage regimen

Treatment of hypersensitivity: Withdraw drug, maintain airway, administer epinephrine, aminophylline, O_2, IV corticosteroids

---

clemastine (℞)

(klem'as-teen)
Contac Allergy 12 Hour, Tavist
Func. class.: Antihistamine
Chem. class.: Ethanolamine derivative, H_1-receptor antagonist

---

Action: Acts on blood vessels, GI, respiratory system by competing with histamine for H_1-receptor site; decreases allergic response by blocking histamine

Uses: Allergy symptoms, rhinitis, angioedema, urticaria, common cold

Dosage and routes:
• *Adult and child >12 yr:* **PO** 1.34-2.68 mg bid-tid, not to exceed 8.04 mg/day

Available forms: Tabs 1.34, 2.68 mg; syr 0.67 mg/ml

Side effects/adverse reactions:

CNS: Dizziness, drowsiness, poor coordination, fatigue, anxiety, euphoria, confusion, paresthesia, neuritis

CV: Hypotension, palpitations, tachycardia

RESP: Increased thick secretions, wheezing, chest tightness

HEMA: Thrombocytopenia, agranulocytosis, hemolytic anemia

GI: Constipation, dry mouth, nausea, vomiting, anorexia, diarrhea

INTEG: Rash, urticaria, photosensitivity

GU: Retention, dysuria, frequency

EENT: Blurred vision, dilated pupils, tinnitus, nasal stuffiness, dry nose, throat, mouth

Contraindications: Hypersensitivity to H_1-receptor antagonists, acute asthma attack, lower respiratory tract disease

Precautions: Increased intraocular pressure, renal disease, cardiac disease, hypertension, bronchial asthma, seizure disorder, stenosed peptic ulcers, hyperthyroidism, prostatic hypertrophy, bladder neck obstruction, pregnancy (B), lactation, elderly

Pharmacokinetics:

PO: Peak 5-7 hr, duration 10-12 hr or more; metabolized in liver, excreted by kidneys

Interactions:
• Increased CNS depression: barbiturates, narcotics, hypnotics, tricyclic antidepressants, alcohol
• Decreased effect of oral anticoagulants, heparin
• Increased effect of clemastine: MAOIs

 Increased CNS depression: kava kava

 Increased anticholinergic effect: henbane leaf

Lab test interferences:

False negative: Skin allergy tests

NURSING CONSIDERATIONS

Assess:
• I&O ratio; be alert for urinary retention, frequency, dysuria; drug should be discontinued
• CBC during long-term therapy
• Blood dyscrasias: thrombocytopenia, agranulocytosis (rare)
• Respiratory status: rate, rhythm, increase in bronchial secretions, wheezing, chest tightness
• Cardiac status: palpitations, increased pulse, hypotension

Administer:
• With meals for GI symptoms; absorption may slightly decrease

---

◆ = Nursing alert   = Herb-drug interaction   ⊘ = Do not crush

Perform/provide:
• Hard candy, gum, frequent rinsing of mouth for dryness
• Storage in tight container at room temp
Evaluate:
• Therapeutic response: absence of running or congested nose or rashes
Teach patient/family:
• All aspects of drug use; to notify prescriber of confusion, sedation, hypotension
• To avoid driving, other hazardous activity if drowsiness occurs
• To avoid concurrent use of alcohol, other CNS depressants
• That drug decreases anticoagulant (oral) effect
• To change position slowly, as drug may cause dizziness, hypotension (elderly)
Treatment of overdose: Administer ipecac syrup or lavage, diazepam, vasopressors, barbiturates (short-acting)

---

clidinium (℞)

(kli di'nee um)
Quarzan
Func. class.: GI anticholinergic
Chem. class.: Synthetic quaternary ammonium antimuscarinic

Action: Inhibits muscarinic actions of acetylcholine at postganglionic parasympathetic neuroeffector sites
Uses: Treatment of peptic ulcer disease in combination with other drugs
Dosage and routes:
• *Adult:* **PO** 2.5-5 mg tid-qid ac, hs
• *Elderly:* **PO** 2.5 mg tid ac
Available forms: Caps 2.5, 5 mg
Side effects/adverse reactions:
CNS: Confusion, stimulation in elderly, headache, insomnia, dizziness, drowsiness, anxiety, weakness, hallucination
GI: Dry mouth, constipation, para-lytic ileus, heartburn, nausea, vomiting, dysphagia, absence of taste
GU: Hesitancy, retention, impotence
CV: Palpitations, tachycardia
EENT: Blurred vision, photophobia, mydriasis, cycloplegia, increased ocular tension
INTEG: Urticaria, rash, pruritus, anhidrosis, fever, allergic reactions
Contraindications: Hypersensitivity to anticholinergics, narrow-angle glaucoma, GI obstruction, myasthenia gravis, paralytic ileus, GI atony, toxic megacolon
Precautions: Hyperthyroidism, coronary artery disease, dysrhythmias, CHF, ulcerative colitis, hypertension, hiatal hernia, hepatic disease, renal disease, pregnancy (C), lactation, urinary retention, prostatic hypertrophy, elderly
Pharmacokinetics:
PO: Onset 1 hr, duration 3 hr; ionized, excreted in urine
Interactions:
• Increased anticholinergic effect: amantadine, tricyclic antidepressants, MAOIs
• Decreased effect of phenothiazines, levodopa, ketoconazole
NURSING CONSIDERATIONS
Assess:
• VS, cardiac status: dysrhythmias, increased rate, palpitations
• I&O ratio; urinary retention or hesitancy, especially elderly
• GI complaints: pain, bleeding (frank or occult), nausea, vomiting, anorexia
Administer:
• ½-1 hr ac for better absorption
• Decreased dose to elderly patients, since their metabolism may be slowed
• Gum, hard candy, frequent rinsing of mouth for dryness of oral cavity
Perform/provide:
• Storage in tight container protected from light

- Increased fluids, bulk, exercise to decrease constipation

Evaluate:
- Therapeutic response: absence of epigastric pain, bleeding, nausea, vomiting

Teach patient/family:
- To avoid driving, other hazardous activities until stabilized on medication

Ⓢ Not to break, crush, or chew caps
- To avoid alcohol, other CNS depressants; will enhance sedating properties of this drug
- To avoid hot environments; stroke may occur, drug suppresses perspiration
- To use sunglasses when outside to prevent photophobia, may cause blurred vision
- To drink plenty of fluids
- To report dysphagia

---

clindamycin (℞)

(klin-da-mye'sin)
Cleocin, Cleocin-T, Clinda-Derm, C/T/S, clindamycin HCl, Dalacin C*, Cleocin Pediatric
Func. class.: Antiinfective, misc
Chem. class.: Lincomycin derivative

Action: Binds to 50S subunit of bacterial ribosomes, suppresses protein synthesis

Uses: Infections caused by staphylococci, streptococci, *Rickettsia, Fusobacterium, Actinomyces, Peptococcus, Bacteroides, Pneumocystis carinii*

Dosage and routes:
- *Adult:* **PO** 150-450 mg q6h; **IM/IV** 1.2-1.8 g/day in 2-4 divided doses, not to exceed 4800 mg/day
- *Child >1 mo:* **PO** 8-25 mg/kg/day in divided doses q6-8h; **IM/IV**

20-40 mg/kg/day in divided doses q6-8h (3-4 equal doses)
- *Child <1 mo:* 15-20 mg/kg/day divided q6-8h
- *PID: Adult:* **IV** 600 mg qid plus gentamicin

Available forms: Inj 150-300 mg/ml; caps 75, 150, 300 mg; oral sol 75 mg/ml

Side effects/adverse reactions:
HEMA: **Leukopenia, eosinophilia, agranulocytosis, thrombocytopenia, polyarthritis**
GI: Nausea, vomiting, abdominal pain, diarrhea, **pseudomembranous colitis,** anorexia, weight loss
GU: Increased AST, ALT, bilirubin, alk phosphatase; jaundice, *vaginitis,* urinary frequency
EENT: Rash, urticaria, pruritus, erythema, pain, abscess at injection site

Contraindications: Hypersensitivity to this drug or lincomycin, ulcerative colitis/enteritis

Precautions: Renal disease, liver disease, GI disease, elderly, pregnancy (B), lactation, tartrazine sensitivity

Pharmacokinetics:
PO: Peak 45 min, duration 6 hr
IM: Peak 3 hr, duration 8-12 hr; half-life 2½ hr; metabolized in liver; excreted in urine, bile, feces as inactive metabolites; crosses placenta; excreted in breast milk

Interactions:
- Increased neuromuscular blockade: nondepolarizing muscle relaxants

Lab test interferences:
Increase: Alk phosphatase, bilirubin, CPK, AST, ALT

NURSING CONSIDERATIONS
Assess:
- Liver studies: AST (SGOT), ALT (SGPT)

◆= Nursing alert   ◉= Herb-drug interaction   Ⓢ= Do not crush

• Blood studies: WBC, RBC, Hct, Hgb, platelets, serum iron, reticulocytes; drug should be discontinued if bone marrow depression occurs

• C&S before drug therapy; drug may be given as soon as culture is taken

• B/P, pulse in patient receiving drug parenterally

• Bowel pattern before, during treatment; if severe diarrhea occurs, drug should be discontinued; may indicate pseudomembranous colitis

• Skin eruptions, itching, dermatitis after administration

• Respiratory status: rate, character, wheezing, tightness in chest

• Allergies before treatment, reaction of each medication

Administer:

• IM deep injection; rotate sites

• Orally with at least 8 oz H_2O

IV

• By infusion only; do not administer bolus dose; dilute 300 mg or less/50 ml or more of D_5W, NS; may be further diluted in greater amounts of D_5W, NS and given as a cont inf in acute PID; give first dose 10 mg/min over ½ hr, then 0.75 mg/min; increased rates may be used to keep serum blood levels higher; run >10 min; no more than 1200 mg in a single 1-hr inf

Additive compatibilities: Amikacin, ampicillin, aztreonam, cefamandole, cefazolin, cefepime, cefonicid, cefoperazone, cefotaxime, cefoxitin, ceftazidime, ceftizoxime, cefuroxime, cephalothin, cimetidine, fluconazole, heparin, hydrocortisone, kanamycin, methylprednisolone, metoclopramide, metronidazole, netilmicin, ofloxacin, penicillin G, piperacillin, potassium chloride, sodium bicarbonate, tobramycin, verapamil, vit B/C

Syringe compatibilities: Amikacin, aztreonam, gentamicin, heparin

Y-site compatibilities: Amifostine, amiodarone, amsacrine, aztreonam, cefpirome, cyclophosphamide, diltiazem, enalaprilat, esmolol, fludarabine, foscarnet, granisetron, heparin, hydromorphone, labetalol, magnesium sulfate, melphalan, meperidine, midazolam, morphine, multivitamins, ondansetron, perphenazine, piperacillin/tazobactam, propofol, sargramostim, tacrolimus, teniposide, theophylline, thiotepa, vinorelbine, vit B/C, zidovudine

Perform/provide:

• Storage at room temp (caps) up to 2 wk (reconstituted)

• Epinephrine, suction, tracheostomy set, endotracheal intubation equipment on unit

• Adequate intake of fluids (2 L) during diarrhea episodes

Evaluate:

• Therapeutic response: decreased temperature, negative C&S

Teach patient/family:

• To take oral drug with full glass H_2O; may give with food to reduce GI symptoms; antiperistaltic drugs may worsen diarrhea

• All aspects of drug therapy: need to complete entire course of medication to ensure organism death (10-14 days); culture may be taken after completed medication course

➤ To report sore throat, fever, fatigue; may indicate superinfection

🚫 Not to break, crush, or chew caps

• That drug must be taken in equal intervals around clock to maintain blood levels

• To notify nurse or prescriber of diarrhea

Treatment of hypersensitivity: Withdraw drug; maintain airway; administer epinephrine, aminophylline, O_2, IV corticosteroids

---

clofazimine (Ŗ)

(kloe-fa'zi-meen)

Lamprene

Func. class.: Leprostatic

Action: Inhibits mycobacterial growth, binds to mycobacterial DNA; exerts antiinflammatory properties in controlling leprosy reactions

Uses: Lepromatous leprosy, dapsone-resistant leprosy, lepromatous leprosy complicated by erythema nodosum leprosum

Dosage and routes:

Erythema nodosum leprosum

• *Adult:* **PO:** 100-200 mg qd × 3 mo, then taper dosage to 100 mg when disease is controlled; do not exceed 200 mg/day

Dapsone-resistant leprosy

• *Adult:* **PO:** 100 mg/day in combination with at least one other antileprosy drug × 3 yr, then 100 mg qd clofazimine (only)

Available forms: Caps 50, 100 mg

Side effects/adverse reactions:

*GI: Diarrhea, nausea, vomiting, abdominal pain, intolerance, **GI bleeding, obstruction,** anorexia, constipation, **hepatitis,** jaundice*

EENT: Pigmentation of cornea, conjunctiva, drying, burning, itching, irritation

INTEG: Pink or brown discoloration, dryness, pruritus, rash, photosensitivity, acne, monilial cheilosis

CNS: Dizziness, headache, fatigue, drowsiness

MISC: Discolored urine, feces, sputum, sweat

Contraindications: Hypersensitivity to this drug

Precautions: Pregnancy (C), lactation, children, abdominal pain, diarrhea, depression

Pharmacokinetics: Deposited in fatty tissue, reticuloendothelial system; half-life 70 days; small amount excreted in feces, sputum, sweat

Lab test interferences:

Increase: Albumin, bilirubin, AST (SGPT), eosinophilia, hypokalemia, glucose, ESR

NURSING CONSIDERATIONS

Assess:

• Liver studies qwk: ALT (SGOT), AST (SGPT), bilirubin

• Renal studies: BUN, creatinine, I&O, specific gravity, urinalysis before, qmo

• Blood level of drug

• Mental status often: affect, mood, behavioral changes; psychosis may occur

• Hepatic status: decreased appetite, jaundice, dark urine, fatigue

Administer:

• With meals to decrease GI symptoms

• Antiemetic if vomiting occurs

• After C&S is completed; qmo to detect resistance

Perform/provide:

• Infants to be kept with mother infected with leprosy; breastfeeding during drug therapy is encouraged

Evaluate:

• Therapeutic response: decreased symptoms of infection

Teach patient/family:

🚫 Not to break, crush, or chew caps

• That therapeutic effects may occur after 3-6 mo of drug therapy

• That compliance with dosage schedule, length is necessary

• That scheduled appointments must be kept or relapse may occur

• That drug must be taken with meals

• That skin, sweat, sputum, urine, feces discoloration, although reversible, may take several months or years to disappear

---

 = Nursing alert   = Herb-drug interaction   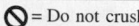 = Do not crush

clomiphene (℞)

(kloe'mi-feen)
Clomid, clomiphene citrate, Milophene, Serophene

Func. class.: Ovulation stimulant

Chem. class.: Nonsteroidal antiestrogenic

Action: Increases LH, FSH release from the pituitary, which increase maturation of ovarian follicle, ovulation, development of corpus luteum

Uses: Female infertility (ovulatory failure)

Dosage and routes:
• *Adult:* **PO** 50-100 mg qd × 5 days or 50-100 mg qd beginning on day 5 of cycle; may be repeated until conception occurs or 3 cycles of therapy have been completed

Available forms: Tabs 50 mg

Side effects/adverse reactions:
CV: Vasomotor flushing, phlebitis, ***deep-vein thrombosis***
EENT: Blurred vision, diplopia, photophobia
CNS: Headache, depression, restlessness, anxiety, nervousness, fatigue, insomnia, dizziness, flushing
GI: Nausea, vomiting, constipation, abdominal pain, bloating
INTEG: Rash, dermatitis, urticaria, alopecia
GU: Polyuria, frequency, birth defects, spontaneous abortions, multiple ovulation, breast pain, oliguria, abnormal uterine bleeding

Contraindications: Hypersensitivity, pregnancy (X), hepatic disease, undiagnosed uterine bleeding, uncontrolled thyroid or adrenal dysfunction, intracranial lesion, ovarian cysts

Precautions: Hypertension, depression, convulsions, diabetes mellitus

Pharmacokinetics: Metabolized in liver, excreted in feces

Lab test interferences:
Increase: FSH/LH, BSP, thyroxine, TBG

NURSING CONSIDERATIONS
Administer:
• After discontinuing estrogen therapy
• At same time qd to maintain drug level

Evaluate:
• Therapeutic response: fertility

Teach patient/family:
• That multiple births are common
• To notify prescriber if low abdominal pain occurs; may indicate ovarian cyst, cyst rupture
• That if dose is missed, to double at next time; if more than one dose is missed, call prescriber
• That response usually occurs 4-10 days after last day of treatment
• The method for taking, recording basal body temp to determine whether ovulation has occurred
• If ovulation can be determined (there is a slight decrease in temp, then a sharp increase for ovulation), to attempt coitus 3 days before and qod until after ovulation
• If pregnancy is suspected, to notify prescriber immediately

clomipramine (℞)

(kloe-mip'ra-meen)
Anafranil

Func. class.: Antidepressant, tricyclic

Chem. class.: Tertiary amine

Action: Not known; potent inhibitor of serotonin uptake; also increases dopamine metabolism; moderate anticholinergic effect

Uses: Depression, dysphoria, phobias, anxiety, agoraphobia, obsessive-compulsive disorder

Dosage and routes:
Obsessive-compulsive disorder
• *Adult:* **PO** 25 mg hs and increase gradually over 4 wk to 75-300 mg/ day in divided doses
• *Child 10-18 yr:* **PO** 25-50 mg/day gradually increased; not to exceed 200 mg/day
Depression
• *Adult:* **PO** 50-150 mg/day in a single or divided dose
Anxiety/agoraphobia
• *Adult:* **PO** 25-75 mg/day
Available forms: Caps 25, 50, 75 mg
Side effects/adverse reactions:
*HEMA: **Agranulocytosis, neutropenia, pancytopenia***
CV: Hypotension, tachycardia, ***cardiac arrest***
*CNS: Dizziness, tremors, mania, **seizures,** aggressiveness, EPS*
ENDO: Galactorrhea, hyperprolactinemia
META: Hyponatremia
GI: Constipation, dry mouth, nausea, dyspepsia
GU: Delayed ejaculation, anorgasmy, retention
INTEG: Diaphoresis, photosensitivity
Contraindications: Hypersensitivity
Precautions: Seizures, suicidal patients, elderly, pregnancy (C), lactation
Pharmacokinetics: Extensively bound to tissue and plasma proteins; demethylated in liver; active metabolites excreted in urine; half-life: 19-37 hr; steady state 1-2 wk
Interactions:
• Hypotensive antagonism: bethanidine
• Toxicity: phenothiazines, cimetidine
• Ethanol reaction: disulfiram, guanadrel increased or decreased effects

• Increased or decreased effects of clomipramine: estrogens
• Delirium: ethchlorvynol
• Hypertensive crisis, convulsions, hypertensive episode: MAOIs
• Decreased seizure threshold: phenytoin, phenobarbital
 Increased CNS depression: kava kava
 Increased anticholinergic effect: belladonna leaf/root, henbane leaf
 Increased action of clomipramine: scopolia root
Lab test interferences:
Increase: Prolactin, TBG
Decrease: Serum thyroid hormone
NURSING CONSIDERATIONS
Assess:
• B/P (lying, standing), pulse q4h; if systolic B/P drops 20 mm Hg, withhold drug, notify prescriber; take vital signs q4h in patients with cardiovascular disease
• Blood studies: CBC, leukocytes, differential, cardiac enzymes if patient is receiving long-term therapy
• Hepatic studies: AST (SGOT), ALT (SGPT), bilirubin
• Mental status: mood, sensorium, affect, suicidal tendencies; increase in psychiatric symptoms: depression, panic
• Urinary retention, constipation; constipation more likely in children
• Withdrawal symptoms: headache, nausea, vomiting, muscle pain, weakness; not usual unless drug discontinued abruptly
• Alcohol consumption; if alcohol consumed, withhold dose until AM
Administer:
• Increased fluids, bulk in diet for constipation, especially elderly
• With food or milk for GI symptoms
• Gum, hard candy, or frequent sips of water for dry mouth

◆ = Nursing alert   = Herb-drug interaction   Ⓝ = Do not crush

Perform/provide:
• Storage in tight container at room temp; do not freeze
• Assistance with ambulation during beginning therapy, since drowsiness/dizziness occurs
• Safety measures, including side rails, primarily in elderly
• Checking to see PO medication swallowed

Evaluate:
• Therapeutic response: decreased anxiety, depression

Teach patient/family:
🚫 Not to break, crush, or chew caps
• That the effects may take 2-3 wk
• To use caution in driving, other activities requiring alertness because of drowsiness, dizziness, blurred vision
• To avoid alcohol ingestion, other CNS depressants
• Not to discontinue medication quickly after long-term use; may cause nausea, headache, malaise
• To wear sunscreen, protective clothing to prevent photosensitivity

Treatment of overdose: ECG monitoring; induce emesis; lavage, activated charcoal; anticonvulsant

---

clonazepam (℞)

(kloe-na'zi-pam)
Klonopin, Syn-Clonazepam*, Rivotril*

Func. class.: Anticonvulsant
Chem. class.: Benzodiazepine derivative

Controlled Substance Schedule IV
Action: Inhibits spike, wave formation in absence seizures (petit mal), decreases amplitude, frequency, duration, spread of discharge in minor motor seizures

Uses: Absence, atypical absence, akinetic, myoclonic seizures, Lennox-Gastaut syndrome

Investigational uses: Parkinsonian dysarthrosis, acute manic episodes, adjunction schizophrenia, neuralgias, multifocal tic disorders, restless leg syndrome

Dosage and routes:
• *Adult:* **PO** not to exceed 1.5 mg/day in 3 divided doses; may be increased 0.5-1 mg q3d until desired response, not to exceed 20 mg/day
• *Child <10 yr or 30 kg:* **PO** 0.01-0.03 mg/kg/day in divided doses q8h, not to exceed 0.05 mg/kg/day; may be increased 0.25-0.5 mg q3d until desired response, not to exceed 0.1-0.2 mg/kg/day

Available forms: Tabs 0.5, 1, 2 mg

Side effects/adverse reactions:
HEMA: **Thrombocytopenia, leukocytosis, eosinophilia**
CNS: Drowsiness, dizziness, confusion, behavioral changes, tremors, insomnia, headache, suicidal tendencies, slurred speech
GI: *Nausea, constipation,* polyphagia, anorexia, xerostomia, diarrhea, gastritis, sore gums
INTEG: Rash, alopecia, hirsutism
EENT: *Increased salivation, nystagmus, diplopia,* abnormal eye movements
RESP: **Respiratory depression,** dyspnea, congestion
CV: Palpitations, bradycardia
GU: Dysuria, enuresis, nocturia, retention

Contraindications: Hypersensitivity to benzodiazepines, acute narrow-angle glaucoma

Precautions: Open-angle glaucoma, chronic respiratory disease, pregnancy (C), lactation, renal, hepatic disease, elderly

Pharmacokinetics:
PO: Peak 1-2 hr; metabolized by liver; excreted in urine; half-life 18-50 hr

---

Interactions:
• Increased CNS depression: alcohol, barbiturates, narcotics, antidepressants, other anticonvulsants, general anesthetics, hypnotics, sedatives
• Decreased effect of levodopa
⫰ Increased CNS depression: kava kava

Lab test interferences:
Increase: AST (SGPT), alk phosphatase

NURSING CONSIDERATIONS
Assess:
• Renal studies: urinalysis, BUN, urine creatinine
• Blood studies: RBC, Hct, Hgb, reticulocyte counts qwk for 4 wk, then qmo
• Hepatic studies: ALT (SGOT), AST (SGPT), bilirubin, creatinine
• Drug levels during initial treatment (therapeutic 20-80 ng/ml)
• Signs of physical withdrawal if medication suddenly discontinued
• Mental status: mood, sensorium, affect, oversedation, behavioral changes; if mental status changes, notify prescriber
• Eye problems: need for ophthalmic exam before, during, after treatment (slit lamp, fundoscopy, tonometry)
• Allergic reaction: red, raised rash; drug should be discontinued
◆ Blood dyscrasias: fever, sore throat, bruising, rash, jaundice
• Toxicity: bone marrow depression, nausea, vomiting, ataxia, diplopia, cardiovascular collapse

Administer:
• With food, milk for GI symptoms
Perform/provide:
• Storage at room temperature
• Assistance with ambulation during early part of treatment; dizziness occurs, especially elderly
Evaluate:
• Therapeutic response: decreased

seizure activity, document on patient's chart
Teach patient/family:
• To carry ID card or Medic Alert bracelet stating name, drugs taken, condition, prescriber's name, phone number
• To avoid driving, other activities that require alertness
• To avoid alcohol ingestion, CNS depressants; increased sedation may occur
• Not to discontinue medication quickly after long-term use; taper off over several wk
Treatment of overdose: Lavage, activated charcoal, monitor electrolytes, VS, administer vasopressors

---

clonidine (℞)
(klon′i-deen)
Catapres, Catapres-TTS, clonidine HCl, Dixarit*, Duraclon
Func. class.: Antihypertensive, analgesic
Chem. class.: Central α-adrenergic agonist

Action: Inhibits sympathetic vasomotor center in CNS, which reduces impulses in sympathetic nervous system; blood pressure, pulse rate, cardiac output decrease
Uses: Mild to moderate hypertension, used alone or in combination; severe pain in cancer patients
Investigational uses: Narcotic withdrawal, prevention of vascular headaches, treatment of menopausal symptoms, dysmenorrhea, attention deficit disorder
Dosage and routes:
Hypertension
• *Adult:* **PO/TRANS** 0.1 mg bid, then increase by 0.1 mg/day or 0.2 mg/day until desired response; range 0.2-0.8 mg/day in divided doses

---

• *Geriatric:* **PO** 0.1 mg hs, may increase gradually

• *Child:* 5-10 µg/kg/day in divided doses q8-12h, max 0.9 mg/day

Opioid withdrawal

• *Adult:* **PO** 0.3-1.2 mg/day; decreased dosage given over several days

Severe pain

• *Adult:* **CONT EPIDURAL INF** 30 µg/hr

ADHD

• *Child:* 0.05 mg/day titrate up to max 0.4 mg/day

Available forms: Tabs 0.1, 0.2, 0.3 mg; TRANS 2.5, 5, 7.5 mg delivering 0.1, 0.2, 0.3 mg/24 hr, respectively

Side effects/adverse reactions:

CNS: Drowsiness, sedation, headache, fatigue, nightmares, insomnia, mental changes, anxiety, depression, hallucinations, delirium

CV: Orthostatic hypotension, palpitations, CHF, ECG abnormalities

EENT: Taste change, parotid pain

ENDO: Hyperglycemia

GI: Nausea, vomiting, malaise, constipation, dry mouth

GU: Impotence, dysuria, *nocturia,* gynecomastia

INTEG: Rash, alopecia, facial pallor, pruritus, hives, edema, burning papules, excoriation (transdermal patches)

MS: Muscle, joint pain; leg cramps

Contraindications: Hypersensitivity

Precautions: MI (recent), diabetes mellitus, chronic renal failure, Raynaud's disease, thyroid disease, depression, COPD, child <12 (patches), asthma, pregnancy (C), lactation, elderly, noncompliant patients

Pharmacokinetics: Absorbed well

PO: Onset ½ to 1 hr, peak 2-4 hr, duration 8 hr; half-life 12-16 hr

TOP: Onset 3 days, duration 1 wk; metabolized by liver (metabolites), excreted in urine (30% unchanged, inactive metabolites), feces; crosses blood-brain barrier, excreted in breast milk

Interactions:

• Increased CNS depression: narcotics, sedatives, hypnotics, anesthetics, alcohol

• Decreased hypotensive effects: tricyclic antidepressants, MAOIs, appetite suppressants, amphetamines

• Increased hypotensive effects: diuretics, other antihypertensive nitrates

• Increased bradycardia: β-blockers, cardiac glycosides

Lab test interferences:

Increase: Blood glucose

Decrease: VMA, catecholamines, aldosterone

NURSING CONSIDERATIONS

Assess:

• Blood studies: neutrophils, decreased platelets

• Renal studies: protein, BUN, creatinine; increased levels may indicate nephrotic syndrome

• Baselines in renal, liver function tests before therapy begins; K levels, although hyperkalemia rare

• Dipstick of urine for protein qd in first morning specimen; if protein is increased, a 24-hr urinary protein should be collected

• B/P, pulse if used for hypertension

• For narcotic withdrawal including fever, diarrhea, nausea, vomiting, cramps, insomnia, shivering, dilated pupils

• Edema in feet, legs daily; monitor I&O; check for falling output

• Allergic reaction: rash, fever, pruritus, urticaria; drug should be discontinued if antihistamines fail to help

- Allergic reaction from patches: rash, urticaria, angioedema; should not continue to use
- Symptoms of CHF: edema, dyspnea, wet rales, B/P
- Renal symptoms: polyuria, oliguria, frequency

Administer:
- SL if patient is unable to swallow
- PO: give last dose at hs
- Topical patch qwk; apply to site without hair; best absorption over chest or upper arm; rotate sites with each application; clean site before application; apply firmly, especially around edges
- Infusion of 0.9% NaCl (as ordered) to expand fluid volume if severe hypotension occurs

Y-site compatibilities: Lorazepam

Perform/provide:
- Storage of patches in cool environment, tablets in tight container

Evaluate:
- Therapeutic response: decrease in B/P in hypertension, decrease in withdrawal symptoms (narcotic), decrease in pain

Teach patient/family:
- To avoid hazardous activities, since drug may cause drowsiness
- To administer 1 hr before meals (PO)
- Not to discontinue drug abruptly, or withdrawal symptoms may occur: anxiety, increased B/P, headache, insomnia, increased pulse, tremors, nausea, sweating
- Not to use OTC (cough, cold, or allergy) products unless directed by prescriber
- To avoid sunlight, wear sunscreen; photosensitivity may occur
- To comply with dosage schedule even if feeling better
- To rise slowly to sitting or standing position to minimize orthostatic hypotension, especially elderly

- To notify prescriber of mouth sores, sore throat, fever, swelling of hands, feet, irregular heartbeat, chest pain, signs of angioedema
- About excessive perspiration, dehydration, vomiting; diarrhea may lead to fall in blood pressure; consult prescriber if these occur
- That drug may cause dizziness, fainting; light-headedness may occur during first few days of therapy
- That drug may cause dry mouth; use hard candy, saliva product, or frequent rinsing of mouth
- That compliance is necessary; not to skip or stop drug unless directed by prescriber
- That drug may cause skin rash or impaired perspiration
- To use patch; patch comes in two parts: drug patch and overlay to keep patch in place
- That response may take 2-3 days if drug is given transdermally; instruct on administration of patch

Treatment of overdose: Supportive treatment; administer tolazoline, atropine, dopamine prn

---

clopidogrel (℞)

(klo-pid′oh-grel)
Plavix

Func. class.: Platelet aggregation inhibitor

Chem. class.: Thienopyridine derivative

Action: Inhibits first and second phases of ADP-induced effects in platelet aggregation

Uses: Reducing the risk of stroke in high-risk patients

Dosage and routes:
- *Adult:* **PO** 75 mg qd with or without food

Available forms: Tabs 75 mg

◆ = Nursing alert　　∥ = Herb-drug interaction　　⊘ = Do not crush

Side effects/adverse reactions:

INTEG: Rash, pruritus

GI: Nausea, vomiting, diarrhea, GI discomfort

HEMA: Epistaxis, purpura

CV: Edema, hypertension

CNS: Headache, dizziness

MS: Arthralgia, back pain

RESP: Upper respiratory tract infection, dyspnea, rhinitis, bronchitis, cough

MISC: UTI, depression, hypercholesterolemia, chest pain, fatigue, *intracranial hemorrhage*

Contraindications: Hypersensitivity, active bleeding

Precautions: Past liver disease, pregnancy (B), lactation, children, increased bleeding risk, neutropenia, agranulocytosis

Pharmacokinetics: Peak 1-3 hr, metabolized by liver, excreted in urine, feces

Interactions:

• Increased bleeding tendencies: anticoagulants, aspirin, NSAIDs

NURSING CONSIDERATIONS

Assess:

• Liver function studies: AST (SGOT), ALT (SGPT), bilirubin, creatinine (long-term therapy)

• Blood studies: CBC, Hct, Hgb, pro-time (long-term therapy)

Administer:

• With food to decrease gastric symptoms

Evaluate:

• Therapeutic response: absence of stroke

Teach patient/family:

• That blood work will be necessary during treatment

• To report any unusual bleeding to prescriber

• To take with food or just after eating to minimize GI discomfort

• To report side effects such as diarrhea, skin rashes, subcutaneous bleeding

clorazepate (℞)

(klor-az′e-pate)

Apo-clorazepate*, clorazepate dipotassium, Gen-XENE, Novo-Clopate*, Tranxene, Tranxene-SD

Func. class.: Antianxiety, anticonvulsant

Chem. class.: Benzodiazepine

Controlled Substance Schedule IV

Action: Potentiates the actions of GABA, especially in limbic system, reticular formation

Uses: Anxiety, acute alcohol withdrawal, adjunct in seizure disorders

Dosage and routes:

Anxiety

• *Adult:* PO 15-60 mg/day

• *Geriatric:* PO 7.5 mg qd-bid

Alcohol withdrawal

• *Adult:* PO 30 mg then 30-60 mg in divided doses; day 2, 45-90 mg in divided doses; day 3, 22.5-45 mg in divided doses; day 4, 15-30 mg in divided doses; then reduce daily dose to 7.5-15 mg

Seizure disorders

• *Adult and child >12 yr:* PO 7.5 mg tid; may increase by 7.5 mg/wk or less, not to exceed 90 mg/day

• *Child 9-12 yr:* PO 7.5 mg bid; may increase by 7.5 mg/wk or less, not to exceed 60 mg/day

Available forms: Caps 3.75, 7.5, 15 mg; tabs 3.75, 7.5, 15 mg; single-dose tab 11.25, 22.5 mg

Side effects/adverse reactions:

CNS: Dizziness, drowsiness, confusion, headache, anxiety, tremors, stimulation, fatigue, depression, insomnia, hallucinations, lethargy

GI: Constipation, dry mouth, nausea, vomiting, anorexia, diarrhea

INTEG: Rash, dermatitis, itching

CV: Orthostatic hypotension, ECG changes, tachycardia, hypotension

EENT: Blurred vision, tinnitus, mydriasis

Contraindications: Hypersensitivity to benzodiazepines, narrow-angle glaucoma, psychosis, pregnancy (D), lactation, child <18 yr

Precautions: Elderly, debilitated, hepatic disease, renal disease

Pharmacokinetics:

PO: Onset 15 min, peak 1-2 hr, duration 4-6 hr; metabolized by liver, excreted by kidneys; crosses placenta, breast milk; half-life 30-100 hr

Interactions:

• Decreased effects of clorazepate: valproic acid

• Increased effects of clorazepate: CNS depressants, alcohol, disulfiram, oral contraceptives, antidepressants, MAOIs, cimetidine

⚭ Increased CNS depression: kava kava

Lab test interferences:

Increase: AST (SGOT), ALT (SGPT), serum bilirubin

Decrease: RAIU

False increase: 17-OHCS

NURSING CONSIDERATIONS

Assess:

• B/P (lying, standing), pulse; if systolic B/P drops 20 mm Hg, hold drug, notify prescriber

• Blood studies: CBC during long-term therapy; blood dyscrasias have occurred rarely

• Hepatic studies: AST (SGOT), ALT (SGPT), bilirubin, creatinine, LDH, alk phosphatase

• I&O; may indicate renal dysfunction

• Mental status: mood, sensorium, affect, sleeping pattern, drowsiness, dizziness

• Physical dependency, withdrawal symptoms: headache, nausea, vomiting, muscle pain, weakness after long-term use

• Suicidal tendencies

Administer:

• With food, milk for GI symptoms

• Crushed if patient cannot swallow whole

• Sugarless gum, hard candy, frequent sips of water for dry mouth

Perform/provide:

• Assistance with ambulation during beginning therapy, for drowsiness/dizziness, especially elderly

• Safety measures, including side rails

• Check to see PO medication has been swallowed

Evaluate:

• Therapeutic response: decreased anxiety, restlessness, insomnia

Teach patient/family:

• That drug may be taken with food

• That drug is not to be used for everyday stress or used longer than 4 mo, unless directed by prescriber; not to take more than prescribed amount; may be habit forming

Ⓢ Not to break, crush, or chew caps

• To avoid OTC preparations unless approved by prescriber

• To avoid driving, activities that require alertness; drowsiness may occur, especially in elderly

• To avoid alcohol ingestion, other psychotropic medications, unless directed by prescriber

• Not to discontinue medication abruptly after long-term use

• To rise slowly or fainting may occur

• That drowsiness may worsen at beginning of treatment

Treatment of overdose: Lavage, VS, supportive care, flumazenil

---

➡ = Nursing alert   **⚭** = Herb-drug interaction   **Ⓢ** = Do not crush

cloxacillin (R)

(klox-a-sill'in)
Apo-Cloxi*, cloxacillin sodium,
Cloxapen, Novo-Cloxin*, Nu-
Clox*, Orbenin*, Tegopen
Func. class.: Broad-spectrum
antiinfective
Chem. class.: Penicillinase-
resistant penicillin

Action: Interferes with cell wall replication of susceptible organisms; the cell wall, rendered osmotically unstable, swells, bursts from osmotic pressure

Uses: Gram-positive cocci (*S. aureus, S. pyogenes, E. pyogenes, S. pneumoniae*), penicillinase-producing staphylococci

Dosage and routes:
• *Adult:* PO 1-4 g/day in divided doses q6h
• *Child:* PO 50-100 mg/kg in divided doses q6h, max 4 g/day
Available forms: Caps 250, 500 mg; powder for oral susp 125 mg/5 ml

Side effects/adverse reactions:
HEMA: Anemia, increased bleeding time, **bone marrow depression, granulocytopenia**
GI: *Nausea, vomiting, diarrhea,* increased AST (SGOT), ALT (SGPT), abdominal pain, glossitis, colitis
GU: **Oliguria, proteinuria,** hematuria, *vaginitis, moniliasis,* **glomerulonephritis**
CNS: Lethargy, hallucinations, anxiety, depression, twitching, **coma, convulsions**

Contraindications: Hypersensitivity to penicillins; neonates, severe renal, hepatic disease

Precautions: Pregnancy (B), lactation, hypersensitivity to cephalosporins

Pharmacokinetics:
PO: Peak 1 hr, duration 6 hr; half-

life 30-60 min; metabolized in liver; excreted in urine, bile, breast milk; crosses placenta, poor penetration in CSF

Interactions:
• Increased cloxacillin concentrations: aspirin, probenecid, disulfiram
• Increased action of anticoagulants
• Decreased action of oral contraceptives

Lab test interferences:
False positive: Urine glucose, urine protein
Decrease: Uric acid

NURSING CONSIDERATIONS
Assess:
• I&O ratio; report hematuria, oliguria, since penicillin in high doses is nephrotoxic
◆ Any patient with compromised renal system, since drug is excreted slowly in poor renal system function; toxicity may occur rapidly
• Liver studies: AST (SGOT), ALT (SGPT)
• Blood studies: WBC, RBC, H&H, bleeding time
• Renal studies: urinalysis, protein, blood
• Culture, sensitivity before drug therapy; drug may be taken as soon as culture is taken
• Bowel pattern before, during treatment
• Skin eruptions after administration of penicillin to 1 wk after discontinuing drug
• Respiratory status: rate, character, wheezing, tightness in chest
• Allergies before initiation of treatment; reaction of each medication; place allergies on chart in bright red

Administer:
• After C&S completed
• Shake suspension well before each dose

---

* = Canada only   Side effects: *italics* = common; ***bold italics*** = life-threatening

Perform/provide:

• Adrenaline, suction, tracheostomy set, endotracheal intubation equipment on unit

• Adequate intake of fluids (2 L) during diarrhea episodes

• Scratch test to assess allergy after securing order from prescriber; usually done when penicillin is only drug of choice

• Storage in tight container; after reconstituting, store in refrigerator for 2 wk, room temp 1 wk

Evaluate:

• Therapeutic response: absence of fever, draining wounds

Teach patient/family:

🚫 Not to break, crush, or chew caps

• All aspects of drug therapy, including need to complete entire course of medication to ensure organism death (10-14 days); culture may be taken after completed course of medication

• To report sore throat, fever, fatigue (may indicate superinfection)

• To wear or carry a Medic Alert ID if allergic to penicillins

• To notify nurse of diarrhea

• To take on an empty stomach with a full glass of water

Treatment of overdose: Withdraw drug; maintain airway; administer epinephrine, aminophylline, O_2, IV corticosteroids for anaphylaxis

---

clozapine (℞)

(kloz′a-peen)
clozapine, Clozaril
Func. class.: Antipsychotic
Chem. class.: Tricyclic dibenzodiazepine derivative

Action: Interferes with dopamine receptor binding with lack of extrapyramidal symptoms; also acts as an adrenergic, cholinergic, his-

taminergic, serotonergic antagonist

Uses: Management of psychotic symptoms in schizophrenic patients for whom other antipsychotics have failed

Dosage and routes:

• *Adult:* **PO** 25 mg qd or bid; may increase by 25-50 mg/day; normal range 300-450 mg/day after 2 wk; do not increase dose more than 2 × per wk; do not exceed 900 mg/day; use lowest dose to control symptoms

Available forms: Tabs 25, 100 mg

Side effects/adverse reactions:

CNS: Sedation, salivation, dizziness, headache, tremors, sleep problems, akinesia, fever, seizures, sweating, akathisia, confusion, fatigue, insomnia, depression, slurred speech, anxiety

GI: Drooling or excessive salivation, constipation, nausea, abdominal discomfort, vomiting, diarrhea, anorexia

MS: Weakness; pain in back, neck, legs; spasm

CV: Tachycardia, hypotension, hypertension, chest pain, ECG changes

GU: Urinary abnormalities, incontinence, ejaculation dysfunction, frequency, urgency, retention

RESP: Dyspnea, nasal congestion, throat discomfort

HEMA: Leukopenia, neutropenia, agranulocytosis, eosinophilia

Contraindications: Hypersensitivity, myeloproliferative disorders, severe granulocytopenia, CNS depression, coma, narrow-angle glaucoma

Precautions: Pregnancy (B); lactation; children <16; hepatic, renal, cardiac disease; seizures; prostatic enlargement; elderly

Pharmacokinetics: Steady state 2.5 hr; 95% protein bound; completely metabolized by liver; excreted in urine and feces (metabolites); half-life 8-12 hr

---

Interactions:
- Increased anticholinergic effects: anticholinergics
- Increased hypotension: antihypertensives
- Increased CNS depression: CNS drugs
- Increased bone marrow suppression: antineoplastics, other drugs suppressing bone marrow
- Increased plasma concentrations: warfarin, digoxin, other highly protein-bound drugs

🍃 Increased CNS depression: kava kava

Lab test interferences:
Increase: Liver function tests, cardiac enzymes, cholesterol, blood glucose, bilirubin, PBI, cholinesterase, [131]I
False positive: Pregnancy tests, PKU
False negative: Urinary steroids, 17-OHCS

NURSING CONSIDERATIONS
Assess:
- Swallowing of PO medication; check for hoarding or giving of medication to other patients
- I&O ratio; obtain baseline before treatment begins; palpate bladder if low urinary output occurs
- Bilirubin, CBC, liver function studies monthly; discontinue treatment if WBC <3000/mm^3 or a granulocyte <1500/mm^3
- Urinalysis is recommended before, during prolonged therapy
- Affect, orientation, LOC, reflexes, gait, coordination, sleep pattern disturbances
- B/P standing and lying; take pulse and respirations q4h during initial treatment; establish baseline before starting treatment; report drops of 30 mm Hg
- Dizziness, faintness, palpitations, tachycardia on rising
- EPS including akathisia (inability to sit still, no pattern to movements), tardive dyskinesia (bizarre movements of the jaw, mouth, tongue, extremities), pseudoparkinsonism (rigidity, tremors, pill rolling, shuffling gait)
- Skin turgor daily
- Constipation, urinary retention daily; if these occur, increase bulk, water in diet, especially elderly

Administer:
- Antiparkinsonian agent for EPS

Perform/provide:
- Decreased noise input by dimming lights, avoiding loud noises
- Supervised ambulation until stabilized on medication; do not involve in strenuous exercise program because fainting is possible; patient should not stand still for long periods
- Increased fluids to prevent constipation
- Storage in tight, light-resistant container

Evaluate:
- Therapeutic response: decrease in emotional excitement, hallucinations, delusions, paranoia, reorganization of patterns of thought, speech

Teach patient/family:
- That orthostatic hypotension occurs often, and to rise from sitting or lying position gradually
- To avoid hot tubs, hot showers, tub baths; hypotension may occur
- To avoid abrupt withdrawal of this drug, or EPS may result; drug should be withdrawn slowly
- To avoid OTC preparations (cough, hay fever, cold) unless approved by prescriber, since serious drug interactions may occur; avoid use with alcohol or CNS depressants, increased drowsiness may occur
- About compliance with drug regimen
- About EPS and necessity for me-

ticulous oral hygiene, since oral candidiasis may occur

• To report sore throat, malaise, fever, bleeding, mouth sores; if these occur, CBC should be drawn and drug discontinued

• That in hot weather, heat stroke may occur; take extra precautions to stay cool

• To avoid driving, other hazardous activities; seizures may occur

• To notify prescriber if pregnant or if pregnancy is intended

Treatment of overdose: Lavage, activated charcoal; provide an airway; do not induce vomiting

---

codeine (℞)

(koe'deen)

Paveral*

Func. class.: Narcotic analgesic, antitussive

Chem. class.: Opiate, phenathrene derivative

Controlled Substance Schedule II, III, IV, V (depends on route)

Action: Depresses pain impulse transmission at the spinal cord level by interacting with opioid receptors, decreases cough reflex, GI motility

Uses: Moderate to severe pain, nonproductive cough

Investigational uses: Diarrhea

Dosage and routes:

Pain

• *Adult:* **PO** 15-60 mg q4h prn; **IM/SC** 15-60 mg q4h prn

• *Child:* **PO** 3 mg/kg/day in divided doses q4h prn

Cough

• *Adult:* **PO** 10-20 mg q4-6h, not to exceed 120 mg/day

• *Child:* **PO** 1-1.5 mg/kg/day in 4 divided doses, not to exceed 60 mg/day

Diarrhea

• *Adult:* **PO** 30 mg; may repeat qid prn

Renal disease

• CrCl 10-50 ml/min 75% of dose; CrCl <10 ml/min 50% of dose

Available forms: Inj 15, 30, 60 mg/ml; tabs 15, 30, 60 mg; oral sol 10 mg/5 ml*, 15 mg/5 ml

Side effects/adverse reactions:

CNS: Drowsiness, sedation, dizziness, agitation, dependency, lethargy, restlessness

GI: Nausea, vomiting, anorexia, constipation

RESP: Respiratory depression, respiratory paralysis

CV: Bradycardia, palpitations, orthostatic hypotension, tachycardia

GU: Urinary retention

INTEG: Flushing, rash, urticaria

Contraindications: Hypersensitivity to opiates, respiratory depression, increased intracranial pressure, seizure disorders, severe respiratory disorders

Precautions: Elderly, cardiac dysrhythmias, pregnancy (C), lactation

Pharmacokinetics: Onset 10-30 min, peak ½-1 hr, duration 4-6 hr; metabolized by liver; excreted by kidneys, in breast milk; crosses placenta; half-life 3 hr

Interactions:

• Effects may be increased with other CNS depressants: alcohol, narcotics, sedative/hypnotics, antipsychotics, skeletal muscle relaxants

🖋 Increased CNS depression: kava kava

NURSING CONSIDERATIONS

Assess:

• I&O ratio; check for decreasing output; may indicate urinary retention, especially elderly

• By using pain-scoring method

• For productive cough

• Cough: type, duration, ability to raise secretion

• CNS changes, dizziness, drowsiness, hallucinations, euphoria, LOC, pupil reaction
• Allergic reactions: rash, urticaria
• Respiratory dysfunction: respiratory depression, character, rate rhythm; notify prescriber if respirations are <10/min, shallow
• Need for pain medication, tolerance

Administer:

IV

• With antiemetic for nausea, vomiting
• When pain is beginning to return; determine dosage interval by patient response

Syringe compatibilities: Glycopyrrolate, hydroxyzine

Y-site compatibilities: Cefinetazole

Perform/provide:

• Storage in light-resistant container at room temp
• Assistance with ambulation if needed
• Safety measures: top side rails, night-light, call bell

Evaluate:

• Therapeutic response: decrease in pain, absence of grimacing, decreased cough

Teach patient/family:

• To report any symptoms of CNS changes, allergic reactions
• That physical dependency may result after extended periods
• To change position slowly; orthostatic hypotension may occur
• To avoid hazardous activities if drowsiness, dizziness occurs
• To avoid alcohol, other CNS depressants unless directed by prescriber

colchicine (℞)

(kol'chi-seen)

Func. class.: Antigout agent
Chem. class.: Colchicum autumnale alkaloid

Action: Inhibits microtubule formation of lactic acid in leukocytes, which decreases phagocytosis and inflammation in joints

Uses: Gout, gouty arthritis (prevention, treatment); to arrest progression of neurologic disability in multiple sclerosis

Investigational uses: Hepatic cirrhosis, familial Mediterranean fever

Dosage and routes:

Prevention

• *Adult:* **PO** 0.5-1.8 mg qd depending on severity; **IV** 0.5-1 mg 1-2 × day

Treatment

• *Adult:* **PO** 0.5-1.2 mg, then 0.5-1.2 mg q1h, until pain decreases or side effects occur

Available forms: Tabs 0.5, 0.6, 1 mg*

Side effects/adverse reactions:

MISC: Myopathy, alopecia, reversible azoospermia, peripheral neuritis

GU: Hematuria, *oliguria, renal damage*

*HEMA: **Agranulocytosis, thrombocytopenia, aplastic anemia, pancytopenia***

GI: Nausea, vomiting, anorexia, malaise, metallic taste, cramps, peptic ulcer, diarrhea

INTEG: Chills, dermatitis, pruritus, purpura, erythema

Contraindications: Hypersensitivity; serious GI, renal, hepatic, cardiac disorders; blood dyscrasias

Precautions: Severe renal disease, blood dyscrasias, pregnancy (C), hepatic disease, elderly, lactation, children

Pharmacokinetics:

PO: Peak ½-2 hr, half-life 20 min; deacetylates in liver; excreted in feces (metabolites/active drug)

Interactions:

• Increased GI effects: NSAIDs

• Increased bone marrow depression: radiation, bone marrow depressants

• Decreased action of vit B_{12}, may cause reversible malabsorption

Lab test interferences:

Increase: Alk phosphatase, AST/ALT

False positive: RBC, Hgb

NURSING CONSIDERATIONS

Assess:

• I&O ratio; observe for decrease in urinary output

• CBC, platelets, reticulocytes before, during therapy (q3mo)

• Coombs' test for Coombs' negative hemolytic anemia

• For toxicity: weakness, abdominal pain, nausea, vomiting, diarrhea

Administer:

• Oral: on empty stomach only, to facilitate absorption

Evaluate:

• Therapeutic response: decreased stone formation on x-ray, decreased pain in kidney region, absence of hematuria, decreased pain in joints

Teach patient/family:

• To increase fluid intake to 3-4 L/day

• To avoid alcohol, OTC preparations that contain alcohol; skin rashes have occurred

• To report any pain, redness, or hard area, usually in legs

• The importance of complying with medical regimen; the possibility of bone marrow depression occurring

Treatment of overdose: D/C medication, may need opioids to treat diarrhea

colestipol (℞)

(koe-les′ti-pole)
Colestid*

Func. class.: Antilipemic

Chem. class.: Bile sequestrant, resin exchange agent

Action: Absorbs, combines with bile acids to form insoluble complex excreted through feces; loss of bile acids lowers cholesterol levels

Uses: Primary hypercholesterolemia, xanthomas, digitalis toxicity, pruritus due to biliary obstruction, diarrhea due to bile acids

Dosage and routes:

• *Adult:* **PO** 15-30 g/day in 2-4 divided doses; 2-8 tabs/day

Available forms: Granules, tabs 1 g

Side effects/adverse reactions:

GI: Constipation, abdominal pain, nausea, fecal impaction, hemorrhoids, flatulence, vomiting, steatorrhea, peptic ulcer

INTEG: Rash, irritation of perianal area, tongue, skin

HEMA: Decreased vit A, D, K, red folate content; **hyperchloremic acidosis, bleeding, decreased pro-time**

Contraindications: Hypersensitivity, biliary obstruction

Precautions: Pregnancy (B), lactation, children, bleeding disorders

Pharmacokinetics:

PO: Excreted in feces

Interactions:

• May reduce action of thiazide, digitalis, warfarin, penicillin G, folic acid, phenylbutazone, tetracycline, corticosteroids, iron, thyroid agents, clindamycin, trimethoprim, chenodiol, fat-soluble vitamins, cephalexin, phenobarbital

Lab test interferences:

Increase: Liver function studies, chloride, PO_4

⬥ = Nursing alert   🖊 = Herb-drug interaction   🚫 = Do not crush

NURSING CONSIDERATIONS
Assess:
• Cardiac glycoside levels, if both drugs are being administered
• For signs of vit A, D, K deficiency
• Serum cholesterol, triglyceride levels, electrolytes (extended therapy)
• Bowel pattern daily; increase bulk, water in diet if constipation develops

Administer:
• Drug ac, hs; give all other medications 1 hr before colestipol or 4 hr after colestipol to avoid poor absorption
• Drug mixed in applesauce or stirred into beverage (2-6 oz); do not take dry; let stand for 2 min
🚫 Tabs should be swallowed whole; do not break, crush, or chew
• Supplemental doses of vit A, D, K if levels are low

Evaluate:
• Therapeutic response: decreased triglycerides, diarrhea, pruritus (excess bile acids)

Teach patient/family:
◆ The symptoms of hypoprothrombinemia: bleeding mucous membranes; dark, tarry stools; hematuria, petechiae; report immediately
• That compliance is needed; toxicity may result if doses are missed
• That risk factors should be decreased: high-fat diet, smoking, alcohol consumption, absence of exercise

corticotropin (ACTH) (R)
(kor-ti-koe-troe'pin)
ACTH, Acthar, ACTH-40, ACTH-80, corticotropin, H.P. Acthar Gel
Func. class.: Pituitary hormone
Chem. class.: Adrenocorticotropic hormone

Action: Stimulates adrenal cortex to produce, secrete corticosterone, cortisol

Uses: Testing adrenocortical function, treatment of adrenal insufficiency caused by administration of corticosteroids (long term), multiple sclerosis, infantile spasms

Dosage and routes:
Testing of adrenocortical function
• *Adult:* **IM/SC** up to 80 U in divided doses; **IV** 10-25 U in 500 ml D₅W given over 8 hr

Inflammation
• *Adult:* **SC/IM** 40 U in 4 divided doses (aqueous) or 40 U q12-24h (gel/repository form)

Infantile spasms
• *Infant:* **IM Gel** 20 U/day × 2 wks, increase if needed

Available forms: Inj SC 40, 80 U/vial; repository inj SC 40, 80/ml

Side effects/adverse reactions:
INTEG: Impaired wound healing, rash, urticaria, hirsutism, petechiae, ecchymoses, sweating, acne, hyperpigmentation
*CNS: **Convulsions,*** dizziness, euphoria, insomnia, headache, mood swings, behavioral changes, depression, psychosis
GI: Nausea, vomiting, ***peptic ulcer perforation,*** pancreatitis, distention, ulcerative esophagitis
GU: Water, sodium retention, hypokalemia
EENT: Cataracts, glaucoma

MS: Weakness, osteoporosis, compression fractures, muscle atrophy, steroid myopathy, myalgia, arthralgia

ENDO: Cushingoid symptoms, diabetes mellitus, antibody formation, growth retardation in children, menstrual irregularities

Contraindications: Hypersensitivity, scleroderma, osteoporosis, CHF, peptic ulcer disease, hypertension, systemic fungal infections, smallpox vaccination, recent surgery, ocular herpes simplex, primary adrenocortical insufficiency/hyperfunction

Precautions: Pregnancy (C), lactation, latent TB, hepatic disease, hypothyroiditis, childbearing age, psychiatric diagnosis, myasthenia gravis, acute gouty arthritis, thromboembolic disorders

Pharmacokinetics:

IV/IM/SC: Onset <6 hr, duration 2-4 hr, repository duration up to 3 days, half-life <20 min, excreted in urine

Interactions:

• Possible ulceration: salicylates, alcohol, corticosteroids

• Hypokalemia: diuretics (K-depleting), amphotericin B

• Hyperglycemia: insulin, oral hypoglycemic agents

NURSING CONSIDERATIONS

Assess:

• Baseline ECG, B/P, chest x-ray, GTT

• Pulse, B/P

• I&O ratio; weight qwk, report gain over 5 lb/wk

• 2 hr postprandial, chest x-ray, serum K, 17 KS, 17-OHCS, cortisol, during long-term treatment

• Dependent edema, moon face, pulmonary edema, cerebral edema

• Infection; drug may mask

• Increased stress in patient's life that may require increased corticosteroids

• Mental status: affect, mood, increased aggressiveness, irritability; change may require decreased steroids

• Growth rate of child

• Hypoadrenalism in neonates if drug was given during pregnancy

• Allergic reaction: rash, urticaria, fever, nausea, vomiting, dyspnea; drug should be discontinued immediately, administer epinephrine 1:1000

Administer:

• Test for hypersensitivity for individuals allergic to pork products

• Decreased Na, increase K for dependent edema

• Increase protein diet for N loss

• Gel at room temp, give deep IM using 21G needle

• May be used to treat edema

IV

IV; give over 2 min; dilute 25 U/1 ml sterile H_2O or NS or 40 U/2 ml; may dilute 10-25 U/500 ml compatible sol; give over 8 hr

Additive compatibilities: Calcium gluconate, chloramphenicol, cytarabine, dimenhydrinate, erythromycin, heparin, hydrocortisone, methicillin, norepinephrine, oxytetracycline, penicillin G potassium, potassium chloride, vancomycin, vit B/C

Perform/provide:

• Storage in refrigerator of unused portion; use within 24 hr

Evaluate:

• Therapeutic response: absence of inflammation, pain, increased muscle strength in myasthenia gravis

Teach patient/family:

• To avoid vaccinations during drug treatment

• To maintain hydration up to 2 L/day unless contraindicated

• To avoid OTC products: salicylates, products with alcohol

• Not to discontinue medication

⬧ = Nursing alert   ▟ = Herb-drug interaction   ⊗ = Do not crush

abruptly; adrenal crisis may occur; should be tapered over several wk
• To wear Medic Alert ID specifying steroid therapy
• That drug does not cure condition, only decreases symptoms
• To notify prescriber of infection: fever, sore throat, muscular pain
• To tell patient to notify anyone involved in dental or medical care that this drug is being taken

---

cortisone (R)

(kor'ti-sone)
Cortone Acetate
Func. class.: Corticosteroid, synthetic
Chem. class.: Glucocorticoid, short-acting

Action: Decreases inflammation by suppression of migration of polymorphonuclear leukocytes, fibroblasts, reversal of increased capillary permeability and lysosomal stabilization

Uses: Inflammation, severe allergy, adrenal insufficiency, collagen disorders, respiratory, dermatologic disorders

Dosage and routes:
• *Adult:* **PO/IM** 25-300 mg qd or q2d, titrated to response
• *Child:* **PO** 2.5-10 mg/kg/day; **IM** 1-5 mg/kg/day
Available forms: Tabs 5, 10, 25 mg; inj 50 mg/ml

Side effects/adverse reactions:
INTEG: Acne, poor wound healing, ecchymosis, bruising, petechiae
CNS: Depression, flushing, sweating, headache, mood changes
*CV: Hypertension, **circulatory collapse, thrombophlebitis, embolism,*** tachycardia, ***necrotizing angiitis,*** *CHF,* edema
*HEMA: **Thrombocytopenia***

MS: Fractures, osteoporosis, weakness
*GI: Diarrhea, nausea, abdominal distention, **GI hemorrhage,*** increased appetite, ***pancreatitis***
EENT: Fungal infections, increased intraocular pressure, blurred vision

Contraindications: Psychosis, hypersensitivity, idiopathic thrombocytopenia, acute glomerulonephritis, amebiasis, fungal infections, nonasthmatic bronchial disease, child <2 yr, AIDS, TB

Precautions: Pregnancy (C), lactation, diabetes mellitus, glaucoma, osteoporosis, seizure disorders, ulcerative colitis, CHF, myasthenia gravis, renal disease, esophagitis, peptic ulcer

Pharmacokinetics:
PO: Peak 2 hr, duration 1½ days
IM: Peak 20-48 hr, duration 1½ days

Interactions:
• Decreased action of cortisone: cholestyramine, colestipol, barbiturates, rifampin, ephedrine, phenytoin, theophylline
• Decreased effects of anticoagulants, anticonvulsants, antidiabetics, ambenonium, neostigmine, isoniazid, toxoids, vaccines, anticholinesterases, salicylates, somatrem
• Increased side effects: alcohol, salicylates, indomethacin, amphotericin B, digitalis, cyclosporine, diuretics
• Increased action of cortisone: salicylates, estrogens, indomethacin, oral contraceptives, ketoconazole, macrolide antibiotics

🍇 Potassium deficiency: chronic use/abuse cascara sagrada bark, aloe, buckthorn bark/berry, rhubarb root, senna leaf/fruits

Lab test interferences:
Increase: Cholesterol, Na, blood glucose, uric acid, Ca, urine glucose
Decrease: Ca, K, T_4, T_3, thyroid

---

^{131}I uptake test, urine 17-OHCS, 17-KS, PBI skin allergy tests

NURSING CONSIDERATIONS
Assess:
• K, blood sugar, urine glucose while on long-term therapy; hypokalemia and hyperglycemia
• Weight daily; notify prescriber of weekly gain >5 lb
• B/P q4h, pulse; notify prescriber if chest pain occurs
• I&O ratio; be alert for decreasing urinary output and increasing edema
• Plasma cortisol levels during long-term therapy (normal level: 138-635 nmol/L SI units if drawn at 8 AM)
• Infection: fever, WBC even after withdrawal of medication; drug masks infection
• K depletion: paresthesias, fatigue, nausea, vomiting, depression, polyuria, dysrhythmias, weakness
• Edema, hypertension, cardiac symptoms
• Mental status: affect, mood, behavioral changes, aggression

Administer:
• After shaking suspension (parenteral)
• Titrated dose; use lowest effective dose
• IM inj deeply in large mass; rotate sites; avoid deltoid; use a 21G needle
• In one dose in AM to prevent adrenal suppression; avoid SC administration; tissue may be damaged
• With food or milk to decrease GI symptoms

Perform/provide:
• Assistance with ambulation in patient with bone tissue disease to prevent fractures

Evaluate:
• Therapeutic response: ease of respirations, decreased inflammation

Teach patient/family:
• That ID as steroid user should be carried at all times

• To notify prescriber if therapeutic response decreases; dosage adjustment may be needed

◆ Not to discontinue abruptly or adrenal crisis can result

• To avoid OTC products: salicylates, alcohol in cough products, cold preparations unless directed by prescriber
• All aspects of drug usage, including cushingoid symptoms
• The symptoms of adrenal insufficiency: nausea, anorexia, fatigue, dizziness, dyspnea, weakness, joint pain

---

cromolyn (OTC, ℞)

(kroe′moe-lin)

Gastrocrom, Intal , Intal p*, Nasalcrom, Rynacrom*

Func. class.: Antiasthmatic
Chem. class.: Mast cell stabilizer

Action: Stabilizes the membrane of the sensitized mast cell, preventing release of chemical mediators after an antigen-IgE interaction

Uses: Allergic rhinitis, severe perennial bronchial asthma, prevention of exercise-induced bronchospasm, acute bronchospasm induced by environmental pollutants, mastocytosis

Dosage and routes:
Allergic rhinitis
• *Adult and child >6 yr:* **NASAL SOL** 1 spray in each nostril tid-qid, not to exceed 6 doses/day
Bronchospasm
• *Adult and child >6 yr:* **INH** 20 mg <1 hr before exercise
Bronchial asthma
• *Adult and child >6 yr:* **INH** 20 mg qid; **NEB** 20 mg qid by nebulization
Systemic mastocytosis
• *Adult and child >12 yr:* **PO** 200 mg qid ac and hs

◆ = Nursing alert   ⫻ = Herb-drug interaction   ⊘ = Do not crush

- *Child 2-12 yr:* **PO** 100 mg qid ½ ac and hs

Available forms: Sol 40 mg/ml; inh, caps for inh, 20 mg; caps for oral sol 100 mg; neb sol 20 mg/2 ml; aerosol 800 µg/actuation

Side effects/adverse reactions:

EENT: Throat irritation, cough, nasal congestion, burning eyes

CNS: Headache, dizziness, neuritis

GU: Frequency, dysuria

GI: Nausea, vomiting, anorexia, dry mouth, bitter taste

INTEG: Rash, urticaria, angioedema

MS: Joint pain/swelling

Contraindications: Hypersensitivity to this drug or lactose, status asthmaticus

Precautions: Pregnancy (B), lactation, renal disease, hepatic disease, child <5 yr

Pharmacokinetics:

INH: Peak 15 min, duration 4-6 hr; excreted unchanged in feces; half-life 80 min

ORAL: Unknown

NURSING CONSIDERATIONS

Assess:

- Eosinophil count during treatment
- Respiratory status: rate, rhythm, characteristics, cough, wheezing, dyspnea

Administer:

- For oral dose, dissolve powder in caps mixed with hot water; further dilute in cold water
- By inhalation/nebulizer only
- Gargle, sip of water to decrease irritation in throat

Evaluate:

- Therapeutic response: decrease in asthmatic symptoms; congested, runny nose

Teach patient/family:

- To clear mucus before using
- Proper inhalation technique: exhale; using inhaler, inhale deeply with head tipped back to open airway; remove; hold breath; exhale; repeat until all of drug is inhaled, use demonstration; return demonstration
- That therapeutic effect may take up to 4 wk
- Not to swallow capsule
- That drug is preventive only, not restorative

---

cyanocobalamin (vit B₁₂)/hydroxocobalamin (vit B₁₂a) (OTC, ℞)

(sye-an-oh-koe-bal'a-min)
Bedoz*, B₁₂Resin, Cobex, Crystamine, Crysti-12, Cyanabin*, Cyanoject, Cyomin, Ener-B, Permavite, Redisol, Rubesol-1000, Rubion*, Rubramin PC, Sytobex, Vitamin B₁₂

Func. class.: Vit B₁₂, water-soluble vitamin

Action: Needed for adequate nerve functioning, protein and carbohydrate metabolism, normal growth, RBC development, cell reproduction

Uses: Vit B₁₂ deficiency, pernicious anemia, vit B₁₂ malabsorption syndrome, Schilling test, increased requirements with pregnancy, thyrotoxicosis, hemolytic anemia, hemorrhage, renal and hepatic disease

Dosage and routes:

- *Adult:* **PO** 25 µg qd × 5-10 days, maintenance 100-200 mg **IM** qmo; **IM/SC** 30-100 µg qd × 5-10 days, maintenance 100-200 µg **IM** qmo
- *Child:* **PO** 30-50 µg qd × 14 days, maintenance 100 µg **IM** qmo or more; **IM/SC** 30-50 µg qd × 14 days, maintenance 100 µg **IM** qmo or more

---

Pernicious anemia/malabsorption syndrome
• *Adult:* **IM** 100-1000 μg qd × 2 wk, then 100-1000 μg **IM** qmo
• *Child:* **IM** 100-500 μg over 2 wk or more given in 100-500 μg doses, then 60 μg **IM/SC** monthly

Schilling test
• *Adult and child:* **IM** 1000 μg in one dose

Available forms: Tabs 25, 50, 100, 250, 500, 1000 μg; inj 100, 120, 1000 μg/ml

Side effects/adverse reactions:
CNS: Flushing, optic nerve atrophy
GI: Diarrhea
CV: **CHF,** peripheral vascular thrombosis, *pulmonary edema*
INTEG: Itching, rash, pain at inj site
META: Hypokalemia
SYST: **Anaphylactic shock**

Contraindications: Hypersensitivity, optic nerve atrophy

Precautions: Pregnancy (A), lactation, children

Pharmacokinetics: Gastric intrinsic factor must be present for absorption to occur; stored in liver, kidneys, stomach; 50%-90% excreted in urine; crosses placenta, excreted in breast milk

Interactions:
• Decreased absorption: aminoglycosides, anticonvulsants, colchicine, chloramphenicol, aminosalicylic acid, K preparation, cimetidine
• Increased absorption: prednisone

Lab test interferences:
False positive: Intrinsic factor

NURSING CONSIDERATIONS
Assess:
• GI function: diarrhea, constipation
• K levels during beginning treatment
• CBC for increase in reticulocyte count during first week of therapy, then increase in RBC and hemoglobin

• Nutritional status: egg yolks, fish, organ meats, dairy products, clams, oysters: good sources of vit B_{12}
• For pulmonary edema, worsening of CHF in cardiac patients

Administer:
• With fruit juice to disguise taste; immediately after mixing
• With meals if possible for better absorption
• By IM inj for pernicious anemia for life unless contraindicated
• IV route not recommended but may be admixed in TPN solution

Additive compatibilities: Ascorbic acid, chloramphenicol, metaraminol, vit B/C

Solution compatibilities: Dextrose/Ringer's or lactated Ringer's combinations, dextrose/saline combinations, D_5W, $D_{10}W$, 0.45% NaCl, Ringer's or lactated Ringer's sol

Y-site compatibilities: Heparin, hydrocortisone, potassium chloride, vit B/C

Perform/provide:
• Protection from light and heat

Evaluate:
• Therapeutic response: decreased anorexia, dyspnea on exertion, palpitations, paresthesias, psychosis, visual disturbances

Teach patient/family:
• That treatment must continue for life for pernicious anemia
• To eat well-balanced diet
• To avoid contact with persons with infection; infections common

Treatment of overdose: Discontinue drug

---

cyclandelate (℞)

(sye-klan′da-late)

Cyclan, Cyclandelate, Cyclospasmol

Func. class.: Peripheral vasodilator

Chem. class.: Nonnitrate

Action: Relaxes vascular smooth muscle, dilates peripheral vascular smooth muscle by direct action

Uses: Intermittent claudication, thrombophlebitis, Raynaud's phenomenon, ischemic cerebrovascular disease, arteriosclerosis obliterans, nocturnal leg cramps

Dosage and routes:

• *Adult:* **PO** 200 mg qid, not to exceed 400 mg qid; maintenance dose 400-800 mg/day in 2-4 divided doses

Available forms: Tabs 200, 400 mg; caps 200, 400 mg

Side effects/adverse reactions:

HEMA: Increased bleeding time (rare)

*CV: **Tachycardia***

CNS: Headache, paresthesias, dizziness, weakness

GI: Heartburn, eructation, nausea, pyrosis

INTEG: Sweating, flushing

Contraindications: Hypersensitivity

Precautions: Glaucoma, pregnancy (C), lactation, recent MI, hypertension, severe obliterative coronary artery or cerebrovascular disease

Pharmacokinetics:

PO: Onset 15 min, peak 1½ hr, duration 4 hr

NURSING CONSIDERATIONS

Assess:

• Bleeding time in individuals with bleeding disorders

• Cardiac status: B/P, pulse, rate, rhythm, character; watch for increasing pulse

Administer:

• With meals for GI symptoms

Perform/provide:

• Storage in air-tight container at room temp

Evaluate:

• Therapeutic response: ability to walk without pain, increased temperature in extremities, increased pulse volume

Teach patient/family:

🚫 Not to break, crush, or chew caps

• That medication is not a cure; it may have to be taken for life

• That it is necessary to quit smoking to prevent excessive vasoconstriction

• That improvement may be sudden but usually occurs gradually over several wk

• To report headache, weakness, increased pulse, as drug may have to be decreased or discontinued

• To avoid hazardous activities until stabilized on medication; dizziness may occur

cyclizine (OTC, ℞)

(sye′kli-zeen)

Marezine

Func. class.: Antiemetic, antihistamine, anticholinergic

Chem. class.: H_2-receptor antagonist, piperazine derivative

Action: Acts centrally by blocking chemoreceptor trigger zone, which in turn acts on vomiting center

Uses: Motion sickness, prevention of postoperative vomiting

Dosage and routes:

Vomiting

• *Adult:* **IM** 25-50 mg ½ hr before termination of surgery, then q4-6h prn (lactate)

• *Child:* **IM** 3 mg/kg divided in 3 equal doses

Motion sickness

• *Adult:* **PO** 50 mg then q4-6h prn, not to exceed 200 mg/day (HCl)

• *Child:* **PO** 25 mg q4-6h prn

Available forms: Tabs 50 mg; inj 50 mg/ml

Side effects/adverse reactions:

CNS: *Drowsiness, dizziness,* vertigo, fatigue, restlessness, headache, insomnia, hallucinations (auditory/visual), hallucinations and *convulsions* in children

GI: Nausea, anorexia

EENT: Dry mouth, blurred vision, tinnitus

Contraindications: Hypersensitivity to cyclizines, shock

Precautions: Children, narrow-angle glaucoma, urinary retention, lactation, prostatic hypertrophy, elderly, pregnancy (B), lactation

Pharmacokinetics:

PO: Duration 4-6 hr; other pharmacokinetics not known

Interactions:

• May increase CNS effect: alcohol, tranquilizers, narcotics

⧸ Increased CNS depression: kava kava

Lab test interferences:

False negative: Allergy skin testing

NURSING CONSIDERATIONS

Assess:

• VS, B/P

• Signs of toxicity of other drugs or masking of symptoms of disease: brain tumor, intestinal obstruction

• Observe for drowsiness/dizziness

Administer:

• IM inj in large muscle mass; aspirate to avoid IV administration

• Tablets may be swallowed whole, chewed, or allowed to dissolve

Evaluate:

• Therapeutic response: absence of motion sickness, vomiting

Teach patient/family:

• That a false-negative result may occur with skin testing; skin testing procedures should not be scheduled for 4 days after discontinuing use

• To avoid hazardous activities or activities requiring alertness; dizziness may occur; instruct patient to request assistance with ambulation

• To avoid alcohol, other depressants

---

cyclobenzaprine (℞)

(sye-kloe-ben′za-preen)
cyclobenzaprine HCl, Cycloflex, Flexeril

Func. class.: Skeletal muscle relaxant, central acting

Chem. class.: Tricyclic amine salt

Action: Unknown; may be related to antidepressant effects

Uses: Adjunct for relief of muscle spasm and pain in musculoskeletal conditions

Dosage and routes:

• *Adult:* **PO** 10 mg tid × 1 wk, not to exceed 60 mg/day × 3 wk

• *Child:* 20-40 mg/kg/day in 2-4 divided doses

Available forms: Tabs 10 mg

Side effects/adverse reactions:

CNS: *Dizziness, weakness, drowsiness,* headache, tremor, depression, insomnia, confusion, paresthesia

EENT: Diplopia, temporary loss of vision

CV: Postural hypotension, tachycardia, *dysrhythmias*

GI: *Nausea,* vomiting, hiccups, dry mouth, constipation

INTEG: Rash, pruritus, fever, facial flushing, sweating

GU: Urinary retention, frequency, change in libido

Contraindications: Acute recovery phase of myocardial infarction,

---

dysrhythmias, heart block, CHF, hypersensitivity, child <12 yr, intermittent porphyria, thyroid disease

Precautions: Renal disease, hepatic disease, addictive personality, pregnancy (B), lactation, elderly

Pharmacokinetics:

PO: Onset 1 hr, peak 3-8 hr, duration 12-24 hr, half-life 1-3 days; metabolized by liver; excreted in urine; crosses placenta; excreted in breast milk

Interactions:

• Decreased effects of guanethidine

• Increased CNS depression: alcohol, tricyclic antidepressants, narcotics, barbiturates, sedatives, hypnotics

• Do not use within 14 days of MAOI

🍴 Increased CNS depression: kava kava

NURSING CONSIDERATIONS
Assess:

• Blood studies: CBC, WBC, differential for blood dyscrasias

• Liver function studies: AST, ALT, alk phosphatase; hepatitis may occur

• ECG in epileptic patients; poor seizure control has occurred

• Allergic reactions: rash, fever, respiratory distress

• Severe weakness, numbness in extremities

• Psychologic dependency: increased need for medication, more frequent requests for medication, increased pain

• CNS depression: dizziness, drowsiness, psychiatric symptoms

Administer:

• With meals for GI symptoms

Perform/provide:

• Storage in tight container at room temp

• Assistance with ambulation if dizziness, drowsiness occur, especially elderly

Evaluate:

• Therapeutic response: decreased pain, spasticity; muscle spasms of acute, painful musculoskeletal conditions generally short term; long-term therapy seldom warranted

Teach patient/family:

• Not to discontinue medication quickly; insomnia, nausea, headache, spasticity, tachycardia will occur; drug should be tapered off over 1-2 wk

• Not to take with alcohol, other CNS depressants

• To avoid hazardous activities if drowsiness/dizziness occurs

• To avoid using OTC medication: cough preparations, antihistamines, unless directed by prescriber

• To use gum, frequent sips of water for dry mouth

Treatment of overdose: Empty stomach with emesis, gastric lavage, then administer activated charcoal; use anticonvulsants if indicated; monitor cardiac function

---

cyclophosphamide (℞)

(sye-kloe-foss'fa-mide)

Cytoxan, Neosar, Procytox*

Func. class.: Antineoplastic alkylating agent

Chem. class.: Nitrogen mustard

Action: Alkylates DNA, RNA; inhibits enzymes that allow synthesis of amino acids in proteins; is also responsible for cross-linking DNA strands; activity is not cell cycle phase specific

Uses: Hodgkin's disease; lymphomas; leukemia; cancer of female reproductive tract, lung, prostate; multiple myeloma; neuroblastoma; retinoblastoma; Ewing's sarcoma

Dosage and routes:
Renal disease
• CrCl 25-50 ml/min 50% of dose; CrCl <25 ml/min avoid use
• *Adult:* **PO** initially 1-5 mg/kg over 2-5 days, maintenance is 1-5 mg/kg; **IV** initially 40-50 mg/kg in divided doses over 2-5 days, maintenance 10-15 mg/kg q7-10d, or 3-5 mg/kg q3d
• *Child:* **PO/IV** 2-8 mg/kg or 60-250 mg/m² in divided doses for 6 or more days; maintenance 10-15 mg/kg q7-10d or 30 mg/kg q3-4wk; dose should be reduced by half when bone marrow depression occurs

Available forms: Inj 100, 200, 500 mg, 1, 2 g; tabs 25, 50 mg

Side effects/adverse reactions:
CV: **Cardiotoxicity** (high doses)
HEMA: **Thrombocytopenia, leukopenia, pancytopenia; myelosuppression**
GI: *Nausea, vomiting, diarrhea, weight loss, colitis, **hepatotoxicity***
GU: **Hemorrhagic cystitis,** *hematuria, neoplasms, amenorrhea, azoospermia, sterility, ovarian fibrosis*
INTEG: *Alopecia,* dermatitis
RESP: **Fibrosis**
ENDO: Syndrome of inappropriate antidiuretic hormone (SIADH)
CNS: Headache, dizziness

Contraindications: Lactation, pregnancy (D)
Precautions: Radiation therapy
Pharmacokinetics: Metabolized by liver; excreted in urine; half-life 4-6½ hr; 50% bound to plasma proteins
Interactions:
• Increased toxicity: aminoglycosides
• Increased metabolism of cyclophosphamide: phenobarbital
• Potentiation of cyclophosphamide: succinylcholine
• Increased bone marrow depression: allopurinol, thiazides
• Decreased digoxin levels: digoxin

Lab test interferences:
Increase: Uric acid
False positive: Pap test
False negative: PPD, mumps, trichophytin, *Candida*
Decrease: Pseudocholinesterase

NURSING CONSIDERATIONS
Assess:
• CBC, differential, platelet count weekly; withhold drug if WBC is <4000 or platelet count is <75,000; notify prescriber of results
• Pulmonary function tests, chest x-ray films before, during therapy; chest film should be obtained q2wk during treatment
• Renal function studies: BUN, serum uric acid, urine CrCl before, during therapy
• I&O ratio; report fall in urine output of <30 ml/hr
• Monitor temp q4h (may indicate beginning infection)
• Liver function tests before, during therapy (bilirubin, AST [SGOT], ALT [SGPT], LDH) as needed or monthly
• Bleeding: hematuria, guaiac, bruising or petechiae, mucosa or orifices q8h
• Dyspnea, rales, unproductive cough, chest pain, tachypnea
• Food preferences; list likes, dislikes
• Effects of alopecia on body image, discuss feelings about body changes
• Yellowing of skin, sclera; dark urine; clay-colored stools; itchy skin; abdominal pain; fever; diarrhea
• Edema in feet, joint pain, stomach pain, shaking
• Inflammation of mucosa, breaks in skin
• Buccal cavity q8h for dryness, sores or ulceration, white patches,

 = Nursing alert   = Herb-drug interaction   = Do not crush

oral pain, bleeding, dysphagia; obtain prescription for viscous lidocaine (Xylocaine)

◆ Symptoms indicating severe allergic reaction: rash, pruritus, urticaria, purpuric skin lesions, itching, flushing

• Tachypnea, ECG changes, dyspnea, edema, fatigue

Administer:

• Topical or systemic analgesics for pain

• Local or systemic drugs for infection

• In AM so drug can be eliminated before hs

• Fluids IV or PO before chemotherapy to hydrate patient

• Antacid before oral agent, give after evening meal, before bedtime

• Antiemetic 30-60 min before giving drug and prn

• Allopurinol or sodium bicarbonate to maintain uric acid levels, alkalinization of urine

• Prevent hyperuricemia

• Antibiotics for prophylaxis of infection

IV

• IV after diluting 100 mg/5 ml of sterile H_2O or bacteriostatic H_2O; shake; let stand until clear; may be further diluted in up to 250 ml D_5 or NS; give 100 mg or less/min through 3-way stopcock of glucose or saline inf

• Using 21, 23, 25G needle; check site for irritation, phlebitis

Additive compatibilities: Cisplatin with etoposide, fluorouracil, hydroxyzine, methotrexate, methotrexate/fluorouracil, mitoxantrone, ondansetron

Solution compatibilities: Amino acids 4.25%/D_{25}, D_5/0.9% NaCl, D_5W, 0.9% NaCl

Syringe compatibilities: Bleomycin, cisplatin, doxapram, doxorubicin, droperidol, fluorouracil, furosemide, heparin, leucovorin, methotrexate, metoclopramide, mitomycin, vinblastine, vincristine

Y-site compatibilities: Allopurinol, amifostine, amikacin, ampicillin, azlocillin, aztreonam, bleomycin, cefamandole, cefazolin, cefepime, cefoperazone, cefotaxime, cefoxitin, cefuroxime, cephalothin, cephapirin, chloramphenicol, chlorpromazine, cimetidine, cisplatin, cladribine, clindamycin, dexamethasone, diphenhydramine, doxorubicin, doxycycline, droperidol, erythromycin, famotidine, filgrastim, fludarabine, fluorouracil, furosemide, gallium, ganciclovir, gentamicin, granisetron, heparin, hydromorphone, idarubicin, kanamycin, leucovorin, lorazepam, melphalan, methotrexate, methylprednisolone, metoclopramide, metronidazole, mezlocillin, minocycline, mitomycin, morphine, moxalactam, nafcillin, ondansetron, oxacillin, paclitaxel, penicillin G potassium, piperacillin, piperacillin/tazobactam, prochlorperazine, promethazine, propofol, ranitidine, sargramostim, sodium bicarbonate, teniposide, thiotepa, ticarcillin, ticarcillin-clavulanate, tobramycin, trimethoprim-sulfamethoxazole, vancomycin, vinblastine, vincristine, vinorelbine

Perform/provide:

• Storage in tight container at room temperature

• Strict medical asepsis, protective isolation if WBC levels are low

• Special skin care

• Deep-breathing exercises with patient tid-qid; place in semi-Fowler's position

• Increase fluid intake to 2-3 L/day to prevent urate deposits, calculi formation, reduce incidence of hemorrhagic cystitis

- Diet low in purines: organ meats (kidney, liver), dried beans, peas to maintain alkaline urine
- Rinsing of mouth tid-qid with water, club soda; brushing of teeth bid-tid with soft brush or cotton-tipped applicators for stomatitis; use unwaxed dental floss
- Warm compresses at injection site for inflammation

Evaluate:
- Therapeutic response: decreased tumor size, spread of malignancy

Teach patient/family:
- About protective isolation
- That amenorrhea can occur; reversible after stopping treatment
- To report any changes in breathing or coughing
- That hair may be lost during treatment; a wig or hairpiece may make patient feel better; new hair may be different in color, texture
- To avoid foods with citric acid, hot or rough texture
- To report any bleeding, white spots, ulcerations in mouth to prescriber; tell patient to examine mouth qd
- To report signs of infection: increased temperature, sore throat, flu symptoms
- To report signs of anemia: fatigue, headache, faintness, shortness of breath, irritability
- To report bleeding: avoid use of razors, commercial mouthwash
- To avoid use of aspirin products, ibuprofen

---

cycloserine (℞)

(sye-kloe-ser'een)
Seromycin Pulvules
Func. class.: Antitubercular
Chem. class.: *S. orchidaceus,* antibiotic

Action: Inhibits cell wall synthesis, analog of D-alanine

Uses: Pulmonary tuberculosis, extrapulmonary as adjunctive

Dosage and routes:
- *Adult:* **PO** 250 mg q12h × 14 days, then 250 mg q8h × 2 wk if no signs of toxicity, then 250 mg q6h if no signs of toxicity, not to exceed 1 g/day
- *Child:* **PO** 10-20 mg/kg/day (max 0.75-1 g) in 2 divided doses

Available forms: Caps 250 mg

Side effects/adverse reactions:
INTEG: Dermatitis, photosensitivity
CV: **CHF,** dysrhythmias
CNS: Headache, anxiety, drowsiness, tremors, ***convulsions,*** lethargy, depression, confusion, psychosis, aggression
HEMA: ***Megaloblastic anemia,*** vit B_{12}, folic acid deficiency, leukocytosis

Contraindications: Hypersensitivity

Precautions: Pregnancy (C), children, seizure disorders, renal disease, alcoholism (chronic), depression, severe anxiety, lactation, anemia

Pharmacokinetics:
PO: Peak 3-8 hr; excreted unchanged in urine; crosses placenta; excreted in breast milk

Interactions:
- Seizures: alcohol
- May increase CNS toxicity: isoniazid, ethionamide

Lab test interferences:
Increase: AST/ALT

 = Nursing alert   = Herb-drug interaction   🚫 = Do not crush

NURSING CONSIDERATIONS
Assess:
- Liver studies qwk: ALT, AST, bilirubin
- CBC
- Renal studies: BUN, creatinine, I&O
- Hepatic status: fatigue, jaundice, dark urine, decreased appetite
- Blood levels of drug; keep <30 µg/ml or toxicity may occur
- Mental status often: affect, mood, behavioral changes, psychosis may occur

Administer:
- Using pipette provided; use glass container to prevent adherence to sides
- After C&S is completed, qmo to detect resistance
- Pyridoxine (200-300 mg/day) if ordered to prevent neurotoxicity

Perform/provide:
- Storage in air-tight container at room temp

Evaluate:
- Therapeutic response: decreased symptoms of TB

Teach patient/family:
- 🚫 Not to break, crush, or chew caps
- To avoid alcohol while taking drug
- That compliance with dosage schedule, length is necessary
- ➦ To report neurotoxicity: confusion, headache, drowsiness, tremors, paresthesias, mental changes
- To avoid hazardous activities if drowsiness or dizziness occurs

Treatment of overdose: Administer vit B_6, anticonvulsants, lavage, O_2, assisted respiration

cyclosporine (℞)
(sye'kloe-spor-een)
Neoral, Sandimmune
Func. class.: Immunosuppressant
Chem. class.: Fungus-derived peptide

Action: Produces immunosuppression by inhibiting lymphocytes (T)

Uses: Organ transplants to prevent rejection

Dosage and routes:
- *Adult and child:* **PO** 15 mg/kg several hr before surgery, daily for 2 wk, reduce dosage by 2.5 mg/kg/wk to 5-10 mg/kg/day; **IV** 5-6 mg/kg several hr before surgery, daily, switch to PO form as soon as possible

Available forms: Oral sol 100 mg/ml; inj 50 mg/ml; soft gelatin caps 25, 100 mg

Side effects/adverse reactions:
GI: Nausea, vomiting, diarrhea, *oral Candida, gum hyperplasia,* **hepatotoxicity,** pancreatitis
INTEG: Rash, acne, *hirsutism*
CNS: Tremors, headache
GU: **Albuminuria, hematuria, proteinuria, renal failure**

Contraindications: Hypersensitivity

Precautions: Severe renal disease, severe hepatic disease, pregnancy (C)

Pharmacokinetics: Peak 4 hr, highly protein bound, half-life (biphasic) 1.2 hr, 25 hr; metabolized in liver; excreted in feces; crosses placenta; excreted in breast milk

Interactions:
- Increased action of cyclosporine: amphotericin B, cimetidine, ketoconazole
- Decreased action of cyclosporine: phenytoin, rifampin

NURSING CONSIDERATIONS

Assess:

- Renal studies: BUN, creatinine at least monthly during treatment, 3 mo after treatment
- Liver function studies: alk phosphatase, AST, ALT, bilirubin
- Drug blood level during treatment
- Hepatotoxicity: dark urine, jaundice, itching, light-colored stools; drug should be discontinued

Administer:

- For several days before transplant surgery
- With corticosteroids
- With meals for GI upset or in chocolate milk
- With oral antifungal for *Candida* infections

IV

- After diluting each 50 mg/20-100 ml of NS or D_5W; run over 2-6 hr; use an infusion pump, glass inf bottles only

Additive compatibilities: Ciprofloxacin

Solution compatibilities: D_5W, NaCl 0.9%

Y-site compatibilities: Cefmetazole, propofol, sargramostim

Evaluate:

- Therapeutic response: absence of rejection

Teach patient/family:

- To report fever, chills, sore throat, fatigue, since serious infections may occur
- To use contraceptive measures during treatment, for 12 wk after ending therapy

🚫 Not to break, crush, or chew caps

---

cyproheptadine (℞)

(si-proe-hep′ta-deen)
cyproheptadine HCl, Periactin
Func. class.: Antihistamine, H_1-receptor antagonist
Chem. class.: Piperidine

Action: Acts on blood vessels, GI, respiratory system by competing with histamine for H_1-receptor site; decreases allergic response by blocking histamine

Uses: Allergy symptoms, rhinitis, pruritus, cold urticaria

Investigational uses: Appetite stimulant, management of vascular headache

Dosage and routes:

- *Adult:* **PO** 4 mg tid-qid, not to exceed 0.5 mg/kg/day
- *Child 7-14 yr:* **PO** 4 mg bid-tid, not to exceed 16 mg/day
- *Child 2-6 yr:* **PO** 2 mg bid-tid, not to exceed 12 mg/day

Available forms: Tabs 4 mg; syr 2 mg/5 ml

Side effects/adverse reactions:

CNS: Dizziness, drowsiness, poor coordination, fatigue, anxiety, euphoria, confusion, paresthesia, neuritis

CV: Hypotension, palpitations, tachycardia

RESP: Increased thick secretions, wheezing, chest tightness

GI: Constipation, dry mouth, nausea, vomiting, anorexia, diarrhea, weight gain

INTEG: Rash, urticaria, photosensitivity

GU: Retention, dysuria, frequency, increased appetite

EENT: Blurred vision, dilated pupils; tinnitus; nasal stuffiness; dry nose, throat, mouth

Contraindications: Hypersensitivity to H_1-receptor antagonist, acute

---

asthma attack, lower respiratory tract disease

Precautions: Increased intraocular pressure, renal disease, cardiac disease, hypertension, bronchial asthma, seizure disorder, stenosed peptic ulcers, hyperthyroidism, prostatic hypertrophy, bladder neck obstruction, pregnancy (B), lactation, elderly

Pharmacokinetics:
PO: Duration 4-6 hr; metabolized in liver; excreted by kidneys; excreted in breast milk

Interactions:
• Increased CNS depression: barbiturates, narcotics, hypnotics, tricyclic antidepressants, alcohol
• Decreased effect of oral anticoagulants, heparin
• Increased effect of cyproheptadine: MAOIs
🌿 Increased CNS depression: kava kava
🌿 Increased anticholinergic effect: henbane leaf

Lab test interferences:
False negative: Skin allergy tests

NURSING CONSIDERATIONS
Assess:
• I&O ratio; be alert for urinary retention, frequency, dysuria; drug should be discontinued
• CBC during long-term therapy
• Respiratory status: rate, rhythm, increase in bronchial secretions, wheezing, chest tightness
• Cardiac status: palpitations, increased pulse, hypotension

Administer:
• With meals for GI symptoms; absorption may slightly decrease

Perform/provide:
• Hard candy, gum, frequent rinsing of mouth for dryness
• Storage in air-tight container at room temp

Evaluate:
• Therapeutic response: absence of running or congested nose, rashes

Teach patient/family:
• All aspects of drug use; to notify prescriber of confusion, sedation, hypotension
• That this drug decreases anticoagulant (oral) effect
• To avoid driving, other hazardous activity if drowsiness occurs, especially elderly
• To avoid concurrent use of alcohol, other CNS depressants

Treatment of overdose: Ipecac syrup or lavage, diazepam, vasopressors, barbiturates (short-acting)

cytarabine (℞)
(sye tare'a-been)
Ara-C, Cytosar*, Cytosar-U, cytosine arabinoside

Func. class.: Antineoplastic, antimetabolite
Chem. class.: Pyrimidine nucleoside

Action: Competes with physiologic substrate of DNA synthesis, thus interfering with cell replication in the S phase of the cell cycle (before mitosis)

Uses: Acute myelocytic leukemia, acute lymphocytic leukemia, chronic myelocytic leukemia, and in combination for non-Hodgkin's lymphomas in children

Dosage and routes:
Acute myelocytic leukemia
• *Adult:* IV INF 200 mg/m^2/day × 5 days; **INTRATHECAL** 5-50 mg/m^2/day × 3 days/wk or 30 mg/m^2/day q4d

In combination
• *Child:* IV INF 100 mg/m^2/day × 5-10 days

Available forms: Inj, intrathecal 100, 500 mg, 1, 2 g

Side effects/adverse reactions:
HEMA: *Thrombophlebitis, bleeding, thrombocytopenia, leukopenia, myelosuppression, anemia*
GI: *Nausea, vomiting, anorexia, diarrhea, stomatitis,* *hepatotoxicity,* abdominal pain, hematemesis, *GI hemorrhage*
EENT: Sore throat, conjunctivitis
GU: Urinary retention, *renal failure, hyperuricemia*
INTEG: *Rash, fever,* freckling, cellulitis
RESP: *Pneumonia,* dyspnea
CV: Chest pain, *cardiopathy*
CNS: Neuritis, dizziness, headache, personality changes, ataxia, mechanical dysphasia, *coma*
CYTARABINE SYNDROME: *Fever,* myalgia, bone pain, chest pain, *rash,* conjunctivitis, malaise (6-12 hr after administration)

Contraindications: Hypersensitivity, infants, pregnancy (1st trimester)

Precautions: Renal disease, hepatic disease, pregnancy (C), lactation

Pharmacokinetics:
INTRATHECAL: Half-life 2 hr; metabolized in liver; excreted in urine (primarily inactive metabolite); crosses blood-brain barrier, placenta
IV: Distribution half-life 10 min, elimination half-life 1-3 hr

Interactions:
• Increased toxicity: radiation or other antineoplastics
• Decreased effects of oral digoxin

NURSING CONSIDERATIONS
Assess:
• CBC (RBC, Hct, Hgb), differential, platelet count weekly; withhold drug if WBC is <4000/mm³, platelet count is <75,000/mm³, or RBC, Hct, Hgb low; notify prescriber of these results
• Renal function studies: BUN, serum uric acid, urine creatinine clearance, electrolytes before and during therapy
• I&O ratio; report fall in urine output to <30 ml/hr
• Monitor temp q4h; fever may indicate beginning infection; no rectal temperatures
• Liver function tests before and during therapy: bilirubin, ALT (SGOT), AST (SGPT), alk phosphatase, as needed or monthly
• Blood uric acid during therapy
◆ Cytarabine syndrome 6-12hr after inf: fever, myalgia, bone pain, chest pain, rash, conjunctivitis, malaise; corticosteroids may be ordered
• Bleeding: hematuria, heme-positive stools, bruising or petechiae, mucosa or orifices q8h
• Dyspnea, rales, unproductive cough, chest pain, tachypnea, fatigue, increased pulse, pallor, lethargy; personality changes, with high doses
• Food preferences; list likes, dislikes
• Edema in feet, joint pain, stomach pain, shaking
• Inflammation of mucosa, breaks in skin
• Yellowing of skin, sclera; dark urine; clay-colored stools; itchy skin; abdominal pain; fever; diarrhea
• Buccal cavity q8h for dryness, sores or ulceration, white patches, oral pain, bleeding, dysphagia
• Local irritation, pain, burning, discoloration at injection site
• GI symptoms: frequency of stools, cramping
• Acidosis, signs of dehydration: rapid respirations, poor skin turgor, decreased urine output, dry skin, restlessness, weakness

Administer:
• Antiemetic 30-60 min before giving drug and prn

• Allopurinol or sodium bicarbonate to maintain uric acid levels and alkalinization of the urine
• Topical or systemic analgesics for pain
• Transfusion for anemia
• Antispasmodic for GI symptoms
IV
• After diluting 100 mg/5 ml of sterile H_2O for inj; given by direct IV over 1-3 min through free-flowing tubing (IV); may be further diluted in 50-100 ml NS or D_5W, given over 30 min to 24 hr depending on dose
Additive compatibilities: Corticotropin, daunorubicin with etoposide, etoposide, hydroxyzine, lincomycin, mitoxantrone, ondansetron, potassium chloride, prednisolone, sodium bicarbonate, vincristine
Solution compatibilities: Amino acids, D_3/I R, $D_5/0.2\%$ NaCl, $D_5/0.9\%$ NaCl, $D_{10}/0.9\%$ NaCl, D_5W, invert sugar 10% in electrolyte #1, Ringer's LR, 0.9% NaCl, sodium lactate ⅙ mol/L, TPN #57
Syringe compatibilities: Metoclopramide
Y-site compatibilities: Amifostine, amsacrine, aztreonam, cefepime, chlorpromazine, cimetidine, cladribine, dexamethasone, diphenhydramine, droperidol, famitodine, filgrastim, fludarabine, gentamicin, granisetron, heparin, hydrocortisone, hydromorphone, idarubicin, lorazepam, melphalan, methotrexate, methylprednisolone, metoclopramide, morphine, ondansetron, paclitaxel, piperacillin/tazobactam, prochlorperazine, promethazine, propofol, ranitidine, sargramostim, sodium bicarbonate, teniposide, thiotepa, vinorelbine
Perform/provide:
• Strict medical asepsis and protective isolation if WBC levels are low

• Increase fluid intake to 2-3 L/day to prevent urate deposits and calculi formation, unless contraindicated
• Diet low in purines: absence of organ meats (kidney, liver), dried beans, peas to prevent increased urate deposits
• Rinsing of mouth tid-qid with water, club soda; brushing of teeth bid-tid with soft brush or cotton-tipped applicators for stomatitis; use unwaxed dental floss
• HOB raised to facilitate breathing if dyspnea or pneumonia
Evaluate:
• Therapeutic response: decreased tumor size, spread of malignancy
Teach patient/family:
• Why protective isolation is necessary
• To report any coughing, chest pain, changes in breathing; may indicate beginning pneumonia
• To avoid foods with citric acid, hot or rough texture if stomatitis is present
• To report stomatitis: any bleeding, white spots, ulcerations in mouth; tell patient to examine mouth qd, report any symptoms
• To report signs of infection: increased temperature, sore throat, flu symptoms
• To report signs of anemia: fatigue, headache, faintness, shortness of breath, irritability
• To report bleeding; avoid use of razors, commercial mouthwash
• To avoid use of aspirin products or ibuprofen

dacarbazine (R)

(da-kar′ba-zeen)
DTIC-Dome
Func. class.: Antineoplastic alkylating agent
Chem. class.: Cytotoxic triazine

Action: Alkylates DNA, RNA; inhibits enzymes that allow synthesis of amino acids in proteins; also responsible for cross-linking DNA strands; activity is not cell cycle phase specific

Uses: Hodgkin's disease, sarcomas, neuroblastoma, malignant melanoma

Dosage and routes:
• *Adult:* **IV** 2-4.5 mg/kg or 250 mg/m^2 qd × 5 days; repeat q3wk depending on response

Available forms: Inj 100, 200 mg

Side effects/adverse reactions:
*HEMA: **Thrombocytopenia, leukopenia,** anemia*
*GI: Nausea, anorexia, vomiting, **hepatotoxicity***
CNS: Facial paresthesia, flushing, fever, malaise
INTEG: Alopecia, dermatitis, pain at injection site

Contraindications: Lactation
Precautions: Radiation therapy, pregnancy (1st trimester) (C)
Pharmacokinetics: Metabolized by liver; excreted in urine; half-life 35 min, terminal 5 hr, 5% protein bound

Interactions:
• Decreased effectiveness of dacarbazine: phenytoin, phenobarbital

NURSING CONSIDERATIONS
Assess:
• CBC, differential, platelet count weekly; withhold drug if WBC <4000 or platelet count <75,000; notify prescriber of results

• Monitor temp q4h (may indicate beginning infection)
• Liver function tests before, during therapy (bilirubin, AST, ALT, LDH) as needed or monthly
• Bleeding: hematuria, guaiac, bruising or petechiae, mucosa or orifices q8h
• Food preferences; list likes, dislikes
• Effects of alopecia on body image, discuss feelings about body changes
• Yellowing of skin, sclera; dark urine; clay-colored stools; itchy skin; abdominal pain; fever; diarrhea
• Inflammation of mucosa, breaks in skin

Administer:
• Antiemetic 30-60 min before giving drug to prevent vomiting
• Antibiotics for prophylaxis of infection
IV
• After diluting 100 mg/9.9 ml of sterile H$_2$O for inj (10 mg/ml), give by direct IV over 1 min through Y-tube or 3-way stopcock; may be further diluted in 50-250 ml D$_5$W or NS for inj, given as an inf over ½ hr
• Watch for extravasation; give Na thiosulfate 10% 4 ml plus sterile H$_2$O 5 ml, 3-5 ml SC if needed

Additive compatibilities: Bleomycin, carmustine, cyclophosphamide, cytarabine, dactinomycin, doxorubicin, fluorouracil, mercaptopurine, methotrexate, ondansetron, vinblastine

Additive incompatibilities: Hydrocortisone sodium succinate, cysteine

Y-site compatibilities: Amifostine, aztreonam, filgrastim, fludarabine, granisetron, melphalan, ondansetron, paclitaxel, sargramostim, teniposide, thiotepa, vinorelbine

Perform/provide:

• Storage in light-resistant container, dry area

• Strict medical asepsis, protective isolation if WBC levels are low

• Increase fluid intake to 2-3 L/day to prevent urate deposits, calculi formation

• Warm compresses at infusion site for inflammation

Evaluate:

• Therapeutic response: decreased tumor size, spread of malignancy

Teach patient/family:

• About protective isolation

• That patient should avoid prolonged exposure to sun

• That hair may be lost during treatment; a wig or hairpiece may make the patient feel better; new hair may be different in color, texture

• To report signs of infection: fever, sore throat, flu symptoms

• To report signs of anemia: fatigue, headache, faintness, shortness of breath, irritability

• To report bleeding; avoid use of razors, commercial mouthwash

• To avoid use of aspirin products or ibuprofen

---

dactinomycin (℞)

(dak-ti-noe myc'sin)

Cosmegen

Func. class.: Antineoplastic, antibiotic

Action: Inhibits DNA, RNA, protein synthesis; derived from *S. parvullus;* replication is decreased by binding to DNA, which causes strand splitting; cell cycle nonspecific; a vesicant

Uses: Sarcomas, melanomas, trophoblastic tumors in women, testicular cancer, Wilms' tumor, rhabdomyosarcoma

Dosage and routes:

• *Adult:* IV 500 µg/m²/day × 5 days; stop drug for 2-4 wk; then repeat cycle

• *Child:* IV 15 µg/kg/day × 5 days, not to exceed 500 µg/day; stop drug until bone marrow recovery, then repeat cycle

Available forms: Inj 0.5 mg/vial

Side effects/adverse reactions:

HEMA: **Thrombocytopenia, leukopenia, aplastic anemia**

GI: Nausea, vomiting, anorexia, stomatitis, *hepatotoxicity,* abdominal pain, diarrhea

INTEG: Rash, alopecia, pain at injection site, folliculitis, acne, desquamation, *extravasation*

EENT: Chelitis, dysphagia, esophagitis

CNS: Malaise, fatigue, lethargy, fever

MS: Myalgia

Contraindications: Hypersensitivity, herpes infection, child <6 mo

Precautions: Renal disease, hepatic disease, pregnancy (C), lactation, bone marrow depression

Pharmacokinetics: Half-life 36 hr; IV onset 2-5 min; concentrates in kidneys, liver, spleen; does not cross blood-brain barrier; excreted in feces and urine

Interactions:

• Increased toxicity: other antineoplastics, radiation

Lab test interferences:

Increase: Uric acid

NURSING CONSIDERATIONS

Assess:

• CBC, differential, platelet count weekly; withhold drug if WBC is <4000/mm³ or platelet count is <75,000/mm³; notify prescriber

• Renal function studies: BUN, serum uric acid, urine CrCl, electrolytes before, during therapy

• I&O ratio; report fall in urine output to <30 ml/hr

- Monitor temp q4h; fever may indicate beginning infection
- Liver function tests before, during therapy: bilirubin, AST, ALT, alk phosphatase, as needed or monthly
- Bleeding: hematuria, guaiac stools, bruising, petechiae, mucosa or orifices q8h
- Food preferences; list likes, dislikes
- Effects of alopecia on body image; discuss feelings about body changes
- Inflammation of mucosa, breaks in skin
- Yellowing of skin, sclera; dark urine; clay-colored stools; itchy skin; abdominal pain; fever; diarrhea
- Buccal cavity q8h for dryness, sores, ulceration, white patches, oral pain, bleeding, dysphagia
- Local irritation, pain, burning at injection site
- ⬥ Symptoms indicating severe allergic reaction: rash, pruritus, urticaria, purpuric skin lesions, itching, flushing
- GI symptoms: frequency of stools, cramping, nausea, vomiting, anorexia
- Acidosis, signs of dehydration: rapid respirations, poor skin turgor, decreased urine output, dry skin, restlessness, weakness, sunken eyeball in children

Administer:
- Antiemetic 30-60 min before giving drug to prevent vomiting
- Topical or systemic analgesics for pain
- Local or systemic drugs for infection
- Antispasmodic for GI symptoms: cramping, diarrhea, nausea, vomiting

IV
- After diluting 0.5 mg/1.1 ml of sterile H_2O for inj without preservative; use 2.2 ml (0.25 mg/ml),

give by direct IV at 0.5 mg or less/min through Y-tube or 3-way stopcock if inf in progress; may be further diluted if required in 50 ml D_5W or NS for infusion; run over 10-15 min; change needles between reconstitution and direct IV administration
- Hydrocortisone, sodium thiosulfate to infiltration area, and ice compress after stopping infusion

Y-site compatibilities: Allopurinol, amifostine, aztreonam, cefepime, fludarabine, granisetron, melphalan, ondansetron, sargramostim, teniposide, thiotepa, vinorelbine

Perform/provide:
- Strict hand-washing technique, gloves and protective covering
- Liquid diet: carbonated beverages; gelatin may be added if patient is not nauseated or vomiting
- Rinsing of mouth tid-qid with water, club soda; brushing of teeth bid-qid with soft brush or cotton-tipped applicators for stomatitis; use unwaxed dental floss to prevent injury
- Storage in cool, dark environment; do not expose to bright light or freeze

Evaluate:
- Therapeutic response: decreased tumor size, spread of malignancy

Teach patient/family:
- That contraception is needed during treatment and for 4-6 mo after discontinuing therapy
- To avoid vaccinations without order by prescriber
- That hair may be lost during treatment after 1-2 wk and that wig or hairpiece may make patient feel better; that new hair may be different in color, texture
- To avoid foods with citric acid, hot or rough texture when stomatitis is present
- To report any bleeding, white spots,

⬥ = Nursing alert   ⫸ = Herb-drug interaction   ⊘ = Do not crush

ulcerations in mouth to prescriber; tell patient to examine mouth qd
• To avoid crowds, persons with known infection when granulocyte count is low

---

dalteparin (R)

(dahl'ta-pear-in)
Fragmin
Func. class.: Anticoagulant
Chem. class.: Low molecular weight heparin

Action: Prevents conversion of fibrinogen to fibrin and prothrombin to thrombin by enhancing inhibitory effects of antithrombin III
Uses: Prevention of deep vein thrombosis in abdominal surgery patients
Dosage and routes:
• *Adult:* SC 2500 IU each day starting 1-2 hr prior to surgery and repeat qd × 5-10 days postoperatively; to be used SC only
Available forms: Prefilled syringes, 2500 antifactor-Xa IU/0.2 ml
Side effects/adverse reactions:
CNS: Intracranial bleeding
SYST: Hypersensitivity, *hemorrhage, anaphylaxis* possible
HEMA: Thrombocytopenia
INTEG: Pruritus, superficial wound infection
Contraindications: Hypersensitivity to this drug, heparin, or other anticoagulants; hemophilia, leukemia with bleeding, thrombocytopenic purpura, cerebrovascular hemorrhage, cerebral aneurysm, severe hypertension, other severe cardiac disease
Precautions: Elderly, pregnancy (B), hepatic disease, severe renal disease, blood dyscrasias, subacute bacterial endocarditis, acute nephritis, lactation, child, recent childbirth, peptic ulcer disease, pericarditis, pericardial effusion, recent lumbar puncture, vasculitis, other diseases where bleeding is possible
Pharmacokinetics: Excreted by kidneys, half-life 2 hr, peak 4 hr onset and duration unknown
Interactions:
• Increased risk of bleeding: aspirin, oral anticoagulants, platelet inhibitors
🍃 Possible increased risk of bleeding: bromelain, cinchona bark
NURSING CONSIDERATIONS
Assess:
• For blood studies (Hct, occult blood in stools) during treatment since bleeding can occur
◆ For bleeding gums, petechiae, ecchymosis, black tarry stools, hematuria, epistaxis, decrease in Hct, B/P; may indicate bleeding, possible hemorrhage; notify prescriber immediately, drug should be discontinued
• For hypersensitivity: fever, skin rash, urticaria; notify prescriber immediately
• For needed dosage change q1-2wk; dose may need to be decreased if bleeding occurs
Administer:
• Do not give IM or IV drug route; approved is SC only
• By SC only; have patient sit or lie down; SC inj may be 2 in from umbilicus in a U-shape, upper outer side of thigh or upper outer quadrangle of the buttocks; rotate inj sites
• Changing needles is not recommended
Evaluate:
• Therapeutic response: absence of deep-vein thrombosis
Teach patient/family:
• To avoid OTC preparations that contain aspirin; other anticoagulants, serious drug interaction may occur
• To use soft-bristle toothbrush to avoid bleeding gums, avoid contact

sports, use electric razor, avoid IM injection

• To report any signs of bleeding: gums, under skin, urine, stools; unusual bruising

Treatment of overdose: Protamine sulfate 1% given IV; 1 mg protamine/ 100 anti-Xa IU of dalteparin given

---

danaparoid (℞)

(dan-a-pair′oid)
Orgaran
Func. class.: Anticoagulant
Chem. class.: Low molecular weight heparin

Action: Prevents conversion of fibrinogen to fibrin and prothrombin to thrombin by enhancing inhibitory effects of antithrombin III

Uses: Prevention of vein thrombosis in hemodialysis, stroke, elective surgery for malignancy or total hip replacement, hip fracture surgery

Dosage and routes:

Prevention of venous thrombosis/ elective surgery

• *Adult:* SC 750 anti-Xa units bid × 7-10 days

Hip fracture surgery

• *Adult:* SC 750 anti-Xa units bid until postoperative days 10-12 has been effective

Hemodialysis

• *Adult:* SC 2400-4800 anti-Xa units given predialysis

Available forms: Inj 2500/5000 anti-Xa units/0.2 ml

Side effects/adverse reactions:

SYST: Hypersensitivity, *hemorrhage*

HEMA: **Thrombocytopenia**

INTEG: Rash

Contraindications: Hypersensitivity to this drug, sulfites, pork; hemophilia, leukemia with bleeding, thrombocytopenia, purpura, cerebrovascular hemorrhage, cerebral aneurysm, severe hypertension, other severe cardiac disease

Precautions: Hypersensitivity to heparin, elderly, pregnancy (C), hepatic disease, severe renal disease, blood dyscrasias, subacute bacterial endocarditis, acute nephritis, lactation, child, recent childbirth, peptic ulcer disease, pericarditis, pericardial effusion, recent lumbar puncture, vasculitis, other diseases where bleeding is possible

Pharmacokinetics: Excreted by kidneys, half-life 2-3 hr, peak 4 hr

Interactions:

• Increased risk of bleeding: aspirin, oral anticoagulants, platelet inhibitors

 Increased risk of bleeding: bromelain, cinchona bark

NURSING CONSIDERATIONS

Assess:

• For blood studies (Hct, occult blood in stools) during treatment since bleeding can occur; aPTT, ACT, antifactor Xa test, platelets

• For bleeding gums, petechiae, ecchymosis, black tarry stools, hematuria, epistaxis, decrease in Hct, B/P; may indicate bleeding, possible hemorrhage; notify prescriber immediately, drug should be discontinued

• For hypersensitivity: fever, skin, rash, urticaria; notify prescriber immediately

• For needed dosage change q1-2wk; dose may need to be decreased if bleeding occurs

Administer:

• By SC, have patient sit or lie down; SC inj may be around the navel in a U-shape, upper outer side of thigh or upper outer quadrangle of the buttocks; rotate inj sites

• Changing needles is not recommended

Evaluate:
• Therapeutic response: absence of deep-vein thrombosis

Teach patient/family:
• To avoid OTC preparations that may cause serious drug interactions unless directed by prescriber; may contain aspirin, other anticoagulants
• To use soft bristle toothbrush to avoid bleeding gums, avoid contact sports, use electric razor, avoid IM injection
• To report any signs of bleeding: gums, under skin, urine, stools; unusual bruising

Treatment of overdose: Protamine sulfate 1% given IV; 1 mg protamine/100 anti-Xa IU of danaparoid given

---

danazol (Ŗ)

(da′na-zole)

Cyclomen*, danazol, Danocrine

Func. class.: Androgen

Chem. class.: α-Ethinyl testosterone derivative

Action: Atrophy of endometrial tissue; decreases FSH, LH, which are controlled by pituitary; this leads to amenorrhea/anovulation

Uses: Endometriosis, prevention of hereditary angioedema, fibrocystic breast disease

Dosage and routes:

Endometriosis
• *Adult:* PO initial dose 500 mg bid, then decreased to 400 mg bid × 3-9 mo

Fibrocystic breast disease
• *Adult:* PO 100-400 mg qd in 2 divided doses × 2-6 mo

Hereditary angioedema
• *Adult:* PO 200 mg bid-tid until desired response, then decrease dose to 100 mg at 1-3 mo intervals

Available forms: Caps 50, 100, 200 mg

Side effects/adverse reactions:
INTEG: Rash, acneiform lesions, oily hair, skin, flushing, sweating, acne vulgaris, alopecia, hirsutism, pruritis

CNS: Dizziness, headache, fatigue, tremors, paresthesias, flushing, sweating, anxiety, lability, insomnia, carpal tunnel syndrome

MS: Cramps, spasms

CV: Increased B/P

GU: Hematuria, amenorrhea, atrophic vaginitis, decreased libido, decreased breast size, clitoral hypertrophy, testicular atrophy

GI: Nausea, vomiting, constipation, weight gain, *__cholestatic jaundice__*

EENT: Conjunctival edema, nasal congestion

ENDO: Abnormal GTT

Contraindications: Severe renal, severe cardiac, severe hepatic disease, hypersensitivity, genital bleeding (abnormal)

Precautions: Migraine headaches, seizure disorders, pregnancy (C)

Interactions:
• Increased effects of oral antidiabetics, oxyphenbutazone
• Increased prothrombin time: anticoagulants
• Increased edema: ACTH, adrenal steroids
• Decreased effects of: insulin

Lab test interferences:
Increase: Cholesterol
Decrease: Cholesterol, T_4, T_3, thyroid ^{131}I uptake test, 17-KS, PBI
Interference: GTT

NURSING CONSIDERATIONS

Assess:
• K, blood sugar, urine glucose while on long-term therapy
• Weight daily; notify prescriber if weekly weight gain is >5 lb; drug should be decreased or discontinued
• I&O ratio; be alert for decreasing urinary output, increasing edema

---

• Edema, hypertension, cardiac symptoms, jaundice
• Mental status: affect, mood, behavioral changes, aggression, sleep disorders, depression, anxiety, lability
• Signs of virilization: deepening of voice, decreased libido, facial hair that may not be reversible
• Hypercalcemia: GI symptoms, polydipsia, polyuria, increased calcium levels above 11 mg/dl, loss of muscle tone

Administer:
• With food or milk to decrease GI symptoms (i.e., nausea, vomiting, anorexia, dyspepsia)

Perform/provide:
• Storage in air-tight container at room temp; do not freeze
• ROM exercise for patients who are immobile to relieve cramps and spasms

Evaluate:
• Therapeutic response: decreased pain in endometriosis; decreased size, pain in fibrocystic breast disease

Teach patient/family:
🚫 Not to break, crush, or chew caps
• To notify prescriber if therapeutic response decreases
• Not to discontinue medication abruptly; to taper over several wk
• To report menstrual irregularities; that amenorrhea usually occurs but menstruation resumes 2-3 mo after termination of therapy without medical intervention
• About routine breast self-exam and to report any increase in nodule size
• That drug should induce anovulation; reversible within 60-90 days after drug is discontinued and treatment will need to be resumed
• That endometriosis tends to recur after drug is discontinued

dantrolene (℞)

(dan'troe-leen)
Dantrium, Dantrium Intravenous
Func. class.: Skeletal muscle relaxant, direct acting
Chem. class.: Hydantoin

Action: Interferes with intracellular release of calcium from the sarcoplasmic reticulum necessary to initiate contraction; slows catabolism in malignant hyperthermia

Uses: Spasticity in multiple sclerosis, stroke, spinal cord injury, cerebral palsy, malignant hyperthermia

Dosage and routes:
Spasticity
• *Adult:* **PO** 25 mg/day; may increase by 25-100 mg bid-qid, not to exceed 400 mg/day × 1 wk
• *Child:* **PO** 1 mg/kg/day given in divided doses bid-tid; dosage may increase gradually, not to exceed 100 mg qid

Prevention of malignant hyperthermia
• *Adult and child:* **PO** 4-8 mg/kg/day in 3-4 divided doses × 1-2 days prior to procedures, give last dose 4 hr preop; **IV** 2.5 mg/kg prior to anesthesia

Malignant hyperthermia
• *Adult and child:* **IV** 1 mg/kg, may repeat to total dose of 10 mg/kg; **PO** 4-8 mg/kg/day in 4 divided doses × 3 days to prevent further hyperthermia; post-crisis follow-up 4-8 mg/kg/day for 1-3 days

Available forms: Caps 25, 50, 100 mg; powder for inj 20 mg/vial

Side effects/adverse reactions:
CNS: Dizziness, weakness, fatigue, drowsiness, headache, disorientation, insomnia, paresthesias, tremors

---

◆ = Nursing alert   ∥ = Herb-drug interaction   🚫 = Do not crush

EENT: Nasal congestion, blurred vision, mydriasis

HEMA: **Eosinophilia**

CV: Hypotension, chest pain, palpitations

GI: **Hepatic injury**, *nausea,* constipation, vomiting, increased AST (SGOT), alk phosphatase, abdominal pain, dry mouth, anorexia, hepatitis, dyspepsia

GU: Urinary frequency, nocturia, impotence, crystalluria

INTEG: Rash, pruritus, photosensitivity

Contraindications: Hypersensitivity, compromised pulmonary function, active hepatic disease, impaired myocardial function

Precautions: Peptic ulcer disease, renal disease, hepatic disease, stroke, seizure disorder, diabetes mellitus, pregnancy (C), lactation, elderly

Pharmacokinetics:

PO: Peak 5 hr; highly protein bound; half-life 8 hr; metabolized in liver; excreted in urine (metabolites)

Interactions:

• Dysrhythmias: verapamil

• Increased CNS depression: alcohol, tricyclic antidepressants, narcotics, barbiturates, sedatives, hypnotics, magnesium sulfate, antihistamines

• Increased action: warfarin, clofibrate

• Hepatotoxicity: estrogens

• Considered incompatible in sol or syringe; compatibility unknown

NURSING CONSIDERATIONS

Assess:

• For increased seizure activity, ECG in epilepsy patient; poor seizure control has occurred

• I&O ratio; check for urinary retention, frequency, hesitancy, especially elderly

• Hepatic function by frequent determination of AST (SGOT), ALT (SGPT), renal function studies, BUN, creatinine, CBC

• Allergic reactions: rash, fever, respiratory distress

• Severe weakness, numbness in extremities; prescriber should be notified and drug discontinued

• Tolerance: increased need for medication, more frequent requests for medication, increased pain

• CNS depression: dizziness, drowsiness, insomnia, psychiatric symptoms

◆ Signs of hepatotoxicity: jaundice, yellow sclera, pain in abdomen, nausea, fever; prescriber should be notified, drug should be discontinued

Administer:

• With meals for GI symptoms, caps may be opened and mixed with food/liquid

• IV after diluting 20 mg/60 ml sterile H_2O for inj without bacteriostatic agent (333 µg/ml); shake until clear; give by rapid IV push through Y-tube or 3-way stopcock; follow by prescribed doses immediately

Perform/provide:

• Storage in tight container at room temp; protect diluted sol from light, use within 6 hr

• Gum, frequent sips of water for dry mouth

• Assistance with ambulation if dizziness/drowsiness occurs

Evaluate:

• Therapeutic response: decreased pain, spasticity

Teach patient/family:

• Not to discontinue medication quickly; hallucinations, spasticity, tachycardia will occur; drug should be tapered off over 1-2 wk; notify prescriber of abdominal pain, jaundiced sclera, clay-colored stools, change in color of urine

- Not to take with alcohol, other CNS depressants
- That if improvement does not occur within 6 wk, prescriber may discontinue
- To avoid hazardous activities if drowsiness, dizziness occurs
- To avoid using OTC medication: cough preparations, antihistamines, unless directed by prescriber

 Not to break, crush, or chew caps

Treatment of overdose: Induce emesis of conscious patient; lavage, dialysis

---

dapsone (DDS) (℞)

(dap'sone)
Avlosulfon*, Dapsone
Func. class.: Leprostatic
Chem. class.: Sulfone

Action: Bactericidal and bacteriostatic against *M. leprae*

Uses: Hansen's disease, PCP (*Pneumocystis carinii* pneumonia), malaria, dermatitis herpetiformis

Dosage and routes:
Hansen's disease
- *Adult:* **PO** 100 mg qd with rifampin 600 mg qd × 6 mo, then dapsone alone for 3-10 yr
- *Child:* **PO** 1-2 mg/kg/day
PCP
- *Adult:* **PO** 50-100 mg/day usually given with trimethoprim 20 mg/kg/day in 4 divided doses for 3 wk
- *Child:* **PO** 2 mg/kg/day
Available forms: Tabs 25, 100 mg

Side effects/adverse reactions:
INTEG: Exfoliative dermatitis, photosensitivity
CNS: Peripheral neuropathy, headache, anxiety, drowsiness, tremors, *convulsions,* lethargy, depression, confusion, psychosis, aggression

GI: Nausea, vomiting, abdominal pain, anorexia
GU: Proteinuria, nephrotic syndrome, renal papillary necrosis
EENT: Blurred vision, optic neuritis, photophobia
HEMA: Megaloblastic anemia

Contraindications: Hypersensitivity to sulfones, severe anemia

Precautions: Renal disease, hepatic disease, G6PD deficiency, pregnancy (C), lactation

Pharmacokinetics: Rapid complete absorption; half-life 25-31 hr; highly bound to plasma protein; metabolized in liver; excreted in urine

Interactions:
- Increased side effects: hemolytic agents
- Increased action of dapsone: probenecid, folic acid antagonists
- Decreased blood levels of dapsone: rifampin, didanosine
- Decreased bactericidal action: PABA
- Decreased GI absorption of dapsone: activated charcoal

NURSING CONSIDERATIONS
Assess:
- Temp; if >101° F (38.3° C), drug should be reduced
- Liver studies qwk: ALT (SGPT), AST (SGOT), bilirubin
- Renal status: BUN, creatinine, output, specific gravity, urinalysis before; qmo
- Blood levels of drug
- For anemia: Hct, Hgb, fatigue; for peripheral neuritis; or exfoliative dermatitis
- Mental status often: affect, mood, behavioral changes; psychosis may occur
- Hepatic status: decreased appetite, jaundice, dark urine, fatigue

Administer:
- With meals for GI symptoms
- Antiemetic if vomiting occurs

 = Nursing alert   = Herb-drug interaction   = Do not crush

• After C&S is completed; qmo to detect resistance

Perform/provide:
• Infants kept with mothers infected with leprosy; breastfeeding during drug therapy encouraged

Evaluate:
• Therapeutic response: decreased symptoms of Hansen's disease

Teach patient/family:
• That therapeutic effects may occur after 3-6 mo of drug therapy
• That compliance with dosage schedule, duration is necessary
• To avoid hazardous machinery if drowsiness occurs

---

daunorubicin (℞)

(daw-noe-roo'bi-sin)
Cerubidine
Func. class.: Antineoplastic, antibiotic
Chem. class.: Anthracycline glycoside

Action: Inhibits DNA synthesis, primarily; derived from *S. verticillus;* replication is decreased by binding to DNA, which causes strand splitting; cell cycle specific (S phase); a vesicant

Uses: Myelogenous, monocytic leukemia, acute nonlymphocytic leukemia, Ewing's sarcoma, Wilms' tumor, neuroblastoma, rhabdomyosarcoma

Dosage and routes:
Single agent
• *Adult:* IV 60 mg/m²/day × 3-5 days q4wk
In combination
• *Adult:* IV 45 mg/m²/day × 3 days, then 2 days of subsequent courses in combination
• *Child:* IV 25-60 mg/m² depending on cycle

Available forms: Inj 20 mg pwd/vial; inj 5 mg/ml

Side effects/adverse reactions:
HEMA: **Thrombocytopenia, leukopenia, anemia**
GI: Nausea, vomiting, anorexia, mucositis, **hepatotoxicity**
GU: Impotence, sterility, amenorrhea, gynecomastia, hyperuricemia
INTEG: Rash, **extravasation,** dermatitis, reversible alopecia, cellulitis, thrombophlebitis at injection site
CV: **Dysrhythmias, CHF, pericarditis, myocarditis,** peripheral edema
CNS: Fever, chills

Contraindications: Hypersensitivity, pregnancy (1st trimester) (D), lactation, systemic infections, cardiac disease

Precautions: Renal, hepatic disease; gout; bone marrow depression

Pharmacokinetics: Half life 18½ hr; metabolized by liver; crosses placenta; excreted in breast milk, urine, bile

Interactions:
• Increased toxicity: other antineoplastics, radiation
• Incompatible with dexamethasone, heparin

Lab test interferences:
Increase: Uric acid

NURSING CONSIDERATIONS
Assess:
• CBC, differential, platelet count weekly; withhold drug if WBC is <4000/mm³ or platelet count is <75,000/mm³; notify prescriber
• Blood, urine uric acid levels
• Renal function studies: BUN, serum uric acid, urine CrCl, electrolytes before, during therapy
• I&O ratio; report fall in urine output to <30 ml/hr
• Monitor temp q4h; fever may indicate beginning infection
• Liver function tests before, during

therapy: bilirubin, AST (SGOT), ALT (SGPT), alk phosphatase as needed or monthly

• ECG; watch for ST-T wave changes, low QRS and T, possible dysrhythmias (sinus tachycardia, heart block, PVCs)

• Bleeding: hematuria, guaiac stools, bruising or petechiae, mucosa or orifices q8h

• Food preferences; list likes, dislikes

• Effects of alopecia on body image; discuss feelings about body changes

• Inflammation of mucosa, breaks in skin

• Yellowing of skin, sclera; dark urine; clay-colored stools; itchy skin; abdominal pain; fever; diarrhea

• Buccal cavity q8h for dryness, sores or ulceration, white patches, oral pain, bleeding, dysphagia

• Local irritation, pain, burning at injection site

• GI symptoms: frequency of stools, cramping

• Acidosis, signs of dehydration: rapid respirations, poor skin turgor, decreased urine output, dry skin, restlessness, weakness

• Cardiac status: B/P, pulse, character, rhythm, rate

Administer:

• Antiemetic 30-60 min before giving drug and 6-10 hr after treatment to prevent vomiting

• Allopurinol or sodium bicarbonate to reduce uric acid levels, alkalinization of urine

• Transfusion for anemia

• Antispasmodic for GI symptoms

IV

• After diluting 20 mg/4 ml sterile H_2O for inj (5 mg/ml), rotate, further dilute in 10-15 ml NS; give over 3-5 min by direct IV through Y-tube or 3-way stopcock of inf of D_5 or NS

• Hydrocortisone for extravasation; apply ice compress after stopping infusion

Additive compatibilities: Cytarabine/etoposide, hydrocortisone; not recommended for admixing

Solution compatibilities: $D_{3.3}$/0.3% NaCl, D_5W, Normosol R, Ringer's, 0.9% NaCl

Y-site compatibilities: Amifostine, filgrastim, granisetron, melphalan, methotrexate, ondansetron, sodium bicarbonate, teniposide, thiotepa, vinorelbine

Perform/provide:

• Strict hand-washing technique, gloves, protective clothing

• Liquid diet: carbonated beverages, gelatin may be added if patient is not nauseated or vomiting

• Increased fluid intake to 2-3 L/day to prevent urate and calculi formation

• Diet low in purines: absence of organ meats (kidney, liver), dried beans, peas to reduce uric acid level

• Rinsing of mouth tid-qid with water, club soda; brushing of teeth bid-qid with soft brush or cotton-tipped applicators for stomatitis; use unwaxed dental floss

• Storage at room temp 24 hr after reconstituting or 48 hr refrigerated

Evaluate:

• Therapeutic response: decreased tumor size, spread of malignancy

Teach patient/family:

• To report any complaints, side effects to nurse or prescriber

• That hair may be lost during treatment and wig or hairpiece may make patient feel better; tell patient that new hair may be different in color, texture

• To avoid foods with citric acid, hot or rough texture

• To report any bleeding, white spots, ulcerations in mouth; tell patient to examine mouth qd

---

◆ = Nursing alert   ✿ = Herb-drug interaction   Ⓢ = Do not crush

• That urine and other body fluids may be red-orange for 48 hr

---

deferoxamine (℞)

(de-fer-ox′a-meen)
Desferal
Func. class.: Heavy metal antagonist
Chem. class.: Chelating agent

Action: Binds iron ions (ferric ions) to form water-soluble complex that is removed by kidneys

Uses: Acute, chronic iron intoxication, hemochromatosis, hemosiderosis

Dosage and routes:
Acute iron toxicity
• *Adult and child:* **IM/IV** 1 g, then 500 mg q4h × 2 doses, then 500 mg q4-12h × 2 doses, not to exceed 15 mg/kg/hr or 6 g/24 hr
Chronic iron toxicity
• *Adult and child:* **IM** 500 mg-1 g/day plus **IV INF** 2 g given by separate line with each blood transfusion, not to exceed 15 mg/kg/hr or 6 g/24 hr; **SC** 1-2 g over 8-24 hr by SC infusion pump
Available forms: Powder for inj 500 mg/vial

Side effects/adverse reactions:
CNS: Flushing, ***shock following rapid IV***
INTEG: Urticaria, erythema, pruritus, pain at injection site, fever
CV: Hypotension, tachycardia
GI: Diarrhea, abdominal cramps
EENT: Blurred vision, cataracts, decreased healing, *ototoxicity*
MS: Leg cramps
GU: Dysuria, pyelonephritis
SYST: ***Anaphylaxis***

Contraindications: Hypersensitivity, anuria, severe renal disease, child <3 yr

Precautions: Pregnancy (C), lactation

Pharmacokinetics: Primarily forms a complex excreted by kidneys as complex, unchanged drug

Interactions:
• Incompatible with other drugs in sol or syringe

NURSING CONSIDERATIONS
Assess:
• Poisoning; type of agent, time, amount ingested
◆ Acute, early iron toxicity: nausea, vomiting, abdominal cramping, bloody diarrhea
• Acute later iron toxicity: loss of consciousness, shock, metabolic acidosis
• Inj site for redness, inflammation, pain
• For blood in stools
• Vision and hearing periodically
• VS
• I&O, kidney function studies: BUN, creatinine, CrCl, serum iron levels
• Allergic reactions: rash, urticaria; drug should be discontinued

Administer:
• IV (used for shock) after diluting 500 mg/2 ml H_2O for inj; when dissolved, must be further diluted with D_5W or LR or NS; run at <15 mg/kg/hr; 2 g/1000 ml usually given over 24 hr; to be used only for short time; IM is preferred route
• IM after diluting with 2 ml sterile water for injection per 500 mg of drug; rotate injection sites
• SC route use abdominal SC tissue by infusion pump × 8-24 hr/treatment
• Only when epinephrine 1:1000 is on unit for anaphylaxis

Evaluate:
• Therapeutic response: decreased symptoms of heavy metal intoxication

---

Teach patient/family:
- That urine may turn red
- To avoid vit C preparations

---

demeclocycline (℞)

(dem-e-kloe-sye′kleen)
Declomycin
Func. class.: Antiinfective
Chem. class.: Tetracycline

Action: Inhibits protein synthesis, phosphorylation in microorganisms by binding to 30S ribosomal subunits, reversibly binding to 50S ribosomal subunits; bacteriostatic

Uses: Uncommon gram-positive/gram-negative bacteria, protozoa, *Rickettsia, Mycoplasma*, SIADH

Dosage and routes:
- *Adult:* PO 150 mg q6h or 300 mg q12h
- *Child >8 yr:* PO 6-12 mg/kg/day in divided doses q6-12h

Gonorrhea
- *Adult:* PO 600 mg, then 300 mg q12h × 4 days, total 3 g

SIADH
- *Adult:* PO 3.25-3.75 mg/kg q6h

Available forms: Tabs 150, 300 mg; caps 150 mg

Side effects/adverse reactions:

CNS: Fever, headache, paresthesia

*HEMA: **Eosinophilia, neutropenia, thrombocytopenia, leukocytosis, hemolytic anemia***

EENT: Dysphagia, glossitis, decreased calcification of deciduous teeth, abdominal pain, oral candidiasis

GI: Nausea, vomiting, diarrhea, anorexia, enterocolitis, ***hepatotoxicity,*** flatulence, abdominal cramps, epigastric burning, stomatitis, ***pseudomembranous colitis***

CV: Pericarditis

GU: Increased BUN, polyuria, polydipsia, ***renal failure, nephrotoxicity***

*INTEG: Rash, urticaria, photosensitivity, increased pigmentation, **exfoliative dermatitis,*** pruritus, angioedema

Contraindications: Hypersensitivity to tetracyclines, children <8 yr, pregnancy (D)

Precautions: Renal disease, hepatic disease, lactation, nephrogenic diabetes insipidus

Pharmacokinetics:
PO: Peak 3-6 hr, duration 48-72 hr, half-life 10-17 hr; excreted in urine; crosses placenta; excreted in breast milk; 41%-50% bound to serum protein

Interactions:
- Decreased effect of demeclocycline: antacids, NaHCO₃, dairy, alkali products, iron, kaolin/pectin, cimetidine, barbiturates, carbamazepine, phenytoin, warfarin
- Increased effect: warfarin
- Decreased effect: penicillins, oral contraceptives
- Nephrotoxicity: methoxyflurane
- *Increased action: bromelain*

Lab test interferences:
False negative: Urine glucose with Clinistix or Tes-Tape
False increase: Urinary catecholamines, AST (SGOT), ALT (SGPT), BUN

NURSING CONSIDERATIONS
Assess:
- I&O ratio
- Blood studies: PT, CBC, AST, ALT, BUN, creatinine
- Urine specific gravity, Na
- Signs of infection
- Allergic reactions: rash, itching, pruritus, angioedema
- Nausea, vomiting, diarrhea; administer antiemetic, antacids as ordered

---

• Overgrowth of infection: increased temp, malaise, redness, pain, swelling, drainage, perineal itching, diarrhea, changes in cough, sputum
Administer:
• On empty stomach 1 hr ac or 2 hr pc with 8 oz H_2O
• After C&S
• 2 hr before or after laxative or ferrous products; 3 hr after antacid or kaolin-pectin products
Perform/provide:
• Storage in tight, light-resistant container at room temp
Evaluate:
• Therapeutic response: decreased temp, absence of lesions, negative C&S
Teach patient/family:
• To avoid sun exposure; sunscreen does not seem to decrease photosensitivity
• If diabetic, to avoid use of Clinistix, Diastix, or Tes-Tape for urine glucose testing
🚫 Not to break, crush, or chew caps
• To take all prescribed medication to prevent superinfection; to discard when expires, may be toxic
• To avoid milk products; take with full glass of water

---

desmopressin (℞)

(des-moe-press'in)
DDAVP, Stimate
Func. class.: Pituitary hormone
Chem. class.: Synthetic antidiuretic hormone

Action: Promotes reabsorption of water by action on renal tubular epithelium; causes smooth muscle constriction, increase in plasma factor VIII levels, which increases platelet aggregation resulting in vasopressor effect, similar to vasopressin

Uses: Hemophilia A, von Willebrand's disease type 1, nonnephrogenic diabetes insipidus, symptoms of polyuria/polydipsia caused by pituitary dysfunction, nocturnal enuresis
Dosage and routes:
Primary nocturnal enuresis
• *Child ≥6 yr:* **INTRANASAL** 20 µg (10 µg in each nostril) hs, may increase to 40 µg
Diabetes insipidus
• *Adult:* **INTRANASAL** 0.1-0.4 ml qd in divided doses (1-4 sprays with pump); **IV/SC** 0.5-1 ml qd in divided doses
• *Child 3 mo to 12 yr:* **INTRANASAL** 0.05-0.3 ml qd in divided doses
Hemophilia/von Willebrand's disease
• *Adult and child >3 mo:* **IV** 0.3 µg/kg in NaCl over 15-30 min; may repeat if needed
Available forms: Intranasal pipets 0.01 mg/ml, inj 4 µg/ml, Rhihal Tube del 2.5 mg/vial; tabs 0.1, 0.2 mg
Side effects/adverse reactions:
EENT: Nasal irritation, congestion, rhinitis
CNS: Drowsiness, headache, lethargy, flushing
GU: Vulval pain
GI: Nausea, heartburn, cramps
CV: Increased B/P
SYST: Anaphylaxis (IV)
Contraindications: Hypersensitivity, nephrogenic diabetes insipidus
Precautions: Pregnancy (B), CAD, lactation, hypertension
Pharmacokinetics:
NASAL: Onset 1 hr, peak 1-2 hr, duration 8-20 hr, half-life 8 min, 76 min (terminal)
Interactions:
• Increased response: carbamazepine, chlorpropamide, clofibrate

• Decreased response; lithium, alcohol, demeclocyclines, heparin, large doses of epinephrine

• Compatibility not known

NURSING CONSIDERATIONS
Assess:

• Pulse, B/P when giving IV or SC

• I&O ratio, weight daily; check for edema in extremities; if water retention is severe, diuretic may be prescribed

• Water intoxication: lethargy, behavioral changes, disorientation, neuromuscular excitability

• Intranasal use: nausea, congestion, cramps, headache; usually decreased with decreased dose

⬥ For severe allergic reaction including anaphylaxis (IV route)

• For nasal mucosa changes: congestion, edema, discharge, scarring (nasal route)

• Urine vol/osmolality and plasma osmolality (diabetes insipidus)

• Factor VIII coagulant activity before using for hemostasis

Administer:

• Undiluted over 1 min in diabetes insipidus

• Diluted, one single dose/50 ml of NS (adult & child >10 kg), a single dose/10 ml as an IV INF over 15-30 min in von Willebrand's disease or hemophilia A

Perform/provide:

• Storage in refrigerator or cool environment

Evaluate:

• Therapeutic response: absence of severe thirst, decreased urine output, osmolality

Teach patient/family:

• The proper technique for nasal instillation: to insert tube into nostril to instill drug

• To avoid OTC products: cough, hay fever products, since these preparations may contain epinephrine, decrease drug response; do not use with alcohol

• To wear Medic Alert ID specifying therapy

• That if dose is missed, take when remembered up to 1 hr before next dose; do not double dose

---

dexamethasone/ dexamethasone acetate/dexamethasone sodium phosphate (℞)

(dex-a-meth′a-sone)

Aeroseb-Dex, Dalalone, Dalalone D.P., Dalalone L.A., Decaderm, Decadron-LA, Decadron Phosphate, Decadron Phosphate Respihaler, Decaject, Decaject-L.A. , Decaspray, Dexacen LA-8, Dexacen-4, Dexamethasone Acetate, Dexamethasone Sodium Phosphate, Dexasone, Dexasone L.A., Dexone, Dexone LA, Hexadrol Phosphate, Solurex, Solurex LA

Func. class.: Corticosteroid

Chem. class.: Glucocorticoid, long-acting

Action: Decreases inflammation by suppression of migration of polymorphonuclear leukocytes, fibroblasts, reversal of increased capillary permeability and lysosomal stabilization

Uses: Inflammation, allergies, neoplasms, cerebral edema, septic shock, collagen disorders

Dosage and routes:

Inflammation

• *Adult:* **PO** 0.25-4 mg bid-qid, **IM** 4-16 mg q1-3wk (acetate)

• *Child:* **PO** 0.08-0.3 mg/kg/day in divided doses q6-12h

⬥ = Nursing alert   🌿 = Herb-drug interaction   ⊘ = Do not crush

Shock
- *Adult:* **IV** 1-6 mg/kg or 40 mg q2-6h (phosphate)

Cerebral edema
- *Adult:* **IV** 10 mg, then 4-6 mg **IM** q6h × 2-4 days, then taper over 1 wk
- *Child:* **PO** 0.2 mg/kg/day in divided doses

Available forms: Tabs 0.25, 0.5, 0.75, 1, 1.5, 3, 4, 6 mg; inj acetate 8, 16 mg/ml; inj phosphate 4, 10 mg/ml; elix 0.5 mg/5 ml; oral sol 0.5 mg/5 ml, 0.5 mg/1 ml

Side effects/adverse reactions:

INTEG: Acne, poor wound healing, ecchymosis, petechiae

CNS: Depression, flushing, sweating, headache, mood changes, euphoria, psychosis

*CV: Hypertension, **circulatory collapse, thrombophlebitis, embolism,*** tachycardia, edema

*HEMA: **Thrombocytopenia***

MS: Fractures, osteoporosis, weakness

*GI: Diarrhea, nausea, abdominal distention, **GI hemorrhage,** increased appetite, **pancreatitis***

EENT: Fungal infections, increased intraocular pressure, blurred vision

ENDO: HPA suppression

META: Hypokalemia

Contraindications: Psychosis, hypersensitivity, idiopathic thrombocytopenia, acute glomerulonephritis, amebiasis, fungal infections, nonasthmatic bronchial disease, child <2 yr, AIDS, TB

Precautions: Pregnancy (C), lactation, diabetes mellitus, glaucoma, osteoporosis, seizure disorders, ulcerative colitis, CHF, myasthenia gravis, renal disease, peptic ulcer, esophagitis

Pharmacokinetics:

PO: Peak 1-2 hr, duration 2⅓ days

IM: Peak 8 hr, duration 6 days
Half-life 3-4½ hr

Interactions:
- Decreased action of dexamethasone: cholestyramine, colestipol, barbiturates, rifampin, ephedrine, phenytoin, theophylline, antacids
- Decreased effects of anticoagulants, anticonvulsants, antidiabetics, ambenonium, neostigmine, isoniazid, toxoids, vaccines, anticholinesterases, salicylates, somatrem
- Increased side effects: alcohol, salicylates, indomethacin, amphotericin B, digitalis, cyclosporine, diuretics
- Increased action of dexamethasone: salicylates, estrogens, indomethacin, oral contraceptives, ketoconazole, macrolide antibiotics

�ません Potassium deficiency: aloe, buckthorn bark/berry, cascara sagrada bark, ephedra, senna pod/leaf

Lab test interferences:

Increase: Cholesterol, Na, blood glucose, uric acid, Ca, urine glucose

Decrease: Ca, K, T_4, T_3, thyroid ^{131}I uptake test, urine 17-OHCS, 17-KS, PBI skin allergy tests

NURSING CONSIDERATIONS

Assess:
- K, blood sugar, urine glucose while on long-term therapy; hypokalemia and hyperglycemia
- Weight daily; notify prescriber of weekly gain >5 lb
- B/P q4h, pulse; notify prescriber of chest pain
- I&O ratio; be alert for decreasing urinary output, increasing edema
- Plasma cortisol levels during long-term therapy (normal: 138-635 nmol/L SI units when drawn at 8 AM)
- Infection: fever, WBC even after withdrawal of medication; drug masks infection
- Potassium depletion: paresthesias, fatigue, nausea, vomiting, depression, polyuria, dysrhythmias, weakness

322   dexchlorpheniramine

- Edema, hypertension, cardiac symptoms
- Mental status: affect, mood, behavioral changes, aggression

Administer:
- Titrated dose; use lowest effective dose
- IM inj deeply in large muscle mass; rotate sites; avoid deltoid; use 21G needle
- In one dose in AM to prevent adrenal suppression; avoid SC administration, may damage tissue
- With food or milk to decrease GI symptoms

IV
- Undiluted direct over 1 min or less or diluted with NS or D_5W and give as an IV INF at prescribed rate
- After shaking suspension (parenteral); do not give suspension IV

Additive compatibilities: Aminophylline, bleomycin, cimetidine, floxacillin, furosemide, granisetron, lidocaine, meropenem, mitomycin, nafcillin, netilmicin, ondansetron, prochlorperazine, ranitidine, verapamil

Syringe compatibilities: Granisetron, metoclopramide, ranitidine, sufentanil

Y-site compatibilities: Acyclovir, allopurinol, amifostine, amikacin, amsacrine, aztreonam, cefepime, cefpirome, cisplatin, cladribine, cyclophosphamide, cytarabine, doxorubicin, famotidine, filgrastim, fluconazole, fludarabine, foscarnet, granisetron, heparin, lorazepam, melphalan, meperidine, meropenem, morphine, ondansetron, paclitaxel, piperacillin/tazobactam, potassium chloride, propofol, sargramostim, sodium bicarbonate, sufentanil, tacrolimus, teniposide, theophylline, thiotepa, vinorelbine, vit B/C, zidovudine

Perform/provide:
- Assistance with ambulation in patient with bone tissue disease to prevent fractures

Evaluate:
- Therapeutic response: ease of respirations, decreased inflammation

Teach patient/family:
- That ID as steroid user should be carried
- To notify prescriber if therapeutic response decreases; dosage adjustment may be needed
- ◆ Not to discontinue abruptly or adrenal crisis can result
- Symptoms of adrenal insufficiency: nausea, anorexia, fatigue, dizziness, dyspnea, weakness, joint pain
- To avoid OTC products: salicylates, alcohol in cough products, cold preparations unless directed by prescriber
- To teach patient all aspects of drug usage, including cushingoid symptoms; to notify health-care provider of infection

---

dexchlorpheniramine (℞)
(dex-klor-fen-eer′a-meen)
Dexchlor, Dexchlorpheniramine Maleate, Poladex, Polaramine
Func. class.: Antihistamine
Chem. class.: Alkylamine derivative, H_1-receptor antagonist

Action: Acts on blood vessels, GI, respiratory system by competing with histamine for H_1-receptor site; decreases allergic response by blocking histamine
Uses: Allergy symptoms, rhinitis, pruritus, contact dermatitis

---

◆= Nursing alert   ∥= Herb-drug interaction   ⊘= Do not crush

Dosage and routes:
• *Adult:* **PO** 1-2 mg tid-qid; **RE-PEAT ACTION** 4-6 mg bid-tid
• *Child 6-11 yr:* **PO** 1 mg q4-6h, or **TIME REL** 4 mg hs
• *Child 2-5 yr:* **PO** 0.5 mg q4-6h; do not use repeat action form
Available forms: Tabs 2 mg; repeat-action tabs 4, 6 mg; syr 2 mg/5 ml

Side effects/adverse reactions:

CNS: Dizziness, drowsiness, poor coordination, fatigue, anxiety, euphoria, confusion, paresthesia, neuritis
CV: Hypotension, palpitations, tachycardia
RESP: Increased thick secretions, wheezing, chest tightness
GI: Constipation, dry mouth, nausea, vomiting, anorexia, diarrhea
INTEG: Rash, urticaria, photosensitivity
GU: Retention, dysuria, frequency
EENT: Blurred vision, dilated pupils, tinnitus, nasal stuffiness, dry nose, throat, mouth

Contraindications: Hypersensitivity to H_1-receptor antagonist; acute asthma attack, lower respiratory tract disease

Precautions: Increased intraocular pressure, renal disease, cardiac disease, hypertension, bronchial asthma, seizure disorder, stenosed peptic ulcers, hyperthyroidism, prostatic hypertrophy, bladder neck obstruction, pregnancy (B), lactation, elderly

Pharmacokinetics:

PO: Onset 15 min, peak 3 hr, duration 3-6 hr; metabolized in liver; excreted by kidneys (inactive metabolites); excreted in breast milk (small amounts)

Interactions:
• Increased CNS depression: barbiturates, narcotics, hypnotics, tricyclic antidepressants, alcohol
• Decreased effect: oral anticoagulants, heparin
• Increased effect of dexchlorpheniramine: MAOIs
🖋 Increased anticholinergic effect: henbane leaf

Lab test interferences:
False negative: Skin allergy tests

NURSING CONSIDERATIONS
Assess:
• I&O ratio; be alert for urinary retention, frequency, dysuria; drug should be discontinued
• CBC during long-term therapy
• Respiratory status: rate, rhythm, increase in bronchial secretions, wheezing, chest tightness
• Cardiac status: palpitations, increased pulse, hypotension

Administer:
• With meals for GI symptoms; absorption may slightly decrease

Perform/provide:
• Hard candy, gum, frequent rinsing of mouth for dryness
• Storage in tight container at room temp

Evaluate:
• Therapeutic response: absence of running or congested nose or rashes

Teach patient/family:
• All aspects of drug use; to notify prescriber of confusion/sedation/hypotension
• To avoid driving, other hazardous activity if drowsiness occurs, especially elderly
• That this drug decreases anticoagulant (oral) effect
• To avoid concurrent use of alcohol, other CNS depressants

Treatment of overdose: Ipecac syrup or lavage, diazepam, vasopressors, barbiturates (short-acting)

dextran 40 (℞)

(deks'tran)

Dextran 40, Gentran 40, LMD
10%, Rheomacrodex

Func. class.: Plasma volume expander

Chem. class.: Low molecular weight polysaccharide

Action: Similar to human albumin, which expands plasma volume by drawing fluid from interstitial space to intravascular space

Uses: Expand plasma volume, prophylaxis of embolism, thrombosis

Dosage and routes:

Shock

• *Adult:* **IV INF** 500 ml over 15-30 min, total dose in 24 hr not to exceed 20 ml/kg; subsequent doses given slowly; if given >24 hr, not to exceed 10 ml/kg/day; not to exceed therapy >5 days

Thrombosis/embolism

• *Adult:* **IV INF** 500-1000 ml, then 500 ml/day × 3 days, then 500 ml q2-3 days × 2 wk if needed

Available forms: 10% dextran 40/5% dextrose, 10% dextran 40/0.9% NaCl

Side effects/adverse reactions:

HEMA: Decreased hematocrit, platelet function; *increased bleeding/coagulation times*

INTEG: Rash, urticaria, pruritus, *angioedema,* chills, fever, flushing

RESP: Wheezing, dyspnea, *bronchospasm, pulmonary edema*

CV: Hypotension, *cardiac arrest*

GU: Osmotic nephrosis, renal failure, stasis, hyponatremia

GI: Nausea, vomiting, increased AST, ALT

SYST: Anaphylaxis

Contraindications: Hypersensitivity, renal failure, CHF (severe), extreme dehydration

Precautions: Active hemorrhage, pregnancy (C)

Pharmacokinetics:

IV: Expands blood vol 1-2 × amount infused; excreted in urine and feces

Interactions:

• Incompatible with chlortetracycline, phytonadione, promethazine

Lab test interferences:

False increase: Blood glucose, urinary protein, bilirubin, total protein

Interference: Rh test, blood typing/crossmatching

NURSING CONSIDERATIONS

Assess:

• VS q5min × 30 min

• CVP during infusion (5-10 cm H_2O—normal range)

• Urine output q1h; watch for increase in urinary output (common); if output does not increase, decrease or discontinue infusion

• I&O ratio and specific gravity, urine osmolarity; if specific gravity is very low, renal clearance is low; drug should be discontinued

• Allergy: rash, urticaria, pruritus, wheezing, dyspnea, bronchospasm, drug should be discontinued immediately

◆ Circulatory overload: increased pulse, respirations, SOB, wheezing, chest tightness, chest pain

• Dehydration after infusion: decreased output, decreased specific gravity of urine, increased temp, poor skin turgor, increased specific gravity, dry skin

Administer:

IV

• After prescribed dilution; may give inital 500 mg at 15-30 min; distribute remainder of daily dose over 8-24 hr

• After crossmatch is drawn, if blood is to be given also

• Dextran 1 (Promit) to prevent anaphylaxis if ordered

◆ = Nursing alert   ∥ = Herb-drug interaction   ⊘ = Do not crush

Additive compatibilities: Cloxacillin

Y-site compatibilities: Enalaprilat, famotidine

Perform/provide:
• Storage at constant temp 15°-30° C (59°-86° F); discard unused portions, protect from freezing

Evaluate:
• Therapeutic response: increased plasma volume

---

dextran 70/75 (R)

(deks′tran)

Dextran 70, Dextran 75, Gentran 75, Macrodex

Func. class.: Plasma volume expander

Chem. class.: High molecular weight polysaccharide

Action: Similar to human albumin, which expands plasma volume by drawing fluid from interstitial spaces to intravascular space

Uses: Expand plasma volume in hypovolemic shock or impending shock

Dosage and routes:
• *Adult:* **IV INF** 500-1000 ml not to exceed 20-40 ml/min, not to exceed 10 ml/kg/24 hr if therapy >24 hr

Available forms: 70/75 dextran in 0.9% NaCl, D_5%

Side effects/adverse reactions:

HEMA: Decreased hematocrit, platelet function; *increased bleeding/coagulation times*

INTEG: Rash, urticaria, pruritus, *angioedema,* chills, fever, flushing

RESP: Wheezing, dyspnea, *bronchospasm, pulmonary edema*

CV: Hypotension, *cardiac arrest*

GU: Osmotic nephrosis, renal failure, stasis, hypernatremia

GI: Nausea, vomiting, increased AST, ALT

SYST: Anaphylaxis

Contraindications: Hypersensitivity, renal failure, CHF (severe), extreme dehydration

Precautions: Active hemorrhage, pregnancy (C)

Pharmacokinetics:
IV: Expands blood vol 1-2 × amount infused; excreted in urine, feces

Lab test interferences:
False increase: Blood glucose, urinary protein, bilirubin, total protein
Interference: Rh test, blood typing/crossmatching

NURSING CONSIDERATIONS

Assess:
• VS q5min × 30 min
• CVP during infusion (5-10 cm H_2O—normal range)
• Urine output q1h; watch for increase in urinary output (common); if output does not increase, decrease or discontinue infusion
• I&O ratio and specific gravity urine osmolarity; if specific gravity is very low, renal clearance is low; drug should be discontinued
• Allergy: rash, urticaria, pruritus, wheezing, dyspnea, bronchospasm; drug should be discontinued immediately

➧ Circulatory overload: increased pulse, respirations, SOB, wheezing, chest tightness, chest pain

• Dehydration after infusion: decreased output, increased temp, poor skin turgor, increased specific gravity, dry skin

Administer:
• After prescribed dilution, may give inital 500 mg at 20-40 ml/min, reduce flow to lowest rate
• After crossmatch is drawn, if blood is to be given also
• Dextran 1 (Promit) to prevent anaphylaxis

Perform/provide:
• Storage at constant temp <25° C (77° F); discard unused portions; do not use unless clear

---

Evaluate:
• Therapeutic response: increased plasma volume

---

dextroamphetamine (℞)

(dex-troe-am-fet′a-meen)
Dexedrine, Dexedrine Spansules, dextroamphetamine sulfate, Ferndex, Oxydess II, Spancap #1
Func. class.: Cerebral stimulant
Chem. class.: Amphetamine

Controlled Substance Schedule II
Action: Increases release of norepinephrine, dopamine in cerebral cortex to reticular activating system
Uses: Narcolepsy, attention deficit disorder with hyperactivity
Dosage and routes:
Narcolepsy
• **Adult: PO** 5-60 mg qd in divided doses
• *Child >12 yr:* **PO** 10 mg qd increasing by 10 mg/day at weekly intervals
• *Child 6-12 yr:* **PO** 5 mg qd increasing by 5 mg/wk (max 60 mg/day)
Attention deficit disorder
• *Child >6 yr:* **PO** 5 mg qd-bid increasing by 5 mg/day at weekly intervals
• *Child 3-6 yr:* **PO** 2.5 mg qd increasing by 2.5 mg/day at weekly intervals
Available forms: Tabs 5, 10 mg; caps sus rel 5, 10, 15 mg; elix 5 mg/5 ml
Side effects/adverse reactions:
CNS: Hyperactivity, insomnia, restlessness, talkativeness, dizziness, headache, chills, stimulation, dysphoria, irritability, aggressiveness, tremor, dependence, addiction
GI: Anorexia, dry mouth, diarrhea, constipation, weight loss, metallic taste
GU: Impotence, change in libido
CV: Palpitations, tachycardia, hypertension, decrease in heart rate, *dysrhythmias*
INTEG: Urticaria
Contraindications: Hypersensitivity to sympathomimetic amines, hyperthyroidism, hypertension, glaucoma, severe arteriosclerosis, drug abuse, cardiovascular disease, anxiety
Precautions: Gilles de la Tourette's disorder, pregnancy (C), lactation, child <3 yr
Pharmacokinetics:
PO: Onset 30 min, peak 1-3 hr, duration 4-20 hr; metabolized by liver; urine excretion pH dependent; crosses placenta, breast milk; half-life 10-30 hr
Interactions:
• Hypertensive crisis: MAOIs or within 14 days of MAOIs, furazolidine
• Increased effect of dextroamphetamine: acetazolamide, antacids, sodium bicarbonate, phenothiazines, haloperidol
• Decreased effect of dextroamphetamine: barbiturates, ascorbic acid, ammonium chloride, tricyclics
• Decreased effect: guanethidine
NURSING CONSIDERATIONS
Assess:
• VS, B/P; this drug may reverse antihypertensives; check patients with cardiac disease often
• CBC, urinalysis; in diabetes: blood sugar, urine sugar; insulin changes may be required, since eating will decrease
• Height, growth rate in children; growth rate may be decreased
• Mental status: mood, sensorium, affect, stimulation, insomnia, irritability

---

➡ = Nursing alert   ⫽ = Herb-drug interaction   ⊘ = Do not crush

• Tolerance or dependency: an increased amount may be used to get same effect; will develop after long-term use
• Overdose: pain, fever, dehydration, insomnia, hyperactivity
Administer:
• At least 6 hr before hs to avoid sleeplessness
• Gum, hard candy, frequent sips of water for dry mouth
Evaluate:
• Therapeutic response: increased CNS stimulation, decreased drowsiness
Teach patient/family:
🚫 Not to break, crush, or chew sus rel forms
• To decrease caffeine consumption (coffee, tea, cola, chocolate); may increase irritability, stimulation
• To avoid OTC preparations unless approved by prescriber
• To taper drug over several wk; depression, increased sleeping, lethargy
• To avoid alcohol ingestion
• To avoid hazardous activities until stabilized on medication
• To get needed rest; patient will feel more tired at end of day
Treatment of overdose: Administer fluids, hemodialysis or peritoneal dialysis; antihypertensive for increased B/P, ammonium Cl for increased excretion

---

dextromethorphan
(OTC)
(dex-troe-meth-or'fan)
Balminil DM*, Benylin DM*, Broncho-Grippol-DM*, Children's Hold, Delsym, Dextromethorphan, Hold DM, Koffex*, Neo-DM*, Orex DM*, Pertussin, Pertussin ES, Robidex*, Robitussin Cough Calmers, Robitussin Pediatric, Sedatuss*, St. Joseph Cough Suppressant, Sucrets Cough Control, Suppress, Trocal, Vicks Formula 44
Func. class.: Antitussive, nonnarcotic
Chem. class.: Levorphanol derivative

Action: Depresses cough center in medulla by direct effect
Uses: Nonproductive cough
Dosage and routes:
• *Adult:* **PO** 10-20 mg q4h, or 30 mg q6-8h, not to exceed 120 mg/day; **SUS-REL LIQ** 60 mg bid, not to exceed 120 mg/day
• *Child 6-12 yr:* **PO** 5-10 mg q4h, **SUS-REL LIQ** 30 mg bid, not to exceed 60 mg/day
• *Child 2-6 yr:* **PO** 2.5-5 mg q4h, or 7.5 mg q6-8h, not to exceed 30 mg/day
Available forms: Loz 2.5, 5 mg; sol 3.5, 5, 7.5, 10, 15 mg/5 ml; syrup 15 mg/15 ml, 10 mg/5 ml; sus-action liq 30 mg/5 ml
Side effects/adverse reactions:
CNS: Dizziness
GI: Nausea
Contraindications: Hypersensitivity, asthma/emphysema, productive cough
Precautions: Nausea/vomiting, fever, persistent headache, pregnancy (C)

Pharmacokinetics:

PO: Onset 15-30 min, duration 3-6 hr

SUS: Duration 12 hr

Interactions:

• Do not give with MAOIs or within 2 wk of MAOIs

NURSING CONSIDERATIONS
Assess:

• Cough: type, frequency, character, including sputum

Administer:

• Decreased dose to elderly patients; metabolism may be slowed

Perform/provide:

• Increased fluids to liquefy secretions

• Humidification of patient's room

Evaluate:

• Therapeutic response: absence of cough

Teach patient/family:

• To avoid driving, other hazardous activities until patient is stabilized on this medication

• To avoid smoking, smoke-filled rooms, perfumes, dust, environmental pollutants, cleaners that increase cough

• To avoid alcohol, other CNS depressants

• To notify prescriber if cough persists over a few days

---

dextrose
(D-glucose) (℞)
Glucose, Glutose, Insta-Glucose, Insulin Reaction
Func. class.: Caloric

Action: Needed for adequate utilization of amino acids; decreases protein, nitrogen loss; prevents ketosis

Uses: Increases intake of calories; increases fluids in patients unable to take adequate fluids, calories orally

Investigational uses: Varicose veins, acute alcohol intoxication

Dosage and routes:

• *Adult and child:* **IV** depends on individual requirements

Available forms: Inj 2.5%, 5%, 10%, 20%, 40%, 50%, 60%, 70%; oral gel 40%; chew tab 5 g

Side effects/adverse reactions:

CNS: Confusion, *loss of consciousness,* dizziness

CV: Hypertension, *CHF, pulmonary edema*

GU: Glycosuria, osmotic diuresis

ENDO: Hyperglycemia, rebound hypoglycemia, hyperosmolar syndrome, hyperglycemic nonketotic syndrome

INTEG: Chills, flushing, warm feeling, rash, urticaria, extravasation necrosis

Contraindications: Hyperglycemia, delirium tremens, hemorrhage (cranial/spinal), CHF

Precautions: Renal, liver, cardiac disease, diabetes mellitus

NURSING CONSIDERATIONS
Assess:

• Electrolytes (K, Na, Ca, Cl, Mg), blood glucose, ammonia, phosphate

• Injection site for extravasation: redness along vein, edema at site, necrosis, pain; hard, tender area; site should be changed immediately

• Monitor temp q4h for increased fever, indicating infection; if infection suspected, infusion is discontinued, tubing, bottle, catheter tip cultured

• Serum glucose in patients receiving hypotonic glucose 50% and over

• Nutritional status: calorie count by dietitian

Administer:

• Only (4%) protein and dextrose (up to 12.5%) via peripheral vein; stronger sol: central IV administration

• May be given undiluted via prepared sol; give 10% sol, 5 ml/15

◆ = Nursing alert   🖊 = Herb-drug interaction   🚫 = Do not crush

sec; 10% sol, 1000 ml/3 hr or more; 20% sol, 500 ml/½-1 hr; 50% sol, 10 ml/min

• Oral glucose preparations (gel, chew tabs) are to be used in conscious patients only; check serum blood glucose after first dose

• After changing IV catheter, dressing q24h with aseptic technique

Evaluate:

• Therapeutic response: increased weight

Teach patient/family:

• The reason for dextrose infusion

• To review hypoglycemia/hyperglycemia symptoms

• To review blood glucose monitoring procedure

---

dezocine (℞)

(dez'oh-seen)

Dalgan

Func. class.: Narcotic agonist-antagonist analgesic

Chem. class.: Opioid, synthetic

Action: Depresses pain impulse transmission at the spinal cord level by interacting with opioid receptors

Uses: Severe pain

Dosage and routes:

• *Adult:* **IM** 5-20 mg q3-6h, not to exceed 120 mg/day; **IV** 2.5-10 mg q2-4h

Available forms: Inj 5, 10, 15 mg/ml single-dose vials, multiple dose 10 mg/ml

Side effects/adverse reactions:

CV: Hypotension, pulse irregularity, hypertension, chest pain, pallor, edema, thrombophlebitis

CNS: Drowsiness, dizziness, confusion, sedation, anxiety, headache, depression, delirium, sleep disturbances, dependency

GI: Nausea, vomiting, anorexia, constipation, cramps, abdominal pain, dry mouth, diarrhea

INTEG: Injection site reactions, pruritus, rash, sweating, chills

RESP: **Respiratory depression,** hiccups

GU: Urinary frequency, hesitancy, retention

EENT: Blurred vision, slurred speech, diplopia

Contraindications: Hypersensitivity

Precautions: Addictive personality, pregnancy (C), lactation, increased intracranial pressure, respiratory depression, hepatic disease, renal disease, child <18 yr, elderly, biliary surgery, COPD, sulfite sensitivity

Pharmacokinetics:

IM: Onset 30 min, peak 50-90 min, duration 2-4 hr

IV: Onset 10 min, peak 30 min, duration 2-4 hr

Metabolized by liver; excreted by kidneys; may cross placenta

Interactions:

• Incompatibility: not known

• Increased CNS depression: alcohol, narcotics, sedative/hypnotics, antipsychotics, skeletal muscle relaxants, general anesthetics, tranquilizers

NURSING CONSIDERATIONS

Assess:

• I&O ratio; decreasing output may indicate urinary retention

• CNS changes: dizziness, drowsiness, hallucinations, euphoria, LOC, pupil reaction

• Allergic reactions: rash, urticaria

• Respiratory dysfunction: respiratory depression, character, rate, rhythm of respirations; notify prescriber if <10/min, shallow

• Need for pain medication, physical dependence

Administer:

• Undiluted 5 mg or less over 2-3 min

• With antiemetic if nausea, vomiting occur

• When pain is beginning to return; determine dosage interval by patient response

Perform/provide:

• Storage in light-resistant area at room temp

• Assistance with ambulation

• Safety measures: top side rails, night-light, call bell in easy reach

Evaluate:

• Therapeutic response: decrease in pain

Teach patient/family:

• To report any symptoms of CNS changes, allergic reactions

• That physical dependency may result after extended use

• That withdrawal symptoms may occur: nausea, vomiting, cramps, fever, faintness, anorexia

Treatment of overdose: Naloxone 0.2-0.8 mg IV, O_2, IV fluids, vasopressors

---

diazepam (R)

(dye-az'-e-pam)

Diastat, Diazemuls*, diazepam, Diazepam Intensol, Dizac, D-Tran*, E-Pam*, Meval*, Novodipam*, Stress-Pam*, Valium, Valrelease, Vivol*, Vazepam, Zetran

Func. class.: Antianxiety

Chem. class.: Benzodiazepine

Controlled Substance Schedule IV

Action: Potentiates the actions of GABA, especially in limbic system, reticular formation; enhances presympathetic inhibition, inhibits spinal polysynaptic afferent paths

Uses: Anxiety, acute alcohol withdrawal, adjunct in seizure disorders; preoperatively as a relaxant, skeletal muscle relaxation; rectally for acute repetitive seizures

Investigational uses: Panic attacks

Dosage and routes:

Anxiety/convulsive disorders

• *Adult:* **PO** 2-10 mg bid-qid; **EXT REL** 15-30 mg qd

• *Geriatric:* **PO** 1-2 mg qd-bid, increase slowly as needed

• *Child >6 mo:* **PO** 1-2.5 mg tid-qid

Muscle relaxation

• *Geriatric:* **PO** 2-5 mg bid-qid

Tetanic muscle spasms

• *Child <5 yr:* **IM/IV** 5-10 mg q3-4h prn

• *Infant >30 days:* **IM/IV** 1-2 mg q3-4h prn

Status epilepticus

• *Adult:* **IV BOL** 5-20 mg, 2 mg/min, may repeat q5-10min, not to exceed 60 mg; may repeat in 30 min if seizures reappear

• *Child:* **IV BOL** 0.1-0.3 mg/kg (1 mg/min over 3 min); may repeat q15min × 2 doses

• *Adult:* **RECT** 0.2 mg/kg, may repeat 4-12 hr later

• *Child 6-11 yr:* **RECT** 0.3 mg/kg, may repeat 4-12 hr later

• *Child 2-5 yr:* **RECT** 0.5 mg/kg, may repeat 4-12 hr later

Available forms: Tabs 2, 5, 10 mg; caps ext rel 15 mg; inj emulsified 5 mg/ml; oral sol 5 mg/5 ml, 5 mg/ml; gel, rectal delivery system 10, 15, 20 mg, twin packs

Side effects/adverse reactions:

CNS: Dizziness, drowsiness, confusion, headache, anxiety, tremors, stimulation, fatigue, depression, insomnia, hallucinations

CV: Orthostatic hypotension, ECG changes, tachycardia, hypotension

EENT: Blurred vision, tinnitus, mydriasis

GI: Constipation, dry mouth, nausea, vomiting, anorexia, diarrhea

INTEG: Rash, dermatitis, itching

Contraindications: Hypersensitivity to benzodiazepines, narrow-angle glaucoma, psychosis, pregnancy (D), lactation

Precautions: Elderly, debilitated, hepatic disease, renal disease

Pharmacokinetics:

PO: Rapidly absorbed; onset ½ hr, duration 2-3 hr

IM: Onset 15-30 min, duration 1-1½ hr; absorption slow and erratic

IV: Onset 1-5 min, duration 15 min Metabolized by liver, excreted by kidneys, crosses placenta, excreted in breast milk, crosses the blood-brain barrier; half-life 20-50 hr, more effective by mouth

Interactions:

• Decreased effects of diazepam: oral contraceptives, rifampin, valproic acid, cimetidine, disulfiram, narcotic analgesics, propoxyphene, isoniazid, propranolol

• Increased CNS depression: CNS depressants, alcohol

• Increased action of diazepam: kava kava

Lab test interferences:

Increase: AST (SGOT)/ALT (SGPT), serum bilirubin

False increase: 17-OHCS

Decrease: RAIU

NURSING CONSIDERATIONS

Assess:

• B/P (lying, standing), pulse; respiratory rate; if systolic B/P drops 20 mm Hg, hold drug, notify prescriber; respirations q5-15min if given IV

• Blood studies: CBC during long-term therapy; blood dyscrasias (rare)

• Degree of anxiety; what precipitates anxiety and whether drug controls symptoms

• For alcohol withdrawal symptoms, including hallucinations (visual, auditory), delirium, irritability, agitation, fine to coarse tremors

• For seizure control and type, duration, intensity of convulsions

• Hepatic studies: AST (SGOT), ALT (SGPT), bilirubin, creatinine, LDH alk phosphatase

• IV site for thrombosis or phlebitis, which may occur rapidly

• Mental status: mood, sensorium, affect, sleeping pattern, drowsiness, dizziness

• Physical dependency, withdrawal symptoms: headache, nausea, vomiting, muscle pain, weakness after long-term use

• Suicidal tendencies

Administer:

• With food or milk for GI symptoms; crushed if patient is unable to swallow medication whole; do not crush ext rel capsules

• Sugarless gum, hard candy, frequent sips of water for dry mouth

• Reduced narcotic dose by ⅓ if given concomitantly with diazepam

IV

• Into large vein; give IV 5 mg or less/1 min or total dose over 3 min or more (children, infants); continuous infusion is not recommended; Dizac; IV only

Additive compatibilities: Netilmicin, verapamil

Syringe compatibilities: Cimetidine

Y-site compatibilities: Cefmetazole, dobutamine, nafcillin, quinidine, sufentanil

Perform/provide:

• Assistance with ambulation during beginning therapy, for drowsiness, dizziness

• Safety measures, including side rails

• Check to see PO medication has been swallowed

Evaluate:

• Therapeutic response: decreased anxiety, restlessness, insomnia

Teach patient/family:

• That drug may be taken with food
• That drug is not to be used for everyday stress or used longer than 4 mo unless directed by prescriber; no more than prescribed amount; may be habit forming
• To avoid OTC preparations unless approved by prescriber
• To avoid driving, activities that require alertness; drowsiness may occur
• To avoid alcohol, other psychotropic medications unless directed by prescriber
• Not to discontinue medication abruptly after long-term use
• To rise slowly or fainting may occur, especially in elderly
• That drowsiness may worsen at beginning of treatment
🚫 Not to break, crush, or chew ext rel caps

Treatment of overdose: Lavage, VS, supportive care, flumazenil

---

diazoxide (℞)

(dye-az-ox′ide)
diazoxide parenteral, Hyperstat IV

Func. class.: Antihypertensive
Chem. class.: Vasodilator

Action: Vasodilates arteriolar smooth muscle by direct relaxation; a reduction in blood pressure with concomitant increases in heart rate, cardiac output; inhibits release of insulin from the pancreas

Uses: Hypertensive crisis when urgent decrease of diastolic pressure required; increase blood glucose levels in hyperinsulinism

Dosage and routes:
• *Adult:* IV BOL 1-3 mg/kg rapidly up to a max of 150 mg in a single injection; dose may be repeated at 5-15 min intervals until desired response is achieved; give IV in 30 sec or less
• *Child:* **IV BOL** 1-2 mg/kg rapidly; administration same as adult, not to exceed 150 mg

Available forms: Inj 15 mg/ml

Side effects/adverse reactions:

CV: **Hypotension,** T-wave changes, angina pectoris, palpitations, *supraventricular tachycardia, edema,* rebound hypertension
CNS: *Headache,* sleepiness, euphoria, anxiety, EPS, confusion, tinnitus, blurred vision, dizziness, weakness
GI: Nausea, vomiting, dry mouth
INTEG: Rash
HEMA: Decreased hemoglobin, hematocrit, *thrombocytopenia*
GU: Breast tenderness; increased BUN, fluid, electrolyte imbalances; Na, water retention
ENDO: Hyperglycemia in diabetics, transient hyperglycemia in nondiabetics

Contraindications: Hypersensitivity to thiazides, sulfonamides, hypertension of aortic coarctation or AV shunt, pheochromocytoma, dissecting aortic aneurysm

Precautions: Tachycardia, fluid, electrolyte imbalances, pregnancy (C), lactation, impaired cerebral or cardiac circulation, children

Pharmacokinetics:
IV: Onset 1-2 min, peak 5 min, duration 3-12 hr; half-life 20-36 hr, excreted slowly in urine, crosses blood-brain barrier, placenta

Interactions:
• Increased hyperuricemic, antihypertensive effects of diazoxide: thiazide diuretics
• Hyperglycemia: sulfonylureas
• Decreased anticonvulsant effect: hydantoins

NURSING CONSIDERATIONS
Assess:
• B/P q5min until stabilized, then q1h × 2 hr, then q4h
• Pulse, jugular venous distention q4h
• Electrolytes, blood studies: K, Na, Cl, CO_2, CBC, serum glucose
• Weight daily, I&O
• Edema in feet, legs daily
• Skin turgor, dryness of mucous membranes for hydration status
• Rales, dyspnea, orthopnea
• IV site for extravasation, rate
• Signs of CHF: dyspnea, edema, wet rales
• Postural hypotension, take B/P sitting, standing
Administer:
• Undiluted; give over ½ min or less
• To patient in recumbent position; keep in that position for 1 hr after administration
Syringe compatibilities: Heparin
Perform/provide:
• Protection from light
Evaluate:
• Therapeutic response: decreased B/P, primarily diastolic pressure
Treatment of overdose: Dopamine, or norepinephrine for hypotension, Trendelenburg maneuver

---

diazoxide (oral) (℞)
(dye-az-ox′ide)
Proglycem
Func. class.: Hyperglycemic
Chem. class.: Benzothiadiazine

Action: Decreases release of insulin from β-cells in pancreas, increasing blood glucose
Uses: Hypoglycemia caused by hyperinsulinism
Dosage and routes:
• *Adult and child:* **PO** 3-8 mg/kg/day in 2-3 divided doses q8-12h

• *Infant and neonate:* **PO** 8-15 mg/kg/day in 2-3 divided doses q8-12h
Available forms: Caps 50 mg; oral susp 50 mg/ml
Side effects/adverse reactions:
GU: Reversible nephrotic syndrome, decreased urinary output, hematuria
CNS: Headache, weakness, malaise, anxiety, dizziness, insomnia, paresthesia
EENT: Diplopia, cataracts, ring scotoma, subconjunctival hemorrhage, lacrimation
HEMA: **Thrombocytopenia, leukopenia,** eosinophilia, decreased Hgb, Hct
INTEG: Increased hair growth or loss of scalp hair, rash, dermatitis, herpes
GI: Nausea, vomiting, anorexia, abdominal pain, transient loss of taste, diarrhea
CV: Tachycardia, palpitations, hypotension, transient hypertension
META: Hyperuricemia, sodium/fluid retention, ketoacidosis, hyperglycemia, azotemia
Contraindications: Hypersensitivity to this drug or thiazides, functional hypoglycemia
Precautions: Pregnancy (C), lactation, renal disease, diabetes mellitus, CV disease, gout
Pharmacokinetics:
PO: Onset 1 hr, duration 8 hr, half-life 28 hr; excreted unchanged by kidneys; crosses blood-brain barrier, placenta
Interactions:
• Increased effects of diazoxide: phenothiazines, thiazide diuretics
• Decreased effects of phenytoin
• Increased effects of antihypertensives, oral anticoagulants
• Decreased effects of diazoxide: α-adrenergic blockers, sulfonylureas, insulin

---

Side effects: *italics* = common; ***bold italics*** = life-threatening

Lab test interferences:
Increase: Bilirubin, uric acid, blood glucose
Decrease: Creatinine, Hgb, Hct, plasma-free fatty acids

NURSING CONSIDERATIONS
Assess:
• I&O ratio, weight weekly
• Electrolytes (K, Na, Cl), glucose, Hct, Hgb, platelets, differential
• Urine for glucose, ketones qd
Administer:
• Shake susp before using
Perform/provide:
• Susp storage: protect from light
Evaluate:
• Therapeutic response: adequate blood, urine glucose, absence of ketones in urine
Teach patient/family:
• That if not effective within 2-3 wk, drug may be discontinued
• That any hirsutism is reversible after discontinuing treatment

---

diclofenac (℞)

(dye-kloe'fen-ak)
Cataflam, Voltaren, Voltaren SR
Func. class.: Nonsteroidal antiinflammatory
Chem. class.: Phenylacetic acid

Action: Inhibits prostaglandin synthesis by decreasing enzyme needed for biosynthesis; analgesic, antiinflammatory, antipyretic
Uses: Acute, chronic rheumatoid arthritis, osteoarthritis; ankylosing spondylitis, analgesia, primary dysmenorrhea; ophth: postoperative inflammation after cataract extraction
Dosage and routes:
Osteoarthritis
• *Adult:* PO 100-150 mg/day in 2-3 divided doses
Rheumatoid arthritis
• *Adult:* PO 150-200 mg/day in 2-4 divided doses

Ankylosing spondylitis
• *Adult:* PO 100-125 mg/day in 4-5 divided doses, give 25 mg qid and 25 mg hs if needed
Postcataract surgery
• *Adult:* OPHTH 1 gtt of 0.1% sol qid × 2 wk 24 hr post surgery
Analgesia/primary dysmenorrhea
• *Adult:* PO 50 mg tid, max 150 mg/day (potassium tab only)
Available forms: Tabs enteric coated 25, 50, 75 mg tabs, del rel 25, 50, 75, 100 mg; tabs 50 mg (potassium); ophth sol 1%
Side effects/adverse reactions:
GI: Nausea, anorexia, vomiting, diarrhea, *jaundice, cholestatic hepatitis,* constipation, flatulence, cramps, dry mouth, peptic ulcer, GI bleeding
CNS: Dizziness, drowsiness, fatigue, tremors, confusion, insomnia, anxiety, depression, nervousness, paresthesia, muscle weakness
CV: *CHF,* tachycardia, peripheral edema, palpitations, *dysrhythmias,* hypotension, hypertension, fluid retention
INTEG: Purpura, rash, pruritus, sweating, erythema, petechiae, photosensitivity, alopecia
GU: *Nephrotoxicity: dysuria, hematuria, oliguria, azotemia, cystitis, UTI*
HEMA: *Blood dyscrasias,* epistaxis, bruising
EENT: Tinnitus, hearing loss, blurred vision
RESP: Dyspnea, hemoptysis, pharyngitis, *bronchospasm, laryngeal edema,* rhinitis, shortness of breath
Contraindications: Hypersensitivity to aspirin, iodides, other nonsteroidal antiinflammatory agents, asthma
Precautions: Pregnancy (B) 1st, 2nd trimester; lactation, children, bleeding disorders, GI disorders, cardiac disorders, hypersensitivity to other

---

antiinflammatory agents, CrCl <30 ml/min

Pharmacokinetics:

PO: Peak 2-3 hr, elimination half-life 1-2 hr, 90% bound to plasma proteins, metabolized in liver to metabolite, excreted in urine

Interactions:

• Decreased antihypertensive effect: β-blockers, diuretics

• Increased anticoagulant effect: coumadin

• Increased toxicity: phenytoin, sulfonamides, sulfonylurea, digoxin, lithium

• Increased GI side effects: alcohol, aspirin, other NSAIDs, colchicine, glucocorticoids

• Increased plasma levels of diclofenac: probenecid, K-sparing diuretics

NURSING CONSIDERATIONS
Assess:

• Blood counts during therapy; watch for decreasing platelets; if low, therapy may need to be discontinued, restarted after hematologic recovery

• LFTs and uric acid periodically

◆ Blood dyscrasias (thrombocytopenia): bruising, fatigue, bleeding, poor healing

Evaluate:

• Therapeutic response: decreased inflammation in joints

Teach patient/family:

• That drug must be continued for prescribed time to be effective

• To report bleeding, bruising, fatigue, malaise; blood dyscrasias do occur

Ⓧ Not to break, crush, or chew enteric products

• To avoid aspirin, alcoholic beverages

• To take with food, milk, or antacids to avoid GI upset, to swallow whole

• To use caution when driving; drowsiness, dizziness may occur

• To take with a full glass of water to enhance absorption

---

dicloxacillin (℞)

(dye-klox-a-sill'-in)
Dicloxacillin sodium, Dycill, Dynapen, Pathocil
Func. class.: Antiinfective
Chem. class.: Penicillinase-resistant penicillin

Action: Interferes with cell wall replication of susceptible organisms; osmotically unstable cell wall swells, bursts from osmotic pressure

Uses: Effective for gram-positive cocci *(S. aureus, S. pyogenes, S. viridans, S. faecalis, S. bovis, S. pneumoniae)*, infections caused by penicillinase-producing *Staphylococcus*

Dosage and routes:

• *Adult:* PO 0.5-4 g/day in divided doses q6h

• *Child:* PO 12.5-50 mg/kg in divided doses q6h, max 4 g/day

Available forms: Caps 125, 250, 500 mg; powder for oral susp 62.5 mg/5 ml

Side effects/adverse reactions:

HEMA: Anemia, increased bleeding time, ***bone marrow depression, granulocytopenia***

GI: Nausea, vomiting, diarrhea, increased AST (SGOT), ALT (SGPT), abdominal pain, glossitis, pseudomembranous colitis

*GU: **Oliguria, proteinuria, hematuria,** vaginitis, moniliasis, **glomerulonephritis***

CNS: Lethargy, hallucinations, anxiety, depression, twitching, ***coma, convulsions***

*SYST: **Anaphylaxis***

Contraindications: Hypersensitivity to penicillins; neonates

Precautions: Hypersensitivity to cephalosporins, pregnancy (B), lactation, severe renal or hepatic disease

Pharmacokinetics:

PO: Peak 1 hr, duration 4-6 hr, half-life 30-60 min; metabolized in liver; excreted in urine, bile, breast milk; crosses placenta

Interactions:

• Increased dicloxacillin concentrations: aspirin, probenecid, disulfiram

• Increased effect of anticoagulants

• Decreased action of oral contraceptives

Lab test interferences:

False positive: Urine glucose, urine protein

NURSING CONSIDERATIONS

Assess:

• I&O ratio; report hematuria, oliguria, since penicillin in high doses is nephrotoxic

◆▶ Any patient with compromised renal system, since drug is excreted slowly in poor renal system function; toxicity may occur rapidly

• Blood studies: WBC, RBC, Hgb, Hct, bleeding time

• Renal studies: urinalysis, protein, blood

• C&S before drug therapy; drug may be given as soon as culture is taken

• WBC and differential, ALT (SGOT), AST (SGPT), BUN, creatinine for patients on long-term therapy

• Bowel pattern before, during treatment

• Skin eruptions after administration of penicillin to 1 wk after discontinuing drug

• Respiratory status: rate, character, wheezing, tightness in chest

• Allergies before initiation of treatment, reaction of each medication; highlight allergies on chart in red

Administer:

• Drug after C&S

• On an empty stomach with a full glass of water

• Susp after shaking well before each dose

Perform/provide:

• Adrenalin, suction, tracheostomy set, endotracheal intubation equipment

• Adequate fluid intake (2 L) during diarrhea episodes

• Scratch test to assess allergy after securing order from prescriber; usually done when penicillin is only drug of choice

• Storage in tight container; after reconstituting, store in refrigerator up to 2 wk

Evaluate:

• Therapeutic response: absence of fever, draining wounds

Teach patient/family:

• All aspects of drug therapy, including need to complete course of medication to ensure organism death (10-14 days); culture may be taken after completed course

• To report sore throat, fever, fatigue; may indicate superinfection

🚫 Not to break, crush, or chew caps

• To wear or carry Medic Alert ID if allergic to penicillins

• To notify nurse of diarrhea

Treatment of anaphylaxis: Withdraw drug; maintain airway; administer epinephrine, aminophylline, O_2, IV corticosteroids

---

dicyclomine (℞)

(dye-sye′kloe-meen)
Antispas, Bentyl, Bentylol*, Byclomine, Dibent, Dicyclomine HCL, Di-Spaz, Formulex*, Neoquess, OR-Tyl, Spasmoject, Viserol

Func. class.: Gastrointestinal anticholinergic

Chem. class.: Synthetic tertiary amine

Action: Inhibits muscarinic actions of acetylcholine at postganglionic parasympathetic neuroeffector sites

Uses: Treatment of peptic ulcer disease in combination with other drugs; infant colic, urinary incontinence

Dosage and routes:
• *Adult:* PO 10-20 mg tid-qid; IM 20 mg q4-6h
• *Child >2 yr:* PO 10 mg tid-qid
• *Child 6 mo-2 yr:* PO 5 mg tid-qid
Available forms: Caps 10, 20 mg; tabs 20 mg; syr 10 mg/5 ml; inj 10 mg/ml

Side effects/adverse reactions:

CNS: Confusion, stimulation in elderly, headache, insomnia, dizziness, drowsiness, anxiety, weakness, hallucination; *seizures, coma* (child <3 mo)

GI: Dry mouth, constipation, paralytic ileus, heartburn, nausea, vomiting, dysphagia, absence of taste

GU: Hesitancy, retention, impotence

CV: Palpitations, tachycardia

EENT: Blurred vision, photophobia, mydriasis, cycloplegia, increased ocular tension

INTEG: Urticaria, rash, pruritus, anhidrosis, fever, allergic reactions

Contraindications: Hypersensitivity to anticholinergics, narrow-angle glaucoma, GI obstruction, myasthenia gravis, paralytic ileus, GI atony, toxic megacolon

Precautions: Hyperthyroidism, coronary artery disease, dysrhythmias, CHF, ulcerative colitis, hypertension, hiatal hernia, hepatic disease, renal disease, pregnancy (B), lactation, urinary retention, prostatic hypertrophy

Pharmacokinetics:

PO: Onset 1-2 hr, duration 3-4 hr; metabolized by liver; excreted in urine

Interactions:
• Increased anticholinergic effect: amantadine, tricylic antidepressants, MAOIs, H_1-antihistamines
• Decreased effect of phenothiazines, levodopa, ketoconazole

NURSING CONSIDERATIONS

Assess:
• VS, cardiac status: checking for dysrhythmias, increased rate, palpitations
• I&O ratio, check for urinary retention or hesitancy
• GI complaints: pain, bleeding (frank or occult), nausea, vomiting, anorexia
• Anticholinergic effects in the elderly: urinary retention, constipation, delirium

Administer:
• ½-1 hr ac for better absorption
• Decreased dose to elderly patients; metabolism may be slowed
• Gum, hard candy, frequent rinsing of mouth for dry oral cavity

Perform/provide:
• Storage in tight container protected from light
• Increased fluids, bulk, exercise to decrease constipation

Evaluate:
• Therapeutic response: absence of epigastric pain, bleeding, nausea, vomiting

Teach patient/family:

🚫 Not to break, crush, or chew caps

• To avoid driving, other hazardous activities until stabilized on medication; may cause blurred vision

• To avoid alcohol, other CNS depressants; will enhance sedating properties of this drug

• To avoid hot environments; stroke may occur; drug suppresses perspiration

• To use sunglasses when outside to prevent photophobia

• To drink plenty of fluids

• To report dysphagia

---

didanosine (℞)

(dye-dan′oh-seen)

ddI, Dideoxyinosine, Videx

Func. class.: Antiviral

Chem. class.: Synthetic purine nucleoside of deoxyadenosine

Action: Nucleoside analog incorporating into cellular DNA by viral reverse transcriptase, thereby terminating the cellular DNA chain

Uses: Advanced HIV, AIDS infections in adults and children who have been unable to use zidovudine or who have not responded to treatment

Dosage and routes:

• Reduce dosage CrCl <60 ml/min

• *Adult:* **PO** >75 kg, 300 mg bid tabs, or 375 mg bid buffered pwd; 50-74 kg, 200 mg bid tabs, or 250 mg bid buffered pwd; 35-49 kg, 125 mg bid tabs, or 167 mg bid buffered pwd

• *Child:* **PO** tabs 90-120 mg/m^2 q12h; buffered pwd packets 112.5-150 mg/m^2 q12h; **PO** (child BSA 1.1-1.4 m^2) tab 100 mg q8-12h; recon pedi pwd 125 mg q8-12h; **PO** (child BSA 0.8-1 m^2) tabs 75 mg

q8-12h; recon pedi pwd 94 mg q8-12h; **PO** (child BSA 0.5-0.7 m^2) tabs 50 mg q8-12h; recon pedi pwd 62 mg q8-12h; **PO** (child BSA <0.4 m^2) tabs 25 mg q8-12h; recon pedi pwd 31 mg q8-12h

Available forms: Tabs, buffered, chewable/dispersible 25, 50, 100, 150 mg; pwd for oral sol, buffered 100, 167, 250, 375 mg; pwd for oral sol, pedi 2, 4 g

Side effects/adverse reactions:

*GI: **Pancreatitis**, diarrhea, nausea, vomiting, abdominal pain,* constipation, stomatitis, dyspepsia, liver abnormalities, flatulence, taste perversion, dry mouth, oral thrush, melena, increased ALT, AST, alk phosphatase, amylase

GU: Increased bilirubin, uric acid

*CNS: **Peripheral neuropathy, seizures**, confusion, anxiety,* hypertonia, abnormal thinking, asthenia, *insomnia, **CNS depression**, pain,* dizziness, chills, fever

RESP: Cough, pneumonia, dyspnea, asthma, epistaxis, hypoventilation, sinusitis

INTEG: Rash, pruritus, alopecia, ecchymosis, hemorrhage, petechiae, sweating

MS: Myalgia, arthritis, myopathy, muscular atrophy

CV: Hypertension, vasodilation, dysrhythmia, syncope, CHF, palpitation

EENT: Ear pain, otitis, photophobia, visual impairment, retinal depigmentation

*HEMA: **Leukopenia, granulocytopenia, thrombocytopenia, anemia***

Contraindications: Hypersensitivity

Precautions: Renal, hepatic disease, pregnancy (B), lactation, children, sodium-restricted diets, elevated amylase, preexistant peripheral neuropathy, phenylketonuria, hyperuricemia

---

➡ = Nursing alert   ⬦ = Herb-drug interaction   🚫 = Do not crush

Pharmacokinetics:
PO: Elimination half-life 1.62 hr, extensive metabolism is thought to occur; administration within 5 min of food will decrease absorption

Interactions:
• Decreased absorption: ketoconazole, dapsone, food
• Do not give with tetracyclines
• Decreased concentrations of fluoroquinolone antibiotics

NURSING CONSIDERATIONS
Assess:
• Peripheral neuropathy: tingling or pain in hands and feet, distal numbness
• Pancreatitis: abdominal pain, nausea, vomiting, elevated liver enzymes; drug should be discontinued, since condition can be fatal
• Children by dilated retinal examination q6mo to rule out retinal depigmentation
• CBC, differential, platelet count qmo; withhold drug if WBC is <1000 or platelet count is <75,000; notify prescriber of results; alk phosphatase, monitor amylase
• Renal function studies: BUN, serum uric acid, urine CrCl before, during therapy
• Temp q4h, may indicate beginning infection
• Liver function tests before, during therapy (bilirubin, AST [SGOT], ALT [SGPT]) as needed or qmo

Administer:
• Antibiotics for prophylaxis of infection

Perform/provide:
• Strict medical asepsis, protective isolation if WBC levels are low
• Cleanup of powdered products; use wet mop or damp sponge

Evaluate:
• Therapeutic response: absence of infection; symptoms of HIV

Teach patient/family:
• To take on an empty stomach; not to take dapsone at same time as ddI; do not mix powder with fruit juice; chew tab or crush and dissolve in water; drink powder immediately after mixing
• To report signs of infection: increased temp, sore throat, flu symptoms
• To report signs of anemia: fatigue, headache, faintness, shortness of breath, irritability
• To report bleeding; avoid use of razors, commercial mouthwash
• That hair may be lost during therapy (rare); a wig or hairpiece may make patient feel better

---

dienestrol (Ⓡ)
(dye-en-ess'trole)
DV, Ortho Dienestrol
Func. class.: Estrogen
Chem class.: Nonsteroidal synthetic estrogen

Action: Needed for adequate functioning of female reproductive system, it affects release of pituitary gonadotropins, inhibits ovulation, adequate calcium use in bone structures

Uses: Atrophic vaginitis, kraurosis vulvae

Dosage and routes:
• *Adult:* **VAG CREAM** 1-2 applications qd × 2 wk, then ½ dose × 2 wk, then 1 application
Available forms: Vag cream 0.01%

Side effects/adverse reactions:
CNS: Dizziness, headache, migraines, depression
CV: Hypotension, thrombophlebitis, edema, ***thromboembolism, stroke, pulmonary embolism, myocardial infarction***
GI: Nausea, vomiting, diarrhea, anorexia, pancreatitis, cramps, constipation, increased appetite, increased weight, ***cholestatic jaundice***

EENT: Contact lens intolerance, increased myopia, astigmatism

GU: Amenorrhea, cervical erosion, breakthrough bleeding, dysmenorrhea, vaginal candidiasis, breast changes, gynecomastia, testicular atrophy, impotence

INTEG: Rash, urticaria, acne, hirsutism, alopecia, oily skin, seborrhea, purpura, melasma

META: Folic acid deficiency, hypercalcemia, hyperglycemia

Contraindications: Breast cancer, thromboembolic disorders, reproductive cancer, genital bleeding (abnormal, undiagnosed), pregnancy (X), lactation

Precautions: Hypertension, asthma, blood dyscrasias, gallbladder disease, CHF, diabetes mellitus, bone disease, depression, migraine headache, convulsive disorders, hepatic disease, renal disease, family history of cancer of the breast or reproductive tract

Pharmacokinetics:

TOP: Degraded in liver; excreted in urine; crosses placenta; excreted in breast milk

Interactions:

• Decreased action of anticoagulants, oral hypoglycemics

• Toxicity: tricyclic antidepressants

• Decreased action of dienestrol: anticonvulsants, barbiturates, phenylbutazone, rifampin

• Increased action of: corticosteroids

NURSING CONSIDERATIONS

Assess:

• Weight daily; notify prescriber of weekly weight gain >5 lb

• B/P q4h

• I&O ratio; be alert for decreasing urinary output and increasing edema

• Liver function studies including ALT (SGOT), AST (SGPT), bilirubin

• Edema, hypertension, cardiac symptoms, jaundice

• Mental status: affect, mood, behavioral changes, aggression

• Hypercalcemia

Administer:

• At hs for better absorption

• Titrated dose; use lowest effective dose to prevent adverse reactions

• Dosage reduction should continue at 3-6 mo intervals

Perform/provide:

• Storage in tight, light-resistant container in refrigerator

Evaluate:

• Therapeutic response: decreased symptoms of vaginitis, kraurosis

Teach patient/family:

• How to fill applicator and insert cream

• To check with prescriber before using any OTC drugs

• To report breast lumps, vaginal bleeding, edema, jaundice, dark urine, clay-colored stools, dyspnea, headache, blurred vision, abdominal pain, numbness or stiffness in legs, chest pain

• To stop using product and report to prescriber if pregnancy is suspected

---

diethylstilbestrol/diethylstilbestrol diphosphate (℞)

(dye-eth-il-stil-bess′trole)

DES, diethylstilbestrol, Honvol*, Stilphostrol

Func. class.: Estrogen

Chem. class.: Nonsteroidal synthetic estrogen

Action: Needed for adequate functioning of female reproductive sys-

---

 = Nursing alert   = Herb-drug interaction   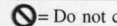 = Do not crush tem, it affects release of pituitary gonadotropins, inhibits ovulation, adequate calcium use in bone structures

Uses: Breast cancer, prostatic cancer, vasomotor symptoms of menopause

Dosage and routes:

Prostatic cancer
• *Adult:* PO 1-3 mg qd, then 1 mg qd; PO 50-200 mg tid (diphosphate); IM 5 mg 2×/wk, then 4 mg 2×/wk; IV 500 mg-1 g qd × 5 days, then 250-500 mg 1-2×/wk

Breast cancer (postmenopausal)
• *Adult:* PO 15 mg qd

Available forms: Tabs 1, 5 mg; diethylstilbestrol diphosphate tab 50 mg; inj 0.25 g

Side effects/adverse reactions:

CNS: Dizziness, headache, migraines, depression

CV: Hypotension, thrombophlebitis, edema, ***thromboembolism, stroke, pulmonary embolism, myocardial infarction***

GI: Nausea, vomiting, diarrhea, anorexia, pancreatitis, cramps, constipation, increased appetite, increased weight, ***cholestatic jaundice***

EENT: Contact lens intolerance, increased myopia, astigmatism

GU: Amenorrhea, cervical erosion, breakthrough bleeding, dysmenorrhea, vaginal candidiasis, breast changes, gynecomastia, testicular atrophy, impotence, ***endometrial cancer***

INTEG: Rash, urticaria, acne, hirsutism, alopecia, oily skin, seborrhea, purpura, melasma

META: Folic acid deficiency, hypercalcemia, hyperglycemia

Contraindications: Premenopausal breast cancer, thromboembolic disorders, reproductive cancer, genital bleeding (abnormal, undiagnosed), pregnancy (X), lactation

Precautions: Hypertension, asthma, blood dyscrasias, gallbladder disease, CHF, diabetes mellitus, bone disease blocking agents, MI

Interactions:
• Decreased action of anticoagulants, oral hypoglycemics
• Toxicity: tricyclic antidepressants
• Decreased action of diethylstilbestrol: anticonvulsants, barbiturates, phenylbutazone, rifampin
• Increased action of corticosteroids
🍴 Possible additive hormonal effect: alfalfa

Lab test interferences:

Increase: BSP retention test, PBI, T_4, serum Na, platelet aggregability, thyroxine-binding globulin (TBG), prothrombin; factors VII, VIII, IX, X; triglycerides

Decrease: Serum folate, serum triglyceride, T_3 resin uptake test, glucose tolerance test, antithrombin III, pregnanediol, metyrapone test

False positive: LE prep, antinuclear antibodies

NURSING CONSIDERATIONS

Assess:
• Urine glucose in patient with diabetes; urine glucose may rise
• If female patient has an intact uterus
• Weight daily, notify prescriber of weekly weight gain >5 lb; if increase, diuretic may be ordered
• B/P q4h, watch for increase caused by H_2O and Na retention
• I&O ratio; be alert for decreasing urinary output and increasing edema
• Liver function studies, including AST (SGOT), ALT (SGPT), bilirubin, alk phosphatase
• Edema, hypertension, cardiac symptoms, jaundice
• Mental status: affect, mood, behavioral changes, aggression

Administer:
• IV after diluting in 300 ml dextrose or NS sol; give at 1-2 ml/min

× 15 min; may increase rate to complete infusion 1 hr after starting

• Titrated dose; use lowest effective dose

• In one dose in AM for prostatic cancer

• With food, milk for GI symptoms

• With a progesterone for 10-13 day/mo for female patients with an intact uterus

Evaluate:

• Therapeutic response: absence of breast engorgement, reversal of menopause or decrease in tumor size in prostatic cancer

Teach patient/family:

• To weigh weekly, report gain >5 lb

• To report breast lumps, vaginal bleeding, edema, jaundice, dark urine, clay-colored stools, dyspnea, headache, blurred vision, abdominal pain, numbness or stiffness in legs, chest pain; male to report impotence or gynecomastia

• To check with prescriber before taking any OTC drugs

---

difenoxin/atropine sulfate diphenoxylate/ atropine (℞)

(dye-fen-ox′in)

Diphenatol, Lofene, Logene, Lomanate, Lomotil, Lo-Trol, Motofen, Nor-Mil

Func. class.: Antidiarrheal

Chem. class.: Phenylpiperidine derivative opiate agonist

Controlled Substance Schedule IV (difenoxin); V diphenoxylate

Action: Inhibits gastric motility by acting on mucosal receptors responsible for peristalsis

Uses: Acute nonspecific and acute exacerbations of chronic functional diarrhea

Dosage and routes:

• *Adult:* **PO** 2.5-5 mg qid titrated to patient response needed, not to exceed 8 tabs/24 hr

• *Child 2-12 yr:* **PO** 0.3-0.4 mg/kg/ day in divided dose

Available forms: Tabs 1 mg difenoxin HCl, 0.025 mg atropine; tabs 2.5 mg diphenoxylate/0.025 mg atropine; liq 2.5 mg diphenoxylate/ 0.025 mg atropine/5 ml

Side effects/adverse reactions:

CNS: Dizziness, drowsiness, lightheadedness, headache, fatigue, nervousness, insomnia, confusion

GI: Nausea, vomiting, dry mouth, epigastric distress, constipation

EENT: Burning eyes, blurred vision

Contraindications: Hypersensitivity, pseudomembranous enterocolitis, jaundice, glaucoma, child <2 yr, severe electrolyte imbalances, diarrhea associated with organisms that penetrate intestinal mucosa

Precautions: Hepatic disease, renal disease, ulcerative colitis, pregnancy (C), lactation, severe liver disease

Pharmacokinetics:

PO: Onset 40-60 min, peak 2 hr, duration 3-4 hr, terminal half-life 12-14 hr; metabolized in liver to inactive metabolite; excreted in urine, feces

Interactions:

• Do not use with MAOIs; hypertensive crisis may occur

• Increased action of alcohol, narcotics, barbiturates, other CNS depressants, anticholinergics

NURSING CONSIDERATIONS

Assess:

• Electrolytes (K, Na, Cl) if on long-term therapy

• Bowel pattern before; for rebound constipation after termination of medication; bowel sounds

---

• Response after 48 hr; if none, drug should be discontinued
• Abdominal distention, toxic megacolon, which may occur in ulcerative colitis

Administer:
• For 48 hr only; if no response, drug should be discontinued

Evaluate:
• Therapeutic response: decreased diarrhea

Teach patient/family:
• To avoid OTC products unless directed by prescriber; may contain alcohol
• Not to exceed recommended dose
• That drug may be habit forming
• Not to engage in hazardous activities; drowsiness may occur

---

diflunisal (R)

(dye-floo'ni-sal)
Diflunisal, Dolobid
Func. class.: Nonsteroidal antiinflammatory/analgesic (nonopioid)
Chem. class.: Salicylate derivative

Action: May block pain impulses in CNS that occur in response to inhibition of prostaglandin synthesis; antipyretic action results from inhibition of hypothalamic heatregulating center to produce vasodilation to allow heat dissipation

Uses: Mild to moderate pain or fever including arthritis; 3-4 times more potent than aspirin

Dosage and routes:
Pain/fever
• *Adult:* PO loading dose 1 g; then 500-1000 mg/day in 2 divided doses, q12h, not to exceed 1500 mg/day
Available forms: Tabs 250, 500 mg

Side effects/adverse reactions:
HEMA: Thrombocytopenia, agranu-locytosis, leukopenia, neutropenia, hemolytic anemia, increased protime
CNS: Stimulation, drowsiness, dizziness, confusion, *convulsions,* headache, flushing, hallucinations, coma
GI: Nausea, vomiting, GI bleeding, diarrhea, heartburn, anorexia, *hepatitis*
INTEG: Rash, urticaria, bruising
EENT: Blurred vision, decreased acuity, corneal deposits
CV: Rapid pulse, *pulmonary edema*
RESP: Wheezing, hyperpnea
ENDO: Hypoglycemia, hyponatremia, hypokalemia

Contraindications: Hypersensitivity to salicylates, GI bleeding, bleeding disorders, children <12 yr, vit K deficiency

Precautions: Anemia, hepatic disease, renal disease, Hodgkin's disease, pregnancy (C), lactation

Pharmacokinetics:
PO: Onset 15-30 min, peak 2-3 hr, half-life 10-12 hr; metabolized by liver; excreted by kidneys; crosses placenta; 99% protein bound; excreted in breast milk

Interactions:
• Decreased effects of diflunisal: antacids, steroids, urinary alkalizers
• Increased blood loss: alcohol, heparin
• Increased effects of anticoagulants, insulin, methotrexate, hydrochlorothiazide, acetaminophen
• Decreased effects of probenecid, spironolactone, sulfinpyrazone, sulfa drugs
• Toxic effects: PABA
• Decreased blood sugar levels: salicylates

Lab test interferences:
Increase: Coagulation, liver function studies, serum uric acid, amylase, CO_2, urinary protein

---

Decrease: Serum K, PBI, cholesterol

Interference: Urine catecholamines, pregnancy test

NURSING CONSIDERATIONS
Assess:

• Pain: frequency, intensity, characteristics, relief after med
• Liver function studies: AST (SGOT), ALT (SGPT), bilirubin, creatinine (long-term therapy)
• Renal function studies: BUN, urine creatinine (long-term therapy)
• Blood studies: CBC, Hct, Hgb, pro-time (long-term therapy)
• I&O ratio; decreasing output may indicate renal failure (long-term therapy)
• For asthma, aspirin hypersensitivity, nasal polyps that may develop hypersensitivity reactions
• Hepatotoxicity: dark urine; clay-colored stools; yellowing of skin, sclera; itching; abdominal pain; fever; diarrhea (long-term therapy)
• Allergic reactions: rash, urticaria; drug may have to be discontinued
• Renal dysfunction: decreased urine output
• Ototoxicity: tinnitus, ringing, roaring in ears; audiometric testing is needed before, after long-term therapy
• Visual changes: blurring, halos, corneal, retinal damage
• Edema in feet, ankles, legs
• Drug history; many interactions

Administer:

• To patient whole
• With food, milk for gastric symptoms

Evaluate:

• Therapeutic response: decreased pain, stiffness of joints

Teach patient/family:

◆ To report any symptoms of hepatotoxicity, renal toxicity, visual changes, ototoxicity, allergic reactions (long-term therapy)

• Not to exceed recommended dosage; acute poisoning may result
• To read label on other OTC drugs; many contain aspirin
• That therapeutic response takes 2 wk (arthritis)
• To avoid alcohol ingestion; GI bleeding may occur

Treatment of overdose: Lavage, activated charcoal, monitor electrolytes, VS

---

digitoxin (℞)
(di-ji-tox′in)
Crystodigin, digitoxin
Func. class.: Antidysrhythmic, cardiac glycoside, cardiotonic
Chem. class.: Digitalis preparation

Action: Inhibits sodium-potassium ATPase, which makes more calcium available for contractile proteins, resulting in increased cardiac output

Uses: CHF, atrial fibrillation, atrial flutter, atrial tachycardia

Dosage and routes:

• *Adult and child >12 yr:* **PO** 1.2-1.6 mg initially (loading); give in divided doses over 24 hr; 150 µg qd; maintenance dose: 0.05-0.3 mg qd, usual 0.15 mg qd; rapid loading dose 0.6 mg, then 0.4 mg, then 0.2 mg q4-6h; slow loading dose 0.2 mg/bid × 4 days, then maintenance
• *Child <1 yr:* 0.045 mg/kg
• *Child 1-2 yr:* 0.04 mg/kg
• *Child >2 yr:* 0.03 mg/kg (0.75 mg/m²); maintenance: 10% of digitalizing dose

Available forms: Tabs 100 (0.1 mg), 200 µg (0.2 mg)

Side effects/adverse reactions:
CNS: Headache, drowsiness, apa-

thy, confusion, disorientation, fatigue, depression, hallucinations

CV: **Dysrhythmias,** *hypotension, bradycardia,* **AV block**

GI: Nausea, vomiting, anorexia, abdominal pain, diarrhea

EENT: Blurred vision, yellow-green halos, photophobia, diplopia

MS: Muscular weakness

Contraindications: Hypersensitivity to digitalis, ventricular fibrillation, ventricular tachycardia, carotid sinus syndrome, 2nd- or 3rd-degree heart block

Precautions: Hepatic disease, acute MI, AV block, hypokalemia, hypomagnesemia, sinus node disease, lactation, severe respiratory disease, hypothyroidism, elderly, pregnancy (C), lactation

Pharmacokinetics:
PO: Onset 1-4 hr, peak 4-12 hr; duration 2-3 wk, half-life 4-20 days; metabolized in liver; excreted in urine

Interactions:
• Hypokalemia: thiazides
• Increased blood levels: spironolactone
• Decreased effects: hydantoins, aminoglutethimide, rifampin, phenylbutazone, barbiturates, cholestyramine, colestipol
• Toxicity: adrenergics, diuretics, succinylcholine, quinidine, thioamines
• Decreased level of digitoxin: thyroid agents
🌿 Increased action: aloe, buckthorn bark/berry, cascara sagrada bark, senna pod/leaf
🌿 Dysrhythmias: ephedra
🌿 Bradycardia: Indian snakeroot

Lab test interferences:
Increase: CPK

NURSING CONSIDERATIONS
Assess:
• Apical pulse for 1 min before giving drug; if pulse <60, take again in 1 hr; if <60, call prescriber
• Electrolytes: K, Na, Cl, Ca; renal function studies: BUN, creatinine; blood studies: ALT (SGOT), AST (SGPT), bilirubin
• Monitor drug levels (therapeutic level 9-25 ng/ml)
• Cardiac status: apical pulse, character, rate, rhythm

Administer:
• K supplements if ordered for K levels <3.0 mg/dl

Evaluate:
• Therapeutic response: decreased weight, edema, pulse, respiration and increased urine output

Teach patient/family:
• Not to stop drug abruptly; teach all aspects of drug, digitalis toxicity; to keep tabs in container protected from light
• To avoid OTC medications; many adverse interactions
• To notify prescriber of loss of appetite, lower stomach pain, diarrhea, weakness, drowsiness, headache, blurred or yellow vision, rash, depression

Treatment of overdose: Discontinue drug, administer K, digoxin immune FAB, monitor ECG

---

digoxin (℞)
(di-jox'in)
digoxin, Lanoxicaps, Lanoxin
Func. class.: Inotropic, antidysrhythmic, cardiac glycoside
Chem. class.: Digitalis preparation

Action: Inhibits the sodium-potassium ATPase, which makes more calcium available for contractile proteins, resulting in increased cardiac output

---

Uses: CHF, atrial fibrillation, atrial flutter, atrial tachycardia, cardiogenic shock, paroxysmal atrial tachycardia, rapid digitalization in these disorders

Dosage and routes:

• *Adult:* **IV** *digitalizing dose* 0.6-1.0 mg (10-15 µg/kg) given as 50% of the dose initially, additional fractions given at 4-8 hr intervals; **PO** *digitalizing dose* 0.75-1.25 mg (10-15 mg/kg) given as 50% of the dose initially, additional fractions given at 4-8 hr intervals; *maintenance* 0.063-0.5 mg/day (tabs), or 0.350-0.5 mg/day (gelatin cap)

• *Child >10 yr:* **IV** *digitalizing dose* 8-12 µg/kg given as 50% of the dose initially, additional fractions given at 4-8 hr intervals; **PO** *digitalizing dose* 10-15 µg/kg given as 50% of the dose initially, additional fractions given at 6-8 hr intervals; *maintenance* 25%-35% of the loading dose qd as a single dose

• *Child 5-10 yr:* **IV** *digitalizing dose* 15-30 µg/kg given as 50% of the dose initially, additional fractions given at 4-8 hr intervals; **PO** *digitalizing dose* 20-35 µg/kg given as 50% of the dose initially, additional fractions given at 6-8 hr intervals; *maintenance* 25%-35% of the loading dose qd in 2 divided doses

• *Child 2-5 yr:* **IV** *digitalizing dose* 25-35 µg/kg given as 50% of the dose initially, additional fractions given at 4-8 hr intervals; **PO** *digitalizing dose* 30-40 µg/kg given as 50% of the dose initially, additional fractions given at 6-8 hr intervals; *maintenance* 25%-35% of the loading dose qd in 2 divided doses

• *Child 1-2 yr:* **IV** *digitalizing dose* 30-50 µg/kg given as 50% of the dose initially, additional fractions given at 4-8 hr intervals; **PO** *digitalizing dose* 35-60 µg/kg given as 50% of the dose initially, additional fractions given at 4-8 hr intervals; *maintenance* 25%-35% of the loading dose qd in 2 divided doses

• *Infants:* **IV** *digitalizing dose* 20-30 µg/kg given as 50% of the dose initially, additional fractions given at 4-8 hr intervals; **PO** *digitalizing dose* 25-35 µg/kg given as 50% of the dose initially, additional fractions given at 6-8 hr intervals; *maintenance* 25%-35% of the loading dose qd in 2 divided doses

• *Infants, premature:* **IV** *digitalizing dose* 15-25 µg/kg given as 50% of the dose initially, additional fractions given at 4-8 hr intervals; **PO** *digitalizing dose* 20-30 µg/kg given as 50% of the dose initially, additional fractions given at 6-8 hr intervals; *maintenance* 20%-30% of the loading dose qd in 2 divided doses

Available forms: Caps 50, 100, 200 µg; elix 50 µg/ml; tabs 125, 250, 500 µg; inj 250 µg/ml: pediatric inj 100 µg/ml

Side effects/adverse reactions:

CNS: **Headache**, drowsiness, apathy, confusion, disorientation, fatigue, depression, hallucinations

CV: **Dysrhythmias,** *hypotension,* bradycardia, **AV block**

EENT: Blurred vision, yellow-green halos, photophobia, diplopia

GI: Nausea, vomiting, anorexia, abdominal pain, diarrhea

Contraindications: Hypersensitivity to digitalis, ventricular fibrillation, ventricular tachycardia, carotid sinus syndrome, 2nd or 3rd degree heart block

Precautions: Renal disease, acute MI, AV block, severe respiratory disease, hypothyroidism, elderly, pregnancy (C), sinus nodal disease, lactation, hypokalemia

Pharmacokinetics:

PO: Onset ½-2 hr, peak 6-8 hr, duration 3-4 days

 = Nursing alert   = Herb-drug interaction   = Do not crush

IV: Onset 5-30 min, peak 1-5 hr, duration variable

Half-life 1.5 days, excreted in urine

Interactions:

• Hypokalemia: diuretics, amphotericin B, carbenicillin, ticarcillin, corticosteroids, piperacillin

• Decreased digoxin level: thyroid agents

• Increased blood levels: propantheline, spironolactone quinidine, verapamil, aminoglycosides PO, amiodarone, anticholinergics, quinine, diltiazem

• Increased bradycardia: β-adrenergic blockers, antidysrythmics

• Toxicity: adrenergics, amphotericin, corticosteroids, diuretics, glucose, insulin, reserpine, succinylcholine, quinidine, thioamines

🌢 Increased action: aloe, buckthorn bark/berry, cascara sagrada bark, senna pod/leaf

🌢 Dysrhythmias. Ephedra

🌢 Bradycardia: Indian snakeroot

Lab test interferences:

Increase: CPK

NURSING CONSIDERATIONS

Assess:

• Apical pulse for 1 min before giving drug; if pulse <60 in adult or <90 in an infant, take again in 1 hr; if <60 in adult, call prescriber; note rate, rhythm, character; monitor ECG continuously during parenteral loading dose

• Electrolytes: K, Na, Cl, Mg, Ca; renal function studies: BUN, creatinine; blood studies: ALT (SGOT), AST (SGPT), bilirubin, Hct, Hgb before initiating treatment and periodically thereafter

• I&O ratio, daily weights; monitor turgor, lung sounds, edema

• Monitor drug levels (therapeutic level 0.5-2 ng/ml)

• Cardiac status: apical pulse, character, rate, rhythm

Administer:

PO

• PO with or without food; may crush tabs, mix with food/fluids

• K supplements if ordered for K levels <3, or foods high in K: bananas, orange juice

IV

• Undiluted or 1 ml of drug/4 ml sterile H_2O, D_5, or NS; give >5 min through Y-tube or 3-way stopcock; during digitalization close monitoring is necessary

Additive compatibilities: Bretylium, cimetidine, floxacillin, furosemide, lidocaine, ranitidine, verapamil

Syringe compatibilities: Heparin, milrinone

Y-site compatibilities: Amrinone, cefmetazole, ciprofloxacin, diltiazem, famotidine, heparin/hydrocortisone, meperidine, meropenem, midazolam, milrinone, morphine, potassium chloride, propofol, tacrolimus, vit B/C

Perform/provide:

• Storage protected from light

Evaluate:

• Therapeutic response: decreased weight, edema, pulse, respiration, rales; increased urine output; serum digoxin level (0.5-2 ng/ml)

Teach patient/family:

• Not to stop drug abruptly; teach all aspects of drug, to take exactly as ordered

• To avoid OTC medications, since many adverse drug interactions may occur; do not take antacid at same time

• To notify prescriber of loss of appetite, lower stomach pain, diarrhea, weakness, drowsiness, headache, blurred or yellow vision, rash, depression, toxicity

• The toxic symptoms of this drug and when to notify prescriber

• To maintain a sodium-restricted diet as ordered

🚫 Not to break, crush, or chew caps

• To report shortness of breath, difficulty breathing, weight gain, edema, persistent cough

Treatment of overdose: Discontinue drug; give K; monitor ECG; give adrenergic-blocking agent, digoxin immune FAB

---

digoxin immune FAB (ovine) (℞)

(di-jox'in im-myoon' FAB)
Digibind
Func. class.: Antidote—digoxin specific

Action: Antibody fragments bind to free digoxin to reverse digoxin toxicity by not allowing digoxin to bind to sites of action

Uses: Life-threatening digoxin or digitoxin toxicity

Dosage and routes:
Digoxin toxicity
• *Adult:* IV dose (mg) = dose ingested (mg) × serum digoxin conc × 5.6 × wt in kg ÷ 1000; if ingested amount is unknown, give 800 mg **IV;** if digoxin liquid caps, **IV,** do not multiply ingested dose by 0.8
Digitoxin
• Body load in mg = serum digitoxin conc × 0.56 × wt in kg ÷ 1000
Available forms: Inj 38 mg/vial (binds 0.5 mg digoxin or digitoxin)
Side effects/adverse reactions:
CV: CHF, ventricular rate increase, *atrial fibrillation,* low cardiac output
RESP: Impaired respiratory function, rapid respiratory rate
META: Hypokalemia
INTEG: Hypersensitivity, allergic reactions, facial swelling, redness

Contraindications: Mild digoxin toxicity, hypersensitivity
Precautions: Children, lactation, cardiac disease, renal disease, pregnancy (C)
Pharmacokinetics:
IV: Peaks after completion of infusion, onset 30 min (variable); not known if crosses placenta, breast milk; half-life biphasic—14-20 hr; prolonged in renal disease; excreted by kidneys
Interactions:
• Considered incompatible with all drugs in syringe or sol
Lab test interferences:
Interference: Immunoassay digoxin
NURSING CONSIDERATIONS
Assess:
• Hypokalemia: ST depression, flat T waves, presence of U wave, ventricular dysrhythmia; K levels may decrease rapidly
Administer:
• After diluting 38 mg/4 ml of sterile H_2O for inj 10 mg/ml mix; may be further diluted with normal saline, sol should be clear, colorless
• By bolus if cardiac arrest is imminent or IV over 30 min using a 0.22 µm filter
Perform/provide:
• Storage of reconstituted sol for up to 4 hr in refrigerator
Evaluate:
• Therapeutic response: correction of digoxin toxicity; check digoxin levels 0.5-2 ng/ml; digitoxin level 9-25 ng/ml
Teach patient/family:
• The purpose of medication; to report fever, chills, itching, swelling, dyspnea
• To tell patient to notify anyone in dental or medical care that this drug is being taken

---

◆ = Nursing alert   🖊 = Herb-drug interaction   🚫 = Do not crush

dihydroergotamine (R̥)
(dye-hye-droe-er-got′a-meen)
D.H.E. 45
Func. class.: α-Adrenergic blocker
Chem. class.: Ergot alkaloid (dihydrogenated)

Action: Constricts smooth muscle in periphery, cranial blood vessels; inhibits norepinephrine uptake

Uses: Vascular headache (migraine or histamine)

Dosage and routes:
• *Adult:* IM/IV 1 mg; may repeat q1-2h if needed, not to exceed 3 mg/day or 6 mg/wk; nasal: 1 spray in each nostril, repeat after 15 min, max 3 mg/24 hr
Available forms: Inj 1 mg/ml; nasal 4 mg/ml

Side effects/adverse reactions:
CNS: Numbness in fingers, toes, weakness
CV: Transient tachycardia, chest pain, bradycardia, increase or decrease in B/P, **gangrene**
GI: Nausea, vomiting
MS: Muscle pain

Contraindications: Hypersensitivity to ergot preparations, occlusion (peripheral, vascular), CAD, hepatic disease, pregnancy (X), renal disease, peptic ulcer, hypertension, lactation, children, uremia

Pharmacokinetics:
IM: Onset 15-30 min, peak 2 hr, duration 3-4 hr
IV: Onset 5 min, peak 45 min, duration 3-4 hr; half-life 1.3-4 hr

Interactions:
• Increased vasoconstriction: β-blockers
• Incompatible with any drug in syringe or sol

NURSING CONSIDERATIONS
Assess:
• Weight daily, check for peripheral edema in feet, legs
• For stress level, activity, recreation, coping mechanisms
• Neurologic status: LOC, blurring vision, nausea, vomiting, tingling in extremities that precede headache
• Ingestion of tyramine (pickled products, beer, wine, aged cheese), food additives, preservatives, colorings, artificial sweeteners, chocolate, caffeine; may precipitate these headaches

Administer:
• IV undiluted; give 1 mg or less/min
• At beginning of headache; dose must be titrated to patient response
• Only to women who are not pregnant; harm to fetus may occur

Perform/provide:
• Storage in dark area; do not use discolored solutions
• Quiet, calm environment with decreased stimulation for noise, bright light, excessive talking

Evaluate:
• Therapeutic response: decrease in frequency, severity of headache

Teach patient/family:
• Not to use OTC medications; serious drug interactions may occur
• To report side effects: increased vasoconstriction starting with cold extremities, then paresthesia, weakness
• That an increase in headaches may occur when this drug is discontinued after long-term use
• To keep drug out of reach of children; death may occur

dihydrotachysterol (℞)

(dye-hye-droh-tak-iss'ter-ole)
DHT, DHT Intensol, Hytakerol
Func. class.: Parathyroid agent
(calcium regulator)
Chem. class.: Vitamin D analog

Action: Increases intestinal absorption of calcium for bones, increases renal tubular absorption of phosphate; regulates calcium levels by regulating calcitonin, parathyroid hormone

Uses: Renal osteodystrophy, hypoparathyroidism, pseudohypoparathyroidism, familial hypophosphatemia, postoperative tetany

Dosage and routes:

Hypophosphatemia
• *Adult and child:* **PO** 0.5-2 mg qd, maintenance 0.3-1.5 mg qd

Hypoparathyroidism/pseudohypoparathyroidism
• *Adult:* **PO** 0.8-2.4 mg qd × 4 days, maintenance 0.2-2 mg qd regulated by serum calcium levels
• *Child:* **PO** 1-5 mg qd × 1 wk, maintenance 0.2-1 mg qd regulated by serum Ca levels

Renal osteodystrophy
• *Adult:* **PO** 0.1-0.25 mg qd, then 0.2-1 mg/day

Available forms: Tabs 0.125, 0.2, 0.4 mg; caps 0.125 mg; oral sol 0.2, 0.25 mg/5 ml

Side effects/adverse reactions:

EENT: Tinnitus
CNS: Drowsiness, headache, vertigo, fever, lethargy
GI: Nausea, diarrhea, vomiting, jaundice, anorexia, dry mouth, constipation, cramps, metallic taste
MS: Myalgia, arthralgia, decreased bone development
GU: **Polyuria,** hypercalciuria, hyperphosphatemia, *hematuria*

Contraindications: Hypersensitivity, renal disease, hyperphosphatemia, hypercalcemia

Precautions: Pregnancy (C), renal calculi, lactation, CV disease

Pharmacokinetics:
PO: Onset 2 wk; metabolized by liver, excreted in feces (active/inactive)

Interactions:
• Decreased absorption of dihydrotachysterol: cholestyramine, colestipol mineral oil
• Hypercalcemia: thiazide diuretics, calcium supplements
• Cardiac dysrhythmias: cardiac glycosides, verapamil
• Decreased effect of dihydrotachysterol: corticosteroids, phenytoin, barbiturates

Lab test interferences:
False increase: Cholesterol

NURSING CONSIDERATIONS

Assess:
• BUN, urinary Ca, AST (SGOT), ALT (SGPT), cholesterol, creatinine, alk phosphatase, uric acid, chlorine, magnesium, electrolytes, urine pH, phosphate; may increase calcium, should be kept at 9-10 mg/dl, vit D 50-135 IU/dl, phosphate 70 mg/dl
• Alk phosphatase; may be decreased
• For increased blood level, since toxic reactions may occur rapidly
• For dry mouth, metallic taste, polyuria, bone pain, muscle weakness, headache, fatigue, tinnitus, change in LOC, irregular pulse, dysrhythmias, increased respirations, anorexia, nausea, vomiting, cramps, diarrhea, constipation; may indicate hypercalcemia
• Renal status: decreased urinary output (oliguria, anuria), edema in extremities, weight gain >5 lb, periorbital edema
• Nutritional status, diet for sources of vit D (milk, some seafood), Ca

(dairy products, dark green vegetables), phosphates (dairy products) must be avoided

Administer:
• PO, may be increased q4wk depending on blood level

Perform/provide:
• Storage in tight, light-resistant containers at room temp
• Restriction of Na, K if required
• Restriction of fluids if required for chronic renal failure

Evaluate:
• Therapeutic response: prevention of bone deficiencies

Teach patient/family:
• The symptoms of hypercalcemia
• About foods rich in calcium, vit D
• ⊘ Not to break, crush, or chew caps

Pharmacokinetics:
PO: Onset 20-40 min, excreted in feces

Interactions:
• Decreased effectiveness of: tetracyclines, ketoconazole, isoniazid, phenothiazines, iron salts, digitalis
• Constipation; increase bulk in the diet if needed

NURSING CONSIDERATIONS
Administer:
• Laxatives or stool softeners if constipation occurs

Evaluate:
• Therapeutic response: absence of pain, decreased acidity

Teach patient/family:
• To increase fluids to 2 L/day unless contraindicated
• To avoid long-term use; high sodium content

---

dihydroxyaluminum sodium carbonate (OTC)

(dye-hye-drox'ee-a-loom a-nium)
Rolaids Antacid
Func. class.: Antacid
Chem. class.: Aluminum product

Action: Neutralizes gastric acidity, reduces pepsin

Uses: Antacid

Dosage and routes:
• *Adult:* **PO** 1-2 as needed; may give up to 2-4 tabs

Available forms: Chewable tab 334 mg

Side effects/adverse reactions:
*GI: Constipation, **obstruction***

Contraindications: Hypersensitivity to aluminum products

Precautions: Elderly, sodium/fluid restriction, decreased GI motility, GI obstruction, dehydration, severe renal disease, CHF, pregnancy (C)

---

diltiazem (℞)

(dil-tye'a zem)
Apo-Diltiaz*, Cardizem, Cardizem CD, Cardizem SR, Cartia XT, Dilacor-XR, diltiazem, Tiamate
Func. class.: Calcium channel blocker
Chem. class.: Benzothiazepine

Action: Inhibits calcium ion influx across cell membrane during cardiac depolarization; produces relaxation of coronary vascular smooth muscle, dilates coronary arteries, slows SA/AV node conduction times, dilates peripheral arteries

Uses: Angina pectoris due to coronary insufficiency, hypertension, vasospasm; parenteral: atrial fibrillation, flutter, paroxysmal supraventricular tachycardia

Dosage and routes:
• *Adult:* **PO** 30 mg qid, increasing dose gradually to 180-360 mg/day

in divided doses or 60-120 mg bid; may increase to 240-360 mg/day
• *Adult:* **IV BOL** 0.25 mg/kg over 2 min initially, then 0.35 mg/kg may be given after 15 min; if no response, may give **CONT INF** 5-15 mg/hr for up to 24 hr
• *Adult:* **PO** (Cardizem CD) qd
Available forms: Tabs 30, 60, 90, 120 mg; caps sus rel 60, 90, 120, 180, 240, 300 mg; inj 5 mg/ml (5, 10 ml)

Side effects/adverse reactions:

CV: Dysrhythmia, edema, **CHF,** bradycardia, hypotension, palpitations, *heart block*
GI: Nausea, vomiting, diarrhea, gastric upset, *constipation,* increased liver function studies
GU: Nocturia, polyuria, **acute renal failure**
INTEG: Rash, pruritus, flushing, photosensitivity
CNS: Headache, fatigue, drowsiness, dizziness, depression, weakness, insomnia, tremor, paresthesia

Contraindications: Sick sinus syndrome, 2nd- or 3rd-degree heart block, hypotension less than 90 mm Hg systolic, acute MI, pulmonary congestion

Precautions: CHF, hypotension, hepatic injury, pregnancy (C), lactation, children, renal disease

Pharmacokinetics: Onset 30-60 min; peak 2-3 hr, immediate rel, 6-11 sus rel; half-life 3 ½-9 hr; metabolized by liver; excreted in urine (96% as metabolites)

Interactions:
• Increased effects of β-blockers, digitalis, lithium, carbamazepine, cyclosporine
• Increased effects of diltiazem: cimetidine

NURSING CONSIDERATIONS
Assess:
• Cardiac status: B/P, pulse, respiration, ECG and intervals PR, QRS, QT

Administer:
• Before meals, hs (PO)
IV
• IV undiluted over 2 min or diluted 125 mg/100 ml, 250 mg/250 ml of D₅W, 0.9% NaCl, D₅/0.45% NaCl, give 10 mg/hr, may increase by 5 mg/hr to 15 mg/hr, continue infusion up to 24 hr

Y-site compatibilities: Albumin, amikacin, amphotericin B, aztreonam, bretylium, bumetanide, cefazolin, cefotaxime, cefotetan, cefoxitin, ceftazidime, ceftriaxone, cefuroxime, cimetidine, ciprofloxacin, clindamycin, digoxin, dobutamine, dopamine, doxycycline, epinephrine, erythromycin, esmolol, fentanyl, fluconazole, gentamicin, hetastarch, hydromorphone, imipenem-cilastatin, labetalol, lidocaine, lorazepam, meperidine, metoclopramide, metronidazole, midazolam, milrinone, morphine, multivitamins, nicardipine, nitroglycerin, norepinephrine, oxacillin, penicillin G potassium, pentamidine, piperacillin, potassium chloride, potassium phosphates, ranitidine, sodium nitroprusside, theophylline, ticarcillin, ticarcillin/clavulanate, tobramycin, trimethoprim-sulfamethoxazole, vancomycin, vecuronium

Perform/provide:
• Storage in tight container at room temp

Evaluate:
• Therapeutic response: decreased anginal pain, decreased B/P

Teach patient/family:
• How to take pulse before taking drug; record or graph should be kept
• To avoid hazardous activities until stabilized on drug, dizziness is no longer a problem
• To limit caffeine consumption

 = Nursing alert   = Herb-drug interaction   = Do not crush

D

• To avoid OTC drugs unless directed by prescriber
• The importance of complying with all areas of medical regimen: diet, exercise, stress reduction, drug therapy
🚫 Not to break, crush, or chew sus rel caps or tabs
• To report dizziness, shortness of breath, palpitations
• Not to discontinue abruptly
• To take with a full glass of water
Treatment of overdose: Defibrillation, atropine for AV block, vasopressor for hypotension

---

dimenhydrinate
(OTC, ℞)

(dye-men-hye′dri-nate)
Calm-X, dimenhydrinate, Dimetabs, Dinate, Dumnmanate, Dramamine, Dramanate, Dramocen, Dramoject, Dymenate, Gravol*, Hydrate, Marmine, Nauseal*, Nauseatol*, Nico-Vert, Novodimenate*, Travamine*, Triptone Caplets, Wehamine
Func. class.: Antiemetic, antihistamine, anticholinergic
Chem. class.: H$_1$-receptor antagonist, ethanolamine derivative

Action: Vestibular stimulation is decreased
Uses: Motion sickness, nausea, vomiting
Dosage and routes:
• *Adult:* PO 50-100 mg q4h; **RECT** 100 mg qd or bid; **IM/IV** 50 mg q4h as needed
• *Child:* **IM/PO** 5 mg/kg divided in 4 equal doses
Available forms: Tabs 50 mg; inj 50 mg/ml; liq 12.5 mg/4 ml; supp 50, 100 mg; chew tabs 50 mg; caps 50 mg
Side effects/adverse reactions:
CNS: Drowsiness, restlessness, headache, dizziness, insomnia, confusion, nervousness, tingling, vertigo; hallucinations and ***convulsions*** in young children
GI: Nausea, anorexia, vomiting, *constipation*
CV: Hypertension, *hypotension,* palpitation
INTEG: Rash, urticaria, fever, chills, flushing
EENT: Dry mouth, blurred vision, diplopia, nasal congestion, photosensitivity
Contraindications: Hypersensitivity to narcotics, shock
Precautions: Children, cardiac dysrhythmias, elderly, asthma, pregnancy (B), lactation, prostatic hypertrophy, bladder-neck obstruction, narrow-angle glaucoma, stenosing peptic ulcer, pyloroduodenal obstruction
Pharmacokinetics:
IM/PO: Duration 4-6 hr
Interactions:
• Increased effect: alcohol, other CNS depressants
• May mask ototoxic symptoms associated with aminoglycosides
🖋 Increased anticholinergic effect: henbane leaf
Lab test interferences:
False negative: Allergy skin testing
NURSING CONSIDERATIONS
Assess:
• VS, B/P; check patients with cardiac disease more often
• Signs of toxicity of other drugs or masking of symptoms of disease: brain tumor, intestinal obstruction
• Observe for drowsiness, dizziness
Administer:
• IM injection in large muscle mass; aspirate to avoid IV administration

---

• Tablets may be swallowed whole, chewed, or allowed to dissolve

IV

• After diluting 50 mg/10 ml of NaCl inj; give 50 mg or less over 2 min

Additive compatibilities: Amikacin, calcium gluconate, chloramphenicol, corticotropin, erythromycin, heparin, hydroxyzine, methicillin, norepinephrine, penicillin G potassium, pentobarbital, phenobarbital, potassium chloride, prochlorperazine, vancomycin, vit B/C

Syringe compatibilities: Atropine, diphenhydramine, droperidol, fentanyl, heparin, hydromorphone, meperidine, metoclopramide, morphine, pentazocine, perphenazine, ranitidine, scopolamine

Y-site compatibilities: Acyclovir

Evaluate:

• Therapeutic response: absence of nausea, vomiting

Teach patient/family:

• That a false-negative result may occur with skin testing; these procedures should not be scheduled for 4 days after discontinuing use

• To avoid hazardous activities, activities requiring alertness; dizziness may occur; instruct patient to request assistance with ambulation

• To avoid alcohol, other depressants

---

dinoprostone ($\mathbb{R}$)

(dye-noe-prost′one)
Cervidil, Prepidil, Prostin E_2
Func. class.: Oxytocic, abortifacient
Chem. class.: Prostaglandin E_2

Action: Stimulates uterine contractions, causing abortion; acts within 30 hr for complete abortion

Uses: Abortion during 2nd trimester, benign hydatidiform mole, expulsion of uterine contents in fetal deaths to 28 wk, missed abortion, to efface and dilate the cervix in pregnancy at term

Dosage and routes:

• *Adult:* **VAG SUPP** 20 mg, repeat q3-5h until abortion occurs, max dose is 240 mg

• *Adult:* **GEL** warm up to room temp, choose correct length shielded catheter (10 or 20 mm), fill catheter by pushing plunger; patient should remain recumbent for 15-30 min

• *Adult:* **INSERT** 10 mg, remove upon onset of active labor or 12 hr of insertion

Available forms: Vag supp 20 mg; gel 0.5 mg/3 g (prefilled syringe); vaginal insert 10 mg

Side effects/adverse reactions:

CNS: Headache, dizziness, chills, fever

CV: Hypotension

GI: Nausea, vomiting, diarrhea

GU: Vaginitis, vaginal pain, vulvitis, vaginismus

INTEG: Rash, skin color changes

MS: Leg cramps, joint swelling, weakness

EENT: Blurred vision

INSERT: Uterine hyperstimulation, fever, nausea, vomiting, diarrhea, abdominal pain

GEL: Uterine contractile abnormality, GI side effects, back pain, fever

FETAL: Bradycardia (i.e., deceleration)

Contraindications: Hypersensitivity, uterine fibrosis, cervical stenosis, pelvic surgery, pelvic inflammatory disease, respiratory disease

Precautions: Hepatic disease, renal disease, cardiac disease, asthma, anemia, jaundice, diabetes mellitus, convulsive disorders, hypertension, hypotension

Interactions

 Hypertension: Ephedra

 = Nursing alert   = Herb-drug interaction   = Do not crush

Pharmacokinetics:
SUPP: Onset 10 min, duration 2-3 hr; metabolized in spleen, kidney, lungs; excreted in urine

NURSING CONSIDERATIONS

Assess:
• Dilation, effacement of cervix and uterine contraction, fetal heart tones, check for contractions over 1 min
• For fever that occurs ½ hr after suppository insertion (abortion)
• Respiratory rate, rhythm, depth; notify prescriber of abnormalities, pulse, B/P, temp
• Vaginal discharge: check for itching, irritation; indicates vaginal infection
• For fever, chills: increase fluids or give tepid sponge bath or blanket

Administer:
• By insert: transversely in the posterior fornix of the vagina immediately after insertion from foil package; do not insert without retrieval system
• By gel: after warming to room temp, remove seal from end of syringe, and remove the protective end cap and insert into plunger stopper assembly; make sure patient is in dorsal position
• Antiemetic/antidiarrheal before administration of this drug

Evaluate:
• Therapeutic response; expulsion of fetus

Teach patient/family:
• To remain supine for 10-15 min after insertion
• To report excessive cramping, bleeding, chills, fever
• Some methods of pain, comfort control

diphenhydramine
(OTC, ℞)

(dye-fen-hye'dra-meen)
Allerdryl*, AllerMax*, Banophen, Belix, Bena-D 10, Bena-D 50, Benadryl, Benadryl 25, Benadryl Kapseals, Benahist 10, Benahist 50, Ben-Allergin-50, Benoject, Benoject-10, Benoject-50, Benylin Cough, Bydramine, Compōz, Dermamycin, Diahist, Diphenacen-50, Diphen Cough, Diphenhist, Diphenhydramine HCl, Dormarex 2, Dormin, Dyrexin, Genahist, Hydramine, Hydramyn, Hyrexin-50, Insomnal*, Nidryl, Nordryl, Nordryl Cough, Nytol, Phendry, Scot-Tussin Allergy, Silphen Cough, Sleep-Eze 3, Sleepinal, Sominex 2, Sominex Caplets, Tusstat, Twilite, Uni-Bent Cough, Wehdryl

Func. class.: Antihistamine

Chem. class.: Ethanolamine derivative, H_1-receptor antagonist

Action: Acts on blood vessels, GI, respiratory system by competing with histamine for H_1-receptor site; decreases allergic response by blocking histamine

Uses: Allergy symptoms, rhinitis, motion sickness, antiparkinsonism, nighttime sedation, infant colic, nonproductive cough

Dosage and routes:

Renal disease
• CrCl 10-50 ml/min dose q6-12h; CrCl <10 ml/min dose q12-18h
• *Adult:* **PO** 25-50 mg q4-6h, not to exceed 400 mg/day; **IM/IV** 10-50 mg, not to exceed 400 mg/day
• *Child >12 kg:* **PO/IM/IV** 5 mg/kg/day in 4 divided doses, not to exceed 300 mg/day

Available forms: Caps 25, 50 mg; tabs 25, 50 mg; elix 12.5 mg/5 ml; syr 12.5 mg/5 ml; inj 50 mg/ml; cream 1, 2%; lotion 1%

Side effects/adverse reactions:

CNS: Dizziness, drowsiness, poor coordination, fatigue, anxiety, euphoria, confusion, paresthesia, neuritis
RESP: Increased thick secretions, wheezing, chest tightness
HEMA: Thrombocytopenia, agranulocytosis, hemolytic anemia
GI: Dry mouth, nausea, anorexia, diarrhea
INTEG: Photosensitivity
GU: Retention, dysuria, frequency
EENT: Blurred vision, dilated pupils, tinnitus, nasal stuffiness, dry nose, throat, mouth

Contraindications: Hypersensitivity to H_1-receptor antagonist, acute asthma attack, lower respiratory tract disease

Precautions: Increased intraocular pressure, renal disease, cardiac disease, hypertension, bronchial asthma, seizure disorder, stenosed peptic ulcers, hyperthyroidism, prostatic hypertrophy, bladder neck obstruction, pregnancy (C), lactation

Pharmacokinetics:

PO: Peak 1-3 hr, duration 4-7 hr;
IM: Onset ½ hr, peak 1-4 hr, duration 4-7 hr; *IV:* Onset immediate, duration 4-7 hr; metabolized in liver, excreted by kidneys; crosses placenta, excreted in breast milk; half-life 2-7 hr

Interactions:

• Increased CNS depression: barbiturates, narcotics, hypnotics, tricyclic antidepressants, alcohol
• Decreased effect of: oral anticoagulants, heparin
• Increased effect of: diphenhydramine: MAOIs
🍃 Increased anticholinergic effect: henbane leaf

Lab test interferences:

False negatives: Skin allergy tests

NURSING CONSIDERATIONS

Assess:

• I&O ratio; be alert for urinary retention, frequency, dysuria; drug should be discontinued
• CBC during long-term therapy; blood dyscrasias
• Respiratory status: rate, rhythm, increase in bronchial secretions, wheezing, chest tightness

Administer:

• With meals for GI symptoms; absorption may slightly decrease
• Deep IM in large muscle; rotate site
• Hs only if using for sleep aid

IV

• Undiluted; give 25 mg/1 min

Additive compatibilities: Amikacin, aminophylline, ascorbic acid, bleomycin, cephapirin, erythromycin, hydrocortisone, lidocaine, methicillin, methyldopa, nafcillin, netilmicin, penicillin G potassium, penicillin G sodium, polymyxin B, vit B/C

Syringe compatibilities: Atropine, butorphanol, chlorpromazine, cimetidine, dimenhydrinate, droperidol, fentanyl, fluphenazine, glycopyrrolate, hydromorphone, hydroxyzine, meperidine, metoclopramide, midazolam, morphine, nalbuphine, pentazocine, perphenazine, prochlorperazine, promazine, promethazine, ranitidine, scopolamine, sufentanil, thiothixene

Y-site compatibilities: Acyclovir, aldesleukin, amifostine, amsacrine, aztreonam, ciprofloxacin, cisplatin, cladribine, cyclophosphamide, cytarabine, doxorubicin, famotidine, filgrastim, fluconazole, fludarabine, gallium, granisetron, heparin, hydrocortisone, idarubicin, melphalan,

◥ = Nursing alert   🍃 = Herb-drug interaction   🚫 = Do not crush meperidine, meropenem, methotrexate, ondansetron, paclitaxel, piperacillin/tazobactam, potassium chloride, propofol, sargramostim, sufentanil, tacrolimus teniposide, thiotepa, vinorelbine, vit B/C

Perform/provide:

• Hard candy, gum, frequent rinsing of mouth for dryness

• Storage in tight container at room temp

Evaluate:

• Therapeutic response: absence of running or congested nose or rashes, improved sleep

Teach patient/family:

• All aspects of drug use; to notify prescriber of confusion, sedation, hypotension

• To avoid driving, other hazardous activity if drowsiness occurs

• That this drug may decrease anticoagulant (oral)

• To avoid concurrent use of alcohol, other CNS depressants

Treatment of overdose: Administer ipecac syrup or lavage, diazepam, vasopressors, barbiturates (short-acting)

---

diphenidol (R̶)

(dye-fen'i-dole)
Vontrol

Func. class.: Antiemetic
Chem. class.: Trihexyphenidyl derivative

Action: May act as dopamine antagonist at chemoreceptor trigger zone to inhibit vomiting

Uses: Nausea, vomiting, peripheral dizziness

Dosage and routes:

• *Adult:* **PO** 25-50 mg q4h

• *Child >23 kg:* **PO** 25 mg q4h prn; do not exceed 5.5 mg/kg/24hr

Available forms: Tabs 25 mg

Side effects/adverse reactions:

CNS: Drowsiness, fatigue, restlessness, tremor, headache, stimulation, dizziness, insomnia, twitching, disorientation, confusion, sleep disturbance, auditory or visual hallucination, depression

GI: Nausea, indigestion

CV: Hypotension

INTEG: Rash

EENT: Dry mouth, blurred vision

Contraindications: Hypersensitivity, psychosis, anuria

Precautions: Children, prostatic hypertrophy, glaucoma, pyloric and duodenal stenosis, elderly, pregnancy (C), lactation

Pharmacokinetics:

PO: Onset 30-45 min, duration 3-6 hr, metabolized by liver, excreted by kidneys

NURSING CONSIDERATIONS

Assess:

• VS, B/P; check patients with cardiac disease more often

• Observe for CNS adverse effects: confusion, hallucination

• Monitor I&O (90% excreted in urine)

• Signs of toxicity of other drugs or masking of symptoms of disease: brain tumor, intestinal obstruction

• Drowsiness, dizziness

Administer:

• Tabs may be swallowed whole, chewed, or allowed to dissolve

Evaluate:

• Therapeutic response: absence of nausea, vomiting

Teach patient/family:

• To avoid alcohol, other depressants

• That drug should be used only under close supervision

---

diphtheria and tetanus toxoids and pertussis vaccine (DPT) (℞)

Diphtheria and Tetanus Toxoids and Pertussis Vaccine, Tri-Immunol

Func. class.: Vaccine, toxoid

Action: Provide immunity to diphtheria, tetanus, pertussis by stimulating antibody/antitoxin production

Uses: Prevention of diphtheria, tetanus, pertussis

Dosage and routes:
• *Adult:* booster dose q10yr
• *Child >6 wk-6 yr:* **IM** 0.5 ml at 2, 4, 6 mo, 1 ½ yr; booster needed 0.5 ml at age 6

Available forms: Inj diphtheria 12.5 LfU, tetanus 5 LfU, pertussis 4 U/0.5 ml

Side effects/adverse reactions:
GI: Nausea, vomiting, anorexia
INTEG: Skin abscess, urticaria, itching, swelling, erythema, edema at site
CV: Tachycardia, hypotension
SYST: Lymphadenitis, *anaphylaxis,* fever, chills, malaise
CNS: Crying, fretfulness, fever, drowsiness, *seizures*
MS: Osteomyelitis

Contraindications: Hypersensitivity, active infection, poliomyelitis outbreak, immunosuppression, febrile illness

Precautions: Pregnancy

Interactions:
• Decreased response to toxoid: immunosuppressive agents: antineoplastics, corticosteroids, radiation therapy; alkylating agents

NURSING CONSIDERATIONS
Assess:
• For skin reactions: swelling, rash, urticaria

• For anaphylaxis: inability to breathe, bronchospasm

Administer:
• At least 4 wk apart × 3 doses
• Only with epinephrine 1:1000 on unit to treat laryngospasm
• IM only; not to be given SC (vastus lateralis in infants)

Perform/provide:
• Storage in refrigerator, do not freeze
• Written record of immunization

Evaluate:
• For history of allergies, skin conditions (eczema, psoriasis, dermatitis), reactions to vaccinations

Teach patient/family:
• That doses are given at least 4 wk apart × 3 doses; booster needed at 10 yr intervals, diphtheria/tetanus

dipyridamole (℞)

(dye-peer-id′a-mole)
Apo-Dipyridamole*, dipyridamole*, Persantine, Persantine IV

Func. class.: Coronary vasodilator, antiplatelet
Chem. class.: Nonnitrate

Action: Inhibits adenosine uptake, which produces coronary vasodilation; increases oxygen saturation in coronary tissues, coronary blood flow; acts on small resistance vessels with little effect on vascular resistance; may increase development of collateral circulation; decreases platelet aggregation by the inhibition of phosphodiesterase (an enzyme)

Uses: Prevention of transient ischemic attacks, inhibition of platelet adhesion to prevent myocardial reinfarction, thromboembolism, with warfarin in prosthetic heart valves, prevention of coronary bypass graft

◆ = Nursing alert   ⫟ = Herb-drug interaction   ⊘ = Do not crush

occlusion with aspirin; possibly effective for long-term therapy of chronic angina pectoris
Dosage and routes:
TIA
• *Adult:* **PO** 50 mg tid, 1 hr ac, not to exceed 400 mg qd
Inhibition of platelet adhesion
• *Adult:* **PO** 50-75 mg qid in combination with aspirin or warfarin; **IV** 570 µg/kg
Available forms: Tabs 25, 50, 75 mg; inj 5 mg/ml, 10 mg/2 ml
Side effects/adverse reactions:
CV: Postural hypotension
CNS: Headache, dizziness, weakness, fainting, syncope
GI: Nausea, vomiting, anorexia, diarrhea
INTEG: Rash, flushing
Contraindications: Hypersensitivity, hypotension
Precautions: Pregnancy (C), lactation
Pharmacokinetics:
PO: Peak 2-2½ hr, duration 6 hr; therapeutic response may take several months; metabolized in liver; excreted in bile; undergoes enterohepatic recirculation
Interactions:
• Incompatibility not known
• Additive antiplatelet effects: ASA, NSAID
• Increased bleeding: warfarin
NURSING CONSIDERATIONS
Assess:
• B/P, pulse during treatment until stable; take B/P lying, standing; orthostatic hypotension is common
• Cardiac status: chest pain, what aggravates or ameliorates condition
Administer:
• IV after diluting each 5 mg/2 ml or more D₅W, 0.45% NaCl, or 0.9% NaCl to a total vol of 20-50 ml; give over 4 min; do not give undiluted

• On an empty stomach: 1 hr before meals or 2 hr after; give with 8 oz water for better absorption
Perform/provide:
• Storage at room temp
Evaluate:
• Therapeutic response: decreased chest pain (angina), decreased platelet adhesion
Teach patient/family:
• That medication is not cure; may have to be taken continuously in evenly spaced doses only as directed
• That it is necessary to quit smoking to prevent excessive vasoconstriction
• To avoid hazardous activities until stabilized on medication; dizziness may occur
• To rise slowly from sitting or lying to prevent orthostatic hypotension
• Not to use alcohol or OTC medications unless approved by prescriber
Treatment of overdose: Administer IV phenylephrine

dirithromycin (R)
(dye-rith-roe-mye'sin)
Dynabac
Func. class.: Antiinfective
Chem. class.: Macrolide

Action: Binds to 50S ribosomal subunits of susceptible bacteria, suppresses protein synthesis
Uses: Infections of the respiratory tract caused by *Moraxella catarrhalis, Streptococcus* sp., (*S. pneumoniae, S. agalactiae, S. viridans), Legionella pneumophilia, Mycoplasma pneumoniae, S. pyogenes, Staphylococcus aureus, Bordetella pertussis, Propionibacterium acnes*

Dosage and routes:
• *Adult:* PO 500 mg qd, given for 7-14 days depending on infections
Available forms: Tabs, enteric coated 250 mg
Side effects/adverse reactions:
GI: Abdominal pain, *nausea*, *diarrhea*, *vomiting*, *dyspepsia*, GI disorders, flatulence, abnormal stools, anorexia, constipation, ***pseudomembranous colitis***
CNS: Headache, *dizziness*, *insomnia*
HEMA: Increased platelet count, increased eosinophils
RESP: Cough, dyspnea
INTEG: Pruritus, urticaria
Contraindications: Hypersensitivity to this drug or any other macrolide, or erythromycin, bacteremias
Precautions: Pregnancy (C), lactation, children, hepatic, renal disease
Pharmacokinetics: Rapidly absorbed, widely distributed, no hepatic metabolism, excreted in bile, feces (up to 97%), plasma half-life 8 hr, terminal 44 hr
Interactions:
• Absorption of dirithromycin slightly enhanced: antacids, H_2-antagonists
NURSING CONSIDERATIONS
Assess:
• I&O ratio; report hematuria, oliguria in renal disease
• Liver studies: AST, ALT
• Renal studies: Urinalysis, protein, blood
• C&S before drug therapy; drug may be given as soon as culture is taken; C&S may be repeated after treatment
• Bowel pattern before, during treatment; pseudomembranous colitis may occur
• Skin eruptions, itching
• Respiratory status: rate, character, wheezing, tightness in chest; discontinue drug

• Allergies before treatment, reaction of each medication; place allergies on chart, notify all people giving drugs
Administer:
• Adequate intake of fluids (2 L) during diarrhea episodes
🚫 Whole; do not break, crush, or chew tablets
• With food or within 1 hr of food at same time each day
Perform/provide:
• Storage at room temp, in tight container
Evaluate:
• Therapeutic response: C&S negative for infection
Teach patient/family:
• To take with full glass of water; to give with food
• To report sore throat, fever, fatigue; may indicate superinfection
• To notify prescriber of diarrhea stools, dark urine, pale stools, yellow discoloration of eyes or skin, severe abdominal pain
• To take at evenly spaced intervals; complete dosage regimen
Treatment of hypersensitivity:
Withdraw drug, maintain airway, administer epinephrine, aminophylline, O_2, IV corticosteroids

---

disopyramide (℞)

(dye-soe-peer'a-mide)
disopyramide, Napamide, Norpace, Norpace CR, Rhythmodan
Func. class.: Antidysrhythmic (Class IA)
Chem. class.: Nonnitrate

Action: Prolongs duration of action potential and effective refractory period; reduces disparity in refractory between normal and infarcted myocardium; prevents increased myo-

---

◆ = Nursing alert   ∥ = Herb-drug interaction   🚫 = Do not crush

cardial excitability and conduction contractility

Uses: PVCs, ventricular tachycardia, supraventricular tachycardia, atrial flutter, fibrillation

Investigational uses: Supraventricular tachycardia (prevention, treatment)

Dosage and routes:

Renal disease
• CrCl 30-40 ml/min dose q8h; CrCl 15-30 ml/min dose q12h; CrCl <15 ml/min dose q24h
• *Adult:* **PO** 100-200 mg q6h, in renal dysfunction 100 mg q6h; **SUS REL CAPS** 200 mg q12h
• *Child 12-18 yr:* **PO** 6-15 mg/kg/day, in divided doses q6h
• *Child 4-12 yr:* **PO** 10-15 mg/kg/day in divided doses q6h
• *Child 1-4 yr:* **PO** 10-20 mg/kg/day in divided doses q6h
• *Child <1 yr:* **PO** 10-30 mg/kg/day, in divided doses q6h

Available forms: Caps 100, 150 mg (as phosphate); sus rel caps, 100, 150 mg

Side effects/adverse reactions:

GU: Retention, hesitancy, impotence
CNS: Headache, dizziness, psychosis, fatigue, depression, paresthesias, anxiety, insomnia
GI: Dry mouth, constipation, nausea, anorexia, flatulence, diarrhea, vomiting
CV: Hypotension, bradycardia, angina, PVCs, tachycardia, increased QRS, QT segments, *cardiac arrest,* edema, weight gain, AV block, *CHF,* syncope, chest pain
META: Hypoglycemia
INTEG: Rash, pruritus, urticaria
MS: Weakness, pain in extremities
EENT: Blurred vision; dry nose, throat, eyes; narrow-angle glaucoma
HEMA: Thrombocytopenia, agranulocytosis, anemia (rare), decreased Hgb, Hct

Contraindications: Hypersensitivity, 2nd- or 3rd-degree block, cardiogenic shock, CHF (uncompensated), sick sinus syndrome, QT prolongation

Precautions: Pregnancy (C), lactation, diabetes mellitus, renal disease, children, hepatic disease, myasthenia gravis, narrow-angle glaucoma, cardiomyopathy, conduction abnormalities

Pharmacokinetics:
PO: Peak 30 min-3 hr, duration 6-12 hr; half-life 4-10 hr; metabolized in liver; excreted in feces, urine, breast milk; crosses placenta

Interactions:
• Increased effects of disopyramide: quinidine, procainamide, propranolol, lidocaine, atenolol, other antidysrhythmics, erythromycin
• Do not administer within 48 hr of verapamil
• Increased side effects of disopyramide: anticholinergics
• Decreased effects of disopyramide: phenytoin, rifampin, phenobarbital
🍴 Increased action: aloe, buckthorn bark/berry, cascara sagrada bark, senna pod/leaf

Lab test interferences:
Increase: Liver enzymes, lipids, BUN, creatinine
Decrease: Hgb/Hct, blood glucose

NURSING CONSIDERATIONS
Assess:
• Apical pulse for 1 min; if less than 60, check again in 1 hr; if still less than 60, notify prescriber
• ECG; check for increased QT, widening QRS; drug should be discontinued
• Blood level during treatment (therapeutic level 2-8 µg/ml); ANA titer
• Weight daily; a rapid weight gain should be reported
• For dehydration or hypovolemia, I&O ratio, electrolytes (Na, K, Cl)

• Liver, kidney function studies (AST [SGOT], ALT [SGPT], bilirubin, BUN, creatinine) during treatment
• Diabetics for signs of hypoglycemia
• B/P continuously for hypotension, hypertension
• Increase in QRS, QT; drug should be discontinued
• For rebound hypertension after 1-2 hr
• Constipation: increased bulk in diet, water, stool softeners, or laxatives needed
• Cardiac rate, respiration: rate, rhythm, character
• Urinary hesitancy, frequency, or a change in I&O ratio; check for edema daily; check for toxicity

Administer:
🚫 Do not break, crush, or chew sus rel cap; give 1 hr before or 2 hr after meals
• Sugar-free gum, frequent sips of water for dry mouth
• Reduced dosage slowly with ECG monitoring

Evaluate:
• Therapeutic response: decreased dysrhythmias

Teach patient/family:
• To take drug exactly as prescribed; if dose is missed, take within 3-4 hr of next dose; do not double dose
• To avoid alcohol, or severe hypotension may occur; to avoid OTC drugs, or serious drug interactions may occur
• To make position change slowly during early therapy to prevent orthostatic hypotension
• To avoid hazardous activities if dizziness or blurred vision occurs
• The importance of complying with drug regimen; tell patient that this drug does not cure condition

Treatment of overdose: O₂, artificial ventilation, ECG, dopamine for circulatory depression, diazepam or thiopental for convulsions, gastric lavage

---

DNase (dornase alfa) (℞)
Pulmozyme
Func. class.: Cystic fibrosis agent (orphan drug)

Action: May break down molecules in large amounts of infected sputum; improves air flow, lessens chance of bacterial infection

Uses: Management of cystic fibrosis

Dosage and routes:
• *Adult/child >5 yr:* **INH** 2.5 mg qd
Available forms: Neb 2.5 mg

Side effects/adverse reactions:
RESP: Possibly laryngitis, hoarseness, hemoptysis, transient decrease in pulmonary function

Contraindications: Hypersensitivity

NURSING CONSIDERATIONS
Assess:
• Resp function: B/P, pulse, lung sounds

Administer:
• By nebulization only

Evaluate:
• Therapeutic response: decreased thick tenacious secretions, ease of respirations

Teach patient/family:
• To rinse mouth after use
• About all aspects of drug; avoid smoking, smoke-filled rooms, persons with respiratory infections

---

dobutamine (℞)

(doe-byoo'ta-meen)
dobutamine, Dobutrex
Func. class.: Adrenergic direct-acting β_1-agonist
Chem. class.: Catecholamine

Action: Causes increased contractility, increased coronary blood flow and heart rate by acting on β_1-receptors in heart; minor α and β_2 effects

Uses: Cardiac surgery, refractory heart failure, cardiac decompensation

Investigational uses: Cardiogenic shock in children

Unlabeled uses: Congenital heart disease in children undergoing cardiac cath

Dosage and routes:
• *Adult:* IV INF 2.5-10 μg/kg/min; may increase to 40 μg/kg/min if needed
• *Child:* IV INF 5-20 μg/kg/min over 10 min for cardiac cath

Available forms: Inj 12.5 mg/ml

Side effects/adverse reactions:
CNS: Anxiety, headache, dizziness
CV: Palpitations, tachycardia, hypertension, PVCs, angina
GI: Heartburn, nausea, vomiting
MS: Muscle cramps (leg)

Contraindications: Hypersensitivity, idiopathic hypertrophic subaortic stenosis

Precautions: Pregnancy (C), lactation, children, hypertension

Pharmacokinetics:
IV: Onset 1-2 min, peak 10 min, half-life 2 min; metabolized in liver (inactive metabolites); excreted in urine

Interactions:
• Severe hypertension: guanethidine
• Dysrhythmias: general anesthetics, bretylium

• Decreased action of dobutamine: other β-blockers
• Increased B/P: oxytocics
• Increased pressor effect and dysrhythmias: tricyclic antidepressant, MAOIs

NURSING CONSIDERATIONS
Assess:
• Hypovolemia; if present, correct first
• Oxygenation/perfusion deficit (check B/P, chest pain, dizziness, loss of consciousness)
• Heart failure: S_3 gallop, dyspnea, neck vein distention, bibasilar crackles in patients with CHF, cardiomyopathy
• I&O ratio
• ECG during administration continuously; if B/P increases, drug is decreased; CVP or PWP during infusion if possible
• B/P and pulse q5min after parenteral route
• Sulfite sensitivity, which may be life-threatening

Administer:
IV
• Diluting each 250 mg/10 ml of sterile H_2O or D_5W for inj; may be further diluted to 50 ml or more given at prescribed rate; should be gradually increased to desired rate
• Plasma expanders for hypovolemia

Additive compatibilities: Amiodarone, atracurium, atropine, dopamine, enalaprilat, epinephrine, flumazenil, hydralazine, isoproterenol, lidocaine, meperidine, meropenem, metaraminol, morphine, nitroglycerin, norepinephrine, phentolamine, phenylephrine, procainamide, propranolol, ranitidine

Syringe compatibilities: Heparin, ranitidine

Y-site compatibilities: Amifostine, amiodarone, amrinone, atracurium, aztreonam, bretylium, calcium

chloride, calcium gluconate, ciprofloxacin, cladribine, diazepam, diltiazem, dopamine, enalaprilat, epinephrine, famotidine, fentanyl, fluconazole, granisetron, haloperidol, hydromorphone, insulin (regular), labetalol, lidocaine, lorazepam, magnesium sulfate, meperidine, milrinone, morphine, nicardipine, nitroglycerin, norepinephrine, pancuronium, potassium chloride, propofol, ranitidine, sodium nitroprusside, streptokinase, tacrolimus, theophylline, thiotepa, tolazoline, vecuronium, verapamil, zidovudine
Perform/provide:

• Storage of reconstituted solution if refrigerated for <24 hr
Evaluate:

• Therapeutic response: increased B/P with stabilization, increased urine output
Teach patient/family:

• The reason for drug administration
Treatment of overdose: Administer a β_1-adrenergic blocker; reduce IV or discontinue, ensure oxygenation/ventilation; for severe tachydysrhythmias (ventricular) give lidocaine or propranolol

docusate calcium/ docusate potassium/ docusate sodium (℞)

(dok'yoo-sate)
Correctol Extra Gentle, DC Softgels, Diocto, Diocto-K, Dioeze, Disonate, Docusate Calcium, Docusate Sodium, DOK, DOS Softgel, Doxinate, D-S-S, Kasof/Colace, Modane Soft, Pro-Cal-Sof, Regulex SS, Regutol, Sulfalax Calcium, Surfak/Dialose
Func. class.: Laxative, emollient

Chem. class.: Anionic surfactant

Action: Increases water, fat penetration in intestine; allows for easier passage of stool
Uses: To soften stools
Dosage and routes:

• *Adult:* **PO** 50-300 mg qd (sodium) or 240 mg (calcium or potassium) prn; **ENEMA** 5 ml (sodium)
• *Child >12 yr:* **ENEMA** 2 ml (sodium)
• *Child 6-12 yr:* **PO** 40-120 mg qd (sodium)
• *Child 3-6 yr:* **PO** 20-60 mg qd (sodium)
• *Child <3 yr:* **PO** 10-40 mg qd (sodium)
Available forms: Calcium: caps 50, 240 mg; *potassium:* caps 100 mg; *sodium:* caps 50, 100, 240, 250 mg; tabs 100 mg; syr 20 mg/5 ml; liquid 150 mg/15 ml; sol 50 mg/ml; enema 283 mg/3.9 cap
Side effects/adverse reactions:

GI: Nausea, anorexia, cramps, diarrhea
INTEG: Rash
EENT: Bitter taste, throat irritation
Contraindications: Hypersensitivity, obstruction, fecal impaction, nausea/vomiting

Precautions: Pregnancy (C), lactation

Pharmacokinetics: Onset 24-72 hr

NURSING CONSIDERATIONS

Assess:

• Cause of constipation; identify whether fluids, bulk, or exercise are missing from lifestyle

• Cramping, rectal bleeding, nausea, vomiting; if these symptoms occur, drug should be discontinued

Administer:

• Alone with 8 oz H_2O only for better absorption; do not take within 1 hr of other drugs or within 1 hr of antacids, milk, or H_2 blockers

• In morning or evening (oral dose)

Perform/provide:

• Storage in cool environment; do not freeze

Evaluate:

• Therapeutic response: decrease in constipation

Teach patient/family:

🚫 To swallow tabs whole; do not break, crush, or chew

• That normal bowel movements do not always occur daily

• Not to use in presence of abdominal pain, nausea, vomiting

• To notify prescriber if constipation unrelieved or if symptoms of electrolyte imbalance occur: muscle cramps, pain, weakness, dizziness, excessive thirst

• To keep out of children's reach

---

dolasetron (℞)

(do-la'se-tron)

Anzemet

Func. class.: Antiemetic

Chem. class.: 5-HT3 receptor antagonist

Action: Prevents nausea, vomiting by blocking serotonin peripherally, centrally, and in the small intestine

Uses: Prevention of nausea, vomiting associated with cancer chemotherapy, radiotherapy, and prevention of postoperative nausea, vomiting

Investigational uses: Radiotherapy-induced nausea/vomiting

Dosage and routes:

Prevention of nausea/vomiting of cancer chemotherapy

• *Adult and child 2-16 yr:* **IV** 1.8 mg/kg as a single dose, ½ hr prior to chemotherapy

• *Adult:* **PO** 100 mg/hr prior to chemotherapy

• *Child 2-16 yr:* **PO** 1.8 mg/kg/hr prior to chemotherapy

Prevention of postoperative nausea/vomiting

• *Adult:* **IV** 12.5 mg as a single dose, 15 min before cessation of anesthesia; **PO** 100 mg 2 hr before surgery (prevention only)

• *Child 2-16 yr:* **IV** 0.35 mg/kg as a single dose, 15 min before cessation of anesthesia; **PO** 1.2 mg/kg 2 hr before surgery (prevention only)

Available forms: Tabs 50, 100 mg; inj 20 mg/ml

Side effects/adverse reactions:

GI: Diarrhea, constipation, increased AST, ALT

CNS: Headache

MISC: Rash, **bronchospasm**

Contraindications: Hypersensitivity

Precautions: Pregnancy (B), lactation, children, elderly

Pharmacokinetics: Unknown

NURSING CONSIDERATIONS

Assess:

• For absence of nausea, vomiting during chemotherapy

• Hypersensitivity reaction: rash, bronchospasm

Perform/provide:

• Storage at room temp 48 hr after dilution

Evaluate:

• Therapeutic response: absence of

nausea, vomiting during cancer chemotherapy

Teach patient/family:
• To report diarrhea, constipation, rash, or changes in respirations

---

donepezil (℞)

(don-ep-ee′zill)
Aricept
Func. class.: Reversible cholinesterase

Action: Elevates acetylcholine concentrations (cerebral cortex) by slowing degradation of acetylcholine released in cholinergic neurons; does not alter underlying dementia

Uses: Treatment of mild to moderate dementia in Alzheimer's disease

Dosage and routes:
• *Adult:* **PO** 5-10 mg qd hs
Available forms: Tabs 5, 10 mg

Side effects/adverse reactions:
CNS: Dizziness, insomnia, somnolence, headache, fatigue, abnormal dreams, syncope
CV: Hypotension or hypertension
GI: Nausea, vomiting, anorexia
GU: Frequency, UTI, incontinence
INTEG: Rash, flushing
RESP: Rhinitis, URI, cough, pharyngitis
MS: Cramps, arthritis

Contraindications: Hypersensitivity to this drug or piperidine derivatives

Precautions: Sick sinus syndrome, history of ulcers, GI bleeding, hepatic disease, bladder obstruction, asthma, pregnancy (C), lactation, children, seizures, asthma, COPD

Pharmacokinetics: Well absorbed PO, metabolized to metabolites, elimination half-life 10 hr

Interactions:
• Decreased activity of anticholinergics

• Synergistic effects: succinylcholine, cholinesterase inhibitors, cholinergic agonists
• Increased gastric acid secretions: NSAIDs

NURSING CONSIDERATIONS
Assess:
• B/P: hypotension, hypertension
• Mental status: affect, mood, behavioral changes, depression, complete suicide assessment
• GI status: nausea, vomiting, anorexia, diarrhea
• GU status: urinary frequency, incontinence

Administer:
• Between meals; may be given with meals for GI symptoms
• Dosage adjusted to response no more than q6wk

Perform/provide:
• Assistance with ambulation during beginning therapy; dizziness, ataxia may occur

Evaluate:
• Therapeutic response: decrease in confusion, improved mood

Teach patient/family:
• To report side effects: twitching, nausea, vomiting, sweating; indicates overdose
• To use drug exactly as prescribed; at regular intervals, preferably between meals; may be taken with meals for GI upset
• To notify prescriber of nausea, vomiting, diarrhea (dose increase or beginning treatment), or rash
• Not to increase or abruptly decrease dose; serious consequences may result
• That drug is not a cure

Treatment of overdose: Withdraw drug, administer tertiary anticholinergics, provide supportive care

---

◆ = Nursing alert   ⫽ = Herb-drug interaction   ⊘ = Do not crush

dopamine (℞)

(doe'pa-meen)

dopamine HCl, Dopastat, Intropin, Revimine*

Func. class.: Adrenergic
Chem. class.: Catecholamine

Action: Causes increased cardiac output; acts on β_1- and α-receptors, causing vasoconstriction in blood vessels; low dose causes renal and mesenteric vasodilation; β_1 stimulation produces inotropic effects with increased cardiac output

Uses: Shock; increased perfusion; hypotension

Unlabeled uses: COPD, RDS in infants

Dosage and routes:
• *Adult:* **IV INF** 2-5 µg/kg/min, not to exceed 50 µg/kg/min, titrate to patient's response
• *Child:* **IV** 5-20 µg/kg/min adjust depending on response

COPD
• *Adult:* **IV** 4 µg/kg/min
CHF
• *Adult:* **IV** 2-5 µg/kg/min
RDS
• *Infant:* **IV** 5 µg/kg/min

Available forms: Inj 0.8, 1.6, 40, 80, 160 mg/ml

Side effects/adverse reactions:
CNS: Headache
CV: Palpitations, tachycardia, hypertension, ectopic beats, angina, wide QRS complex, peripheral vasoconstriction
GI: Nausea, vomiting, diarrhea
INTEG: Necrosis, tissue sloughing with extravasation, ***gangrene***
RESP: Dyspnea

Contraindications: Hypersensitivity, ventricular fibrillation, tachydysrhythmias, pheochromocytoma

Precautions: Pregnancy (C), lactation, arterial embolism, peripheral vascular disease

Pharmacokinetics:
IV: Onset 5 min, duration <10 min; metabolized in liver, kidney, plasma, excreted in urine (metabolites), half-life 2 min

Interactions:
• Do not use within 2 wk of MAOIs, phenytoin; hypertensive crisis may result
• Dysrhythmias: general anesthetics
• Decreased action of dopamine: other β-blockers
• Increased B/P: oxytocics
• Increased pressor effect: tricyclic antidepressant, MAOIs
• Additive effect: diuretics

NURSING CONSIDERATIONS
Assess:
• Hypovolemia; if present, correct first
• Oxygenation/perfusion deficit (check B/P, chest pain, dizziness, loss of consciousness)
• Heart failure: S_3 gallop, dyspnea, neck vein distention, bibasilar crackles in patients with CHF, cardiomyopathy
• I&O ratio
• ECG during administration continuously; if B/P increases, drug is decreased
• B/P and pulse q5min after parenteral route
• CVP or PWP during infusion if possible
• Paresthesias and coldness of extremities; peripheral blood flow may decrease
• Injection site: tissue sloughing; if this occurs, administer phentolamine mixed with NS

Administer:
IV
• Plasma expanders or whole blood for hypovolemia

• IV after diluting 200-400 mg/250-500 ml of D_5W, D_5 0.45% NaCl, D_5 0.9% NaCl, D_5LR, LR
• Parenteral IV dose slowly; after reconstituting, use infusion pump; flush line before infusing; infuse as secondary IV line

Additive compatibilities: Aminophylline, atracurium, bretylium, calcium chloride, cephalothin, chloramphenicol, dobutamine, enalaprilat, flumazenil, heparin, hydrocortisone, kanamycin, lidocaine, meropenem, methylprednisolone, nitroglycerin, oxacillin, potassium chloride, ranitidine, verapamil

Syringe compatibilities: Doxapram, heparin, ranitidine

Y-site compatibilities: Aldesleukin, amifostine, amiodarone, amrinone, atracurium, aztreonam, cefmetazole, cefpirome, ciprofloxacin, cladribine, diltiazem, dobutamine, enalaprilat, epinephrine, esmolol, famotidine, fentanyl, fluconazole, foscarnet, granisetron, haloperidol, heparin, hydrocortisone, hydromorphone, labetalol, lidocaine, lorazepam, meperidine, methylprednisolone, metronidazole, midazolam, milrinone, morphine, nicardipine, nitroglycerin, norepinephrine, ondansetron, pancuronium, piperacillin/tazobactam, potassium chloride, propofol, ranitidine, sargramostim, sodium nitroprusside, streptokinase, tacrolimus, theophylline, thiotepa, tolazoline, vecuronium, verapamil, vit B/C, warfarin, zidovudine

Perform/provide:
• Storage of reconstituted sol if refrigerated no longer than 24 hr
• Do not use discolored sol; protect from light

Evaluate:
• Therapeutic response: increased B/P with stabilization; increased urine output

Teach patient/family:
• The reason for drug administration

Treatment of overdose: Discontinue IV, may give a short-acting α-adrenergic blocker (phentolamine)

---

doxacurium (℞)
(dox-a-cure′ee-um)
Nuromax
Func. class.: Neuromuscular blocker (nondepolarizing)

Action: Inhibits transmission of nerve impulses by binding with cholinergic receptor sites, antagonizing action of acetylcholine

Uses: Facilitation of endotracheal intubation, skeletal muscle relaxation during mechanical ventilation, surgery, or general anesthesia

Dosage and routes:
• *Adult:* **IV** 0.05 mg/kg; 0.08 mg/kg is used for prolonged neuromuscular blockade; maintenance 0.025 mg/kg
• *Child 2-12 yr:* **IV** 0.03-0.05 mg/kg; may decrease for maintenance dose

Available forms: Inj 1 mg/ml

Side effects/adverse reactions:
CV: Decreased B/P, ventricular fibrillation, myocardial infarction, cardiovascular accident
RESP: Prolonged apnea, bronchospasm, wheezing, respiratory depression
EENT: Diplopia
MS: Weakness, prolonged skeletal muscle relaxation, *paralysis*
INTEG: Rash, urticaria

Contraindications: Hypersensitivity

Precautions: Pregnancy (C), renal, hepatic disease, lactation, children <3 mo, fluid and electrolyte imbal-

---

ances, neuromuscular disease, respiratory disease, obesity, elderly, severe burns

Pharmacokinetics: Not metabolized; excretion of unchanged drug in urine and bile

Interactions:
• Increased neuromuscular blockade: aminoglycosides, quinidine, local anesthetics, polymyxin antibiotics, enflurane, isoflurane, tetracyclines, halothane, magnesium, colistin, procainamide, bacitracin, lincomycin, clindamycin, lithium
• Longer onset and shorter duration of doxacurium: phenytoin, carbamazepine

NURSING CONSIDERATIONS
Assess:
• For electrolyte imblances (K, Mg); may lead to increased action of this drug
• Vital signs (B/P, pulse, respirations, airway) until fully recovered; rate, depth, pattern of respirations, strength of hand grip
• I&O ratio; check for urinary retention, frequency, hesitancy
• Recovery: decreased paralysis of face, diaphragm, leg, arm, rest of body
• Allergic reactions: rash, fever, respiratory distress, pruritus; drug should be discontinued

Administer:
IV
• Using nerve stimulator by anesthesiologist to determine neuromuscular blockade
• After succinylcholine effects subside
• Anticholinesterase to reverse neuromuscular blockade
• By slow IV over 1-2 min (only by qualified persons, usually an anesthesiologist)
• Only fresh sol

Solution compatibilities: LR, D$_5$/LR, D$_5$/0.9% NaCl

Y-site compatibilities: Etomidate, thiopental

Perform/provide:
• Storage at room temp; do not freeze
• Reassurance if communication is difficult during recovery from neuromuscular blockade
• Use reconstituted sol within 24 hr
• Frequent (q2h) instillation of artificial tears and covering eyes to prevent drying of cornea

Evaluate:
• Therapeutic response: paralysis of jaw, eyelid, head, neck, rest of body

Treatment of overdose: Neostigmine; monitor VS; may require mechanical ventilation

---

doxapram (R)
(dox'a-pram)
Dopram
Func. class.: Analeptic

Action: Respiratory stimulation through activation of peripheral carotid chemoreceptor; with higher doses, medullary respiratory centers are stimulated; general CNS stimulation

Uses: Chronic obstructive pulmonary disease (COPD), postanesthesia respiratory stimulation, prevention of acute hypercapnia, drug-induced CNS depression

Dosage and routes:
Postanesthesia
• *Adult:* IV inj 0.5-1 mg/kg, not to exceed 1.5 mg/kg total as a single injection; **IV INF** 250 mg in 250 ml sol, not to exceed 4 mg/kg; run at 1-3 mg/min

Drug-induced CNS depression
• *Adult:* IV priming dose of 2 mg/kg, repeated in 5 min; repeat q1-2h till patient awakes; **IV INF** priming dose 2 mg/kg at 1-3 mg/min, not to exceed 3 g/day

---

COPD (Hypercapnia)
• *Adult:* IV INF 1-2 mg/min, not to exceed 3 mg/min for no longer than 2 hr

Apnea of premature infant
• *Infant:* 2.5-3 mg/kg loading dose followed by infusion of 1 mg/kg/hr

Available forms: Inj 20 mg/ml

Side effects/adverse reactions:

CNS: **Convulsions,** (clonus/generalized), *headache,* restlessness, dizziness, confusion, paresthesias, flushing, sweating, bilateral Babinski's sign, rigidity, depression

GI: Nausea, vomiting, diarrhea, hiccups

GU: Retention, incontinence

CV: Chest pain, hypertension, change in heart rate, lowered T waves, tachycardia, dysrhythmias

INTEG: Pruritus, irritation at injection site

EENT: Pupil dilation, sneezing

RESP: **Laryngospasm, bronchospasm,** rebound hypoventilation, dyspnea, cough, tachypnea, hiccoughs

Contraindications: Hypersensitivity, seizure disorders, severe hypertension, severe bronchial asthma, severe dyspnea, severe cardiac disorders, pneumothorax, pulmonary embolism, severe respiratory disease, newborns

Precautions: Bronchial asthma, pheochromocytoma, severe tachycardia, dysrhythmias, pregnancy (B), hypertension, lactation, children

Pharmacokinetics:

IV: Onset 20-40 sec, peak 1-2 min, duration 5-10 min; metabolized by liver; excreted by kidneys (metabolites); half-life 2.5-4 hr

Interactions:
• Synergistic pressor effect: MAOIs, sympathomimetics
• Cardiac dysrhythmias: halothane, cyclopropane, enflurane

NURSING CONSIDERATIONS

Assess:
• BP, heart rate, deep tendon reflexes, ABGs, LOC before administration, q30min
• Po_2, Pco_2, O_2 saturation during treatment
• Hypertension, dysrhythmias, tachycardia, dyspnea, skeletal muscle hyperactivity; may indicate overdosage; discontinue drug
• Respiratory stimulation: increased rate, abnormal rhythm
• Extravasation; change IV site q48h

Administer:

IV
• Undiluted or diluted with equal parts of sterile H_2O for inj; may be diluted 250 mg/250 ml of D_5W, $D_{10}W$ and run as infusion
• IV undiluted over 5 min; IV inf at 1-3 mg/min; adjust for desired respiratory response, using infusion pump IV; if an inf is used after initial dose, start at 1-3 mg/min depending on patient response; D/C after 2 hr; wait 1-2 hr and repeat
• Only after adequate airway is established
• After O_2, IV barbiturates, resuscitative equipment available

Syringe compatibilities: Amikacin, bumetadine, chlorpromazine, cimetidine, cisplatin, cyclophosphamide, dopamine, doxycycline, epinephrine, hydroxyzine, imipramine, isoniazid, lincomycin, methotrexate, netilmicin, phytonadione, pyridoxine, terbutaline, thiamine, tobramycin, vincristine

Perform/provide:
• Placing patient in Sims' position to prevent aspiration of vomitus
• Discontinue infusion if side effects occur; narrow margin of safety

Evaluate:
• Therapeutic response: increased breathing capacity

◆ = Nursing alert   ∅ = Herb-drug interaction   ⊘ = Do not crush

Teach patient/family:
• Purpose of medication
Treatment of overdose: Lavage, activated charcoal; monitor electrolytes, vital signs

---

doxazosin (R̶)

(dox-ay´zoe-sin)
Cardura
Func. class.: Peripheral α₁-adrenergic blocker
Chem. class.: Quinazoline

Action: Peripheral blood vessels are dilated, peripheral resistance lowered; reduction in blood pressure results from α_1-adrenergic receptors being blocked

Uses: Hypertension, urinary outflow obstruction, symptoms of benign prostatic hyperplasia
Investigational uses: CHF with digoxin and diuretics

Dosage and routes:
BPH
• *Adult:* **PO** 1 mg qd, increase in stepwise manner to 2, 4, 8 mg qd as needed, max 8 mg
• *Adult:* **PO** 1 mg qd, increasing up to 16 mg qd if required; usual range 4-16 mg/day
HTN
• *Geriatric:* **PO** 0.5 mg qhs, gradually increase
Available forms: Tabs 1, 2, 4, 8 mg

Side effects/adverse reactions:
CV: Palpitations, *orthostatic hypotension,* tachycardia, edema, dysrhythmias, chest pain
CNS: Dizziness, headache, drowsiness, anxiety, depression, vertigo, weakness, fatigue, asthenia
GI: Nausea, vomiting, diarrhea, constipation, abdominal pain
GU: Incontinence, polyuria
EENT: Epistaxis, tinnitus, dry mouth, red sclera, pharyngitis, rhinitis

Contraindications: Hypersensitivity to quinazolines
Precautions: Pregnancy (C), children, lactation, hepatic disease
Pharmacokinetics:
PO: Onset 2 hr, peak 2-6 hr, duration 6-12 hr; half-life 22 hr; metabolized in liver; excreted via bile/feces (<63%) and in urine (9%); extensively protein bound (98%)
Interactions:
• Increased hypotensive effects: β-blockers, verapamil
• Decreased hypotensive effects: indomethacin, NSAIDs
• Decreased effects of clonidine
🌿 Increased doxazosin effect: angelica

NURSING CONSIDERATIONS
Assess:
• B/P (lying, standing) and pulse 2-6 hr after each dose and with each increase; postural effects may occur, rales, dyspnea, orthopnea with B/P; pulse, jugular venous distention q4h
• BUN, uric acid if on long-term therapy
• I&O, weight daily
• Edema in feet, legs daily
• Skin turgor, dryness of mucous membranes for hydration status
Administer:
• Tablets broken, crushed or chewed; if chewed, will be bitter
Perform/provide:
• Storage in tight container in cool environment
Evaluate:
• Therapeutic response: decreased B/P; decreased symptoms of BPH
Teach patient/family:
• That fainting occasionally occurs after first dose; do not drive or operate machinery for 4 hr after first dose or after dosage increase or take first dose hs

---

• To take 1st dose at hs to decrease orthostatic B/P changes

Treatment of overdose: Administer volume expanders or vasopressors; discontinue drug; place in supine position

---

doxepin (℞)

(dox'e-pin)

Adepin, doxepin HCl, Sinequan, Sinequan Concentrate, Triadapin*, Zonolon Topical Cream

Func. class.: Antidepressant, tricyclic

Chem. class.: Dibenzoxepin, tertiary amine

Action: Blocks reuptake of norepinephrine, serotonin into nerve endings, increasing action of norepinephrine, serotonin in nerve cells

Uses: Major depression, anxiety

Investigational uses: Chronic pain management

Dosage and routes:
• *Adult:* PO 75 mg/day, may increase to 300 mg/day for severely ill
• Oral conc should be diluted with 120 ml of water, milk, orange, grapefruit, tomato, prune, pineapple juice. Do not mix with grape juice
• *Geriatric:* PO 10-25 mg hs, increase qwk by 10-25 mg to desired dose

Available forms: Caps 10, 25, 50, 75, 100, 150 mg; oral conc 10 mg/ml

Side effects/adverse reactions:

*HEMA: **Agranulocytosis, thrombocytopenia, eosinophilia, leukopenia***

CNS: Dizziness, drowsiness, confusion, headache, anxiety, tremors, stimulation, weakness, insomnia, nightmares, EPS (elderly), increased psychiatric symptoms, paresthesia

GI: Diarrhea, dry mouth, nausea, vomiting, ***paralytic ileus,*** increased appetite, cramps, epigastric distress, jaundice, ***hepatitis,*** stomatitis, constipation

*GU: Retention, **acute renal failure***

INTEG: Rash, urticaria, sweating, pruritus, photosensitivity

*CV: Orthostatic hypotension, ECG changes, tachycardia, **hypertension,*** palpitations

EENT: Blurred vision, tinnitus, mydriasis, ophthalmoplegia, glossitis

Contraindications: Hypersensitivity to tricyclic antidepressants, urinary retention, narrow-angle glaucoma, prostatic hypertrophy

Precautions: Suicidal patients, elderly, pregnancy (C), lactation

Pharmacokinetics:

PO: Steady state 2-8 days; metabolized by liver; excreted by kidneys; crosses placenta; excreted in breast milk; half-life 8-24 hr

Interactions:
• Decreased effects of guanethidine, clonidine, indirect-acting sympathomimetics (ephedrine)
• Increased effects of direct-acting sympathomimetics (epinephrine), alcohol, barbiturates, benzodiazepines, CNS depressants
• Hyperpyretic crisis, convulsions, hypertensive episode: MAOI (pargyline [Eutonyl])

🖋 Increased anticholinergic effect: belladonna leaf/root, henbane leaf

🖋 Increased action of doxepin: scopolia root, kava kava

Lab test interferences:

Increase: Serum bilirubin, blood glucose, alk phosphatase

False increase: Urinary catecholamines

Decrease: VMA, 5-HIAA

◆ = Nursing alert   🖋 = Herb-drug interaction   🚫 = Do not crush

NURSING CONSIDERATIONS
Assess:

• B/P (lying, standing), pulse q4h; if systolic B/P drops 20 mm Hg, hold drug, notify prescriber; take vital signs q4h in patients with cardiovascular disease

• Blood studies: CBC, leukocytes, differential, cardiac enzymes if patient is receiving long-term therapy

• Hepatic studies: AST (SGOT), ALT (SGPT), bilirubin

• Weight qwk; appetite may increase with drug

• ECG for flattening of T wave, bundle branch block, AV block, dysrhythmias in cardiac patients

• EPS primarily in elderly: rigidity, dystonia, akathisia

• Mental status: mood, sensorium, affect, suicidal tendencies, an increase in psychiatric symptoms: depression, panic

• Urinary retention, constipation; constipation most likely in children, elderly

• Withdrawal symptoms: headache, nausea, vomiting, muscle pain, weakness; not usual unless drug is discontinued abruptly

• Alcohol consumption; if alcohol is consumed, hold dose until morning

Administer:

• Increased fluids, bulk in diet for constipation

• With food, milk for GI symptoms

• Dosage hs for oversedation during day; may take entire dose hs; elderly may not tolerate qd dosing

• Gum, hard candy, or frequent sips of water for dry mouth

Perform/provide:

• Storage in tight container protected from direct sunlight

• Assistance with ambulation during beginning therapy, since drowsiness/dizziness occurs

• Safety measures primarily for elderly

• Checking to see PO medication swallowed

Evaluate:

• Therapeutic response: decreased anxiety, depression

Teach patient/family:

• That therapeutic effects may take 2-3 wk

• To use caution in driving, other activities requiring alertness, because of drowsiness, dizziness, blurred vision

• To avoid alcohol ingestion, other CNS depressants

• Not to discontinue medication quickly after long-term use; may cause nausea, headache, malaise

• To wear sunscreen or large hat, since photosensitivity occurs

Treatment of overdose: ECG monitoring, induce emesis; lavage, activated charcoal; administer anticonvulsant

doxorubicin (℞)
(dox-oh-roo′bi-sin)
Adriamycin, Adriamycin PFS, Adriamycin RDF, Doxorubicin HCl, Rubex
Func. class.: Antineoplastic, antibiotic
Chem. class.: Anthracycline glycoside

Action: Inhibits DNA synthesis primarily; derived from *Streptomyces peucetius;* replication is decreased by binding to DNA, which causes strand splitting; active throughout entire cell cycle; a vesicant

Uses: Wilms' tumor; bladder, breast, cervical, head, neck, liver, lung, ovarian, prostatic, stomach, testicular, thyroid cancer; Hodgkin's disease; acute lymphoblastic leukemia; myeloblastic leukemia; neuroblastomas; lymphomas; sarcomas

Dosage and routes:
• *Adult:* IV 60-75 mg/m^2 q3wk, or 30 mg/m^2 on days 1-3 of 4-wk cycle, not to exceed 550 mg/m^2 cumulative dose; Doxil: Adult **IV** 20 mg/m^2 q3wk
• *Child:* IV 30 mg/m^2/day × 3 days, may repeat q4wk

Available forms: Inj 10, 20, 50, 100, 150 mg; Doxil: liposomal dispersion for inj: 20 mg/ml

Side effects/adverse reactions:

HEMA: ***Thrombocytopenia, leukopenia, anemia***

GI: Nausea, vomiting, anorexia, mucositis, ***hepatotoxicity***

GU: Impotence, sterility, amenorrhea, gynecomastia, hyperuricemia

INTEG: *Rash, necrosis at injection site,* dermatitis, reversible alopecia, cellulitis, thrombophlebitis at injection site

CV: Increased B/P, ***sinus tachycardia, PVCs,*** chest pain, ***bradycardia, extrasystoles***

Contraindications: Hypersensitivity, pregnancy (1st trimester) (D), lactation, systemic infections

Precautions: Renal, hepatic, cardiac disease; gout, bone marrow depression (severe)

Pharmacokinetics: Triphasic pattern of elimination; half-life 12 min, 3⅓ hr, 29⅔ hr; metabolized by liver; crosses placenta; excreted in urine, bile, breast milk

Interactions:
• Increased toxicity: other antineoplastics or radiation
• Decreased serum digoxin levels: digoxin
• Decreased antibody response: live virus vaccine

Lab test interferences:
Increase: Uric acid

NURSING CONSIDERATIONS
Assess:
• CBC, differential, platelet count weekly; withhold drug if WBC is <4000/mm^3 or platelet count is <75,000/mm^3; notify prescriber of these results
• Blood, urine uric acid levels
• Renal function studies: BUN, serum uric acid, urine CrCl, electrolytes before, during therapy
• I&O ratio; report fall in urine output to <30 ml/hr
• Monitor temp q4h; fever may indicate beginning infection
• Liver function tests before, during therapy: bilirubin, AST (SGOT), ALT (SGPT), alk phosphatase as needed or monthly
• ECG; watch for ST-T wave changes, low QRS and T, possible dysrhythmias (sinus tachycardia, heart block, PVCs)
• Bleeding: hematuria, guaiac, bruising, or petechiae, mucosa or orifices q8h
• Food preferences; list likes, dislikes
• Effects of alopecia on body image; discuss feelings about body changes
• Inflammation of mucosa, breaks in skin
• Yellowing of skin and sclera, dark urine, clay-colored stools, itchy skin, abdominal pain, fever, diarrhea
• Buccal cavity q8h for dryness, sores, ulceration, white patches, oral pain, bleeding, dysphagia
• Alkalosis if severe vomiting is present
• Local irritation, pain, burning at injection site
• GI symptoms: frequency of stools, cramping
• Acidosis, signs of dehydration: rapid respirations, poor skin turgor, decreased urine output, dry skin, restlessness, weakness

---

◆ = Nursing alert   ⫻ = Herb-drug interaction   Ⓝ = Do not crush

- Cardiac status: B/P, pulse, character, rhythm, rate, ABGs, ECG

Administer:
- Antiemetic 30-60 min before giving drug to prevent vomiting
- Allopurinol or sodium bicarbonate to maintain uric acid levels, alkalinization of urine
- Topical or systemic analgesics for pain
- Transfusion for anemia
- Antispasmodic for GI symptoms

IV
- Hydrocortisone, dexamethasone, or sodium bicarbonate (1 mEq/1 ml) for extravasation; apply ice compresses
- IV after diluting 10 mg/5 ml of NaCl for inj; another 5 ml of diluent/10 mg is recommended; shake; give over 3-5 min; give through Y-tube of free-flowing 5% dextrose INF or NS

Additive compatibilities: Ondansetron

Syringe compatibilities: Bleomycin, cisplatin, cyclophosphamide, droperidol, leucovorin, methotrexate, metoclopramide, mitomycin, vincristine

Y-site compatibilities: Amifostine, aztreonam, bleomycin, chlorpromazine, cimetidine, cisplatin, cladribine, cyclophosphamide, dexamethasone, diphenhydramine, droperidol, famotidine, filgrastim, fludarabine, fluorouracil, granisetron, hydromorphone, leucovorin, lorazepam, melphalan, methotrexate, methylprednisolone, metoclopramide, mitomycin, morphine, ondansetron, paclitaxel, prochlorperazine, promethazine, propofol, ranitidine, sargramostim, sodium bicarbonate, teniposide, thiotepa, vinblastine, vincristine, vinorelbine
- IV (Doxil): dilute dose up to 90 mg/250 ml D_5W, give over ½ hr; do not admix with other sol or meds

Perform/provide:
- Strict hand-washing technique, gloves, protective clothing
- Liquid diet: carbonated beverages, geletin may be added if patient is not nauseated or vomiting
- Increased fluid intake to 2-3 L/day to prevent urate, calculi formation
- Diet low in purines: absence of organ meats (kidney, liver), dried beans, peas to maintain alkaline urine
- Rinsing of mouth tid-qid with water, club soda; brushing of teeth bid-tid with soft brush or cotton-tipped applicators for stomatitis; use unwaxed dental floss
- Storage at room temp for 24 hr after reconstituting or 48 hr refrigerated

Evaluate:
- Therapeutic response: decreased tumor size, spread of malignancy

Teach patient/family:
- To report any complaints, side effects to nurse or prescriber
- That hair may be lost during treatment and wig or hairpiece may make patient feel better; tell patient that new hair may be different in color, texture
- To avoid foods with citric acid, hot or rough texture
- To report any bleeding, white spots, ulcerations in mouth to prescriber; tell patient to examine mouth qd
- That urine and other body fluids may be red-orange for 48 hr
- To avoid crowds and persons with infections when granulocyte count is low
- That contraceptive measures are recommended during therapy
- To avoid vaccinations; reactions may occur

doxycycline (Ŗ)

(dox-i-sye'kleen)
Apo-Doxy*, Atridox, Doryx, Doxy 100, Doxy 200, Doxy-Caps, Doxychel Hyclate, Doxycin*, Doxycycline, Monodox, Novodoxyclin*, Vibramycin, Vibramycin IV, Vibra-Tabs, Vovox

Func. class.: Antiinfective
Chem. class.: Tetracycline

Action: Inhibits protein synthesis, prosphorylation in microorganisms by binding to 30S ribosomal subunits, reversibly binding to 50S ribosomal subunits; bacteriostatic

Uses: Syphilis, *Chlamydia trachomatis,* gonorrhea, *Rickettsia,* lymphogranuloma venereum, uncommon gram-negative/positive organisms, malaria prophylaxis, chronic periodontitis

Investigational uses: Traveler's diarrhea, Lyme disease, prevention of chronic bronchitis

Dosage and routes:
• *Adult:* **PO/IV** 100 mg q12h on day 1, then 100 mg/day; **IV** 200 mg in 1-2 inf on day 1, then 100-200 mg/day; delivery syst: 10% for cont rel
• *Child >8 yr (<45 kg):* **PO/IV** 2.2-4.4 mg/kg/day in divided doses q12h
Gonorrhea (uncomplicated) in patients allergic to penicillin
• *Adult:* **PO** 200 mg, then 100 mg hs and 100 mg bid × 3d or 300 mg, then 300 mg in 1 hr; disseminated; 100 mg **PO** bid × at least 7 days
Malaria prophylaxis
• *Adult:* 100 mg qd 1-2 days prior to travel and daily during travel
C. trachomatis
• *Adult:* **PO** 100 mg bid × 7 days

Syphilis
• *Adult:* **PO** 300 mg/day in divided doses × 10 days
Available forms: Tabs 50, 100 mg; caps 50, 100 mg; syr 50 mg/ml; pwd for inj 100, 200 mg; pwd for oral susp 25 mg/5 ml; Atrigel del syst 10%
Side effects/adverse reactions:
CNS: Fever
*HEMA: **Eosinophilia, neutropenia, thrombocytopenia, hemolytic anemia***
EENT: Dysphagia, glossitis, decreased calcification of deciduous teeth, oral candidiasis
GI: Nausea, abdominal pain, vomiting, diarrhea, anorexia, enterocolitis, **hepatotoxicity,** flatulence, abdominal cramps, gastric burning, stomatitis
CV: Pericarditis
GU: Increased BUN
*INTEG: Rash, urticaria, photosensitivity, increased pigmentation, **exfoliative dermatitis,** pruritus, **angioedema***
Contraindications: Hypersensitivity to tetracyclines, children <8 yr, pregnancy (D)
Precautions: Hepatic disease, lactation
Pharmacokinetics:
PO: Peak 1½-4 hr, half-life 15-22 hr; excreted in bile, 90% protein bound
Interactions:
• Decreased effects of doxycycline: antacids, $NaHCO_3$, dairy products, alkali products, iron, kaolin/pectin, barbiturates, carbamazepine, phenytoin, cimetidine
• Increased effect: warfarin
• Decreased effects: penicillins, oral contraceptives
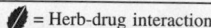 Increased action: bromelain
Lab test interferences:
False negative: Urine glucose with Clinistix or Tes-Tape

 = Nursing alert   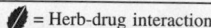 = Herb-drug interaction   🚫 = Do not crush

False increase: Urinary catecholamines; ALT, AST

NURSING CONSIDERATIONS
Assess:
• I&O ratio
• Blood studies: PT, CBC, AST, ALT, BUN, creatinine
• Signs of infection
• Allergic reactions: rash, itching, pruritus, angioedema
• Nausea, vomiting, diarrhea; administer antiemetic, antacids as ordered
• Overgrowth of infection: fever, malaise, redness, pain, swelling, drainage, perineal itching, diarrhea, changes in cough or sputum
• IV site for phlebitis/thrombosis; drug is highly irritating

Administer:
• After C&S
• 2 hr before or after laxative or iron products; 3 hr after antacid or kaolin-pectin products

IV
• After diluting 100 mg or less/10 ml of sterile H_2O or NS for inj; further dilute with 100-1000 ml of NaCl, D_5, Ringer's LR D_5LR, Normosol-M, Normosol-R in D_5W, run 100 mg or less over 1-4 hr; do not give IM/SC; inf must be completed in 6 hr, when diluted in LR sol, or 12 hr in other sol

Additive compatibilities: Ranitidine

Syringe compatibilities: Doxapram

Y-site compatibilities: Acyclovir, amifostine, amiodarone, aztreonam, cyclophosphamide, diltiazem, filgrastim, fludarabine, granisetron, hydromorphone, magnesium sulfate, melphalan, meperidine, morphine, ondansetron, perphenazine, propofol, sargramostim, tacrolimus, teniposide, theophylline, thiotepa, vinorelbine

Perform/provide:
• Storage in tight, light-resistant container at room temp

Evaluate:
• Therapeutic response: decreased temp, absence of lesions, negative C&S

Teach patient/family:
• To avoid sun, since burns may occur; sunscreen does not seem to decrease photosensitivity
• That all prescribed medication must be taken to prevent superinfection
🚫 Not to break, crush, or chew caps
• To take with a full glass of water; may take with food

D-penicillamine (℞)
(pen-i-sill'a-meen)
Cuprimine, Depen
Func. class.: Heavy metal antagonist
Chem. class.: Chelating agent (thiol compound)

Action: Binds with ions of lead, mercury, copper, iron, zinc to form a water-soluble complex excreted by kidneys

Uses: Wilson's disease, rheumatoid arthritis, cystinuria, lead poisoning

Dosage and routes:
Cystinuria
• *Adult:* PO 250 mg qid ac, not to exceed 5 g/day
• *Child:* PO 30 mg/kg/day in divided doses qid ac

Wilson's disease
• *Adult:* PO 250 mg qid ac
• *Child:* PO 20 mg/kg/day in divided doses ac

Rheumatoid arthritis
• *Adult:* PO 125-250 mg/day, then increased 250 mg q2-3mo if needed, not to exceed 1 g/day

• *Child:* **PO** 3 mg/kg/day, increase to max 10 mg/kg/day
Available forms: Caps 125, 250 mg; tabs 250 mg

Side effects/adverse reactions:
HEMA: **Thrombocytopenia, granulocytopenia, leukopenia, hemolytic anemia, aplastic anemia, eosinophilia,** lupus syndrome, increased sedimentation rate
INTEG: Urticaria, erythema, pruritus, fever, ecchymosis, alopecia
CV: Hypotension, tachycardia
GI: Diarrhea, abdominal cramping, nausea, vomiting, **hepatotoxicity,** anorexia, pain, peptic ulcer
EENT: Tinnitus, optic neuritis
MS: Arthralgia
GU: **Proteinuria, nephrotic syndrome, glomerulonephritis**
SYST: **Anaphylaxis**
RESP: Pneumonitis, **asthma, pulmonary fibrosis**

Contraindications: Hypersensitivity to penicillins, anuria, agranulocytosis, severe renal disease, pregnancy (D), lactation

Pharmacokinetics:
PO: Peak 1 hr, metabolized in liver, excreted in urine

Interactions:
• Increased side effects: oxyphenbutazone, phenylbutazone, gold salts, antimalarials, cytotoxics
• Decreased absorption of D-penicillamine: oral iron, antacids, food

NURSING CONSIDERATIONS
Assess:
• Monitor hepatic, renal studies: AST/ALT, alk phosphatase, BUN, creatinine
• Monitor I&O, temp
• Monitor platelet, neutropenia, WBC, H&H; if WBC <3500/mm³ or if platelets <100,000/mm³, drug should be discontinued
• Allergic reactions (rash, urticaria); if these occur, drug should be discontinued

Administer:
• On an empty stomach, ½-1 hr before meals; at least 2 hr after meals
• Vit B_6 daily, depleted when this drug is used
• Only when epinephrine 1:1000 is on unit for anaphylaxis
• Fluids to 3 L/day to prevent renal failure

Evaluate:
• Therapeutic response: absence of pain, rigidity in joints (rheumatoid arthritis)

Teach patient/family:
• That urine may be red
• That therapeutic effect may take 1-3 mo
◆ To report sore throat, easy bruising, bleeding from mucous membranes; may indicate bone marrow depression
🚫 Not to break, crush, or chew caps

---

droperidol (℞)
(droe-per′i-dole)
Droperidol, Inapsine
Func. class.: Neuroleptic
Chem. class.: Butyrophenone derivative

Action: Acts on CNS at subcortical levels, produces tranquilization, sleep; antiemetic

Uses: Premedication for surgery; induction, maintenance in general anesthesia; postoperatively for nausea, vomiting

Dosage and routes:
Induction
• *Adult:* **IV/IM** 0.22-0.275 mg/kg given with analgesic or general anesthetic; may give 1.25-2.5 mg additionally
• *Child 2-12 yr:* **IV** 88-165 µg/kg, titrated to response needed

Premedication
• *Adult:* **IM** 2.5-10 mg ½-1 hr before surgery
• *Child 2-12 yr:* **IM** 1-1.5 mg/20-25 lb

Maintaining general anesthesia
• *Adult:* **IV** 1.25-2.5 mg

Regional anesthesia adjunct
• *Adult:* **IV/IM** 2.5-5 mg

Diagnostic procedures without general anesthesia
• *Adult:* **IM** 2.5-10 mg ½-1 hr prior to procedure; 1.25-2.5 mg may be needed

Available forms: Inj 2.5 mg/ml

Side effects/adverse reactions:
*RESP: **Laryngospasm, bronchospasm***
CNS: Dystonia, akathisia, flexion of arms, fine tremors, dizziness, anxiety, drowsiness, restlessness, hallucination, depression
CV: Tachycardia, hypotension
EENT: Upward rotation of eyes, oculogyric crisis
INTEG: Chills, facial sweating, shivering

Contraindications: Hypersensitivity, child <2 yr, pregnancy (C), lactation

Precautions: Elderly, cardiovascular disease (hypotension, bradydysrhythmias), renal disease, liver disease, Parkinson's disease

Pharmacokinetics:
IM/IV: Onset 3-10 min, peak ½ hr, duration 3-6 hr; metabolized in liver; excreted in urine as metabolites; crosses placenta

Interactions:
• Increased CNS depression: alcohol, narcotics, barbiturates, antipsychotics, or other CNS depressants
• Decreased effects of amphetamines, anticonvulsants, anticoagulants when given with this drug
• Increased intraocular pressure: anticholinergics, antiparkinsonian drugs
• Increased side effects of lithium
🍃 Increased action: kava kava

NURSING CONSIDERATIONS
Assess:
• VS q10min during IV administration, q30min after IM dose
• EPS: dystonia, akathisia
◆ For increasing heart rate or decreasing B/P, notify prescriber at once; do not place patient in Trendelenburg position, or sympathetic blockade may occur, causing respiratory arrest

Administer:
• Anticholinergics (benztropine, diphenhydramine) for EPS
• Only with crash cart, resuscitative equipment nearby
• IM deep in large muscle mass
IV
• Undiluted; give through Y-tube at 10 mg or less/min; titrate to patient response; may be given as an infusion by adding dose to 250 ml LR, D_5W, 0.9% NaCl

Syringe compatibilities: Atropine, bleomycin, butorphanol, chlorpromazine, cimetidine, cisplatin, cyclophosphamide, dimenhydrinate, diphenhydramine, doxorubicin, fentanyl, glycopyrrolate, hydroxyzine, meperidine, metoclopramide, midazolam, mitomycin, morphine, nalbuphine, pentazocine, perphenazine, prochlorperazine, promazine, promethazine, scopolamine, vinblastine, vincristine

Y-site compatibilities: Amifostine, aztreonam, bleomycin, cladribine, cisplatin, cyclophosphamide, cytarabine, doxorubicin, famotidine, filgrastim, fluconazole, fludarabine, granisetron, hydrocortisone, idarubicin, melphalan, meperidine, metoclopramide, mitomycin, ondansetron, paclitaxel, potassium chloride, propofol, sargramostim, teniposide, thiotepa, vinblastine, vincristine, vinorelbine, vit B/C

Perform/provide:
• Slow movement of patient to avoid orthostatic hypotension

Evaluate:
• Therapeutic response: decreased anxiety, absence of vomiting during and after surgery
• To rise slowly from sitting or standing to minimize orthostatic hypotension

---

dyphylline (℞)
(dye'fi-lin)
Dilor, Dyflex-200, Dyflex-400, Dylline, Dyphylline, Lufyllin, Lufyllin-400, Neothylline, Protophylline*

Func. class.: Bronchodilator
Chem. class.: Xanthine, ethylenediamide

Action: Relaxes smooth muscle of respiratory system by blocking phosphodiesterase, which increases cyclic AMP; cyclic AMP results in positive inotropic, chronotropic effects, bronchodilation, stimulation of CNS

Uses: Bronchial asthma, bronchospasm in chronic bronchitis, COPD

Dosage and routes:
• *Adult:* **PO** 200-800 mg q6h; **IM** 250-500 mg q6h injected slowly
• *Child >6 yr:* **PO** 4-7 mg/kg/day in 4 divided doses

Available forms: Tabs 200, 400 mg; elix 100, 160 mg/15 ml; inj 250 mg/ml

Side effects/adverse reactions:
CNS: Anxiety, restlessness, insomnia, dizziness, convulsions, headache, light-headedness, muscle twitching
CV: Palpitations, sinus tachycardia, hypotension, flushing, dysrhythmias
GI: Nausea, vomiting, anorexia, dyspepsia, epigastric pain

INTEG: Flushing, urticaria
RESP: Tachypnea
OTHER: Fever, dehydration, *albuminuria,* hyperglycemia

Contraindications: Hypersensitivity to xanthines, tachydysrhythmias

Precautions: Elderly, CHF, cor pulmonale, hepatic disease, active peptic ulcer disease, diabetes mellitus, hyperthyroidism, hypertension, children, renal disease, pregnancy (C), lactation, glaucoma

Pharmacokinetics: Peak 1 hr, half-life 2 hr, excreted in urine unchanged

Interactions:
• Do not mix in syringe with other drugs
• Increased action of dyphylline: cimetidine, propranolol, erythromycin, troleandomycin
• May increase effects of anticoagulants
• Cardiotoxicity: β-blockers
• Increased metabolism: barbiturates, phenytoin
• Decreased elimination of dyphylline: uricosurics

NURSING CONSIDERATIONS
Assess:
• Dyphylline blood levels; toxicity may occur with small increase above 20 µg/ml
• Monitor I&O; diuresis occurs; dehydration may result in elderly or children
• Whether theophylline was given recently
• Auscultate lung fields bilaterally; notify prescriber of abnormalities
• Allergic reactions: rash, urticaria; drug should be discontinued

Administer:
• PO after meals to decrease GI symptoms; absorption may be affected
• Avoid IM injection; pain occurs

Perform/provide:
• Storage protected from light, at room temp

◆ = Nursing alert   ⫻ = Herb-drug interaction   ⊘ = Do not crush

Evaluate:
• Therapeutic response: decreased dyspnea, respiratory rate, rhythm

Teach patient/family:
• To check OTC medications, current prescription medications for ephedrine; will increase stimulation; not to drink alcohol or caffeine
• To avoid hazardous activities; dizziness, drowsiness, blurred vision may occur
• For GI upset, to take drug with 8 oz water; avoid taking with food, since absorption may be decreased

---

edetate disodium (℞)

(ee′de-tate)

Chealamide, Disodium EDTA, Disotate, Endrate

Func. class.: Metal antagonist
Chem. class.: Chelating agent

Action: Binds with ions of calcium, zinc, magnesium to form a water-soluble complex excreted from kidneys

Uses: Hypercalcemic crisis, control of ventricular dysrhythmias associated with digitalis toxicity

Dosage and routes:
• *Adult and child:* IV INF 15-50 mg/kg/day in 2 divided doses, diluted in 500 ml D₅W or 0.9% NaCl, given over 3-4 hr, not to exceed 3 g/day (adult) or 70 mg/kg/day (child); allow 5 days between courses (child), 2 days (adult)

Available forms: Inj conc 150 mg/ml

Side effects/adverse reactions:
*CNS: Headache, paresthesia, **numbness***
INTEG: Urticaria, **exfoliative dermatitis,** erythema, pain at injection site
CV: Hypotension, thrombophlebitis
GI: Nausea, vomiting, diarrhea
GU: Dysuria, pyelonephritis, **neph-**

rotoxicity, hyperuricemia, hypomagnesemia, polyuria, ***proteinuria, renal tubular necrosis, hypocalcemia***

Contraindications: Hypersensitivity, anuria, hepatic insufficiency, poisoning of other metals, severe renal disease, child <3 yr, seizure disorders, active/inactive TB

Precautions: Hypertension, pregnancy (C), lactation

Pharmacokinetics: Excreted in urine as calcium chelate

Interactions:
• Incompatible in 5% alcohol

Lab test interferences:
False decrease: Calcium
Decrease: Magnesium, alk phosphatase

NURSING CONSIDERATIONS

Assess:
• VS, B/P, pulse; if hypotension occurs, drug should be discontinued
• Monitor I&O, kidney function studies: BUN, creatinine, CrCl, Ca (must be done following each administration)
• Hypocalcemia: numbness of feet, hands, tongue, lips; positive Chvostek's, Trousseau's signs; convulsions; stupor
• Cardiac abnormalities: dysrhythmias, hypotension, tachycardia
• Allergic reactions (rash, urticaria); if these occur, drug should be discontinued

Administer:
• IV inf after diluting in 500 ml dextrose, or isotonic saline sol, not to exceed 15 mg of actual medication/min, total dose is usually given over 3-4 hr
• Only when IV Ca preparation is on unit for emergency use
• EDTA, BAL separately
• IV use infusion pump, rotate infusion sites, observe site for redness, inflammation

---

- IV fluids to ensure adequate hydration before administration of drug

Perform/provide:
- Assistance with ambulation

Evaluate:
- Therapeutic response: Ca levels 9-10 mg/dl; absence of hypercalcemic symptoms

Teach patient/family:
- To remain recumbent for ½ hr to prevent postural hypotension
- To make position changes slowly to prevent fainting
- That dosage schedule must be followed
- That breath may be odorous

---

edrophonium (℞)

(ed-roe-fone′ee-um)
Enlon, Reversol, Tensilon
Func. class.: Cholinergics, anticholinesterase
Chem. class.: Quaternary ammonium compound

Action: Inhibits destruction of acetylcholine, which increases concentration at sites where acetylcholine is released; this facilitates transmission of impulses across myoneural junction

Uses: To diagnose myasthenia gravis; curare antagonist; differentiation of myasthenic crisis from cholinergic crisis

Dosage and routes:
Tensilon test (myasthenia gravis diagnosis)
- *Adult:* **IV** 1-2 mg over 15-30 sec, then 8 mg if no response; **IM** 10 mg; if cholinergic reaction occurs, retest after ½ hr with 2 mg **IM**
- *Child >34 kg:* **IV** 2 mg; if no response in 45 sec, then 1 mg q45sec, not to exceed 10 mg; **IM** 5 mg
- *Child <34 kg:* **IV** 1 mg; if no response in 45 sec, then 1 mg q45sec, not to exceed 5 mg; **IM** 2 mg

- *Infant:* **IV** 0.5 mg

Reversal of nondepolarizing neuromuscular blockers
- *Adult:* **IV** 10 mg over 30-45 sec, may repeat, not to exceed 40 mg

Differentiation of myasthenic crisis from cholinergic crisis
- *Adult:* **IV** 1 mg, if no response in 1 min, may repeat

Available forms: Inj 10 mg/ml

Side effects/adverse reactions:
INTEG: Rash, urticaria
CNS: Dizziness, headache, sweating, weakness, *convulsions,* incoordination, *paralysis,* drowsiness, *loss of consciousness*
GI: Nausea, diarrhea, vomiting, cramps, increased salivary and gastric secretions, dysphagia, increased peristalsis
CV: Dysrhythmias, bradycardia, hypotension, *AV block,* ECG changes, *cardiac arrest,* syncope
GU: Frequency, incontinence, urgency
RESP: **Respiratory depression, bronchospasm, constriction, laryngospasm, respiratory arrest,** dyspnea, increased bronchial secretions
EENT: Miosis, blurred vision, lacrimation, visual changes

Contraindications: Obstruction of intestine, renal system, hypersensitivity

Precautions: Seizure disorders, bronchial asthma, coronary occlusion, hyperthyroidism, dysrhythmias, peptic ulcer, megacolon, poor GI motility, pregnancy (C), bradycardia, hypotension

Pharmacokinetics:
IV: Onset 30-60 sec, duration 6-15 min
IM: Onset 2-10 min, duration 12-45 min

Interactions:
- Decreased action of edrophonium: procainamide, quinidine, atropine, anesthetics, mecamylamine, poly-

---

◆ = Nursing alert   ∥ = Herb-drug interaction   ⊘ = Do not crush

myxin, magnesium, corticosteroids, antidysrhythmics

• Bradycardia: digitalis

• Increased action of edrophonium: aminoglycosides

NURSING CONSIDERATIONS

Assess:

• VS, respiration during test; muscle strength

• Diabetic patient carefully, since this drug lowers blood glucose

Administer:

◆ Only with atropine sulfate available for cholinergic crisis

• Only after all other cholinergics have been discontinued

IV, direct

• 2 mg or less over 15-30 sec; as a curare antagonist, over 30-45 sec; or given as continuous infusion in myasthenic crisis

Y-site compatibilities: Heparin, hydrocortisone, potassium chloride, vit B/C

Perform/provide:

• Storage at room temp

Evaluate:

• Therapeutic response: increased muscle strength, hand grasp; improved gait; absence of labored breathing (if severe)

Teach patient/family:

• To wear Medic Alert ID specifying myasthenia gravis, drugs taken

Treatment of overdose: Respiratory support, atropine 1-4 mg (IV)

---

enalapril/ enalaprilat (℞)

(e-nal′a-pril)/(e-nal′a-pril-at)
Vasotec, Vasotec IV

Func. class.: Antihypertensive
Chem. class.: Angiotensin-converting enzyme inhibitor

Action: Selectively suppresses renin-angiotensin-aldosterone system; inhibits ACE; prevents conversion of angiotensin I to angiotensin II, dilation of arterial, venous vessels

Uses: Hypertension, systolic CHF, diabetic neuropathy, post MI, left ventricular dysfunction

Dosage and routes:

Hypertension

• *Adult:* **PO** 5 mg/day, may increase or decrease to desired response range 10-40 mg/day; **IV** 1.25 mg q6h over 5 min

• *Child:* **PO** 0.1 mg/kg/day in 1-2 divided doses, max 0.5 mg/kg/day

• *Child:* **IV** 5-10 μg/kg/dose q8-24h

Patients on diuretics

• *Adult:* **IV** 0.625 mg over 5 min, may give additional doses of 1.25 mg q6h

Renal impairment

• *Adult:* **PO** 2.5 mg qd (CrCl <30 ml/min) increase gradually; **IV** CrCl >30 ml/min 1.25 mg q6h; CrCl <30 ml/min 0.625 mg as one time dose, increase as per B/P

CHF

• *Adult:* **PO** 5-20 mg/day in 2 divided doses

Available forms: Tabs 2.5, 5, 10, 20 mg; tabs, ext rel inj 1.25 mg/ml

Side effects/adverse reactions:

CV: Hypotension, chest pain, tachycardia, dysrhythmias, syncope

CNS: Insomnia, dizziness, paresthesias, headache, fatigue, anxiety

GI: Nausea, vomiting, colitis, cramps, diarrhea, constipation, flatulence, dry mouth, loss of taste

INTEG: Rash, purpura, alopecia, hyperhidrosis

*HEMA: **Agranulocytosis, neutropenia***

EENT: Tinnitus, visual changes, sore throat, double vision, dry burning eyes

*GU: **Proteinuria, renal failure,*** increased frequency of polyuria or oliguria

RESP: Dyspnea, dry cough, rales, angioedema

META: Hyperkalemia

Contraindications: Hypersensitivity, history of angioedema

Precautions: Renal disease, hyperkalemia, pregnancy (C), lactation, hepatic failure, dehydration, bilateral renal artery stenosis

Pharmacokinetics:

PO: Peak 4-6 hr; half-life 1½ hr; metabolized by liver to active metabolite, excreted in urine

IV: Onset 5-15 min, peak up to 4 hr

Interactions:

• Hypersensitivity: allopurinol
• Severe hypotension: diuretics, other antihypertensives
• Decreased effects of enalapril: aspirin, antacids
• Increased K levels: salt substitutes, K-sparing diuretics, K supplements
• May increase effects of ergots, neuromuscular blocking agents, antihypertensives, hypoglycemics, barbiturates, reserpine, levodopa, lithium
• Effects may be increased by phenothiazines, diuretics, phenytoin, quinidine, nifedipine

Lab test interferences:

Interference: Glucose/insulin tolerance tests

NURSING CONSIDERATIONS

Assess:

• B/P, pulse q4h; note rate, rhythm, quality
• Electrolytes: K, Na, Cl during 1st 2 wk of therapy
• Baselines in renal, liver function tests before therapy begins and 1 wk into therapy
• Edema in feet, legs daily
• Skin turgor, dryness of mucous membranes for hydration status
• Symptoms of CHF: edema, dyspnea, wet rales

Administer:

IV, direct/int inf

• Undiluted over 5 min, use diluent provided or 50 ml D_5W, 0.9% NaCl, 0.9% NaCl in D_5W or LR, Isolyte E, give through Y-tube of free-flowing inf of 0.9% NaCl, D_5W, LR, Isolyte E

Additive compatibilities: Dobutamine, dopamine, heparin, meropenem, nitroglycerin, nitroprusside, potassium chloride

Y-site compatibilities: Allopurinol, amifostine, amikacin, aminophylline, ampicillin, ampicillin/sulbactam, aztreonam, butorphanol, calcium gluconate, cefazolin, cefoperazone, ceftazidime, ceftizoxime, chloramphenicol, cimetidine, cladribine, clindamycin, dextran 40, dobutamine, dopamine, erythromycin, esmolol, famotidine, fentanyl, filgrastim, ganciclovir, gentamicin, granisetron, heparin, hetastarch, hydrocortisone, labetalol, lidocaine, magnesium sulfate, melphalan, meropenem, methylprednisolone, metronidazole, morphine, nafcillin, nicardipine, nitroprusside, penicillin G potassium, phenobarbital, piperacillin, piperacillin/tazobactam, potassium chloride, potassium phosphate, propofol, ranitidine, sodium acetate, teniposide, thiotepa, tobramycin, trimethoprim/sulfamethoxazole, vancomycin, vinorelbine

Evaluate:

• Therapeutic response: decreased B/P

Teach patient/family:

• Not to use OTC (cough, cold, or allergy) products unless directed by prescriber; to avoid salt substitutes
• To avoid sunlight or wear sunscreen for photosensitivity
• To comply with dosage schedule, even if feeling better

◆ = Nursing alert   ▮ = Herb-drug interaction   ⊘ = Do not crush

• To notify prescriber of mouth sores, sore throat, fever, swelling of hands or feet, irregular heartbeat, chest pain, signs of angioedema
• That excessive perspiration, dehydration, vomiting, diarrhea may lead to fall in blood pressure; consult prescriber if these occur
• That drug may cause dizziness, fainting; light-headedness may occur during 1st few days of therapy
• That drug may cause skin rash or impaired perspiration; angioedema may occur and to D/C if it occurs
• Not to discontinue drug abruptly
• That CV adverse reactions may reoccur
• To rise slowly to sitting or standing position to minimize orthostatic hypotension

Treatment of overdose: Lavage, IV atropine for bradycardia, IV theophylline for bronchospasm, digitalis, O_2, diuretic for cardiac failure

---

enoxacin (℞)

(e-nox′a-sin)
Penetrex
Func. class.: Antiinfective
Chem. class.: Fluoroquinolone

Action: Inhibits the enzyme that repairs bacterial DNA, thereby preventing bacterial replication; DNA-gyrase inhibitor

Uses: Uncomplicated urethral or cervical gonorrhea, uncomplicated and complicated UTI; effective against staphylococci, *Aeromonas* sp., *Citrobacter* sp., *Enterobacter* sp., *Escherichia coli*, *Hemophilus ducreyi*, *Klebsiella* sp., *Moranella morganii*, *Neisseria gonorrhoeae*, *Proteus vulgaris*, *Proteus mirabilis*, *Providencia* sp., *Pseudomonas aeruginosa*, *Serratia*

Dosage and routes:
Gonorrhea
• *Adult:* **PO** 400 mg as a single dose
Uncomplicated UTI
• *Adult:* **PO** 200 mg bid × 7 days
Complicated UTI
• *Adult:* **PO** 400 mg bid × 14 days
Renal disease
• CrCl <30 ml/min give initial dose, then give 50% of dose q12h
Available forms: Tabs 200, 400 mg
Side effects/adverse reactions:

CNS: Dizziness, headache, fatigue, somnolence, depression, insomnia, anxiety
GI: Diarrhea, nausea, vomiting, anorexia, flatulence, heartburn, abdominal pain, dry mouth, increased AST (SGOT), ALT (SGPT)
INTEG: Rash, pruritus, photosensitivity
EENT: Visual disturbances, dizziness

Contraindications: Hypersensitivity to quinolones
Precautions: Pregnancy (C), lactation, children, elderly, renal disease, seizure disorders
Pharmacokinetics:
PO: Peak 1 hr, half-life 3-6 hr, steady state 2 days; excreted in urine as unchanged drug, metabolites
Interactions:
• Decreased effects of enoxacin: antacids, nitrofurantoin, iron salts, sucralfate, antineoplastics, zinc, bismuth salts
• Increased enoxacin levels: probenecid, cimetidine
• Increased toxicity: theophylline, cyclosporine, caffeine/warfarin
NURSING CONSIDERATIONS
Assess:
• Kidney, liver function studies: BUN, creatinine, AST (SGOT), ALT (SGPT)
• I&O ratio, urine pH; <5.5 is ideal

Side effects: *italics* = common; ***bold italics*** = life-threatening

• CNS symptoms: insomnia, vertigo, headache, agitation, confusion
• Allergic reactions: rash, flushing, urticaria, pruritus

Administer:

• After clean-catch urine for C&S
• 2 hr before or 2 hr after antacids, zinc, iron, calcium

Perform/provide:

• Limited intake of alkaline foods, drugs; milk, dairy products, peanuts, vegetables, alkaline actacids, sodium bicarbonate

Evaluate:

• Therapeutic response: negative C&S, absence of symptoms of infection

Teach patient/family:

• That fluids must be increased to 3 L/day to avoid crystallization in kidneys
• If dizziness occurs, to ambulate, perform activities with assistance
• Not to take within 2 hr of antacids, calcium, iron, milk, sucralfate
• To use sunscreen, protective clothing for photosensitivity
• To complete full course of drug therapy, take 1 hr ac or 2 hr pc
• To contact prescriber if adverse reactions occur or if inflammation or pain of tendon occurs

---

enoxaparin (℞)

(ee-nox′a-par-in)
Lovenox
Func. class.: Anticoagulant
Chem. class.: Unfractionated porcine heparin

Action: Prevents conversion of fibrinogen to fibrin and prothrombin to thrombin by enhancing inhibitory effects of antithrombin III; produces higher ratio of antifactor Xa to antifactor IIa

Uses: Prevention of deep-vein thrombosis, pulmonary emboli in hip and knee replacement

Dosage and routes:

Hip/knee replacement
• *Adult:* SC 30 mg bid given 12-24 hr post-op for 7-10 days, provided that hemostasis has been established

Abdominal surgery
Adult: SC 40 mg qd × 7-10 days to prevent thromboembolic complications

Available forms: Inj 30 mg/0.3 ml, 40 mg/0.4 ml, prefilled syringes

Side effects/adverse reactions:

CNS: Fever, confusion
GI: Nausea
GU: Edema, peripheral edema
HEMA: **Hypochromic anemia, thrombocytopenia,** bleeding
INTEG: Ecchymosis

Contraindications: Hypersensitivity to this drug, heparin, or pork; hemophilia, leukemia with bleeding, peptic ulcer disease, thrombocytopenic purpura, heparin-induced thrombocytopenia

Precautions: Alcoholism, elderly, pregnancy (C), hepatic disease (severe), renal disease (severe), blood dyscrasias, severe hypertension, subacute bacterial endocarditis, acute nephritis, lactation, children

Pharmacokinetics:

SC: Maximum antithrombin activity (3-5 hr), elimination half-life 4½ hr

Interactions:

• Increased action of enoxaparin: oral anticoagulants, salicylates
• Do not mix with other drugs or infusion fluids
🌿 Increased risk of bleeding: bromelain, cinchona bark

NURSING CONSIDERATIONS

Assess:

• Blood studies (Hct, platelets, occult blood in stools), anti-Xa; thrombocytopenia may occur

---

◆ = Nursing alert   🌿 = Herb-drug interaction   🚫 = Do not crush

• Bleeding gums, petechiae, ecchymosis, black tarry stools, hematuria
Administer:
• Only after screening patient for bleeding disorders
• SC only; do not give IM
• To recumbent patient; give SC; rotate inj sites (left/right anterolateral, left/right posterolateral abdominal wall)
• Insert whole length of needle into skin fold held with thumb and forefinger
◆ Only this drug when ordered; not interchangeable with heparin
• At same time each day to maintain steady blood levels
• Do not massage area or aspirate when giving SC injection
• Avoiding all IM injections that may cause bleeding
Perform/provide:
• Storage at 77° F (25° C); do not freeze
Evaluate:
• Therapeutic response: prevention of deep vein thrombosis
Teach patient/family:
• To use soft-bristle toothbrush to avoid bleeding gums, to use electric razor
• To report any signs of bleeding: gums, under skin, urine, stools
Treatment of overdose: Protamine SO₄ 1% sol; dose should equal dose of enoxaparin

ephedrine (℞)

(e-fed′rin)
Ephedrine, Ephedrine sulfate, Neorespin
Func. class.: Bronchodilator, adrenergic, mixed direct and indirect effects
Chem. class.: Phenylisopropylamine

Action: Causes increased contractility and heart rate by acting on β-receptors in the heart; also acts on α-receptors, causing vasoconstriction in blood vessels
Uses: Shock; increased perfusion; hypotension, bronchodilation
Dosage and routes:
Vasopressor
• *Adult:* **IM/SC** 25-50 mg, not to exceed 150 mg/24 hr; **IV** 10-25 mg, not to exceed 150 mg/24 hr
• *Child:* **SC/IV** 3 mg/kg/day or 25-100 mg/m²/day in divided doses q4-6h
Bronchodilator
• *Adult:* **PO** 25-50 mg bid-qid, not to exceed 400 mg/day; **IM/SC** 12.5-25 mg
• *Child:* **PO** 2-3 mg/kg/day or 100 mg/m²/day in 4-6 divided doses
Orthostatic hypotension
• *Adult:* **PO** 25 mg qd-qid
• *Child:* **PO** 3 mg/kg/day in 4-6 divided doses
Stimulation
• *Adult:* **PO** 25-50 mg q3-4h prn
• *Child:* **PO** 3 mg/kg/day or 100 mg/m²/day in divided doses
Labor
• *Adult:* Administer **IV** dose to maintain B/P at or <1³⁰⁄₈₀ mm Hg
Available forms: Inj 25, 50 mg/ml; caps 25, 50 mg; syr 11, 20 mg/5 ml
Side effects/adverse reactions:
CNS: Tremors, anxiety, insomnia, headache, dizziness, confusion, hal-

lucinations, ***convulsions, CNS depression***

GU: Dysuria, urinary retention

CV: Palpitations, tachycardia, hypertension, chest pain, ***dysrhythmias***

GI: Anorexia, nausea, vomiting

*RESP: **Dyspnea***

Contraindications: Hypersensitivity to sympathomimetics, narrow-angle glaucoma

Precautions: Pregnancy (C), lactation, cardiac disorders, hyperthyroidism, diabetes mellitus, prostatic hypertrophy

Pharmacokinetics:

PO: Onset 15-60 min, duration 2-4 hr

IV: Onset 5 min, duration 2 hr
Metabolized in liver; excreted in urine (unchanged), breast milk; crosses blood-brain barrier, placenta

Interactions:

• Severe hypertension: oxytocics

• Do not use with MAOIs or tricyclic antidepressants; hypertensive crisis may occur

• Decreased effect of ephedrine: methyldopa, urinary acidifiers, rauwolfia alkaloids

• Increased effect of this drug: urinary alkalizers

• Dysrhythmia: halothane anesthetics, digitalis

• Decreased effect of guanethidine

 Increased action of ephedrine: ephedra

NURSING CONSIDERATIONS

Assess:

• I&O ratio

• ECG continuously during administration; if B/P increases, drug is decreased

• B/P and pulse q5min after parenteral route

• CVP or PWP during infusion if possible

• For paresthesias and coldness of extremities; peripheral blood flow may decrease

• Injection site: tissue sloughing; if this occurs, administer phentolamine mixed with 0.9% NaCl

Administer:

IV, direct

• Through Y-tube or 3-way stopcock; give 10 mg or less over 1 min

• Plasma expanders for hypovolemia

Additive compatibilities: Chloramphenicol, lidocaine, metaraminol, nafcillin, penicillin G potassium

Solution compatibilities: D_5W, $D_{10}W$, ionosol, LR, 0.9% NaCl, 0.45% NaCl, Ringer's

Syringe compatibilities: Pentobarbital

Y-site compatibilities: Etomidate, propofol

Perform/provide:

• Storage of reconstituted sol refrigerated no longer than 24 hr

• Do not use discolored sol

Evaluate:

• Therapeutic response: increased B/P with stabilization

Teach patient/family:

• The reason for drug administration

Treatment of overdose: Administer phentolamine for hypertension, diazepam for convulsions

---

epinephrine (℞)

(ep-i-nef'rin)

Adrenalin Chloride, Adrenalin Chloride Solution, Asthma Haler, Asthma Nefrin, Bronitin Mist, Bronkaid Mist, Epinal, Epinephrine, Epinephrine HCl, Epinephrine Pediatric, Epipen Jr., Epitrate, Eppy/N, Glaucon, Medihaler-Epi, Micro-Nefrin, Nephron Inhalant, Primatene Mist, S-2 Inhalant, Sus-Phrine, Vaponefrin

Func. class.: Bronchodilator-adrenergic

Chem. class.: Catecholamine

Action: β_1- and β_2-agonist causing increased levels of cyclic AMP producing bronchodilation, cardiac, and CNS stimulation; large doses cause vasoconstriction; small doses can cause vasodilation via β_2-vascular receptors

Uses: Acute asthmatic attacks, hemostasis, bronchospasm, anaphylaxis, allergic reactions, cardiac arrest, adjunct in anesthesia

Dosage and routes:

Asthma

• *Adult and child:* **INH** 1-2 puffs of 1:100 or 2.25% racemic q15min

Bronchodilator

• *Adult:* **SC** 0.2-0.5 mg q20min-4h, max 1 mg/dose

Anaphylactic shock/vasopressor

• *Adult:* **SC/IM** 0.5 mg, repeat q5min if needed, then **IV; IV** 0.1-0.25 mg, repeat q5-15min or inf 1 μg/min, increase to 4 μg/min if needed

• *Child:* **SC/IM/IV** 10 μg/kg, repeat q5-15min up to 0.3 mg

Anaphylactic reaction/asthma

• *Adult:* **SC/IM** 0.1-0.5 mg, repeat q10-15min, do not exceed 1 mg/dose; epinephrine susp 0.5 mg **SC,** may repeat 0.5-1.5 mg q6h

• *Child:* **SC** 0.01 mg/kg, repeat q15min, × 2 doses, then q4h, max 0.5 mg/dose; epinephrine susp 0.025 mg/kg **SC,** may repeat q6h, max 0.75 mg in child ≤30 kg

Cardiac arrest

• *Adult:* **IC, IV,** endotracheal 0.1-1 mg, repeat q5min prn

• *Child:* **IC, IV,** endotracheal 5-10 μg q5min, may use 0.1 μg/kg/min **IV INF** after initial dose

Available forms: Aerosol 0.16 mg/spray, 0.2 mg/spray, 0.25 mg/spray; inj 1:1000 (1 mg/ml), 1:200 (5 mg/ml), 0.01 mg/ml (1:100,000), 0.1 mg/ml (1:10,000), 0.5 mg/ml (1:2000); sol for nebulization 1:100, 1.25%, 2.25% (base)

Side effects/adverse reactions:

GU: Urinary retention

CNS: Tremors, anxiety, insomnia, headache, dizziness, confusion, hallucinations, ***cerebral hemorrhage***

CV: Palpitations, tachycardia, hypertension, *dysrhythmias,* increased T wave

GI: Anorexia, nausea, vomiting

RESP: Dyspnea

Contraindications: Hypersensitivity to sympathomimetics, narrow-angle glaucoma

Precautions: Pregnancy (C), lactation, cardiac disorders, hyperthyroidism, diabetes mellitus, prostatic hypertrophy

Pharmacokinetics:

SC: Onset 3-5 min, duration 20 min

PO, INH: Onset 1 min

Crosses placenta; metabolized in liver

Interactions:

• Do not use with MAOIs or tricyclic antidepressants; hypertensive crisis may occur

• Toxicity: sympathomimetics

• Decreased hypertensive effects: α-adrenergic blockers

E

• Dysrhythmias: bretylium cardiac glycosides, anesthetics
• Decreased vascular response: diuretics, ergot alkaloids, phenothiazines
• Increased pressor response: guanethidine, antihistamines, levothyroxine
• Severe hypertension: oxytocics
🍃 Increased action of epinephrine: ephedra

NURSING CONSIDERATIONS
Assess:
• ECG during administration continuously; if B/P increases, drug is decreased
• B/P and pulse q5min after parenteral route
• CVP, ISVR, PCWP during infusion if possible
• Injection site: tissue sloughing; administer phentolamine with NS
• Sulfite sensitivity, which may be life-threatening
Administer:
• Increased dose of insulin in diabetic patients
IV
• Parenteral dose slowly, after reconstituting 1 mg (1:1000 sol)/10 ml or more NS; to prepare a 1:10,000 sol for maintenance, may be further diluted in 500 ml D_5W; give 1 mg or less over 1 min or more through Y-tube or 3-way stopcock; 1 mg = 1 ml of 1:1000 or 10 ml of 1:10,000
Additive compatibilities: Amikacin, cimetidine, dobutamine, floxacillin, furosemide, metaraminol, ranitidine, verapamil
Syringe compatibilities: Doxapram, heparin, milrinone
Y-site compatibilities: Amrinone, atracurium, calcium chloride, calcium gluconate, diltiazem, dobutamine, dopamine, famotidine, fentanyl, furosemide, heparin, hydrocortisone sodium succinate, hy-

dromorphone, labetalol, lorazepam, midazolam, milrinone, morphine, nicardipine, nitroglycerin, norepinephrine, pancuronium, phytonadione, potassium chloride, propofol, ranitidine, vecuronium, vit B/C, warfarin
Perform/provide:
• Storage of reconstituted sol refrigerated no longer than 24 hr
• Do not use discolored sol
Evaluate:
• Therapeutic response: increased B/P with stabilization or ease of breathing
Teach patient/family:
• The reason for drug administration
• To rinse mouth after use to prevent dryness after inhalation
• Not to take OTC preparations
Treatment of overdose: Administer an α-blocker and a β-blocker

---

epoetin (℞)
(ee-poe'e-tin)
EPO, Epogen, erythropoietin, Procrit
Func. class.: Biologic modifier, hormone
Chem. class.: Amino acid polypeptide

Action: Erythropoietin is one factor controlling rate of red cell production; drug is developed by recombinant DNA technology
Uses: Anemia caused by reduced endogenous erythropoietin production, primarily end-stage renal disease; to correct hemostatic defect in uremia; anemia due to AZT treatment in HIV patients; anemia due to chemotherapy; reduction of allogeneic blood transfusion in surgery patients

---

◆ = Nursing alert   🍃 = Herb-drug interaction   🚫 = Do not crush

Dosage and routes:

Anemia secondary to chemotherapy
• *Adult:* SC 150 U/kg 3 ×/wk, may increase after 2 mo up to 300 U/kg 3 ×/wk

Anemia in chronic renal failure
• *Adult:* SC/IV 50-100 U/kg 3 ×/wk, then adjust dose by 25 U/kg/dose to maintain Hct; maintenance: 12.5-25 U/kg, titrate to target Hct

Anemia secondary to zidovudine treatment
• *Adult:* SC/IV 100 U/kg 3 ×/wk × 2 mo, may increase by 50-100 U/kg q1-2mo, up to 300 U/kg 3 ×/wk

Available forms: Inj 2000, 3000, 4000, 10,000, 20,000 U/ml

Side effects/adverse reactions:
*CV: Hypertension, **hypertensive encephalopathy,** headache*
*CNS: **Seizures,** coldness, sweating*
MS: Bone pain

Contraindications: Hypersensitivity to mammalian cell-derived products, or human albumin

Precautions: Seizure disorder, uncontrolled hypertension, porphyria

Pharmacokinetics:
IV: Metabolized in body; extent of metabolism unknown; onset of increased reticulocyte count 1-2 wk

NURSING CONSIDERATIONS
Assess:
• Renal studies: urinalysis, protein, blood, BUN, creatinine
• Blood studies: ferritin, transferrin monthly; Hct 2 ×/wk until stabilized in target range (30%-33%) then at regular intervals
• I&O; report drop in output to <50 ml/hr
• CNS symptoms: coldness, sweating
• CV status: B/P; hypertension may occur rapidly leading to hypertensive encephalopathy

Administer:
IV
• Do not shake

• Decrease dose by 25 U/kg, if Hct increases by 4% in 2 wk

Solution compatibilities: NaCl 0.9%, $D_{10}W$, $D_{10}W$/albumin, sterile water for inj, TPN

Evaluate:
• Therapeutic response: increase in reticulocyte count in 1-2 wk, Hgb/Hct; increased appetite, enhanced sense of well-being

---

ergoloid (Ŗ)

(er'goe-loid)
Ergoloid Mesylates, Gerimal, Hydergine, Hydergine LC
Func. class.: Migraine agent
Chem. class.: Ergot alkaloid—amino acid

Action: May increase cerebral metabolism and blood flow

Uses: Dementias: senile, Alzheimer's, multiinfarct, primary progressive

Dosage and routes:
• *Adult:* PO/SL 1 mg tid, may increase to 4.5-12 mg/day

Available forms: Tabs SL 0.5, 1 mg; tabs 1 mg; caps 1 mg; liquid 1 mg/ml

Side effects/adverse reactions:
GI: Nausea, vomiting, sublingual irritation

Contraindications: Hypersensitivity to ergot preparations; psychosis

Precautions: Acute intermittent porphyria, pregnancy (C), lactation

Pharmacokinetics:
PO: Peak 1 hr; metabolized in liver; excreted as metabolites in feces; crosses blood-brain barrier; half-life 3½ hr

NURSING CONSIDERATIONS
Assess:
• Weight daily; check for peripheral edema in feet, legs
• B/P and pulse, check regularly

• Neurologic status: LOC, blurring vision, nausea, vomiting, tingling in extremities; underlying and reversible causes of dementia
• Toxicity: dyspnea; hypotension or hypertension; rapid, weak pulse; delirium; nausea; vomiting; bradycardia

Administer:

• With or after meals to avoid GI symptoms

🚫 SL tabs whole; do not break, crush, or chew

• For 6 mo, if no improvement at max dose, D/C drug should be considered

Perform/provide:

• Storage in well-closed container at room temp

Evaluate:

• Therapeutic response: decreased forgetfulness, increased mental alertness and ability for self-care

Teach patient/family:

• To change positions slowly and to move extremities before walking
• To maintain dosage at approved level; not to increase drug
• To report side effects, including increased vasoconstriction starting with cold extremities, then paresthesia, weakness
• That 6 mo treatment may be required; some improvement occurs in 1 mo
• To keep drug out of reach of children; death may occur

Treatment of overdose: Induce emesis if orally ingested, or gastric lavage; administer saline cathartic, keep warm

---

ergonovine (℞)
(er-goe-noe′veen)
ergonovine maleate, Ergotrate Maleate
Func. class.: Oxytocic
Chem. class.: Ergot alkaloid

Action: Stimulates uterine contractions and vascular smooth muscle, decreases bleeding

Uses: Postpartum or postabortion hemorrhage

Investigational uses: To induce a coronary artery spasm

Dosage and routes:

Oxytocic
• *Adult:* **PO** 0.2-0.4 mg q6-12h; **IM** 0.2 mg q2-4h, not to exceed 5 doses; **IV** 0.2 mg given over 1 min

Induced coronary artery spasm
• *Adult:* **IV** 50 µg q5min up to 400 µg or when chest pain occurs

Available forms: Inj 0.2 mg/ml; tab 0.2 mg

Side effects/adverse reactions:

CNS: Headache, dizziness, fainting
CV: Hypertension, chest pain
GI: Nausea, vomiting
INTEG: Sweating
RESP: Dyspnea
EENT: Tinnitus
GU: Cramping

Contraindications: Hypersensitivity to ergot medication, augmentation of labor, before delivery of placenta, spontaneous abortion (threatened), pelvic inflammatory disease

Precautions: Hepatic disease, renal disease, cardiac disease, asthma, anemia, convulsive disorders, hypertension, glaucoma, obliterative vascular disease

Pharmacokinetics:
IM: Onset 2-5 min, duration 3 hr
IV: Onset immediate, duration 45 min

◆ = Nursing alert   = Herb-drug interaction   🚫 = Do not crush

Metabolized in liver, excreted in urine

Interactions:

• Hypertension: sympathomimetics, ergots

🥄 Hypertension: ephedra

NURSING CONSIDERATIONS
Assess:

• Ergotism: nausea, vomiting, weakness, muscular pain, insensitivity to cold, paresthesias of extremities; drug should be discontinued

• B/P, pulse; watch for change that may indicate hemorrhage

• Respiratory rate, rhythm, depth; notify prescriber of abnormalities

• Fundal tone, nonphasic contractions; check for relaxation

Administer:

• IM inj deep in large muscle mass; rotate injection sites if additional doses are given

• With emergency equipment available

IV, direct

• Through Y-tube or 3-way stopcock

Additive compatibilities: Amikacin, cephapirin, sodium bicarbonate

Evaluate:

• Therapeutic response: decreased blood loss, severe cramping

Teach patient/family:

• To report increased blood loss, increased temp, or foul-smelling lochia; that cramping is normal

Treatment of overdose: Stop drug, give vasodilators, heparin, dextran

---

ergotamine (℞)

(er-got′a-meen)
Ergostat Ergomar*
Func. class.: α-Adrenergic blocker
Chem. class.: Ergot alkaloid—amino acid

E

Action: Constricts smooth muscle in peripheral, cranial blood vessels, relaxes uterine muscle; blocks serotonin release

Uses: Vascular headache (migraine, cluster histamine)

Dosage and routes:

• *Adult:* **PO** 2 mg, then 1-2 mg qh or q½h for **SL,** not to exceed 6 mg/day or 10 mg/wk; **INH** 1 puff, may repeat in 5 min, not to exceed 6/24 hr or 15 sprays/wk

Available forms: SL tabs 2 mg; tabs 1 mg; oral inh 360 μg/dose

Side effects/adverse reactions:

CNS: Numbness in fingers, toes, headache, weakness

CV: Transient tachycardia, chest pain, bradycardia, edema, claudication, increase or decrease in B/P

GI: Nausea, vomiting, diarrhea, abdominal cramps

MS: Muscle pain

Contraindications: Hypersensitivity to ergot preparations, occlusion (peripheral, vascular), CAD, hepatic disease, renal disease, peptic ulcer, hypertension, pregnancy (X), Raynaud's disease, peripheral vascular disease, intermittent claudication

Precautions: Lactation, children, anemia, elderly

Pharmacokinetics:

PO: Peak 30 min-3 hr; metabolized in liver; excreted as metabolites in feces; crosses blood-brain barrier; excreted in breast milk

---

Interactions:

• Increased effects: troleandomycin
• Increased vasoconstriction: β-blockers

NURSING CONSIDERATIONS
Assess:

• Ergotism: nausea, vomiting, weakness, muscular pain, insensitivity to cold, paresthesia of extremities; drug should be discontinued
• Weight daily, check for peripheral edema in feet, legs
• For stress level, activity, recreation, coping mechanisms
• Neurologic status: LOC, blurring vision, nausea, vomiting, tingling in extremities that occurs preceding the headache
• Ingestion of tyramine foods (pickled products, beer, wine, aged cheese), food additives, preservatives, colorings, artificial sweeteners, chocolate, caffeine; may precipitate headaches
• Toxicity: dyspnea, hypotension or hypertension, rapid, weak pulse, delirium, nausea, vomiting

Administer:

• At beginning of headache; dose must be titrated to patient response
• By SL route if possible for better, faster absorption
• With or after meals to avoid GI symptoms (PO route only)
• Not to pregnant women; harm to fetus may occur

Perform/provide:

• Quiet, calm environment with decreased stimulation for noise, bright light, or excessive talking

Evaluate:

• Therapeutic response: decrease in frequency, severity of headache

Teach patient/family:

• Not to use OTC medications; serious drug interactions may occur
• To maintain dose at approved level; not to increase even if drug does not relieve headache
• To report side effects including increased vasoconstriction starting with cold extremities, then paresthesia, weakness
• That an increase in headaches may occur when this drug is discontinued after long-term use
• To keep drug out of reach of children; death may occur
• How to use inhaler, protect ampules from heat/light

Treatment of overdose: Induce emesis or gastric lavage if orally ingested; administer saline cathartic; keep warm

---

erythrityl (℞)

(e-ri'thri-till)
Cardilate
Func. class.: Vasodilator, coronary
Chem. class.: Nitrate

Action: Decreases preload, afterload, which is responsible for decreasing left ventricular end diastolic pressure, systemic vascular resistance; improves exercise tolerance

Uses: Chronic stable angina pectoris, prophylaxis of angina pain, pulmonary arteriolar dilation

Dosage and routes:

• *Adult:* **PO** 10-30 mg tid; **SL** 5-15 mg before stressful activity

Available forms: Chew tabs 10 mg; tabs 5, 10 mg

Side effects/adverse reactions:

CV: Postural hypotension, tachycardia, *collapse,* syncope, edema
GI: Nausea, vomiting
INTEG: Pallor, sweating, rash
CNS: Headache, flushing, dizziness weakness, fainting
MISC: Twitching, hemolytic anemia, *methemoglobinemia*

Contraindications: Hypersensitivity to this drug or nitrites, severe

---

◆ = Nursing alert   ✒ = Herb-drug interaction   🚫 = Do not crush

• Respiratory status: rate, character, wheezing, tightness in chest; discontinue drug if these occur

• Allergies before treatment, reaction of each medication; place allergies on chart in bright red; notify all people giving drugs

Administer:

• Do not give by IM or IV push

• Enteric-coated tablets may be given with food

🚫 Do not break, crush, or chew

• Chewable tabs should be chewed only

IV

• After diluting 500 mg or less/10 ml sterile H_2O without preservatives; dilute further in 80-250 ml of 0.9% NaCl, LR, Normosol-R; may be further diluted to 1 mg/ml and given as continuous infusion; run 1 g or less/100 ml over ½-1 hr; continuous infusion over 6 hr, may require buffers to neutralize pH if dilution is <250 ml, use infusion pump

Additive compatibilities: *Gluceptate:* Calcium gluconate, corticotropin, dimenhydrinate, heparin, hydrocortisone, methicillin, penicillin G potassium, potassium chloride, sodium bicarbonate

Lactobionate: Aminophylline, ampicillin, cimetidine, diphenhydramine, hydrocortisone, lidocaine, methicillin, penicillin G potassium or sodium, pentobarbital, polymyxin B, potassium chloride, prednisolone, prochlorperazine, promazine, ranitidine, sodium bicarbonate, verapamil

Syringe compatibilities: *Lactobionate:* Methicillin

Y-site compatibilities: Acyclovir, amiodarone, cyclophosphamide, diltiazem, enalaprilat, esmolol, famotidine, foscarnet, heparin, hydromorphone, idarubicin, labetalol, lorazepam, magnesium sulfate, meperidine, midazolam, morphine, multivitamins, perphenazine, tacrolimus, theophylline, vit B/C, zidovudine

Perform/provide:

• Storage at room temp; store susp in refrigerator

• Adequate intake of fluids (2 L) during diarrhea episodes

Evaluate:

• Therapeutic response: decreased symptoms of infection

Teach patient/family:

• To take oral drug with full glass of water; with food for GI symptoms

• Not to take with fruit juice

• To report sore throat, fever, fatigue (could indicate superinfection)

• To notify nurse of diarrhea stools, dark urine, pale stools, yellow discoloration of eyes or skin, and severe abdominal pain

• To take at evenly spaced intervals; complete dosage regimen

Treatment of hypersensitivity: Withdraw drug; maintain airway; administer epinephrine, aminophylline, O_2, IV corticosteroids

---

esmolol (℞)

(ez′moe-lole)

Brevibloc

Func. class.: β-Adrenergic blocker (antidysrhythmic II)

Action: Competitively blocks stimulation of β_1-adrenergic receptors in the myocardium; produces negative chronotropic, inotropic activity (decreases rate of SA node discharge, increases recovery time), slows conduction of AV node, decreases heart rate, decreases O_2 consumption in myocardium; also decreases renin-aldosterone-angiotensin system at high doses; inhibits β_2-receptors in bronchial system slightly

Uses: Supraventricular tachycardia,

noncompensatory tachycardia, hypertensive crisis

Dosage and routes:

• *Adult:* **IV** loading dose 500 μg/kg/min over 1 min; maintenance 50 μg/kg/min for 4 min; if no response in 5 min, give 2nd loading dose; then increase inf to 100 μg/kg/min for 4 min; if no response, repeat loading dose, then increase maintenance inf by 50 μg/kg/min (max of 200 μg/kg/min), titrate to patient response

• *Child:* **IV** 50 μg/kg/min, may increase q10min (max 300 μg/kg/min)

Available forms: Inj 10 mg, 250 mg/ml

Side effects/adverse reactions:

INTEG: Induration, inflammation at site, discoloration, edema, erythema, burning pallor, flushing, rash, pruritus, dry skin, alopecia

CNS: Confusion, light-headedness, paresthesia, somnolence, fever, dizziness, fatigue, headache, depression, anxiety

GI: Nausea, vomiting, anorexia, gastric pain, flatulence, constipation, heartburn, bloating

CV: Hypotension, bradycardia, chest pain, peripheral ischemia, shortness of breath, *CHF,* conduction disturbances

GU: Urinary retention, impotence, dysuria

RESP: Bronchospasm, dyspnea, cough, wheeziness, nasal stuffiness

Contraindications: 2nd- or 3rd-degree heart block, cardiogenic shock, CHF, cardiac failure, hypersensitivity

Precautions: Hypotension, pregnancy (C), peripheral vascular disease, diabetes, hypoglycemia, thyrotoxicosis, renal disease, lactation

Pharmacokinetics:

Onset very rapid, duration short, half-life 9 min; metabolized by hydrolysis of the ester linkage; excreted via kidneys

Interactions:

• Increased digoxin levels: digoxin

• Increased esmolol levels: morphine

• Reversal of esmolol effects: isoproterenol, norepinephrine, dopamine, dobutamine

• Increased effects of both drugs: disopyramide

• Increased effects of lidocaine

 Potassium deficiency: aloe, buckthorn bark/berry, cascara sagrada bark, senna pod/leaf

Lab test interferences:

Interference: Glucose/insulin tolerance test

NURSING CONSIDERATIONS

Assess:

• I&O ratio, weight daily

• B/P, pulse q4h; note rate, rhythm, quality; rapid changes can cause shock; if systolic <100 or diastolic <60, notify prescriber before giving drug

• Apical/radial pulse before administration; notify prescriber if <60 bpm

• Baselines in renal, liver function tests before therapy begins

• Breath sounds and respiratory pattern

• Respiratory pattern: wheezing from bronchospasm

• Edema in feet, legs daily

• Skin turgor, dryness of mucous membranes for hydration status

Administer:

• Reduced dosage in cool environment

IV

• IV diluted 5 g/20 ml of D_5W, D_5R, D_5 0.9% NaCl, 0.45% NaCl, LR, D_5 0.45% NaCl, 0.9% NaCl further dilute in the remaining 480 ml (10 mg/ml) and give as infusion; give loading dose over 1 min, then maintenance over 4 min; may repeat loading dose q5min with increased maintenance dose; maintenance dose should not be >200 μg/kg/min and be given up to 48 hr; dose should be tapered at 25 μg/kg/min; use infusion pump

Additive compatibilities: Aminophylline, atracurium, bretylium, heparin

Y-site compatibilities: Amikacin, aminophylline, amiodarone, ampicillin, atracurium, butorphanol, calcium chloride, cefazolin, cefmetazole, cefoperazone, ceftazidime, ceftizoxime, chloramphenicol, cimetidine, clindamycin, diltiazem, dopamine, enalaprilat, erythromycin, famotidine, fentanyl, gentamicin, heparin, hydrocortisone, insulin (regular), labetalol, magnesium sulfate, methyldopate, metronidazole, midazolam, morphine, nafcillin, nitroglycerin, norepinephrine, nitroprusside, pancuronium, penicillin G potassium, phenytoin, piperacillin, polymyxin B, potassium chloride, potassium phosphate, propofol, ranitidine, sodium acetate, streptomycin, tacrolimus, tobramycin, trimethoprim-sulfamethoxazole, vancomycin, vecuronium

Perform/provide:
• Storage protected from light, moisture; in cool environment

Evaluate:
• Therapeutic response: lower B/P immediately, lower heart rate

Treatment of overdose: Discontinue drug

---

esoprostenol
(e-soh-proh′sti-nole)
Flolan
Func. class.: Antihypertensive

Action: Produces decrease in B/P by direct vasodilation of pulmonary and systemic arterial vascular beds, inhibition of platelet aggregation

Uses: Pulmonary hypertension; long-term IV treatment (NYHA Class III, IV)

Dosage and routes:
Hypertension
• *Adult:* IV via central-line catheter; 4 ng/kg/min (continuous chronic infusion) or 8.6 ng/kg/min (acute dose ranging)

Available forms: Powder for reconstitution 0.5, 1.5 mg

Side effects/adverse reactions:
CV: Hypotension, bradycardia, tachycardia, flushing, heart failure, syncope, shock, chest pain
CNS: Dizziness, headache, anxiety, depression, paresthesias
GI: Nausea, vomiting, diarrhea
INTEG: Rash, pruritus
RESP: Dyspnea, cough, hypoxia
MS: MS pain, back pain, jaw pain, myalgia

Contraindications: Hypersensitivity, CHF

Precautions: Pregnancy (B), lactation, children, elderly

Pharmacokinetics: Half-life 6½ min; metabolized by liver (metabolites inactive); excreted in urine

Interactions:
• Increased hypotension; diuretics, other antihypertensives
• Increased bleeding: antiplatelet agents, anticoagulants

NURSING CONSIDERATIONS
Assess:
• I&O, weight daily
• B/P during beginning treatment, periodically thereafter; pulse q4h; note rate, rhythm, quality
• Apical/radial pulse; notify prescriber of any significant changes
• Baselines in renal, liver function tests before therapy begins
• Edema in feet, legs daily
• Skin turgor, dryness of mucous membranes for hydration status

Administer:
• IV in diluent only; for 3,000 ng/ml

E

dissolve vial of 0.5 mg/5 ml diluent, withdraw 3 ml, add sufficient diluent to make 100 ml
• Use following calculation:

$$\text{INF rate (ml/hr)} = \frac{\text{dose (ng/kg/min)} \times \text{weight (kg)} \times 60}{\text{Final conc. (ng/ml)}}$$

Perform/provide:
• Storage in dry area at room temp
Evaluate:
• Therapeutic response: decreased B/P
Teach patient/family:
• Not to discontinue drug abruptly; taper over 2 wk; may cause precipitate angina
• Not to use OTC products unless directed by prescriber
• To report bradycardia, dizziness, depression
• To comply with weight control, dietary adjustment, modified exercise program
• To carry Medic Alert ID to identify drug, allergies
• To report symptoms of CHF: difficult breathing, especially on exertion or when lying down, night cough, swelling of extremities

---

estazolam (℞)

(ess-taz'oh-lam)
ProSom
Func. class.: Sedative, hypnotic
Chem. class.: Benzodiazepine derivative

Controlled Substance Schedule IV (US)
Action: Produces CNS depression at the limbic, thalamic, hypothalamic levels of the CNS; may be mediated by neurotransmitter γ-aminobutyric acid (GABA); results are sedation, hypnosis, skeletal muscle relaxation, anxiolytic action
Uses: Insomnia

Dosage and routes:
• *Adult:* **PO** 1-2 mg hs
• *Elderly:* **PO** 0.5 mg hs
Available forms: Tabs 1, 2 mg
Side effects/adverse reactions:
INTEG: Dermatitis, allergy, sweating, flushing, pruritus
HEMA: **Leukopenia, granulocytopenia (rare)**
CNS: Lethargy, drowsiness, daytime sedation, dizziness, confusion, lightheadedness, headache, anxiety, irritability, weakness, tremors, depression, lack of coordination
GI: Nausea, vomiting, diarrhea, heartburn, abdominal pain, constipation, anorexia, taste alteration
CV: Chest pain, pulse changes, palpitations, tachycardia
MISC: Joint pain, congestion
Contraindications: Hypersensitivity to benzodiazepines, pregnancy (X), sleep apnea
Precautions: Hepatic disease, renal disease, suicidal individuals, drug abuse, elderly, psychosis, child <18, lactation, depression, pulmonary insufficiency
Pharmacokinetics: Onset 15-45 min, peak 1½-2 hr, duration 7-8 hr, half-life 10-24 hr; metabolized by liver; excreted by kidneys (inactive/active metabolites); crosses placenta; excreted in breast milk
Interactions:
• Increased effects of estazolam: cimetidine, disulfiram, isoniazid, probenecid, oral contraceptives
• Increased CNS depression: alcohol, CNS depressants
• Decreased effect of estazolam: theophylline, rifampin, smoking, caffeine
🗲 Increased CNS depression: kava kava

NURSING CONSIDERATIONS
Assess:
• Blood studies: Hct, Hgb, RBCs (if on long-term therapy)

◆ = Nursing alert　　🗲 = Herb-drug interaction　　🚫 = Do not crush

• For REM rebound if abruptly discontinued after 3 wk of use
• Hepatic studies: AST (SGOT), ALT (SGPT), bilirubin
• Mental status: mood, sensorium, affect, memory (long, short)
• Blood dyscrasias: fever, sore throat, bruising, rash, jaundice, epistaxis (rare)
• Type of sleep problem: falling asleep, staying asleep

Administer:
• After removal of cigarettes to prevent fire
• After trying conservative measures for insomnia
• ½-1 hr before hs for sleeplessness
• On empty stomach for fast onset; with food for GI symptoms

Perform/provide:
• Assistance with ambulation after receiving dose
• Safety measures: side rails, nightlight, call bell within easy reach
• Checking to see PO medication has been swallowed
• Storage in tight container in cool environment

Evaluate:
• Therapeutic response: ability to sleep at night, fewer early AM awakenings

Teach patient/family:
• To avoid driving, other activities requiring alertness until drug is stabilized
• To report palpitations, chest pain

---

esterified estrogens (℞)

Climestrone*, Estratab*, Menest, Neo-Estrone*

Func. class.: Estrogen
Chem. class.: Nonsteroidal synthetic estrogen

Action: Needed for adequate functioning of female reproductive system; affects release of pituitary gonadotropins, inhibits ovulation, adequate calcium use in bone

Uses: Menopause, prostatic cancer, hypogonadism, female castration, primary ovarian failure, atropic vaginitis, kraurosis vulvae, osteoporosis, advanced inoperable breast cancer

Dosage and routes:
Menopause
• *Adult:* PO 0.3-3.75 mg qd 3 wk on, 1 wk off
Hypogonadism/castration/ovarian failure
• *Adult:* PO 2.5 mg qd-tid 3 wk on, 1 wk off
Prostatic cancer
• *Adult:* PO 1.25-2.5 mg tid
Breast cancer
• *Adult:* PO 10 mg tid × 3 mo or longer
Available forms: Tabs 0.3, 0.625, 1.25, 2.5 mg

Side effects/adverse reactions:
CNS: Dizziness, headache, migraines, depression
CV: Hypotension, thrombophlebitis, edema, ***thromboembolism, stroke, pulmonary embolism, myocardial infarction***
GI: Nausea, vomiting, diarrhea, anorexia, pancreatitis, cramps, constipation, increased appetite, increased weight, ***cholestatic jaundice***
EENT: Contact lens intolerance, increased myopia, astigmatism
GU: Amenorrhea, cervical erosion, breakthrough bleeding, dysmenorrhea, vaginal candidiasis, breast changes, *gynecomastia, testicular atrophy, impotence*
INTEG: Rash, urticaria, acne, hirsutism, alopecia, oily skin, seborrhea, purpura, melasma
META: Folic acid deficiency, hypercalcemia, hyperglycemia
Contraindications: Breast cancer, thromboembolic disorders, repro-

E

ductive cancer, genital bleeding (abnormal, undiagnosed), pregnancy (X)

Precautions: Hypertension, asthma, blood dyscrasias, gallbladder disease, CHF, diabetes mellitus, bone disease, depression, migraine headache, convulsive disorders, hepatic disease, renal disease, family history of cancer of breast or reproductive tract

Pharmacokinetics:
PO: Degraded in liver; excreted in urine; crosses placenta; excreted in breast milk

Interactions:
• Decreased action of anticoagulants, oral hypoglycemics
• Toxicity: tricyclic antidepressants
• Decreased action of estrogens: anticonvulsants, barbiturates, phenylbutazone, rifampin
• Increased action of corticosteroids

NURSING CONSIDERATIONS
Assess:
• Blood glucose in patient with diabetes
• Weight daily; notify prescriber of weekly weight gain >5 lb; if increase, diuretic may be ordered
• B/P q4h; watch for increase caused by H_2O and Na retention
• I&O ratio; be alert for decreasing urinary output and increasing edema
• Liver function studies, including AST (SGOT), ALT (SGPT), bilirubin, alk phosphatase
• Edema, hypertension, cardiac symptoms, jaundice
• Mental status: affect, mood, behavioral changes, aggression
• Hypercalcemia
• Female patient for intact uterus, if so, progesterone should be added to estrogen therapy to decrease the risk of endometrial cancer

Administer:
• Titrated dose; use lowest effective dose

• With food or milk to decrease GI symptoms

Evaluate:
• Therapeutic response: reversal of menopause or decrease in tumor size in prostatic cancer

Teach patient/family:
• To weigh weekly, report gain >5 lb
• To check with prescriber before using OTC drugs
• To report breast lumps, vaginal bleeding, edema, jaundice, dark urine, clay-colored stools, dyspnea, headache, blurred vision, abdominal pain, numbness or stiffness in legs, chest pain; male to report impotence or gynecomastia

---

estradiol/estradiol cypionate/estradiol valerate/estradiol transdermal system (℞)

(ess-tra-dye'ole)

Alora, Cypionate, Delestrogen, dep-Gynogen, Depo Estradiol, Depogen, Dioval 40, Dioval XX, Dura-Estrin, Duragen-10, Duragen-20, Duragen-40, Esclim, Estra-D, Estraderm/Deladiol-40, Estraderm TTS, Estradiol Cypionate, Estradiol Valerate, Estra-L 20, Estra-L 40, Estro-Cyp, Estroject-LA, Estronol-LA/Estrace, FemPatch, Gynogen L.A. "10," Gynogen L.A. "20," Gynogen L.A. "40," L.A.E. 20, Valergen 10, Valergen 20, Valergen 40/Estrace

Func. class.: Estrogen

Chem. class.: Nonsteroidal synthetic estrogen

Action: Needed for adequate functioning of female reproductive system; affects release of pituitary go-

---

nadotropins, inhibits ovulation, adequate calcium use in bone

Uses: Menopause, inoperable breast cancer, prostatic cancer, atrophic vaginitis, kraurosis vulvae, hypogonadism, primary ovarian failure, prevention of osteoporosis

Dosage and routes:
Hormone replacement
• *Adult:* **TD** 0.05-0.1 mg/24 hr, apply 2 ×/wk
Menopause/hypogonadism/castration/ovarian failure
• *Adult:* **PO** 1-2 mg qd 3 wk on, 1 wk off or 5 days on, 2 days off **IM** 1-5 mg q3-4wk (cyprionate); 10-20 mg q4wk (valerate)
• *Adult:* **TOP** Estraderm 0.05 mg/24 hr applied 2 ×/wk Climera 0.05 mg/hr applied 1 ×/wk in a cyclic regimen; women with hysterectomy may use continuously
Prostatic cancer
• *Adult:* **IM** 30 mg q1-2wk (valerate); **PO** 1-2 mg tid (oral estradiol)
Breast cancer
• *Adult:* **PO** 10 mg tid × 3 mo or longer
Atropic vaginitis/kraurosis vulvae
• *Adult:* **VAG CREAM** 2-4 g qd × 1-2 wk, then 1 g 1-3 ×/wk cycled
Available forms: Estradiol tabs 0.5, 1, 2 mg; cypionate inj 5 mg/ml; valerate inj 10, 20, 40 mg/ml; transderm 0.025, 0.0375, 0.05, 0.075, 0.1 mg/24 hr release rate; vag cream 100 μg/g

Side effects/adverse reactions:
CNS: Dizziness, headache, migraines, depression
CV: Hypotension, thrombophlebitis, edema, ***thromboembolism, stroke, pulmonary embolism, myocardial infarction***
GI: Nausea, vomiting, diarrhea, anorexia, pancreatitis, cramps, constipation, increased appetite, increased weight, ***cholestatic jaundice***

EENT: Contact lens intolerance, increased myopia, astigmatism
GU: Amenorrhea, cervical erosion, breakthrough bleeding, dysmenorrhea, vaginal candidiasis, breast changes, *gynecomastia, testicular atrophy, impotence*
INTEG: Rash, urticaria, acne, hirsutism, alopecia, oily skin, seborrhea, purpura, melasma
META: Folic acid deficiency, hypercalcemia, hyperglycemia

Contraindications: Breast cancer, thromboembolic disorders, reproductive cancer, genital bleeding (abnormal, undiagnosed), pregnancy (X)

Precautions: Hypertension, asthma, blood dyscrasias, gallbladder disease, CHF, diabetes mellitus, bone disease, depression, migraine headache, convulsive disorders, hepatic disease, renal disease, family history of cancer of breast or reproductive tract

Pharmacokinetics:
PO/INJ/TD: Degraded in liver; excreted in urine; crosses placenta; excreted in breast milk

Interactions:
• Decreased action of anticoagulants, oral hypoglycemics
• Toxicity: tricyclic antidepressants
• Decreased action of estradiol: anticonvulsants, barbiturates, phenylbutazone, rifampin, milk products, calcium
• Increased action of: corticosteroids

Lab test interferences:
Increase: BSP retention test, PBI, T_4, serum sodium, platelet aggregation, thyroxine-binding globulin (TBG), prothrombin, factors VII, VIII, IX, X, triglycerides
Decrease: Serum folate, serum triglyceride, T_3 resin uptake test, glucose tolerance test, antithrombin III, pregnanediol, metyrapone test

---

* = Canada only   Side effects: *italics* = common; ***bold italics*** = life-threatening

False positive: LE prep, antinuclear antibodies

NURSING CONSIDERATIONS
Assess:
- Blood glucose of diabetic patient
- Weight daily, notify prescriber of weekly weight gain >5 lb; if increase, diuretic may be ordered
- B/P q4h, watch for increase caused by H_2O and Na retention
- I&O ratio; decreasing urinary output, increasing edema
- Liver function studies, including AST (SGOT), ALT (SGPT), bilirubin, alk phosphatase
- Hypertension, cardiac symptoms, jaundice, hypercalcemia
- Mental status: affect, mood, behavioral changes, aggression
- Female patient for intact uterus, if so, progesterone should be added to estrogen therapy to decrease risk of endometrial cancer

Administer:
- Titrated dose; use lowest effective dose
- IM inj deeply in large muscle mass
- With food or milk to decrease GI symptoms (oral)
- Apply to trunk of body 2 ×/wk (transdermal)
- On intermittent cycle schedule: 3 wk on, then 1 wk off; if patch falls off, reapply (transdermal)

Evaluate:
- Therapeutic response: reversal of menopause or decrease in tumor size in prostatic cancer

Teach patient/family:
- To weigh weekly, report gain >5 lb
- To report breast lumps, vaginal bleeding, edema, jaundice, dark urine, clay-colored stools, dyspnea, headache, blurred vision, abdominal pain, numbness or stiffness in legs, chest pain; male to report impotence or gynecomastia

---

estrogenic substances, conjugated (R)
C.E.S*, conjugated estrogens*, Conjugated Estrogens C.S.D*, Premarin, Premarin Intravenous

Func. class.: Estrogen
Chem. class.: Nonsteroidal synthetic estrogen

Action: Needed for adequate functioning of female reproductive system; it affects release of pituitary gonadotropins, inhibits ovulation, adequate calcium use in bone

Uses: Menopause, inoperable breast cancer, prostatic cancer, abnormal uterine bleeding, hypogonadism, primary ovarian failure, osteoporosis

Dosage and routes:
Menopause
- *Adult:* **PO** 0.3-1.25 mg qd 3 wk on, 1 wk off

Osteoporosis
- *Adult:* **PO** 0.625 mg qd or in cycle

Atrophic vaginitis
- *Adult:* **VAG CREAM** 2-4 g ml qd × 21 days, off 7 days, repeat

Prostatic cancer
- *Adult:* **PO** 1.25-2.5 mg tid

Breast cancer
- *Adult:* **PO** 10 mg tid × 3 mo or longer

Abnormal uterine bleeding
- *Adult:* **IV/IM** 25 mg, repeat in 6-12 hr

Castration/primary ovarian failure
- *Adult:* **PO** 1.25 mg qd 3 wk on, 1 wk off

Hypogonadism
- *Adult:* **PO** 2.5 mg bid-tid × 20 days/mo

Available forms: Tabs 0.3, 0.625, 0.9, 1.25, 2.5 mg; inj 25 mg/vial; vag cream 0.625 mg/g

---

 = Nursing alert   = Herb-drug interaction   ⊘ = Do not crush

Side effects/adverse reactions:
CNS: Dizziness, headache, migraine, depression
CV: Hypotension, thrombophlebitis, edema, **thromboembolism, stroke, pulmonary embolism, myocardial infarction**
GI: Nausea, vomiting, diarrhea, anorexia, pancreatitis, cramps, constipation, increased appetite, increased weight, **cholestatic jaundice**
EENT: Contact lens intolerance, increased myopia, astigmatism
GU: Amenorrhea, cervical erosion, breakthrough bleeding, dysmenorrhea, vaginal candidiasis, breast changes, *gynecomastia, testicular atrophy, impotence*
INTEG: Rash, urticaria, acne, hirsutism, alopecia, oily skin, seborrhea, purpura, melasma
META: Folic acid deficiency, hypercalcemia, hyperglycemia
Contraindications: Breast cancer, thromboembolic disorders, reproductive cancer, genital bleeding (abnormal, undiagnosed), pregnancy (X), lactation
Precautions: Hypertension, asthma, blood dyscrasias, gallbladder disease, CHF, diabetes mellitus, bone disease, depression, migraine headache, convulsive disorders, hepatic disease, renal disease, family history of cancer of breast or reproductive tract
Pharmacokinetics:
PO/IV/IM: Degraded in liver, excreted in urine, crosses placenta, excreted in breast milk
Interactions:
• Decreased action of anticoagulants, oral hypoglycemics
• Toxicity: tricyclic antidepressants
• Decreased action of estrogens: anticonvulsants, barbiturates, phenylbutazone, rifampin
• Increased action of corticosteroids

NURSING CONSIDERATIONS
Assess:
• Blood glucose if diabetic patient
• Weight daily; notify prescriber of weekly weight gain >5 lb; if increase, diuretic may be ordered
• B/P q4h; watch for increase caused by H_2O and Na retention
• I&O ratio; be alert for decreasing urinary output, increasing edema
• Liver function studies: AST (SGOT), ALT (SGPT), bilirubin, alk phosphatase
• Hypertension, cardiac symptoms, jaundice, hypercalcemia
• Mental status: affect, mood, behavioral changes, aggression
• Female patient for intact uterus, if so, progesterone should be added to estrogen therapy to decrease risk of endometrial cancer
Administer:
• Titrated dose, use lowest effective dose
• IM reconstitute after withdrawing >5 ml of air from container and inject sterile diluent on vial side, rotate to dissolve; give injection deep in large muscle mass
• With food or milk to decrease GI symptoms (PO)
IV, direct
• IV, after reconstituting as for IM, inject into distal port of running IV line of D_5W, 0.9% NaCl, LR at 5 mg/min or less
Y-site compatibilities: Heparin/hydrocortisone, potassium chloride, vit B/C
Evaluate:
• Therapeutic response: absence of breast engorgement, reversal of menopause, or decrease in tumor size in prostatic cancer
Teach patient/family:
• To avoid breastfeeding, since drug is excreted in breast milk

E

- To weigh weekly, report gain >5 lb
- To report breast lumps, vaginal bleeding, edema, jaundice, dark urine, clay-colored stools, dyspnea, headache, blurred vision, abdominal pain, numbness or stiffness in legs, chest pain; male to report impotence or gynecomastia
- To avoid sunlight or wear sunscreen; burns may occur

---

estrone (℞)
(ess'trone)
Aquest, Estrone Aqueous, Estrone-5, Estronol, Femogen Forte*, Kestrone-5, Theelin Aqueous
Func. class.: Estrogen
Chem. class.: Nonsteroidal synthetic estrogen

Action: Needed for adequate functioning of female reproductive system; affects release of pituitary gonadotropins, inhibits ovulation, promotes adequate calcium use in bone structures

Uses: Menopause, prostatic cancer, atrophic vaginitis, hypogonadism, primary ovarian failure, kraurosis vulvae, female castration, osteoporosis

Dosage and routes:
Menopause/atrophic vaginitis
- *Adult:* IM 0.1-0.5 mg 2-3 ×/wk
Prostatic cancer
- *Adult:* IM 2-4 mg 2-3 ×/wk
Female hypogonadism/primary ovarian failure
- *Adult:* IM 0.1-1 mg qwk in one dose or divided doses
Available forms: Inj 2, 5 mg/ml
Side effects/adverse reactions:
CNS: Dizziness, headache, migraine, depression
CV: Hypotension, thrombophle-

bitis, edema, ***thromboembolism, stroke, pulmonary embolism, myocardial infarction***
GI: Nausea, vomiting, diarrhea, anorexia, pancreatitis, cramps, constipation, increased appetite, increased weight, *cholestatic jaundice*
EENT: Contact lens intolerance, increased myopia, astigmatism
GU: Amenorrhea, cervical erosion, breakthrough bleeding, dysmenorrhea, vaginal candidiasis, breast changes, *gynecomastia, testicular atrophy, impotence*
INTEG: Rash, urticaria, acne, hirsutism, alopecia, oily skin, seborrhea, purpura, melasma
META: Folic acid deficiency, hypercalcemia, hyperglycemia
Contraindications: Breast cancer, thromboembolic disorders, reproductive cancer, genital bleeding (abnormal, undiagnosed), pregnancy (X)
Precautions: Hypertension, asthma, blood dyscrasias, gallbladder disease, CHF, diabetes mellitus, bone disease, depression, migraine headache, convulsive disorders, hepatic disease, renal disease, family history of cancer of the breast or reproductive tract
Pharmacokinetics:
IM: Degraded in liver; excreted in urine, breast milk; crosses placenta
Interactions:
- Decreased action of anticoagulants, oral hypoglycemics
- Toxicity: tricyclic antidepressants
- Decreased action of estrone: anticonvulsants, barbiturates, phenylbutazone, rifampin
- Increased action of corticosteroids
NURSING CONSIDERATIONS
Assess:
- Blood glucose in diabetic patient
- Weight daily, notify prescriber of

◆ = Nursing alert   🌿 = Herb-drug interaction   ⊘ = Do not crush

weekly weight gain >5 lb; if increase, diuretic may be ordered
• B/P q4h, watch for increase caused by H_2O, Na retention
• I&O ratio; be alert for decreasing urinary output, increasing edema
• Liver function studies, including AST (SGOT), ALT (SGPT), bilirubin, alk phosphatase
• Hypertension, cardiac symptoms, jaundice, hypercalcemia
• Mental status: affect, mood, behavioral changes, aggression
• Female patient for intact uterus, if so, progesterone should be added to estrogen therapy to decrease risk of endometrial cancer

Administer:
• Titrated dose; use lowest effective dose
• IM injection deep in large muscle mass

Evaluate:
• Therapeutic response: absence of breast engorgement, reversal of menopause, or decrease in tumor size in prostatic cancer

Teach patient/family:
• To weigh weekly, report gain >5 lb
• To report breast lumps, vaginal bleeding, edema, jaundice, dark urine, clay-colored stools, dyspnea, headache, blurred vision, abdominal pain, numbness or stiffness in legs, chest pain; male to report impotence or gynecomastia
• To avoid sunlight or wear sunscreen, burns may occur

---

ethacrynate/ethacrynic (R)
(eth-a-kri'nate)
Edecrin, Edecrin Sodium
Func. class.: Loop diuretic
Chem. class.: Ketone derivative

E

Action: Acts on loop of Henle by inhibiting reabsorption of chloride, sodium
Uses: Pulmonary edema, edema in CHF, liver disease, nephrotic syndrome, ascites
Investigational uses: Glaucoma
Dosage and routes:
• *Adult:* **PO** 50-200 mg/day; may give up to 200 mg bid
• *Child:* **PO** 25 mg, increased by 25 mg/day until desired effect occurs
Pulmonary edema
• *Adult:* **IV** 50-100 mg given over several min or 0.5-1 mg/kg
Available forms: Tabs 25, 50 mg; powder for inj 50 mg
Side effects/adverse reactions:
GU: Polyuria, **renal failure,** glycosuria
ELECT: Hypokalemia, hypochloremic alkalosis, hypomagnesemia, hyperuricemia, hypocalcemia, hyponatremia, decreased glucose tolerance
CNS: Headache, fatigue, weakness, vertigo
GI: Nausea, **severe diarrhea,** dry mouth, vomiting, anorexia, cramps, upset stomach, abdominal pain, **acute pancreatitis,** jaundice, **GI bleeding;** abdominal distention
EENT: Loss of hearing, ear pain, tinnitus, blurred vision
INTEG: Photosensitivity, *rash*
ENDO: Hyperglycemia
HEMA: **Thrombocytopenia, agranulocytosis, leukopenia, neutropenia**
Contraindications: Hypersensitivity to sulfonamides, anuria, hypo-

volemia, lactation, electrolyte depletion, infants

Precautions: Dehydration, ascites, severe renal disease, pregnancy (D), hypoproteinemia

Pharmacokinetics:

PO: Onset ½ hr, peak 2 hr, duration 6-8 hr

IV: Onset 5 min, peak 15-30 min, duration 2 hr

Excreted by kidneys; crosses placenta; half-life 30-70 min

Interactions:

• Increased hypotension: antihypertensives

• Decreased diuretic effect: indomethacin, NSAIDs

• Increased ototoxicity: cisplatin, aminoglycosides, vancomycin

• Increased toxicity: lithium, nondepolarizing skeletal muscle relaxants, digitalis

• Increased anticoagulant activity: warfarin

NURSING CONSIDERATIONS

Assess:

• Weight, I&O daily to determine fluid loss; effect of drug may be decreased if used qd

• Rate, depth, rhythm of respiration, effect of exertion

• B/P lying, standing; postural hypotension may occur

• Electrolytes: K, Na, Cl; include BUN, blood sugar, CBC, serum creatinine, blood pH, ABGs, uric acid, Ca, Mg

• Glucose in urine if diabetic

• Hearing if high IV doses

• Improvement in CVP q8h

• Signs of metabolic alkalosis: drowsiness, restlessness

• Signs of hypokalemia: postural hypotension, malaise, fatigue, tachycardia, leg cramps, weakness

• Rashes, fever qd

• Confusion, especially in elderly; take safety precautions if needed

Administer:

• In AM to avoid interference with sleep if using drug as a diuretic

• K replacement if K less than 3 mg/dl

• With food if nausea occurs; absorption may be decreased slightly

• PO, IV only; do not give IM/SC

IV

• After diluting with 50 ml NaCl inj; give through Y-tube or 3-way stopcock or heplock; give 10 mg or less over 1 min or run infusion over ½ hr; do not add to IV sol

Additive compatibilities: Chlorpromazine, cimetidine, prochlorperazine, promazine

Y-site compatibilities: Heparin/hydrocortisone, potassium chloride, vit B/C

Evaluate:

• Therapeutic response: improvement in edema of feet, legs, sacral area daily if being used in CHF

Teach patient/family:

• To increase fluid intake to 2-3 L/day unless contraindicated; to rise slowly from lying or sitting position

• About adverse reactions: muscle cramps, weakness, nausea, dizziness

• To take with food or milk for GI symptoms

• To take early in day to prevent nocturia

• To use sunscreen for photosensitivity

Treatment of overdose: Lavage if taken orally; monitor electrolytes; give dextrose in saline; monitor hydration, CV, renal status

---

◆ = Nursing alert   ✎ = Herb-drug interaction   ⊘ = Do not crush

ethambutol (℞)

(e-tham'byoo-tole)
Etibi*, Myambutol*
Func. class.: Antitubercular
Chem. class.: Diisopropylethylene diamide derivative

Action: Inhibits RNA synthesis, decreases tubercle bacilli replication

Uses: Pulmonary tuberculosis, as an adjunct, other mycobacterial infections

Dosage and routes:
• *Adult and child >13 yr:* **PO** 15-25 mg/kg/day as a single dose

Renal disease
• CrCl 10-50 ml/min dose q24-36h; CrCl <10 ml/min dose q48h

Retreatment
• *Adult:* **PO** 25 mg/kg/day as single dose × 2 mo with at least 1 other drug, then decrease to 15 mg/kg/day as single dose, max 2.5 g/day
• *Child:* 15 mg/kg/day

Available forms: Tabs 100, 400 mg

Side effects/adverse reactions:
GI: Abdominal distress, anorexia, nausea, vomiting
INTEG: Dermatitis, pruritus
CNS: Headache, confusion, fever, malaise, dizziness, *disorientation,* hallucinations
EENT: Blurred vision, optic neuritis, photophobia, decreased visual acuity
META: Elevated uric acid, acute gout, liver function impairment
MISC: **Thrombocytopenia,** joint pain, bloody sputum

Contraindications: Hypersensitivity, optic neuritis, child <13 yr

Precautions: Pregnancy (B), lactation, renal disease, diabetic retinopathy, cataracts, ocular defects, hepatic and hematopoietic disorders

Pharmacokinetics:
PO: Peak 2-4 hr, half-life 3 hr; metabolized in liver; excreted in urine (unchanged drug/inactive metabolites, unchanged drug in feces)

Interactions:
• Increased renal toxicity: aminoglycosides, cisplatin
• Delayed absorption of ethambutol: aluminum salts

NURSING CONSIDERATIONS

Assess:
• Liver studies qwk: ALT (SGOT), AST (SGPT), bilirubin
• Signs of anemia: Hct, Hgb, fatigue
• Mental status often: affect, mood, behavioral changes; psychosis may occur
• Hepatic status: decreased appetite, jaundice, dark urine, fatigue
• C&S, including sputum, before treatment

Administer:
PO
• With meals to decrease GI symptoms
• Antiemetic if vomiting occurs
• After C&S is completed; qmo to detect resistance
• 2 hr before antacids

Evaluate:
• Therapeutic response: decreased symptoms of TB

Teach patient/family:
• To avoid alcohol products
• That compliance with dosage schedule, duration is necessary
• That scheduled appointments must be kept or relapse may occur
• To report any visual changes or rash to physician

E

ethchlorvynol (℞)

(eth-klor-vi′nole)
Placidyl
Func. class.: Sedative/hypnotic
Chem. class.: Tertiary acetylenic alcohol

Controlled Substance Schedule IV (USA), Schedule F (Canada)

Action: Produces cerebral depression; exact action is unknown

Uses: Sedation, insomnia

Dosage and routes:

Sedation
• *Adult:* **PO** 100-200 mg bid or tid

Insomnia
• *Adult:* **PO** 500 mg-1g ½ hr before hs; may repeat 100-200 mg prn
• *Elderly:* **PO** 200 mg ½ hr before hs

Renal disease
• CrCl <50 ml/min avoid use

Medication for EEG
• *Child:* **PO** 25 mg/kg in one dose not to exceed 1 g

Available forms: Caps 100, 200, 500, 750 mg

Side effects/adverse reactions:

HEMA: Thrombocytopenia
CNS: Fatigue, drowsiness, dizziness, sedation, ataxia, nightmares, hangover, giddiness, weakness, hysteria
GI: Nausea, vomiting
INTEG: Rash, urticaria
EENT: Blurred vision, bitter aftertaste
CV: Hypotension

Contraindications: Hypersensitivity to this drug, severe pain, porphyria

Precautions: Depression, hepatic disease, renal disease, suicidal individual, pregnancy (C) (3rd trimester), lactation, elderly

Pharmacokinetics:
PO: Onset 15-30 min, peak 1-1½ hr,

duration 5 hr; metabolized by liver; excreted by kidneys; half-life 10-20 hr, 21-100 hr terminal

Interactions:
• Decreased hypoprothrombinemic effect: dicumarol, warfarin
• Increased CNS effects of ETOH, barbiturates, other CNS depressants, MAOIs

 Increased action: kava kava

Lab test interferences: Clinitest

NURSING CONSIDERATIONS

Assess:
• Blood studies: Hct, Hgb, RBCs before and after treatment if blood dyscrasias are suspected
• Renal function studies: creatinine clearance, BUN; before initiating therapy
• Hepatic studies: AST (SGOT), ALT (SGPT), bilirubin if hepatic disease is present
• Mental status: mood, sensorium, affect, memory (long, short)
• Physical tolerance: more frequent requests for medication, shakes, anxiety

 Toxicity: hypotension, hypothermia, weakness, poor muscle coordination, visual problems; drug should be discontinued
• Respiratory dysfunction: depression, character, rate, rhythm; hold drug if respirations <10/min or if pupils dilated (rare)
• Blood dyscrasias: fever, sore throat, bruising, rash, jaundice, epistaxis (rare)
• Allergy to tartrazine: this drug contains tartrazine and should not be used by patients allergic to this dye

Administer:
• After removal of cigarettes to prevent fires
• After trying conservative measures for insomnia
• ½-1 hr before hs for sleeplessness
• With food or meals to decrease dizziness, giddiness

 = Nursing alert   = Herb-drug interaction   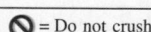 = Do not crush

• For only 1 wk; not intended for long-term treatment

Perform/provide:

• Assistance with ambulation after receiving dose, especially elderly

• Safety measures: side rails, night-light, call bell within easy reach

• Checking to see if PO medication swallowed

• Storage in tight, light-resistant container in cool environment

Evaluate:

• Therapeutic response: ability to sleep at night, less early AM awakening if taking for insomnia

Teach patient/family:

• To avoid driving, other activities requiring alertness

• To avoid alcohol ingestion, CNS depressants; serious CNS depression may result

• That effects may take 2 nights for benefits to be noticed

• Alternative measures to improve sleep: reading, exercise several hr before hs, warm bath, warm milk, TV, self-hypnosis, deep breathing

🚫 Not to break, crush, or chew caps

Treatment of overdose: Lavage, activated charcoal; monitor electrolytes, vital signs

---

ethinyl estradiol (℞)

(eth′in-il ess-tra-dye′ole)
Estinyl, Feminone
Func. class.: Estrogen
Chem. class.: Nonsteroidal synthetic estrogen

Action: Needed for adequate functioning of female reproductive system; affects release of pituitary gonadotropins, inhibits ovulation, promotes adequate calcium use in bone structures

Uses: Menopause, prostatic cancer, atropic vaginitis, kraurosis vulvae, osteoporosis, breast cancer (5 yr or more after menopause), breast engorgement, hypogonadism

Dosage and routes:

Menopause

• *Adult:* PO 0.02-0.5 mg qd 3 wk on, 1 wk off

Prostatic cancer

• *Adult:* PO 0.15-2 mg qd

Hypogonadism

• *Adult:* PO 0.05 mg qd-tid × 2 wk/mo, then 2 wk progesterone, then 3-6 mo cycles, then 2 mo off

Breast cancer

• *Adult:* PO 1 mg tid

Breast engorgement

• *Adult:* PO 0.5-1 mg qd × 3 days, then tapered off over 7 days

Available forms: Tabs 0.02, 0.05, 0.5 mg

Side effects/adverse reactions:

CNS: Dizziness, headache, migraine, depression

CV: Hypotension, thrombophlebitis, edema, ***thromboembolism, stroke, pulmonary embolism, myocardial infarction***

GI: Nausea, vomiting, diarrhea, anorexia, pancreatitis, cramps, constipation, increased appetite, increased weight, ***cholestatic jaundice***

EENT: Contact lens intolerance, increased myopia, astigmatism

GU: Amenorrhea, cervical erosion, breakthrough bleeding, dysmenorrhea, vaginal candidiasis, breast changes, *gynecomastia, testicular atrophy, impotence*

INTEG: Rash, urticaria, acne, hirsutism, alopecia, oily skin, seborrhea, purpura, melasma

META: Folic acid deficiency, hypercalcemia, hyperglycemia

Contraindications: Thromboembolic disorders, reproductive cancer, genital bleeding (abnormal, undiagnosed), pregnancy (X)

E

Precautions: Hypertension, asthma, blood dyscrasias, gallbladder disease, CHF, diabetes mellitus, bone disease, depression, migraine headache, convulsive disorders, hepatic disease, renal disease, family history of cancer of breast or reproductive tract

Pharmacokinetics:

PO: Degraded in liver; excreted in urine, breast milk; crosses placenta

Interactions:

• Decreased action of anticoagulants, oral hypoglycemics
• Toxicity: tricyclic antidepressants
• Decreased action of estradiol: anticonvulsants, barbiturates, phenylbutazone, rifampin
• Increased action of corticosteroids

NURSING CONSIDERATIONS

Assess:

• Blood glucose of diabetic patient
• Weight daily, notify prescriber of weekly weight gain >5 lb; if increase, diuretic may be ordered
• B/P q4h; watch for increase caused by H_2O, Na retention
• I&O ratio; be alert for decreasing urinary output, increasing edema
• Liver function studies: AST (SGOT), ALT (SGPT), bilirubin, alk phosphatase
• Hypertension, cardiac symptoms, jaundice, hypercalcemia
• Mental status: affect, mood, behavioral changes, aggression
• Female patients for intact uterus, if so, progesterone should be added to decrease risk of endometrial cancer

Administer:

• Titrated dose; use lowest effective dose
• With food or milk to decrease GI symptoms

Evaluate:

• Therapeutic response: absence of breast engorgement, reversal of menopause, or decrease in tumor size in prostatic cancer

Teach patient/family:

• To weigh weekly, report gain >5 lb
• To report breast lumps, vaginal bleeding, edema, jaundice, dark urine, clay-colored stools, dyspnea, headache, blurred vision, abdominal pain, numbness or stiffness in legs, chest pain; male to report impotence or gynecomastia

---

ethionamide (℞)

(e-thye-on-am′ide)
Trecator-SC
Func. class.: Antitubercular
Chem. class.: Thiomine derivative

Action: Bacteriostatic against *M. tuberculosis*

Uses: Pulmonary, extrapulmonary TB when other antitubercular drugs have failed

Dosage and routes:

Renal disease

• CrCl <50 ml/min 50% dose
• *Adult:* **PO** 500 mg-1 g qd in divided doses, with another antitubercular drug and pyridoxine
• *Child:* **PO** 15-20 mg/kg/day in 3-4 doses, not to exceed 1g

Available forms: Tabs 250 mg

Side effects/adverse reactions:

INTEG: Dermatitis, alopecia, acne
CV: Severe postural hypotension
CNS: Headache, *drowsiness*, tremors, **convulsions**, depression, psychosis, dizziness, peripheral neuritis
GI: **Anorexia, nausea, vomiting,** *diarrhea, metallic taste,* **hepatitis**, jaundice
EENT: Blurred vision, optic neuritis

HEMA: ***Thrombocytopenia,*** purpura
MISC: Gynecomastia, impotence, menorrhagia, difficulty managing diabetes mellitus
Contraindications: Hypersensitivity, severe hepatic disease
Precautions: Pregnancy (D), lactation, renal disease, diabetic retinopathy, cataracts, ocular defects, child <13 yr
Pharmacokinetics:
PO: Peak 3 hr, duration 9 hr, half-life 3 hr; metabolized in liver; excreted in urine (unchanged drug/inactive); crosses placenta
Interactions:
• Increased neurotoxicity: cycloserine, ethyl alcohol
• Increased adverse reactions: TB test agents, anti-TB drugs
NURSING CONSIDERATIONS
Assess:
• Signs of anemia: Hgb, Hct, fatigue
• Liver studies qwk: ALT (SGOT), AST (SGPT), bilirubin
• Mental status often: affect, mood, behavioral changes; psychosis may occur
• Hepatic status: decreased appetite, jaundice, dark urine, fatigue
Administer:
• With meals or antacids to decrease GI symptoms
• Antiemetic if vomiting occurs
• After C&S is completed, qmo to detect resistance
• Pyridoxine to prevent neuritis
Evaluate:
• Therapeutic response: decreased symptoms of TB
Teach patient/family:
• That compliance with dosage schedule, duration are necessary
• To avoid alcohol while taking this drug
• To notify prescriber of depression, mood changes, loss of appetite, which are symptoms of toxicity

---

ethosuximide (℞)
(eth-oh-sux′i-mide)
Zarontin
Func. class.: Anticonvulsant
Chem. class.: Succinimide

E

Action: Inhibits spike, wave formation in absence seizures (petit mal), decreases amplitude, frequency, duration, spread of discharge in minor motor seizures
Uses: Absence seizures, partial seizures, tonic-clonic seizures
Dosage and routes:
• *Adult and child >6 yr:* **PO** 250 mg bid initially; may increase by 250 mg q4-7d, not to exceed 1.5 g/day
• *Child 3-6 yr:* **PO** 250 mg/day or 125 mg bid; may increase by 250 mg q4-7d, not to exceed 1.5 g/day
Available forms: Caps 250 mg, syr 250 mg/5 ml
Side effects/adverse reactions:
HEMA: ***Agranulocytosis, aplastic anemia, thrombocytopenia, leukocytosis, eosinophilia, pancytopenia***
CNS: Drowsiness, dizziness, fatigue, euphoria, lethargy, anxiety, aggressiveness, irritability, depression, insomnia, headache
GI: Nausea, vomiting, heartburn, anorexia, diarrhea, abdominal pain, cramps, dry mouth, constipation, hiccups, weight loss, gum hypertrophy, tongue swelling
GU: Vaginal bleeding; pink, brown urine
INTEG: Urticaria, pruritic erythema, hirsutism, ***Stevens-Johnson syndrome***
EENT: Myopia, blurred vision
Contraindications: Hypersensitivity to succinimide derivatives
Precautions: Lactation, pregnancy (C), hepatic disease, renal disease
Pharmacokinetics:
PO: Peak 1-7 hr, steady state 4-7

---

days; metabolized by liver; excreted in urine, bile, feces; half-life 24-60 hr

Interactions:

• Increased hydantoin levels

• Decreased primidone, phenobarbital levels

Lab test interferences:

False positive: Direct Coombs' test

NURSING CONSIDERATIONS

Assess:

• Renal studies: urinalysis, BUN, urine creatinine

• Blood studies: CBC, Hct, Hgb, reticulocyte counts qwk for 4 wk, then qmo

• Hepatic studies: AST (SGOT), ALT (SGPT), bilirubin

• Drug levels during treatment; therapeutic range (40-100 µg/ml)

• Mental status: mood, sensorium, affect, behavioral changes; if mental status changes, notify prescriber

• Eye problems: need for ophthalmic examinations before, during, after treatment (slit lamp, fundoscopy, tonometry)

• Allergic reaction: red, raised rash; exfoliative dermatitis; if these occur, drug should be discontinued

• Blood dyscrasias: fever, sore throat, bruising, rash, jaundice

◆ Toxicity: bone marrow depression, nausea, vomiting, ataxia, diplopia, cardiovascular collapse, Stevens-Johnson syndrome

Administer:

• With food, milk to decrease GI symptoms

Perform/provide:

• Hard candy, frequent rinsing, gum for dry mouth

• Assistance with ambulation early in treatment; dizziness occurs

• Seizure precautions: padded side rails, move objects that could harm patient

Evaluate:

• Therapeutic response: decreased seizure activity; document on patient's chart

Teach patient/family:

• To carry ID card or Medic Alert bracelet stating patient's name, drugs taken, condition, prescriber's name, phone number

• To avoid driving, other activities that require alertness

• To avoid alcohol ingestion, CNS depressants; increased sedation may occur

🚫 Not to break, crush, or chew caps

• Not to discontinue medication quickly after long-term use; absence seizures may occur

• To continue regular dental checkups to identify gingival hyperplasia

• Symptoms of thrombocytopenia, leukopenia; notify prescriber if these occur

Treatment of overdose: Lavage, activated charcoal; monitor electrolytes, VS

ethotoin (℞)

(eth'oh-to-in)

Peganone

Func. class.: Anticonvulsant

Chem. class.: Hydantoin derivative

Action: Inhibits nerve impulses in the motor cortex by decreasing sodium ion influx, limiting tetanic stimulation

Uses: Generalized tonic-clonic or complex-partial seizures

Dosage and routes:

• *Adult:* PO 250 mg qid pc initially; may increase over several days to 3 g/day in divided doses

• *Child:* PO 250 mg bid; may increase by 250 mg qid

Available forms: Tabs 250, 500 mg

Side effects/adverse reactions:
*HEMA: **Agranulocytosis, thrombocytopenia, leukopenia, pancytopenia, megaloblastic anemia,** lymphadenopathy*
CNS: Fatigue, insomnia, numbness, fever, headache, dizziness
GI: Nausea, vomiting, diarrhea, gingival hypertrophy
INTEG: Rash
EENT: Nystagmus, diplopia
CV: Chest pain

Contraindications: Hypersensitivity to hydantoins, blood dyscrasias, hematologic disease, hepatic disease, pregnancy (D), lactation

Pharmacokinetics: Metabolized by liver; excreted in urine; half-life 3-9 hr

Interactions:
- Decreased ethotoin effects: rifampin, chronic alcohol, barbiturates, antacids, other anticonvulsants, antineoplastics, folic acid, oxacillin
- Increased ethotoin effects: benzodiazepines, cimetidine, salicylates, sulfonamide, pyrazolones, phenothiazines, disulfiram, chloramphenicol
- Seizures: valproic acid
- Paranoia: phenacemide
- Myocardial depressions: lidocaine, propranolol, sympathomimetics
- Decreased effects: valproic acid, oral contraceptives, dicumarol, corticosteroids, cardiac glycosides, estrogens, quinidine, sulfonylureas
- Increased toxic effects: lithium, primidone

Lab test interferences:
Increase: Serum glucose, urine glucose, BSP, alk phosphatase
Decrease: Urinary steroids, PBI, dexamethasone/metyrapone tests

NURSING CONSIDERATIONS
Assess:
- Renal studies: urinalysis, BUN, urine creatinine
- Blood studies: RBC, Hct, Hgb, reticulocyte counts qwk for 4 wk then qmo
- Hepatic studies: AST (SGOT), ALT (SGPT), bilirubin, creatinine periodically
- For signs, symptoms of infection: sore throat, fever, bruising, petechiae
- Drug levels during initial treatment, therapeutic level (15-50 µg/ml)
- Mental status: mood, sensorium, affect, behavioral changes; if mental status changes, notify prescriber
- Eye problems: need for ophthalmic examinations before, during, after treatment (slit lamp, fundoscopy, tonometry)
- Allergic reaction: red, raised rash; drug should be discontinued
- Blood dyscrasias: fever, sore throat, bruising, rash, jaundice
◆ Toxicity: bone marrow depression, nausea, vomiting, ataxia, diplopia, cardiovascular collapse, Stevens-Johnson syndrome, lupus-like syndrome

Administer:
- With food, milk for GI symptoms
- After meals

Perform/provide:
- Hard candy, frequent rinsing, gum for dry mouth
- Assistance with ambulation early in treatment; dizziness occurs
- Seizure precautions: padded side rails, removing items that may harm patient

Evaluate:
- Therapeutic response: decreased seizure activity, document on patient's chart

Teach patient/family:
- To carry ID card or Medic Alert bracelet stating patient's name, drugs taken, condition, prescriber's name, phone number

---

Side effects: *italics* = common; ***bold italics*** = life-threatening

• To avoid driving, other activities that require alertness
• To avoid alcohol ingestion, CNS depressants; increased sedation may occur
• To notify dentist; use good oral hygiene; monitor gums
• Not to discontinue medication quickly after long-term use; taper off over several wk

Treatment of overdose: Lavage, activated charcoal; monitor electrolytes, VS

---

ethylnorepinephrine (R)

(eth-il-nor-ep-i-nef'rin)
Bronkephrine
Func. class.: Adrenergic
Chem. class.: Catecholamine

Action: α-Stimulation with vasoconstriction, pressor response, nasal decongestion and β₂-stimulation with vasodilation and bronchial dilation

Uses: Bronchospasm

Dosage and routes:
• *Adult:* **IM/SC** 0.5-1 ml
• *Child:* **IM/SC** 0.1-0.5 ml

Available forms: Inj 2 mg/ml

Side effects/adverse reactions:

CNS: Tremors, anxiety, insomnia, headache, dizziness, confusion,

CV: Palpitations, tachycardia, hypertension, chest pain, ***dysrhythmias***

GI: Anorexia, nausea, vomiting

Contraindications: Hypersensitivity to sympathomimetics, narrow-angle glaucoma

Precautions: Pregnancy (C), lactation, cardiac disorders, hyperthyroidism, diabetes mellitus, prostatic hypertrophy

Pharmacokinetics:

IM/SC: Onset 6-12 min, duration 1-2 hr

Interactions:
• Do not use with MAOIs or tricyclic antidepressants; hypertensive crisis may occur
• Decreased effect of ethylnorepinephrine when used with methyldopa, urinary acidifiers, rauwolfia alkaloids
• Increased effect of ethylnorepinephrine when used with urinary alkalizers

NURSING CONSIDERATIONS

Assess:
• B/P and pulse q5min after parenteral route

Perform/provide:
• Storage of reconstituted sol refrigerated no longer than 24 hr
• Do not use discolored sol

Evaluate:
• Therapeutic response: ease of breathing after several min

Teach patient/family:
• The reason for drug administration

---

etidronate (R)

(eh-tih-droe'nate)
Didronel, Didronel IV
Func. class.: Parathyroid agent (calcium regulator)
Chem. class.: Diphosphate

Action: Decreases bone resorption and new bone development (accretion)

Uses: Paget's disease, heterotopic ossification, hypercalcemia of malignancy

Dosage and routes:

Paget's disease
• *Adult:* **PO** 5-10 mg/kg/day 2 hr ac with H₂O, not to exceed 20 mg/kg/day, max 6 mo or 11-20 mg/kg/day for max of 3 mo

Heterotopic ossification
• *Adult:* **PO** 20 mg/kg qd × 2 wk,

◆ = Nursing alert   ✍ = Herb-drug interaction   ⊘ = Do not crush

then 10 mg/kg/day for 10 wk, total 12 wk
Hypercalcemia
• *Adult:* **IV** 7.5 mg/kg/day × 3 days, then **PO** 20 mg/kg/day
Heterotopic ossification/hip replacement
• *Adult:* **PO** 20 mg/kg/day × 4 wk before and 3 mo after surgery
Available forms: Tabs 200, 400 mg; inj 50 mg/ml
Side effects/adverse reactions:
GI: Nausea, diarrhea
MS: Bone pain, hypocalcemia, decreased mineralization of nonaffected bones
GU: Nephrotoxicity
Contraindications: Pathologic fractures, children, colitis, severe renal disease with creatinine >5 mg/dl
Precautions: Pregnancy (B), renal disease, lactation, restricted vit D/calcium
Pharmacokinetics: Not metabolized; excreted in urine/feces; therapeutic response: 1-3 mo
NURSING CONSIDERATIONS
Assess:
• I&O ratio; check for decreased output in renal patients
• BUN, creatinine, uric acid, phosphate chloride, albumin, pH, urine Ca, Mg, alk phosphatase, urinalysis; Ca should be kept at 9-10 mg/dl, vit D 50-135 IU/dl
• Muscle spasm, laryngospasm, paresthesias, facial twitching, colic; may indicate hypocalcemia
• Nutritional status, diet for sources of vit D (milk, some seafood), Ca (dairy products, dark green vegetables), phosphates—adequate intake is necessary
• Persistent nausea or diarrhea
Administer:
• On empty stomach with H_2O 2 hr ac
• Drug therapy should not last longer than 6 mo

• IV after diluting in 250 ml or more NS; give over 2 hr or longer
• Food, especially high in Ca; vitamins with mineral supplements or antacids high in metals should not be given within 2 hr of dose
Evaluate:
• Therapeutic response: prevention of bone deficiencies
Teach patient/family:
• To avoid OTC products
• That therapeutic response may take 1-3 mo; effects persist for months after drug is discontinued
• That adequate intake of Ca^+, vit D is necessary

etodolac (℞)
(ee-toe'doe-lak)
Lodine, Lodine XL
Func. class.: Nonsteroidal antiinflammatory/nonopioid analgesic

Action: Inhibits prostaglandin synthesis by decreasing an enzyme needed for biosynthesis; analgesic, antiinflammatory, antipyretic
Uses: Mild to moderate pain, osteoarthritis
Dosage and routes:
Osteoarthritis
• *Adult:* **PO** 800-1200 mg/day in divided doses q6-8h initially, then adjust dose to 600-1200 mg/day in divided doses; do not exceed 1200 mg/day; patients <60 kg not to exceed 20 mg/kg
Analgesia
• *Adult:* **PO** 200-400 mg q6-8h prn for acute pain; do not exceed 1200 mg/day; patients <60 kg, not to exceed 20 mg/kg
Available forms: Caps 200, 300 mg; tabs 400, 500 mg; ext rel 400, 600 mg
Side effects/adverse reactions:
CV: Tachycardia, peripheral edema,

fluid retention, palpitations, dysrhythmias, CHF

GU: ***Nephrotoxicity: dysuria, hematuria, oliguria, azotemia,*** cystitis, urinary tract infection

HEMA: ***Blood dyscrasias***

INTEG: Erythema, urticaria, purpura, rash, pruritus, sweating

GI: Nausea, anorexia, vomiting, diarrhea, jaundice, ***cholestatic hepatitis,*** constipation, flatulence, cramps, dry mouth, peptic ulcer, dyspepsia, ***GI bleeding***

CNS: Dizziness, headache, drowsiness, fatigue, tremors, confusion, insomnia, anxiety, depression, lightheadedness, vertigo

EENT: Tinnitus, hearing loss, blurred vision, photophobia

Contraindications: Hypersensitivity; patients in whom aspirin, iodides, or other nonsteroidal antiinflammatories have produced asthma, rhinitis, urticaria, nasal polyps, angioedema, bronchospasm

Precautions: Pregnancy (C); lactation; children; bleeding; GI, cardiac disorders; elderly; renal, hepatic disorders

Pharmacokinetics:

PO: Peak 1-2 hr, serum protein binding >90%, half-life 7 hr; metabolized by liver (metabolites excreted in urine)

Interactions:

• Increased action of warfarin, phenytoin, cyclosporine, lithium
• Decreased antihypertensive effects: β-blockers, diuretics
• Decreased plasma concentration of etodolac: salicylates
• Increased concentration and toxicity of etodolac: probenecid

NURSING CONSIDERATIONS
Assess:

• Pain: location, frequency, characteristics; relief after med

• Blood, renal, liver studies: BUN, creatinine, AST (SGOT), ALT (SGPT), Hgb, before treatment, periodically thereafter
• For GI bleeding: black stools, hematemesis
• Audiometric, ophthalmic examination before, during, after treatment
• For eye, ear problems: blurred vision, tinnitus; may indicate toxicity
• For asthma, aspirin hypersensitivity, nasal polyps that may be hypersensitive to etodolac

Administer:
PO

• With food to decrease GI symptoms, since extent of absorption is not affected by food

Perform/provide:

• Storage at room temp

Evaluate:

• Therapeutic response: decreased pain, stiffness, swelling in joints, ability to move more easily

Teach patient/family:

• To report blurred vision or ringing, roaring in ears; may indicate toxicity

🚫 Not to break, crush, or chew ext rel tabs

• To avoid driving, other hazardous activities if dizziness or drowsiness occurs

◆ To report change in urine pattern, weight increase, edema, pain increase in joints, fever, blood in urine; indicates nephrotoxicity

• That therapeutic effects may take up to 1 mo
• To avoid aspirin, alcoholic beverages while taking this medication

---

◆ = Nursing alert   ⫻ = Herb-drug interaction   🚫 = Do not crush

etomidate (R)

(e-tom'i-date)
Amidate
Func. class.: General anesthetic
Chem. class.: Nonbarbiturate hypnotic

Action: Acts at level of reticular-activating system to produce anesthesia

Uses: Induction of general anesthesia

Dosage and routes:
• *Adult and child >10 yr:* **IV** 0.2-0.6 mg/kg over ½-1 min

Available forms: Inj 2 mg/ml

Side effects/adverse reactions:

GI: Nausea, vomiting (postoperatively)

CNS: Tonic movements, myoclonic movements, averting movements

CV: Tachycardia, hypotension, hypertension, bradycardia

ENDO: Decreases steroid production

RESP: Laryngospasm

INTEG: Pain on administration

Contraindications: Hypersensitivity, labor/delivery

Precautions: Pregnancy (C), child <10 yr, lactation, liver disease

Pharmacokinetics:

IV: Onset 20 sec, peak 1 min, duration 3-5 min; half-life 75 min; metabolized in liver; excreted in urine

NURSING CONSIDERATIONS

Assess:
• I&O ratio for increasing urine output
• VS q10min during IV administration
• Plasma cortisol levels if administered over several hr (5-20 µg/100 ml normal level of cortisol)
• Increasing or decreasing heart rate or dysrhythmias shown on ECG

Administer:
• Corticosteroids for severe hypotension
• Only with crash cart, resuscitative equipment nearby

IV
• IV slowly only; muscular twitching is reduced with fentanyl before anesthesia induction

Y-site compatibilities: Alfentanil, atracurium, atropine, doxacurium, ephedrine, fentanyl, lidocaine, lorazepam, midazolam, mivacurium, morphine, pancuronium, phenylephrine, succinylcholine, sufentanil

Evaluate:
• Therapeutic response: induction of anesthesia

etoposide (R)

(e-toe-poe'side)
Etopophos, VePesid
Func. class.: Antineoplastic-misc.
Chem. class.: Semisynthetic podophyllotoxin

Action: Inhibits mitotic activity through metaphase to mitosis; also inhibits cells from entering mitosis, depresses DNA, RNA synthesis

Uses: Leukemias, lung, testicular cancer, lymphomas, neuroblastoma, melanoma, ovarian cancer

Dosage and routes:
• *Adult:* **IV** 45-75 mg/m^2/day × 3-5 days given q3-5wk or 200-250 mg/m^2/wk, or 125-140 mg/m^2/day 3 × wk, q5wk

Available forms: Inj 20 mg/ml; powder for inj (lyophilized) 119.3 mg/300 mg dextran; caps 50 mg

Side effects/adverse reactions:

HEMA: Thrombocytopenia, leukopenia, myelosuppression, anemia

GI: Nausea, vomiting, anorexia, hepatotoxicity

INTEG: Rash, alopecia, phlebitis at IV site

RESP: **Bronchospasm**

CV: Hypotension

CNS: Headache, *fever*

GU: **Nephrotoxicity**

Contraindications: Hypersensitivity, bone marrow depression, severe hepatic disease, severe renal disease, bacterial infection, pregnancy (D)

Precautions: Renal disease, hepatic disease, lactation, children, gout

Pharmacokinetics: Half-life 3 hr, terminal 15 hr; metabolized in liver; excreted in urine; crosses placental barrier

Interactions:
• Increased pro-time: warfarin

NURSING CONSIDERATIONS
Assess:
• CBC, differential, platelet count weekly; withhold drug if WBC is <4000 or platelet count is <75,000; notify prescriber
• Renal function studies: BUN, serum uric acid, urine CrCl, electrolytes before, during therapy
• I&O ratio; report fall in urine output to <30 ml/hr; check blood pressure bid and report any significant decrease
• Monitor temp q4h; may indicate beginning infection
• Liver function tests before, during therapy (bilirubin, AST [SGOT], ALT [SGPT], LDH) as needed or monthly
• RBC, Hct, Hgb; may be decreased
• Bleeding: hematuria, guaiac stools, bruising or petechiae, mucosa or orifices q8h
• Food preferences; list likes, dislikes
• Effects of alopecia on body image; discuss feelings about body changes

• Yellowing of skin and sclera, dark urine, clay-colored stools, itchy skin, abdominal pain, fever, diarrhea
• Buccal cavity q8h for dryness, sores or ulceration, white patches, oral pain, bleeding, dysphagia
• Local irritation, pain, burning, discoloration at injection site
• Symptoms indicating severe allergic reaction: rash, pruritus, urticaria, purpuric skin lesions, itching, flushing

 Symptoms of anaphylaxis: flushing, restlessness, coughing, difficulty breathing
• Frequency of stools, characteristics: cramping, acidosis; signs of dehydration: rapid respirations, poor skin turgor, decreased urine output, dry skin, restlessness, weakness

Administer:
• Antiemetic 30-60 min before giving drug and prn to prevent vomiting
• Allopurinol or sodium bicarbonate to maintain uric acid levels, alkalinization of urine
• Hyaluronidase 150 U/ml to 1 ml NaCl to infiltration area, ice compress for vesicant activity
• Transfusion for anemia
• Antispasmodic

IV (VePesid)
• After diluting 100 mg/250 ml or more D_5W or NaCl to 0.2-0.4 mg/ml, infuse over 30-60 min

Additive compatibilities: Carboplatin, cisplatin, cytarabine, floxuridine, fluorouracil, hydroxyzine, ifosfamide, ondansetron

Y-site compatibilities: Allopurinol, amifostine, aztreonam, cladribine, fludarabine, granisetron, melphalan, ondansetron, paclitaxel, piperacillin/tazobactam, sargramostim, sodium bicarbonate, teniposide, thiotepa, vinorelbine

---

 = Nursing alert   = Herb-drug interaction   🚫 = Do not crush

Perform/provide:
• Liquid diet: carbonated beverages, Jell-O; dry toast or crackers may be added if patient is not nauseated or vomiting
• Increase fluid intake to 2-3 L/day to prevent urate deposits, calculi formation
• Diet low in purines: organ meats (kidney, liver), dried beans, peas to maintain alkaline urine
• Nutritious diet with iron, vitamin supplements
• HOB raised to facilitate breathing

Evaluate:
• Therapeutic response: decreased tumor size, spread of malignancy

Teach patient/family:
• To report any complaints or side effects to nurse or prescriber
• To report any changes in breathing or coughing
• That hair may be lost during treatment; a wig or hairpiece may make patient feel better; tell patient that new hair may be different in color, texture
• To make position changes slowly to prevent fainting

---

factor IX complex (human)/factor IV (human) (Ŗ)

Alpha-Nine SD, Benefix, Konyne 80, Mononine, Profilnine/Alpha Nine, Proplex SX-T, Proplex T

Func. class.: Hemostatic
Chem. class.: Factors II, VII, IX, X

Action: Causes an increase in blood levels of clotting factors II, VII, IX, X; factor IX (human) has IX activity

Uses: Hemophilia B (Christmas disease), factor IX deficiency, antico-agulant reversal, control of bleeding in patients with factor VIII inhibitors, reversal of overdose of anticoagulants in emergencies

Dosage and routes:
Factor IX complex (human) bleeding in hemophilia B
• *Adult and child:* **IV** establish 25% of normal factor IX or 60-75 U/kg, then 10-20 U/kg/day 1-2 ×/wk

Prophylaxis for bleeding in hemophilia B
• *Adult and child:* **IV** 10-20 U/kg 1-2 ×/wk

Bleeding in hemophilia A/inhibitors of factor VIII (Proplex T, Konyne 80)
• *Adult and child:* **IV** 75 U/kg, repeat in 12 hr

Oral anticoagulant reversal
• *Adult and child:* **IV** 15 U/kg

Factor VII deficiency (use Proplex T only)
• *Adult and child:* **IV** 0.5 U/kg × weight (kg) × desired factor IX increase (% of normal); repeat q4-6h if needed

Factor IX (human) minor-moderate hemorrhage
Use only Alpha Nine, Alpha-Nine SD
• *Adult and child:* **IV** dose to increase factor IX level to 20%-30% in one dose

Serious hemorrhage
• *Adult and child:* **IV** dose to increase factor IX to 30%-50% as daily inf

Minor hemorrhage (mononine only)
• *Adult and child:* **IV** dose to increase factor IX to 15%-25% (20-30 U/kg), repeat in 24 hr if needed

Major hemorrhage
• *Adult and child:* **IV** dose to increase factor IX to 25%-50% (75 U/kg) q18-30h × 10 days or less

Available forms: Inj (number of units noted on label)

Side effects/adverse reactions:

GI: Nausea, vomiting, abdominal cramps, jaundice, ***viral hepatitis***

INTEG: Rash, flushing, *urticaria*

CNS: Headache, dizziness, malaise, paresthesia, *lethargy, chills, fever, flushing*

HEMA: ***Thrombosis, hemolysis, AIDS, DIC***

CV: Hypotension, tachycardia, *MI,* ***venous thrombosis, pulmonary embolism***

RESP: ***Bronchospasm***

Contraindications: Hypersensitivity, hepatic disease, DIC, elective surgery, mild factor IX deficiency

Precautions: Neonates/infants, pregnancy (C)

Pharmacokinetics:

IV: Half-life factor VII–3-6 hr, factor IX–24-36 hr; rapidly cleared from plasma

Interactions:

• Incompatible with protein products

• Increased risk of thrombosis: aminocaproic acid; do not administer

NURSING CONSIDERATIONS

Assess:

• Blood studies (coagulation factors assays by % normal: 5% prevents spontaneous hemorrhage, 30%-50% for surgery, 80%-100% for severe hemorrhage)

• Increased B/P, pulse

• For bleeding q15-30min, immobilize and apply ice to affected joints

• I&O; if urine becomes orange or red, notify prescriber

• Allergic or pyrogenic reaction: fever, chills, rash, itching, slow infusion rate if not severe

◆ DIC: bleeding, ecchymosis, hypersensitivity, changes in coagulation tests

Administer:

• IV after warming to room temp 3 ml/min or less, with plastic syringe only; do not admix

• After dilution with provided diluent, 50 U/ml or 25 U/ml; do not exceed 10 ml/min; decrease rate if fever, headache, flushing, tingling occur

• After crossmatch if patient has blood type A, B, AB, to determine incompatibility with factor

Perform/provide:

• Storage of reconstituted sol for 3 hr at room temp or up to 2 yr refrigeration (powder); check expiration date

Evaluate:

• Therapeutic response: prevention of hemorrhage

Teach patient/family:

• To report any signs of bleeding: gums, under skin, urine, stools, emesis

• The risk of viral hepatitis, AIDS; to be tested q2-3mo for HIV

• That immunization for hepatitis B may be given first

• To carry ID identifying disease; avoid salicylates, inform other health professionals of condition

---

famciclovir (℞)

(fam-cy′clo-veer)
Famvir

Func. class.: Antiviral
Chem. class.: Guanosine nucleoside

Action: Inhibits DNA polymerase and viral DNA synthesis by conversion of this guanosine nucleoside to penciclovir

Uses: Treatment of acute herpes zoster, genital herpes

Dosage and routes:

• *Adult:* **PO** 500 mg q8h; in renal disease, if CrCl is ≥60 ml/min, 500 mg q8h; if 40-59 ml/min, 500 mg q12h; if 20-39 ml/min, 500 mg q24h

Available forms: Tabs 125, 250, 500 mg

◆ = Nursing alert   🔏 = Herb-drug interaction   🚫 = Do not crush

Side effects/adverse reactions:
MS: Back pain, arthralgia
GU: Decreased sperm count
CNS: Headache, fatigue, dizziness, paresthesia, somnolence, fever
RESP: Pharyngitis, sinusitis
GI: Nausea, vomiting, diarrhea, constipation, *abdominal pain, anorexia*
INTEG: Pruritus

Contraindications: Hypersensitivity to this drug, penciclovir

Precautions: Renal disease, pregnancy (B), hypersensitivity to acyclovir, ganciclovir, lactation

Pharmacokinetics: Unknown

Interactions:

• Decreased renal excretion: theophylline, probenecid, digoxin

• Decreased metabolism: cimetidine

NURSING CONSIDERATIONS
Assess:

• For number, distribution of lesions; burning, itching, pain, which are early symptoms of herpes infection

• Renal function studies: urine CrCl, BUN before and during treatment if decreased renal function; dose may have to be lowered

• Bowel pattern before, during treatment; diarrhea may occur

Administer:

• With or without meals; absorption does not appear to be lowered when taken with food

• Within 72 hr of the appearance of rash in herpes zoster

Evaluate:

• Therapeutic response: decreased size, spread of lesions

Teach patient/family:

• How to recognize beginning infection

• How to prevent spread of infection

• The reason for medication, expected results

famotidine (OTC, ℞)
(fa-moe′ti-deen)
Mylanta AR, Pepcid, Pepcid AC, Pepcid IV
Func. class.: H$_2$-histamine receptor antagonist

Action: Competitively inhibits histamine at histamine H$_2$-receptor site, decreasing gastric secretion while pepsin remains at a stable level

Uses: Short-term treatment of active duodenal ulcer, maintenance therapy for duodenal ulcer, Zollinger-Ellison syndrome, multiple endocrine adenomas, gastric ulcers; gastroesophageal reflux disease, heartburn

Dosage and routes:
Renal disease
• CrCl <10 ml/min 20 mg hs
Duodenal ulcer
• *Adult:* PO 40 mg qd hs × 4-8 wk, then 20 mg qd hs if needed (maintenance); IV 20 mg q12h if unable to take PO
Hypersecretory conditions
• *Adult:* PO 20 mg q6h; may give 160 mg q6h if needed; IV 20 mg q12h if unable to take PO
Heartburn relief/prevention
• *Adult:* PO 10 mg with water or 1 hr before eating

Available forms: Tabs 10, 20, 40 mg; powder for oral susp 40 mg/5 ml; inj 10 mg/ml, 20 mg/50 ml 0.9% NaCl

Side effects/adverse reactions:
*HEMA: **Thrombocytopenia***
CNS: Headache, dizziness, paresthesia, **seizure,** depression, anxiety, somnolence, insomnia, fever
EENT: Taste change, tinnitus, orbital edema
GI: Constipation, nausea, vomiting,

F

anorexia, cramps, abnormal liver enzymes
INTEG: Rash
MS: Myalgia, arthralgia
RESP: **Bronchospasm**
Contraindications: Hypersensitivity
Precautions: Pregnancy (B), lactation, children <12 yr, severe renal disease, severe hepatic function, elderly
Pharmacokinetics: Absorption 50% (PO)
PO: Onset 30-60 min, duration 6-12 hr, peak 1-3 hr
IV: Onset immediate, peak 30-60 min, duration 6-12 hr, plasma protein-binding 15%-20%; metabolized in liver 30% (active metabolites), 70% excreted by kidneys, half-life 2½-3½ hr
Interactions:
• Decreased absorption: ketoconazole
• Decreased absorption of famotidine: antacids
NURSING CONSIDERATIONS
Assess:
• Blood counts during therapy; watch for decreasing platelets; if low, therapy may have to be discontinued and restarted after hematologic recovery
• For bleeding, hematuria, hematuresis, occult blood in stools
• Blood dyscrasias (thrombocytopenia): bruising, fatigue, bleeding, poor healing
Administer:
• Antacids 1 hr before or 2 hr after famotidine; may be given with foods or liquids
• After shaking oral suspension
IV, direct
• After diluting 2 ml of drug (10 mg/ml) in 0.9% NaCl to total volume of 5-10 ml; inject over 2 min to prevent hypotension

IV, int inf
• After diluting 2 mg of drug in 100 ml of LR, 0.9% NaCl, D_5W, $D_{10}W$; run over 15-30 min
Additive compatibilities: Cefazolin, cefmetazole, flumazenil
Y-site compatibilities: Acyclovir, allopurinol, amifostine, aminophylline, amphotericin, ampicillin, ampicillin/sulbactam, amrinone, amsacrine, atropine, aztreonam, bretylium, calcium gluconate, cefazolin, cefoperazone, cefotaxime, cefotetan, cefoxitin, ceftazidime, ceftizoxime, ceftriaxone, cefuroxime, cephalothin, cephapirin, chlorpromazine, cisplatin, cladribine, cyclophosphamide, cytarabine, dexamethasone, dextran 40, digoxin, diphenhydramine, dobutamine, dopamine, doxorubicin, droperidol, enalaprilat, epinephrine, erythromycin, esmolol, filgrastim, fluconazole, fludarabine, folic acid, gentamicin, granisetron, haloperidol, heparin, hydrocortisone, hydromorphone, hydroxyzine, imipenem/cilastatin, insulin (regular), isoproterenol, labetalol, lidocaine, lorazepam, magnesium sulfate, melphalan, meperidine, methotrexate, methylprednisolone, metoclopramide, mezlocillin, midazolam, morphine, nafcillin, nitroglycerin, nitroprusside, norepinephrine, ondansetron, oxacillin, paclitaxel, perphenazine, phenylephrine, phenytoin, phytonadione, piperacillin, potassium chloride, potassium phosphate, procainamide, propofol, sargramostim, sodium bicarbonate, teniposide, theophylline, thiamine, thiotepa, ticarcillin, ticarcillin/clavulanate, verapamil, vinorelbine
Perform/provide:
• Storage in cool environment (oral); IV sol is stable for 48 hr at room temp; do not use discolored sol; discard unused oral sol after 1 mo

---

◆ = Nursing alert   ✒ = Herb-drug interaction   ⊘ = Do not crush

Evaluate:
• Therapeutic response: decreased abdominal pain

Teach patient/family:
• That drug must be continued for prescribed time in prescribed method to be effective; do not double dose
• To report bleeding, bruising, fatigue, malaise, since blood dyscrasias occur
• About possibility of decreased libido, reversible after discontinuing therapy
• To avoid irritating foods, alcohol, aspirin, and extreme temp of foods that may irritate GI system
• That smoking should be avoided; diminishes effectiveness of drug
• To avoid tasks requiring alertness; dizziness, drowsiness may occur
• To increase bulk and fluids in the diet to prevent constipation

---

fat emulsions (R)

Intralipid 10%, Intralipid 20%, Liposyn II 10%, Liposyn II 20%, Liposyn III 10%, Liposyn III 20%, Soyacal 20%

Func. class.: Caloric

Chem class.: Fatty acid, long chain

Action: Needed for energy, heat production; consist of neutral triglycerides, primarily unsaturated fatty acids

Uses: Increase calorie intake, fatty acid deficiency, prevention

Dosage and routes:
Deficiency
• *Adult and child:* IV 8%-10% of required calorie intake (intralipid)

Adjunct to TPN
• *Adult:* IV 1 ml/min over 15-30 min (10%) or 0.5 ml/min over 15-30 min (20%); may increase to 500 ml

over 4-8 hr if no adverse reactions occur; not to exceed 2.5 g/kg
• *Child:* IV 0.1 ml/min over 10-15 min (10%) or 0.05 ml/min over 10-15 min (20%); may increase to 1 g/kg over 4 hr if no adverse reactions occur; not to exceed 4 g/kg

Prevention of deficiency
• *Adult:* IV 500 ml 2 ×/wk (10%), given 1 ml/min for 30 min, not to exceed 500 ml over 6 hr
• *Child:* IV 5-10 ml/kg/day (10%), given 0.1 ml/min for 30 min, not to exceed 100 ml/hr

Available forms: Inj 10% (50, 100, 200, 250, 500 ml), 20% (50, 100, 200, 250, 500 ml)

Side effects/adverse reactions:
CNS: Dizziness, headache, drowsiness, *focal seizures*
CV: Shock
GI: Nausea, vomiting, *hepatomegaly*
RESP: Dyspnea, *fat in lung tissue*
HEMA: Hyperlipemia, hypercoagulation, thrombocytopenia, leukopenia, leukocytosis

Contraindications: Hypersensitivity, hyperlipemia, lipid necrosis, acute pancreatitis accompanied by hyperlipemia, hyperbilirubinemia of the newborn

Precautions: Severe liver disease, diabetes mellitus, thrombocytopenia, gastric ulcers, premature and term newborns, pregnancy (C), sepsis

NURSING CONSIDERATIONS
Assess:
• Triglycerides, free fatty acid levels, platelet counts daily to prevent fat overload, thrombocytopenia
• Liver function studies: AST (SGOT), ALT (SGPT) Hct, Hgb; notify prescriber if abnormal
• Nutritional status: calorie count by dietitian; monitor weight daily

---

Administer:
IV, int inf
• At 10% (1 ml/min); 20% (0.5 ml/min) initially × 15-30 min, may increase 10% (120 ml/hr); 20% (62.5 ml/hr) if no adverse reaction; do not give more than 500 ml on first day
• After changing IV tubing at each infusion: infection may occur with old tubing
• With infusion pump at prescribed rate; do not use in-line filter sized for lipid emulsion; clogging will occur

Additive compatibilities: Cefamandole, chloramphenicol, cimetidine, cyclosporine, diphenhydramine, famotidine, heparin, hydrocortisone, multivitamins, nizatidine, penicillin G potassium

Y-site compatibilities: Ampicillin, cefamandole, cefazolin, cefoxitin, cephapirin, clindamycin, digoxin, dopamine, erythromycin, furosemide, gentamicin, IL-2, isoproterenol, kanamycin, lidocaine, norepinephrine, oxacillin, penicillin G potassium, ticarcillin, tobramycin

Perform/provide:
• Do not use mixed sol separated or oily looking

Evaluate:
• Therapeutic response: increased weight

Teach patient/family:
• The reason for use of lipids

---

felbamate (℞)

(fell′ba-mate)
Felbatol
Func. class.: Anticonvulsant
Chem. class.: Carbamate derivative

Action: Mechanism of action unknown; may increase seizure threshold; has weak inhibitory effects on GABA-receptor and benzodiazepine-receptor binding

Uses: Partial seizures, with or without generalization in adults; partial and generalized seizures in children with Lennox-Gastaut syndrome

Dosage and routes:
Adjunctive therapy
• *Adult:* **PO** add 1.2 g/day in 3-4 divided doses; reduce other anticonvulsants (valproic acid, phenytoin, carbamazepine and derivatives) by 20% to control plasma concentrations; may increase felbamate 1.2 g/day increments qwk, up to 3.6 g/day

Monotherapy
• *Adult:* **PO** 1.2 g/day in 3-4 divided doses; titrate with close supervision; increase dose by 600-mg increments q2wk to 3.6 g/day if needed

Lennox-Gastaut syndrome adjunctive therapy
• *Child 2-14 yr:* **PO** add 15 mg/kg/day in 3-4 divided doses; reduce other anticonvulsants (valproic acid, phenytoin, carbamazepine and derivatives) by 20% to control plasma concentrations; may increase felbamate 15 mg/kg/day qwk up to 45 mg/day

Available forms: Tabs 400, 600 mg; susp 600 mg/5 ml

Side effects/adverse reactions:
CNS: Headache, insomnia, anxiety
CV: Chest pain
EENT: Dry mouth, blurred vision, diplopia
GI: Nausea, *constipation, diarrhea,* anorexia, *vomiting, increased liver enzymes,* **hepatic failure**
GU: Intramenstrual bleeding, UTI
HEMA: Purpura, **leukopenia, aplastic anemia**
INTEG: Rash, acne
RESP: Upper respiratory tract infection, rhinitis, sinusitis, pharyngitis, coughing

---

◆ = Nursing alert   🌿 = Herb-drug interaction   🚫 = Do not crush

Contraindications: Hypersensitivity to this drug, other carbamates, blood dyscrasia, hepatic disease

Precautions: Renal, cardiac disease; psychosis, pregnancy (C), lactation, child <6 yr, elderly

Pharmacokinetics:

PO: Well absorbed, metabolized by liver, excreted in urine >90%; crosses placenta, excreted in breast milk, terminal half-life 20-23 hr; protein binding (22%-25% to albumin)

Interactions:

• Increased levels: phenytoin, valproic acid, methsuximide

• Decreased levels: carbamazepine, phenobarbital

• Increased felbamate levels: phenytoin, carbamazepine

• Decreased felbamate levels: phenobarbital

NURSING CONSIDERATIONS
Assess:

• Renal studies: urinalysis, BUN, urine creatinine q3mo; hepatic studies: ALT (SGPT), AST (SGOT), bilirubin

• Description of seizures

• Mental status: mood, sensorium, affect, behavioral changes; if mental status changes, notify prescriber

• Eye problems: need for ophthalmic examinations before, during, after treatment (slit lamp, fundoscopy, tonometry)

• Allergic reaction: purpura; red, raised rash; drug should be discontinued

Administer:

• With food, milk to decrease GI symptoms

• Shake susp well

Perform/provide:

• Storage at room temp away from heat and light

• Hard candy, frequent rinsing of mouth, gum for dry mouth

• Assistance with ambulation during early part of treatment; dizziness occurs

• Seizure precautions: padded side rails, move objects that may harm patient

Evaluate:

• Therapeutic response: decreased seizure activity; document on patient's chart

Teach patient/family:

• To carry Medic Alert ID stating patient's name, drugs taken, condition, prescriber's name, phone number

• To avoid driving, other activities that require alertness

• Not to discontinue medication quickly after long-term use

Treatment of overdose: Lavage, VS

F

---

felodipine (℞)

(fell-oh′di-peen)

Plendil

Func. class.: Antihypertensive, calcium channel blocker

Chem. class.: Dihydropyridine

Action: Inhibits calcium ion influx across cell membrane, resulting in dilation of peripheral arteries

Uses: Essential hypertension, alone or with other antihypertensives

Dosage and routes:

• *Adult:* **PO** 5 mg qd initially, usual range 5-10 mg qd; do not exceed 20 mg qd; do not adjust dosage at intervals of <2 wk

• *Geriatric:* **PO** 2.5 mg qd

Hepatic disease

• **PO** 2.5 mg, max 10 mg/day

Available forms: Ext rel tabs 2.5, 5, 10 mg

Side effects/adverse reactions:

CV: Dysrhythmia, edema, CHF, hypotension, palpitations, *MI, pulmo-*

---

nary edema, tachycardia, syncope, AV block, angina

GI: Nausea, vomiting, diarrhea, gastric upset, constipation, increased liver function studies, dry mouth

GU: Nocturia, polyuria

INTEG: Rash, pruritus

MISC: Flushing, sexual difficulties, cough, nasal congestion, shortness of breath, wheezing, epistaxis, respiratory infection, chest pain

CNS: Headache, fatigue, drowsiness, dizziness, anxiety, depression, nervousness, insomnia, lightheadedness, paresthesia, tinnitus, psychosis, somnolence

HEMA: Anemia

Contraindications: Hypersensitivity, sick sinus syndrome, 2nd- or 3rd-degree heart block

Precautions: CHF, hypotension <90 mm Hg systolic, hepatic injury, pregnancy (C), lactation, children, renal disease, elderly

Pharmacokinetics: Peak plasma levels 2.5-5 hr; highly protein bound, >99% metabolized in liver, 0.5% excreted unchanged in urine; elimination half-life 11-16 hr

Interactions:
• Increased effects of β-blockers, antihypertensives, digitalis
• Increased felodipine level: cimetidine, ranitidine

NURSING CONSIDERATIONS
Assess:
• Cardiac status: B/P, pulse, respiration, ECG

Administer:
• Once daily as whole tab

Evaluate:
• Therapeutic response: decreased B/P

Teach patient/family:
🚫 To swallow whole; do not break, crush, or chew
• To avoid hazardous activities until stabilized on drug, dizziness is no longer a problem
• To avoid OTC drugs unless directed by a prescriber, to limit caffeine consumption
• The importance of complying with all areas of medical regimen: diet, exercise, stress reduction, drug therapy

Treatment of overdose: Defibrillation, atropine for AV block, vasopressor for hypotension

---

fenofibrate (℞)

(fen-oh-fee'brate)

Lipidil

Func. class.: Antilipemic

Chem. class.: Aryloxisobutyric acid derivative

Action: Inhibits biosynthesis of low-density and very low-density lipoproteins, which are responsible for triglyceride development; mobilizes triglycerides from tissue; increases excretion of neutral sterols

Uses: Types IV, V hyperlipidemia

Dosage and routes:
• *Adult:* PO 100 mg/day

Available forms: Caps 100 mg

Side effects/adverse reactions:
CNS: Fatigue, weakness, drowsiness, dizziness

CV: Angina, dysrhythmias, thrombophlebitis, *pulmonary emboli*

GI: Nausea, vomiting, dyspepsia, increased liver enzymes, stomatitis, flatulence, hepatomegaly, gastritis, increased cholelithiasis, weight gain

GU: Decreased libido, impotence, dysuria, proteinuria, oliguria, *hematuria*

HEMA: Leukopenia, anemia, *eosinophilia,* bleeding

INTEG: Rash, urticaria, pruritus, dry hair and skin, alopecia

---

➤ = Nursing alert   🔬 = Herb-drug interaction   🚫 = Do not crush

MISC: Polyphagia, weight gain
MS: Myalgias, arthralgias
Contraindications: Severe hepatic disease, severe renal disease, primary biliary cirrhosis
Precautions: Peptic ulcer, pregnancy (C), lactation
Pharmacokinetics: Not known
Interactions:
• Increased effects of sulfonylureas, insulin
• Increased toxicity of fenofibrate: probenecid
• Increased anticoagulant effects of oral anticoagulants
• Decreased effects of fenofibrate: rifampin
Lab test interferences:
Increase: Liver function studies, CPK, BSP, thymol turbidity
NURSING CONSIDERATIONS
Assess:
• Renal and hepatic levels if patient is on long-term therapy
Administer:
• Drug with meals if GI symptoms occur
Evaluate:
• Therapeutic response: decreased triglycerides, diarrhea, pruritus (excess bile acids)
• Bowel pattern daily; increase bulk, water in diet if constipation develops
Teach patient/family:
• That compliance is needed, since toxicity may result if doses are missed
• That risk factors should be decreased: high-fat diet, smoking, alcohol consumption, absence of exercise
• That birth control should be practiced while on this drug
• To report GU symptoms: decreased libido, impotence, dysuria, proteinuria, oliguria, hematuria
🚫 Not to break, crush, or chew caps

fenoprofen (℞)

(fen-oh-proe′fen)
fenoprofen, Nalfon
Func. class.: Nonsteroidal antiinflammatory/nonopioid analgesic
Chem. class.: Propionic acid derivative

Action: Inhibits prostaglandin synthesis by decreasing enzyme needed for biosynthesis; analgesic, antiinflammatory, antipyretic
Uses: Mild to moderate pain, osteoarthritis, rheumatoid arthritis, acute gout, arthritis, ankylosing spondylitis, inflammation, dysmenorrhea
Dosage and routes:
Pain
• *Adult:* PO 200 mg q4-6h prn
Arthritis
• *Adult:* PO 300-600 mg qid, not to exceed 3.2 g/day
Available forms: Caps 200, 300 mg; tabs 600 mg
Side effects/adverse reactions:
GI: Nausea, anorexia, vomiting, diarrhea, jaundice, *cholestatic hepatitis,* constipation, flatulence, cramps, dry mouth, peptic ulcer
CNS: Dizziness, headache, drowsiness, fatigue, tremors, confusion, insomnia, anxiety, depression
CV: Tachycardia, peripheral edema, palpitations, *dysrhythmias*
INTEG: Purpura, rash, pruritus, sweating
GU: Nephrotoxicity: dysuria, hematuria, oliguria, azotemia
HEMA: Blood dyscrasias
EENT: Tinnitus, hearing loss, blurred vision
Contraindications: Hypersensitivity, asthma, severe renal disease, severe hepatic disease
Precautions: Pregnancy (B) 1st and

F

2nd trimester, lactation, children, bleeding disorders, GI disorders, cardiac disorders, hypersensitivity to other antiinflammatory agents, elderly, CrCl <30 ml/min, hypertension

Pharmacokinetics:

PO: Peak 2 hr, half-life 3-3½ hr; metabolized in liver; excreted in urine (metabolites), breast milk; 99% plasma protein binding

Interactions:

• May increase the action of warfarin, sulfonamides, salicylates

• May decrease effects of fenoprofen: phenobarbital, probenecid

NURSING CONSIDERATIONS

Assess:

• Renal, liver, blood studies: BUN, creatinine, AST (SGOT), ALT (SGPT), Hgb, before treatment, periodically thereafter

• Audiometric, ophthalmic examination before, during, after treatment

• For eye, ear problems: blurred vision, tinnitus; may indicate toxicity

Administer:

• With food for GI symptoms; however, best to take on empty stomach to facilitate absorption

Perform/provide:

• Storage at room temp

Evaluate:

• Therapeutic response: decreased pain, stiffness in joints, decreased swelling in joints, ability to move more easily

Teach patient/family:

• To report blurred vision, ringing, roaring in ears; may indicate toxicity

• To avoid driving, other hazardous activities if dizziness, drowsiness occurs

• To report change in urine pattern, increased weight, edema, increased pain in joints, fever, blood in urine; indicates nephrotoxicity

• That therapeutic effects may take up to 1 mo, to take as prescribed

• To take with a full glass of water to enhance absorption

• To avoid concurrent use of alcohol, aspirin, acetaminophen, other OTC meds without consulting prescriber

Ⓢ Not to break, crush, or chew caps

---

fentanyl (℞)

(fen′ta-nill)

Fentanyl, Sublimaze

Func. class.: Narcotic analgesic

Chem. class.: Opiate, synthetic phenylpiperidine derivative

Controlled Substance Schedule II

Action: Inhibits ascending pain pathways in CNS, increases pain threshold, alters pain perception by binding to opiate receptors

Uses: Preoperatively, postoperatively; adjunct to general anesthetic, when combined with droperidol

Dosage and routes:

Anesthetic

• *Adult:* **IV** 0.05-0.1 mg q2-3min prn

Preoperatively

• *Adult:* **IM** 0.05-0.1 mg q30-60 min before surgery

Postoperatively

• *Adult:* **IM** 0.05-0.1 mg q1-2h prn

Available forms: Inj 0.05 mg/ml

Side effects/adverse reactions:

CNS: Dizziness, delirium, euphoria

GI: Nausea, vomiting

MS: Muscle rigidity

EENT: Blurred vision, miosis

CV: **Bradycardia, arrest,** hypotension or hypertension

RESP: **Respiratory depression, arrest, laryngospasm**

Contraindications: Hypersensitivity to opiates, myasthenia gravis

---

◆ = Nursing alert   ⚗ = Herb-drug interaction   Ⓢ = Do not crush

Precautions: Elderly, respiratory depression, increased intracranial pressure, seizure disorders, severe respiratory disorders, cardiac dysrhythmias, pregnancy (C), lactation

Pharmacokinetics:

IM: Onset 7-8 min, peak 30 min, duration 1-2 hr

IV: Onset immediate, peak 3-5 min, duration ½-1 hr; metabolized by liver; excreted by kidneys; crosses placenta; excreted in breast milk; half-life 1½-6 hr; 80% bound to plasma proteins

Interactions:

• Effects may be increased with other CNS depressants: alcohol, narcotics, sedative/hypnotics, antipsychotics, skeletal muscle relaxants

✗ Increased action: kava kava

NURSING CONSIDERATIONS

Assess:

• VS after parenteral route; note muscle rigidity, drug history, liver, kidney function test

• CNS changes: dizziness, drowsiness, hallucinations, euphoria, LOC, pupil reaction

• Allergic reactions: rash, urticaria

• Respiratory dysfunction: respiratory depression, character, rate, rhythm; notify prescriber if respirations are <10/min

Administer:

• By injection (IM, IV); give slowly to prevent rigidity

• Only with resuscitative equipment available

IV

• IV undiluted by anesthesiologist or diluted with 5 ml or more sterile H$_2$O or 0.9% NaCl given through Y-tube or 3-way stopcock at 0.1 mg or less/1-2 min

Additive compatibilities: Bupivacaine

Solution compatibilities: D$_5$W, 0.9% NaCl

Syringe compatibilities: Atracurium, atropine, bupivacaine/ketamine, butorphanol, chlorpromazine, cimetidine, clonidine/lidocaine, dimenhydrinate, diphenhydramine, droperidol, heparin, hydromorphone, hydroxyzine, meperidine, metoclopramide, midazolam, morphine, pentazocine, perphenazine, prochlorperazine, promazine, promethazine, ranitidine, scopolamine

Y-site compatibilities: Atracurium, diltiazem, dobutamine, dopamine, enalaprilat, epinephrine, esmolol, etomidate, furosemide, heparin, hydrocortisone, hydromorphone, labetalol, lorazepam, midazolam, milrinone, morphine, nafcillin, nicardipine, nitroglycerin, norepinephrine, pancuronium, potassium chloride, propofol, ranitidine, sargramostim, thiopental, vecuronium, vit B/C

Perform/provide:

• Storage in light-resistant area at room temp

• Coughing, turning, deep breathing for postoperative patients

• Safety measures: side rails, nightlight, call bell within reach

Evaluate:

• Therapeutic response: induction of anesthesia

---

fentanyl/droperidol combination (R)

(fen′ta-nil)/(droe-per′i-dole)

Innovar

Func. class.: General anesthetic, narcotic analgesic

Chem. class.: Phenylpiperone derivative

Controlled Substance Schedule II

Action: Action at subcortical levels to reduce motor activity, produces analgesia

Uses: Premedication, adjunct to general anesthesia, maintenance of anesthesia

Dosage and routes:
Induction
- *Adult:* **IV** 1 ml/20-25 lb
- *Child:* **IV** 0.5 ml/20 lb

Premedication
- *Adult:* **IM** 0.5-2 ml 45-60 min before surgery or procedure
- *Child:* **IM** 0.25 ml/20 lb 45-60 min before surgery or procedure

Available forms: Inj 0.05 mg fentanyl, 2.5 mg droperidol/ml

Side effects/adverse reactions:
RESP: Laryngospasm, bronchospasm, respiratory arrest
CNS: Dystonia, akathisia, flexion of arms, fine tremors, dizziness, anxiety, drowsiness, restlessness, hallucination, depression, muscular rigidity, EPS
CV: Tachycardia, hypotension, circulatory depression
EENT: Upward rotation of eyes, oculogyric crisis, blurred vision
INTEG: Chills, facial sweating, shivering, diaphoresis
GI: Nausea, vomiting

Contraindications: Hypersensitivity, child <2 yr, myasthenia gravis
Precautions: Elderly, increased intracranial pressure, cardiovascular disease (bradydysrhythmias), renal disease, liver disease, Parkinson's disease, COPD, pregnancy (C)

Pharmacokinetics:
IV: Onset 20 sec, peak 2-10 min, duration ½-2 hr; tranquilizing effect may last up to 12 hr
IM: Onset 7 min, duration 1-2 hr; metabolized in liver; excreted in urine metabolites (90%)

Interactions:
- Increased CNS depression: alcohol, narcotics, barbiturates, antipsychotics, other CNS depressants
- Decreased effects of amphetamines, anticonvulsants, anticoagulants
- Increased intraocular pressure: anticholinergics, antiparkinson drugs
- Increased side effects of lithium

� Increased action: kava kava

NURSING CONSIDERATIONS
Assess:
- VS q10min during IV administration, q30min after IM dose
- Liver functions test and BUN, creatinine, $Paco_2$
- Rigidity of skeletal muscles
- EPS: dystonia, akathisia
- Increasing heart rate or decreasing B/P by >10% from baseline; notify prescriber at once; do not place patient in Trendelenburg position or sympathetic blockade may occur, causing respiratory arrest

Administer:
- Anticholinergics (benztropine, diphenhydramine) for EPS
- Only with crash cart, resuscitative equipment nearby; narcotic antagonist for severe respiratory depression, cardiac monitor

IV
- IV direct undiluted through Y-tube or 3-way stopcock; give each 1 ml undiluted drug/1min or more; 0.1 ml/kg may be diluted in 250 ml D_5W and given as IV INF over 5-10 min; titrate to response

Additive compatibilities: Sodium bicarbonate
Syringe compatibilities: Benzquinamide, glycopyrrolate
Y-site compatibilities: Hydrocortisone, potassium chloride, vit B/C

Perform/provide:
- Slow movement of patient to avoid orthostatic hypotension

Evaluate:
- Therapeutic response: decreased anxiety, absence of vomiting, maintenance of anesthesia

---

Teach patient/family:
• To use deep breathing, turning, coughing after surgery to prevent increased secretions in lungs

fentanyl transdermal (℞)
Duragesic-25, Duragesic-50, Duragesic-75, Duragesic-100
Func. class.: Narcotic analgesic
Chem. class.: Opiate, synthetic phenylpiperidine

Controlled Substance Schedule II
Action: Inhibits ascending pain pathways in CNS, increases pain threshold, alters pain perception by binding to opiate receptors
Uses: Management of chronic pain for those requiring opioid analgesia
Dosage and routes:
• *Adult:* 25 µg/hr; may increase until pain relief occurs; apply patch to flat surface on upper torso and wear for 72 hr; apply new patch on different site for continued relief
Available forms: Patch 2.5, 5, 7.5, 10 mg/hr
Side effects/adverse reactions:
CNS: Dizziness, delirium, euphoria, light-headedness, sedation, dysphoria, agitation, anxiety
GI: Nausea, vomiting, diarrhea, cramps
EENT: Blurred vision, miosis
CV: Bradycardia, *cardiac arrest,* hypotension or hypertension, facial flushing, chills
*RESP: **Respiratory depression, laryngospasm, bronchospasm;*** depresses cough; hypoventilation
Contraindications: Hypersensitivity to opiates, myasthenia gravis, children <12 yr, patient <18 yr with weight <110 lb
Precautions: Elderly, respiratory depression, increased intracranial pressure, seizure disorders, severe respiratory disorders, cardiac dysrhythmias, pregnancy (C), fever
Interactions:
• Effects may be increased with other CNS depressants: alcohol, narcotics, sedative/hypnotics, antipsychotics, skeletal muscle relaxants
🍃 Increased action: kava kava
NURSING CONSIDERATIONS
Assess:
• Pain control; check for duration, site, character of pain, fever; use pain and sedation scoring
• CNS changes: dizziness, drowsiness, hallucinations, euphoria, LOC, pupil reaction
• Allergic reactions: rash, urticaria
• Respiratory dysfunction: respiratory depression, character, rate, rhythm; notify prescriber if respirations are <10/min
Administer:
• q72h for continuous pain relief; dosage is adjusted after at least two applications
• Give short-acting analgesics until patch takes effect (24 hr)
Perform/provide:
• Safety measures: side rails, nightlight, call bell within reach
Evaluate:
• Therapeutic response: decreased pain
Teach patient/family:
• To avoid activities that require alertness

ferrous fumarate/ ferrous gluconate/ ferrous sulfate (OTC, ℞)

(fer'us)

Femiron, Feosol, Feostat, Feratab, Fergon, Fer-In-Sol, Fer-Iron, Fero-Gradumet, Ferospace, Ferralet, Ferralet S.R., Ferralyn, Ferra-TD, Ferrets, Ferrous Fumarate, Ferrous Gluconate, Ferrous Sulfate, Fumasorb, Fumerin, Hemocyte, Ircon, Mol-Iron, Nephro-Fer, Simron, Slow-Fe, Span-FF

Func. class.: Hematinic
Chem. class.: Iron preparation

Action: Replaces iron stores needed for red blood cell development, energy and O_2 transport, utilization; fumarate contains 33% elemental iron; gluconate, 12%; sulfate, 20%; iron, 30%; ferrous sulfate exsiccated

Uses: Iron deficiency anemia, prophylaxis for iron deficiency in pregnancy

Dosage and routes:
Fumarate
• *Adult:* **PO** 200 mg tid-qid
• *Child 2-12 yr:* **PO** 3 mg/kg/day (elemental iron) tid-qid
• *Child 6 mo-2 yr:* **PO** up to 6 mg/kg/day (elemental iron) tid-qid; **PO** 6 mg/kg/day in 3-4 divided doses
• *Infant:* **PO** 10-25 mg/day (elemental iron) in 3-4 divided doses
Gluconate
• *Adult:* **PO** 200-600 mg tid
• *Child 6-12 yr:* **PO** 300-900 mg qd
• *Child <6 yr:* **PO** 100-300 mg qd
Sulfate
• *Adult:* **PO** 0.75-1.5 g/day in divided doses tid
• *Child 6-12 yr:* **PO** 600 mg/day in divided doses

Pregnancy
• *Adult:* **PO** 300-600 mg/day in divided doses
Available forms:
Fumarate
Tabs 63, 195, 200, 324, 325 mg; tabs chewable 100 mg; tabs cont rel 300 mg; oral susp 100 mg/5 ml, 45 mg/0.6 ml
Gluconate
Tabs 300, 320, 325 mg; caps 86, 325, 435 mg; tabs film-coated 300 mg; elix 300 mg/5 ml
Sulfate
Tabs, 195, 300, 325 mg; tabs enteric-coated 325 mg; tabs ext rel, time-rel caps, 525 mg
Side effects/adverse reactions:
GI: Nausea, constipation, epigastric pain, black and red tarry stools, vomiting, diarrhea
INTEG: Temporarily discolored tooth enamel and eyes
Contraindications: Hypersensitivity, ulcerative colitis/regional enteritis, hemosiderosis/hemochromatosis, peptic ulcer disease, hemolytic anemia, cirrhosis
Precautions: Anemia (long-term), pregnancy (A)
Pharmacokinetics:
PO: Excreted in feces, urine, skin, breast milk; enters bloodstream; bound to transferrin; crosses placenta
Interactions:
• Decreased absorption of: penicillamine, levodopa, methyldopa, quinolone, tetracycline
• Decreased absorption of iron preparations: antacids, tetracycline, vit E
• Increased absorption of iron preparation: ascorbic acid, chloramphenicol
Lab test interferences:
False positive: Occult blood
NURSING CONSIDERATIONS
Assess:
• Blood studies: Hct, Hgb, reticu-

locytes, bilirubin before treatment, at least monthly

◆ Toxicity: nausea, vomiting, diarrhea (green, then tarry stools), hematemesis, pallor, cyanosis, shock, coma

• Elimination; if constipation occurs, increase water, bulk, activity

• Nutrition: amount of iron in diet (meat, dark green leafy vegetables, dried beans, dried fruits, eggs)

• Cause of iron loss or anemia, including salicylates, sulfonamides, antimalarials, quinidine

Administer:

• Between meals for best absorption; may give with juice; do not give with antacids or milk, delay at least 1 hr; if GI symptoms occur, give pc even if absorption is decreased; eggs, milk products, chocolate, caffeine interfere with absorption

• Liquid through plastic straw to avoid discoloration of tooth enamel; dilute thoroughly

• At least 1 hr before hs, since corrosion may occur in stomach

• For <6 mo for anemia

Perform/provide:

• Storage in tight, light-resistant container

Evaluate:

• Therapeutic response: improvement in Hct, Hgb, reticulocytes; decreased fatigue, weakness

Teach patient/family:

• That iron will change stools black or dark green

• That iron poisoning may occur if increased beyond recommended level

🚫 To swallow tab whole; not to break, crush, or chew

• To keep out of reach of children

• Not to substitute one iron salt for another; elemental iron content differs (e.g., 300 mg ferrous fumarate contains about 100 mg elemental

iron; 300 mg ferrous gluconate contains only about 30 mg elemental iron)

• To avoid reclining position for 15-30 min after taking drug to avoid esophageal corrosion

• To follow diet high in iron

Treatment of overdose: Induce vomiting; give eggs, milk until lavage can be done

F

---

fexofenadine (℞)

(fex-oh-fi′na-deen)

Allegra

Func. class.: Antihistamine

Chem. class.: Piperidine, peripherally selective

Action: Acts on blood vessels, GI, respiratory system by competing with histamine for H_1-receptor site; decreases allergic response by blocking pharmacologic effects of histamine

Uses: Rhinitis, allergy symptoms

Dosage and routes:

• *Adult and child >12 yr:* 60 mg bid

• CrCl <80 ml/min 60 mg qd

Available forms: Caps 60 mg

Side effects/adverse reactions:

GU: Frequency, dysuria, urinary retention, impotence

HEMA: **Hemolytic anemia, thrombocytopenia, leukopenia, agranulocytosis, pancytopenia**

RESP: Thickening of bronchial secretions, dry nose, throat

GI: Nausea, diarrhea, abdominal pain, vomiting, constipation

CNS: Headache, stimulation, drowsiness, sedation, fatigue, confusion, blurred vision, tinnitus, restlessness, tremors, paradoxical excitation in children or elderly

INTEG: Rash, eczema, photosensitivity, urticaria

V: Hypotension, palpitations, ‚radycardia, tachycardia, *dysrhyth-‚ias (rare)*

Contraindications: Hypersensitiv-ıty, newborn or premature infants, lactation, severe hepatic disease

Precautions: Pregnancy (C), el-derly, children, respiratory disease, narrow-angle glaucoma, prostatic hypertrophy, bladder neck obstruc-tion, asthma, elderly

Pharmacokinetics: Well absorbed; onset 3-5 min, peak 1-2 hr, duration 8-12 hr

Interactions:
• Increased CNS depression: alco-hol, other CNS depressants, procar-bazine
• Increased anticholinergic effects: MAOIs
• Decreased action of: oral antico-agulants
• Serious CV reactions: ketocona-zole, itraconazole, erythromycin
• Avoid use with antifungals, mac-rolide antibiotics
📕 Increased anticholinergic effect: henbane leaf

Lab test interferences:
False negative: Skin allergy tests

NURSING CONSIDERATIONS
Assess:
• I&O ratio: be alert for urinary re-tention, frequency, dysuria, espe-cially elderly; drug should be dis-continued if these occur
• Respiratory status: rate, rhythm, increase in bronchial secretions, wheezing, chest tightness

Administer:
• On empty stomach 1 hr before or 2 hr after meals

Perform/provide:
• Hard candy, gum, frequent rinsing of mouth for dryness
• Storage in tight, light-resistant con-tainer

Evaluate:
• Therapeutic response: absence of running or congested nose or rashes

Teach patient/family:
• All aspects of drug use; to notify prescriber if confusion, sedation, hy-potension occur
• To avoid driving, other hazardous activity if drowsiness occurs
• To avoid alcohol, other CNS de-pressants
• Not to exceed recommended dose; dysrhythmias may occur
🚫 Not to break, crush, or chew caps

Treatment of overdose: Adminis-ter ipecac syrup or lavage, diaz-epam, vasopressors, barbiturates (short-acting)

fibrinolysin/ desoxyri- bonuclease (℞)

(fye-brin-oh-lye′sin)/(dez-ox-ee-rye-boo-nuke′lee-ase)
Elase
Func. class.: Enzyme
Chem. class.: Proteolytic, bo-vine

Action: Dissolves fibrin in clots and fibrinous exudates; attacks DNA in areas of disintegrating cells

Uses: Debridement of wounds, vaginitis, cervicitis, ulcerative coli-tis; 2nd-, 3rd-degree burns; irrigat-ing wounds, topically

Dosage and routes:
Debridement/intravaginally
• *Adult:* **OINT** 5 g × 5 applications
Irrigating
• *Adult:* **IRIG** dilution depends on type of wound

Available forms: Fibrinolysin with desoxyribonuclease 666.6 U/g; pow-der for reconstitution fibrinolysin 25 U/desoxyribonuclease 15,000 U

◆ = Nursing alert　　📕 = Herb-drug interaction　　🚫 = Do not crush

Side effects/adverse reactions:
INTEG: Hyperemia
Contraindications: Hypersensitivity to bovine or mercury products, hematoma
Precautions: Pregnancy (C)
NURSING CONSIDERATIONS
Assess:
• For signs of irritation and inflammation; drug should be discontinued
• Wound: drainage, color, odor, size, depth
Administer:
• After reconstituting with 10 ml sterile NaCl sol; use only fresh sol
• After removing necrotic debris, dry eschar
• Wet dressing by mixing 1 vial elase/10-50 ml NS; saturate gauze with sol; pack area; remove in 6-8 hr; repeat tid-qid
Perform/provide:
• Cleansing of wound using aseptic technique; cover with drug, then dressing; change at least qid
Evaluate:
• Therapeutic response: decrease in wound scarring, tissue necrosis

---

filgrastim (℞)

(fill-grass'stim)
G-CSF, granulocyte colony stimulator, Neupogen
Func. class.: Biologic modifier
Chem. class.: Granulocyte colony-stimulating factor

Action: Stimulates proliferation and differentiation of neutrophils
Uses: To decrease infection in patients receiving antineoplastics that are myelosuppressive; to increase WBC in patients with drug-induced neutropenia; bone marrow transplantation
Dosage and routes:
• *Adult and child:* IV/SC 5 µg/kg/ day in a single dose; may increase by 5 µg/kg in each chemotherapy cycle; give qd for up to 2 wk until the absolute neutrophil count (ANC) 10,000/mm^3; response to G-CSF is much greater with **SC** than **IV** therapy
Available forms: Inj 300 µg/ml
Side effects/adverse reactions:
RESP: Respiratory distress syndrome
CNS: Fever
*HEMA: **Thrombocytopenia***
INTEG: Alopecia, exacerbation of skin conditions
MS: Osteoporosis, skeletal pain
GI: Nausea, vomiting, diarrhea, mucositis, anorexia
Contraindications: Hypersensitivity to proteins of *E. coli*
Precautions: Pregnancy (C), lactation, cardiac conditions, children, myeloid malignancies
Pharmacokinetics: Metabolism, excretion, distribution not known
Interactions:
• Do not use this drug concomitantly with antineoplastics
Lab test interferences:
Increase: Uric acid, lactate dehydrogenase, alk phosphatase
NURSING CONSIDERATIONS
Assess:
• Blood studies: CBC, platelet count before treatment and twice weekly; neutrophil counts may be increased for 2 days after therapy
Administer:
• Using single-use vials; after dose is withdrawn, do not reenter vial
• For 2 wk or until ANC is 10,000/ mm^3 after the expected chemotherapy neutrophil nadir
Cont IV inf
• Dilute in D$_5$W to a conc of >15 µg/ml, vial is for one-time use; give over 15-30 min (chemotherapy); over 4-24 hr (bone marrow transplantation)
Y-site compatibilities: Acyclovir,

allopurinol, amikacin, aminophylline, ampicillin, ampicillin/sulbactam, aztreonam, bleomycin, bumetanide, buprenorphine, butorphanol, calcium gluconate, carboplatin, carmustine, cefazolin, cefotetan, ceftazidime, chlorpromazine, cimetidine, cisplatin, cyclophosphamide, cytarabine, dacarbazine, daunorubicin, dexamethasone, diphenhydramine, doxorubicin, doxycycline, droperidol, enalaprilat, famotidine, floxuridine, fluconazole, fludarabine, gallium, ganciclovir, granisetron, haloperidol, hydrocortisone, hydromorphone, hydroxyzine, idarubicin, ifosfamide, leucovorin, lorazepam, mechlorethamine, melphalan, meperidine, mesna, methotrexate, metoclopramide, miconazole, minocycline, mitoxantrone, morphine, nalbuphine, netilmicin, ondansetron, plicamycin, potassium chloride, promethazine, ranitidine, sodium bicarbonate, streptozocin, ticarcillin, ticarcillin/clavulanate, tobramycin, trimethoprim-sulfamethoxazole, vancomycin, vinblastine, vincristine, vinorelbine, zidovudine

Perform/provide:
• Storage in refrigerator; do not freeze; may store at room temp up to 6 hr
• Avoid shaking

Evaluate:
• Therapeutic response: absence of infection

Teach patient/family:
• The technique for self-administration: dose, side effects, disposal of containers and needles; provide instruction sheet

finasteride (R̲)

(fin-ass′te-ride)
Proscar, Propecia
Func. class.: Androgen hormone inhibitor
Chem. class.: 5-α-reductase inhibitor

Action: Inhibits 5-α-reductase and reduction in DHT; DHT induces androgenic effects by binding to androgen receptors in the cell nuclei of the prostate gland, liver, skin; prevents development of BHP

Uses: Symptomatic benign prostatic hyperplasia (Proscar); male-pattern baldness (Propecia)

Dosage and routes:
Proscar
• *Adult:* PO 5 mg qd × 6-12 mo
Propecia
• *Adult:* PO 1 mg qd
Available forms: Tabs 5 mg

Side effects/adverse reactions:
GU: Impotence, decreased libido, decreased volume of ejaculate

Contraindications: Hypersensitivity, children, women who are pregnant or may become pregnant should not handle tabs

Precautions: Large residual urinary volume, severely diminished urinary flow, liver function abnormalities

Pharmacokinetics: Bioavailability 63%, plasma protein binding 90%; metabolized in the liver; excreted in urine (metabolites) 39%, feces (57%); crosses blood-brain barrier

Interactions:
• Increases theophylline clearance

NURSING CONSIDERATIONS
Assess:
• Urinary patterns, residual urinary volume, severely diminished urinary flow

• PSA levels and digital rectal exam prior to initiating therapy and periodically thereafter

• Liver function studies prior to treatment; extensively metabolized in liver

Administer:

• Without regard to meals

Perform/provide:

• Storage <86° F (30° C); protect from light; keep container tightly closed

Evaluate:

• Therapeutic response: increased urinary flow, decreased postvoiding dribbling, frequency, nocturia

Teach patient/family:

• Pregnant women or women who may become pregnant should not touch crushed tabs or come into contact with semen of a patient taking this drug; may adversely affect developing male fetus

• That volume of ejaculate may be decreased during treatment; impotence and decreased libido may also occur

• Propecia results may not occur for 3 mo

• Proscar results may not occur for 6-12 mo

---

flavoxate (R)

(fla-vox′ate)
Urispas
Func. class.: Spasmolytic
Chem. class.: Flavone derivative

Action: Relaxes smooth muscles in urinary tract

Uses: Relief of nocturia, incontinence, suprapubic pain, dysuria, frequency associated with urologic conditions (symptomatic only)

Dosage and routes:

• *Adult and child >12 yr:* **PO** 100-200 mg tid-qid

Available forms: Tabs 100 mg

Side effects/adverse reactions:

HEMA: **Leukopenia, eosinophilia**

CNS: Anxiety, restlessness, dizziness, **convulsions,** headache, drowsiness, confusion, decreased concentration

CV: Palpitations, sinus tachycardia, hypotension

GI: Nausea, vomiting, anorexia, abdominal pain, constipation

GU: Dysuria

INTEG: Urticaria, dermatitis

EENT: Blurred vision, increased intraocular tension, dry mouth, throat

Contraindications: Hypersensitivity, GI obstruction, GI hemorrhage, GU obstruction

Precautions: Pregnancy (B), lactation, suspected glaucoma, children <12 yr, elderly

Pharmacokinetics: Excreted in urine

NURSING CONSIDERATIONS

Assess:

• Urinary status: dysuria, frequency, nocturia, incontinence

• Allergic reactions: rash, urticaria; drug should be discontinued

Evaluate:

• Therapeutic response: decreased dysuria

Teach patient/family:

• To avoid hazardous activities; dizziness may occur

---

flecainide (R)

(flek-ay′nide)
Tambocor
Func. class.: Antidysrhythmic (Class IC)

Action: Decreases conduction in all parts of the heart, with greatest effect on His-Purkinje system, which stabilizes cardiac membrane

Uses: Life-threatening ventricular dysrhythmias, sustained ventricular tachycardia, supraventricular tachy-dysrhythmias

Dosage and routes:
• *Adult:* **PO** 50-100 mg q12h; may increase q4d by 50 mg q12h to desired response, not to exceed 400 mg/day
Renal disease
• CrCl <35 ml/min dose 50%-75%
Available forms: Tabs 50, 100, 150 mg

Side effects/adverse reactions:
CNS: Headache, dizziness, involuntary movement, confusion, psychosis, restlessness, irritability, paresthesias, ataxia, flushing, somnolence, depression, anxiety, malaise
EENT: Tinnitus, blurred vision, hearing loss
GI: Nausea, vomiting, anorexia, constipation, abdominal pain, flatulence, change in taste
CV: Hypotension, bradycardia, angina, PVCs, **heart block, cardiovascular collapse, arrest,** dysrhythmias, **CHF, fatal ventricular tachycardia**
RESP: Dyspnea, **respiratory depression**
INTEG: Rash, urticaria, edema, swelling
HEMA: Leukopenia, thrombocytopenia
GU: Impotence, decreased libido, polyuria, urinary retention

Contraindications: Hypersensitivity, severe heart block, cardiogenic shock, nonsustained ventricular dysrhythmias, frequent PVCs, non-life-threatening dysrhythmias

Precautions: Pregnancy (C), lactation, children, renal disease, liver disease, CHF, respiratory depression, myasthenia gravis

Pharmacokinetics:
PO: Peak 3 hr; half-life 12-27 hr; metabolized by liver; excreted unchanged by kidneys (10%); excreted in breast milk

Interactions:
• Increased levels of both drugs: propranolol
• Increased level of flecainide: amiodarone, cimetidine
• Increased negative inotropic effects: disopyramide, verapamil
• Increased digoxin level: digoxin
 Potassium deficiency: aloe, buckthorn bark/berry, cascara sagrada bark, senna pod/leaf

Lab test interferences:
Increase: CPK

NURSING CONSIDERATIONS
Assess:
• For hypokalemia, hyperkalemia before administration; correct electrolytes
• Blood levels: trough (0.2-1 µg/ml)
• B/P, ECG continuously for fluctuations
 Malignant hyperthermia: tachypnea, tachycardia, changes in B/P, increased temp
• Cardiac rate, respiration: rate, rhythm, character, continuously
• Respiratory status: rate, rhythm, lung fields for rales
• CNS effects: dizziness, confusion, psychosis, paresthesias, convulsions; drug should be discontinued
• Increased respiration, increased pulse; drug should be discontinued

Administer:
• Reduced dosage as soon as dysrhythmia is controlled

Evaluate:
• Therapeutic response: decreased dysrhythmias

Teach patient/family:
• To change position slowly from lying or sitting to standing to minimize orthostatic hypotension
• To take as prescribed, not to skip or double dose
• To avoid hazardous activities that require alertness until response is known

---

 = Nursing alert   = Herb-drug interaction   = Do not crush

Treatment of overdose: O_2, artificial ventilation, ECG, dopamine for circulatory depression, diazepam or thiopental for convulsions, treat ventricular dysrhythmias

---

fluconazole (R)
(floo-kon′a-zole)
Diflucan
Func. class.: Antifungal

Action: Inhibits ergosterol biosynthesis, causes direct damage to membrane phospholipids
Uses: Oropharyngeal candidiasis in AIDS patients, chronic mucocutaneous candidiasis, urinary candidiasis, cryptococcal meningitis
Dosage and routes:
Renal disease
• CrCl 11-50 ml/min dose 50%
Vaginal candidiasis
• *Adult:* PO 150 mg as a single dose
Serious fungal infections
• *Adult:* **PO/IV** 50-400 mg initially, then 200 mg qd for 4 wk
• *Child:* 6-12 mg/kg/day
Oropharyngeal candidiasis
• *Adult:* **PO/IV** 200 mg initially, then 100 mg qd for at least 2 wk
• *Child:* 3 mg/kg/day
Available forms: Tabs 50, 100, 200 mg; inj 200, 400 mg; powder for oral susp 10 mg, 40 mg/ml
Side effects/adverse reactions:
GI: Nausea, vomiting, diarrhea, cramping, flatus, increased AST, ALT, *hepatotoxicity*
CNS: Headache
INTEG: Stevens-Johnson syndrome
Contraindications: Hypersensitivity
Precautions: Renal disease, pregnancy (C), lactation
Pharmacokinetics: Peak 2-4 hr, bioavailability (PO) 90%, excreted unchanged in urine 80%

Interactions:
• Potentiation of anticoagulation: warfarin
• Increased renal dysfunction: cyclosporines
• Decreased effect of fluconazole: rifampin, cimetidine
• Decreased effect: oral contraceptives
• Increased effect: phenytoin, theophylline, zidovudine, sulfonylureas
NURSING CONSIDERATIONS
Assess:
• VS q15-30min during first infusion; note changes in pulse, B/P
• I&O ratio; watch for decreasing urinary output, change in specific gravity; discontinue drug to prevent renal damage
• Weight weekly; if weight gain >2 lb/wk and edema is present, renal damage should be considered
◆ Renal toxicity: increasing BUN, serum creatinine; if BUN is >40 mg/dl or if serum creatinine is >3 mg/dl, drug may be discontinued or dosage reduced
• For hepatotoxicity: increasing AST (SGOT), ALT (SGPT), alk phosphatase, bilirubin
Administer:
• Drug only after C&S confirms organism, drug needed to treat condition
IV
• After diluting according to package directions; run at 200 mg/hr or less; do not use plastic containers in connections; check for bag leaks
• Using an infusion pump check for extravasation and necrosis q2h
Additive compatibilities: Acyclovir, amikacin, amphotericin B, cefazolin, ceftazidime, clindamycin, gentamicin, heparin, meropenem, metronidazole, morphine, piperacillin, potassium chloride, theophylline

Y-site compatibilities: Acyclovir, aldesleukin, allopurinol, amifostine, amikacin, aminophylline, ampicillin/sulbactam, aztreonam, benztropine, cefazolin, cefepime, cefotetan, cefoxitin, cefpirome, chlorpromazine, cimetidine, dexamethasone, diphenhydramine, dobutamine, dopamine, droperidol, famotidine, filgrastim, fludarabine, foscarnet, gallium, ganciclovir, gentamicin, granisetron, heparin, hydrocortisone, immune globulin, leucovorin, lorazepam, melphalan, meperidine, meropenem, metoclopramide, metronidazole, midazolam, morphine, nafcillin, nitroglycerin, ondansetron, oxacillin, paclitaxel, pancuronium, penicillin G potassium, phenytoin, piperacillin/tazobactam, prochlorperazine, promethazine, propofol, ranitidine, sargramostim, tacrolimus, teniposide, theophylline, thiotepa, ticarcillin/clavulanate, tobramycin, vancomycin, vecuronium, vinorelbine, zidovudine

Perform/provide:

• Storage protected from moisture and light, diluted sol is stable 24 hr

Evaluate:

• Therapeutic response: decreasing oral candidiasis, fever, malaise, rash; negative C&S for infection organism

Teach patient/family:

• That long-term therapy may be needed to clear infection

• That medication may be taken with food to reduce GI effects

• To consider using alternative contraception if using oral contraceptives

---

flucytosine (℞)

(floo-sye'toe-seen)

Ancobon, Ancotil*, 5-FC

Func. class.: Antifungal

Chem. class.: Pyrimidine (fluorinated)

Action: Converted to fluorouracil after entering fungi; inhibits RNA, DNA synthesis; synergistic action when used with amphotericin B in some fungal infections

Uses: *Candida* infections (septicemia, endocarditis, pulmonary, UTI), *Cryptococcus* (meningitis, pulmonary, urinary tract infections)

Dosage and routes:

Renal disease

• CrCl 10-50 ml/min give q16h; CrCl <10 ml/min give q24h

• *Adult and child >50 kg:* **PO** 50-150 mg/kg/day q6h

• *Adult and child <50 kg:* **PO** 1.5-4.5 g/m²/day or 50-100 mg/kg/day in 4 divided doses

Available forms: Caps 250, 500 mg

Side effects/adverse reactions:

INTEG: Rash

CNS: Headache, confusion, dizziness, sedation, vertigo

GI: Nausea, vomiting, anorexia, diarrhea, abdominal distention, cramps, enterocolitis; increased AST (SGOT), ALT (SGPT), alk phosphatase; ***bowel perforation*** (rare)

*HEMA: **Thrombocytopenia, agranulocytosis, anemia, leukopenia, pancytopenia***

GU: Increased BUN, creatinine

Contraindications: Hypersensitivity

Precautions: Renal disease, impaired hepatic function, bone marrow depression, blood dyscrasias, radiation/chemotherapy, pregnancy (C), lactation

---

◆ = Nursing alert   ⫸ = Herb-drug interaction   ⊘ = Do not crush

Pharmacokinetics:
PO: Peak 2½-6 hr, half-life 3-6 hr, excreted in urine (unchanged), well distributed to CSF, aqueous humor, joints

Interactions:
• Synergism: amphotericin B

Lab test interferences:
False increase: Creatinine

NURSING CONSIDERATIONS
Assess:
• VS q15-30min during first infusion; note changes in pulse, B/P
• Blood studies: CBC, including platelets
• Drug level during treatment (therapeutic level 25-100 µg/ml); if renal impairment is present, level usually kept <100 µg/ml
➡ For renal toxicity: increasing BUN, serum creatinine; if serum creatinine >1.7 mg/100 ml, dosage may be reduced
• For hepatotoxicity: increasing AST (SGOT), ALT (SGPT), alk phosphatase
• For allergic reaction: dermatitis, rash; drug should be discontinued, antihistamines (mild reaction) or epinephrine (severe reaction) administered
• For blood dyscrasias, fatigue, bruising, malaise, dark urine

Administer:
• Drug only after C&S confirms organism, drug needed to treat condition
• Few caps at a time with fluid to decrease nausea, vomiting over 15 min

Perform/provide:
• Symptomatic treatment as ordered for adverse reactions: aspirin, antihistamines, antiemetics, antispasmodics
• Storage in tight, light-resistant container at room temp

Evaluate:
• Therapeutic response: decreased fever, malaise, rash, negative C&S for infecting organism

Teach patient/family:
• That long-term therapy may be needed to clear infection (1-2 mo depending on type of infection)
• To report symptoms of blood dyscrasias: fatigue, bruising, malaise, dark urine
🚫 Not to break, crush, or chew caps

F

---

fludrocortisone (℞)
(floo droe-kor′ti sone)
Florinef, Acetate
Func. class.: Corticosteroid
Chem. class.: Mineralocorticoid

Action: Promotes increased reabsorption of sodium and loss of potassium, water, hydrogen from distal renal tubules

Uses: Adrenal insufficiency, salt-losing adrenogenital syndrome

Dosage and routes:
• *Adult:* PO 0.1-0.2 mg qd
• *Child:* PO 0.05-0.1 mg/day
Available forms: Tabs 0.1 mg

Side effects/adverse reactions:
CNS: Flushing, sweating, headache
CV: Hypertension, circulatory collapse, thrombophlebitis, embolism, tachycardia
MS: Fractures, osteoporosis, weakness

Contraindications: Hypersensitivity, acute glomerulonephritis, amebiasis

Precautions: Pregnancy (C), osteoporosis, CHF, lactation

Pharmacokinetics:
PO: Half-life 3.5 hr, metabolized by liver, excreted in urine

Interactions:
• Decreased action of fludrocorti-

---

sone: cholestyramine, colestipol, barbiturates, rifampin, ephedrine, phenytoin, theophylline
• Decreased effects of: diuretics, potassium-sparing diuretics, potassium supplements
• Increased side effects: sodium-containing food or medication, digitalis preparations

🌿 Potassium deficiency: aloe, buckthorn bark/berry, cascara sagrada bark, senna pod/leaf

Lab test interferences:
Increase: Potassium, sodium
Decrease: Hematocrit

NURSING CONSIDERATIONS
Assess:
• Weight daily; notify prescriber of weekly gain >5 lb
• B/P q4h, pulse; notify prescriber if chest pain occurs
• I&O ratio; be alert for decreasing urinary output, increasing edema
• K depletion: paresthesias, fatigue, nausea, vomiting, depression, polyuria, dysrhythmias, weakness
• Edema, hypertension, cardiac symptoms

Administer:
• Titrated dose; use lowest effective dose
• With food or milk to decrease GI symptoms

Perform/provide:
• Assistance with ambulation in patient with bone tissue disease to prevent fractures

Evaluate:
• Therapeutic response: correction of adrenal insufficiency

Teach patient/family:
• That ID as steroid user should be carried
• Not to discontinue this medication abruptly
• To notify health-care provider of muscle cramps, weight gain, edema, nausea

---

flumazenil (R)
(flu-maz′e-nill)
Anexate*, Romazicon
Func. class.: Antidote: Benzodiazepine receptor antagonist
Chem. class.: Imidazobenzodiazepine derivative

Action: Antagonizes actions of benzodiazepines on CNS, competitively inhibits activity at benzodiazepine recognition site on GABA/benzodiazepine receptor complex

Uses: Reversal of sedative effects of benzodiazepines

Dosage and routes:
Reversal of conscious sedation or in general anesthesia
• *Adult:* **IV** 0.2 mg given over 15 sec; wait 45 sec, then give 0.2 mg if consciousness does not occur; may be repeated at 60-sec intervals prn (max 3 mg/hr)
• *Child:* **IV** 10 μg (0.01 mg)/kg; cumulative dose of 1 mg or less

Management of suspected benzodiazepine overdose
• *Adult:* **IV** 0.2 mg given over 30 sec; wait 30 sec, then give 0.3 mg over 30 sec if consciousness does not occur; further doses of 0.5 mg can be given over 30 sec at intervals of 1 min up to cumulative dose of 3 mg
• *Child:* **IV** 100 μg (0.1 mg)/kg; cumulative dose of 1 mg or less

Available forms: Inj 0.1 mg/ml

Side effects/adverse reactions:
EENT: Abnormal vision, blurred vision, tinnitus
CV: Hypertension, palpitations, cutaneous vasodilation, dysrhythmias, bradycardia, tachycardia, chest pain
GI: Nausea, vomiting, hiccups
CNS: Dizziness, agitation, emotional lability, confusion, ***convulsions,*** somnolence

---

◆ = Nursing alert   🌿 = Herb-drug interaction   ⊘ = Do not crush

SYST: Headache, injection site pain, increased sweating, fatigue, rigors

Contraindications: Hypersensitivity to this drug or benzodiazepines, serious cyclic antidepressant overdose, patients given benzodiazepine for control of life-threatening condition

Precautions: Pregnancy (C), lactation, children, elderly, renal disease, seizure disorders, head injury, labor/delivery, hepatic disease, hypoventilation, panic disorder, drug & alcohol dependency, ambulatory patients

Pharmacokinetics: Terminal half-life 41-79 min; metabolized in liver

Interactions:
• Toxicity: mixed drug overdosage
• Ingestion of food during IV INF: increased flumazenil clearance

NURSING CONSIDERATIONS
Assess:
• Cardiac status using continuous monitoring
• For seizures; protect patient from injury
• GI symptoms: nausea, vomiting; place in side-lying position to prevent aspiration
• Allergic reactions: flushing, rash, urticaria, pruritus

Administer:
• Check airway and IV access before administration

IV, direct
• Give undiluted or diluted with 0.9% NaCl, D_5W, LR, give over 15 sec

Additive compatibilities: Aminophylline, cimetidine, dobutamine, dopamine, famotidine, heparin, lidocaine, procainamide, ranitidine

Solution compatibilities: D_5W

Evaluate:
• Therapeutic response: decreased sedation, respiratory depression, toxicity

Teach patient/family:
• That amnesia may continue

• Not to engage in hazardous activities for 18-24 hr after discharge
• Not to take any alcohol or nonprescription drugs for 18-24 hr

---

flunisolide (℞)

(floo-nis'oh-lide)
AeroBid, Nasalide

Func. class.: Misc. respiratory drug

Chem. class.: Glucocorticoid

Action: Decreases inflammation by suppression of migration of polymorphonuclear leukocytes, fibroblasts, reversal of increased capillary permeability and lysosomal stabilization; does not depress hypothalamus

Uses: Rhinitis, allergies, nasal polyps

Dosage and routes:
• *Adult and child >6 yr:* **SPRAY** 2 puffs bid, not to exceed 4 puffs bid

Available forms: Nasal sol 25 μg/metered dose (Nasalide), 250 μg/metered dose (AeroBid)

Side effects/adverse reactions:

CNS: Headache, nervousness, restlessness

EENT: Hoarseness, *Candida* infection of oral cavity, sore throat

GI: Nausea, vomiting, dry mouth

Contraindications: Hypersensitivity, child <6 yr

Precautions: Nonasthmatic bronchial disease; bacterial, fungal, viral infections of mouth, throat, lungs; respiratory TB; untreated fungal, bacterial, or viral infections; pregnancy (C), glaucoma

Pharmacokinetics:
INH: Duration 1 hr

NURSING CONSIDERATIONS
Assess:
• Infection: increased temp, WBC, even after withdrawal of medication; drug masks infection

Administer:
- Titrated dose; use lowest effective dose

Evaluate:
- Therapeutic response: ease of respirations, decreased inflammation

Teach patient/family:
- To use gum: rinse mouth after each dose
- That ID as steroid user should be carried
- To notify prescriber if therapeutic response decreases; dosage adjustment may be needed
- The proper administration technique; shake well before use
- The importance of compliance to therapy
- Teach patient about cushingoid symptoms
- The symptoms of adrenal insufficiency: nausea, anorexia, fatigue, dizziness, dyspnea, weakness, joint pain

---

fluoride

(floor′ide)

ACT, Checkmate, Fluor-A-Day*, Fluorigard, Fluorinse, Fluoritab, Fluotic*, Flura, Flura-Drops, Flura-Loz, Gel II, Gel-Kam, Gel-Tin, Karidium, Karigel , Karigel-N, Listermint with Fluoride, Loz-Tabs, Luride, Luride Lozi-Tabs, Luride 0.25 Lozi-Tabs, Luride 0.5 Lozi-Tabs, Luride-SF, Minute-Gel, Pediaflor, Pharmaflur, Pharmaflur 1.1, Pharmaflur df, Phos-Flur, Point-Two, Prevident, Sodium Fluoride, Stop, Thera-Flur, Thera-Flur-N

Func. class.: Trace elements
Chem. class.: Fluoride ion

Action: Needed for hard tooth enamel and for resistance to periodontal disease; reduces acid production by dental bacteria

Uses: Prevention of dental caries, osteoporosis

Dosage and routes:
- *Adult and child >12 yr:* **TOP** 10 ml 0.2% sol qd after brushing teeth, rinse mouth for >1 min with sol
- *Child 6-12 yr:* **TOP** 5 ml 0.2% sol
- *Child >3 yr:* **PO** 1 mg qd
- *Child <3 yr:* **PO** 0.5 mg qd

Available forms: Tabs chewable 0.55, 1.1, 2.2 mg; tabs 2.2 mg, tabs effervescent 10 mg; drops 0.125, 0.25, 0.5 mg/ml; rinse supplements 0.2 mg/ml, rinse 0.01%, 0.02%, 0.09%; gel 0.1%, 0.5%, 1.23%

Side effects/adverse reactions:
*ACUTE OVERDOSE: **Black tarry stools, bloody vomit, diarrhea, decreased respiration, increased salivation, watery eyes***
*CHRONIC OVERDOSE: **Hypocalcemia and tetany, respiratory arrest, sores in mouth, constipation, loss of appetite, nausea, vomiting, weight loss, discoloration of teeth** (white, black, brown)*

Contraindications: Hypersensitivity, pregnancy (D)

Precautions: Child <6 yr

Pharmacokinetics:
PO: Excreted in urine and feces; crosses placenta, breast milk

Interactions:
- Avoid use with dairy products

NURSING CONSIDERATIONS
Assess:
- Use in children
- Nutritional status: increase fluoride content of water, decrease carbohydrate snacks, increase fish, tea, mineral water

Administer:
- Drops after meals with fluids or undiluted tabs; may be chewed; do not swallow whole; may be given with water or juice; avoid milk

---

 = Nursing alert   = Herb-drug interaction   = Do not crush

Evaluate:
• Therapeutic response: absence of dental caries

Teach patient/family:
• To monitor children using gel or rinse; not to be swallowed
• Not to drink, eat, or rinse mouth for at least ½ hr
• Not to use during pregnancy
• To apply after brushing and flossing hs
• To store out of children's reach

---

fluorouracil (5-fluorouracil) (℞)

(flure-oh-yoor'a-sil)
Adrucil, Efudex, Fluoroplex, 5-FU

Func. class.: Antineoplastic, antimetabolite
Chem. class.: Pyrimidine antagonist

Action: Inhibits DNA synthesis; interferes with cell replication by competitively inhibiting thymidylate synthesis, S phase of cell cycle–specific vesicant

Uses: Cancer of breast, colon, rectum, stomach, pancreas

Dosage and routes:
• *Adult:* IV 12 mg/kg/day × 4 days not to exceed 800 mg/day; may repeat with 6 mg/kg on day 6, 8, 10, 12; maintenance is 10-15 mg/kg/wk as a single dose, not to exceed 1 g/wk

Available forms: Inj 50 mg/ml
Side effects/adverse reactions:
CV: Myocardial ischemia, angina
HEMA: **Thrombocytopenia, leukopenia, myelosuppression, anemia, agranulocytosis**
GI: *Anorexia, stomatitis,* diarrhea, nausea, vomiting, **hemorrhage,** enteritis glossitis
GU: **Renal failure**

EENT: Epistaxis
INTEG: *Rash,* fever
CNS: Lethargy, malaise, weakness
Contraindications: Hypersensitivity, myelosuppression, pregnancy (D), poor nutritional status, serious infections

Precautions: Renal disease, hepatic disease, bone marrow depression, angina, lactation, children

Pharmacokinetics: Half-life 10-20 min, 20 hr terminal; metabolized in the liver; excreted in the urine; crosses blood-brain barrier

Interactions:
• Increased toxicity: radiation or other antineoplastics

Lab test interferences:
Increase: Liver function studies, 6-HIAA
Decrease: Albumin

NURSING CONSIDERATIONS

Assess:
• CBC, differential, platelet count weekly; withhold drug if WBC is <3500/mm^3 or platelet count is <100,000/mm^3; notify prescriber of these results; drug should be discontinued
• Renal function studies: BUN, serum uric acid, urine CrCl, electrolytes before, during therapy
• I&O ratio; report fall in urine output to <30 ml/hr
• Temp q4h; fever may indicate beginning infection
• Liver function tests before, during therapy: bilirubin, alk phosphatase, AST (SGOT), ALT (SGPT), LDH; prn or q mo
• Bleeding: hematuria, guaiac, bruising or petechiae, mucosa or orifices q8h
• Food preferences: list likes, dislikes
• Inflammation of mucosa, breaks in skin
• Buccal cavity q8h for dryness,

Side effects: *italics* = common; **bold italics** = life-threatening

sores or ulceration, white patches, oral pain, bleeding, dysphagia
• Symptoms indicating severe allergic reaction: rash, urticaria, itching, flushing
• GI symptoms: frequency of stools, cramping
• Acidosis, signs of dehydration: rapid respirations, poor skin turgor, decreased urine output, dry skin, restlessness, weakness

Administer:
• Antiemetic 30-60 min before giving drug to prevent vomiting and for several days thereafter
• Antibiotics for prophylaxis of infection
• Topical or systemic analgesics for pain
• Transfusion for anemia
• Antispasmodic for diarrhea

IV
• Undiluted; may inject through Y-tube or 3-way stopcock; give over 1-3 min; may be diluted in NS, D_5W, given over 2-8 hr as IV INF

Additive compatibilities: Bleomycin, cephalothin, cyclophosphamide, etoposide, floxuridine, hydromorphone, ifosfamide, methotrexate, mitoxantrone, prednisolone, vincristine

Solution compatibilities: Amino acids 4.25%/D_{25}, D_5/LR, $D_{3.3}$/0.3 NaCl, D_5W, 0.9% NaCl, TPN #23

Syringe compatibilities: Bleomycin, cisplatin, cyclophosphamide, furosemide, heparin, leucovorin, methotrexate, metoclopramide, mitomycin, vinblastine, vincristine

Y-site compatibilities: Allopurinol, amifostine, aztreonam, bleomycin, cefepime, cisplatin, cyclophosphamide, doxorubicin, fludarabine, furosemide, granisetron, heparin, hydrocortisone, leucovorin, mannitol, melphalan, methotrexate, metoclopramide, mitomycin, paclitaxel, piperacillin/tazobactam, potassium chloride, propofol, sargramostim, teniposide, thiotepa, vinblastine, vincristine, vit B/C

Perform/provide:
• Protection from light
• Strict asepsis, protective isolation if WBC levels are low
• Increase fluid intake to 2-3 L/day to prevent dehydration, unless contraindicated
• Changing of IV site q48h
• Rinsing of mouth tid-qid with water, club soda; brushing of teeth bid-tid with soft brush or cotton-tipped applicator for stomatitis; use unwaxed dental floss
• Nutritious diet with iron, vitamin supplements, low fiber, few dairy products, especially when combined with radiotherapy as ordered

Evaluate:
• Therapeutic response: decreased tumor size, spread of malignancy

Teach patient/family:
• Why protective isolation is necessary
• To avoid foods with citric acid, hot or rough texture if stomatitis is present; to drink adequate fluids
• To report stomatitis: any bleeding, white spots, ulcerations in mouth; tell patient to examine mouth qd, report symptoms
• To report signs of infection: fever, sore throat, flu symptoms
• To report signs of anemia: fatigue, headache, faintness, shortness of breath, irritability
• To report bleeding: avoid use of razors, commercial mouthwash
• To avoid use of aspirin products or ibuprofen
• To use contraception during therapy (men and women)

◆ = Nursing alert   ✏ = Herb-drug interaction   Ⓝ = Do not crush

fluoxetine (℞)

(floo-ox'eh-teen)

Prozac

Func. class.: Antidepressant, bicyclic

Action: Inhibits CNS neuron uptake of serotonin but not of norepinephrine

Uses: Major depressive disorder, obsessive-compulsive disorder, bulimia nervosa

Investigational uses: Alcoholism, anorexia nervosa, ADHD, bipolar II affective disorder, borderline personality disorder, cataplexy, narcolepsy, kleptomania, migraine, obesity, post-traumatic stress disorder, schizophrenia, Tourette syndrome, trichotillomania, levodopa-induced dyskinesia, social phobia

Dosage and routes:

Depression/obsessive-compulsive disorder

• *Adult:* PO 20 mg qd in AM; after 4 wk if no clinical improvement is noted, dose may be increased to 20 mg bid in AM, PM, not to exceed 80 mg/day

• *Geriatric:* PO 10 mg/day, increase as needed

• *Child 5-18 yr:* PO 5-10 mg/kg/day, max 20 mg/day

Bulimia nervosa

• *Adult:* PO 60 mg/day in AM

Available forms: Pulvules 10, 20 mg; liquid 20 mg/5 ml

Side effects/adverse reactions:

*CNS: Headache, nervousness, insomnia, drowsiness, anxiety, tremor, dizziness, fatigue, sedation, poor concentration, abnormal dreams, agitation, **convulsions,** apathy, euphoria, hallucinations, delusions, psychosis*

GI: Nausea, diarrhea, dry mouth, anorexia, dyspepsia, constipation, cramps, vomiting, taste changes, flatulence, decreased appetite

INTEG: Sweating, rash, pruritus, acne, alopecia, urticaria

RESP: Infection, pharyngitis, nasal congestion, sinus headache, sinusitis, cough, dyspnea, bronchitis, asthma, hyperventilation, pneumonia

CV: Hot flashes, palpitations, angina pectoris, **hemorrhage,** hypertension, *tachycardia,* first-degree AV block, **bradycardia, MI, thrombophlebitis**

MS: Pain, arthritis, twitching

GU: Dysmenorrhea, decreased libido, urinary frequency, UTI, amenorrhea, cystitis, impotence, urine retention

EENT: Visual changes, ear/eye pain, photophobia, tinnitus

SYST: Asthenia, viral infection, fever, allergy, chills

Contraindications: Hypersensitivity

Precautions: Pregnancy (B), lactation, children, elderly, diabetes mellitus

Pharmacokinetics:

PO: Peak 6-8 hr; metabolized in liver; excreted in urine; half-life 1-384 hr; steady state 28-35 days, protein binding 94%

Interactions:

• Do not use with MAOIs

• Increased side effects: highly protein-bound drugs

• Increased half-life of diazepam

• Hallucinations may occur with dextromethorphan

• Increased hydantoin when used with phenytoin

• Toxicity: carbamazepine, lithium, L-tryptophan

• Increased tricyclic antidepressant levels: tricyclic antidepressants

• Paradoxical worsening of OCD: buspirone

F

• Increased clozapine levels: clozapine

/ Increased action: kava kava

Lab test interferences:

Increase: Serum bilirubin, blood glucose, alk phosphatase

Decrease: VMA, 5-HIAA

False increase: Urinary catecholamines

NURSING CONSIDERATIONS
Assess:

• Mental status: mood, sensorium, affect, suicidal tendencies, increase in psychiatric symptoms, depression, panic

• B/P (lying/standing), pulse q4h; if systolic B/P drops 20 mm Hg, hold drug, notify prescriber; take vital signs q4h in patients with cardiovascular disease

• Blood studies: CBC, leukocytes, differential, cardiac enzymes if patient is receiving long-term therapy; check platelets; bleeding can occur

• Hepatic studies: AST (SGOT), ALT (SGPT), bilirubin, creatinine

• Weight qwk; appetite may decrease with drug

• ECG for flattening of T wave, bundle branch, AV block, dysrhythmias in cardiac patients

• EPS primarily in elderly: rigidity, dystonia, akathisia

• Urinary retention, constipation

➡ Withdrawal symptoms: headache, nausea, vomiting, muscle pain, weakness; not usual unless drug discontinued abruptly

• Alcohol consumption; if alcohol is consumed, hold dose until AM

Administer:

• Increased fluids, bulk in diet if constipation, urinary retention occur

• With food or milk for GI symptoms

• Crushed if patient is unable to swallow medication whole

• Dosage hs if oversedation occurs during the day; may take entire dose hs; elderly may not tolerate once/day dosing

• Gum, hard candy, frequent sips of water for dry mouth

Perform/provide:

• Storage at room temp; do not freeze

• Assistance with ambulation during therapy, since drowsiness, dizziness occur

• Safety measures including side rails, primarily in elderly

• Checking to see if PO medication swallowed

Evaluate:

• Therapeutic response: decreased depression

Teach patient/family:

• That therapeutic effect may take 2-3 wk

• To use caution in driving, other activities requiring alertness because of drowsiness, dizziness, blurred vision

• Not to discontinue medication quickly after long-term use; may cause nausea, headache, malaise

• To avoid alcohol ingestion, other CNS depressants

• To notify prescriber if pregnant or plan to become pregnant or breastfeed

---

fluoxymesterone (R)

(floo-ox-ee-mess'te-rone)

fluoxymesterone, *Halotestin*

Func. class.: Androgenic anabolic steroid

Chem. class.: Halogenated testosterone derivative

Action: Increases weight by building body tissue, increases potassium, phosphorus, chloride, nitrogen levels, bone development

Uses: Impotence from testicular deficiency, hypogonadism; breast en-

---

➡ = Nursing alert   / = Herb-drug interaction   🚫 = Do not crush gorgement; palliative treatment of female breast cancer

Dosage and routes:
Hypogonadism/impotence
• *Adult:* **PO** 2-10 mg qd
Breast engorgement
• *Adult:* **PO** 2.5 mg qd, then 5-10 mg qd × 5 days
Breast cancer
• *Adult:* **PO** 15-30 mg qd in divided doses until therapeutic effect occurs, then dosage should be reduced
Available forms: Tabs 2, 5, 10 mg

Side effects/adverse reactions:
INTEG: Rash, acneiform lesions; oily hair, skin; flushing, sweating, acne vulgaris, alopecia, hirsutism
CNS: Dizziness, headache, fatigue, tremors, paresthesias, flushing, sweating, anxiety, lability, insomnia, carpal tunnel syndrome
MS: Cramps, spasms
CV: Increased B/P
GU: **Hematuria,** amenorrhea, vaginitis, decreased libido, decreased breast size, clitoral hypertrophy, testicular atrophy
GI: Nausea, vomiting, constipation, weight gain, **cholestatic jaundice**
EENT: Conjunctival edema, nasal congestion
ENDO: Abnormal GTT

Contraindications: Severe renal, severe cardiac, severe hepatic disease, hypersensitivity, pregnancy (X), lactation, genital bleeding (abnormal), children

Precautions: Diabetes mellitus, CV disease, MI

Pharmacokinetics:
PO: Metabolized in liver; excreted in urine; crosses placenta; excreted in breast milk

Interactions:
• Increased effects of oral antidiabetics, oxyphenbutazone
• Increased PT: anticoagulants
• Edema: ACTH, adrenal steroids
• Decreased effects of insulin

Lab test interferences:
Increase: Serum cholesterol, blood glucose, urine glucose
Decrease: Serum Ca; serum K, T_4, T_3; thyroid ^{131}I uptake test, urine 17-OHCS, 17-KS, PBI, BSP

NURSING CONSIDERATIONS
Assess:
• Weight daily; notify prescriber if weekly weight gain is >5 lb
• B/P q4h
• I&O ratio; be alert for decreasing urinary output, increasing edema
• Growth rate in children; growth rate may be uneven (linear/bone growth) if used for extended periods
• Electrolytes: K, Na, Cl, cholesterol
• Liver function studies: ALT (SGPT), AST (SGOT), bilirubin
• Edema, hypertension, cardiac symptoms, jaundice
• Mental status: affect, mood, behavioral changes, aggression
• Signs of masculinization in female: increased libido, deepening of voice, breast tissue, enlarged clitoris, menstrual irregularities; male: gynecomastia, impotence, testicular atrophy
• Hypercalcemia: lethargy, polyuria, polydipsia, nausea, vomiting, constipation; drug may have to be decreased
• Hypoglycemia in diabetics, since oral antidiabetic action is increased

Administer:
• Titrated dose, use lowest effective dose
• With food or milk to decrease GI symptoms

Perform/provide:
• Diet with increased calories, protein; decrease Na if edema occurs

Evaluate:
• Therapeutic response: increased appetite, stamina

F

Teach patient/family:
- That drug must be combined with complete health plan: diet, rest, exercise
- To notify prescriber if therapeutic response decreases
- Not to discontinue abruptly
- About change in gender characteristics
- That females need to report menstrual irregularities
- That 1-3 mo course is necessary for response in breast cancer
- That steroids should not be used for bodybuilding

---

fluphenazine (R)

(floo-fen'a-zeen)
fluphenazine decanoate, fluphenazine HCl, Permitil, Prolixin, Prolixin Decanoate, Prolixin Enanthate

Func. class.: Antipsychotic, neuroleptic

Chem. class.: Phenothiazine, piperazine

Action: Depresses cerebral cortex, hypothalamus, limbic system, which control activity and aggression; blocks neurotransmission produced by dopamine at synapse; exhibits strong α-adrenergic and anticholinergic blocking action; mechanism for antipsychotic effects is unclear

Uses: Psychotic disorders, schizophrenia

Dosage and routes:
Enanthate, decanoate
- *Adult and child >12 yr:* SC 12.5-25 mg q1-3wk

HCl
- *Adult:* PO 2.5-10 mg, in divided doses q6-8h, not to exceed 20 mg qd; IM initially 1.25 mg then 2.5-10 mg in divided doses q6-8h
- *Child:* PO 0.25-3.5 mg qd in divided doses q4-6h, max 10 mg/qd

Available forms: HCl tabs 1, 2.5, 5, 10 mg; elix 2.5 mg/5 ml; conc 5 mg/ml; inj 2.5 mg/ml; enanthate, decanoate, inj 25 mg/ml

Side effects/adverse reactions:
RESP: **Laryngospasm,** dyspnea, **respiratory depression**

CNS: EPS: pseudoparkinsonism, akathisia, dystonia, tardive dyskinesia, drowsiness, headache, seizures, neuroleptic malignant syndrome

HEMA: Anemia, **leukopenia, leukocytosis, agranulocytosis**

INTEG: Rash, photosensitivity, dermatitis

EENT: Blurred vision, glaucoma, dry eyes

GI: Dry mouth, nausea, vomiting, anorexia, constipation, diarrhea, jaundice, weight gain, **paralytic ileus, hepatitis**

GU: Urinary retention, urinary frequency, enuresis, impotence, amenorrhea, gynecomastia

CV: Orthostatic hypotension, hypertension, **cardiac arrest,** ECG changes, **tachycardia**

Contraindications: Hypersensitivity, circulatory collapse, liver damage, cerebral arteriosclerosis, coronary disease, severe hypertension/hypotension, blood dyscrasias, coma, child <12 yr, brain damage, bone marrow depression, alcohol and barbiturate withdrawal

Precautions: Pregnancy (C), lactation, seizure disorders, hypertension, hepatic disease, cardiac disease, elderly

Pharmacokinetics:
PO/IM (HCl): Onset 1 hr, peak 2-4 hr, duration 6-8 hr

SC (enanthate): Onset 1-2 days, peak 2-3 days, duration 1-3 wk, half-life 3.5-4 days; decanoate: onset 1-3 days, peak 1-2 days, duration over 4 wk, single-dose half-life 6.8-9.6

◆ = Nursing alert   ∥ = Herb-drug interaction   ⊘ = Do not crush

days; multiple dose, 14.3 days; metabolized by liver; excreted in urine (metabolites); crosses placenta; enters breast milk

Interactions:

• Oversedation: other CNS depressants, alcohol, barbiturate anesthetics

• Toxicity: epinephrine

• Decreased effects of levodopa, lithium

• Decreased effects of fluphenazine: smoking, phenobarbital

• Increased effects of both drugs: β-adrenergic blockers, alcohol

• Increased effects: anticholinergics

🖋 Increased anticholinergic effect: henbane leaf

🖋 Possible increased action: kava kava

Lab test interferences:

Increase: Liver function tests, cardiac enzymes, cholesterol, blood glucose, prolactin, bilirubin, PBI, cholinesterase

Decrease: Hormones (blood and urine)

False positive: Pregnancy tests, PKU urinary steroids, 17-OHCS, pregnancy tests

NURSING CONSIDERATIONS

Assess:

• Swallowing of PO medication; check for hoarding, giving of medication to other patients

• I&O ratio; palpate bladder if low urinary output occurs

• Bilirubin, CBC, liver function studies monthly

• Urinalysis is recommended before and during prolonged therapy

• Affect, orientation, LOC, reflexes, gait, coordination, sleep pattern disturbances

• B/P standing and lying; take pulse and respirations q4h during initial treatment; establish baseline before starting treatment; report drops of 30 mm Hg

• Dizziness, faintness, palpitations, tachycardia on rising

• EPS including akathisia (inability to sit still, no pattern to movements), tardive dyskinesia (bizarre movements of jaw, mouth, tongue, extremities), pseudoparkinsonism (rigidity, tremors, pill rolling, shuffling gait)

• Skin turgor qd

• Constipation, urinary retention qd; if these occur, increase bulk, H_2O in diet

Administer:

• Concentrate with juice, milk, or uncaffeinated drinks

• Antiparkinsonian agent if EPS occur

• IM inj into large muscle mass; to minimize postural hypotension, give injection and have patient remain seated or recumbent for ½ hr

• Use dry needle, or solution will become cloudy; use 21/G or larger due to viscosity

Syringe compatibilities: Benztropine, diphenhydramine, hydroxyzine

Perform/provide:

• Decreased noise input by dimming lights, avoiding loud noises

• Supervised ambulation until stabilized on medication; do not involve in strenuous exercise; fainting is possible; patient should not stand still for long periods

• Increased fluids to prevent constipation

• Sips of water, candy, gum for dry mouth

• Storage in tight, light-resistant container in cool environment

Evaluate:

• Therapeutic response: decrease in emotional excitement, hallucinations, delusions, paranoia, reorganization of patterns of thought, speech

Teach patient/family:
• That orthostatic hypotension occurs often; to rise from sitting or lying position gradually; avoid hazardous activities until stabilized on medication
• To avoid hot tubs, hot showers, tub baths, since hypotension may occur; that in hot weather, heat stroke may occur; take extra precautions to stay cool
 To avoid abrupt withdrawal of this drug, or EPS may result; drug should be withdrawn slowly
• To avoid OTC preparations (cough, hay fever, cold) unless approved by prescriber; serious drug interactions may occur; avoid use with alcohol, CNS depressants; increased drowsiness may occur
• To use a sunscreen to prevent burns
• About importance of compliance with drug regimen
• About EPS and necessity for meticulous oral hygiene, since oral candidiasis may occur
• To report sore throat, malaise, fever, bleeding, mouth sores; if these occur, CBC should be drawn and drug discontinued
• That urine may turn pink to reddish-brown
Treatment of overdose: Lavage; if orally ingested, provide an airway; *do not induce vomiting*

---

flurazepam (℞)
(flure-az'e-pam)
Dalmane, flurazepam, Somnol*
Func. class.: Sedative/hypnotic
Chem. class.: Benzodiazepine derivative

Controlled Substance Schedule IV (USA), Schedule F (Canada)
Action: Produces CNS depression at the limbic, thalamic, hypothalamic levels of CNS; may be mediated by neurotransmitter γ-aminobutyric acid (GABA); results are sedation, hypnosis, skeletal muscle relaxation, anticonvulsant activity, anxiolytic action
Uses: Insomnia
Dosage and routes:
• *Adult:* **PO** 15-30 mg hs; may repeat dose once if needed
• *Elderly:* **PO** 15 mg hs; may increase if needed
Available forms: Caps 15, 30 mg
Side effects/adverse reactions:
HEMA: **Leukopenia, granulocytopenia** (rare)
CNS: Lethargy, drowsiness, daytime sedation, dizziness, confusion, lightheadedness, headache, anxiety, irritability
GI: Nausea, vomiting, diarrhea, heartburn, abdominal pain, constipation
CV: Chest pain, pulse changes
Contraindications: Hypersensitivity to benzodiazepines, pregnancy, lactation, intermittent porphyria, uncontrolled pain
Precautions: Anemia, hepatic disease, renal disease, suicidal individuals, drug abuse, elderly, psychosis, child <15 yr
Pharmacokinetics:
PO: Onset 15-45 min, duration 7-8 hr; metabolized by liver; excreted by kidneys (inactive/active metabolites); crosses placenta; excreted in breast milk; half-life 47-100 hr, additional 100 hr for active metabolites
Interactions:
• Increased effects of flurazepam: cimetidine, disulfiram, probenicid, isoniazid
• Increased action of both drugs: alcohol, CNS depressants
• Decreased effect of flurazepam: antacids, theophylline, rifampin, smoking

---

 = Nursing alert   = Herb-drug interaction   = Do not crush

✐ Increased action: kava kava

Lab test interferences:

Increase: AST (SGOT), ALT (SGPT), serum bilirubin

False increase: Urinary 17-OHCS

Decrease: RAI uptake

NURSING CONSIDERATIONS

Assess:

• Blood studies: Hct, Hgb, RBC (if on long-term therapy)

• Hepatic studies: AST (SGOT), ALT (SGPT), bilirubin

• Mental status: mood, sensorium, affect, memory (long, short)

◆ Blood dyscrasias: fever, sore throat, bruising, rash, jaundice, epistaxis (rare)

• Type of sleep problem: falling asleep, staying asleep

Administer:

• After removal of cigarettes to prevent fires

• After trying conservative measures for insomnia

• ½-1 hr before hs for sleeplessness

• On empty stomach for fast onset, but may be taken with food if GI symptoms occur

Perform/provide:

• Assistance with ambulation after receiving dose

• Safety measure: nightlight, call bell within easy reach

• Checking to see if PO medication has been swallowed

• Storage in tight container in cool environment

Evaluate:

• Therapeutic response: ability to sleep at night, decreased amount of early morning awakening if taking drug for insomnia

Teach patient/family:

• To avoid driving or other activities requiring alertness until drug is stabilized

• To avoid alcohol ingestion or CNS depressants; serious CNS depression may result

• That effects may take 2 nights for benefits to be noticed

• Alternative measures to improve sleep: reading, exercise several hr before hs, warm bath, warm milk, TV, self-hypnosis, deep breathing

• That hangover is common in elderly

🚫 Not to break, crush, or chew caps

Treatment of overdose: Lavage, activated charcoal; monitor electrolytes, vital signs

---

flutamide (℞)

(floo′-ta-mide)

Eulexin

Func. class.: Antineoplastic, hormone

Chem. class.: Antiandrogen

Action: Interferes with testosterone uptake in the nucleus or testosterone activity in target tissues; arrests tumor growth in androgen-sensitive tissue, i.e., prostate gland

Uses: Metastatic prostatic carcinoma, stage D2 in combination with LHRH agonist analogs (leuprolide)

Dosage and routes:

• *Adult:* **PO** 250 mg q8h tid, for a daily dosage of 750 mg

Available forms: Caps 125 mg

Side effects/adverse reactions:

CNS: Hot flashes, drowsiness, confusion, depression, anxiety

GU: Decreased libido, impotence, gynecomastia

GI: Diarrhea, nausea, vomiting, increased liver function studies, ***hepatitis,*** anorexia

INTEG: Irritation at site, rash, photosensitivity

MISC: Edema, hematopoietic symptoms, neuromuscular and pulmonary symptoms, hypertension

---

Contraindications: Hypersensitivity, pregnancy (D)

Pharmacokinetics: Rapidly and completely absorbed; excreted in urine and feces as metabolites; half-life 6 hr, geriatric half-life 8 hr; 94% bound to plasma proteins

NURSING CONSIDERATIONS
Assess:
• Liver function studies: AST (SGOT), ALT (SGPT), alk phosphatase, which may be elevated
• For CNS symptoms including: drowsiness, confusion, depression, anxiety

Evaluate:
• Therapeutic response: decrease in prostatic tumor size, decrease in spread of cancer

Teach patient/family:
🚫 Not to break, crush, or chew caps
• To report side effects: decreased libido, impotence, breast enlargement, hot flashes, diarrhea
• That this drug is taken with leuprolide

Treatment of overdose: Induce vomiting, provide supportive care

---

fluvastatin (℞)
(flu'vah-stay-tin)
Lescol
Func. class.: Antilipidemic
Chem. class.: Synthetically derived fermentation product

Action: Inhibits HMG-CoA reductase enzyme, which reduces cholesterol synthesis

Uses: As an adjunct in primary hypercholesterolemia (types Ia, Ib)

Dosage and routes:
• *Adult:* PO 20-40 mg qd in PM initially, usual range 20-80 mg, not to exceed 80 mg; should be given in 2 doses (40 mg AM, 40 mg PM); dosage adjustments may be made in 4 wk intervals or more

Available forms: Caps 20, 40 mg

Side effects/adverse reactions:
INTEG: Rash, pruritus
GI: Nausea, constipation, diarrhea, dyspepsia flatus, *liver dysfunction,* pancreatitis
EENT: Lens opacities
MS: Myalgia, *myositis, rhabdomyolysis*
CNS: Headache, dizziness, insomnia
MISC: Fatigue, influenza
RESP: Upper respiratory infection, rhinitis, cough, pharyngitis, sinusitis

Contraindications: Hypersensitivity, pregnancy (X), lactation, active liver disease

Precautions: Past liver disease, alcoholism, severe acute infections, trauma, hypotension, uncontrolled seizure disorders, severe metabolic disorders, electrolyte imbalance

Pharmacokinetics: Metabolized in liver, highly protein bound, excreted primarily in feces, half-life <1 hr

Interactions:
• Increased effects of warfarin
• Increased myalgia, myositis: cyclosporine, gemfibrozil, niacin, erythromycin
• Increased serum level of digoxin
• Decreased effects of fluvastatin: bile acid sequestrants, propranolol, nicotinic acid, digoxin, rifampin; alcohol after a meal within 1 hr of taking drug

NURSING CONSIDERATIONS
Assess:
• Fasting lipid profile (cholesterol, LDL, HDL, TG) q8wk, then q3-6 mo when stable
• Liver function studies q1-2mo during the first 1½ yr of treatment; AST (SGOT), ALT (SGPT), liver function tests may be increased

---

◆ = Nursing alert   ⫻ = Herb-drug interaction   🚫 = Do not crush

• Renal studies in patients with compromised renal system: BUN, I&O ratio, creatinine

• Eyes with slit lamp before, 1 mo after treatment begins, annually; lens opacities may occur

Perform/provide:

• Storage in cool environment in tight container protected from light

Evaluate:

• Therapeutic response: decrease in cholesterol to desired level after 8 wk

Teach patient/family:

• That treatment is chronic

• That blood work and eye exam will be necessary during treatment

• To report severe GI symptoms, headache

• That previously prescribed regimen will continue: low-cholesterol diet, exercise program

🚫 Not to break, crush, or chew caps

---

fluvoxamine (℞)

(flu-vox′a-meen)

Luvox

Func. class.: Antidepressant-SSRI

Action: Inhibits CNS neuron uptake of serotonin but not of norepinephrine

Uses: Obsessive-compulsive disorder

Investigational uses: Depression

Dosage and routes:

• *Adult:* **PO** 50 mg hs, increase by 50 mg at 4-7 day intervals

Available forms: Tabs 50, 100 mg

Side effects/adverse reactions:

CNS: Headache, drowsiness, dizziness, convulsions, sleep disorders

GI: Nausea, anorexia, constipation, hepatotoxicity, vomiting, diarrhea

INTEG: Rash, sweating

GU: Decreased libido

Contraindications: Hypersensitivity

Precautions: Pregnancy (B), lactation, child, elderly

Pharmacokinetics: Crosses blood-brain barrier, 77% protein binding, metabolism by the liver, terminal half-life 16.9 hr, peak 2-8 hr

Interactions:

• Increased CNS depression: alcohol, barbiturates, benzodiazepines

• Increased toxicity: tricyclic antidepressants, theophylline, lithium

• Fatal reaction: MAO inhibitors, astemizole, cisapride

• Drug/smoking: Increased metabolism, decreased effects

🌿 Increased effect, possible fatal reaction: St. John's wort

🌿 Increased effect: kava kava

NURSING CONSIDERATIONS

Assess:

• Hepatic studies: AST (SGOT), ALT (SGPT), bilirubin

• Mental status: mood, sensorium, affect, suicidal tendencies; increase in psychiatric symptoms: depression, panic

• Constipation; most likely in elderly

⬧ For withdrawal symptoms: headache, nausea, vomiting, muscle pain, weakness; not usual unless discontinued abruptly

Administer:

• With food, milk for GI symptoms

Perform/provide:

• Storage at room temp; do not freeze

Evaluate:

• Therapeutic response: decrease in depression

Teach patient/family:

• That therapeutic effects may take 2-3 wk

• To use caution in driving, other activities requiring alertness because of drowsiness, dizziness that may occur

• Not to discontinue medication

---

quickly after long-term use: may cause nausea, headache, malaise
• To increase bulk in diet if constipation occurs, especially elderly
• To take gum; hard, sugarless candy; or frequent sips of water for dry mouth

---

folic acid (vit B₉) (OTC)

(foe'lik a'sid)
Apo-Folic*, Folate, Folvite, Novofolacid*, Vitamin B₉
Func. class.: Vit B complex group

Action: Needed for erythropoiesis; increases RBC, WBC, platelet formation in megaloblastic anemias

Uses: Megaloblastic or macrocytic anemia caused by folic acid deficiency; liver disease, alcoholism, hemolysis, intestinal obstruction, pregnancy

Dosage and routes:
Therapeutic dose
• *Adult/child:* **PO/IM/SC/IV** up to 1 mg qd
Maintenance dose
• *Adult/child >4 yr:* **PO/IM/IV/SC** 0.4 mg/day
• *Pregnant/lactating:* **PO/IM/IV/ SC** 0.8 mg/day
• *Child <4 yr:* **PO/IM/IV/SC** 0.3 mg/day
Available forms: Tabs 0.1, 0.4, 0.8, 1 mg; inj 5, 10 mg/ml

Side effects/adverse reactions:
RESP: **Bronchospasm**
INTEG: Flushing

Contraindications: Hypersensitivity, anemias other than megaloblastic/macrocytic anemia, vit B₁₂ deficiency anemia, uncorrected pernicious anemia

Precautions: Pregnancy (A)

Pharmacokinetics:
PO: Peak ½-1 hr; bound to plasma proteins; excreted in breast milk; metabolized by liver; excreted in urine (small amounts)

Interactions:
• Decreased folate levels: chloramphenicol
• Increased metabolism of phenobarbital, hydantoins
• Do not use with methotrexate unless leucovorin rescue is available

NURSING CONSIDERATIONS
Assess:
• For fatigue, dyspnea, weakness, SOB that are signs of megaloblastic anemia
• Hgb, Hct, and reticulocyte count
• Folate levels: 6-15 μg/ml
• Nutritional status: bran, yeast, dried beans, nuts, fruits, fresh vegetables, asparagus
• Drugs currently taken: alcohol, oral contraceptives, hydantoins, trimethoprim; these drugs may cause increased folic acid use by body and contribute to a deficiency

Administer:
IV
• Direct undiluted 5 mg or less/1 min or may be added to most IV sol or TPN

Solution compatibilities: D₂₀W
Y-site compatibilities: Famotidine

Perform/provide:
• Storage in light-resistant container

Evaluate:
• Therapeutic response: increased weight, oriented well-being; absence of fatigue

Teach patient/family:
• To take drug exactly as prescribed
• To notify prescriber of side effects

follitropin alfa/
follitropin beta (℞)

(fol'ee-tro-pin)
Gonal-F/Follistim
Func. class.: Ovulation stimulant
Chem. class.: Gonadotropin

Action: Stimulates ovarian follicular growth in primary ovarian failure

Uses: Induction of ovulation, assisted reproductive technologies (in vitro fertilization)

Dosage and routes:
Ovulation induction
• **SC** 75 IU, may increase by 37.5 IU after 2 wk, may increase again after 1 wk by 37.5 IU; treatment should not exceed 35 days unless a serum estradiol rise indicates imminent follicular development
Follicle stimulation
• *Adult:* **SC** 150 IU/day on day 2 or 3 of the follicular phase, should not exceed 10 days
Available forms: Gonal-F: 75 IU, 150 IU; Follistim: powder for inj 75 IU

Side effects/adverse reactions:
CNS: Malaise
GI: Nausea, vomiting, constipation, increased appetite, abdominal pain
INTEG: Rash, dermatitis, urticaria, alopecia
GU: Polyuria, frequency, birth defects, spontaneous abortions, multiple ovulation, breast pain

Contraindications: Hypersensitivity, pregnancy (X), undiagnosed vaginal bleeding, intracranial lesion, ovarian cyst not caused by polycystic ovarian disease

Precautions: Lactation, arterial thromboembolism

Pharmacokinetics: Metabolized in liver, excreted in feces, stored in fat

NURSING CONSIDERATIONS
Administer:
• At same time qd to maintain drug level
• After dissolving contents of ampule in 1-2 ml of sterile saline, give immediately, discard unused portion

Evaluate:
• Therapeutic response: ovulation, pregnancy

Teach patient/family:
• That multiple births are common after taking this drug
• To notify prescriber of low abdominal pain; may indicate ovarian cyst, cyst rupture
• The proper method of taking, recording basal body temp to determine whether ovulation has occurred
• That if ovulation can be determined (there is a slight decrease, then a sharp increase for ovulation), to attempt coitus 3 days before and qod until after ovulation
• That if pregnancy is suspected, to notify prescriber immediately

foscarnet (℞)

(foss-kar'net)
Foscavir
Func. class.: Antiviral
Chem. class.: Inorganic pyrophosphate organic analog

Action: Antiviral activity is produced by selective inhibition at the pyrophosphate binding site on virus-specific DNA polymerases and reverse transcriptases at concentrations that do not affect cellular DNA polymerases

Uses: Treatment of CMV retinitis, HSV infections, used with ganciclovir for relapsing patients

Dosage and routes:
• *Adult:* **IV INF** 60 mg/kg given over at least 1 hr, q8h × 2-3 wk

initially, then 90-120 mg/kg/day over 2 hr, usually give with at least 750-1000 ml **NS** qd

In renal abnormalities:

• *Adult:* **IV**

Male:

$$\frac{140 - \text{age}}{\text{serum creatinine} \times 72} = \text{Ccr}$$

Female: 0.85 × above value Dose based on table provided in package insert

Available forms: Inj 24 mg/ml

Side effects/adverse reactions:

CNS: Fever, dizziness, *headache, seizures, fatigue,* neuropathy, tremor, ataxia, dementia, stupor, EEG abnormalities, vertigo, *coma,* abnormal gait, hypertonia, EPS, hemiparesis, *paralysis,* hyperreflexia, paraplegia, *tetany,* hyporeflexia, neuralgia, neuritis, cerebral edema, *paresthesia,* depression, *confusion, anxiety,* insomnia, somnolence, amnesia, hallucinations, agitation

GI: Nausea, vomiting, diarrhea, anorexia, abdominal pain, constipation, dysphagia, rectal hemorrhage, dry mouth, melena, flatulence, ulcerative stomatitis, pancreatitis, enteritis, enterocolitis, glossitis, proctitis, stomatitis, increased amylases, gastroenteritis, *pseudomembranous colitis,* duodenal ulcer, *paralytic ileus, esophageal ulceration,* abnormal A-G ratio, increased AST (SGOT), ALT (SGPT), cholecystitis, *hepatitis,* dyspepsia, tenesmus, hepatosplenomegaly, jaundice

INTEG: Rash, sweating, pruritus, skin ulceration, seborrhea, skin discoloration, alopecia, acne, dermatitis, pain/inflammation at injection site, facial edema, dry skin, urticaria

HEMA: Anemia, granulocytopenia, leukopenia, thrombocytopenia, platelet abnormalities, *thrombosis, pulmonary embolism, coagulation disorders, decreased prothrombin, hypochromic anemia, pancytopenia, hemolysis, leukocytosis,* lymphadenopathy, epistaxis, lymphopenia

SYST: Hypokalemia, hypocalcemia, hypomagnesemia; increased alk phosphatase, LDH, BUN; acidosis, hypophosphatemia, hyperphosphatemia, dehydration, glycosuria, increased CPK, hypervolemia, infection, *sepsis, death, ascites,* hyponatremia, hypochloremia, hypercalcemia

GU: Acute renal failure, decreased CrCl and increased serum creatinine, *glomerulonephritis, toxic nephropathy, nephrosis, renal tubular disorders, pyelonephritis, uremia, hematuria, albuminuria,* dysuria, polyuria

RESP: Coughing, dyspnea, pneumonia, sinusitis, pharyngitis, *pulmonary infiltration,* stridor, *pneumothorax, hemoptysis, bronchospasm,* bronchitis, *respiratory depression, pleural effusion, pulmonary hemorrhage,* rhinitis

EENT: Visual field defects, vocal cord paralysis, speech disorders, taste perversion, eye pain, conjunctivitis, tinnitus, otitis

CV: Hypertension, palpitations, ECG abnormalities, 1st degree AV block, nonspecific ST-T segment changes, hypotension, cerebrovascular disorder, cardiomyopathy, *cardiac arrest,* bradycardia, dysrhythmias

MS: Arthralgia, myalgia

Contraindications: Hypersensitivity, CrCl <0.4 ml/min/kg

Precautions: Pregnancy (C), lactation, children, elderly, renal disease, seizure disorders, electrolyte/mineral imbalances, severe anemia

Pharmacokinetics: 14%-17% plasma protein bound, half-life 2-8 hr in normal renal function

Interactions:

• Nephrotoxicity: aminoglycosides, amphotericin B, IV pentamidine

---

 = Nursing alert   = Herb-drug interaction   = Do not crush

- Hypocalcemia: pentamidine
- Seizures: ciprofloxacin
- Increased anemia: zidovudine

NURSING CONSIDERATIONS
Assess:
- Culture should be done prior to treatment (blood, urine, throat)
- Ophthalmic exam should confirm diagnosis
- Kidney, liver function studies: BUN, creatinine, AST (SGOT), ALT (SGPT)
- I&O ratio, urine pH
- Blood counts q2wk; watch for decreasing granulocytes, Hgb; if low, therapy may have to be discontinued and restarted after hematologic recovery; blood transfusions may be required
- GI symptoms: nausea, vomiting, diarrhea; severe symptoms may necessitate discontinuing drug
- Electrolytes and minerals: Ca, P, Mg, Na, K; watch closely for tetany during first administration
- ◆ Blood dyscrasias (anemia, granulocytopenia); bruising, fatigue, bleeding, poor healing
- Allergic reactions: flushing, rash, urticaria, pruritus

Administer:
- Increased fluids before and during drug administration to induce diuresis and minimize renal toxicity

IV, int inf
- Using infusion device, at no more than 1 mg/kg/min; do not give by rapid or bolus IV; give by CVP or peripheral vein; standard 24 mg/ml sol may be used without dilution if using by CVP; dilute the 24 mg/ml sol to 12 mg/ml with D_5W or NS if using peripheral vein

Y-site compatibilities: Aldesleukin, amikacin, aminophylline, ampicillin, aztreonam, benzquinamide, cefazolin, cefoperazone, cefoxitin, ceftazidime, ceftizoxime, ceftriaxone, cefuroxime, chloramphenicol, cimetidine, clindamycin, dexamethasone, dopamine, erythromycin, fluconazole, flucytosine, furosemide, gentamicin, heparin, hydrocortisone, hydromorphone, hydroxyzine, imipenem-cilastatin, metoclopramide, metronidazole, miconazole, morphine, nafcillin, oxacillin, penicillin G potassium, phenytoin, piperacillin, ranitidine, ticarcillin/clavulanate, tobramycin

Perform/provide:
- Regular ophthalmologic exams
- Close monitoring during therapy if tingling, numbness, paresthesias; if these occur, stop infusion, obtain lab sample for electrolytes

Evaluate:
- Therapeutic response: improvement in CMV retinitis

Teach patient/family:
- To call prescriber if sore throat, swollen lymph nodes, malaise, fever occur, since other infections may occur
- To report perioral tingling, numbness in extremities, and paresthesias
- That serious drug interactions may occur if OTC products are ingested; check first with prescriber
- That drug is not a cure but will control symptoms

---

fosfomycin (℞)

(foss-foe-mye'sin)
Monurol
Func. class.: Urinary antiinfective

Action: Interferes with protein synthesis in bacterial cell by binding to ribosomal subunit, causing misreading of the genetic code; inaccurate peptide sequence forms in protein chain, causing bacterial death

Uses: Infections of the urinary tract caused by *E. faecalis, E. coli*

Dosage and routes:
• *Adult >18 yr:* 1 sachet with or without food, always mix with water before ingesting
Available forms: Single-dose sachet (3 g fosfomycin), orange flavored

Side effects/adverse reactions:
GU: Vaginitis, dysuria, hematuria, menstrual disorder
CNS: Headache, dizziness, fever, insomnia, somnolence, migraine, asthenia, nervousness
GI: Nausea, vomiting, anorexia, constipation, dry mouth, flatulence, increased SGPT; *diarrhea,* dyspepsia
INTEG: Rash, pruritus

Contraindications: Hypersensitivity

Precautions: Pregnancy (B), child <12 yr, lactation, renal disease

Pharmacokinetics: Rapidly absorbed, not bound to plasma proteins, excreted unchanged in urine/feces, half-life 4-8 hr

Interactions:
• Increased urinary excretion of fosfomycin: metoclopramide
• Decreased absorption of fosfomycin: food, antacids, calcium

NURSING CONSIDERATIONS
Assess:
• Urine pH, urine should be kept alkaline
• Overgrowth of infections: fever, pain
• C&S before starting treatment to identify infecting organism

Administer:
• PO, pour contents of sachet into 3-4 oz (½ cup) of water, stir to dissolve, use cold water, take immediately
• Only a single dose is necessary
• 1 hr ac or 2 hr pc antacids or calcium

Perform/provide:
• Adequate fluids of 2-3 L/day, unless contraindicated

• Storage at 59-86° F
Evaluate:
• Therapeutic response: absence of fever, negative C&S after treatment

Teach patient/family:
• Give patient directions to dissolve sachet, caution patient not to take in dry form
• Not to take with antacids or calcium products

---

fosinopril (℞)
(foss'in-oh-pril)
Monopril
Func. class.: Antihypertensive
Chem. class.: Angiotensin-converting enzyme (ACE) inhibitor

Action: Selectively suppresses renin-angiotensin-aldosterone system; inhibits ACE; prevents conversion of angiotensin I to angiotensin II; results in dilation of arterial, venous vessels

Uses: Hypertension, alone or in combination with thiazide diuretics, systolic CHF

Dosage and routes:
• *Adult:* **PO** 10 mg qd initially, then 20-40 mg/day divided bid or qd
Available forms: Tabs 10, 20, 40 mg

Side effects/adverse reactions:
CV: Hypotension, chest pain, palpitations, angina, orthostatic hypotension
GU: Proteinuria, increased BUN, creatinine, decreased libido
HEMA: Decreased Hct, Hgb; *eosinophilia, leukopenia, neutropenia*
INTEG: Angioedema, rash, flushing, sweating, photosensitivity, pruritus
RESP: Cough, sinusitis, dyspnea, *bronchospasm*
META: Hyperkalemia

◆ = Nursing alert   🖊 = Herb-drug interaction   ⊘ = Do not crush

GI: Nausea, constipation, vomiting, diarrhea

CNS: Insomnia, paresthesia, headache, dizziness, fatigue, memory disturbance, tremor, mood change

MS: Arthralgia, myalgia

Contraindications: Hypersensitivity to ACE inhibitors, pregnancy (D), lactation, children

Precautions: Impaired liver function, hypovolemia, blood dyscrasias, CHF, COPD, asthma, elderly

Pharmacokinetics:

PO: Peak 3 hr; serum protein binding 97%; half-life 12 hr; metabolized by liver (metabolites excreted in urine, feces)

Interactions:

• Increased hypotension: diuretics, other antihypertensives, ganglionic blockers, adrenergic blockers

• Increased toxicity: vasodilators, hydralazine, prazosin, K-sparing diuretics, sympathomimetics

• Decreased absorption: antacids

• Decreased antihypertensive effect: indomethacin

• Increased serum levels of digoxin, lithium

• Increased hypersensitivity: allopurinol

Lab test interferences:

False positive: Urine acetone

NURSING CONSIDERATIONS

Assess:

• Blood studies: neutrophils, decreased platelets

• B/P, orthostatic hypotension, syncope

• Renal studies: protein, BUN, creatinine; increased levels may indicate nephrotic syndrome; daily urine for protein

• Baselines in renal, liver function tests before therapy begins

• K levels, although hyperkalemia rarely occurs

• Edema in feet, legs daily

• Allergic reactions: rash, fever, pruritus, urticaria; drug should be discontinued if antihistamines fail to help

• Renal symptoms: polyuria, oliguria, frequency, dysuria

Administer:

• IV infusion of 0.9% NaCl (as ordered) to expand fluid volume if severe hypotension occurs

Perform/provide:

• Storage in tight container at 86° F (30° C) or less

• Supine or Trendelenburg position for severe hypotension

Evaluate:

• Therapeutic response: decrease in B/P

Teach patient/family:

• Not to discontinue drug abruptly

• Not to use OTC products (cough, cold, allergy) unless directed by prescriber; not to use salt substitutes containing potassium without consulting prescriber

• The importance of complying with dosage schedule, even if feeling better

• To rise slowly to sitting or standing position to minimize orthostatic hypotension

• To notify prescriber of mouth sores, sore throat, fever, swelling of hands or feet, irregular heartbeat, chest pain

• To report excessive perspiration, dehydration, vomiting, diarrhea; may lead to fall in B/P

• That drug may cause dizziness, fainting, light-headedness during first few days of therapy

• That drug may cause skin rash or impaired perspiration

• How to take B/P; normal readings for age group

Treatment of overdose: 0.9% NaCl IV INF, hemodialysis

fosphenytoin (R)

(foss-fen′i-toy-in)
Cerebyx
Func. class.: Anticonvulsant
Chem. class.: Hydantoin

Action: Inhibits spread of seizure activity in motor cortex by altering ion transport; increases AV conduction

Uses: Generalized tonic-clonic seizures; status epilepticus

Dosage and routes:

Status epilepticus
• *Adult and child:* IV loading dose 15-20 mg PE/kg given at 100-150 mg PE/min

Nonemergent/maintenance dosing
• *Adult and child:* IV loading dose 10-20 mg PE/kg; maintenance dosing 4-6 mg PE/kg/day given at a rate of <150 mg PE/min

Available forms: Inj 150 mg (100 mg phenytoin equiv), 750 mg (500 mg phenytoin equiv)

Side effects/adverse reactions:

CNS: Drowsiness, dizziness, insomnia, paresthesias, depression, suicidal tendencies, aggression, headache, confusion

CV: Hypotension, ventricular fibrillation

EENT: Nystagmus, diplopia, blurred vision

GI: Nausea, vomiting, constipation, anorexia, weight loss, hepatitis, jaundice, gingival hyperplasia

*GU: **Nephritis,*** urine discoloration

*HEMA: **Agranulocytosis, leukopenia, aplastic anemia, thrombocytopenia, megaloblastic anemia***

INTEG: Rash, lupus erythematosus, *Stevens-Johnson syndrome,* hirsutism

SYST: Hypocalcemia

Contraindications: Hypersensitivity, psychiatric conditions, pregnancy (D), bradycardia, SA and AV block, Stokes-Adams syndrome

Precautions: Allergies, hepatic disease, renal disease

Pharmacokinetics: Metabolized by liver, excreted by kidneys

Interactions:
• Decreased effects of fosphenytoin: alcohol (chronic use), antihistamines, antacids, antineoplastics, CNS depressants, rifampin, folic acid

Lab test interferences:

Decrease: Dexamethasone, metyrapone test serum, PBI, urinary steroids

Increase: Glucose, alk phosphatase

NURSING CONSIDERATIONS

Assess:
• Drug level: toxic level 30-50 μg/ml
• Blood studies: CBC, platelets q2 wk until stabilized, then qmo × 12 mo, then q3mo; discontinue drug if neutrophils <1600/mm^3
• Mental status: mood, sensorium, affect, memory (long, short)
• Respiratory depression; rate, depth, character of respirations
• Blood dyscrasias: fever, sore throat, bruising, rash, jaundice
• Continuous monitoring of ECG, B/P, respiratory function

Administer:

IV
• Dilute in D$_5$ or 0.9% NaCl 1.5-25 mg PE/ml, give <150 mg PE/min

Y-site compatibilities: Esmolol, famotidine, foscarnet

Evaluate:
• Therapeutic response: decrease in severity of seizures

Teach patient/family:
• The reason for and expected outcome of treatment

 = Nursing alert   = Herb-drug interaction   = Do not crush

furosemide (℞)

(fur-oh′se-mide)
Fumide, Furomide M.D., furo-
semide, Lasix, Luramide,
Novosemide*, Uritol*
Func. class.: Loop diuretic
Chem. class.: Sulfonamide de-
rivative

Action: Inhibits reabsorption of sodium and chloride at proximal and
distal tubule and in the loop of Henle
Uses: Pulmonary edema; edema in
CHF, liver disease, nephrotic syndrome, ascites, hypertension
Investigational uses: Hypercalcemia in malignancy
Dosage and routes:
• *Adult:* **PO** 20-80 mg/day in AM;
may give another dose in 6 hr up to
600 mg/day; **IM/IV** 20-40 mg, increased by 20 mg q2h until desired
response
• *Child:* **PO/IM/IV** 2 mg/kg; may
increase by 1-2 mg/kg/q6-8h up to
6 mg/kg
Pulmonary edema
• *Adult:* **IV** 40 mg given over several min, repeated in 1 hr; increase
to 80 mg if needed
*Hypertensive crisis/acute renal fail-
ure*
• *Adult:* **IV** 100-200 mg over 1-2
min
Available forms: Tabs 20, 40, 80
mg; oral sol 10 mg/ml, 40 mg/5 ml;
inj 10 mg/ml
Side effects/adverse reactions:
CNS: Headache, fatigue, weakness,
vertigo, paresthesias
CV: Orthostatic hypotension, chest
pain, ECG changes, *circulatory collapse*
EENT: **Loss of hearing,** ear pain,
tinnitus, blurred vision
ELECT: Hypokalemia, hypochloremic alkalosis, hypomagnesemia,
hyperuricemia, hypocalcemia, hyponatremia, metabolic alkalosis
ENDO: Hyperglycemia
GI: Nausea, diarrhea, dry mouth,
vomiting, anorexia, cramps, oral,
gastric irritations, pancreatitis
*GU: Polyuria, **renal failure,*** glycosuria
HEMA: **Thrombocytopenia, agranulocytosis, leukopenia, neutropenia,
anemia**
INTEG: Rash, pruritus, purpura,
Stevens-Johnson syndrome, sweating, photosensitivity, urticaria
MS: Cramps, stiffness
Contraindications: Hypersensitivity to sulfonamides, anuria, hypovolemia, infants, lactation, electrolyte depletion
Precautions: Diabetes mellitus, dehydration, severe renal disease, pregnancy (C), cirrhosis, ascites
Pharmacokinetics:
PO: Onset 1 hr, peak 1-2 hr, duration
6-8 hr; absorbed 70%
IV: Onset 5 min, peak ½ hr, duration
2 hr (metabolized by the liver 30%)
Excreted in urine, some as unchanged drug, feces; crosses placenta; excreted in breast milk; half-
life ½-1 hr
Interactions:
• Increased toxicity: lithium, nondepolarizing skeletal muscle relaxants, digitalis
• Increased K action of antihypertensives, oral anticoagulants, nitrates
• Increased ototoxicity: aminogly-
cosides, cisplatin, vancomycin
• Decreased antihypertensive effect
of furosemide: indomethacin, metolazone
Lab test interferences:
Interference: GTT
NURSING CONSIDERATIONS
Assess:
• Signs of metabolic alkalosis:
drowsiness, restlessness

F

- Signs of hypokalemia: postural hypotension, malaise, fatigue, tachycardia, leg cramps, weakness
- Rashes, temp elevation qd
- Confusion, especially in elderly; take safety precautions if needed
- Hearing, including tinnitus and hearing loss, when giving high doses for extended periods
- Weight, I&O qd to determine fluid loss; effect of drug may be decreased if used qd
- Rate, depth, rhythm of respiration, effect of exertion, lung sounds
- B/P lying, standing; postural hypotension may occur
- Electrolytes: K, Na, Cl; include BUN, blood sugar, CBC, serum creatinine, blood pH, ABGs, uric acid, Ca, Mg
- Skin turgor, edema, condition of mucous membranes in mouth and nose
- Glucose in urine if patient is diabetic
- Allergies to sulfonamides, thiazides

Administer:
- In AM to avoid interference with sleep if using drug as a diuretic
- K replacement if K <3
- PO with food if nausea occurs; absorption may be decreased slightly; tabs may be crushed

IV
- Undiluted; may be given through Y-tube or 3-way stopcock; give 20 mg or less/min; may be added to NS or D$_5$W if large doses are required and given as IV INF, not to exceed 4 mg/min; use infusion pump

Additive compatibilities: Amikacin, aminophylline, ampicillin, atropine, bumetanide, calcium gluconate, cefamandole, cefoperazone, cefuroxime, cimetidine, cloxacillin, dexamethasone, diamorphine, digoxin, epinephrine, heparin, isosorbide, kanamycin, lidocaine, meropenem, morphine, nitroglycerin, penicillin G, potassium chloride, ranitidine, scopolamine, sodium bicarbonate, theophylline, tobramycin, verapamil

Syringe compatibilities: Bleomycin, cisplatin, cyclophosphamide, fluorouracil, heparin, leucovorin, methotrexate, mitomycin

Y-site compatibilities: Allopurinol, amifostine, amikacin, aztreonam, bleomycin, cefepime, cefmetazole, cisplatin, cladribine, cyclophosphamide, cytarabine, epinephrine, fentanyl, fludarabine, fluorouracil, foscarnet, gallium, granisetron, heparin, hydrocortisone, hydromorphone, indomethacin, kanamycin, leucovorin, lorazepam, melphalan, meropenem, methotrexate, mitomycin, nitroglycerin, norepinephrine, paclitaxel, piperacillin/tazobactam, potassium chloride, propofol, ranitidine, sargramostim, tacrolimus, teniposide, thiotepa, tobramycin, tolazoline, vit B/C

Evaluate:
- Therapeutic response: improvement in edema of feet, legs, sacral area daily if medication is being used for CHF

Teach patient/family:
- To discuss the need for a high-K diet or K replacement with prescriber
- To increase fluid intake 2-3 L/day unless contraindicated
- To rise slowly from lying or sitting position; orthostatic hypotension may occur
- To recognize adverse reactions that may occur: muscle cramps, weakness, nausea, dizziness
- Regarding entire regimen, including exercise, diet, stress relief for hypertension
- To take with food or milk for GI symptoms

◆ = Nursing alert   ∥ = Herb-drug interaction   ⊘ = Do not crush

• To use sunscreen or protective clothing to prevent photosensitivity
• To take early in day to prevent sleeplessness
• To avoid OTC medication unless directed by prescriber

Treatment of overdose: Lavage if taken orally; monitor electrolytes; administer dextrose in saline; monitor hydration, CV, renal status

---

gabapentin (R)

(gab'a-pen-tin)
Neurontin
Func. class.: Anticonvulsant

Action: Mechanism unknown; may increase seizure threshold; structurally similar to GABA; gabapentin binding sites in neocortex, hippocampus

Uses: Adjunct treatment of partial seizures, with or without generalization in adults

Investigational uses: Chronic pain

Dosage and routes:
• *Adult:* PO 900-1800 mg/day in 3 divided doses; may titrate by giving 300 mg on the first day, 300 mg bid on second day, 300 mg tid on third day; may increase to 1800 mg/day by adding 300 mg on subsequent days

Available forms: Caps 100, 300, 400 mg

Side effects/adverse reactions:
CNS: Dizziness, fatigue, anxiety, somnolence, ataxia, amnesia, abnormal thinking, unsteady gait, depression
CV: Vasodilation
EENT: Dry mouth, blurred vision, diplopia
GI: Constipation, increased appetite, dental abnormalities
GU: Impotence, bleeding, *UTI*
HEMA: **Leukopenia,** decreased WBC
INTEG: Pruritus, abrasion

MS: Myalgia
RESP: Rhinitis, pharyngitis, coughing

Contraindications: Hypersensitivity to this drug

Precautions: Hepatic disease, renal disease, pregnancy (C), lactation, child <12 yr, elderly

Pharmacokinetics: Largely unbound to plasma proteins; not metabolized; excreted in urine (unchanged); elimination half-life 5-7 hr

Interactions:
• Decreased levels of gabapentin: antacids

NURSING CONSIDERATIONS
Assess:
• Renal studies: urinalysis, BUN, urine creatinine q3mo
• Hepatic studies: ALT (SGPT), AST (SGOT), bilirubin
• Description of seizures
• Mental status: mood, sensorium, affect, behavioral changes; if mental status changes, notify prescriber
• Eye problems, need for ophthalmic examinations before, during, after treatment (slit lamp, fundoscopy, tonometry)
• Allergic reaction: purpura, red raised rash; if these occur, drug should be discontinued

Administer:
• At least 2 hr pc with antacid

Perform/provide:
• Storage at room temp away from heat and light
• Hard candy, frequent rinsing of mouth, gum for dry mouth
• Assistance with ambulation during early part of treatment; dizziness occurs
• Seizure precautions: padded side rails; move objects that may harm patient
• Increased fluids, bulk in diet for constipation

Evaluate:
• Therapeutic response: decreased seizure activity; document on patient's chart

Teach patient/family:
• To carry Medic Alert ID stating patient's name, drugs taken, condition, prescriber's name and phone number
• To avoid driving, other activities that require alertness
• Not to discontinue medication quickly after long-term use
🚫 Not to break, crush, or chew caps

Treatment of overdose: Lavage, VS

---

gallamine (℞)
(gal′a-meen)
Flaxedil
Func. class.: Neuromuscular blocker (nondepolarizing)

Action: Inhibits transmission of nerve impulses by binding with cholinergic receptor sites, antagonizing action of acetylcholine

Uses: Facilitation of endotracheal intubation, skeletal muscle relaxation during mechanical ventilation, surgery, general anesthesia

Dosage and routes:
• *Adult and child >1 mo:* **IV** 1 mg/kg, not to exceed 100 mg, then 0.5-1 mg/kg q30-40min
• *Child <1 mo, >5 kg:* **IV** 0.25-0.75 mg/kg, then 0.01-0.05 mg/kg q30-40min

Available forms: Inj 20 mg/ml

Side effects/adverse reactions:
CV: Bradycardia, tachycardia, increased, decreased B/P
*RESP: **Prolonged apnea, bronchospasm, cyanosis, respiratory depression***
EENT: Increased secretions
INTEG: Rash, flushing, pruritus, urticaria

*CNS: **Malignant hyperthermia***
GI: Decreased motility

Contraindications: Hypersensitivity to iodides

Precautions: Pregnancy (C), thyroid disease, collagen disease, cardiac disease, lactation, children <2 yr, electrolyte imbalances, dehydration, neuromuscular disease (myasthenia gravis), respiratory disease, renal disease

Pharmacokinetics:
IV: Onset 2 min, duration 20-30 min; half-life 2 min, 29 min (terminal); excreted in urine, feces (metabolites); crosses placenta

Interactions:
• Increased neuromuscular blockade: aminoglycosides, clindamycin, lincomycin, quinidine, local anesthetics, polymyxin antibiotics, lithium, narcotic analgesics, thiazides, enflurane, isoflurane; used with cyclopropane, may provoke ventricular dysrhythmias
• Dysrhythmias: theophylline
• Incompatible with anesthetics, barbiturates in sol; incompatible with any other drug in syringe

NURSING CONSIDERATIONS
Assess:
• For electrolyte imbalances (K, Mg); may lead to increased action of this drug
• Vital signs (B/P, pulse, respirations, airway) q15min until fully recovered; rate, depth, pattern of respirations, strength of hand grip
• I&O ratio; check for urinary retention, frequency, hesitancy
• Recovery: decreased paralysis of face, diaphragm, leg, arm, rest of body
• Allergic reactions: rash, fever, respiratory distress, pruritus; drug should be discontinued

Administer:
• Using nerve stimulator by anes-

◆ = Nursing alert   🌿 = Herb-drug interaction   🚫 = Do not crush

thesiologist to determine neuromuscular blockade
• Anticholinesterase to reverse neuromuscular blockade
• IV undiluted over 1-2 min (only by qualified person, usually an anesthesiologist)
• Only slightly discolored sol
Perform/provide:
• Storage in light-resistant, cool area
• Reassurance if communication is difficult during recovery from neuromuscular blockade
Evaluate:
• Therapeutic response: paralysis of jaw, eyelid, head, neck, rest of body
Treatment of overdose: Edrophonium or neostigmine, atropine; monitor VS; may require mechanical ventilation

---

gallium (℞)

(gal'ee-um)
Ganite
Func. class.: Electrolyte modifier
Chem. class.: Hypocalcemic drug

Action: Lowers serum calcium levels by inhibiting calcium resorption from bone
Uses: Cancer-related hypercalcemia
Dosage and routes:
• *Adult:* IV 100-200 mg/m^2 qd × 5 days; infuse over 24 hr
Available forms: 25 mg/ml inj
Side effects/adverse reactions:
HEMA: **Anemia, leukopenia**
CV: Tachycardia
EENT: Blurred vision, optic neuritis, hearing loss
GU: **Nephrotoxicity,** increased BUN, creatinine
META: *Hypophosphatemia,* hypo-

calcemia, decreased serum bicarbonate
Contraindications: Hypersensitivity, severe renal disease
Precautions: Pregnancy (C), lactation, children, mild renal disease
Pharmacokinetics:
IV: Onset 12-24 hr, peak 5 days, duration 8 days
Interactions:
• Increased nephrotoxicity: aminoglycosides, amphotericin B
NURSING CONSIDERATIONS
Assess:
• Renal status: BUN, creatinine, urine output; if creatinine level is 2.5 mg/dl or more, drug should be discontinued
• Monitor Ca, phosphate, bicarbonate, since all levels may be decreased and supplements of phosphate may be needed
• For hypercalcemia: nausea, vomiting, fatigue, weakness, thirst, dehydration, dysrhythmias, change in mental status
• For hypocalcemia: dysrhythmias; paresthesia; twitching; colic; laryngospasm; Trousseau's, Chvostek's sign; tremors
• For hypophosphatemia: confusion, decreased reflexes, joint stiffness and pain, portal hypotension
Administer:
IV
• Adequate hydration with IV saline, 2 L/day during treatment
• After dilution of dose/1 L 0.9% NaCl or D$_5$W, run over 24 hr, use infusion pump
Y-site compatibilities: Acyclovir, allopurinol, amifostine, aminophylline, ampicillin/sulbactam, aztreonam, cefazolin, ceftazidime, ceftriaxone, cimetidine, ciprofloxacin, cladribine, cyclophosphamide, dexamethasone, diphenhydramine, filgrastim, fluconazole, furosemide, granisetron, heparin, hydro-

cortisone, ifosfamide, magnesium sulfate, mannitol, melphalan, meperidine, mesna, methotrexate, metoclopramide, ondansetron, piperacillin, piperacillin/tazobactam, potassium chloride, ranitidine, sodium bicarbonate, teniposide, thiotepa, ticarcillin/clavulanate, trimethoprimsulfamethoxazole, vancomycin, vinorelbine

Perform/provide:
• Storage of solution 48 hr at room temp, 1 wk in refrigerator

Evaluate:
• Therapeutic response: decreased serum Ca levels

Teach patient/family:
• To follow dietary guidelines given by prescriber, including adequate Ca (dairy products, broccoli) and vit D (fortified milk, grain products, fish oil)

---

ganciclovir (DHPG) ℞
(gan-sye′kloe-vir)
Cytovene
Func. class.: Antiviral
Chem. class.: Synthetic nucleoside analog

Action: Inhibits replication of herpesviruses in vitro, in vivo by selective inhibition of the human CMV DNA polymerase and by direct incorporation into viral DNA

Uses: Cytomegalovirus (CMV) retinitis in immunocompromised persons, including those with AIDS, after indirect ophthalmoscopy confirms diagnosis

Dosage and routes:
• Reduce dose in renal disease CrCl <70 ml/min

Prevention of CMV
• *Adult:* **IV** 5 mg/kg q12h × 1-2 wk,
then 5 mg/kg/day or 6 mg/kg × 5 days/wk

Induction treatment
• *Adult:* **IV** 5 mg/kg given over 1 hr, q12h × 2-3 wk

Maintenance treatment
• *Adult:* **IV INF** 5 mg/kg given over 1 hr, qd × 7 days/wk; or 6 mg/kg qd ×5 days/wk; **INTRAVITERAL** 200 µg qwk; **PO** 1000 mg tid with food or 500 mg q3h while awake
• Dosage must be reduced in renal impairment

Available forms: Powder 500 mg/vial; caps 250 mg; implant, intraviteral 4.5 mg

Side effects/adverse reactions:
HEMA: **Granulocytopenia, thrombocytopenia, irreversible neutropenia, anemia, eosinophilia**
GI: Abnormal LFTs, nausea, vomiting, anorexia, diarrhea, abdominal pain, hemorrhage
INTEG: Rash, alopecia, *pruritus*, urticaria, pain at site, phlebitis
CNS: Fever, chills, **coma,** *confusion*, abnormal thoughts, dizziness, bizarre dreams, *headache*, psychosis, tremors, somnolence, *paresthesia, weakness*
CV: Dysrhythmia, hypertension/hypotension
RESP: Dyspnea
EENT: Retinal detachment in CMV retinitis
GU: **Hematuria,** increased creatinine, BUN

Contraindications: Hypersensitivity to acyclovir or ganciclovir, absolute neutrophil count <500, platelet count <25,000

Precautions: Preexisting cytopenias, renal function impairment, pregnancy (C), lactation, children <6 mo, elderly

Pharmacokinetics: Half-life 3-4½ hr; excreted by the kidneys (unchanged drug); crosses blood-brain barrier, CSF

◆ = Nursing alert   ⫽ = Herb-drug interaction   ⊘ = Do not crush

Interactions:
• Decreased renal clearance of ganciclovir: probenecid
• Increased toxicity: dapsone, pentamidine, flucytosine, vincristine, vinblastine, adriamycin, doxorubicin, amphotericin B, trimethoprim-sulfa combinations, or other nucleoside analogs, cyclosporine
• Severe granulocytopenia: zidovudine; do not give together
• Increased seizures: imipenem/cilastatin

NURSING CONSIDERATIONS
Assess:
• For leukopenia/neutropenia/thrombocytopenia: WBCs, platelets q2d during 2 ×/d dosing and q1wk thereafter
• For leukopenia with qd WBC count in patients with prior leukopenia with other nucleoside analogs or for whom leukopenia counts are <1000 cells/mm^3 at start of treatment
• Serum creatinine or CrCl at least q2wk

Administer:
IV
• Mixed in biologic cabinet, using gown, gloves, mask
• IV after diluting 500 mg/10 ml sterile H$_2$O for injection (50 mg/ml); shake; further dilute in 100 ml D$_5$W, 0.9% NaCl, LR and run over 1 hr; use infusion pump
• Slowly; do not give by bolus IV, IM, SC injection
• Using diluted sol within 12 hr; do not refrigerate or freeze

Y-site compatibilities: Allopurinol, cisplatin, cyclophosphamide, enalaprilat, filgrastim, fluconazole, granisetron, melphalan, methotrexate, paclitaxel, propofol, tacrolimus, teniposide, thiotepa

Evaluate:
• Therapeutic response: decreased symptoms of CMV

Teach patient/family:
• That drug does not cure condition, that regular ophthalmologic examinations are necessary
• That major toxicities may necessitate discontinuing drug
• To use contraception during treatment and that infertility may occur; men should use barrier contraception for 90 days after treatment

Treatment of overdose: Discontinue drug, use hemodialysis, and increase hydration

---

gemcitabine (R)

(jem-sit′a-been)
Gemzar
Func. class.: Misc. antineoplastic
Chem. class.: Nucleoside analog

Action: Exhibits antitumor activity by killing cells undergoing DNA synthesis (S-phase) and blocking G1/S-phase boundary

Uses: Adenocarcinoma of the pancreas (nonresectable Stage II, III, or metastatic Stage IV); non–small cell lung cancer (Stage IIIA or B, IV)

Dosage and routes:
• *Adult:* **IV** 1000 mg/m^2 given over ½ hr qwk × 7 wk, then 1 wk rest period; subsequent cycles should be infused once qwk × 3 wk out of every 4 wk

Available forms: Lyophilized powder 20 mg/ml

Side effects/adverse reactions:
GI: Diarrhea, nausea, vomiting, anorexia, constipation, stomatitis
INTEG: Irritation at site, rash, alopecia
HEMA: **Leukopenia, anemia, neutropenia, thrombocytopenia**
OTHER: Dyspnea, fever, **hemorrhage,** infection

Contraindications: Hypersensitivity, pregnancy (D)

Precautions: Lactation, children, elderly, myelosuppression, irradiation

Pharmacokinetics: Half-life 42-79 min

Interactions:

• Increased myelosuppression, diarrhea: other antineoplastics

NURSING CONSIDERATIONS

Assess:

• CBC, differential, platelet count weekly; withhold drug if WBC is <3500/mm^3, or platelet count <100,000/mm^3; notify prescriber of these results; drug should be discontinued

• Food preferences: list likes, dislikes

• Buccal cavity q8h for dryness, sores, or ulceration, white patches, oral pain, bleeding, dysphagia

• GI symptoms: frequency of stools; cramping

• Signs of dehydration: rapid respirations, poor skin turgor, decreased urine output, dry skin, restlessness, weakness

Perform/provide:

• Increased fluid intake to 2-3 L/day to prevent dehydration, unless contraindicated

• Changing of IV site q48h

• Rinsing of mouth tid-qid with water, club soda; brushing of teeth bid-tid with soft brush or cotton-tipped applicator for stomatitis; use unwaxed dental floss

• Nutritious diet with iron, vitamin supplement, low fiber, few dairy products

Evaluate:

• Therapeutic response: decrease in tumor size, decrease in spread of cancer

Teach patient/family:

• To avoid foods with citric acid or hot or rough texture if stomatitis is present; to drink adequate fluids

• To report stomatitis; any bleeding, white spots, ulcerations in mouth; tell patient to examine mouth qd, report symptoms

• To report signs of anemia: fatigue, headache, faintness, shortness of breath, irritability

• To use contraception during therapy

Treatment of overdose: Induce vomiting, provide supportive care

---

gemfibrozil (℞)

(jem-fi'broe-zil)

Lopid

Func. class.: Antilipemic

Chem. class.: Aryloxyisobutyric acid derivative

Action: Inhibits biosynthesis of VLDL, decreases triglycerides, increases HDL

Uses: Type II, III/IV, V hyperlipidemia as adjunct with diet therapy

Dosage and routes:

• *Adult:* **PO** 1200 mg in divided doses bid 30 min before meals

Available forms: Tabs 600 mg

Side effects/adverse reactions:

GI: Nausea, vomiting, dyspepsia, diarrhea, abdominal pain

INTEG: Rash, urticaria, pruritus

HEMA: **Leukopenia, anemia, eosinophilia, thrombocytopenia**

CNS: Dizziness, blurred vision

MISC: Taste perversion

Contraindications: Severe hepatic disease, preexisting gallbladder disease, severe renal disease, primary biliary cirrhosis, hypersensitivity

Precautions: Monitor hematologic and hepatic function, pregnancy (C), lactation

Pharmacokinetics:

PO: Peak 1-2 hr; plasma protein bind-

 = Nursing alert   = Herb-drug interaction   Ⓝ = Do not crush ing >90%; half-life 1½ hr; excreted in urine; metabolized in liver

Interactions:
• May increase anticoagulant properties: oral anticoagulants
• Increased risk of myositis, myalgia: lovastatin

Lab test interferences:
Increase: Liver function studies, CPK, BSP, thymol turbidity, glucose
Decrease: Hgb, Hct, WBC

NURSING CONSIDERATIONS
Assess:
• Triglycerides, cholesterol; if cholesterol increases, drug should be discontinued
• Renal studies, LFTs, CBC if patient is on long-term therapy
• Bowel pattern daily; increase bulk, water in diet if constipation develops, especially elderly

Administer:
PO
• 30 min before morning and evening meals

Evaluate:
• Therapeutic response: decreased cholesterol, triglyceride levels

Teach patient/family:
• That compliance is needed for positive results; do not double or skip dose
• That risk factors should be decreased: high-fat diet, smoking, alcohol consumption, absence of exercise
• To notify prescriber of diarrhea, nausea, vomiting, chills, fever, sore throat
🚫 Not to break, crush, or chew caps

gentamicin (℞)
(jen-ta-mye′sin)
Alcomicin*, Apogen*, Cidomycin*, Garamycin, Garamycin Intrathecal, Garamycin IV Piggyback, Garamycin Pediatric, gentamicin sulfate, Gentamicin Sulfate IV Piggyback, Jenamicin, Pediatric Gentamicin Sulfate
Func. class.: Antiinfective
Chem. class.: Aminoglycoside

G

Action: Interferes with protein synthesis in bacterial cell by binding to ribosomal subunit, causing misreading of genetic code; inaccurate peptide sequence forms in protein chain, causing bacterial death

Uses: Severe systemic infections of CNS, respiratory, GI, urinary tract, bone, skin, soft tissues caused by susceptible strains of *P. aeruginosa, Proteus, Klebsiella, Serratia, E. coli, Enterobacter, Citrobacter, Staphylococcus, Shigella, Salmonella, Acinetobacter*, acute PID

Dosage and routes:
Severe systemic infections
• *Adult:* **IV INF** 3-5 mg/kg/day in 3 divided doses q8h; dilute in 50-200 ml **NS** or D_5W given over 30 min-1 hr; **IM** 3 mg/kg/day in divided doses q8h
• *Adult:* **INTRATHECAL** 4-8 mg qd
• *Child:* **IV/IM** 2-2.5 mg/kg q8h
• *Neonate and infant:* **IV/IM** 2.5 mg/kg q8-12h
• *Neonate <1 wk:* 2.5 mg/kg q12-24h
• *Infant and child >3 mo:* **INTRATHECAL** 1-2 mg qd
Once daily dosing/extended interval dosing
• *Adult:* **IV** 5-7 mg/kg/dose, adjust according levels

Dental/respiratory procedures, GI/GU surgery (prophylaxis endocarditis)
• *Adult:* IM 1.5 mg/kg ½-1 hr before procedure with ampicillin
• *Child:* IM 2.5 mg/kg ½-1 hr before procedure with ampicillin
Available forms: Inj 10, 40, 60, 80, 100 mg; intrathecal 2 mg/ml

Side effects/adverse reactions:
GU: Oliguria, hematuria, renal damage, azotemia, renal failure, nephrotoxicity
CNS: Confusion, depression, numbness, tremors, *convulsions,* muscle twitching, *neurotoxicity,* dizziness, vertigo
EENT: Ototoxicity, deafness, visual disturbances, tinnitus
HEMA: Agranulocytosis, thrombocytopenia, leukopenia, eosinophilia, anemia
GI: Nausea, vomiting, anorexia; increased ALT, AST, bilirubin; hepatomegaly, *hepatic necrosis,* splenomegaly
CV: Hypotension, hypertension, palpitations
INTEG: Rash, burning, urticaria, dermatitis, alopecia

Contraindications: Severe renal disease, hypersensitivity

Precautions: Neonates, mild renal disease, pregnancy (C), hearing deficits, myasthenia gravis, lactation, elderly, Parkinson's disease

Pharmacokinetics:
IM: Onset rapid, peak 1-2 hr
IV: Onset immediate, peak 1-2 hr; plasma half-life 1-2 hr, infants 6-7 hr; duration 6-8 hr; not metabolized; excreted unchanged in urine; crosses placental barrier; poor penetration into CSF

Interactions:
• Increased ototoxicity, neurotoxicity, nephrotoxicity: other aminoglycosides, amphotericin B, polymyxin, vancomycin, ethacrynic acid, furosemide, mannitol, methoxyflurane, cisplatin, cephalosporins, bacitracin, enflurane, penicillins
• Increased effects: nondepolarizing neuromuscular blockers

NURSING CONSIDERATIONS
Assess:
• Weight before treatment; calculation of dosage is usually based on ideal body weight, but may be calculated on actual body weight
• I&O ratio, urinalysis daily for proteinuria, cells, casts; report sudden change in urine output; toxicity is increased in patients with decreased renal function if high doses are given
• VS during infusion; watch for hypotension, change in pulse
• IV site for thrombophlebitis, including pain, redness, swelling, q30min, change site if needed; apply warm compresses to discontinued site
• Serum peak, drawn at 30-60 min after IV INF or 60 min after IM inj, and trough level drawn just before next dose; blood level should be 2-4 times bacteriostatic level; peak = 4-12 µg/ml, trough = 1-2 µg/ml
• Urine pH if drug is used for UTI; urine should be kept alkaline
• Renal impairment by securing urine for CrCl testing, BUN, serum creatinine; lower dosage should be given in renal impairment (CrCl <80 ml/min)
• Deafness by audiometric testing, ringing, roaring in ears, vertigo; assess hearing before, during, after treatment
• Dehydration: high specific gravity, decrease in skin turgor, dry mucous membranes, dark urine
• Overgrowth of infection including fever, malaise, redness, pain, swelling, perineal itching, diarrhea, stomatitis, change in cough or sputum

 = Nursing alert　　　 = Herb-drug interaction　　　 = Do not crush

• C&S before starting treatment to identify infecting organism

• Vestibular dysfunction: nausea, vomiting, dizziness, headache; drug should be discontinued if severe

• Injection sites for redness, swelling, abscesses; use warm compresses at site

Administer:

• IM inj in large muscle mass; rotate injection sites

• Drug in evenly spaced doses to maintain blood level

• Bicarbonate to alkalinize urine if ordered for UTI, as drug is most active in alkaline environment

IV

• After diluting in 50-200 ml NS or D_5W; sol concentration should be 1 mg/ml or less; decrease vol of diluent in child; maintain 0.1% sol run over ½-1 hr (adults) or up to 2 hr (children); flush IV line with NS or D_5W after administration

Additive compatibilities: Atracurium, aztreonam, bleomycin, cefoxitin, cimetidine, ciprofloxacin, fluconazole, meropenem, methicillin, metronidazole, ofloxacin, penicillin G sodium, ranitidine, verapamil

Syringe compatibilities: Clindamycin, methicillin, penicillin G sodium

Y-site compatibilities: Acyclovir, amifostine, amiodarone, amsacrine, atracurium, aztreonam, cefpirome, ciprofloxacin, cyclophosphamide, cytarabine, diltiazem, enalaprilat, esmolol, famotidine, filgrastim, fluconazole, fludarabine, foscarnet, granisetron, hydromorphone, IL-2, insulin, labetalol, lorazepam, magnesium sulfate, melphalan, meperidine, meropenem, midazolam, morphine, multivitamins, ondansetron, paclitaxel, pancuronium, perphenazine, sargramostim, tacrolimus, teniposide, theophylline, thiotepa, tola-zine, vecuronium, vinorelbin, B/C, zidovudine

Perform/provide:

• Adequate fluids of 2-3 L/day, un less contraindicated, to prevent irritation of tubules

• Supervised ambulation, other safety measures with vestibular dysfunction

Evaluate:

• Therapeutic response: absence of fever, draining wounds, negative C&S after treatment

Teach patient/family:

• To report headache, dizziness, symptoms of overgrowth of infection, renal impairment

• To report loss of hearing, ringing, roaring in ears or feeling of fullness in head

Treatment of overdose: Hemodialysis; monitor serum levels of drug

---

glatiramer (℞)

(glah-tear′a-meer)
Copaxone
Func. class.: MS agent

Action: Unknown, may modify the immune responses responsible for multiple sclerosis

Uses: Reduction of the frequency of relapses in patients with relapsing-remitting multiple sclerosis

Dosage and routes:

• *Adult:* SC 20 mg/day

Available forms: Inj 20 mg/ml

Side effects/adverse reactions:

CV: Migraine, palpitations, syncope, tachycardia, vasodilation

GI: Nausea, vomiting, diarrhea, anorexia, gastroenteritis

HEMA: Ecchymosis, lymphadenopathy

META: Edema, weight gain

MS: Arthralgia

CNS: Anxiety, hypertonia, tremor,

, speech disorder, agitation,
sion

SP: Bronchitis, dyspnea

INTEG: Pruritus, rash, sweating, urticaria, erythema

EENT: Ear pain

GU: Urgency, dysmenorrhea, vaginal moniliasis

Contraindications: Hypersensitivity to this drug or mannitol

Precautions: Immune disorders, renal disease, pregnancy (B), lactation

Pharmacokinetics: Unknown

NURSING CONSIDERATIONS

Assess:

• Blood, renal, hepatic studies: prior to treatment

• For CNS symptoms: anxiety, confusion, vertigo

• GI status: diarrhea, vomiting, abdominal pain, gastroenteritis

• Cardiac status: tachycardia, palpitations, vasodilation

Administer:

• SC route

• Using a sterile syringe/needle to transfer the supplied diluent into the vial, rotate vial gently, do not shake; withdraw medication using a syringe with 27 G needle; administer SC into hip, thigh, arm; discard unused portion

• Use SC route only; do not give IM or IV

• Do not use sol that contains precipitate or is discolored

Evaluate:

• Therapeutic response: decreased symptoms of multiple sclerosis

Teach patient/family:

• Give written, detailed instructions about the drug; provide initial and return demonstrations on inj procedure; give information on use and disposal of drug

• That blurred vision, sweating may occur

• That irregular menses, dysmenorrhea, or metrorrhagia as well as breast pain may occur; use contraception during treatment

• That if pregnancy is suspected, or if nursing, notify prescriber

• Not to change dosing or to stop taking drug without advice of prescriber

---

glipizide (℞)

(glip-i′zide)

Glucotrol, Glucotrol XL

glimepiride

(glye-me′pi-ride)

Amaryl

Func. class: Antidiabetic

Chem. class.: Sulfonylurea (2nd generation)

Action: Causes functioning β-cells in pancreas to release insulin, leading to drop in blood glucose levels; may improve insulin binding to insulin receptors or increase the number of insulin receptors with prolonged administration; may also reduce basal hepatic glucose secretion; not effective if patient lacks functioning β-cells

Uses: Stable adult-onset diabetes mellitus (type II) NIDDM

Dosage and routes:

Glipizide

• *Adult:* **PO** 5 mg initially, then increase to desired response; max 40 mg/day in divided doses or 15 mg/dose

• *Elderly/hepatic disease:* **PO** 2.5 mg initially, then increase to desired response; max 40 mg/day in divided doses or 15 mg/dose

Glimepiride

• *Adult:* **PO** 1-2 mg qd, then increase q1-2wk up to 8 mg/day

Available forms: glipizide: tabs 5,

◆ = Nursing alert　　🌿 = Herb-drug interaction　　🚫 = Do not crush

10 mg scored; ext rel tab 10 mg; glimepiride: tabs 1, 2, 4 mg

Side effects/adverse reactions:

CNS: Headache, weakness, dizziness, drowsiness, tinnitus, fatigue, vertigo

GI: Hepatotoxicity, cholestatic jaundice, nausea, vomiting, diarrhea, heartburn

HEMA: Leukopenia, thrombocytopenia, agranulocytosis, aplastic anemia; increased AST, ALT, alk phosphatase; *pancytopenia, hemolytic anemia*

INTEG: Rash, allergic reactions, pruritus, urticaria, eczema, photosensitivity, erythema

ENDO: Hypoglycemia

Contraindications: Hypersensitivity to sulfonylureas, juvenile or brittle diabetes

Precautions: Pregnancy (C), elderly, cardiac disease, severe renal disease, severe hepatic disease, thyroid disease

Pharmacokinetics:

PO: Completely absorbed by GI route, onset 1-1½ hr, peak 1-3 hr, duration 10-24 hr, half-life 2-4 hr; metabolized in liver; excreted in urine; 90%-95% is plasma protein bound

Interactions:

• Increased hypoglycemic effects: insulin, MAOIs, cimetidine, chloramphenicol, guanethidine, methyldopa, nonsteroidal antiinflammatories, salicylates, probenecid

• Effectiveness may be decreased: calcium channel blockers, corticosteroids, oral contraceptives, thiazide diuretics, thyroid preparations, estrogens, phenothiazines, phenytoin, rifampin, isoniazid, phenobarbital, sympathomimetics

• Disulfiram-like reaction: alcohol

• Decreased effects of both drugs: diazoxide

NURSING CONSIDERATIONS

Assess:

• Blood, urine glucose levels during treatment to determine diabetes control

• Hypo/hyperglycemic reaction that can occur soon after meals

Administer:

• Drug 30 min before meals

Perform/provide:

• Storage in tight, light-resistant container at room temp

Evaluate:

• Therapeutic response: decrease in polyuria, polydipsia, polyphagia, clear sensorium, absence of dizziness, stable gait

Teach patient/family:

• Not to drink alcohol; explain disulfiram reaction

• To check for symptoms of cholestatic jaundice: dark urine, pruritus, yellow sclera; prescriber should be notified

• To use a capillary blood glucose test while on this drug

• To test blood glucose levels tid

• The symptoms of hypo/hyperglycemia, what to do about each; to have glucagon emergency kit available

• That drug must be continued on daily basis; explain consequence of discontinuing drug abruptly

• To take drug in morning to prevent hypoglycemic reactions at night

• To avoid OTC medications unless ordered by prescriber

• That diabetes is a lifelong illness; drug will not cure disease

• That all food in diet plan must be eaten to prevent hypoglycemia

• To carry Medic Alert ID for emergency purposes

• To test urine for glucose/ketones tid if this drug is replacing insulin

• To continue weight control, dietary restrictions, exercise, hygiene

G

Treatment of overdose: Glucose 25 g IV via dextrose 50% solution 50 ml or 1 mg glucagon

---

glyburide (℞)

(glye'byoor-ide)
DiaBeta*, Glynase PresTab, Micronase
Func. class.: Antidiabetic
Chem. class.: Sulfonylurea (2nd generation)

Action: Causes functioning β-cells in pancreas to release insulin, leading to drop in blood glucose levels; may improve insulin binding to insulin receptors and increase number of insulin receptors with prolonged administration; may also reduce basal hepatic glucose secretion; not effective if patient lacks functioning β-cells

Uses: Stable adult-onset diabetes mellitus (type II) NIDDM

Dosage and routes:
DiaBeta/micronase
• *Adult:* **PO** 2.5-5 mg initially, then increased to desired response
• *Elderly:* **PO** 1.25 mg initially, then increased to desired response; max 20 mg/day, maintenance 1.25-20 mg/qd; tabs, micronized
Glynase PresTab
• *Adult:* **PO** 1.5-3 mg/day initially, may increase by 1.5 mg/wk
• *Elderly:* **PO** 0.75-3 mg/day, may increase by 1.5 mg/wk
Available forms: Micronized tabs 1.25, 1.5, 2.5, 3, 4.5, 5, 6 (Glynase PresTab) 1.5, 3, 6 mg

Side effects/adverse reactions:
CNS: Headache, weakness, paresthesia, tinnitus, fatigue, vertigo
GI: Nausea, fullness, heartburn, *hepatotoxicity, cholestatic jaundice,* vomiting, diarrhea
HEMA: Leukopenia, thrombocytopenia, agranulocytosis, aplastic anemia, increased AST, ALT, alk phosphatase
INTEG: Rash, allergic reactions, pruritus, urticaria, eczema, photosensitivity, erythema
ENDO: Hypoglycemia
MS: Joint pain

Contraindications: Hypersensitivity to sulfonylureas, juvenile or brittle diabetes

Precautions: Pregnancy (B), elderly, cardiac disease, severe renal disease, severe hepatic disease, thyroid disease, severe hypoglycemic reactions

Pharmacokinetics:
PO: Completely absorbed by GI route; onset 2-4 hr, peak 2-8 hr, duration 24 hr; half-life 10 hr; metabolized in liver; excreted in urine, feces (metabolites); crosses placenta; 90%-95% is plasma protein bound

Interactions:
• Both drugs' effects may be decreased: diazoxide
• Decreased digoxin level: digoxin
• Increased hypoglycemic effects: insulin, MAOIs, cimetidine, oral anticoagulants, chloramphenicol, guanethidine, methyldopa, nonsteroidal antiinflammatories, salicylates, probenecid
• Decreased action of glyburide: calcium channel blockers, corticosteroids, oral contraceptives, thiazide diuretics, thyroid preparations, estrogens, phenothiazines, phenytoin, rifampin, isoniazid, phenobarbital, sympathomimetics
• Disulfiram-like reaction: alcohol

NURSING CONSIDERATIONS
Assess:
• Hypo/hyperglycemic reaction that can occur soon after meals
Administer:
• With breakfast

◆ = Nursing alert   ▰ = Herb-drug interaction   ⊘ = Do not crush

Perform/provide:
• Storage in tight container in cool environment
Evaluate:
• Therapeutic response: decrease in polyuria, polydipsia, polyphagia, clear sensorium, absence of dizziness, stable gait
Teach patient/family:
• Not to drink alcohol; explain disulfiram reaction
• To check for symptoms of cholestatic jaundice: dark urine, pruritus, yellow sclera; if these occur, notify prescriber
• To use a capillary blood glucose test while on this drug
• The symptoms of hypo/hyperglycemia, what to do about each
• That drug must be continued on daily basis; explain consequence of discontinuing drug abruptly
• To take drug in morning to prevent hypoglycemic reactions at night
• To avoid OTC medications unless ordered by prescriber
• That diabetes is a lifelong illness; drug will not cure disease
• That all food included in diet plan must be eaten to prevent hypoglycemia; to have glucagon emergency kit available
• To carry a Medic Alert ID for emergency purposes
Treatment of overdose: Glucose 25 g IV via dextrose 50% sol, 50 ml or 1 mg glucagon

---

glycerin (OTC)

(gli′ser-in)
Fleet Babylax, Glycerin USP, Glycerol, Osmoglyn, Sani-Supp
Func. class.: Laxative, hyperosmotic
Chem. class.: Trihydric alcohol

Action: Increases osmotic pressure, draws fluid into colon, lumen from extravascular spaces to intravascular
Uses: Constipation
Dosage and routes:
Laxative
• *Adult and child >6 yr:* **RECT SUPP** 3 g; **ENEMA** 5-15 ml
• *Child <6 yr:* **RECT SUPP** 1-1.5 g; **ENEMA** 2-5 ml
Intraocular pressure reduction
• *Adult:* **PO** 1-1.5 g/kg once, then may be given 500 mg/kg q6h
• *Child:* **PO** 1-1.5 g/kg once, then 500 mg/kg 4-8 hr after first dose
Available forms: Rec sol 4 ml/applicator; supp; oral sol 0.6 g/ml
Side effects/adverse reactions:
CNS: Headache, confusion, ***convulsions***
GI: Nausea, vomiting, diarrhea
META: Dehydration
Contraindications: Hypersensitivity
Precautions: Pregnancy (C)
NURSING CONSIDERATIONS
Assess:
• Cause of constipation; identify whether fluids, bulk, or exercise is missing from lifestyle
• Cramping, rectal bleeding, nausea, vomiting; if these symptoms occur, drug should be discontinued
Administer:
• Insert supp; may cause evacuation in ½ hr
• Enema: use 4 ml applicator; patient should be in side-lying position
• Pour oral sol over cracked ice and sip through a straw
• To prevent cerebral dehydration, headache, patient should be recumbent during and after administration
Perform/provide:
• Storage in cool environment; do not freeze
Evaluate:
• Therapeutic response: decrease in constipation

Teach patient/family:
• Not to use laxatives for long-term therapy; bowel tone will be lost
• That normal bowel movements do not always occur daily
• Not to use in presence of abdominal pain, nausea, vomiting
• To notify prescriber if constipation unrelieved or if symptoms of electrolyte imbalance occur: muscle cramps, pain, weakness, dizziness, excessive thirst

---

glycopyrrolate (℞)

(glye-koe-pye'roe-late)
glycopyrrolate, Robinul, Robinul Forte
Func. class.: Cholinergic blocker
Chem. class.: Quaternary ammonium compound

Action: Inhibits the action of acetylcholine at receptor sites in autonomic nervous system, which controls secretions, free acids in stomach

Uses: Decreased secretions before surgery, reversal of neuromuscular blockade, peptic ulcer disease, irritable bowel syndrome

Dosage and routes:
Preoperatively
• *Adult:* IM 0.002 mg/kg ½-1 hr before surgery
• *Child 2-12 yr:* IM 0.002-0.004 mg/kg
• *Child <2 yr:* IM 0.004 mg/kg
Control of secretions
• *Child:* PO 40-100 μg/kg/dose q3-4×/day
Reversal of neuromuscular blockade
• *Adult and child:* IV 0.2 mg for each 1 mg of neostigmine or 5 mg IV of pyridostigmine simultaneously
GI disorders
• *Adult:* PO 1-2 mg bid-tid; IM/IV

0.1-0.2 mg tid-qid, titrated to patient response
Available forms: Tabs 1, 2 mg; inj 0.2 mg/ml

Side effects/adverse reactions:
INTEG: Urticaria, allergic reactions
MISC: Suppression of lactation, nasal congestion, decreased sweating
CNS: Confusion, anxiety, restlessness, irritability, delusions, hallucinations, headache, sedation, depression, incoherence, dizziness, lethargy, flushing, weakness
EENT: Blurred vision, photophobia, dilated pupils, difficulty swallowing, increased intraocular pressure, mydriasis, cycloplegia
CV: Palpitations, tachycardia, postural hypotension, paradoxical bradycardia
GI: Dryness of mouth, constipation, nausea, vomiting, abdominal distress, paralytic ileus, altered taste perception
GU: Hesitancy, retention, impotence

Contraindications: Hypersensitivity, narrow-angle glaucoma, myasthenia gravis, GI/GU obstruction, child <3 yr, tachycardia, myocardial ischemia, hepatic disease, ulcerative colitis, toxic megacolon

Precautions: Pregnancy (C), elderly, lactation, prostatic hypertrophy, renal disease, CHF, pulmonary disease, hyperthyroidism

Pharmacokinetics:
PO: Peak 1 hr, duration 8-12 hr
IM: Peak 30-45 min, duration 2-7 hr
IV: Peak 10-15 min, duration 2-7 hr; excreted in urine (50%), (unchanged); half-life 1-2 hr

Interactions:
• Increased anticholinergic effect: alcohol, antihistamines, phenothiazines, amantadine, tricyclics
• Decreased absorption of glycopyrrolate: antacids, antidiarrheals

---

NURSING CONSIDERATIONS
Assess:
• I&O ratio; retention commonly causes decreased urinary output
• Urinary hesitancy, retention: palpate bladder if retention occurs
• Constipation; increase fluids, bulk, exercise if this occurs
• For tolerance over long-term therapy; dose may have to be increased or changed
• Mental status: affect, mood, CNS depression, worsening of mental symptoms during early therapy
Administer:
• Parenteral dose with patient recumbent to prevent postural hypotension
• Parenteral dose slowly; keep in bed for at least 1 hr after dose; monitor vital signs
• After checking dose carefully; even slight overdose may lead to toxicity
• With or after meals to prevent GI upset; may give with fluids other than water

IV
• Undiluted, give through a Y-tube or 3-way stopcock; give 0.2 mg or less over 1-2 min
Syringe compatibilities: Atropine, benzquinamide, chlorpromazine, cimetidine, codeine, diphenhydramine, droperidol, droperidol/fentanyl, hydromorphone, hydroxyzine, levorphanol, lidocaine, meperidine, meperidine/promethazine, midazolam, morphine, nalbuphine, neostigmine, oxymorphone, procaine, prochlorperazine, promazine, promethazine, pyridostigmine, ranitidine, scopolamine, triflupromazine, trimethobenzamide
Y-site compatibilities: Propofol
Perform/provide:
• Storage at room temp
• Hard candy, frequent drinks, sugarless gum to relieve dry mouth

Evaluate:
• Therapeutic response: decreased secretions
Teach patient/family:
• Not to discontinue this drug abruptly; to taper off over 1 wk
• To avoid driving, other hazardous activities; drowsiness may occur
• To avoid OTC medication: cough, cold preparations with alcohol, antihistamines unless directed by prescriber

G

---

gonadorelin HCl (R)
(goe-nad-oh-rell'in)
Factrel
Func. class.: Gonadotropin hormone
Chem. class.: Synthetic luteinizing hormone-releasing hormone

---

Action: Combination luteinizing hormone (releasing hormone) that acts on anterior pituitary
Uses: Evaluation of response of gonadotropic hormone
Dosage and routes:
• *Women:* SC/IV 100 µg usually given between day 1-7 of menstrual cycle
Available forms: Powder for inj 100, 500 µg/vial
Side effects/adverse reactions:
CNS: Dizziness, headache, flushing
GI: Nausea
INTEG: Inflammation at injection site
SYST: Anaphylaxis, antibody formation (large doses)
Contraindications: Hypersensitivity
Precautions: Pregnancy (B)
Pharmacokinetics: Metabolized to inactive compound; excreted by kidneys; half-life up to 40 min
Interactions:
• Increased level of gonadorelin: levodopa, spironolactone

~reased level of gonadorelin: ~n, oral contraceptives, phe~ines, dopamine antagonists ~t interferences:
~esults when used with androgens, glucocorticoids, estrogens, progestins

NURSING CONSIDERATIONS
Assess:
• Test result: pituitary/hypothalamus dysfunction (decreased LH); postmenopausal (increased LH)
Administer:
• After reconstituting with sterile diluent (1 ml)/100 μg or 500 μg/2 ml enclosed in package; give over 30 sec
• Repeat doses if necessary to elevate pituitary gonadotropin reserve
Perform/provide:
• Discard unused portions
Teach patient/family:
• To report rash, hives, difficult breathing, flushing

---

goserelin (℞)
(goe′se-rel-lin)
Zoladex

Func. class.: Gonadotropin-releasing hormone

Chem. class.: Synthetic decapeptide analog of LHRH

Action: Inhibitor of pituitary gonadotropin secretion; initially increases LH and FSH, with increases in testosterone, reduction in sex steroid levels

Uses: Advanced prostate cancer
Dosage and routes:
• *Adult:* **SC** 3.6 mg q28d
Available forms: Depot inj 3.6 mg
Side effects/adverse reactions:
CNS: Headaches, **spinal cord compression,** anxiety, depression
CV: **Dysrhythmia, cerebrovascular accident,** hypertension, **MI,** chest pain

ENDO: Gynecomastia, breast tenderness, hot flashes
GI: Nausea, vomiting, constipation, diarrhea, ulcer
GU: Spotting, breakthrough bleeding, decreased libido, renal insufficiency, urinary obstruction, urinary tract infection
INTEG: Rash, pain on injection
MS: Osteoneuralgia
Contraindications: Hypersensitivity, pregnancy (X)
Pharmacokinetics: Peak serum concentrations in 14-28 days; half-life 4½ hr
Lab test interferences:
Increase: Alk phosphatase, estradiol, FSH, LH, testosterone levels
Decrease: Testosterone levels, progesterone

NURSING CONSIDERATIONS
Assess:
• I&O ratios; palpate bladder for distention in urinary obstruction
• For relief of bone pain (back pain)
Administer:
• SC using implant, inserted by qualified person into upper subcutaneous tissue in abdominal wall q28d
Evaluate:
• Therapeutic response: more normal levels of prostate-specific antigen, acid phosphatase, alk phosphatase; testosterone level of <25 ng/dl
Teach patient/family:
• That gynecomastia and postmenopausal symptoms may occur but will decrease after treatment is discontinued

---

◆ = Nursing alert   ▟ = Herb-drug interaction   ⊘ = Do not crush

granisetron (℞)
(grane-iss′e-tron)
Kytril
Func. class.: Antiemetic
Chem. class.: 5-HT$_3$ receptor antagonist

Action: Prevents nausea, vomiting by blocking serotonin peripherally, centrally, and in the small intestine

Uses: Prevention of nausea, vomiting associated with cancer chemotherapy including high-dose cisplatin

Dosage and routes:
• *Adult and child:* **IV** 10 µg/kg over 5 min, 30 min before the start of cancer chemotherapy; *adult* **PO** 1 mg bid, give first dose 1 hr before chemotherapy and next dose 12 hr after first

Available forms: Inj 1 mg/ml; tab 1 mg

Side effects/adverse reactions:
CNS: Headache
GI: Diarrhea, constipation, increased AST (SGOT), ALT (SGPT)
MISC: Rash, ***bronchospasm***

Contraindications: Hypersensitivity

Precautions: Pregnancy (B), lactation, children, elderly

Pharmacokinetics: Metabolized in liver to an active metabolite, half-life 10-12 hr

NURSING CONSIDERATIONS
Assess:
• For absence of nausea, vomiting during chemotherapy
• Hypersensitive reaction: rash, bronchospasm

Administer:
IV, direct
• Over 5 min

Additive compatibilities: Dexamethasone, methylprednisolone

Solution compatibilities: D$_5$W, 0.9% NaCl

Y-site compatibilities: Acyclovir, allopurinol, amifostine, amikacin, aminophylline, ampicillin, ampicillin/sulbactam, amsacrine, aztreonam, bleomycin, bumetanide, buprenorphine, butorphanol, calcium gluconate, carboplatin, carmustine, cefazolin, cefepime, cefonicid, cefoperazone, cefotaxime, cefotetan, cefoxitin, ceftazidime, ceftizoxime, ceftriaxone, cefuroxime, chlorpromazine, cimetidine, ciprofloxacin, cisplatin, cladribine, clindamycin, cyclophosphamide, cytarabine, dacarbazine, dactinomycin, daunorubicin, dexamethasone, diphenhydramine, dobutamine, dopamine, doxarubicin, doxycycline, droperidol, enalaprilat, etoposide, famotidine, filgrastim, fluconazole, fluorouracil, floxuridine, fludarabine, furosemide, gallium, ganciclovir, gentamicin, haloperidol, heparin hydrocortisone, hydromorphone, hydroxyzine, idarubicin, ifosfamide, imipenem-cilastatin, leucovorin, lorazepam, magnesium sulfate, melphalan, meperidine, mesna, methotrexate, methylprednisolone, metoclopramide, metronidazole, mezlocillin, miconazole, minocycline, mitomycin, mitoxantrone, morphine, nalbuphine, netilmicin, ofloxacin, paclitaxel, piperacillin, piperacillin/tazobactam, plicamycin, potassium chloride, prochlorperazine, promethazine, propofol, ranitidine, sargramostim, sodium bicarbonate, streptozocin, teniposide, thiotepa, ticarcillin, ticarcillin/clavulanate, tobramycin, trimethoprim-sulfamethoxazole, vancomycin, vinblastine, vincristine, vinorelbine, zidovudine

Perform/provide:
• Storage at room temp for 48 hr after dilution

Evaluate:

• Therapeutic response: absence of nausea, vomiting during cancer chemotherapy

Teach patient/family:

• To report diarrhea, constipation, rash, changes in respirations

---

grepafloxacin (℞)

(gre-pa-floks′a-sin)
Raxar
Func. class.: Antiinfective
Chem. class.: Fluoroquinolone

Action: Interferes with conversion of intermediate DNA fragments into high-molecular-weight DNA in bacteria; DNA gyrase inhibitor

Uses: Acute sinusitis, acute chronic bronchitis, community-acquired pneumonia, nongonococcal urethritis, cervicitis, uncomplicated gonorrhea caused by *S. pneumoniae, H. influenzae, H. parainfluenzae, M. catarrhalis*

Dosage and routes:

• *Adult:* **PO** 200-400 mg qd × 7-10 days

Uncomplicated gonorrhea

• **PO** 400 mg as a single dose

Available forms: Tabs 200 mg

Side effects/adverse reactions:

CNS: Headache, dizziness, insomnia, anxiety

GI: Nausea, flatulence, vomiting, diarrhea, abdominal pain, ***pseudomembranous colitis***

GU: Vaginitis, crystalluria

INTEG: Rash, pruritus, photosensitivity

Contraindications: Hypersensitivity to quinolones, photosensitivity, hepatic failure, prolonged QT

Precautions: Pregnancy (C), lactation, children

Pharmacokinetics: Peak 2-5 hr metabolized in the liver, excreted in urine unchanged

Lab test interferences:

Decrease: Glucose, lymphocytes

NURSING CONSIDERATIONS

Assess:

• For previous sensitivity reaction

• For signs and symptoms of infection: characteristics of sputum, WBC >10,000, fever; obtain baseline information before and during treatment

• C&S before beginning drug therapy to identify if correct treatment has been initiated

• For allergic reactions: rash, urticaria, pruritus, chills, fever, joint pain; may occur a few days after therapy begins; epinephrine and resuscitation equipment should be available for anaphylactic reaction

• Bowel pattern qd; if severe diarrhea occurs, drug should be discontinued

• For overgrowth of infection: perineal itching, fever, malaise, redness, pain, swelling, drainage, rash, diarrhea, change in cough, sputum

Evaluate:

• Therapeutic response: absence of signs/symptoms of infection (WBC <10,000/mm^3, temp WNL)

Teach patient/family:

• To contact prescriber if vaginal itching, loose, foul-smelling stools, furry tongue occur; may indicate superinfection; report itching, rash, pruritus, urticaria

• To notify prescriber of diarrhea with blood or pus

◆ = Nursing alert   🌿 = Herb-drug interaction   🚫 = Do not crush

griseofulvin microsize/ griseofulvin ultramicrosize (℞)

(gris-ee-oh-ful'vin)
Fulvicin P/G, Fulvicin-U/F, Grifulvin V, Grisactin, Grisactin 500, Grisactin-Ultra, Gris-PEG
Func. class.: Antifungal
Chem. class.: Penicillium griseofulvum derivative

Action: Arrests fungal cell division at metaphase; binds to human keratin, making it resistant to disease
Uses: Mycotic infections: tinea corporis, tinea pedis, tinea cruris, tinea barbae, tinea capitis, tinea unguium if caused by *Epidermophyton, Microsporum, Trichophyton*

Dosage and routes:
• *Adult:* **PO** 500-1000 mg qd in single or divided doses (microsize), 125-165 mg bid (ultramicrosize) or 250-330 mg qd; may need 500-660 mg in divided doses for severe infections
• *Child:* **PO** 10 mg/kg/day or 30 mg/m^2/day (microsize) or 5 mg/kg/day (ultramicrosize)
Available forms: Microcaps 125, 250 mg; tabs 250, 500 mg; oral susp 125 mg/ml; ultratabs 125, 165, 250, 330 mg

Side effects/adverse reactions:
INTEG: Rash, urticaria, photosensitivity, lichen planus
CNS: Headache, peripheral neuritis, paresthesias, confusion, dizziness, fatigue
EENT: Transient hearing loss
GU: Proteinuria, cylinduria, precipitate porphyria, increased thirst
GI: Nausea, vomiting, anorexia, diarrhea, cramps, dry mouth, flatulence
HEMA: Leukopenia, granulocytopenia, neutropenia, monocytosis

Contraindications: Hypersensitivity, porphyria, hepatic disease, lupus erythematosus
Precautions: Penicillin sensitivity, pregnancy (C)
Pharmacokinetics:
PO: Peak 4 hr, half-life 9-24 hr, metabolized in liver; excreted in urine (inactive metabolites), feces, perspiration
Interactions:
• Tachycardia: alcohol
• Decreased action of griseofulvin: barbiturates
• Decreased action of warfarin, cyclosporine, salicylates

NURSING CONSIDERATIONS
Assess:
• I&O ratio
• Liver studies qwk (ALT [SGPT], AST [SGOT], bilirubin, alk phosphatase)
• Renal studies: BUN, serum creatinine
• Blood studies: CBC, platelets, q2wk
• Drug level during treatment
• For history of penicillin allergy; may be cross-sensitive to this drug
⬥ For renal toxicity: increasing BUN, serum creatinine, proteinuria, cylinduria
• For hepatotoxicity: increasing ALT (SGPT), AST (SGOT), bilirubin, alk phosphatase
• For blood dyscrasias: fatigue, malaise, dark urine, bruising
Administer:
• Drug carefully, making sure there is no confusion with dosage form (microsize vs ultramicrosize)
• With meals to decrease GI symptoms; fatty meals for better absorption
• Until three separate cultures are negative for infective organism
Perform/provide:
• Storage in tight, light-resistant containers at room temp

G

---

aluate:

...erapeutic response: decreased
...malaise, rash, negative C&S
for infecting organism

Teach patient/family:
• That long-term therapy may be
needed to clear infection (2 wk-6
mo depending on organism)
• Proper hygiene: hand-washing
technique, nail care, use of concomitant topical agents if prescribed
• The importance of compliance
even after feeling better
• To avoid alcohol, since nausea,
vomiting, hypertension may occur
• To use sunscreen or avoid direct
sunlight to prevent photosensitivity
• To notify prescriber of sore throat,
fever, skin rash, which may indicate
overgrowth of organisms
• To use nonhormonal contraception

---

guaifenesin (OTC, R)

(gwye-fen′e-sin)

Amonidrin, Anti-tuss, Balminil*,
Breonesin, Fenesin, Gee-Gee,
Genatuss, GG-Cen, Glyate, Gly-
cotuss, Glytuss, Guaifenesin,
Guiatuss, Halotussin, Humibid,
Humibid L.A., Hytuss, Hytuss
ZX, Malotuss, Monafed, My-
tussin, Naldecon Senior EX,
Resyl*, Robitussin, Scot-Tussin
Expectorant, Sinumist-SR, Uni-
Tussin

Func. class.: Expectorant

Action: Acts as an expectorant by
stimulating a gastric mucosal reflex
to increase the production of lung
mucus

Uses: Dry, nonproductive cough

Dosage and routes:
• *Adult:* PO 100-400 mg q4-6h, not
to exceed 1.2 g/day; **SUS REL** 600-
1200 mg q12h, not to exceed 2.4
g/day

• *Child 6-12 yr:* PO 100-200 mg
q4h; 600 mg q12h (**SUS REL**) not
to exceed 1.2 g/day
• *Child 2-6 yr:* PO 50-100 mg q4h;
not to exceed 600 mg/day
Available forms: Tabs 100, 200 mg;
tabs, sus rel 600 mg; caps 200 mg;
syr 100 mg/5 ml

Side effects/adverse reactions:
CNS: Drowsiness
GI: Nausea, anorexia, vomiting

Contraindications: Hypersensitivity, persistent cough

Precautions: Pregnancy (C)

NURSING CONSIDERATIONS

Assess:
• Cough: type, frequency, character, including sputum; fluids should
be increased to 2 L/day

Perform/provide:
• Storage at room temp
• Increased fluids, room humidifi-
cation to liquefy secretions

Evaluate:
• Therapeutic response: absence of
cough

Teach patient/family:
• To avoid driving, other hazardous
activities if drowsiness occurs (rare)
• To avoid smoking, smoke-filled
room, perfumes, dust, environmental pollutants, cleansers

---

guanabenz (R)

(gwan′a-benz)

Wytensin

Func. class.: Antihypertensive
Chem. class.: Central α₂-
adrenergic agonist

Action: Stimulates central α₂-
adrenergic receptors in the CNS resulting in decreased sympathetic outflow from brain with decreased peripheral resistance

Uses: Hypertension

Dosage and routes:
• *Adult:* PO 4 mg bid, increasing in

---

increments of 4-8 mg/day q1-2wk, not to exceed 32 mg bid
Available forms: Tabs 4, 8 mg
Side effects/adverse reactions:
RESP: Dyspnea
*CV: **Severe rebound hypertension,** chest pain, **dysrhythmias,** palpitations, hypotension*
CNS: Drowsiness, dizziness, sedation, headache, depression, weakness
EENT: Nasal congestion, blurred vision
GI: Nausea, diarrhea, constipation, dry mouth, anorexia, abnormal taste
GU: Impotence, frequency, gynecomastia
MS: Backache, extremities pain
Contraindications: Hypersensitivity to guanabenz
Precautions: Pregnancy (C), lactation, children <12 yr, severe coronary insufficiency, recent myocardial infarction, cerebrovascular disease, severe hepatic or renal failure, elderly
Pharmacokinetics:
PO: Onset 1 hr, peak 2-4 hr; half-life 4-14 hr; excreted in urine
Interactions:
• Increased sedation: CNS depressants
NURSING CONSIDERATIONS
Assess:
• Renal studies: protein, BUN, creatinine; watch for increased levels
• Baselines in renal, liver function tests before therapy begins
• B/P during beginning treatment, periodically thereafter
• Edema in feet and legs daily
• Allergic reaction: rash, fever, pruritus, urticaria; drug should be discontinued if antihistamines fail to help
• Renal symptoms: polyuria, oliguria, frequency
Administer:
• In AM, at hs

Evaluate:
• Therapeutic response: decrease in B/P
Teach patient/family:
• To avoid hazardous activities; sedation may occur
• Not to discontinue drug abruptly, or withdrawal symptoms may occur: anxiety, increased B/P, headache, insomnia, increased pulse, tremors, nausea, sweating
• Not to use OTC (cough, cold, or allergy) products unless directed by prescriber
• The importance of complying with dosage schedule even if feeling better
• To notify prescriber of swelling of hands or feet, irregular heartbeat, chest pain
• About excessive perspiration, dehydration, vomiting, diarrhea; may lead to fall in blood pressure; consult prescriber if these occur
• That drug may cause dizziness, fainting; light-headedness may occur during first few days of therapy
• That compliance is necessary; not to skip or stop drug unless directed by prescriber
• That drug may cause skin rash or impaired perspiration
Treatment of overdose: Administer vasopressor, discontinue drug; supine position

G

---

guanadrel (℞)
(gwahn'a-drel)
Hylorel
Func. class.: Antihypertensive
Chem. class.: Adrenergic blocker, peripheral guanethidine derivative

Action: Inhibits sympathetic vasoconstriction by inhibiting release of norepinephrine, depletes norepinephrine stores in adrenergic nerve endings, adrenal medulla

Uses: Hypertension (moderate to severe as an adjunct)

Dosage and routes:

• *Adult:* **PO** 5 mg bid, adjusted to desired response weekly or monthly; may need 20-75 mg/day in divided doses; higher doses are given tid or qid

• *Geriatric:* **PO** 5 mg/day, titrate as needed

Renal dose

• CrCl 10-50 ml/min dose q12-24h; CrCl <10 ml/min dose q24-48h

Available forms: Tabs 10, 25 mg

Side effects/adverse reactions:

*CV: Orthostatic hypotension, **bradycardia, CHF,** palpitations, chest pain, **tachycardia, dysrhythmias***

CNS: Drowsiness, fatigue, weakness, feeling of faintness, insomnia, dizziness, mental changes, memory loss, hallucinations, depression, anxiety, confusion, paresthesias, headache

GI: Nausea, cramps, diarrhea, constipation, dry mouth, anorexia, indigestion

INTEG: Rash, purpura, alopecia

EENT: Nasal stuffiness, tinnitus, visual changes, sore throat, double vision, dry, burning eyes

GU: Ejaculation failure, impotence, dysuria, nocturia, frequency

*RESP: **Bronchospasm,** dyspnea,* cough, rales, SOB

MS: Leg cramps, aching, pain, inflammation

Contraindications: Hypersensitivity, pheochromocytoma, lactation, CHF, child <18 yr

Precautions: Elderly, pregnancy (B), bronchial asthma, peptic ulcer, electrolyte imbalances, vascular disease

Pharmacokinetics:

PO: Onset 0.5-2 hr, peak 4-6 hr, duration 8 hr; half-life 10-12 hr; metabolized in liver 50%; excreted in urine (50% unchanged)

Interactions:

• Increased hypotension: diuretics, other antihypertensives

• Do not use with MAOIs

• Increased orthostatic hypotension: alcohol, opioids

• Decreased hypotensive effect: tricyclic antidepressants, phenothiazines, ephedrine, phenylpropanolamine

NURSING CONSIDERATIONS

Assess:

• Renal function studies in renal impairment (BUN, creatinine)

• Bleeding time; check for ecchymosis, thrombocytopenia, purpura

• I&O in renal disease patient

• Cardiac status: B/P lying and standing, pulse; watch for hypotension

• Edema in feet, legs daily; take weight daily

• Skin turgor, dryness of mucous membranes for hydration status

• Symptoms of CHF: edema, dyspnea, wet rales

Perform/provide:

• Storage in air-tight container

Evaluate:

• Therapeutic response: decreased B/P

Teach patient/family:

• To avoid driving and performing hazardous activities if drowsiness occurs

• Not to discontinue drug abruptly

• Not to use OTC cough, cold preparations unless directed by prescriber

• To report bradycardia, dizziness, confusion, depression, fever, or sore throat

• That impotence, gynecomastia may occur but are reversible

• To rise slowly to sitting or stand-

 = Nursing alert   = Herb-drug interaction   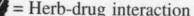 = Do not crush

ing position to minimize orthostatic hypotension
• That therapeutic effect may take 2-4 wk

---

guanethidine (℞)

(gwahn-eth'i-deen)
Apo-Guanethidine*, guanethidine sulfate*, Ismelin
Func. class.: Antihypertensive
Chem. class.: Antiadrenergic agent, peripheral

Action: Inhibits norepinephrine release, depleting norepinephrine stores in adrenergic nerve endings

Uses: Moderate to severe hypertension

Dosage and routes:
• *Adult:* **PO** 10-12.5 mg qd, increase by 10 mg qwk; may require 25-50 mg qd
• *Adult:* (hospitalized) 25-50 mg; may increase by 25-50 mg/day or every other day
• *Child:* **PO** 0.2 mg/kg/day; (6 mg/m²/day) increase q7-10d, 0.2 mg/kg or 6 mg/m²/day not to exceed 3000 µg/kg/24 hr

Available forms: Tabs 10, 25 mg

Side effects/adverse reactions:
CV: Orthostatic hypotension, dizziness, weakness, bradycardia, **CHF,** fatigue, angina, heart block, chest paresthesia
CNS: Depression
GI: Nausea, vomiting, *diarrhea,* constipation, dry mouth, weight gain, anorexia, abdominal pain
INTEG: Dermatitis, loss of scalp hair
EENT: Nasal congestion, ptosis, blurred vision
GU: Ejaculation failure, impotence, nocturia, edema, *retention,* increased BUN, *frequency*

RESP: Dyspnea, cough, shortness of breath

Contraindications: Hypersensitivity, pheochromocytoma, recent MI, CHF, cardiac failure, sinus bradycardia

Precautions: Pregnancy (B), lactation, peptic ulcer, asthma

Pharmacokinetics:
PO: Therapeutic level 1-3 wk; half-life 5 days; metabolized by liver; excreted in urine (metabolites), breast milk

Interactions:
• Increased hypotension: diuretics, other antihypertensives
• Do not use with MAOIs
• Increased orthostatic hypotension: alcohol
• Decreased hypotensive effect: tricyclic antidepressants, phenothiazines, ephedrine, phenylpropanolamine, oral contraceptives, thiothixene, doxepin, haloperidol, amphetamines

Lab test interferences:
Increase: BUN
Decrease: Blood glucose, VMA excretion, urinary norepinephrine

NURSING CONSIDERATIONS
Assess:
• Renal function studies in renal impairment (BUN, creatinine)
• Bleeding time; check for ecchymosis, thrombocytopenia, purpura
• I&O in renal disease patient
• Cardiac status: B/P, pulse; watch for hypotension
• Edema in feet, legs daily; take weight daily
• Skin turgor, dryness of mucous membranes for hydration status
• Symptoms of CHF: edema, dyspnea, wet rales

Evaluate:
• Therapeutic response: decreased B/P

Teach patient/family:

• To avoid driving, hazardous activities if drowsiness occurs

• Not to discontinue drug abruptly

• Not to use OTC cough, cold preparations unless directed by prescriber

• To report bradycardia, dizziness, confusion, depression, fever, sore throat

• That impotence, gynecomastia may occur but are reversible

• To rise slowly to sitting or standing position to minimize orthostatic hypotension; more common in AM, hot weather, during exercise, or when using alcohol

• That therapeutic effect may take 2-4 wk

• To notify prescriber of severe diarrhea

Treatment of overdose: Lavage, vasopressors given cautiously

---

guanfacine (℞)

(gwahn'fa-seen)
Tenex
Func. class.: Antihypertensive
Chem. class.: α₂-adrenergic receptor agonist

Action: Stimulates central α-adrenergic receptors, resulting in decreased sympathetic outflow from brain

Uses: Hypertension in individual using a thiazide diuretic

Dosage and routes:

• *Adult:* **PO** 1 mg/day hs; may increase dose in 2-3 wk to 2-3 mg/day

Available forms: Tabs 1 mg

Side effects/adverse reactions:

GI: Dry mouth, constipation, cramps, nausea, diarrhea

CNS: Somnolence, dizziness, headache, fatigue

GU: Impotence, urinary incontinence

EENT: Taste change, tinnitus, vision change, rhinitis, nasal congestion

MS: Leg cramps

RESP: Dyspnea

INTEG: Dermatitis, pruritus, purpura

CV: Bradycardia, chest pain

Contraindications: Hypersensitivity

Precautions: Pregnancy (B), lactation, children <12 yr, severe coronary insufficiency, recent MI, renal or hepatic disease, CVA, elderly

Pharmacokinetics: Peak 1-4 hr; 70% bound to plasma proteins; half-life 17 hr; eliminated via kidneys unchanged and as metabolites

Interactions:

• Increased sedation: CNS depressants, other antihypertensives

• Decreased hypotensive effect: tricyclic antidepressants

NURSING CONSIDERATIONS

Assess:

• Blood studies: neutrophils, decrease in platelets

• Baselines in renal, liver function tests before therapy begins

• B/P before, during, after treatment; notify prescriber of significant changes

• Edema in feet, legs daily

• Allergic reaction: rash, fever, pruritus, urticaria; drug should be discontinued if antihistamines fail to help

• Symptoms of CHF: edema, dyspnea, wet rales, B/P

• Renal symptoms: polyuria, oliguria, frequency

Perform/provide:

• Storage of tablets in tight container

Evaluate:

• Therapeutic response: decreased B/P in hypertension

◆ = Nursing alert   ⚕ = Herb-drug interaction   ⊘ = Do not crush

Teach patient/family:
• To avoid hazardous activities
• Not to discontinue drug abruptly or withdrawal symptoms may occur: anxiety, increased B/P, headache, insomnia, increased pulse, tremors, nausea, sweating
• Not to use OTC (cough, cold, or allergy) products unless directed by prescriber
• To avoid sunlight or to wear sunscreen; photosensitivity may occur
• The importance of complying with dosage schedule even if feeling better

---

haemophilus b vaccines (℞)

(hee-moef'ih-lus)
b-Capsa 1, Hib-Imune, HibVAX (polysaccharide), HibTITER, Pedvax-HIB, ProHIBit (conjugate)
Func. class.: Vaccine
Chem. class.: H. influenzae capsular polysaccharide

Action: Stimulates antibody production to *H. influenzae b*
Uses: Polysaccharide immunization of children 2-6 yr against *H. influenzae b,* conjugate immunization of child 2, 4, 6 mo; 6 mo dose not needed in Pedvax HIB; booster at 12-18 mo against invasive disease of *H. influenzae b*
Dosage and routes:
• *Child:* **SC** 0.5 ml (polysaccharide), **IM** 0.5 mg (conjugate)
Available forms: Polysaccharide powder for injection 25 µg/0.5 ml after reconstituting; conjugate powder for inj 25 µg polysaccharide and 18 µg conjugated diphtheria toxoid/0.5 ml

Side effects/adverse reactions:
INTEG: Redness, soreness at injection site, rash
SYST: Low-grade fever, acute febrile reactions
Contraindications: Hypersensitivity, febrile illness, active infection
Precautions: Pregnancy (C)
Lab test interferences:
Interference: Latex agglutination, countercurrent immunoelectrophoresis
NURSING CONSIDERATIONS
Assess:
• For skin reactions: swelling, rash, urticaria
• For anaphylaxis: inability to breathe, bronchospasm
Administer:
• After diluting with 0.6 ml diluent, which will yield 10 doses of 0.5 ml
• Only with epinephrine 1:1000 on unit to treat laryngospasm
• Only by SC or IM route
Perform/provide:
• Storage in refrigerator
• Written record of immunization
Evaluate:
• For history of allergies, skin conditions (eczema, psoriasis, dermatitis), reactions to vaccinations

---

halazepam (℞)

(hal-az'e-pam)
Paxipam
Func. class.: Sedative-hypnotic
Chem. class.: Benzodiazepine

Controlled Substance Schedule IV
Action: Depresses subcortical levels of CNS, including limbic system, reticular formation
Uses: Anxiety
Dosage and routes:
• *Adult:* **PO** 20-40 mg tid-qid
• *Elderly:* **PO** 20 mg qd-bid
Available forms: Tabs 20, 40 mg

Side effects/adverse reactions:

CNS: Dizziness, drowsiness, confusion, headache, anxiety, tremors, stimulation, fatigue, depression, insomnia, hallucinations
GI: Constipation, dry mouth, nausea, vomiting, anorexia, diarrhea
INTEG: Rash, dermatitis, itching
CV: Orthostatic hypotension, ECG changes, tachycardia, hypotension
EENT: Blurred vision, tinnitus, mydriasis

Contraindications: Hypersensitivity to benzodiazepines, narrow-angle glaucoma, psychosis, pregnancy (D), lactation, child <18 yr

Precautions: Elderly, debilitated, hepatic disease, renal disease

Pharmacokinetics:

PO: Peak 1-3 hr, duration 3-6 hr; metabolized by liver; excreted by kidneys; crosses placenta, breast milk; half-life 14 hr; half-life active metabolite 50-400 hr

Interactions:

• Decreased effects of halazepam: oral contraceptives, valproic acid
• Increased effects of halazepam: CNS depressants, alcohol, disulfiram, oral contraceptives, cimetidine
• Increased risk of digoxin toxicity: digoxin
🍃 Increased action: kava kava

Lab test interferences:

Increase: AST (SGOT), ALT (SGPT), serum bilirubin
False increase: 17-OHCS
Decrease: RAIU

NURSING CONSIDERATIONS
Assess:

• B/P (lying, standing), pulse; if systolic B/P drops 20 mm Hg, hold drug, notify prescriber
• Blood studies: CBC during long-term therapy; blood dyscrasias have occurred rarely

• Hepatic studies: AST (SGOT), ALT (SGPT), bilirubin, creatinine, LDH, alk phosphatase
• Mental status: mood, sensorium, affect, sleeping pattern, drowsiness, dizziness
• Physical dependency, withdrawal symptoms: headache, nausea, vomiting, muscle pain, weakness after long-term use
• Suicidal tendencies

Administer:

• With food or milk for GI symptoms
• Crushed if patient is unable to swallow medication whole
• Sugarless gum, hard candy, frequent sips of water for dry mouth

Perform/provide:

• Assistance with ambulation during beginning therapy, since drowsiness/dizziness occurs
• Check to see if PO medication has been swallowed

Evaluate:

• Therapeutic response: decreased anxiety, restlessness, sleeplessness

Teach patient/family:

• That drug may be taken with food
• That medication is not to be used for everyday stress or used longer than 4 mo unless directed by prescriber; not to take more than prescribed amount; may be habit forming
• To avoid OTC preparations (hay fever, cough, cold) unless approved by prescriber
• To avoid driving or other activities that require alertness; drowsiness may occur
• To avoid alcohol ingestion or other psychotropic medications unless prescribed by prescriber
• Not to discontinue medication abruptly after long-term use
• To rise slowly or fainting may occur

◆ = Nursing alert   🍃 = Herb-drug interaction   🚫 = Do not crush

• That drowsiness may worsen at beginning of treatment

Treatment of overdose: Lavage, VS, supportive care, flumazenil

---

halofantrine (℞)

(hal-o-fan'treen)
Halfan

Func. class.: Antimalarial
Chem. class.: Synthetic 4-amino-quinoline derivative

Action: Inhibits parasite replications, transcription of DNA to RNA by forming complexes with DNA of parasite

Uses: Malaria caused by *P. vivax, P. malariae, P. ovale, P. falciparum* (multidrug resistant)

Dosage and routes:
• *Adult:* 500 mg **PO** q6h × 3 doses
• *Children <40 kg:* **PO** 8 mg/kg q6h × 3 doses

Available forms: Tabs 500 mg

Side effects/adverse reactions:

CV: Hypotension, heart block, ***asystole with syncope,*** ECG changes

INTEG: Pruritus, pigmentary changes, skin eruptions, lichen planus-like eruptions, eczema, exfoliative dermatitis, alopecia

CNS: Headache, stimulation, fatigue, irritability, ***convulsion,*** bad dreams, dizziness, confusion, psychosis, decreased reflexes

EENT: Blurred vision, corneal changes, retinal changes, difficulty focusing, tinnitus, vertigo, deafness, photophobia, corneal edema

GI: Nausea, vomiting, anorexia, diarrhea, cramps, weight loss, stomatitis

HEMA: ***Thrombocytopenia, agranulocytosis, hemolytic anemia, leukopenia***

Contraindications: Hypersensitivity, retinal field changes, porphyria, children (long-term)

Precautions: Pregnancy (C), children, blood dyscrasias, severe GI disease, neurologic disease, alcoholism, hepatic disease, G6PD deficiency, psoriasis, eczema

Pharmacokinetics:

PO: Peak 1-2 hr, half-life 3-5 days; metabolized in liver; excreted in urine, feces, breast milk; crosses placenta

Interactions:
• Decreased action of chloroquine, magnesium, aluminum compounds, kaolin

NURSING CONSIDERATIONS

Assess:
• Ophthalmic test if long-term treatment or drug dosage 150 mg/day
• Liver studies qwk: AST (SGOT), ALT (SGPT), bilirubin
• Blood studies: CBC, since blood dyscrasias occur
• For decreased reflexes: knee, ankle
• ECG during therapy
• Watch for depression of T waves, widening of QRS complex
• Allergic reactions: pruritus, rash, urticaria
• Blood dyscrasias: malaise, fever, bruising, bleeding (rare)
• For ototoxicity (tinnitus, vertigo, change in hearing); audiometric testing should be done before, after treatment
➤ For toxicity: blurring vision, difficulty focusing, headache, dizziness, knee, ankle reflexes; drug should be discontinued immediately

Administer:
• Before or after meals at same time each day to maintain drug level

Perform/provide:
• Storage in tight, light-resistant containers at room temp; injection should be kept in cool environment

---

Evaluate:
• Therapeutic response: decreased symptoms of infection

Teach patient/family:
• To use sunglasses in bright sunlight to decrease photophobia
• That urine may turn rust or brown
• To report hearing, visual problems, fever, fatigue, bruising, bleeding, which may indicate blood dyscrasias

Treatment of overdose: Induce vomiting; gastric lavage; administer barbiturate (ultrashort-acting), vasopressin; tracheostomy may be necessary

---

haloperidol (℞)

(ha-loe-per′ih-dole)
Apo-Haloperidol*, Haldol*, Haldol L.A.*, haloperidol, Haloperidol Decanoate 50, Haloperidol 100, Novoperidol*, Peridol*

Func. class.: Antipsychotic, neuroleptic
Chem. class.: Butyrophenone

Action: Depresses cerebral cortex, hypothalamus, limbic system, which control activity and aggression; blocks neurotransmission produced by dopamine at synapse; exhibits strong α-adrenergic, anticholinergic blocking action; mechanism for antipsychotic effects unclear

Uses: Psychotic disorders, control of tics, vocal utterances in Gilles de la Tourette's syndrome, short-term treatment of hyperactive children showing excessive motor activity, prolonged parenteral therapy in chronic schizophrenia, control of severe nausea and vomiting in chemotherapy, organic mental syndrome with psychotic features, hiccups (short-term)

Dosage and routes:
Psychosis
• *Adult:* PO 0.5-5 mg bid or tid initially depending on severity of condition; dose is increased to desired dose, max 100 mg/day; IM 2-5 mg q1-8h
• *Geriatric:* 0.25-0.5 mg qd-bid, titrate q3-4 days by 0.25-0.5 mg/dose
• *Child 3-12 yr:* PO/IM 0.05-0.15 mg/kg/day
• *Decanoate:* Initial dose IM is 10-15 × daily oral dose at 4 wk interval; do not administer IV; not to exceed 100 mg
Chronic schizophrenia
• *Adult:* IM 10-15 times PO dose q4wk (decanoate)
• *Child 3-12 yr:* PO/IM 0.05-0.15 mg/kg/day
Tics/vocal utterances
• *Adult:* PO 0.5-5 mg bid or tid, increased until desired response occurs
• *Child 3-12 yr:* PO 0.05-0.075 mg/kg/day
Hyperactive children
• *Child 3-12 yr:* PO 0.05-0.075 mg/kg/day
Available forms: Tabs 0.5, 1, 2, 5, 10, 20 mg; conc 2 mg/ml; inj 5 mg/ml, 50 mg base/ml, 100 mg base/ml

Side effects/adverse reactions:
RESP: **Laryngospasm,** dyspnea, *respiratory depression*
CNS: EPS: *pseudoparkinsonism, akathisia, dystonia, tardive dyskinesia, drowsiness, headache,* **seizures, neuroleptic malignant syndrome,** confusion
INTEG: Rash, photosensitivity, dermatitis
EENT: Blurred vision, glaucoma, dry eyes
GI: Dry mouth, nausea, vomiting, anorexia, constipation, diarrhea, jaundice, weight gain, *ileus,* **hepatitis**

◆ = Nursing alert   ◢ = Herb-drug interaction   ⊗ = Do not crush

GU: Urinary retention, urinary frequency, enuresis, impotence, amenorrhea, gynecomastia

CV: Orthostatic hypotension, hypertension, *cardiac arrest,* ECG changes, *tachycardia*

Contraindications: Hypersensitivity, blood dyscrasias, coma, child <3 yr, brain damage, bone marrow depression, alcohol and barbiturate withdrawal states, Parkinson's disease, angina, epilepsy, urinary retention, narrow-angle glaucoma

Precautions: Pregnancy (C), lactation, seizure disorders, hypertension, hepatic disease, cardiac disease, elderly

Pharmacokinetics:

PO: Onset erratic, peak 2-6 hr, half-life 24 hr

IM: Onset 15-30 min, peak 15-20 min, half-life 21 hr

IM (Decanoate): Peak 4-11 days, half-life 3 wk

Metabolized by liver; excreted in urine, bile; crosses placenta; enters breast milk

Interactions:

• Oversedation: other CNS depressants, alcohol, barbiturate anesthetics

• Toxicity: epinephrine

• Toxicity: lithium, neurotoxicity and brain damage possible

• Decreased effects of lithium, levodopa

• Increased effects of both drugs: β-adrenergic blockers, alcohol

• Increased anticholinergic effects: anticholinergics

• Decreased effects of haloperidol: phenobarbital

⚡ Increased action: kava kava

Lab test interferences:

Increase: Liver function tests, cardiac enzymes, cholesterol, blood glucose, prolactin, bilirubin, PBI, cholinesterase

Decrease: Hormones (blood, urine)

False positive: Pregnancy tests, PKU

False negative: Urinary steroids

NURSING CONSIDERATIONS

Assess:

• Swallowing of PO medication; check for hoarding or giving of medication to other patients

• I&O ratio; palpate bladder if low urinary output occurs

• Bilirubin, CBC, liver function studies monthly

• Urinalysis is recommended before and during prolonged therapy

• For depression in bipolar patients; rapid mood swings may occur with this drug

• Affect, orientation, LOC, reflexes, gait, coordination, sleep pattern disturbances

• B/P standing and lying; take pulse and respirations q4h during initial treatment; establish baseline before starting treatment; report drops of 30 mm Hg

• Dizziness, faintness, palpitations, tachycardia on rising

• EPS including akathisia (inability to sit still, no pattern to movements), tardive dyskinesia (bizarre movements of jaw, mouth, tongue, extremities), pseudoparkinsonism (rigidity, tremors, pill rolling, shuffling gait)

• Skin turgor daily

➡ For neuroleptic malignant syndrome: hyperthermia, muscle rigidity, altered mental status, increased CPK

• Constipation, urinary retention daily; if these occur, increase bulk, water in diet

Administer:

• Reduced dose to elderly

• Antiparkinsonian agent, to be used if EPS occur

• IM inj into large muscle mass, use 21 G, 2″ needle; give no more than

3 ml/inj site; patient should remain recumbent for ½ hr
• Oral liquid: use calibrated dropper; do not mix in coffee or tea
• PO with food or milk

Solution compatibilities: D$_5$W

Syringe compatibilities: Hydromorphone, sufentanil

Y-site compatibilities: Amifostine, amsacrine, aztreonam, cimetidine, cladribine, dobutamine, dopamine, famotidine, filgrastim, fludarabine, granisetron, lidocaine, lorazepam, melphalan, midazolam, nitroglycerin, norepinephrine, ondansetron, paclitaxel, phenylephrine, propofol, sufentanil, tacrolimus, teniposide, theophylline, thiotepa, vinorelbine

Perform/provide:
• Decreased noise input by dimming lights, avoiding loud noises
• Supervised ambulation until stabilized on medication; do not involve in strenuous exercise program because fainting is possible; patient should not stand still for long periods
• Increased fluids to prevent constipation
• Sips of water, candy, gum for dry mouth
• Storage in tight, light-resistant container

Evaluate:
• Therapeutic response: decrease in emotional excitement, hallucinations, delusions, paranoia, reorganization of patterns of thought, speech, improvement in specific behaviors

Teach patient/family:
• That orthostatic hypotension occurs often and to rise from sitting or lying position gradually
• To avoid hazardous activities until stabilized on medication
• To remain lying down after IM inj for at least 30 min
• To avoid hot tubs, hot showers, tub baths, since hypotension may occur
• To avoid abrupt withdrawal of this drug, or EPS may result; drug should be withdrawn slowly
• To avoid OTC preparations (cough, hay fever, cold) unless approved by prescriber, since serious drug interactions may occur; avoid use with alcohol, CNS depressants; increased drowsiness may occur
• To use a sunscreen to prevent burns
• Regarding compliance with drug regimen
• About EPS and necessity for meticulous oral hygiene, since oral candidiasis may occur
• To report impaired vision, jaundice, tremors, muscle twitching
• That in hot weather, heat stroke may occur; take extra precautions to stay cool

Treatment of overdose: Activated charcoal lavage if orally ingested; provide an airway; do not induce vomiting

---

heparin (℞)

(hep′a-rin)
Calcilean*, Calciparine*, Hepalean*, Heparin Leo*, Heparin Lock Flush, heparin sodium, Heparin Sodium and 0.45% Sodium Chloride, Heparin Sodium and 0.9% Sodium Chloride , Hep-Lock, Hep-Lock U/P, Liquaemin Sodium

Func. class.: Anticoagulant

Action: Prevents conversion of fibrinogen to fibrin and prothrombin to thrombin by enhancing inhibitory effects of antithrombin III

Uses: Deep-vein thrombosis, pulmonary emboli, myocardial infarction, open heart surgery, disseminated intravascular clotting syndrome, atrial fibrillation with embolization, as an anticoagulant in transfusion and dialysis procedures, prevention of DVT/PE

Dosage and routes:

Deep-vein thrombosis/MI
• *Adult:* IV PUSH 5000-7000 U q4h then titrated to PTT or ACT level; IV BOL 5000-7500 U, then IV INF; IV INF after bolus dose, then 1000 U/hr titrated to PTT or ACT level
• *Child:* IV INF 50 U/kg, maintenance 100 U/kg q4h or 20,000 U/m² qd

Pulmonary embolism
• *Adult:* IV PUSH 7500-10,000 U q4h then titrated to PTT or ACT level; IV BOL 7500-10,000, then IV INF; IV INF after bolus dose, then 1000 U/hr titrated to PTT or ACT level
• *Child:* IV INF 50 U/kg, maintenance 100 U/kg q4h or 20,000 U/m² qd

Open heart surgery
• *Adult:* IV INF 150-300 U/kg

Prophylaxis for DVT/PE
• *Adult:* SC 5,000 U q8-12h

Heparin flush
• *Adult and child:* IV 10-100 U

Available forms: Heparin sodium inj 10, 1000, 5000, 10,000, 20,000, 40,000 U/ml; heparin calcium inj 5000 U/0.2 ml

Side effects/adverse reactions:
CNS: Fever, chills
GI: Diarrhea, nausea, vomiting, anorexia, stomatitis, abdominal cramps, *hepatitis*
GU: Hematuria
HEMA: Hemorrhage, thrombocytopenia
INTEG: Rash, dermatitis, urticaria, alopecia, pruritus

Contraindications: Hypersensitivity, hemophilia, leukemia with bleeding, peptic ulcer disease, thrombocytopenic purpura, hepatic disease (severe), renal disease (severe), blood dyscrasias, severe hypertension, subacute bacterial endocarditis, acute nephritis

Precautions: Alcoholism, elderly, pregnancy (C)

Pharmacokinetics: Well absorbed (SC)
IV: Peak 5 min, duration 2-6 hr
SC: Onset 20-60 min, duration 8-12 hr
Half-life 1½ hr, excreted in urine, 95% bound to plasma proteins, does not cross placenta or alter breast milk; removed from the system via the lymph and spleen

Interactions:
• Decreased action of corticosteroids
• Increased action of diazepam
• Decreased action of heparin: digitalis, tetracyclines, antihistamines
• Increased action of heparin: oral anticoagulants, salicylates, dextran, steroids, nonsteroidal antiinflammatories
🝙 Increased risk of bleeding: bromelain, cinchona bark

Lab test interferences:
False increase: T₃ uptake, serum thyroxine, BSP
Decrease: Uric acid
False negative: ¹²⁵I fibrinogen uptake

NURSING CONSIDERATIONS
Assess:
• Blood studies (Hct, occult blood in stools) q3mo
• Partial prothrombin time, which should be 1.5-2 × control, PTT often done qd, also APTT, ACT
• Platelet count q2-3d; thrombocytopenia may occur on 4th day of treatment
◆ Bleeding gums, petechiae, ecchymosis, black tarry stools, hematuria, epistaxis, decrease in Hct, B/P;

indicate bleeding and possible hemorrhage

• Fever, skin rash, urticaria
• Needed dosage change q1-2wk

Administer:

• At same time each day to maintain steady blood levels
• SC deep with 25G ⅜″ needle; do not massage area or aspirate when giving SC injection; give in abdomen between pelvic bone, rotate sites; do not pull back on plunger, leave in for 10 sec; apply gentle pressure for 1 min
• Changing needles is not recommended
• Avoiding all IM injections that may cause bleeding

IV

• Diluted in 0.9% NaCl, dextrose, Ringer's sol and given by direct, intermittent, or continuous infusion; give 1000 U or less over 1 min; then 5000 U or less over 1 min; infusion may run from 4-24 hr; use infusion pump
• Blood after adding 7500 U/100 ml NaCl inj, add 6-8 ml of this sol/100 ml of whole blood

Additive compatibilities: Aminophylline, amphotericin, ascorbic acid, bleomycin, calcium gluconate, cefepime, cephapirin, chloramphenicol, clindamycin, cloxacillin, colistimethate, dimenhydrinate, dopamine, enalaprilat, erythromycin gluceptate, esmolol, floxacillin, fluconazole, flumazenil, furosemide, hydrocortisone, isoproterenol, lidocaine, lincomycin, magnesium sulfate, meropenem, methyldopa, methylprednisolone, metronidazole/sodium bicarbonate, nafcillin, norepinephrine, octreotide, penicillin G, potassium chloride, prednisolone, promazine, ranitidine, sodium bicarbonate, verapamil, vit B, vit B/C

Syringe compatibilities: Aminophylline, amphotericin B, ampi-

cillin, atropine, azlocillin, bleomycin, cefamandole, cefazolin, cefoperazone, cefotaxime, cefoxitin, chloramphenicol, cimetidine, cisplatin, clindamycin, cyclophosphamide, diazoxide, digoxin, dimenhydrinate, dobutamine, dopamine, epinephrine, fentanyl, fluorouracil, furosemide, leucovorin, lidocaine, lincomycin, methotrexate, metoclopramide, mezlocillin, mitomycin, moxalactam, nafcillin, naloxone, neostigmine, nitroglycerin, norepinephrine, pancuronium, penicillin G, phenobarbital, piperacillin, sodium nitroprusside, succinylcholine, trimethoprim-sulfamethoxazole, verapamil, vincristine

Y-site compatibilities: Acyclovir, aldesleukin, allopurinol, amifostine, aminophylline, ampicillin, ampicillin/sulbactam, atracurium, atropine, aztreonam, betamethasone, bleomycin, calcium gluconate, cefazolin, cefotetan, cefotiam, ceftazidime, ceftriaxone, cephalothin, cephapirin, chlordiazepoxide, chlorpromazine, cimetidine, cisplatin, cladribine, clindamycin, conjugated estrogens, cyanocobalamin, cyclophosphamide, cytarabine, dexamethasone, digoxin, diphenhydramine, dopamine, edrophonium, enalaprilat, epinephrine, erythromycin, esmolol, ethacrynate, famotidine, fentanyl, fluconazole, fludarabine, fluorouracil, foscarnet, furosemide, gallium, granisetron, hydralazine, hydrocortisone, hydromorphone, insulin (regular), isoproterenol, kanamycin, leucovorin, lidocaine, lorazepam, magnesium sulfate, melphalan, menadiol, meperidine, meropenem, methicillin, methotrexate, methoxamine, methyldopa, methylergonovine, metoclopramide, metronidazole, midazolam, milrinone, minocycline, mitomycin, morphine, nafcillin, neostigmine, nitroglyc-

...eathe, bronchospasm, hypoten-
...on, wheezing, diaphoresis, fever,
flushing

Administer:
• After rotating vial; do not shake
• Only with epinephrine 1:1000 on
unit to treat laryngospasm
• In deltoid for better absorption;
give 2 ml dose in two different sites

Perform/provide:
• Written record of immunization
• Comfort measures

Evaluate:
• Prevention of hepatitis B

---

hetastarch (℞)
(het'a-starch)
Hespan
Func. class.: Plasma expander
Chem. class.: Synthetic poly-
mer

Action: Similar to human albumin,
which expands plasma volume by
colloidal osmotic pressure

Uses: Plasma volume expander, leukapheresis

Dosage and routes:
• *Adult:* IV INF 500-1000 ml (30-60
g), total dose not to exceed 1500
ml/day, not to exceed 20 ml/kg/hr
(hemorrhagic shock)

Leukapheresis
• *Adult:* IV INF 250-700 ml infused at 1:8 ratio with whole blood,
may be repeated 2/wk up to 10 treatments

Available forms: 6% hetastarch/
0.9% NaCl inj

Side effects/adverse reactions:
HEMA: Decreased hematocrit, platelet function, increased bleeding/
coagulation times, increased sed rate
INTEG: Rash, urticaria, pruritus, angioedema, chills, fever, flushing, peripheral edema

RESP: Wheezing, dyspnea, ***bron-
chospasm, pulmonary edema***
GI: Nausea, vomiting
EENT: Periorbital edema
SYST: **Anaphylaxis**
CNS: Headache

Contraindications: Hypersensitivity, severe bleeding disorders, renal
failure, CHF (severe)

Precautions: Pregnancy (C), liver
disease, pulmonary edema

Pharmacokinetics:
IV: Expands blood volume 1-2 ×
amount infused, excreted in urine

Lab test interferences:
False increase: Bilirubin

NURSING CONSIDERATIONS
Assess:
• VS q5min × 30 min; CVP during
infusion (5-10 cm H$_2$O normal
range), PCWP
• Monitor CBC with differential,
Hgb, Hct, pro-time, PTT, platelet
count, clotting time during treatment; Hct may drop; do not allow to
drop >30% by vol
• Urine output q1h, watch for increase in urinary output, which is
common; if output does not increase,
infusion should be decreased or discontinued
• I&O ratio and specific gravity,
urine osmolarity; if specific gravity
is very low, renal clearance is low;
drug should be discontinued
• Allergy: rash, urticaria, pruritus,
wheezing, dyspnea, bronchospasm;
drug should be discontinued immediately
 For circulatory overload:
increased pulse, respirations,
SOB, wheezing, chest tightness,
chest pain
• For dehydration after infusion: decreased output, fever, poor skin turgor, increased specific gravity, dry
skin

Administer:
IV
• INF undiluted, run at 20 ml/kg/hr (1.2 g/kg); reduced rate in septic shock, burns
Additive compatibilities: Cloxacillin
Y-site compatibilities: Cimetidine, diltiazem, enalaprilat
Perform/provide:
• Storage at room temp, discard unused portion, do not freeze, do not use if turbid or deep brown or if precipitate forms
Evaluate:
• Therapeutic response: increased plasma volume

---

hexamethylmelamine (R)

(hex-a-meth'ill-mel-a-meen)
Hexalen
Func. class.: Antineoplastic, alkylating agent

Action: Responsible for inhibition of cell DNA and RNA synthesis, cell death; rapidly degraded; cell cycle nonspecific
Uses: Resistant or recurrent ovarian cancer; may be used alone or in combination
Dosage and routes:
• *Adult* **PO** 260 mg/m^2; average dose 400 mg qd × 14 days, then rest for 14 days; cycle should continue until patient no longer responds
Available forms: Caps 50 mg
Side effects/adverse reactions:
EENT: Tinnitus, hearing loss
HEMA: **Thrombocytopenia, leukopenia**
GI: Nausea, vomiting, diarrhea, stomatitis, weight loss, colitis, hepatotoxicity, anorexia
CNS: Headache, dizziness, drowsiness, paresthesia, peripheral neu-

ropathy, coma, hyporeflexia, muscle weakness
INTEG: Alopecia, pruritus, herpes zoster
Contraindications: Lactation, pregnancy (1st trimester) (D), myelosuppression, acute herpes zoster, hypersensitivity
Precautions: Radiation therapy, leukopenia, thrombocytopenia
Pharmacokinetics: Metabolized in liver, excreted in urine
Interactions:
• Increased toxicity: antineoplastics, radiation
• Reduced efficiency: influenza vaccine, pneumococcal vaccine

NURSING CONSIDERATIONS
Assess:
• CBC, differential, platelet count weekly; withhold drug if WBC is <4000 or platelet count is <75,000; notify prescriber
• Renal function studies: BUN serum uric acid, urine CrCl before, during therapy
• I&O ratio; report fall in urine output to <30 ml/hr
• Monitor temp q4h; fever may indicate beginning infection; no rectal temps
• Liver function tests before, during therapy: bilirubin, AST (SGOT), ALT (SGPT), LDH; prn or qmo
• Bleeding: hematuria, guaiac, bruising, petechiae, mucosa or orifices q8h
• Food preferences: list likes, dislikes
• Yellowing of skin and sclera, dark urine, clay-colored stools, itchy skin, abdominal pain, fever, diarrhea
• Effects of alopecia on body image; discuss feelings about body changes
• Inflammation of mucosa, breaks in skin
• Buccal cavity q8h for dryness,

---

ores, or ulceration, white patches, oral pain, bleeding, dysphagia

 Symptoms indicating severe allergic reaction: rash, pruritus, urticaria, purpuric skin lesions, itching, flushing

Administer:

• As divided daily doses 1-2 hr pc and hs

• Antiemetic 30-60 min before giving drug and prn

• Topical or systemic analgesics for pain

• Local or systemic drugs for infection

Perform/provide:

• Storage at room temp in dry form

• Strict medical asepsis, protective isolation if WBC levels are low

• Special skin care

• Increase fluid intake to 2-3 L/day to prevent urate deposits, calculi formation

• Diet low in purines: organ meats (kidney, liver), dried beans, peas to maintain alkaline urine

• Rinsing of mouth tid-qid with water, club soda; brushing of teeth bid-tid with soft brush or cotton-tipped applicators for stomatitis; use unwaxed dental floss

Evaluate:

• Therapeutic response: decreased tumor size, decreased spread of malignancy

Teach patient/family:

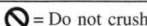 Not to break, crush, or chew caps

• About protective isolation

• That sterility, amenorrhea can occur; reversible after discontinuing treatment

• That hair may be lost during treatment; a wig or hairpiece may make patient feel better; new hair may be different in color, texture

• To avoid foods with citric acid, hot or rough texture

• To report any bleeding, white spots, or ulcerations in mouth to prescriber; tell patient to examine mouth qd

• To report signs of infection: fever, sore throat, flu symptoms

• To report signs of anemia: fatigue, headache, faintness, shortness of breath, irritability

---

hyaluronidase (℞)

(hye-al-yoor-on'i-dase)

Wydase

Func. class.: Enzyme

Action: Hydrolyzes hyaluronic acid within areas filled with exudates

Uses: Hypodermoclysis, subcutaneous urography; adjunct to dispersion of other drugs

Dosage and routes:

Adjunct

• *Adult and child:* **INJ** 150 U with other drug

Urography

• *Adult and child:* **SC** 75 U over scapula, then contrast medium injected at same site

Hypodermoclysis

• *Adult and child >3 yr:* **SC** 150 U/L of clysis sol

Available forms: Inj powder 150, 1500 U; inj sol 150 U/ml

Side effects/adverse reactions:

INTEG: Rash, urticaria, itching

OTHER: Overhydration (hyperdermoclysis)

Contraindications: Hypersensitivity to bovine products, CHF, hypoproteinemia, around infected/inflamed or cancerous area

Precautions: Pregnancy (C)

Interactions:

• Systemic reactions: local anesthetics

NURSING CONSIDERATIONS

Assess:

• Site before administration (hypodermoclysis)

• For overhydration in child <3 yr

 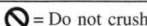

Administer:
• After test dose: 0.02 ml of 150 U/ml sol is injected; if wheal develops or itching occurs, test is positive
• Right after mixing; sol is unstable
• To child <3 yr, not exceeding 200 ml; in neonates, not exceeding 2 ml/min

Additive compatibilities: Amikacin, sodium bicarbonate

Syringe compatibilities: Pentobarbital, thiopental

Evaluate:
• Therapeutic response: absence of swelling, pain after hypodermoclysis

---

hydralazine (Ⓡ)

(hye-dral'a-zeen)
Alazine, Apresoline, Hydralazine HCl, novo-Hylazin*, Pralzine, Rolzine

Func. class.: Antihypertensive, direct-acting peripheral vasodilator

Chem. class.: Phthalazine

Action: Vasodilates arteriolar smooth muscle by direct relaxation; reduction in blood pressure with reflex increases in cardiac function

Uses: Essential hypertension; *parenteral:* severe essential hypertension, CHF

Dosage and routes:
• *Adult:* PO 10 mg qid 2-4 days, then 25 mg for rest of first wk, then 50 mg qid individualized to desired response, not to exceed 300 mg qd; **IV/IM BOL** 20-40 mg q4-6h, administer **PO** as soon as possible; **IM** 20-40 mg q4-6h
• *Child:* PO 0.75-3 mg/kg/day in 4 divided doses, max 7.5 mg/kg/24 hr; **IV BOL** 0.1-0.2 mg/kg q4-6h; **IM** 0.1-0.2 mg/kg q4-6h

Available forms: Inj 20 mg/ml; tabs 10, 25, 50, 100 mg

Side effects/adverse reactions:
MISC: Nasal congestion, muscle cramps, *lupuslike symptoms*
CV: Palpitations, reflex tachycardia, angina, shock, edema, rebound hypertension
CNS: Headache, tremors, dizziness, anxiety, peripheral neuritis, depression
GI: Nausea, vomiting, anorexia, diarrhea, constipation
INTEG: Rash, pruritus
HEMA: Leukopenia, agranulocytosis, anemia
GU: Impotence, urinary retention, Na, H_2O retention

Contraindications: Hypersensitivity to hydralazines, coronary artery disease, mitral valvular rheumatic heart disease, rheumatic heart disease

Precautions: Pregnancy (C), CVA, advanced renal disease, elderly

Pharmacokinetics:
PO: Onset 20-30 min, peak 1 hr, duration 2-4 hr
IM: Onset 5-10 min, peak 1 hr, duration 2-4 hr
IV: Onset 5-20 min, peak 10-80 min, duration 2-6 hr; half-life 2-8 hr; metabolized by liver; less than 10% present in urine

Interactions:
• Increased tachycardia, angina: sympathomimetics (epinephrine, norepinephrine)
• Increased effects of β-blockers
• Use MAOIs with caution in patients receiving hydralazine

NURSING CONSIDERATIONS
Assess:
• B/P q5min × 2 hr, then q1h × 2 hr, then q4h
• Pulse, jugular venous distention q4h

- Electrolytes, blood studies: K, Na, Cl, CO_2, CBC, serum glucose
- Weight daily, I&O
- LE prep, ANA titer before starting therapy
- Edema in feet, legs daily
- Skin turgor, dryness of mucous membranes for hydration status
- Rales, dyspnea, orthopnea
- IV site for extravasation, rate
- Fever, joint pain, tachycardia, palpitations, headache, nausea
- Mental status: affect, mood, behavior, anxiety; check for personality changes

Administer:
- Give with meals (PO) to enhance absorption
- To recumbent patient, keep for 1 hr after administration

IV
- IV undiluted; give through Y-tube or 3-way stopcock each 10 mg or less/min

Additive compatibilities: Dobutamine

Y-site compatibilities: Heparin, hydrocortisone, potassium chloride, verapamil, vit B/C

Evaluate:
- Therapeutic response: decreased B/P

Teach patient/family:
- To take with food to increase bioavailability
- To avoid OTC preparations unless directed by prescriber
- To notify prescriber if chest pain, severe fatigue, fever, muscle or joint pain occurs
- To rise slowly to prevent orthostatic hypotension

Treatment of overdose: Administer vasopressors, volume expanders for shock; if PO, lavage or give activated charcoal, digitalization

hydrochlorothiazide (℞)

(hye-droe-klor-oh-thye'a-zide)
Diaqua, Diuchlor H*, Esidrix, Ezide, Hydro-Chlor, hydrochlorothiazide, HydroDiuril, Hydromal, Hydro-Par, Hydro-T, Hydrozide*, Microzide, Neo-Codema*, Novohydrazide*, Oretic, Thiuretic, Urozide*

Func. class.: Thiazide diuretic, antihypertensive

Chem. class.: Sulfonamide derivative

Action: Acts on distal tubule and cortical thick ascending limb of loop of Henle by increasing excretion of water, sodium, chloride, potassium

Uses: Edema, hypertension, diuresis, CHF; edema in corticosteroid, estrogen therapy

Dosage and routes:
- *Adult:* **PO** 25-100 mg/day
- *Geriatric:* **PO** 12.5 mg/day, initially
- *Child >6 mo:* **PO** 2 mg/kg/day in divided doses
- *Child <6 mo:* **PO** up to 4 mg/kg/day in divided doses

Available forms: Tabs 25, 50, 100 mg; caps 12.5 mg; sol 50 mg/5 ml, 100 mg/ml

Side effects/adverse reactions:

GU: Frequency, polyuria, **uremia, glucosuria,** hyperurecemia

CNS: Drowsiness, paresthesia, depression, headache, *dizziness, fatigue, weakness,* fever

GI: Nausea, vomiting, anorexia, constipation, diarrhea, cramps, pancreatitis, GI irritation, **hepatitis**

EENT: Blurred vision

INTEG: Rash, urticaria, purpura, photosensitivity, alopecia, erythema multiforme

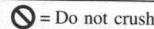

⬥ = Nursing alert   ∅ = Herb-drug interaction   ⊘ = Do not crush

META: Hyperglycemia, hyperuricemia, increased creatinine, BUN

*HEMA: **Aplastic anemia, hemolytic anemia, leukopenia, agranulocytosis, thrombocytopenia, neutropenia***

CV: Irregular pulse, orthostatic hypotension, palpitations, volume depletion, allergic myocarditis

ELECT: Hypokalemia, hypercalcemia, hyponatremia, hypochloremia, hypomagnesemia

Contraindications: Hypersensitivity to thiazides or sulfonamides, anuria, renal decompensation, hypomagnesemia

Precautions: Hypokalemia, renal disease, pregnancy (B), lactation, hepatic disease, gout, COPD, lupus erythematosus, diabetes mellitus, hyperlipidemia, CrCl <25 ml/min

Pharmacokinetics:

PO: Onset 2 hr, peak 4 hr, duration 6-12 hr, half-life 6-15 hr; excreted unchanged by kidneys; crosses placenta; enters breast milk

Interactions:

• Increased toxicity of lithium, nondepolarizing skeletal muscle relaxants, digitalis, allopurinol

• Decreased effects: anticoagulants, antidiabetics, antigout agents

• Decreased absorption of thiazides: cholestyramine, colestipol

• Decreased hypotensive response: indomethacin, NSAIDs

• Hyperglycemia: diazoxide

• Hypokalemia: glucocorticoids, amphotericin B

• Increased effects: loop diuretics

🌿 Potassium deficiency: aloe, buckthorn bark/berry, cascara sagrada bark, licorice root, senna pod/leaf

Lab test interferences:

Increase: BSP retention, amylase, parathyroid test

Decrease: PBI, PSP

NURSING CONSIDERATIONS

Assess:

• Weight, I&O daily to determine fluid loss; effect of drug may be decreased if used qd

• Rate, depth, rhythm of respiration, effect of exertion

• B/P lying, standing; postural hypotension may occur

• Electrolytes: K, Mg, Na, Cl; include BUN, blood sugar, CBC, serum creatinine, blood pH, ABGs, uric acid, Ca; renal function

• Glucose in urine if patient is diabetic

• Signs of metabolic alkalosis: drowsiness, restlessness

• Signs of hypokalemia: postural hypotension, malaise, fatigue, tachycardia, leg cramps, weakness, dehydration

• Rashes, temp qd

• Confusion, especially in elderly; take safety precautions if needed

Administer:

• In AM to avoid interference with sleep if using drug as a diuretic

• K replacement if K <3 mg/dl

• With food; if nausea occurs, absorption may be decreased slightly

Evaluate:

• Therapeutic response: improvement in edema of feet, legs, sacral area qd, decreased B/P

Teach patient/family:

• To increase fluid intake to 2-3 L/day unless contraindicated; to rise slowly from lying or sitting position

• To notify prescriber of muscle weakness, cramps, nausea, dizziness

• That drug may be taken with food or milk

• To use sunscreen for photosensitivity

• That blood sugar may be increased in diabetics

• To take early in day to avoid nocturia

Treatment of overdose: Lavage if taken orally; monitor electrolytes; administer dextrose in saline; monitor hydration, CV, renal status

---

hydrocodone (℞)

(hye-droe-koe'done)
Hycodan, Robidone*
Func. class.: Narcotic analgesic
Chem. class.: Opiate

Controlled Substance Schedule III
Action: Acts directly on cough center in medulla to suppress cough; binds to opiate receptors in CNS to reduce pain
Uses: Hyperactive and nonproductive cough, mild pain
Dosage and routes:
• *Adult:* PO 5 mg q4h prn or 10 mg q12h (long-acting)
• *Child:* PO 1.25-5 mg q4h prn
Available forms: Caps 5 mg; susp 5 mg/ml; tabs 5 mg, 10 mg (long-acting)
Side effects/adverse reactions:
CNS: Drowsiness, dizziness, lightheadedness, confusion, headache, sedation, euphoria, dysphoria, weakness, hallucinations, disorientation, mood changes, dependence, *convulsions*
GI: Nausea, vomiting, anorexia, constipation, cramps, dry mouth
GU: Increased urinary output, dysuria, urinary retention
INTEG: Rash, urticaria, flushing, pruritus
EENT: Tinnitus, blurred vision, miosis, diplopia
CV: Palpitations, tachycardia, bradycardia, change in B/P, *circulatory depression,* syncope
RESP: Respiratory depression
Contraindications: Hypersensitivity, addiction (narcotic)
Precautions: Addictive personality, pregnancy (C), lactation, increased intracranial pressure, MI (acute), severe heart disease, respiratory depression, hepatic disease, renal disease, child <18 yr
Pharmacokinetics: Onset 10-20 min, duration 4-6 hr, half-life 3½-4½ hr; metabolized in liver; excreted in urine; crosses placenta
Interactions:
• Increased CNS depression: alcohol, narcotics, sedative/hypnotics, phenothiazines, skeletal muscle relaxants, general anesthetics, tricyclic antidepressants
Lab test interferences:
Increase: Amylase, lipase
NURSING CONSIDERATIONS
Assess:
• I&O ratio; check for decreasing output; may indicate urinary retention
• CNS changes: dizziness, drowsiness, hallucinations, euphoria, LOC, pupil reaction
• Allergic reactions: rash, urticaria
• Respiratory dysfunction: respiratory depression, character, rate, rhythm; notify prescriber if respirations are <10/min
• Need for pain medication, physical dependence
Administer:
• With antiemetic after meals if nausea or vomiting occurs
Perform/provide:
• Storage in light-resistant area at room temp
• Assistance with ambulation
• Safety measures: side rails, nightlight, call bell within easy reach
Evaluate:
• Therapeutic response: decrease in pain or cough
Teach patient/family:
• To report any symptoms of CNS changes, allergic reactions
• That physical dependency may result when used for extended periods

---

◆ = Nursing alert   ▮ = Herb-drug interaction   🚫 = Do not crush

• That withdrawal symptoms may occur: nausea, vomiting, cramps, fever, faintness, anorexia

🚫 Not to break, crush, or chew caps

Treatment of overdose: Naloxone HCl (Narcan) 0.2-0.8 mg IV, O₂, IV fluids, vasopressors

---

hydrocortisone/hy-drocortisone acetate/ hydrocortisone sodium phosphate/ hydrocortisone sodium succinate (Rx)

(hye-dro-kor'ti-sone)

Cortef, Cortenema, Hydrocortone Acetate/Hydrocortone Phosphate/A-Hydrocort, Hydrocortone/Cortef Acetate, Solu-Cortef

Func. class.: Corticosteroid
Chem. class.: Short-acting glucocorticoid

Action: Decreases inflammation by suppression of migration of polymorphonuclear leukocytes, fibroblasts, reversal of increased capillary permeability and lysosomal stabilization

Uses: Severe inflammation, septic shock, adrenal insufficiency, ulcerative colitis, collagen disorders

Dosage and routes:

Adrenal insufficiency/inflammation

• *Adult:* **PO** 5-30 mg bid-qid; **IM/IV** 100-250 mg (succinate), then 50-100 mg **IM** as needed; **IM/IV** 15-240 mg q12h (phosphate)

Shock

• *Adult:* 500 mg-2 g q2-6h (succinate)

• *Child:* **IM/IV** 0.186-1 mg/kg bid-tid (succinate)

Colitis

• *Adult:* **ENEMA** 100 mg nightly for 21 days

Available forms: Tabs 5, 10, 20 mg; inj 25, 50 mg/ml; enema 100 mg/60 ml; acetate-inj 25*, 50 mg/ml*, enema 10% aerosol foam; supp 25 mg; cypionate-oral susp 10 mg/5 ml; phosphate-inj 50 mg/ml; succinate inj 100 mg*, 250 mg*, 500 mg*, 1000 mg/vial*

Side effects/adverse reactions:

CNS: Depression, flushing, sweating, headache, mood changes

*CV: Hypertension, **circulatory collapse, thrombophlebitis, embolism,*** tachycardia, edema

EENT: Fungal infections, increased intraocular pressure, blurred vision

GI: Diarrhea, nausea, abdominal distention, ***GI hemorrhage,*** increased appetite, ***pancreatitis***

*HEMA: **Thrombocytopenia***

INTEG: Acne, poor wound healing, ecchymosis, petechiae

MS: Fractures, osteoporosis, weakness

Contraindications: Psychosis, hypersensitivity, idiopathic thrombocytopenia, acute glomerulonephritis, amebiasis, fungal infections, nonasthmatic bronchial disease, child <2 yr, AIDS, TB

Precautions: Pregnancy (C), lactation, diabetes mellitus, glaucoma, osteoporosis, seizure disorders, ulcerative colitis, CHF, myasthenia gravis, renal disease, esophagitis, peptic ulcer

Pharmacokinetics:

PO: Onset 1-2 hr, peak 1 hr, duration 1-1½ days

IM/IV: Onset 20 min, peak 4-8 hr, duration 1-1½ days

REC: Onset 3-5 days

Metabolized by liver, excreted in urine (17-OHCS, 17-KS), crosses placenta

H

---

* = Canada only   Side effects: *italics* = common; ***bold italics*** = life-threatening

Interactions:

• Decreased action of hydrocortisone: cholestyramine, colestipol, barbiturates, rifampin, ephedrine, phenytoin, theophylline

• Decreased effects of anticoagulants, anticonvulsants, antidiabetics, ambenonium, neostigmine, isoniazid, toxoids, vaccines, anticholinesterases, salicylates, somatrem

• Increased side effects: alcohol, salicylates, indomethacin, amphotericin B, digitalis, cyclosporine, diuretics

• Increased action of hydrocortisone: salicylates, estrogens, indomethacin, oral contraceptives, ketoconazole, macrolide antibiotics

🌿 Potassium deficiency: aloe, buckthorn bark/berry, cascara sagrada bark, senna pod/leaf

Lab test interferences:

Increase: Cholesterol, Na, blood glucose, uric acid, Ca, urine glucose

Decrease: Ca, K, T_4, T_3, thyroid ^{131}I uptake test, urine 17-OHCS, 17-KS, PBI

False negative: Skin allergy tests

NURSING CONSIDERATIONS
Assess:

• K, blood sugar, urine glucose while on long-term therapy; hypokalemia and hyperglycemia

• Weight daily, notify prescriber of weekly gain >5 lb

• B/P q4h, pulse; notify prescriber of chest pain

• I&O ratio; be alert for decreasing urinary output, increasing edema

• Plasma cortisol levels during long-term therapy (normal level: 138-635 nmol/L SI units when drawn at 8 AM)

• Infection: increased temp, WBC, even after withdrawal of medication; drug masks infection

• K depletion: paresthesias, fatigue, nausea, vomiting, depression, polyuria, dysrhythmias, weakness

• Edema, hypertension, cardiac symptoms

• Mental status: affect, mood, behavioral changes, aggression

Administer:

• Daily dose in AM for better results

• IM inj deep in large muscle mass; rotate sites; avoid deltoid; use 21G needle

• In one dose in AM to prevent adrenal suppression; avoid SC administration; may damage tissue

• With food or milk for GI symptoms

• Rectal: telling patient to retain for 20 min if possible

IV

• Phosphate: IV undiluted or added to dextrose or saline inj and given by infusion; give 25 mg or less/min

• Succinate: IV in mix-o-vial, or reconstitute 250 mg or less/2 ml bacteriostatic H_2O for inj; mix gently; give direct IV over 1 min or more; may be further diluted in 100, 250, 500, or 1000 ml of D_5W, D_5 0.9%, NaCl 0.9% given over ordered rate

Sodium phosphate preparations

Additive compatibilities: Amikacin, amphotericin B, bleomycin, cephapirin, metaraminol, sodium bicarbonate, verapamil

Syringe compatibilities: Metoclopramide

Y-site compatibilities: Allopurinol, amifostine, aztreonam, cefepime, cladribine, famotidine, filgrastim, fluconazole, fludarabine, granisetron, melphalan, ondansetron, paclitaxel, piperacillin/tazobactam, teniposide, thiotepa, vinorelbine

Sodium succinate preparations

Additive compatibilities: Amikacin, aminophylline, amphotericin B, calcium chloride, calcium gluconate, cephalothin, cephapirin, chloramphenicol, clindamycin, cloxacillin, corticotropin, daunorubicin, diphenhydramine, dopamine, eryth-

---

◆ = Nursing alert   🌿 = Herb-drug interaction   ⊘ = Do not crush

romycin, floxacillin, lidocaine, magnesium sulfate, mephentermine, metronidazole/sodium bicarbonate, mitomycin, mitoxantrone, netilmicin, netilmicin/potassium chloride, norepinephrine, penicillin G potassium/sodium, piperacillin, polymyxin B, potassium chloride, sodium bicarbonate, theophylline, thiopental, vancomycin, verapamil, vit B/C

Syringe compatibilities: Metoclopramide, thiopental

Y-site compatibilities: Acyclovir, allopurinol, amifostine, aminophylline, ampicillin, amrinone, amsacrine, atracurium, atropine, aztreonam, betamethasone, calcium gluconate, cefepime, cefmetazole, cephalothin, cephapirin, chlordiazepoxide, chlorpromazine, cladribine, cyanocobalamin, cytarabine, dexamethasone, digoxin, diphenhydramine, dopamine, droperidol, edrophonium, enalaprilat, epinephrine, esmolol, estrogens conjugated, ethacrynate, famotidine, fentanyl, fentanyl/droperidol, filgrastim, fludarabine, fluorouracil, foscarnet, furosemide, gallium, granisetron, heparin, hydralazine, insulin (regular), isoproterenol, kanamycin, lidocaine, lorazepam, magnesium sulfate, melphalan, menadiol, meperidine, methicillin, methoxamine, methylergonovine, minocycline, morphine, neostigmine, norepinephrine, ondansetron, oxacillin, oxytocin, paclitaxel, pancuronium, penicillin G potassium, pentazocine, phytonadione, piperacillin/tazobactam, prednisolone, procainamide, prochlorperazine, propofol, propranolol, pyridostigmine, scopolamine, sodium bicarbonate, succinylcholine, tacrolimus, teniposide, theophylline, thiotepa, trimethaphan, trimethobenzamide, vecuronium, vinorelbine

Perform/provide:
• Assistance with ambulation in patient with bone tissue disease to prevent fractures

Evaluate:
• Therapeutic response: ease of respirations, decreased inflammation

Teach patient/family:
• That ID as steroid user should be carried
• To notify prescriber if therapeutic response decreases; dosage adjustment may be needed; of signs of infection
• Not to discontinue abruptly, or adrenal crisis can result; drug should be tapered off
• To avoid OTC products: salicylates, alcohol in cough products, cold preparations unless directed by prescriber
• About cushingoid symptoms of adrenal insufficiency: nausea, anorexia, fatigue, dizziness, dyspnea, weakness, joint pain

---

hydromorphone (℞)

(hye-droe-mor′fone)
Dilaudid, Dilaudid HP, hydromorphone HCl
Func. class.: Narcotic analgesics
Chem. class.: Opiate, semisynthetic phenanthrene

Controlled Substance Schedule II
Action: Inhibits ascending pain pathways in CNS, increases pain threshold, alters pain perception
Uses: Moderate to severe pain
Dosage and routes:
• *Adult:* PO 1-6 mg q4-6h prn; **IM/SC/IV** 2-4 mg q4-6h; **RECT** 3 mg hs prn
• *Geriatric:* PO 1-2 mg q4-6h
• *Child:* 0.5 mg q3-4h prn

Available forms: Inj 1, 2, 3, 4, 10 mg/ml; tabs 1, 2, 3, 4, 8 mg; rec supp 3 mg; oral sol 5 mg/5 ml

Side effects/adverse reactions:

CNS: Drowsiness, dizziness, confusion, headache, sedation, euphoria

GI: Nausea, vomiting, anorexia, constipation, cramps

GU: Increased urinary output, dysuria, urinary retention

INTEG: Rash, urticaria, bruising, flushing, diaphoresis, pruritus

EENT: Tinnitus, blurred vision, miosis, diplopia

CV: Palpitations, bradycardia, change in B/P

RESP: Respiratory depression

Contraindications: Hypersensitivity, addiction (narcotic)

Precautions: Addictive personality, pregnancy (C), lactation, increased intracranial pressure, MI (acute), severe heart disease, respiratory depression, hepatic disease, renal disease, child <18 yr

Pharmacokinetics: Onset 15-30 min, peak ½-1 hr, duration 4-5 hr; metabolized by liver; excreted by kidneys; crosses placenta; excreted in breast milk, half-life 2-3 hr

Interactions:

• Effects may be increased with other CNS depressants: alcohol, narcotics, sedative/hypnotics, antipsychotics, skeletal muscle relaxants

🌿 Increased action: kava kava

Lab test interferences:

Increase: Amylase

NURSING CONSIDERATIONS

Assess:

• I&O ratio; check for decreasing output; may indicate urinary retention

• CNS changes: dizziness, drowsiness, hallucinations, euphoria, LOC, pupil reaction

• Allergic reactions: rash, urticaria

• Respiratory dysfunction: respiratory depression, character, rate, rhythm; notify prescriber if respirations are <10/min

• Need for pain medication, physical dependence

• Pain control, sedation by scoring

Administer:

• With antiemetic if nausea, vomiting occur

• When pain is beginning to return; determine interval by response

IV

• Direct diluted with 5 ml sterile H_2O or NS; give through Y-tube or 3-way stopcock; give 2 mg or less/5 min

• IV INF: Dilute each 0.1-1 mg/ml NS (0.1-1 mg/ml), deliver by narcotic syringe infusor; may be diluted in D_5W, D_5NaCl, 0.45% NaCl, or NS for larger amounts and delivery through an infusion pump

Additive compatibilities: Bupivacaine, fluorouracil, ondansetron, promethazine, verapamil

Solution compatibilities: D_5W, D_5/0.45% NaCl, D_5/0.9% NaCl, D_5/LR, D_5/Ringer's sol, 0.45% NaCl, 0.9% NaCl, Ringer's and lactated Ringer's sol

Syringe compatibilities: Atropine, chlorpromazine, cimetidine, dimenhydrinate, diphenhydramine, fentanyl, glycopyrrolate, haloperidol, hydroxyzine, lorazepam, midazolam, pentazocine, pentobarbital, prochlorperazine, promethazine, ranitidine, scopolamine, tetracaine, thiethylperazine, trimethobenzamide

Y-site compatibilities: Acyclovir, allopurinol, amifostine, amikacin, amsacrine, aztreonam, cefamandole, cefepime, cefmetazole, cefoperazone, cefotaxime, cefoxitin, ceftazidime, ceftizoxime, cefuroxime, cephalothin, cephapirin, chloramphenicol, cisplatin, cladribine, clindamycin, cyclophosphamide, cyt-

---

arabine, diltiazem, dobutamine, dopamine, doxorubicin, doxycycline, epinephrine, erythromycin lactobionate, famotidine, fentanyl, filgrastim, fludarabine, foscarnet, furosemide, gentamicin, granisetron, heparin, kanamycin, labetalol, lorazepam, magnesium sulfate, melphalan, methotrexate, metronidazole, mezlocillin, midazolam, milrinone, morphine, moxalactam, nafcillin, nicardipine, nitroglycerin, norepinephrine, ondansetron, oxacillin, paclitaxel, penicillin G potassium, piperacillin, piperacillin/tazobactam, propofol, ranitidine, teniposide, thiotepa, ticarcillin, tobramycin, trimethoprim/sulfamethoxazole, vancomycin, vecuronium, vinorelbine

Perform/provide:
• Storage in light-resistant area at room temp
• Assistance with ambulation
• Safety measures: side rails, nightlight, call bell within easy reach

Evaluate:
• Therapeutic response: decrease in pain

Teach patient/family:
• To report any symptoms of CNS changes, allergic reactions
• That physical dependency may result when used for extended periods
• That withdrawal symptoms may occur: nausea, vomiting, cramps, fever, faintness, anorexia

Treatment of overdose: Naloxone HCl (Narcan) 0.2-0.8 mg IV, O$_2$, IV fluids, vasopressors

hydromorphone/guaifenesin/alcohol (℞)
(hye-droe-mor′fone)
Dilaudid Cough Syrup
Func. class.: Antitussive, narcotic
Chem. class.: Phenanthrene derivative, guaifenesin

Controlled Substance Schedule II
Action: Increases respiratory tract fluid by decreasing surface tension, adhesiveness, which increases removal of mucus; analgesic, antitussive
Uses: Cough
Dosage and routes:
• *Adult:* PO 1 mg q3-4h prn
Available forms: Syr 1 mg/5 ml
Side effects/adverse reactions:
CNS: Dizziness, drowsiness
GI: Nausea, constipation, vomiting, anorexia
CV: Hypotension
INTEG: Urticaria, rash
RESP: Respiratory depression
Contraindications: Hypersensitivity, increased intracranial pressure, status asthmaticus
Precautions: Hypothyroidism, Addison's disease, CNS depression, brain tumor, asthma, hepatic disease, renal disease, COPD, psychosis, alcoholism, convulsive disorders, pregnancy (C), lactation
Pharmacokinetics: Metabolized by liver; half-life 2-4 hr
Interactions:
• Enhanced CNS depression: barbiturates, narcotics, antipsychotics, antidepressants
⚕ Increased action: kava kava
NURSING CONSIDERATIONS
Assess:
• VS, cardiac status, including hypotension

- Respiratory rate, depth
- Cough: type, frequency, character, including sputum

Administer:
- Decreased dose to elderly patients; metabolism may be slowed

Perform/provide:
- Storage at room temp
- Increased fluids, bulk, exercise to decrease constipation

Evaluate:
- Therapeutic response: absence of cough

Teach patient/family:
- To avoid driving, other hazardous activities until patient stabilized on medication if drowsiness occurs
- To avoid alcohol, other CNS depressants; will enhance sedating properties of this drug

---

hydroxocobalamin (vit B₁₂) ℞

(hye-drox′-o-ko-bal′a-min)

Acti-B₁₂*, Alphamin, Hydrobexan, Hydro-Crysti 12, Hydroxo-12, hydroxycobalamin, LA-12

Func. class.: Vitamin

Chem. class.: B₁₂—water-soluble vitamin

Action: Needed for adequate nerve functioning, protein and carbohydrate metabolism, normal growth, RBC development

Uses: Vit B₁₂ deficiency, pernicious anemia, vit B₁₂ malabsorption syndrome, Schilling test

Dosage and routes:
- *Adult:* IM 30-100 μg qd × 5-10 days, maintenance 100-200 mg **IM** qmo
- *Child:* IM 1-30 μg qd × 5-10 days, maintenance 60 μg **IM** qmo or more often

Pernicious anemia/malabsorption syndrome
- *Adult:* IM 100-1000 μg qd × 2 wk, then 100-1000 μg **IM** qmo
- *Child:* IM 1000-5000 μg × 2 wk or more given in 100-500 μg doses, then 60 μg **IM/SC** qmo

Schilling test
- *Adult and child:* IM 1000 μg in one dose

Available forms: Inj 1000 μg/ml

Side effects/adverse reactions:

CNS: Flushing, optic nerve atrophy

GI: Diarrhea

CV: **CHF,** peripheral vascular thrombosis, *pulmonary edema*

INTEG: Itching, rash

Contraindications: Hypersensitivity, optic nerve atrophy, cardiac disease

Precautions: Pregnancy (A), lactation, children

Pharmacokinetics: Stored in liver, kidneys, stomach; 50%-90% excreted in urine; crosses placenta, breast milk

Interactions:
- Decreased absorption of hydroxocobalamin: aminoglycosides, anticonvulsants, colchicine, chloramphenicol, antineoplastics, cimetidine, alcohol, vit C, K preparations
- Increased absorption of this drug: prednisone

Lab test interferences:

False positive: Intrinsic factor

NURSING CONSIDERATIONS

Assess:
- K levels during beginning treatment
- CBC for increased reticulocyte count during first week of therapy, followed by increase in RBC and hemoglobin
- For pulmonary edema or worsening of CHF in cardiac patients

Administer:
- By IM inj for pernicious anemia unless contraindicated

◆ = Nursing alert   🖉 = Herb-drug interaction   🚫 = Do not crush

Evaluate:
• Therapeutic response: decreased anorexia, dyspnea on excretion, palpitations, paresthesias, psychosis, visual disturbances

Teach patient/family:
• That treatment must continue for life for pernicious anemia
• The importance of a well-balanced diet

---

hydroxychloroquine (℞)

(hye-drox-ee-klor'oh-kwin)
Plaquenil
Func. class.: Antimalarial
Chem. class.: 4-Aminoquinoline derivative

Action: Inhibits parasite replications, transcription of DNA to RNA by forming complexes with DNA in parasite

Uses: Malaria caused by *P. vivax, P. malariae, P. ovale, P. falciparum* (some strains): lupus erythematosus, rheumatoid arthritis

Dosage and routes:
Malaria
• *Adult and child:* **PO** 5 (base) mg/kg/wk on same day of week, not to exceed 400 mg (310 mg base); treatment should begin 2 wk before entering endemic area, continue 8 wk after leaving; if treatment begins after exposure, 800 mg (620 mg base) for adult, 10 mg/kg for children in 2 divided doses 6 hr apart

Lupus erythematosus
• *Adult:* **PO** 400 mg (310 mg base) qd-bid; length depends on patient response; maintenance 200-400 mg (155-310 mg base) qd
• *Child:* **PO** 3-5 mg (base)/kg/day max 400 mg/day

Rheumatoid arthritis
• *Adult:* **PO** 400-600 mg (310-465

mg base) qd, then 200-300 mg (155-310 mg base) qd after good response

Available forms: Tabs 200 mg (base 155 mg)

Side effects/adverse reactions:
CV: Hypotension, heart block, ***asystole with syncope***
INTEG: Pruritus, pigmentation changes, skin eruptions, lichen planus-like eruptions, eczema, ***exfoliative dermatitis,*** alopecia
CNS: Headache, stimulation, fatigue, irritability, ***convulsion,*** bad dreams, dizziness, confusion, psychosis, decreased reflexes
EENT: Blurred vision, corneal changes, retinal changes, difficulty focusing, tinnitus, vertigo, deafness, photophobia, corneal edema
GI: Nausea, vomiting, anorexia, diarrhea, cramps
*HEMA: **Thrombocytopenia, agranulocytosis, hemolytic anemia, leukopenia***

Contraindications: Hypersensitivity, retinal field changes, porphyria, children (long-term)

Precautions: Blood dyscrasias, severe GI disease, neurologic disease, alcoholism, hepatic disease, G6PD deficiency, psoriasis, eczema, pregnancy (C), lactation

Pharmacokinetics:
PO: Peak 1-2 hr, half-life 3-5 days; metabolized in liver; excreted in urine, feces, breast milk; crosses placenta

Interactions:
• Decreased action of hydroxychloroquine: Mg or Al compounds
• Increased levels of digoxin
• Increased antibody titer: rabies vaccine

NURSING CONSIDERATIONS
Assess:
• Ophthalmic test if long-term treatment or drug dosage >150 mg/day

---

• Liver studies qwk: AST (SGOT), ALT (SGPT), bilirubin
• Blood studies: CBC, platelets; WBC, RBC, platelets may be decreased
• For decreased reflexes: knee, ankle
• ECG during therapy
• Watch for depression of T waves, widening of QRS complex
• Allergic reactions: pruritus, rash, urticaria
• Blood dyscrasias: malaise, fever, bruising, bleeding (rare)
• For ototoxicity (tinnitus, vertigo, change in hearing); audiometric testing should be done before, after treatment
◆ For toxicity: blurring vision, difficulty focusing, headache, dizziness, knee, ankle reflexes; drug should be discontinued immediately

Administer:

PO

• Before or after meals or with milk; at same time each day to maintain drug level

Perform/provide:

• Storage in tight, light-resistant container at room temp; keep injection in cool environment

Evaluate:

• Therapeutic response: decreased symptoms of malaria, lupus erythematosus, rheumatoid arthritis

Teach patient/family:

• To use sunglasses in bright sunlight to decrease photophobia
• That urine may turn rust or brown
• To report hearing, visual problems, fever, fatigue, bruising, bleeding, which may indicate blood dyscrasias

Treatment of overdose: Induce vomiting; gastric lavage; administer barbiturate (ultrashort-acting), vasopressor, ammonium chloride; tracheostomy may be necessary

hydroxyurea (Rx)

(hye-drox'ee-yoo-ree-ah)
Hydrea

Func. class.: Antineoplastic, antimetabolite
Chem. class.: Synthetic urea analog

Action: Acts by inhibiting DNA synthesis without interfering with RNA or protein synthesis; incorporates thymidine into DNA, causing direct damage to DNA strands; S phase specific of cell cycle

Uses: Melanoma, chronic myelocytic leukemia, recurrent or metastatic ovarian cancer, squamous cell carcinoma of the head and neck, sickle cell anemia, psoriasis

Dosage and routes:

Renal disease

• CrCl 10-50 ml/min dose 50%; CrCl <10 ml/min dose 20%

Solid tumors

• *Adult:* PO 80 mg/kg as a single dose q3d or 20-30 mg/kg as a single dose qd

In combination with radiation

• *Adult:* PO 80 mg/kg as a single dose q3d; should be started 7 days before irradiation

Resistant chronic myelocytic leukemia

• *Adult:* PO 20-30 mg/kg/day as a single daily dose

Available forms: Caps 500 mg

Side effects/adverse reactions:

HEMA: **Leukopenia, anemia, thrombocytopenia**

GI: Nausea, vomiting, anorexia, diarrhea, stomatitis, constipation

GU: Increased BUN, uric acid, creatinine, temporary renal function impairment

INTEG: Rash, urticaria, pruritus, dry skin

CV: Angina, ischemia

◆ = Nursing alert   ∅ = Herb-drug interaction   ⊘ = Do not crush

CNS: Headache, confusion, hallucinations, dizziness, **convulsions**

Contraindications: Hypersensitivity, leukopenia (<2500/mm³), thrombocytopenia (<100,000/mm³), anemia (severe), pregnancy (D), lactation

Precautions: Renal disease (severe)

Pharmacokinetics: Readily absorbed when taken orally, peak level in 2 hr; degraded in liver; excreted in urine, almost totally eliminated in 24 hr; readily crosses blood-brain barrier

Interactions:
• Increased toxicity: radiation or other antineoplastics

Lab test interferences:
Increase: Renal function studies

NURSING CONSIDERATIONS

Assess:
• CBC, differential, platelet count qwk; withhold drug if WBC is <3500/mm³ or platelet count is <100,000/mm³; notify prescriber; drug should be discontinued
• Renal function studies: BUN, serum uric acid, urine CrCl, electrolytes before, during therapy
• I&O ratio; report fall in urine output to <30 ml/hr
• Monitor temp q4h; fever may indicate beginning infection
• Liver function tests before, during therapy: bilirubin, alk phosphatase, AST (SGOT), ALT (SGPT), LDH; prn or qmo
• B/P q3-4h; check for chest pain; angina, ischemia may occur
• Bleeding: hematuria, guaiac, bruising or petechiae, mucosa or orifices q8h
• Food preferences; list likes, dislikes
• Inflammation of mucosa, breaks in skin
• Buccal cavity q8h for dryness, sores or ulceration, white patches, oral pain, bleeding, dysphagia

• Symptoms indicating severe allergic reaction: rash, urticaria, itching, flushing
• Neurotoxicity: headaches, hallucinations, convulsions, dizziness

Administer:
• Allopurinol or NaHCO₃ concurrently to prevent high uric acid levels; extra fluids
• Antiemetic 30-60 min before giving drug and prn
• Antibiotics for prophylaxis of infection
• Transfusion for anemia

Perform/provide:
• Rinsing of mouth tid-qid with water, club soda; brushing of teeth bid-tid with soft brush or cotton-tipped applicators for stomatitis; use unwaxed dental floss
• Nutritious diet with iron, vitamin supplements as ordered

Evaluate:
• Therapeutic response: decreased tumor size, spread of malignancy

Teach patient/family:
🚫 Not to break, crush, or chew caps
• To report signs of infection: elevated temp, sore throat, flulike symptoms
• To report signs of anemia: fatigue, headache, faintness, shortness of breath, irritability
• To report bleeding: avoid use of razors, commercial mouthwash
• To avoid use of aspirin products, ibuprofen
• To avoid foods with citric acid, hot or rough texture if stomatitis is present
• To report stomatitis: any bleeding, white spots, ulcerations in the mouth; tell patient to examine mouth qd, report symptoms
• That contraceptive measures are recommended during therapy
• To drink 10-12 (8 oz) glasses of fluid/day

H

• To notify prescriber of fever, chills, sore throat, nausea, vomiting, anorexia, diarrhea, bleeding, bruising; may indicate blood dyscrasias

hydroxyzine (R)

(hye-drox'i-zeen)
Apo-Hydroxyzine*, Atarax, Atarax 100, hydroxyzine HCl, hydroxyzine pamoate, Multipax*, Novohydroxyzine*, Vistaril, Vistazine 50

Func. class.: Antianxiety/antihistamine/sedative-hypnotic
Chem. class.: Piperazine derivative

Action: Depresses subcortical levels of CNS, including limbic system, reticular formation
Uses: Anxiety preoperatively, postoperatively to prevent nausea, vomiting, to potentiate narcotic analgesics; sedation; pruritus
Dosage and routes:
• *Adult:* PO 25-100 mg tid-qid
• *Geriatric:* PO 10 mg tid-qid (pruritus)
• *Child >6 yr:* 50-100 mg/day in divided doses
• *Child <6 yr:* 50 mg/day in divided doses
Preoperatively/postoperatively
• *Adult:* IM 25-100 mg q4-6h
• *Child:* IM 0.5-1.1 mg/kg q4-6h
Available forms: Tabs 10, 25, 50, 100 mg; caps 25, 50, 100 mg; syr 10 mg/5 ml; oral susp 25 mg/5 ml; inj 25, 50 mg/ml
Side effects/adverse reactions:
CV: Hypotension
CNS: Dizziness, drowsiness, confusion, headache, tremors, fatigue, depression, ***convulsions***
GI: Dry mouth
Contraindications: Hypersensitivity to this drug or cetirizine, early pregnancy, lactation, acute asthma

Precautions: Elderly, debilitated, hepatic disease, renal disease, narrow-angle glaucoma, COPD, prostatic hypertrophy, pregnancy (C)
Pharmacokinetics:
PO: Onset 15-30 min, duration 4-6 hr, half-life 3 hr, metabolized by liver, excreted by kidneys
Interactions:
• Increased CNS depressant effect: barbiturates, narcotics, analgesics, alcohol
⚕ Increased anticholinergic effect: henbane leaf
⚕ Increased action: kava kava
NURSING CONSIDERATIONS
Assess:
• B/P (lying, standing), pulse; if systolic B/P drops 20 mm Hg, hold drug, notify prescriber
• Mental status: mood, sensorium, affect
• Increased sedation
Administer:
• By Z-track injection in large muscle for IM to decrease pain, chance of necrosis
• With food or milk for GI symptoms
• Crushed if patient is unable to swallow medication whole
• Gum, hard candy, frequent sips of water for dry mouth
Additive compatibilities: Cisplatin, cyclophosphamide, cytarabine, dimenhydrinate, etoposide, lidocaine, mesna, methotrexate, nafcillin
Syringe compatibilities: Atropine, atropine/meperidine, benzquinamide, bupivacaine, butorphanol, chlorpromazine, cimetidine, codeine, diphenhydramine, doxapram, droperidol, fentanyl, fluphenazine, glycopyrrolate, hydromorphone, lidocaine, meperidine, meperidine/atropine, methotrimeprazine, metoclopramide, midazolam, morphine,

◆ = Nursing alert ⚕ = Herb-drug interaction ⊘ = Do not crush

nalbuphine, oxymorphone, penta-zocine, perphenazine, procaine, prochlorperazine, promazine, pro-methazine, scopolamine, sufenta-nil, thiothixene

Y-site compatibilities: Aztreonam, ciprofloxacin, cladribine, famo-tidine, filgrastim, foscarnet, gran-isetron melphalan, ondansetron, propofol, sufentanil, teniposide, thiotepa, vinorelbine

Perform/provide:
• Assistance with ambulation dur-ing beginning therapy, since drowsiness/dizziness occurs
• Safety measures, including side rails
• Checking to see if PO medication has been swallowed

Evaluate:
• Therapeutic response: decreased anxiety

Teach patient/family:
• That medication is not to be used for everyday stress or used longer than 4 mo
• To avoid OTC preparations (cold, cough, hay fever) unless approved by prescriber
• To avoid driving, activities that require alertness
• To avoid alcohol ingestion, other psychotropic medications
• Not to discontinue medication quickly after long-term use
• To rise slowly or fainting may oc-cur

Treatment of overdose: Lavage if orally ingested; VS, supportive care; IV norepinephrine for hypotension

hyoscyamine (℞)

(hye-oh-sye'a-meen)
Anaspaz, Cystospaz, Cysto-spaz-M, Gastrosed, Levsin, Levsin Drops, Levsinex Time-caps, Neoquess

Func. class.: Anticholinergic
Chem. class.: Belladonna alka-loid

Action: Inhibits muscarinic actions of acetylcholine at postganglionic parasympathetic neuroeffector sites

Uses: Treatment of peptic ulcer dis-ease in combination with other drugs; other GI disorders, other spas-tic disorders, urinary incontinence

Dosage and routes:
• *Adult:* PO/SL 0.125-0.25 mg tid-qid ac, hs; TIME REL 0.375 q12h; IM/SC/IV 0.25-0.5 mg q6h
• *Child 2-10 yr:* ½ adult dose
• *Child <2 yr:* ¼ adult dose

Available forms: Tabs 0.125, 0.13, 0.15 mg; caps time rel 0.375 mg; sol 0.125 mg/ml; elix 0.125 mg/5 ml; inj 0.5 mg/ml

Side effects/adverse reactions:

CNS: Confusion, stimulation in el-derly, headache, insomnia, dizzi-ness, drowsiness, anxiety, weak-ness, hallucination

GI: Dry mouth, constipation, paralytic ileus, heartburn, nausea, vomiting, dysphagia, absence of taste

GU: Hesitancy, retention, impotence

CV: Palpitations, tachycardia

EENT: Blurred vision, photophobia, mydriasis, cycloplegia, increased oc-ular tension

INTEG: Urticaria, rash, pruritus, an-hidrosis, fever, allergic reactions

Contraindications: Hypersensitiv-ity to anticholinergics, narrow-angle glaucoma, GI obstruction, myasthe-nia gravis, paralytic ileus, GI atony,

H

ʃxic megacolon, prostatic hyper-
ʃrophy

Precautions: Hyperthyroidism,
coronary artery disease, dysrhythmias, CHF, ulcerative colitis, hypertension, hiatal hernia, hepatic disease, renal disease, pregnancy (C),
urinary retention, elderly

Pharmacokinetics:
PO: Duration 4-6 hr; metabolized
by liver; excreted in urine; half-life
3.5 hr

Interactions:
• Decreased effect of hyoscyamine:
antacids
• Increased anticholinergic effect:
amantadine, tricyclic antidepressants, MAOIs, H_1-antihistamines
• Decreased effect of phenothiazines, levodopa, ketoconazole

NURSING CONSIDERATIONS
Assess:
• VS, cardiac status: checking for
dysrhythmias, increased rate, palpitations
• I&O ratio; check for urinary retention or hesitancy
• GI complaints: pain, bleeding
(frank or occult), nausea, vomiting,
anorexia

Administer:
• ½ hr ac for better absorption
• Decreased dose to elderly patients;
metabolism may be slowed
• Gum, hard candy, frequent rinsing
of mouth for dryness of oral cavity

Perform/provide:
• Storage in tight container protected from light
• Increased fluids, bulk, exercise to
decrease constipation

Evaluate:
• Therapeutic response: absence of
epigastric pain, bleeding, nausea,
vomiting

Teach patient/family:
• To avoid driving, other hazardous
activities until stabilized on medication

• To avoid alcohol or other CNS
depressants; will enhance sedating
properties of this drug
• To avoid hot environments; heat
stroke may occur; drug suppresses
perspiration
• To use sunglasses when outside to
prevent photophobia; may cause
blurred vision
🚫 Not to break, crush, or chew
time rel caps

---

ibuprofen (OTC, ℞)
(eye-byoo-proe'fen)
Aches-N-Pain, Actiprofen*, Ad-
vil, Amersol*, Apo-Ibuprofen*,
Children's Advil, Excedrin IS,
Genpril, Haltran, Ibuprin, ibu-
profen, Ibuprohm, IBU-Tab,
Medipren, Menadol, Midol-
200, Motrin, Motrin IB, Motrin
Junior Streng th, Novoprofen*,
Nuprin, Pamprin-IB, Rufen,
Saleto-200, Saleto-400, Saleto-
600, Saleto-800, Trendar

Func. class.: Nonsteroidal antiinflammatory

Chem. class.: Propionic acid derivative

Action: Inhibits prostaglandin synthesis by decreasing enzyme needed
for biosynthesis; analgesic, antiinflammatory, antipyretic

Uses: Rheumatoid arthritis, osteoarthritis, primary dysmenorrhea, gout,
dental pain, musculoskeletal disorders, fever

Dosage and routes:
Analgesic
• *Adult:* PO 200-400 mg q4-6h, not
to exceed 3.2 g/day
• *Child:* PO 4-10 mg/kg/dose q6-8h
Antipyretic
• *Child 6 mo-12 yr:* PO 5 mg/kg
(temp <102.5° F or 39.2° C), 10
mg/kg, (temp >102.5° F), may re-
peat q4-6h, max 40 mg/kg/day

◆ = Nursing alert   / = Herb-drug interaction   🚫 = Do not crush

Antiinflammatory
- *Adult:* **PO** 300-800 mg tid-qid, max 3.2 g/day
- *Child:* **PO** 30-40 mg/kg/day in 3-4 divided doses, max 50 mg/kg/day

Available forms: Tabs 200, 300, 400, 600, 800 mg; oral susp 40 mg/ml, 100 mg/5 ml; tabs, chew 100 mg

Side effects/adverse reactions:

CV: Tachycardia, peripheral edema, palpitations, dysrhythmias

CNS: Headache, dizziness, drowsiness, fatigue, tremors, confusion, insomnia, anxiety, depression

EENT: Tinnitus, hearing loss, blurred vision

GI: Nausea, anorexia, vomiting, diarrhea, jaundice, ***cholestatic hepatitis,*** constipation, flatulence, cramps, dry mouth, peptic ulcer

*GU: **Nephrotoxicity:*** dysuria, hematuria, oliguria, azotemia

*HEMA: **Blood dyscrasias,*** increased bleeding time

INTEG: Purpura, rash, pruritus, sweating

Contraindications: Hypersensitivity, asthma, severe renal disease, severe hepatic disease

Precautions: Pregnancy (B) 1st and 2nd trimester, lactation, children, bleeding disorders, GI disorders, cardiac disorders, hypersensitivity to other antiinflammatory agents, elderly, CHF, CrCl <25 ml/min

Pharmacokinetics: Well absorbed (PO)

PO: Onset ½ hr; peak 1-2 hr, half-life 2-4 hr, metabolized in liver (inactive metabolites), excreted in urine (inactive metabolites), 90%-99% plasma protein binding, does not enter breast milk

Interactions:
- May increase action of coumadin, phenytoin, sulfonamides
- Decreased action of ibuprofen: salicylates

NURSING CONSIDERATIONS

Assess:
- Renal, liver, blood studies: BUN, creatinine, AST (SGOT), ALT (SGPT), Hgb, before treatment, periodically thereafter
- Pain: note type, duration, location and intensity with ROM
- Audiometric, ophthalmic examination before, during, after treatment; for eye, ear problems: blurred vision, tinnitus; may indicate toxicity
- Cardiac status: edema (peripheral), tachycardia, palpitations; monitor B/P, pulse for character, quality, rhythm
- For history of peptic ulcer disorder; asthma, aspirin, hypersensitivity, check closely for hypersensitivity reactions

Administer:
- With food, milk, or antacid to decrease GI symptoms; however, best to take on empty stomach to facilitate absorption; if nausea and vomiting occur/persist, notify prescriber

Perform/provide:
- Storage at room temp

Evaluate:
- Therapeutic response: decreased pain, stiffness in joints; decreased swelling in joints; ability to move more easily; reduction in fever or menstrual cramping

Teach patient/family:
- To report blurred vision, ringing, roaring in ears; may indicate toxicity; eye and hearing tests should be done during long-term therapy
- To avoid driving, other hazardous activities if dizziness or drowsiness occurs
- To report change in urine pattern, increased weight, edema, increased pain in joints, fever, blood in urine; indicate nephrotoxicity

---

- That therapeutic inflammatory effects may take up to 1 mo
- To avoid alcohol, salicylates; bleeding may occur
- To avoid sun, sunlamp

---

ibutilide (R)
(eye-byoo'tih-lide)
Corvert
Func. class.: Antidysrhythmic
(Class III)

Action: Prolongs duration of action potential and effective refractory period, noncompetitive α- and β-adrenergic inhibition
Uses: Atrial fibrillation/flutter
Dosage and routes:
- *Adult:* **IV INF** (≥60 kg) 1 vial (1 mg) given over 10 min; **IV INF** (<60 kg) 0.01 mg/kg given over 10 min
Available forms: Sol 0.1 mg/ml
Side effects/adverse reactions:
CNS: Headache
GI: Nausea
CV: Hypotension, bradycardia, sinus arrest, CHF, dysrhythmias, hypertension, extrasystoles, ventricular tachycardia, bundle branch block, AV block
Contraindications: Hypersensitivity
Precautions: Sinus node dysfunction, 2nd- or 3rd-degree AV block, electrolyte imbalances, pregnancy (C), bradycardia, lactation, children <18 yr, renal/hepatic disease, elderly
Pharmacokinetics:
PO: Onset 1-3 wk, peak 2-10 hr; half-life 15-100 days; metabolized by liver, excreted by kidneys
Interactions:
- Prodysrhythmia: phenothiazines, tricyclic/tetracycline antidepressants, H₁-receptor antagonists

- Increased levels of digitalis, quinidine, procainamide, flecainide, disopyramide, phenytoin
- Increased action: aloe, buckthorn bark/berry, cascara sagrada bark, senna pod/leaf

NURSING CONSIDERATIONS
Assess:
- I&O ratio; electrolytes: (K, Na, Cl)
- Liver function studies: AST (SGOT), ALT (SGPT), bilirubin, alk phosphatase
- ECG continuously to determine drug effectiveness, measure PR, QRS, QT intervals, check for PVCs, other dysrhythmias
- For dehydration or hypovolemia
- B/P continuously for hypotension, hypertension
- For rebound hypertension after 1-2 hr
- Cardiac rate, respiration: rate, rhythm, character, chest pain
Administer:
- Reduced dosage slowly with ECG monitoring
Evaluate:
- Therapeutic response: decrease in atrial fibrillation/flutter
Teach patient/family:
- To report side effects immediately

---

idarubicin (R)
(eye-dah-roob'ih-sin)
Idamycin
Func. class.: Antineoplastic, antibiotic
Chem. class.: Anthracycline glycoside

Action: Inhibits DNS synthesis by binding to DNA, a vesicant derived from daunorubicin by binding to DNA, which causes strand splitting; cell cycle specific (S phase)
Uses: Used in combination with

◆ = Nursing alert   ◢ = Herb-drug interaction   ⊘ = Do not crush other antineoplastics for acute my-elocytic leukemia in adults

Dosage and routes:

• *Adult:* **IV** 12 mg/m^2/day × 3 days in combination with cytosine arabinoside

Available forms: Inj 5, 10 mg vials

Side effects/adverse reactions:

HEMA: ***Thrombocytopenia, leukopenia, anemia***

GI: Nausea, vomiting, abdominal pain, mucositis, diarrhea, ***hepatotoxicity***

INTEG: Rash, extravasation, dermatitis, reversible alopecia, urticaria, thrombophlebitis at injection site

CV: ***Dysrhythmias, CHF, pericarditis, myocarditis,*** peripheral edema

CNS: Fever, chills, headache

Contraindications: Hypersensitivity, pregnancy (D), lactation

Precautions: Renal and hepatic disease, gout, bone marrow depression, children

Pharmacokinetics: Half-life 22 hr; metabolized by liver; crosses placenta; excreted in bile, urine (primarily as metabolites)

Interactions:

• Increased toxicity: other antineoplastics or radiation

Lab test interferences:

Increase: Uric acid

NURSING CONSIDERATIONS

Assess:

• CBC, differential, platelet count weekly; withhold drug if WBC is <4000/mm^3 or platelet count is <75,000/mm^3; notify prescriber of these results

• Blood, urine, uric acid levels

• Renal function studies: BUN, serum uric acid, urine CrCl, electrolytes before, during therapy

• I&O ratio; report fall in urine output to <30 ml/hr

• Monitor temp q4h; fever may indicate beginning infection

• Liver function tests before, during therapy: bilirubin, AST (SGOT), ALT (SGPT), alk phosphatase prn or qmo

• ECG: watch for ST-T wave changes, low QRS and T, possible dysrhythmias (sinus tachycardia, heart block, PVCs)

• Bleeding: hematuria, guaiac stools, bruising or petechiae, mucosa or orifices q8h

• Food preferences: list likes, dislikes

• Effects of alopecia on body image; discuss feelings about body changes

• Inflammation of mucosa, breaks in skin

• Yellowing of skin, sclera, dark urine, clay-colored stools, itchy skin, abdominal pain, fever, diarrhea

• Buccal cavity q8h for dryness, sores, ulceration, white patches, oral pain, bleeding, dysphagia

• Local irritation, pain, burning at injection site

• GI symptoms: frequency of stools, cramping

• Acidosis, signs of dehydration: rapid respirations, poor skin turgor, decreased urine output, dry skin, restlessness, weakness

• Cardiac status: B/P, pulse, character, rhythm, rate

Administer:

• Allopurinol or sodium bicarbonate to reduce uric acid levels, alkalinization of urine

• Transfusion for anemia

• Hydrocortisone for extravasation; apply ice compress after stopping infusion

IV, direct

• After preparing in biologic cabinet wearing gown, gloves, mask

• Antiemetic 30-60 min before giving drug and 6-10 hr after treatment to prevent vomiting

---

• After reconstituting 5 mg vial with 5 ml 0.9% NaCl (1 mg/1 ml); give over 10-15 min through Y-tube or 3-way stopcock of inf of D_5 or NS; discard unused portion

Solution compatibilities: $D_{3.3}$/0.3% NaCl, D_5/0.9% NaCl, D_5W, LR, 0.9% NaCl

Y-site compatibilities: Amifostine, amikacin, aztreonam, cimetidine, cladribine, cyclophosphamide, cytarabine, diphenhydramine, droperidol, erythromycin, filgrastim, granisetron, imipenem/cisplatin, magnesium sulfate, mannitol, melphalan, metoclopramide, potassium chloride, ranitidine, sargramostim, thiotepa, vinorelbine

Perform/provide:

• Strict hand-washing technique, gloves, protective clothing

• Liquid diet: carbonated beverages, gelatin may be added if patient is not nauseated or vomiting

• Increase fluid intake to 2-3 L/day to prevent urate and calculi formation

• Diet low in purines: absence of organ meats (kidney, liver), dried beans, peas to reduce uric acid level

• Rinsing of mouth tid-qid with water, club soda; brushing of teeth tid-qid with soft brush or cotton-tipped applicators for stomatitis; use unwaxed dental floss

• Storage at room temp for 3 days after reconstituting or 7 days refrigerated

Evaluate:

• Therapeutic response: decreased tumor size, spread of malignancy

Teach patient/family:

• To report any complaints, side effects to nurse or prescriber

• That hair may be lost during treatment and wig or hairpiece may make patient feel better; tell patient that new hair may be different in color, texture

• To avoid foods with citric acid, hot or rough texture

• To report any bleeding, white spots, ulcerations in mouth; tell patient to examine mouth qd

• That urine may be red-orange for 48 hr

---

idoxuridine-IDU (℞)

(eye-dox-yoor'i-deen)
Herplex, Stoxil
Func. class.: Antiviral
Chem. class.: Pyrimidine nucleoside

Action: Inhibits viral replication by interfering with viral DNA synthesis

Uses: Herpes simplex keratitis, CMV, varicella zoster alone or with corticosteroids

Dosage and routes:

• *Adult and child:* INSTILL 1 gtt q1h during day and 2 hr during night

Available forms: Ophth sol 0.1%, ophth oint 0.5%

Side effects/adverse reactions:

EENT: Poor corneal wound healing, temporary visual haze, overgrowth of nonsusceptible organisms

Contraindications: Hypersensitivity

Precautions: Antibiotic hypersensitivity, pregnancy (C)

Interactions:

• Do not use boric acid with this drug

NURSING CONSIDERATIONS
Assess:

• For infection: redness, crusts, drainage, inflammation

• Allergy: itching, lacrimation, redness, swelling

Administer:

• After washing hands; cleanse

 = Nursing alert   = Herb-drug interaction   = Do not crush

crusts or discharge from eye before application

Perform/provide:
• Storage in refrigerator in light-resistant container until used

Evaluate:
• Therapeutic response: absence of redness, inflammation, tearing, photophobia

Teach patient/family:
• To use drug exactly as prescribed
• Not to use eye makeup, towels, washcloths, eye medication of others; reinfection may occur
• That drug container tip should not be touched to eye
• To report itching, increased redness, burning, stinging, swelling; drug should be discontinued
• That drug may cause blurred vision when ointment is applied

---

ifosfamide (℞)

(i-foss'fa-mide)
Ifex
Func. class.: Antineoplastic alkylating agent
Chem. class.: Nitrogen mustard

Action: Alkylates DNA, RNA, inhibits enzymes that allow synthesis of amino acids in proteins; also responsible for cross-linking DNA strands; activity is not cell cycle stage specific

Uses: Testicular cancer

Dosage and routes:
• *Adult:* IV 1.2 g/m^2/day × 5 days, repeat course q3wk, given with mesna

Available forms: Inj 1, 3 g

Side effects/adverse reactions:
CNS: Facial paresthesia, fever, malaise, somnolence, confusion, depression, hallucinations, dizziness, disorientation, *seizures, coma*
GI: Nausea, vomiting, anorexia, *hepatotoxicity,* stomatitis, constipation
INTEG: Dermatitis, alopecia, pain at injection site
GU: **Hematuria, nephrotoxicity, hemorrhagic cystitis,** dysuria, urinary frequency
HEMA: **Thrombocytopenia, leukopenia, anemia**

Contraindications: Hypersensitivity, bone marrow suppression, pregnancy (D)

Precautions: Renal disease, lactation, children

Pharmacokinetics: Metabolized by liver; saturation occurs at high doses; excreted in urine; half-life 7-15 hr

NURSING CONSIDERATIONS

Assess:
• Liver function studies before, during therapy (bilirubin, AST, ALT, LDH) as needed or monthly
• CBC, differential, platelet count weekly; withhold drug if WBC <4000 or platelet count <75,000; notify prescriber
• Monitor temp q4h (may indicate beginning infection)
• Blood dyscrasias (anemia, granulocytopenia); bruising, fatigue, bleeding, poor healing
• Allergic reactions: dermatitis, exfoliative dermatitis, pruritus, urticaria
• Bleeding: hematuria, guaiac, bruising or petechiae, mucosa or orifices q8h
• Food preferences; list likes, dislikes
• Effects of alopecia on body image, discuss feelings about body changes
• Yellowing of skin, sclera, dark urine, clay-colored stools, itchy skin, abdominal pain, fever, diarrhea
• Inflammation of mucosa, breaks in skin

---

* = Canada only   Side effects: *italics* = common; **bold italics** = life-threatening

Administer:

• Antiemetic 30-60 min before giving drug to prevent vomiting

• Antibiotics for prophylaxis of infection

• Always give with mesna to prevent ifosfamide-induced hemorrhagic cystitis

IV

• After diluting 1 g/20 ml sterile or bacteriostatic H_2O for inj with parabens or benzyl only; shake; may be diluted further with D_5W, LR, NS, sterile H_2O for inj; 1 g/20 ml = 50 mg/ml; 1 g/50ml = 20 mg/ml; 1 g/200 ml = 5 mg/ml; give over 30 min

Additive compatibilities: Carboplatin, cisplatin, etoposide, fluorouracil, mesna

Syringe compatibilities: Mesna

Y-site compatibilities: Allopurinol, amifostine, aztreonam, filgrastim, fludarabine, gallium, granisetron, melphalan, ondansetron, paclitaxel, piperacillin/tazobactam, propofol, sargramostim, sodium bicarbonate, teniposide, thiotepa, vinorelbine

Perform/provide:

• Storage of powder at room temp

• Strict medical asepsis, protective isolation if WBC levels are low

• Increase fluid intake to 2-3 L/day to prevent urate deposits, calculi formation

• Warm compresses at injection site for inflammation

Evaluate:

• Therapeutic response: decrease in size and spread of tumor

Teach patient/family:

• To notify prescriber of sore throat, swollen lymph nodes, malaise, fever; other infections may occur

• About protective isolation

• That hair may be lost during treatment; a wig or hairpiece may make the patient feel better; new hair may be different in color, texture

• To report signs of anemia: fatigue, headache, faintness, shortness of breath, irritability

• To report bleeding; avoid use of razors, commercial mouthwash

• To avoid use of aspirin products or ibuprofen

• To use contraceptive measures during therapy

---

imipenem/cilastatin (℞)
(i-me-pen′em sye-la-stat′in)
Primaxin IM, Primaxin IV
Func. class.: Antiinfective-misc. penicillin

Action: Interferes with cell wall replication of susceptible organisms; osmotically unstable cell wall swells, bursts from osmotic pressure; addition of cilastatin prevents renal inactivation that occurs with high urinary concentrations of imipenem

Uses: Serious infections caused by gram-positive: *S. pneumoniae,* group A β-hemolytic streptococci, *S. aureus,* enterococcus; gram-negative: *Klebsiella, Proteus, E. coli, Acinetobacter, Serratia, P. aeruginosa, Salmonella, Shigella*

Dosage and routes:

• Renal adjustment is needed at CrCl <70 ml/min

• *Adult:* **IV** 250-500 mg q6h; severe infections may require 1 g q6h; may give **IM** q12h (total daily **IM** dosage >1500 mg not recommended); mild to moderate infections

Available forms: Inj 250, 500 mg (IV); inj 500, 750 mg (IM)

Side effects/adverse reactions:

CNS: Fever, somnolence, *seizures,* confusion, dizziness, weakness, myoclonia

GI: Diarrhea, nausea, vomiting,

◆ = Nursing alert   ▮ = Herb-drug interaction   ⊘ = Do not crush

pseudomembranous colitis, hepatitis, glossitis
CV: Hypotension, palpitations
*HEMA: **Eosinophilia, neutropenia,*** decreased Hgb, Hct
INTEG: Rash, urticaria, pruritus, pain at injection site, phlebitis, erythema at injection site
*SYST. **Anaphylaxis***
RESP: Chest discomfort, dyspnea, hyperventilation
Contraindications: Hypersensitivity, IM hypersensitivity to local anesthetics of the amide type
Precautions: Pregnancy (C), lactation, elderly, hypersensitivity to penicillins, seizure disorders, renal disease, children
Pharmacokinetics:
IV: Onset immediate, peak ½-1 hr, half-life 1 hr; 70%-80% excreted unchanged in urine
Interactions:
• Increased imipenem plasma levels: probenecid
• Increased toxicity: beta-lactam antibiotics
Lab test interferences:
Increase: AST (SGOT), ALT (SGPT), LDH, BUN, alk phosphatase, bilirubin, creatinine
False positive: Direct Coombs' test
NURSING CONSIDERATIONS
Assess:
• Sensitivity to penicillin, other cephalosporins
• Renal disease: lower dose may be required
• Bowel pattern qd; if severe diarrhea occurs, drug should be discontinued; may indicate pseudomembranous colitis
• Allergic reactions: rash, urticaria, pruritus; may occur few days after therapy begins
• Overgrowth of infection: perineal itching, fever, malaise, redness, pain, swelling, drainage, rash, diarrhea, change in cough, sputum

Administer:
• After C&S is taken
IV
• After reconstitution of 250 or 500 mg with 10 ml of diluent and shake; add to at least 100 ml of same inf sol
• 250-500 mg over 20-30 min; 1 g over 40-60 min; give through Y-tube or 3-way stopcock; do not give by IV bolus or if cloudy
Y-site compatibilities: Acyclovir, amifostine, aztreonam, cefepime, diltiazem, famotidine, fludarabine, foscarnet, granisetron, idarubicin, insulin (regular), melphalan, methotrexate, ondansetron, propofol, tacrolimus, teniposide, thiotepa, vinorelbine, zidovudine
Evaluate:
• Therapeutic response: negative C&S; absence of signs and symptoms of infection
Teach patient/family:
• To report severe diarrhea; may indicate pseudomembranous colitis
• To report sore throat, bruising, bleeding, joint pain; may indicate blood dyscrasias (rare)
Treatment of overdose: Epinephrine, antihistamines; resuscitate if needed (anaphylaxis)

---

imipramine (℞)
(im-ip′ra-meen)
Apo-Imipramine*, imipramine HCl*, Impril*, Janimine, Novo-Pramine*, SK-Pramine, Tofranil, Tofranil PM, Tripramine
Func. class.: Antidepressant—tricyclic
Chem. class.: Dibenzazepine—tertiary amine

Action: Blocks reuptake of norepinephrine, serotonin into nerve endings, increasing action of norepinephrine, serotonin in nerve cells

Uses: Depression, enuresis in children

Investigational uses: Chronic pain, migraine headaches, cluster headaches as adjunct

Dosage and routes:
• *Adult:* **PO/IM** 75-100 mg/day in divided doses, may increase by 25-50 mg to 200 mg, not to exceed 300 mg/day; may give daily dose hs
• *Geriatric:* **PO** 25 mg hs, may increase to 100 mg/day in divided doses
• *Child:* **PO** 25-75 mg/day
Enuresis
• *Child:* **PO** 10 mg at hs, max 50 mg

Available forms: Tabs 10, 25, 50 mg; inj 25 mg/2 ml; caps 75, 100, 125, 150 mg

Side effects/adverse reactions:
HEMA: Agranulocytosis, thrombocytopenia, eosinophilia, leukopenia
CNS: Dizziness, drowsiness, confusion, headache, anxiety, tremors, stimulation, weakness, insomnia, nightmares, EPS (elderly), increased psychiatric symptoms, paresthesia
GI: Diarrhea, dry mouth, nausea, vomiting, *paralytic ileus;* increased appetite; cramps, epigastric distress, jaundice, *hepatitis,* stomatitis
GU: Retention, acute renal failure
INTEG: Rash, urticaria, sweating, pruritus, photosensitivity
CV: Orthostatic hypotension, ECG changes, tachycardia, hypertension, palpitations
EENT: Blurred vision, tinnitus, mydriasis

Contraindications: Hypersensitivity to tricyclic antidepressants, recovery phase of MI, convulsive disorders, prostatic hypertrophy

Precautions: Suicidal patients, severe depression, increased intraocular pressure, narrow-angle glaucoma, urinary retention, cardiac disease, hepatic disease, hyperthyroidism, electroshock therapy, elective surgery, elderly, pregnancy (C), lactation

Pharmacokinetics:
PO: Steady state 2-5 days; metabolized by liver; excreted in urine, breast milk, feces; crosses placenta; half-life 6-20 hr

Interactions:
• Decreased effects of guanethidine, clonidine, indirect-acting sympathomimetics (ephedrine)
• Increased effects of direct-acting sympathomimetics (epinephrine), alcohol, barbiturates, benzodiazepines, CNS depressants
• Hyperpyretic crisis, convulsions, hypertensive episode: MAOI (pargyline [Eutonyl])
 Increased anticholinergic effect: belladonna leaf/root, henbane leaf
 Increased action of imipramine: scopolia root, kava kava

Lab test interferences:
Increase: Serum bilirubin, alk phosphatase, blood glucose
Decrease: 5-HIAA, VMA, urinary catecholamines

NURSING CONSIDERATIONS
Assess:
• B/P (lying, standing), pulse q4h; if systolic B/P drops 20 mm Hg, hold drug, notify prescriber; take vital signs q4h in patients with cardiovascular disease
• Blood studies: CBC, leukocytes, differential, cardiac enzymes if patient is receiving long-term therapy
• Hepatic studies: AST (SGOT), ALT (SGPT), bilirubin
• Weight qwk; appetite may increase with drug
• ECG for flattening of T wave, bundle branch block, AV block, dysrhythmias in cardiac patients
• EPS primarily in elderly: rigidity, dystonia, akathisia
• Mental status: mood, sensorium,

◆ = Nursing alert   = Herb-drug interaction   🚫 = Do not crush

affect, suicidal tendencies, increase in psychiatric symptoms: depression, panic
• Urinary retention, constipation; constipation is more likely to occur in children, elderly
◆ Withdrawal symptoms: headache, nausea, vomiting, muscle pain, weakness; not usual unless drug discontinued abruptly
• Alcohol consumption; if alcohol is consumed, hold dose until morning

Administer:
• Increased fluids, bulk in diet for constipation, urinary retention
• With food or milk for GI symptoms
• Dosage hs if oversedation occurs during day; may take entire dose hs; elderly may not tolerate once/day dosing
• Gum, hard candy, or frequent sips of water for dry mouth
• In IM route after running warm water over ampule to dissolve crystals

Syringe compatibilities: Doxapram
Y-site compatibilities: Cladribine

Perform/provide:
• Storage in tight container at room temp; do not freeze
• Assistance with ambulation during beginning therapy, since drowsiness/dizziness occurs
• Safety measures, including side rails, primarily in elderly
• Checking to see if PO medication swallowed

Evaluate:
• Therapeutic response: decreased depression, enuresis

Teach patient/family:
• That therapeutic effects may take 2-3 wk
• That drug is dispensed in small amounts because of suicide potential, especially in beginning of therapy

• To use caution in driving, other activities requiring alertness because of drowsiness, dizziness, blurred vision
• To avoid alcohol ingestion, other CNS depressants
• Not to discontinue medication quickly after long-term use; may cause nausea, headache, malaise
• To wear sunscreen or large hat, since photosensitivity occurs
🚫 Not to break, crush, or chew caps

Treatment of overdose: ECG monitoring; induce emesis; lavage, activated charcoal; administer anticonvulsant

---

immune globulin (℞)
gamma globulin, Gamimune N, Gammagard S/D, Gammar-P IV, Iveegam, Polygam, Polygam S/D, Sandoglobulin, Venoglobulin-I, Venoglobulin-S
Func. class.: Immune serum
Chem. class.: IgG

Action: Provides passive immunity to hepatitis A, measles, varicella, rubella, immune globulin deficiency; contains gamma globulin antibodies (IgG)

Uses: Immunodeficiency syndrome, B-cell chronic lymphocytic leukemia, Kawasaki syndrome, bone marrow transplantation, pediatric HIV infection, agammaglobulinemia, hepatitis A, B exposure, measles exposure, measles vaccine complications, purpura, rubella exposure, chickenpox exposure

Dosage and routes:
• *Adult:* **IM** 30-50 ml qmo; **IV** 100 mg/kg qmo, 0.01-0.02 ml/kg/min × ½ hr (Gamimune N); **IV** 200 mg/kg qmo, 0.05-1 ml/min × 15-30 min,

then increase to 1.5-2.5 ml/min (Sandoglobulin)
• *Child:* IM 20-40 ml qmo
Hepatitis A exposure
• *Adult and child:* IM 0.02-0.04 ml/kg or 0.1 mg/kg if treatment is delayed
Hepatitis B exposure
• *Adult and child:* IM 0.06 ml/kg within 1 wk, qmo
Measles (postexposure)
• *Child:* IM 0.25 ml/kg within 6 days
Immunoglobulin deficiency
• *Adult and child:* IM 1.3 ml/kg, then 0.66 ml/kg after 2-4 wk and q2-4wk thereafter
Idiopathic thrombocytopenia, purpura
• *Adult and child:* IV 0.4 g/kg × 5 days or 1 g/kg/day × 1-2 days
Kawasaki syndrome
• *Child:* PO 2 g/kg as a single dose
Available forms: Inj 2, 10 ml/vial; 5% sol, 0.5, 1, 2.5, 3, 6, 10 g vials
Side effects/adverse reactions:
INTEG: Pain at injection site, rash, pruritus, chills, chest pain
MS: Arthralgia
SYST: Lymphadenopathy, **anaphylaxis**
CNS: Headache, fatigue, malaise
GI: Abdominal pain
Contraindications: Hypersensitivity
Precautions: Pregnancy (C)
Interactions:
• Do not administer live virus vaccines within 3 mo of this drug
NURSING CONSIDERATIONS
Assess:
• For exposure date: this drug should be given within 6 days of measles, 7 days of hepatitis B, 14 days of hepatitis A
• For anaphylaxis: diaphoresis, wheezing, chest tightness, hypotension

Administer:
• IM ≤3 ml in one site, use large muscle mass
• Only with epinephrine 1:1000, resuscitative equipment available
• Only within 2 wk of exposure to hepatitis A
IV
• Gamimune N: IV undiluted or dilute with D_5; give 0.01 ml/kg/min; may increase to 0.02-0.04 ml/kg/min
• Sandoglobulin: IV diluted with provided diluent; give 0.5-1 ml/min × 15-30 min; may increase to 1.5-2.5 ml/min
• Venoglobulin-I: (50 mg/ml sol) give 0.01-0.02 ml/kg/min; if no adverse reaction in ½ hr, increase to 0.04 ml/kg/min, store at room temp
• Gammagard: reconstitute with sterile H_2O for inj (50 mg protein/ml); give 0.5 ml/kg/hr, may increase to 4 ml/kg/hr, use infusion set provided
• Gammar-IV: give 0.01 ml/kg/min (50 mg/ml sol) × 15-30 min, may increase to 0.02 ml/kg/min, may increase to 0.03-0.06 ml/kg/min
Y-site compatibilities: Fluconazole, sargramostim
Perform/provide:
• Storage at 36°-46° F (2°-8° C)
Evaluate:
• Prevention of infection, increased platelets
Teach patient/family:
• That passive immunity is temporary
• The treatment of anaphylaxis: epinephrine, diphenhydramine, O_2, vasopressors, corticosteroids

---

indapamide (℞)

(in-dap′a-mide)

Lozol

Func. class.: Diuretic—thiazide-like, antihypertensive

Chem. class.: Indoline

Action: Acts on proximal section of distal renal tubule and thick ascending loop of Henle by inhibiting reabsorption of sodium; may act by direct vasodilation caused by blocking of calcium channel

Uses: Edema of CHF, hypertension, diuresis

Dosage and routes:

Edema

• *Adult:* **PO** 2.5 mg qd in AM; may be increased to 5 mg qd if needed

Antihypertensive

• *Adult:* 1.25-5 mg qd; may increase to 5 mg/day over 8 wk

Available forms: Tabs 1.25, 2.5 mg

Side effects/adverse reactions:

GU: Polyuria, nocturia, frequency, impotence

ELECT: Hypochloremic alkalosis, hypomagnesemia, hyperuricemia, hypercalcemia, hyponatremia, hypokalemia, hyperglycemia

CNS: Headache, dizziness, fatigue, weakness, nervousness, agitation, extremity numbness, depression

GI: Nausea, diarrhea, dry mouth, vomiting, anorexia, cramps, constipation, abdominal pain

EENT: Blurred vision, nasal congestion, increased intraocular pressure

INTEG: Rash, pruritus

MS: Cramps

CV: Orthostatic hypotension, volume depletion, palpitations, dysrhythmias, PVCs

Contraindications: Hypersensitivity, anuria, hepatic coma

Precautions: Hypokalemia, dehydration, ascites, hepatic disease, severe renal disease, pregnancy (B), lactation, CrCl <25 ml/min (not effective)

Pharmacokinetics:

PO: Onset 1-2 hr, peak 2 hr, duration up to 36 hr; excreted in urine, feces; half-life 14-18 hr

Interactions:

• Hyperglycemia: diazoxide

• Increased toxicity of: muscle relaxants, steroids, lithium, digitalis

• Decreased K: steroids, amphotericin B

• Decreased effects: antidiabetics, antigout agents, anticoagulants

• Decreased absorption: cholestyramine, colestipol

• Decreased hypotensive effect: indomethacin, NSAIDs

🖉 Potassium deficiency: aloe, buckthorn bark/berry, cascara sagrada bark, licorice root, senna pod/leaf

Lab test interferences:

Increase: Ca, parathyroid test glucose, uric acid

NURSING CONSIDERATIONS

Assess:

• Weight daily, I&O daily to determine fluid loss; effect of drug may be decreased if used qd

• Rate, depth, rhythm of respiration, effect of exertion

• B/P lying, standing; postural hypotension may occur

• Electrolytes: K, Mg, Na, Cl: include BUN, CBC, serum creatinine, blood pH, ABGs, uric acid, Ca, glucose

• Signs of metabolic alkalosis

• Signs of hypokalemia

• Rashes, fever qd

• Confusion, especially in elderly; take safety precautions if needed

• Hydration: skin turgor, thirst, dry mucous membranes

Administer:

• In AM to avoid interference with sleep

• With food; if nausea occurs, absorption may be decreased slightly

Evaluate:

• Therapeutic response: improvement in edema of feet, legs, sacral area daily, decreased B/P

Teach patient/family:

• To increase fluid intake to 2-3 L/day unless contraindicated; diet high in K; to rise slowly from lying or sitting position

• To recognize adverse reactions: muscle cramps, weakness, nausea, dizziness

• To take with food or milk for GI symptoms

• To use sunscreen for photosensitivity

• To take early in day to prevent nocturia

Treatment of overdose: Lavage if taken orally; monitor electrolytes, administer IV fluids; monitor hydration, CV, renal status

---

indinavir (℞)

(en-den′a-veer)
Crixivan
Func. class.: Antiviral
Chem. class.: Synthetic peptide-like substrate analog

Action: Inhibits human immunodeficiency virus (HIV) protease; this prevents maturation of the infectious virus

Uses: HIV alone or in combination

Dosage and routes:

• Reduce dose in mild/moderate hepatic impairment and ketoconazole co-administration

• *Adult:* **PO** 800 mg q8h; if given with ddI, give 1 hr apart on empty stomach

Available forms: Caps 200, 400 mg

Side effects/adverse reactions:

GI: Diarrhea, abdominal pain, nausea, vomiting, anorexia, dry mouth

CNS: Headache, insomnia, dizziness, somnolence

INTEG: Rash

MS: Pain

OTHER: Asthenia

Contraindications: Hypersensitivity

Precautions: Liver disease, pregnancy (C), lactation, children, renal disease

Pharmacokinetics: Unknown

Interactions:

• Increase indinavir levels: ketoconazole

• Decreased indinavir levels: rifamycins

• Increased levels of both drugs: clarithromycin, zidovudine

• Increased levels of astemizole, cisapride, midazolam, triazolam, isoniazid, oral contraceptives when given with saquinavir

NURSING CONSIDERATIONS

Assess:

• Signs of infection, anemia

• Liver studies: ALT, AST

• The presence of other sexually transmitted diseases

• Bowel pattern before, during treatment; if severe abdominal pain with bleeding occurs, drug should be discontinued; monitor hydration

• Skin eruptions; rash, urticaria, itching

• Allergies before treatment, reaction of each medication; place allergies on chart

Administer:

• With water, 1 hr ac or 2 hr pc

Teach patient/family:

• To take as prescribed; if dose is missed, take as soon as remembered up to 1 hr before next dose; do not double dose

🚫 Not to break, crush, or chew caps

◆ = Nursing alert   🖊 = Herb-drug interaction   🚫 = Do not crush

• That drug must be taken in equal intervals around the clock to maintain blood levels for duration of therapy

---

indomethacin (℞)

(in-doe-meth'a-sin)
Apo-Indomethacin*, Indameth*, Indocid*, Indocin, Indocin IV, Indocin PDA*, Indocin SR, Indomethacin, Novomethacin*

Func. class.: Nonsteroidal antiinflammatory (NSAID)

Chem. class.: Propionic acid derivative

Action: Inhibits prostaglandin synthesis by decreasing enzyme needed for biosynthesis; analgesic, antiinflammatory, antipyretic

Uses: Rheumatoid arthritis, ankylosing rheumatoid spondylitis, acute gouty arthritis, closure of patent ductus arteriosus in premature infants

Dosage and routes:
Arthritis/antiinflammatory
• *Adult:* **PO/RECT** 25-50 mg bid; may increase by 25 mg/day qwk, not to exceed 200 mg/day; **SUS REL** 75 mg qd, may increase to 75 mg bid

Acute arthritis
• *Adult:* **PO/RECT** 50 mg tid; use only for acute attack, then reduce dose

Patent ductus arteriosus
• *Infant <2 days:* **IV** 0.2 mg/kg, then 0.1 mg/kg q12-24h
• *Infant 2-7 days:* **IV** 0.2 mg/kg, then 0.2 mg × 2 doses after 12, 24 hr
• *Infant >7 days:* **IV** 0.2 mg/kg, then 0.25 mg/kg × 2 doses after 12, 24 hr

Available forms: Caps 25, 50 mg; caps ext rel 75 mg; susp 25 mg/5 ml; rec supp 50 mg; inj 1 mg vial

Side effects/adverse reactions:
GI: Nausea, anorexia, *vomiting,* diarrhea, jaundice, ***cholestatic hepatitis,*** *constipation,* flatulence, cramps, dry mouth, peptic ulcer, ***ulceration, perforation, GI bleeding***
CNS: Dizziness, drowsiness, fatigue, tremors, confusion, insomnia, anxiety, depression, headache
CV: Tachycardia, peripheral edema, palpitations, dysrhythmias, hypertension
INTEG: Purpura, rash, pruritus, sweating
*GU: **Nephrotoxicity: dysuria, hematuria, oliguria, azotemia***
*HEMA: **Blood dyscrasias***, prolonged bleeding
EENT: Tinnitus, hearing loss, blurred vision

Contraindications: Hypersensitivity, asthma, severe renal disease, severe hepatic disease, ulcer disease

Precautions: Pregnancy, lactation, children, bleeding disorders, GI disorders, cardiac disorders, hypersensitivity to other antiinflammatory agents, pregnancy (B) 1st and 2nd trimesters, lactation, depression

Pharmacokinetics:
PO: Onset 1-2 hr, peak 3 hr, duration 4-6 hr; metabolized in liver, kidneys; excreted in urine, bile, feces; crosses placenta; excreted in breast milk; 99% plasma protein binding

Interactions:
• Increased action of coumadin, phenytoin, sulfonamides
• Toxicity: lithium, methotrexate, cyclosporine
• Decreased action of triamterene
• Do not give with antacids

NURSING CONSIDERATIONS
Assess:
• Renal, liver, blood studies: BUN, creatinine, AST (SGOT), ALT (SGPT), Hgb, before treatment, periodically thereafter

---

• Audiometric, ophthalmic exam before, during, after treatment
• For eye, ear problems: blurred vision, tinnitus; may indicate toxicity
• For confusion, mood changes, hallucinations, especially in elderly
Administer:
PO
• With food to decrease GI symptoms and prevent ulcerations; do not crush, chew, or break sus rel cap
IV
• After diluting 1 mg/ml or more NS or sterile H$_2$O for inj without preservative; give over 5-10 sec
Y-site compatibilities: Furosemide, insulin (regular), potassium chloride, sodium bicarbonate, sodium nitroprusside
Perform/provide:
• Storage at room temp
Evaluate:
• Therapeutic response: decreased pain, stiffness in joints, decreased swelling in joints, ability to move more easily
Teach patient/family:
• To report blurred vision, ringing, roaring in ears; may indicate toxicity
• To avoid driving, other hazardous activities if dizziness, drowsiness occurs
• To report change in urine pattern, increased weight, edema, increased pain in joints, fever, blood in urine; indicate nephrotoxicity; to report mood changes: anxiety, depression
• That therapeutic antiinflammatory effects may take up to 1 mo
• To avoid alcohol, salicylates; bleeding may occur
🚫 Not to break, crush, or chew sus rel or reg caps

influenza virus vaccine, trivalent A & B (whole virus/split virus) (℞)

Fluogen, FluShield, Fluviral*, Fluvirin, Fluzone, Influenza Virus vaccine, Trivalent
Func. class.: Vaccine

Action: Produces antibodies to influenza virus; split virus vaccine causes less adverse reactions
Uses: Prevention of Russian, Chile, Philippine influenza
Dosage and routes:
• *Adult and child >12 yr:* **IM** 0.5 ml in 1 dose
• *Child 3-12 yr:* **IM** 0.5 ml, repeat in 1 mo (split) unless 1978-1985 vaccine was given
• *Child 6 mo to 3 yr:* **IM** 0.25 ml, repeat in 1 mo (split) unless 1978-1985 vaccine was given
Available forms: Inj IM (varies)
Side effects/adverse reactions:
CNS: Fever, Guillain-Barré syndrome
INTEG: Urticaria, induration, erythema
*SYST: **Anaphylaxis,** malaise*
MS: Myalgia
Contraindications: Hypersensitivity, active infection; chicken, egg allergy, Guillain-Barré syndrome
Precautions: Elderly, immunosuppression, pregnancy (B)
NURSING CONSIDERATIONS
Assess:
• For skin reactions: rash, induration, erythema
• For anaphylaxis: inability to breathe, bronchospasm
Administer:
• Only with epinephrine 1:1000 on unit to treat laryngospasm
• Only IM

Perform/provide:
• Written record of immunization
• At least 2 mo after measles virus vaccine; do not administer at same time as DPT
Evaluate:
• For history of allergies, skin conditions (eczema, psoriasis, dermatitis), reactions to vaccinations

insulin, isophane suspension (NPH) (℞)
Humulin N, Iletin NPH*, Iletin II NPH*, Novolin ge NPH*, Novolin N, Novolin N PenFill, Novolin N Prefilled, NPH Iletin I, NPH Iletin II, NPH-N

insulin, isophane suspension and regular insulin (℞)
Humulin 70/30, Humalin 30/70*, Novolin 70/30, Novolin 70/30 PenFill, Novolin 70/30 Prefilled, Novolin ge 30/70*

insulin, regular (℞)
Humulin R*, Iletin I*, Iletin II*, Novolin ge Toronto*, Novolin R, Novolin R Velosulin, Novolin R PenFill, Novolin R Prefilled, Regular Ilentin I, II, Regular Purified Pork Insulin, Velosulin Human BR

insulin, zinc suspension (Lente) (℞)
Humulin L, Iletin*, Iletin II*, Lente Ilentin I, Lente Iletin II, Lente L, Novolin ge Lente*, Novolin L

insulin, zinc suspension extended (Ultralente) (℞)
Humulin U Ultralente, Humulin U*, Novolin ge Ultralente*

insulin, analog injection (℞)
Humalog

isophane insulin suspension and insulin injection (℞)
Humalin 50/50, Novolin 50/50*

Func. class.: Pancreatic hormone

Chem. class.: Exogenous unmodified insulin

Action: Decreases blood sugar; by transport of insulin into cells and the conversion of glucose to glycogen indirectly increases blood pyruvate and lactate, decreases phosphate and potassium; insulin may be beef, pork, human (processed by recombinant DNA technologies)

Uses: Adult-onset diabetes, juvenile diabetes, ketoacidosis types I and II, type II (non–insulin-dependent) diabetes mellitus, type I (insulin-dependent) diabetes mellitus

Dosage and routes:
Insulin, isophane suspension
• *Adult:* SC dosage individualized by blood, urine glucose; usual dose 7-26 U; may increase by 2-10 U/day if needed

Regular insulin (ketoacidosis)
• *Adult:* IV 5-10 U, then 5-10 U/hr until desired response, then switch to SC dose; IV/inf 2-12 U (50 U/500 ml of normal saline)
• *Child:* IV 0.1 U/kg

Replacement
• *Adult and child:* SC 0.5-1 U/kg/ day qid given 30 min ac
• *Adolescent:* SC 0.8-1.2 mg/kg/ day; this dosage is used during rapid growth

Available forms: NPH Inj 100 U/ml; regular inj 100 U/ml; zinc susp 100 U/ml; insulin analog inj 100 U/ml; insulin zinc susp, ext (ultralente) 100 U/ml; isophane insulin/insulin inj 100 U/ml

Side effects/adverse reactions:
EENT: Blurred vision, dry mouth
INTEG: Flushing, rash, urticaria, warmth, *lipodystrophy,* lipohypertrophy, swelling, redness
META: Hypoglycemia, rebound hyperglycemia (Somogyi effect 12-72 hr or longer)
SYST: Anaphylaxis

Contraindications: Hypersensitivity to protamine

Precautions: Pregnancy (B)

Pharmacokinetics:
SC (NPH): Onset 1-2 hr, peak 4-12 hr, duration 18-24 hr
SC (regular susp): Onset ½ hr, peak 4-8 hr, duration 12-24 hr
SC (regular): Onset ½-1 hr, peak 2-4 hr, duration 5-7 hr
IV (regular): Onset 10-30 min, peak 10-30 min, duration ½-1 hr
SC (regular conc): Onset ½-1 hr, peak 2-5 hr, duration 5-7 hr
SC (zinc susp): Onset 1-2 ½ hr, peak 7-15 hr, duration 12-24 hr
SC (zinc susp conc): Onset 4-8 hr, peak 10-30 hr, duration, 7-36 hr
SC (zinc susp prompt): Onset 1-1 ½ hr, peak 5-10 hr, duration 12-16 hr
Metabolized by liver, muscle, kidneys; excreted in urine

Interactions:
• Increased hypoglycemia: salicylate, alcohol, β-blockers, anabolic steroids, fenfluramine, phenylbutazone, sulfinpyrazone, guanethidine, oral hypoglycemics, MAOIs, tetracycline
• Decreased hypoglycemia: thiazides, thyroid hormones, oral contraceptives, corticosteroids, estrogens, dobutamine, epinephrine

Lab test interferences:
Increase: VMA
Decrease: K, Ca
Interference: Liver function studies, thyroid function studies

NURSING CONSIDERATIONS
Assess:
• Fasting blood glucose, 2 hr PP (80-150 mg/dl, normal fasting level; 70-130 mg/dl, normal 2 hr level); also glycosylated Hgb may be drawn to identify treatment effectiveness
• Urine ketones during illness; insulin requirements may increase during stress, illness, surgery
• For hypoglycemic reaction that can occur during peak time (sweating,

weakness, dizziness, chills, confusion, headache, nausea, rapid weak pulse, fatigue, tachycardia, memory lapses, slurred speech, staggering gait, anxiety, tremors, hunger)
• For hyperglycemia: acetone breath, polyuria, fatigue, polydipsia, flushed, dry skin, lethargy
Administer: SC route
SC
• After warming to room temp by rotating in palms to prevent injecting cold insulin; use only insulin syringes with markings or syringe matching U/ml; rotate inj sites within one area: abdomen, upper back, thighs, upper arm, buttocks; keep record of sites
• Increased dosages if tolerance occurs; give human insulin to those allergic to beef or pork
• Do not use if cloudy, thick, or discolored
IV
• IV direct, undiluted via vein, Y-site, 3-way stopcock; give at 50 U/min or less
• By cont inf after diluting with IV sol and run at prescribed rate; use IV inf pump for correct dosing; give reduced dose at serum glucose level of 250 mg/100 ml
Additive compatibilities: Bretylium, cimetidine, lidocaine, meropenem, ranitidine, verapamil
Syringe compatibilities: Metoclopramide
Y-site compatibilities: Amiodarone, ampicillin, ampicillin/sulbactam, aztreonam, cefazolin, cefotetan, dobutamine, esmolol, famotidine, gentamicin, heparin, heparin/hydrocortisone, imipenem/cilastatin, indomethacin, magnesium sulfate, meperidine, meropenem, midazolam, morphine, nitroglycerin, oxytocin, pentobarbital, potassium chloride, propofol, ritodrine, sodium bicarbonate, sodium nitroprus-

side, tacrolimus, terbutaline, ticarcillin, ticarcillin/clavulanate, tobramycin, vancomycin, vit B/C
Perform/provide:
• Store at room temp for <1 mo; keep away from heat and sunlight; refrigerate all other supply; do not use if discolored; do not freeze—IV route, regular only
Evaluate:
• Therapeutic response: decrease in polyuria, polydipsia, polyphagia, clear sensorium, absence of dizziness, stable gait
Teach patient/family:
• That blurred vision occurs; not to change corrective lens until vision is stabilized 1-2 mo
• To keep insulin, equipment available at all times
• That drug does not cure diabetes but controls symptoms
• To carry Medic Alert ID as diabetic
• To recognize hypoglycemia reaction: headache, tremors, fatigue, weakness
• The dosage, route, mixing instructions, if any diet restrictions, disease process
• To carry candy or lump sugar to treat hypoglycemia
• The symptoms of ketoacidosis: nausea, thirst, polyuria, dry mouth, decreased B/P, dry, flushed skin, acetone breath, drowsiness, Kussmaul respirations
• That a plan is necessary for diet, exercise; all food on diet should be eaten; exercise routine should not vary
• About blood glucose testing; make sure patient is able to determine glucose level
• To avoid OTC drugs unless directed by prescriber
Treatment of overdose: Glucose 25g IV, via dextrose 50% sol, 50 ml or glucagon 1 mg

insulin lispro (℞)
Humalog
Func. class.: Pancreatic hormone
Chem. class.: Insulin analog

Action: Decreases blood sugar, indirectly increases blood pyruvate, lactate, decreases phosphate, potassium; rapid onset, shorter duration of action than regular insulin

Uses: Adult-onset diabetes, juvenile diabetes, ketoacidosis type I, II, NIDDM, IDDM

Dosage and routes:
• *Adult and child:* SC dosage individualized by blood, urine glucose levels
Available forms: Inj U 100/ml, 1.5 ml cartridges

Side effects/adverse reactions:
EENT: Blurred vision, dry mouth
INTEG: Flushing, rash, urticaria, warmth, *lipodystrophy,* lipohypertrophy, swelling, redness
*META: **Hypoglycemia,*** rebound hyperglycemia (Somogyi effect)
*SYST: **Anaphylaxis***

Contraindications: Hypersensitivity

Precautions: Pregnancy (B)

Pharmacokinetics:
SC: Onset 15 min, peak 40-60 min, half-life 46 min; metabolized by liver, muscle, kidneys; excreted in urine

Interactions:
• Increased hypoglycemia: salicylate, alcohol, β-blockers, anabolic steroids, fenfluramine, guanethidine, oral hypoglycemics, MAOIs, tetracycline, sulfinpyrazone
• Decreased hypoglycemia: thiazides, thyroid hormones, oral contraceptives, corticosteroids, estrogens, dobutamine, epinephrine, dextrothyroxine, smoking
• Mask signs/symptoms of hypoglycemia: β-blocker

Lab test interferences:
Increase: VMA
Decrease: K, Ca
Interference: Liver function studies, thyroid function studies

NURSING CONSIDERATIONS
Assess:
• Hypoglycemic/hyperglycemic reaction that can occur soon after meals
• Fasting blood glucose, 2 hr PP (60-100 mg/dl normal fasting level); (70-130 mg/dl normal 2 hr level)
• Urine ketones during illness; insulin requirements increase during times of stress, illness

Administer:
• After warming to room temp by rotating in palms to prevent lipodystrophy from injecting cold insulin
• SC at 90-degree angle (½″ needle), 45-degree angle (⅝″ needle); apply pressure; do not massage
• 15 min ac, so peak action coincides with peak sugar level
• Increased doses if tolerance occurs

Perform/provide:
• Storage at room temp for 1 mo; keep in cool area; refrigerate all other supply; do not freeze; do not use discolored or cloudy sol; discard open vials not used in 1 mo
• Rotation of injection sites: abdomen, upper back, thighs, upper arm, buttocks; keep record of sites

Evaluate:
• Therapeutic response: decrease in polyuria, polydipsia, polyphagia; clear sensorium, absence of dizziness, stable gait

Teach patient/family:
• That blurred vision occurs; not to change corrective lenses until vision is stabilized 1-2 mo
• To keep insulin, equipment available at all times; provide instruc-

tions for using automatic injector if needed

• That drug does not cure diabetes, but controls symptoms

• To carry Medic Alert ID as diabetic

• To recognize hypoglycemic reaction: headache, tremors, fatigue, weakness, sweating

• The dosage, route; if any diet restrictions; disease process

• To carry candy or lump sugar to treat hypoglycemia

• The symptoms of ketoacidosis: nausea, thirst, polyuria, dry mouth, decrease in B/P, dry flushed skin, acetone breath, drowsiness, Kussmaul respirations

• That a plan is necessary for diet, exercise; all food on diet should be eaten; exercise routine should not vary

• About blood glucose testing; make sure patient is able to determine glucose level

• That pregnant patients should use glucose oxidase reagents

• To avoid OTC drugs unless directed by prescriber

• To identify lipotrophy; make chart of rotation sites

Treatment of overdose: Glucose 25 g IV, via dextrose 50% sol, 50 ml or 1 mg glucagon

---

interferon alfa-2a/ interferon alfa-2b (Ŗ)

(in-ter-feer'on)
Roferon-a/Intron-a
Func. class.: Misc. antineoplastic
Chem. class.: Protein product

Action: Antiviral action inhibits viral replication by reprogramming virus; antitumor action suppresses cell proliferation; immunomodulating action phagocytizes target cells; may also inhibit virus replication in virus-infested cells

Uses: Hairy cell leukemia in persons >18 yr, condylomata acuminata, malignant melanoma, AIDS (use phase II with zidovudine), chronic hepatitis B, C

Investigational uses: Bladder tumors, carcinoid tumors, non-Hodgkin's lymphoma, essential thrombocytopenia, cytomegaloviruses, herpes simplex

Dosage and routes:
Alfa-2a
• *Adult:* **SC/IM** 3 million IU × 16-24 wk, then 3 million IU 3 × wk maintenance
Alfa-2b
Chronic hepatitis B
• 30-35 million IU/wk **SC/IM** as 5 million IU/day or 10 million IU/3 × /wk × 16 wk
Hairy cell leukemia
• 2 million IU/m^2 3 × wk; if severe adverse reactions occur, dose should be skipped or reduced by ½
Condylomata acuminata
• 1 million IU/lesion 3 × /wk × 3 wk
Kaposi's sarcoma
• 30 million IU/m^2 3 × /wk
Available forms: alfa-2a inj 3, 6, 36 million IU/ml; alfa-2b inj 3, 5, 10, 18, 25 million U/vial, powder for inj 5, 10, 18, 25, 50 million U/vial

Side effects/adverse reactions:
CNS: Dizziness, confusion, numbness, paresthesias, hallucinations, **convulsions, coma,** amnesia, anxiety, mood changes
CV: Edema, hypotension, hypertension, chest pain, palpitations, dysrhythmias, **CHF, MI, CVA**
INTEG: Rash, dry skin, itching, alopecia, flushing, photosensitivity
GI: Weight loss, taste changes
GU: Impotence
MISC: Flu-like syndrome; fever, fatigue, myalgias, headache, chills

---

Contraindications: Hypersensitivity

Precautions: Severe hypotension, dysrhythmia, tachycardia, pregnancy (C), lactation, children, severe renal or hepatic disease, convulsion disorder

Pharmacokinetics: Half-life (interferon alfa-2a) 3.7-8.5 hr, peak 3-4 hr; half-life (interferon alfa-2b) 2-7 hr, peak 6-8 hr

Interferon alpha-2b

Interactions:

• Increased theophylline levels: aminophylline

• Increased neutropenia: zidovudine

Lab test interferences:

Interference: AST (SGOT), ALT (SGPT), LDH, alk phosphatase, WBC, platelets, granulocytes, creatinine

NURSING CONSIDERATIONS

Assess:

• For symptoms of infection; may be masked by drug fever

• CNS reaction: LOC, mental status, dizziness, confusion

Administer:

• IM/SC after reconstituting 3-5 million IU/1 ml, 10 million IU/2 ml, 25 million IU/5 ml, of diluent provided, mix gently

• Intralesional after reconstituting 10 million IU/1 ml bacteriostatic water for inj; no more than 5 lesions can safely be treated at a time

• At hs to minimize side effects

• Acetaminophen as ordered to alleviate fever and headache

Perform/provide:

• Storage of reconstituted sol for 1 mo in refrigerator

• Increased fluid intake to 2-3 L/day

Evaluate:

• Therapeutic response: decrease in size, number of lesions

Teach patient/family:

• To take acetaminophen for fever

• To avoid hazardous tasks, since confusion, dizziness may occur; avoid prolonged sunlight, use sunscreen

• That brands of this drug should not be changed; each form is different, with different doses

• That fatigue is common; activity may have to be altered to take hs to minimize flu-like symptoms

• Not to become pregnant while taking drug; possible mutagenic effects

• To report signs of infection: sore throat, fever, diarrhea, vomiting

• That impotence may occur during treatment but is temporary

• That emotional lability is common; notify prescriber if severe or incapacitating

---

interferon alfacon-1 (℞)

(in-ter-feer'on al'fa-kon)
Infergen
Func. class.: Recombinant type I interferon

Action: Induces biologic responses and has antiviral, antiproliferative and immunomodulatory effects

Uses: Chronic hepatitis C infections

Investigational uses: Hairy cell leukemia when used with G-CSF

Dosage and routes:

• *Adult:* SC 9 µg as a single inj 3×/wk × 24 wk

Available forms: Inj 9 µg, 15 µg

Side effects/adverse reactions:

CNS: Headache, fatigue, fever, rigors, insomnia, dizziness

GI: Abdominal pain, nausea, diarrhea, anorexia, dyspepsia, vomiting, constipation, flatulence, hemorrhoids, decreased salivation

MS: Back, limb, neck skeletal pain

GU: Dysmenorrhea, vaginitis, menstrual disorders

◆ = Nursing alert　　🖋 = Herb-drug interaction　　⊘ = Do not crush

INTEG: Alopecia, pruritus, rash, erythema, dry skin
EENT: Tinnitus, earache, conjunctivitis, eye pain
HEMA: Granulocytopenia, ***thrombocytopenia, leukopenia,*** ecchymosis
CV: Hypertension, palpitation
PSYCH: Nervousness, depression, anxiety, lability, abnormal thinking
RESP: Pharyngitis, upper respiratory infection, cough, sinusitis, rhinitis, respiratory tract congestion, epistaxis, dyspnea, bronchitis
Contraindications: Hypersensitivity to alpha interferons, or products from *E. coli*
Precautions: Thyroid disorders, myelosuppression, hepatic, cardiac disease, lactation, children <18 yr
Pharmacokinetics: Peak 24-36 hr
Interactions:
• None known
NURSING CONSIDERATIONS
Assess:
• Platelet counts, heme concentration, ANC, serum creatinine concentration, albumin, bilirubin, TSH, T4
• For myelosuppression, hold dose if neutrophil count is $<500 \times 10^6/L$ or if platelets are $<50 \times 10^9/L$
• For hypersensitivity: discontinue immediately if hypersensitivity occurs
Evaluate:
• Therapeutic response: decreased chronic hepatitis C signs/symptoms
Teach patient/family:
• Provide patient or family member with written, detailed information about drug

interferon alfa-n 3 (R)

(in-ter-feer'on)
Alferon N
Func. class.: Antineoplastic
Chem. class.: Human interferon α-protein

Action: Binds interferon to membrane receptors on cell surface with high specificity; this produces protein synthesis, inhibition of virus replication, suppression of cell proliferation, increased phagocytosis
Uses: Condylomata acuminata (venereal/genital warts)
Dosage and routes:
• *Adult:* 0.05 ml (250,000 IU) per wart, given 2 × /wk × 8 wk; not to exceed 0.5 ml (2.5 million IU); inject into base of wart
Available forms: Inj 5 m IU/l ml vial with 3.3 mg/ml phenol and 1 mg/ml human albumin
Side effects/adverse reactions:
CNS: Fever, headache, sweating, vasovagal reaction, chills, fatigue, dizziness, insomnia, sleepiness, depression
GI: Nausea, vomiting, heartburn, diarrhea, constipation, anorexia, stomatitis, dry mouth
MS: Myalgias, arthralgia, back pain
INTEG: Pain at injection site, pruritus
CV: Chest pain, hypotension
Contraindications: Hypersensitivity to this product, egg protein, IgG, neomycin
Precautions: Pregnancy (C), lactation, children, CHF, angina (unstable), COPD, diabetes mellitus with ketoacidosis, hemophilia, pulmonary embolism, thrombophlebitis, bone marrow depression, convulsive disorder
Pharmacokinetics: Unable to detect

Lab test interferences:
Interference: AST (SGOT), ALT (SGPT), LDH, alk phosphatase, WBC, platelets, granulocytes, creatinine

NURSING CONSIDERATIONS
Assess:
• For symptoms of infection; may be masked by drug fever
• CNS reaction: LOC, mental status, dizziness, confusion
• For body image disturbance
Administer:
• Acetaminophen to alleviate fever and headache
Perform/provide:
• Storage of reconstituted sol for 1 mo in refrigerator
• Increased fluid intake to 2-3 L/day
Evaluate:
• Therapeutic response: decrease in wart size
Teach patient/family:
• To avoid hazardous tasks, since confusion, dizziness may occur
• That brands of this drug should not be changed; each form is different, with different doses
• That fatigue is common; activity may have to be altered
• Not to become pregnant while taking drug; possible mutagenic effects
• To report signs of infection: sore throat, fever, diarrhea, vomiting
• To recognize the signs of hypersensitivity: liver, urticaria, wheezing, dyspnea; notify prescriber immediately

---

interferon β-1 b (℞)
(in-ter-feer'on)
Betaseron
Func. class.: Multiple sclerosis agent
Chem. class.: E. coli derivative

Action: Antiviral, immunoregulatory; action not clearly understood; biologic response modifying properties mediated through specific receptors on cells, inducing expression of interferon-induced gene products

Uses: Ambulatory patients with relapsing or remitting multiple sclerosis

Investigational uses: May be useful in treatment of AIDS, AIDS-related Kaposi's sarcoma, malignant melanoma, metastatic renal cell carcinoma, cutaneous T cell lymphoma, acute non-A, non-B hepatitis

Dosage and routes:
Relapsing/remitting multiple sclerosis
• *Adult:* SC 0.25 mg (8 IU) qod
Available forms: Powder for inj lyophilized 0.3 mg (9.6 mIU)

Side effects/adverse reactions:
CNS: Headache, fever, pain, chills, mental changes, hypertonia, **suicide attempts**
CV: Migraine, palpitations, hypertension, tachycardia, peripheral vascular disorders
EENT: Conjunctivitis, blurred vision
GI: Diarrhea, constipation, vomiting, abdominal pain
GU: Dysmenorrhea, irregular menses, metrorrhagia, cystitis, breast pain
*HEMA: **Decreased lymphocytes, ANC, WBC;*** *lymphadenopathy*
INTEG: Sweating, inj site reaction
MS: Myalgia, **myasthenia**
RESP: Sinusitis, dyspnea

Contraindications: Hypersensitivity to natural or recombinant interferon-β or human albumin
Precautions: Pregnancy (C), lactation, child <18 yr, chronic progressive MS, depression, mental disorders

NURSING CONSIDERATIONS
Assess:
• Blood, renal, hepatic studies: CBC,

 = Nursing alert *▮* = Herb-drug interaction Ⓢ = Do not crush

differential, platelet counts, BUN, creatinine ALT, urinalysis
- CNS symptoms: headache, fatigue, depression
- GI status: diarrhea or constipation, vomiting, abdominal pain
- Cardiac status: increased B/P, tachycardia

Administer:
- Acetaminophen for fever, headache
- SC only; do not give IM or IV

Perform/provide:
- Storage in refrigerator; do not freeze

Evaluate:
- Therapeutic response: decreased symptoms of multiple sclerosis

Teach patient/family:
- To provide patient or family member with written, detailed information about the drug
- That blurred vision, sweating may occur
- Female patients that irregular menses, dysmenorrhea, or metrorrhagia as well as breast pain may occur

---

interferon gamma-1 b (℞)

(in-ter-feer´on)
Actimmune
Func. class.: Biologic response modifier
Chem. class.: Lymphokine, interleukin type

Action: Species-specific protein synthesized in response to viruses, potent phagocyte-activating effects; can mediate killing of *S. aureus, T. gondii, L. donovani, L. monocytogenes, M. avium-intracellulare;* enhances oxidative metabolism of macrophages, enhances antibody-dependent cellular cytotoxicity

Uses: Serious infections associated with chronic granulomatous disease

Dosage and routes:
- *Adult:* SC 50 µg/m² (1.5 million U/m²) for patients with surface area >0.5 m²; 1.5 µg/kg/dose for patient with surface area <0.5 m²; give Monday, Wednesday, Friday for 3 × /wk dosing

Available forms: Inj 100 µg (3 million U)/single-dose vial

Side effects/adverse reactions:
GI: Nausea, anorexia, abdominal pain, weight loss, diarrhea, vomiting
CNS: Headache, fatigue, depression, fever, chills
INTEG: Rash, pain at injection site
MS: Myalgia, arthralgia

Contraindications: Hypersensitivity to interferon gamma, *E. coli*-derived products

Precautions: Pregnancy (C), cardiac disease, seizure disorders, CNS disorders, myelosuppression, lactation, children

Pharmacokinetics:
SC: Dose absorbed 89%, elimination half-life 5.9 hr, peak 7 hr

Interactions:
- Increased myelosuppression: other myelosuppressive agents

NURSING CONSIDERATIONS
Assess:
- Blood, renal, hepatic studies: CBC, differential, platelet counts, BUN, creatinine, ALT (SGPT), urinalysis
- CNS symptoms: headache, fatigue, depression

Administer:
- At hs to minimize adverse reactions; administer acetaminophen for fever, headache
- 50% of dose if severe reactions occur or discontinue treatment until reactions subside
- In right and left deltoid and anterior thigh

• Warm to room temp before use; do not leave at room temp over 12 hr (unopened vial)

Perform/provide:
• Storage in refrigerator upon receipt; do not freeze; do not shake

Evaluate:
• Therapeutic response: decreased serious infections, improvement in existing infections and inflammatory conditions

Teach patient/family:
• The method of administration if family members will be giving medication
• Provide patient or family member with written, detailed information about drug

---

ipecac syrup (℞, OTC)
(ip'e-kak)

Func. class.: Emetic
Chem. class.: Cephaelis ipecacuanha derivative

Action: Acts on chemoreceptor trigger zone to induce vomiting; irritates gastric mucosa

Uses: In poisoning to induce vomiting

Dosage and routes:
• *Adult:* **PO** 15-30 ml, then 200-300 ml water; repeat 1×, if vomiting does not occur within 20 min
• *Child >1 yr:* **PO** 15 ml, then 200-300 ml water
• *Child 6-12 mo:* **PO** 5-10 ml, then 100-200 ml water; may repeat dose if needed

Available forms: Liq

Side effects/adverse reactions:
CNS: Depression, convulsions, coma
GI: Nausea, vomiting, bloody diarrhea
CV: Circulatory failure, atrial fibrillation, fatal myocarditis, dysrhythmias

Contraindications: Hypersensitivity, unconscious/semiconscious, depressed gag reflex, poisoning with petroleum products or caustic substances, convulsions

Precautions: Lactation, pregnancy (C)

Pharmacokinetics:
PO: Onset 15-30 min

Interactions:
• Do not administer with activated charcoal; effect will be decreased

NURSING CONSIDERATIONS
Assess:
• VS, B/P; check patients with cardiac disease more often
• Type of poisoning; do not administer if petroleum products or caustic substances have been ingested: kerosene, gasoline, lye, Drano
• Respiratory status before, during, after administration; check rate, rhythm, character; respiratory depression can occur rapidly with elderly or debilitated patients

Administer:
⬥ Ipecac syrup, not ipecac, which is 14 times stronger; death may occur
• Activated charcoal after vomiting completed; may begin lavage after 10-15 min after 2 doses of ipecac syrup with no result

Evaluate:
• Therapeutic response: vomiting

---

ipratropium (℞)
(i-pra-troe'pee-um)
Atrovent

Func. class.: Anticholinergic, bronchodilator
Chem. class.: Synthetic quaternary ammonium compound

Action: Inhibits interaction of acetylcholine at receptor sites on the bronchial smooth muscle, resulting

---

⬥ = Nursing alert   ⚕ = Herb-drug interaction   🚫 = Do not crush

in decreased cGMP and bronchodilation

Uses: Bronchodilation during bronchospasm in those with COPD

Dosage and routes:
• *Adult:* 2 **INH** 4 × day, not to exceed 12 **INH**/24 hr

Available forms: Aerosol 18 µg/actuation

Side effects/adverse reactions:
GI: Nausea, vomiting, cramps
EENT: Dry mouth, blurred vision
CNS: Anxiety, dizziness, headache, nervousness
RESP: Cough, worsening of symptoms, **bronchospasms**
INTEG: Rash
CV: Palpitation

Contraindications: Hypersensitivity to this drug, atropine, soya lecithin

Precautions: Pregnancy (B), lactation, children <12 yr, narrow-angle glaucoma, prostatic hypertrophy, bladder neck obstruction

Pharmacokinetics: Half-life 2 hr; does not cross blood-brain barrier

NURSING CONSIDERATIONS
Assess:
• For palpitations; if severe, drug may have to be changed
• For tolerance over long-term therapy; dose may have to be increased or changed

Perform/provide:
• Storage at room temp
• Hard candy, frequent drinks, sugarless gum to relieve dry mouth

Evaluate:
• Therapeutic response: ability to breathe adequately

Teach patient/family:
• That compliance is necessary with number of inhalations/24 hr, or overdose may occur; spacer device in the elderly
• To shake before using
• The correct method of inhalation and cleaning of equipment daily

---

irbesartan (R_x)

(er-be-sar′tan)
Avapro
Func. class.: Antihypertensive
Chem. class.: Angiotensin II receptor blocker (Type AT$_1$)

Action: Blocks the vasoconstrictor and aldosterone-secreting effects of angiotensin II; selectively blocks the binding of angiotensin II to the AT$_1$ receptor found in tissues

Uses: Hypertension, alone or in combination

Investigational uses: Heart failure, hypertensive patients with diabetic nephropathy caused by type II diabetes

Dosages and routes:
• *Adult:* **PO** 150 mg qd; may be increased to 300 mg qd

Available forms: 75, 150, 300 mg

Side effects/adverse reactions:
CNS: Dizziness, anxiety, headache, fatigue
GI: Diarrhea, dyspepsia
RESP: Cough, upper respiratory infection

Contraindications: Hypersensitivity, pregnancy (D) 2nd and 3rd trimester

Precautions: Hypersensitivity to ACE inhibitors; pregnancy (C) 1st trimester, lactation, children, elderly, renal disease

Pharmacokinetics: Extensively metabolized, half-life 11-15 hr, highly bound to plasma proteins, excreted in urine and feces

Interactions: None significant

NURSING CONSIDERATIONS
Assess:
• B/P, pulse q4h; note rate, rhythm, quality
• Electrolytes: K, Na, Cl
• Baselines in renal, liver function tests before therapy begins

---

Side effects: *italics* = common; ***bold italics*** = life-threatening

- Edema in feet, legs qd
- Skin turgor, dryness of mucous membranes for hydration status

Administer:
- Without regard to meals

Evaluate:
- Therapeutic response: decreased B/P

Teach patient/family:
- To comply with dosage schedule, even if feeling better
- That drug may cause dizziness, fainting; light-headedness may occur
- To rise slowly to sitting or standing position to minimize orthostatic hypotension

---

irinotecan (℞)

(ear-een-oh-tee′kan)

Camptosar

Func. class.: Antineoplastic hormone

Chem. class.: Topoisomerase inhibitor

Action: Cytotoxic by producing damage to double-strand DNA during DNA synthesis

Uses: Metastatic carcinoma of the colon or rectum

Dosage and routes:
- *Adult:* **IV** 125 mg/m^2 given over 1½ hr qwk × 4 wk, then 2 wk rest period, may be repeated; 4 wk or 2 wk off, dosage adjustments may be made to 150 mg/m^2 (high) or 50 mg/m^2 (low); adjustments should be made in increments of 25-50 mg/m^2 depending on patient's tolerance

Available forms: Inj 20 mg/ml

Side effects/adverse reactions:

CNS: Fever, headache, chills, dizziness

GI: Diarrhea, nausea, vomiting, anorexia, constipation, cramps, flatus, stomatitis, dyspepsia

INTEG: Irritation at site, rash, sweating

HEMA: **Leukopenia, anemia, neutropenia**

RESP: Dyspnea, increased cough, rhinitis

CV: Vasodilation

MISC: Edema, asthenia, weight loss

Contraindications: Hypersensitivity, pregnancy (D)

Precautions: Lactation, children, elderly, myelosuppression, irradiation

Pharmacokinetics: Rapidly and completely absorbed; excreted in urine and bile as metabolites; half-life 10 hr, bound to plasma proteins 30%-68%

Interactions:
- Increased myelosuppression, diarrhea: other antineoplastics
- Increased lymphocytopenia: dexamethasone
- Increased akathisia: prochlorperazine
- Increased dehydration: diuretics

NURSING CONSIDERATIONS

Assess:
- For CNS symptoms: fever, headache, chills, dizziness
- CBC, differential, platelet count weekly; withhold drug if WBC is <3500/mm^3, or platelet count <100,000/mm^3; notify prescriber of these results; drug should be discontinued
- Food preferences: list likes, dislikes
- Buccal cavity q8h for dryness, sores, or ulceration, white patches, oral pain, bleeding, dysphagia
- GI symptoms: frequency of stools; cramping
- Signs of dehydration: rapid respirations, poor skin turgor, decreased urine output, dry skin, restlessness, weakness

---

◆ = Nursing alert   ✪ = Herb-drug interaction   ⊘ = Do not crush

Perform/provide:
• Increased fluid intake to 2-3 L/day to prevent dehydration, unless contraindicated
• Changing of IV site q48h
• Rinsing of mouth tid-qid with water, club soda; brushing of teeth bid-tid with soft brush or cotton-tipped applicator for stomatitis; use unwaxed dental floss
• Nutritious diet with iron, vitamin supplement, low fiber, few dairy products

Evaluate:
• Therapeutic response: decrease in tumor size, decrease in spread of cancer

Teach patient/family:
• To avoid foods with citric acid or hot or rough texture if stomatitis is present; to drink adequate fluids
• To report stomatitis; any bleeding, white spots, ulcerations in mouth; tell patient to examine mouth qd, report symptoms
• To report signs of anemia: fatigue, headache, faintness, shortness of breath, irritability
• To use contraception during therapy

Treatment of overdose: Induce vomiting, provide supportive care

---

iron dextran (℞)
Imferon, In Fed
Func. class.: Hematinic
Chem. class.: Ferric hydroxide complex with dextran

Action: Iron is carried by transferrin to the bone marrow, where it is incorporated into hemoglobin
Uses: Iron deficiency anemia

Dosage and routes:
• *Adult and child:* IM 0.5 ml as a test dose by Z-track, then no more than the following per day:
• *Adult <50 kg:* IM 100 mg

• *Adult >50 kg:* IM 250 mg
• *Infant <5 kg:* IM 25 mg
• *Child <5-9 kg:* IM 50 mg
• *Adult:* IV 0.5 ml (25 mg) test dose, then 100 mg qd after 2-3 days; give 25 mg test dose, wait 5 min, then infuse over 6-12 hr or use equation that follows:

$$\frac{0.3 \times \text{wt (lb)} \times \frac{100\text{-Hgb (g/dl)} \times 100}{14.8}}{} = \text{mg iron}$$

<30 lb (66 kg) should be given 80% of above formula dose
Available forms: Inj 50 mg/ml

Side effects/adverse reactions:
CNS: Headache, paresthesia, dizziness, shivering, weakness, *seizures*
GI: Nausea, vomiting, metallic taste, abdominal pain
INTEG: Rash, pruritus, urticaria, fever, sweating, chills, brown skin discoloration, pain at injection site, necrosis, sterile abscesses, phlebitis
CV: Chest pain, *shock,* hypotension, tachycardia
RESP: Dyspnea
HEMA: Leukocytosis
OTHER: Anaphylaxis

Contraindications: Hypersensitivity, all anemias excluding iron deficiency anemia, hepatic disease
Precautions: Acute renal disease, children, asthma, lactation, rheumatoid arthritis (IV), infants <4 mo, pregnancy (C)

Pharmacokinetics:
IM: Excreted in feces, urine, bile, breast milk; crosses placenta; most absorbed through lymphatics; can be gradually absorbed over weeks/months from fixed locations

Interactions:
• Not to mix with other drugs in syringe or sol
• Decreased reticulocyte response: chloramphenicol
• Increased toxicity: oral iron—do not use

Lab test interferences:
False increase: Serum bilirubin
False decrease: Serum Ca
False positive: ^{99m}Tc diphosphate bone scan, iron test (large doses >2 ml)

NURSING CONSIDERATIONS
Assess:
• Blood studies: Hct, Hgb, reticulocytes, bilirubin before treatment, at least monthly
• Allergy: anaphylaxis, rash, pruritus, fever, chills, wheezing; notify prescriber immediately
• Cardiac status: anginal pain, hypotension, tachycardia
• Nutrition: amount of iron in diet (meat, dark green leafy vegetables, dried beans, dried fruits, eggs)
• Cause of iron loss or anemia, including use of salicylates, sulfonamides

Administer:
• D/C oral iron before parenteral; give only after test dose of 25 mg by preferred route; wait at least 1 hr before giving remaining portion
• IM deeply in large muscle mass; use Z-track method and a 19-20G 2-3″; needle; ensure needle is long enough to place drug deep in muscle, change needles after withdrawing drug and before injecting to prevent skin, tissue staining
• Only with epinephrine available in case of anaphylactic reaction during dose
IV
• IV after flushing with 10 ml 0.9% NaCl; give undiluted; may be diluted in 50-250 ml NS for infusion; give 1 ml (50 mg) or less over 1 min or more; flush line after use with 10 ml 0.9% NaCl; patient should remain recumbent for ½-1 hr
• IV injection requires single-dose vial without preservative; verify on label IV use is approved

Additive compatibilities: Netilmicin
Perform/provide:
• Storage at room temp in cool environment
• Recumbent position 30 min after IV injection to prevent orthostatic hypotension
Evaluate:
• Therapeutic response: increased serum iron levels, Hct, Hgb
Teach patient/family:
• That iron poisoning may occur if increased beyond recommended level; not to take oral iron preparation
• That delayed reaction may occur 1-2 days after administration and last 3-4 days (IV) 3-7 days (IM); report fever, chills, malaise, muscle, joint aches, nausea, vomiting, backache

Treatment of overdose: Discontinue drug, treat allergic reaction, give diphenhydramine or epinephrine as needed, give iron-chelating drug in acute poisoning

isoetharine (℞)
(eye-soe-eth'a-reen)
Arm-a-Med, isoetharine HCl, Beta-2, Bronkometer, Bronkosol
Func. class.: β_2-adrenergic agonist

Action: Causes bronchodilation by β_2 stimulation, resulting in increased levels of cAMP, causing relaxation of bronchial smooth muscle with very little effect on heart rate
Uses: Bronchospasm, asthma
Dosage and routes:
• *Adult:* INH 3-7 puffs undiluted, **IPPB** 0.5 ml diluted 1:3 with NS
Available forms: Sol for nebulization 0.06%, 0.08%, 0.1%,

◆ = Nursing alert ⫰ = Herb-drug interaction ⊘ = Do not crush

0.125%, 0.17%, 0.2%, 0.25%, 0.5%, 1.0%

Side effects/adverse reactions:

CNS: Tremors, anxiety, insomnia, headache, dizziness, stimulation

CV: Palpitations, tachycardia, hypertension, ***cardiac arrest,*** dysrhythmias

GI: Nausea

META: Hyperglycemia

Contraindications: Hypersensitivity to sympathomimetics, narrow-angle glaucoma

Precautions: Pregnancy (C), cardiac disorders, hyperthyroidism, diabetes mellitus, prostatic hypertrophy

Pharmacokinetics:

INH: Onset immediate, peak 5-15 min, duration 1-4 hr; metabolized in liver, GI tract, lungs; excreted in urine

Interactions:

• Increased effects of both drugs: other sympathomimetics

• Decreased action when used with other β-blockers

• Hypertensive crisis: MAOIs

NURSING CONSIDERATIONS

Assess:

• Respiratory function: vital capacity, forced expiratory volume, ABGs, pulse, B/P

• Paresthesias and coldness of extremities; peripheral blood flow may decrease

Administer:

• 2 hr before hs to avoid sleeplessness

Perform/provide:

• Storage at room temp; do not use sol if brown or contains a precipitate

Evaluate:

• Therapeutic response: ease of breathing

Teach patient/family:

• Not to use OTC medications; extra stimulation may occur

• Use of inhaler; review package insert with patient

• To avoid getting aerosol in eyes

• To wash inhaler in warm water and dry qd

• About all aspects of drug; avoid smoking, smoke-filled rooms, persons with respiratory infections

---

isoniazid (℞)

(eye-soe-nye'a-zid)

INH, isoniazid, Isotamine*, Laniazid, Laniazid C.T., Nydrazid, PMS-Isoniazid*, Tubizid

Func. class.: Antitubercular

Chem. class.: Isonicotinic acid hydrazide

Action: Bactericidal interference with lipid, nucleic acid biosynthesis

Uses: Treatment, prevention of tuberculosis

Dosage and routes:

Treatment

• *Adult:* **PO/IM** 5 mg/kg qd as single dose for 9 mo to 2 yr, not to exceed 300 mg/day

• *Child and infant:* **PO/IM** 10-20 mg/kg qd as single dose for 18-24 mo, not to exceed 300 mg/day

Prevention

• *Adult:* **PO** 300 mg qd as single dose × 12 mo

• *Child and infant:* **PO/IM** 10 mg/kg qd as single dose for 12 mo, not to exceed 300 mg/day

Available forms: Tabs 50, 100, 300 mg; inj 100 mg/ml; powder, syr 50 mg/5 ml

Side effects/adverse reactions:

Hypersensitivity: fever, skin eruptions, lymphadenopathy, vasculitis

CNS: Peripheral neuropathy, dizziness, memory impairment, ***toxic encephalopathy, convulsions,*** psychosis

EENT: Blurred vision, optic neuritis

HEMA: ***Agranulocytosis, hemolytic, aplastic anemia, thrombocytopenia, eosinophilia, methemoglobinemia***

MISC: Dyspnea, B_6 deficiency, pellagra, hyperglycemia, metabolic acidosis, gynecomastia, rheumatic syndrome, SLE-like syndrome

GI: Nausea, vomiting, epigastric distress, ***jaundice, fatal hepatitis***

Contraindications: Hypersensitivity, acute liver disease

Precautions: Pregnancy (C), renal disease, diabetic retinopathy, cataracts, ocular defects, hepatic disease, child <13 yr

Pharmacokinetics:

PO: Peak 1-2 hr, duration 6-8 hr
IM: Peak 45-60 min
Metabolized in liver; excreted in urine (metabolites); crosses placenta; excreted in breast milk

Interactions:

• Increased toxicity: tyramine foods, alcohol, cycloserine, ethionamide, rifampin, carbamazepine, warfarin, phenytoin, benzodiazepines

• Decreased absorption: aluminum antacids

• Decreased effectiveness of BCG vaccine, ketoconazole

NURSING CONSIDERATIONS

Assess:

• Liver studies qwk: ALT (SGPT), AST (SGOT), bilirubin

• Renal status: before, qmo: BUN, creatinine, output, sp gr, urinalysis

• Mental status often: affect, mood, behavioral changes; psychosis may occur

• Hepatic status: decreased appetite, jaundice, dark urine, fatigue

Administer:

• With meals to decrease GI symptoms; better to take on empty stomach 1 hr ac or 2 hr pc

• Antiemetic if vomiting occurs

• After C&S is completed; qmo to detect resistance

• IM deep in large muscle mass, massage, rotate inj site

Evaluate:

• Therapeutic response: decreased symptoms of TB

Teach patient/family:

• That compliance with dosage schedule, duration is necessary, not to skip or double dose

• That scheduled appointments must be kept or relapse may occur

• To avoid alcohol while taking drug

• That if diabetic, use blood glucose monitor to obtain correct result

• To report weakness, fatigue, loss of appetite, nausea, vomiting, yellowing of skin or eyes, tingling/numbness of hands/feet

---

isoproterenol (℞)

(eye-soe-proe-ter'e-nole)
Aerolone, Dispos-a-Medisoproterenol HCl, Isoproterenol HCl, Isuprel, Isuprel Glossets, Isuprel Mistometer, Medihaler-Iso, Vapo-Iso

Func. class.: β-adrenergic agonist

Chem. class.: Catecholamine

Action: Has $β_1$ and $β_2$ action; relaxes bronchial smooth muscle and dilates the trachea and main bronchi by increasing levels of cAMP, which relaxes smooth muscles; causes increased contractility and heart rate by acting on β-receptors in heart

Uses: Bronchospasm, asthma, heart block, ventricular dysrhythmias, shock

Dosage and routes:

Asthma, bronchospasm

• *Adult:* **SL** 10-20 mg q6-8h; **INH** 1 puff, may repeat in 2-5 min, maintenance 1-2 puffs 4-6 × /day; **IV** 10-20 μg during anesthesia

• *Child:* **SL** 5-10 mg q6-8h; **INH** 1

---

puff, may repeat in 2-5 min, maintenance 1-2 puffs 4-6 × /day

Heart block/ventricular dysrhythmias

• *Adult:* **IV** 0.02-0.06, then 0.01-0.2 mg or 5 µg/min HCl; 0.2 mg, then 0.02-1 mg as needed HCl

Shock

• *Adult:* **IV INF** 0.5-5 µg/min 1 mg/500 ml D₅W, titrate to B/P, CVP, hourly urine output

Available forms: Sol for nebulization 1:400 (0.25%), 1:200 (0.5%), 1:100 (1%); aerosol 0.25%, 0.2%; pwd for INH 0.1 mg/cart; inj 1:5000 (0.2 mg/ml); glossets (SL) 10, 15 mg

Side effects/adverse reactions:

CNS: Tremors, anxiety, insomnia, headache, dizziness, stimulation

CV: Palpitations, tachycardia, hypertension, *cardiac arrest*

GI: Nausea, vomiting

RESP: Bronchial irritation, edema, dryness of oropharynx, *bronchospasms* (overuse)

META: Hyperglycemia

Contraindications: Hypersensitivity to sympathomimetics, narrow-angle glaucoma

Precautions: Pregnancy (C), cardiac disorders, hyperthyroidism, diabetes mellitus, prostatic hypertrophy, elderly

Pharmacokinetics:

IV: Onset rapid, duration 10 min

INH/SL: Onset 1-2 hr

RECT: Onset 2-4 hr

Metabolized in liver, lungs, GI tract

Interactions:

• Increased effects of both drugs: other sympathomimetics

• Decreased action when used with β-blockers

NURSING CONSIDERATIONS

Assess:

• Resp function: B/P, pulse, lung sounds

• Blood studies (CBC, WBC, differential), since blood dyscrasias may occur (rare)

• I&O ratio; check for urinary retention, frequency, hesitancy

• For paresthesias and coldness of extremities; peripheral blood flow may decrease

• Injection site: tissue sloughing; administer phentolamine mixed with 0.9% NaCl

Administer:

• With meals for GI symptoms

• SL tab by rectal route if needed

IV

• Direct dilute 0.2 mg/10 ml 0.9% NaCl (1:50,000 sol); give over 1 min; IV INF 2 mg (1:5000 sol)/500 ml of D₅W; run each 1 ml (1:250,000) sol/min; may be increased; use infusion pump, intracardiac, 1:5000 sol undiluted

Additive compatibilities: Atracurium, calcium chloride, calcium gluceptate, cephalothin, cimetidine, dobutamine, floxacillin, heparin, magnesium sulfate, multivitamins, netilmicin, potassium chloride, ranitidine, succinylchloride, verapamil, vit B/C

Syringe compatibilities: Ranitidine

Y-site compatibilities: Amiodarone, amrinone, atracurium, bretylium, famotidine, heparin, hydrocortisone, pancuronium, potassium chloride, propofol, tacrolimus, vecuronium, vit B/C

Perform/provide:

• Storage at room temp; do not use discolored sol

Evaluate:

• Therapeutic response: increased B/P with stabilization, ease of breathing

Teach patient/family:

• To rinse mouth after use

• Use of inhaler; review package insert with patient; to avoid getting

aerosol in eyes; to wash inhaler in warm water and dry qd
- Use of spacer device in elderly
- About all aspects of drug; avoid smoking, smoke-filled rooms, persons with respiratory infections

Treatment of overdose: Administer a β-blocker

---

isosorbide dinitrate (℞)

(eye-soe-sor'bide)

Apo-ISDN*, Cedocard-SR*, Coronex*, Dilatrate-SR, ISDN, Iso-Bid, Isonate, Isorbid, Isordil, Isordil Tembids, Isordil Titradose, Isosorbide Dinitrate, Isotrate Timecelles, Novasorbide, Sorbitrate, Sorbitrate SA

isosorbide mononitrate

(eye-soe-sor'bide)

Imdur, ISMO, Monoket

Func. class.: Antianginal
Chem. class.: Nitrate

Action: Decreases preload, afterload, which is responsible for decreasing left ventricular end-diastolic pressure, systemic vascular resistance and reducing cardiac O_2 demand

Uses: Chronic stable angina pectoris, prophylaxis of angina pain

Dosage and routes:
Dinitrate
- *Adult:* **PO** 5-40 mg qid; **SL** 2.5-10 mg, may repeat q2-3h; **CHEW TAB** 5-10 mg prn or q2-3h as prophylaxis; **SUS REL** 40-80 mg q8-12h
Mononitrate
- *Adult:* **PO** 10-20 mg bid, 7 hr apart; Imdur: initiate at 30-60 mg/day as a single dose, increase q3d as needed

Available forms:
Dinitrate: Caps sus rel 40 mg; tabs 5, 10, 20, 30, 40 mg; chew tabs 5, 10 mg; SL tabs 2.5, 5, 10 mg; ext rel tab 40, 60 mg
Mononitrate: Tabs 20 mg; (ISMO, Monoket) 10, 20 mg; ext rel (Imdur) 30, 60, 120 mg

Side effects/adverse reactions:
MISC: Twitching, hemolytic anemia, *methemoglobinemia*
CV: Postural hypotension, tachycardia, *collapse,* syncope
GI: Nausea, vomiting
INTEG: Pallor, sweating, rash
CNS: Vascular headache, flushing, dizziness, weakness, faintness

Contraindications: Hypersensitivity to this drug or nitrates, severe anemia, increased intracranial pressure, cerebral hemorrhage, acute MI

Precautions: Postural hypotension, pregnancy (C), lactation, children

Pharmacokinetics:
Mononitrate
Sus action: Duration 6-8 hr
Dinitrate
PO: Onset 15-30 min, duration 4-6 hr
SL: Onset 2-5 min, duration 1-4 hr
CHEW TAB: Onset 3 min, duration ½-3 hr
Metabolized by liver, excreted in urine as metabolites (80%-100%)

Interactions:
- Increased effects: β-blockers, diuretics, antihypertensives, alcohol products

NURSING CONSIDERATIONS
Assess:
- B/P, pulse, respirations during beginning therapy
- Pain: duration, time started, activity being performed, character
- Tolerance if taken over long period
- Headache, light-headedness, decreased B/P; may indicate a need for decreased dosage

Administer:
- After checking expiration date

⬦ = Nursing alert   ⬙ = Herb-drug interaction   🚫 = Do not crush

$\bigcirc$ Do not break, crush, or chew caps
• With 8 oz H_2O on empty stomach (oral tablet); do not crush SR or SL drug

Evaluate:
• Therapeutic response: decrease or prevention of anginal pain

Teach patient/family:
• To leave tabs in original container
• To avoid alcohol products
• That drug may cause headache, but tolerance usually develops; taking with meals may reduce or eliminate headache
• That drug may be taken before stressful activity (exercise, sexual activity)
• That SL may sting when drug comes in contact with mucous membranes
• To avoid hazardous activities if dizziness occurs
• The importance of complying with complete medical regimen
• To make position changes slowly to prevent orthostatic hypotension
$\bigcirc$ Not to crush, chew SL or sus rel tabs

---

isradipine (R)

(is-ra′di-peen)
DynaCirc
Func. class.: Antihypertensive, calcium channel blocker
Chem. class.: Dihydropyridine

Action: Inhibits calcium ion influx across cell membrane during cardiac depolarization; produces relaxation of coronary vascular smooth muscle, peripheral vascular smooth muscle; dilates coronary vascular arteries; increases myocardial oxygen delivery in patients with vasospastic angina

Uses: Essential hypertension, angina

Dosage and routes:
• *Adult:* **PO** 2.5 mg bid; increase at 3-4 wk intervals up to 10 mg bid
Available forms: Caps 2.5, 5 mg

Side effects/adverse reactions:
HEMA: ***Thrombocytopenia, leukopenia, anemia***
CV: Peripheral edema, tachycardia, hypotension, chest pain
GI: Nausea, vomiting, diarrhea, gastric upset, constipation, hepatitis
GU: Nocturia, polyuria, ***acute renal failure***
INTEG: Rash, pruritus, urticaria, photosensitivity, hair loss
CNS: Headache, fatigue, dizziness, fainting, sleep disturbances
MISC: Flushing

Contraindications: Sick sinus syndrome, 2nd- or 3rd-degree heart block, hypotension less than 90 mm Hg systolic, hypersensitivity

Precautions: CHF, hypotension, hepatic disease, pregnancy (C), lactation, children, renal disease, elderly

Pharmacokinetics: Metabolized in liver; metabolites excreted in urine, feces; secreted in breast milk, peak plasma levels at 2-3 hr

Interactions:
• Increased effects: digitalis, neuromuscular blocking agents, cyclosporine
• Increased effects of isradipine: cimetidine, carbamazepine

NURSING CONSIDERATIONS

Assess:
• B/P, pulse rate, chest pain; monitor ECG periodically during therapy
• Cardiac status: B/P, pulse, respiration, ECG

Evaluate:
• Therapeutic response: decreased anginal pain, decreased B/P

Teach patient/family:
$\bigcirc$ Not to break, crush, or chew caps

- To avoid hazardous activities until stabilized on drug, dizziness is no longer a problem
- To limit caffeine consumption
- To avoid OTC drugs unless directed by prescriber
- The importance of compliance in all areas of medical regimen: diet, exercise, stress reduction, drug therapy
- To notify prescriber of irregular heartbeat, shortness of breath, swelling of feet and hands, pronounced dizziness, constipation, nausea, hypotension

Treatment of overdose: Defibrillation, β-agonists, IV Ca inotropic agents, diuretics, atropine for AV block, vasopressor for hypotension

---

itraconazole (℞)

(it-ra-con'a-zol)

Sporanox

Func. class.: Antifungal, systemic

Chem. class.: Triazole derivative

Action: Alters cell membranes and inhibits several fungal enzymes

Uses: Systemic candidiasis, chronic mucocandidiasis, oral thrush, candiduria, coccidioidomycosis, histoplasmosis, chromomycosis, paracoccidioidomycosis, blastomycosis (pulmonary and extrapulmonary), onychomycosis

Dosage and routes:
- *Adult:* PO 200 mg qd with food; may increase to 400 mg qd if needed; life-threatening infections may require a loading dose of 200 mg tid × 3 days
- *Child:* PO 3-5 mg/kg/day

Available forms: Caps 100 mg; oral sol 10 mg/ml

Side effects/adverse reactions:

GU: Gynecomastia, impotence, decreased libido

INTEG: Pruritus, fever, rash,

CNS: Headache, dizziness, insomnia, somnolence, depression

GI: Nausea, vomiting, anorexia, diarrhea, cramps, abdominal pain, flatulence, *GI bleeding, hepatotoxicity*

MISC: Edema, fatigue, malaise, hypertension, hypokalemia, tinnitus

Contraindications: Hypersensitivity, lactation, fungal meningitis, coadministration with terfenadine

Precautions: Hepatic disease, achlorhydria or hypochlorhydria (drug-induced), children, pregnancy (C)

Pharmacokinetics:

PO: Peak 3-5 hr, half-life 60 hr; metabolized in liver; excreted in bile, feces; requires acid pH for absorption; distributed poorly to CSF; highly protein bound

Interactions:

- Do not use with terfenadine, astemizole, cisapride: may result in rare instance of life-threatening dysrhythmias and death
- Hepatotoxicity: other hepatotoxic drugs
- Itraconazole increases levels of cyclosporine
- Decreased action of itraconazole: antacids, H_2-receptor antagonists, isoniazid, rifampin, omeprazole, sucralfate
- Increased anticoagulant effect: warfarin
- Severe hypoglycemia: oral hypoglycemics
- Concomitant administration with phenytoin may result in decreased levels of itraconazole; effects of phenytoin may be increased

NURSING CONSIDERATIONS

Assess:
- I&O ratio

◆= Nursing alert   ⫰= Herb-drug interaction   ⊘= Do not crush

• Liver studies (ALT [SGPT], AST [SGOT], bilirubin) if on long-term therapy
• For allergic reaction: rash, photosensitivity, urticaria, dermatitis
◆ For hepatotoxicity: nausea, vomiting, jaundice, clay-colored stools, fatigue

Administer:
• In the presence of acid products only; do not use alkaline products or antacids within 2 hr of drug; may give coffee, tea, acidic fruit juices
• With food for GI symptoms
• With hydrochloric acid if achlorhydria is present
• Oral sol and caps are not interchangeable on a mg/mg basis

Perform/provide:
• Storage in tight container at room temp

Evaluate:
• Therapeutic response: decreased fever, malaise, rash, negative C&S for infecting organism

Teach patient/family:
• That long-term therapy may be needed to clear infection (1 wk-6 mo depending on infection)
• To avoid hazardous activities if dizziness occurs
• To take 2 hr ac administration of other drugs that increase gastric pH (antacids, H₂-blockers, omeprazole, sucralfate, anticholinergics)
• The importance of compliance with drug regimen
• To notify prescriber of GI symptoms, signs of liver dysfunction (fatigue, nausea, anorexia, vomiting, dark urine, pale stools)
🚫 Not to break, crush, or chew caps

kanamycin (℞)

(kan-a-mye′sin)
kanamycin sulfate, Kantrex
Func. class.: Antiinfective
Chem. class.: Aminoglycoside

Action: Interferes with protein synthesis in bacterial cell by binding to the 30s ribosomal subunit, causing inaccurate peptide sequence to form in protein chain, causing bacterial death

Uses: Severe systemic infections of CNS, respiratory, GI, urinary tract, bone, skin, soft tissues caused by *E. coli, Acinetobacter, Proteus, K. pneumoniae, Pseudomonas aeruginosa;* also used as adjunct in hepatic coma, peritonitis, preoperatively to sterilize bowel; decreases ammonia-producing bacteria in bowel and intraperitoneally after fecal spill during surgery

Dosage and routes:
Severe systemic infections
• *Adult and child:* **IV INF** 15 mg/kg/d in divided doses q8-12h; diluted 500 mg/200 ml of NS or D₅W given over 30-60 min, not to exceed 1.5 g/d; **IM** 15 mg/kg/d in divided doses q8-12h, not to exceed 1.5 g/d, irrigation not to exceed 1.5 g/d

Hepatic coma
• *Adult:* **PO** 8-12 g/d in divided doses

Preoperative bowel sterilization
• *Adult:* **PO** 1 g qh × 4 doses, then q6h × 36-72 hr

Available forms: Inj 75, 500 mg/2 ml, 1 g/3 ml; cap 500 mg

Side effects/adverse reactions:
*GU: **Oliguria, hematuria, renal damage, azotemia, renal failure, nephrotoxicity***
CNS: Confusion, depression, numbness, tremors, ***convulsions,*** muscle twitching, ***neurotoxicity***

RESP: Respiratory depression

*EENT: **Ototoxicity,** deafness, visual disturbances, dizziness, vertigo, tinnitus*

*HEMA: **Agranulocytosis, thrombocytopenia, leukopenia, eosinophilia, anemia***

GI: Nausea, vomiting, anorexia, increased ALT, AST, bilirubin, hepatomegaly, ***hepatic necrosis,*** splenomegaly

CV: Hypotension

INTEG: Rash, burning, urticaria, dermatitis, alopecia

Contraindications: Bowel obstruction, severe renal disease, hypersensitivity, pregnancy (D)

Precautions: Neonates, myasthenia gravis, hearing deficits, mild renal disease, lactation, Parkinson's disease

Pharmacokinetics:

PO: Not absorbed

IM: Onset rapid, peak 1-2 hr

IV: Onset immediate, peak 1-2 hr Plasma half-life 2-3 hr; not metabolized; excreted unchanged in urine; crosses placenta; poor penetration into CSF

Interactions:

• Increased ototoxicity, neurotoxicity, nephrotoxicity: other aminoglycosides, amphotericin B, polymyxin, vancomycin, ethacrynic acid, furosemide, mannitol, methoxyflurane, cisplatin, cephalosporins, bacitracin, penicillins

• Increased effects: nondepolarizing muscle relaxants, succinylcholine

• Decreased effects of oral anticoagulants

NURSING CONSIDERATIONS

Assess:

• Weight before treatment; dosage is usually calculated on ideal body weight, but may be calculated on actual body weight

• I&O ratio, urinalysis daily for proteinuria, cells, casts; report sudden change in urine output

• VS during infusion; watch for hypotension, change in pulse

• IV site for thrombophlebitis, including pain, redness, swelling q30min; change site if needed; apply warm compresses to discontinued site

• Serum peak, drawn at 30-60 min after IV infusion or 60 min after IM injection; trough level drawn just before next dose; blood level should be 2-4 × bacteriostatic level; trough = 5-10 mEq/ml, peak = <30 mEq/ml

• Urine pH if drug is used for UTI; urine should be kept alkaline

• Renal impairment by CrCl, BUN, serum creatinine testing of urine; lower dosage should be given in renal impairment (CrCl <80 ml/min)

• Deafness by audiometric testing, ringing, roaring in ears, vertigo; assess hearing before, during, after treatment

• Dehydration: high specific gravity, decrease in skin turgor, dry mucous membranes, dark urine

• Superinfection: fever, malaise, redness, pain, swelling, perineal itching, diarrhea, stomatitis, change in cough, sputum

• C&S before starting treatment to identify infecting organism

• Vestibular dysfunction: nausea, vomiting, dizziness, headache; drug should be discontinued if severe

• Injection sites for redness, swelling, abscesses; use warm compresses at site

Administer:

• IM inj in large muscle mass; rotate injection sites

• Penicillins at least 1 hr before or after this drug

◆ = Nursing alert   ∥ = Herb-drug interaction   ⊘ = Do not crush

• Drug in evenly spaced doses to maintain blood level

• Bicarbonate to alkalinize urine if ordered in treating UTI, as drug is most active in alkaline environment

IV

• After diluting 500 mg or less/100 ml of D_5W, D_5/NaCl, 0.9% NaCl, LR or more; give 3-4 ml/min or less; flush line after use

Additive compatibilities: Ascorbic acid, cefoxitin, chloramphenicol, clindamycin, dopamine, furosemide, penicillin G potassium, penicillin G sodium, polymyxin B, sodium bicarbonate, vit B/C; admixing is not recommended

Syringe compatibilities: Penicillin G sodium

Y-site compatibilities: Cyclophosphamide, furosemide, heparin with hydrocortisone, hydromorphone, magnesium sulfate, meperidine, morphine, perphenazine, potassium chloride, vit B/C

Perform/provide:

• Adequate fluids of 2-3 L/day unless contraindicated to prevent irritation of tubules

• Flush of IV line with NS or D_5W after infusion

• Supervised ambulation, other safety measures with vestibular dysfunction

Evaluate:

• Therapeutic effect: absence of fever, draining wounds, negative C&S after treatment

Teach patient/family:

• To report headache, dizziness, symptoms of overgrowth of infection, renal impairment

• To report loss of hearing, ringing, roaring in ears or feeling of fullness in head

Treatment of overdose: Hemodialysis; monitor serum levels of drug

---

kaolin, pectin (OTC)

(kay′oh-lin, pek′tin)

Kaodene, Kao-Spen, Kapectolin

Func. class.: Antidiarrheal

Chem. class.: Hydrous magnesium aluminum silicate

Action: Decreases gastric motility, H_2O content of stool; adsorbent, demulcent

Uses: Diarrhea (cause undetermined)

Dosage and routes:

• *Adult:* **PO** 60-120 ml (30 ml conc) after each loose BM

• *Child >12 yr:* **PO** 60 ml after each loose BM

• *Child 6-12 yr:* **PO** 30-60 ml (15 ml conc) after each loose BM

• *Child 3-6 yr:* **PO** 15-30 ml (7.5 ml conc) after each loose BM

Available forms: Susp kaolin 0.87 g/5 ml, pectin 43 mg/5 ml; kaolin 0.98 g/5 ml, pectin 21.7 mg/5 ml

Side effects/adverse reactions:

GI: Constipation (chronic use)

Precautions: Pregnancy (C)

Interactions:

• Decreased action of all other drugs

NURSING CONSIDERATIONS

Assess:

• Bowel pattern before; for rebound constipation

• Dehydration in children

Administer:

• After shaking suspension

• For 48 hr only

Evaluate:

• Therapeutic response: decreased diarrhea

Teach patient/family:

• Not to exceed recommended dose

• To shake well before administration

---

ketoconazole (℞)

(kee-toe-koe'na-zole)
Nizoral
Func. class.: Antifungal
Chem. class.: Imidazole derivative

Action: Alters cell membranes and inhibits several fungal enzymes

Uses: Systemic candidiasis, chronic mucocandidiasis, oral thrush, candiduria, coccidioidomycosis, histoplasmosis, chromomycosis, paracoccidioidomycosis, blastomycosis; tinea cruris, tinea corporis, tinea versicolor, *Pityrosporum ovale*

Investigational uses: Cushing's syndrome, advanced prostatic cancer

Dosage and routes:
• *Adult:* **PO** 200-400 mg qd for 1-2 wk (candidiasis), 6 wk (other infections)
• *Child:* **PO:** >2 yr: 3.3-6.6 mg/kg/day as single daily dose; <2 yr, daily dose not established
• *Adult and child:* **TOP** 2% cream applied qd or bid
• *Adult:* Shampoo massage into scalp 1 min, reapply × 3 min, rinse, continue treatment 2 × /wk × 1 mo, no more than q3d

Available forms: Tabs 200 mg; cream 2%; shampoo 2%

Side effects/adverse reactions:
GU: Gynecomastia, impotence
INTEG: Pruritus, fever, chills, photophobia, rash, dermatitis, purpura, urticaria
CNS: Headache, dizziness, somnolence
SYST: Anaphylaxis
GI: Nausea, vomiting, anorexia, diarrhea, abdominal pain, hepatotoxicity
HEMA: Thrombocytopenia, leukopenia, hemolytic anemia

Contraindications: Hypersensitivity, lactation, fungal meningitis; coadministration with terfenadine

Precautions: Renal disease, hepatic disease, achlorhydria (drug-induced), pregnancy (C), children <2 yr, other hepatotoxic agents including terfenadine

Pharmacokinetics:
PO: Peak 1-2 hr, half-life 2 hr, terminal 8 hr; metabolized in liver; excreted in bile, feces; requires acid pH for absorption; distributed poorly to CSF; highly protein bound

Interactions:
• Do not use with terfenadine; may result in rare instances of life-threatening dysrhythmias and death
• Hepatotoxicity: other hepatotoxic drugs (including terfenadine)
• Ketoconazole increases concentration of cyclosporine and corticosteroids
• Decreased action of ketoconazole: antacids, H_2-receptor antagonists, isoniazid, rifampin
• Increased anticoagulant effect: coumadin, anticoagulants
• Ketoconazole may decrease theophylline effect

NURSING CONSIDERATIONS
Assess:
• I&O ratio
• Liver studies (ALT, AST, bilirubin) if on long-term therapy
• For allergic reaction: rash, photosensitivity, urticaria, dermatitis
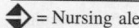 For hepatotoxicity: nausea, vomiting, jaundice, clay-colored stools, fatigue

Administer:
• In the presence of acid products only; do not use alkaline products, proton pump inhibitors, H_2-antagonists, antacids within 2 hr of drug; may give coffee, tea, acidic fruit juices, cola
• With food to decrease GI symptoms

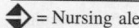

- With HCl if achlorhydria is present

Perform/provide:
- Storage in tight container at room temp

Evaluate:
- Therapeutic response: decreased fever, malaise, rash, negative C&S for infecting organism, absence of scaling

Teach patient/family:
- That long-term therapy may be needed to clear infection (1 wk-6 mo depending on infection)
- To avoid hazardous activities if dizziness occurs
- To take 2 hr ac administration of other drugs that increase gastric pH (antacids, H₂-blockers, omeprazole, sucralfate, anticholinergics)
- The importance of compliance with drug regimen
- To notify prescriber of GI symptoms, signs of liver dysfunction (fatigue, nausea, anorexia, vomiting, dark urine, pale stools)

---

ketoprofen (OTC, ℞)

(ke-toe-proe'ten)

ketoprofen, Orudis, Orudis-E*, Orudis-KT, Oruvail

Func. class.: Nonsteroidal antiinflammatory (NSAID)

Chem. class.: Propionic acid derivative

Action: Inhibits prostaglandin synthesis by decreasing enzyme needed for biosynthesis; analgesic, antiinflammatory, antipyretic

Uses: Mild to moderate pain, osteoarthritis, rheumatoid arthritis, dysmenorrhea

Dosage and routes:

Antiinflammatory
- *Adult:* **PO** 150-300 mg in divided doses tid-qid, not to exceed 300 mg/day

Analgesic
- *Adult:* **PO** 25-50 mg q6-8h

Available forms: Caps 25, 50, 75 mg

Side effects/adverse reactions:

GI: Nausea, anorexia, vomiting, diarrhea, jaundice, *cholestatic hepatitis,* constipation, flatulence, cramps, dry mouth, peptic ulcer

CNS: Dizziness, drowsiness, fatigue, tremors, confusion, insomnia, anxiety, depression, headache

CV: Tachycardia, peripheral edema, palpitations, dysrhythmias, hypertension

INTEG: Purpura, rash, pruritus, sweating

GU: Nephrotoxicity: dysuria, hematuria, oliguria, azotemia

HEMA: Blood dyscrasias

EENT: Tinnitus, hearing loss, blurred vision

Contraindications: Hypersensitivity, asthma, severe renal disease, severe hepatic disease, ulcer disease

Precautions: Pregnancy (B), lactation, children, bleeding disorders, GI disorders, cardiac disorders, hypersensitivity to other antiinflammatory agents, elderly

Pharmacokinetics:
PO: Peak 2 hr, half-life 3-3½ hr; metabolized in liver; excreted in urine (metabolites); excreted in breast milk; 99% plasma protein binding

Interactions:
- Increased action of coumadin, streptokinase, probenecid

NURSING CONSIDERATIONS

Assess:
- Renal, liver, blood studies: BUN, creatinine, AST (SGOT), ALT (SGPT), Hgb, before treatment, periodically thereafter
- Audiometric, ophthalmic examination before, during, after treatment

---

- For eye, ear problems: blurred vision, tinnitus; may indicate toxicity

Administer:

🚫 Whole; do not crush, break, or open caps
- With food to decrease GI symptoms; however, best to take on empty stomach to facilitate absorption

Perform/provide:
- Storage at room temp

Evaluate:
- Therapeutic response: decreased pain, stiffness in joints, decreased swelling in joints, ability to move more easily

Teach patient/family:
- To report blurred vision, ringing, roaring in ears; may indicate toxicity
- To avoid driving, other hazardous activities if dizziness, drowsiness occurs, especially elderly
- To report change in urine pattern, increased weight, edema, increased pain in joints, fever, blood in urine; indicate nephrotoxicity
- That therapeutic effects may take up to 1 mo
- To avoid aspirin, alcohol, steroids

---

ketorolac (Rx)

(kee-toe'role-ak)
Acular, Toradol
Func. class.: Nonsteroidal antiinflammatory/nonopioid analgesic
Chem. class.: Pyrrolo-pyrrole

Action: Inhibits prostaglandin synthesis by decreasing an enzyme needed for biosynthesis; analgesic, antiinflammatory, antipyretic effects

Uses: Mild to moderate pain; seasonal allergic conjunctivitis (ophth)

Dosage and routes:
- *Adult (multiple dosing):* IV **BOL/IM** 30 mg q6h max 120 mg/day, with transition of 20 mg **PO** (1st dose), then 10 mg q4-6h; *≥65 yr, renal impairment, or weight <50 kg:* 15 mg q6h, max 60 mg
- *Adult (single dosing):* **IV BOL/IM** 30 mg **IV** or 60 mg **IM**, then 20 mg transition dose, not to exceed 40 mg/day then 10 mg q4-6h; *≥65 yr, renal impairment, or weight <50 kg:* give 30 mg **IM** or 15 mg **IV**
- *Adult:* **OPHTH** 1 gtt qid

Available forms: Inj 15, 30 mg/ml (prefilled syringes); ophth 0.5% sol; tab 10 mg

Side effects/adverse reactions:

CV: Hypertension, flushing, syncope, pallor, edema, vasodilation

CNS: Dizziness, *drowsiness,* tremors

EENT: Tinnitus, hearing loss, blurred vision

GI: Nausea, anorexia, vomiting, diarrhea, constipation, flatulence, cramps, dry mouth, peptic ulcer, *GI bleeding, perforation*, taste change

GU: **Nephrotoxicity: dysuria, hematuria, oliguria, azotemia**

HEMA: **Blood dyscrasias,** prolonged bleeding

INTEG: Purpura, rash, pruritus, sweating

Contraindications: Hypersensitivity, asthma, severe renal disease, severe hepatic disease, peptic ulcer disease, L&D, lactation, CV bleeding

Precautions: Pregnancy (C), children, bleeding disorders, GI disorders, cardiac disorders, hypersensitivity to other antiinflammatory agents, elderly, CrCl <25 ml/min

Pharmacokinetics:

PO: Peak 2-3 hr, duration 4-6 hr

IM: Peak 50 min, half-life 6 hr enters breast milk, <50% metabolized by liver, excreted by kidneys

---

Interactions:
• Increased action of ketorolac: phenytoin, sulfonamides
• Compatible in 0.9% NaCl, D_5, Ringer's, LR, Plasmalate

NURSING CONSIDERATIONS
Assess:
• Eyes: redness, swelling, tearing, itching (ophth)
• Renal, liver, blood studies: BUN, creatinine, AST (SGOT), ALT (SGPT), Hgb before treatment, periodically thereafter
• Bleeding times; check for bruising, bleeding; test for occult blood in urine
• For eye, ear problems: blurred vision, tinnitus (may indicate toxicity)
⬧ Hepatic dysfunction: jaundice, yellow sclera and skin, clay-colored stools
• Audiometric, ophthalmic exam before, during, after treatment
• GI condition, hypertension, cardiac conditions

Administer:
• IM/IV for 5 days or less

Syringe compatibilities: Sufentanil

Y-site compatibilities: Sufentanil

Perform/provide:
• Storage at room temp

Evaluate:
• Therapeutic response: decreased pain, stiffness, swelling in joints, ability to move more easily; decreased ocular itching (ophth)

Teach patient/family:
• To report blurred vision or ringing, roaring in ears (may indicate toxicity)
• To avoid driving, other hazardous activities if dizziness or drowsiness occurs
• To report change in urine pattern, weight increase, edema, pain increase in joints, fever, blood in urine (indicates nephrotoxicity)
• To avoid alcohol, ASA
• This drug may cause redness, burning if soft contact lenses are worn (ophth)

---

labetalol (℞)
(la-bet'a-lole)
Normodyne, Trandate
Func. class.: Antihypertensive
Chem. class.: α/β-blocker

Action: Produces decreases in B/P without reflex tachycardia or significant reduction in heart rate through mixture of α-blocking, β-blocking effects; elevated plasma renins are reduced

Uses: Mild to moderate hypertension; treatment of severe hypertension (IV)

Investigational uses: Angina pectoris (PO), hypotension during surgery (IV)

Dosage and routes:
Hypertension
• *Adult:* PO 100 mg bid; may be given with a diuretic; may increase to 200 mg bid after 2 days; may continue to increase q1-3 days; max 400 mg bid

Hypertensive crisis
• *Adult:* IV INF 200 mg/160 ml D_5W, run at 2 ml/min; stop infusion at desired response, repeat q6-8h as needed; IV BOL 20 mg over 2 min, may repeat 40-80 mg q10min, not to exceed 300 mg

Available forms: Tabs 100, 200, 300 mg; inj 5 mg/ml in 20 ml amps

Side effects/adverse reactions:
CV: Orthostatic hypotension, bradycardia, **CHF,** *chest pain,* ***ventricular dysrhythmias***, *AV block*
CNS: Dizziness, mental changes,

drowsiness, fatigue, headache, catatonia, depression, anxiety, nightmares, paresthesias, lethargy

GI: Nausea, vomiting, diarrhea

INTEG: Rash, alopecia, urticaria, pruritus, fever

HEMA: Agranulocytosis, thrombocytopenia, purpura (rare)

EENT: Tinnitus, visual changes, sore throat, double vision, dry, burning eyes

GU: Impotence, dysuria, ejaculatory failure

RESP: Bronchospasm, dyspnea, wheezing

Contraindications: Hypersensitivity to β-blockers, cardiogenic shock, heart block (2nd or 3rd degree), sinus bradycardia, CHF, bronchial asthma

Precautions: Major surgery, pregnancy (C), lactation, diabetes mellitus, renal disease, thyroid disease, COPD, well-compensated heart failure, CAD, nonallergic bronchospasm, elderly, hepatic disease

Pharmacokinetics:

PO: Onset ½-2 hr, peak 2-4 hr, duration 8-12 hr

IV: Onset 5 min, peak 15 min, duration 2-4 hr

Half-life 6-8 hr; metabolized by liver (metabolites inactive); excreted in urine; crosses placenta; excreted in breast milk

Interactions:

• Decreased effects of labetalol: glutethimide, thyroid

• Increased bronchodilation: β-adrenergic agonists

• Increased hypotension: diuretics, other antihypertensives, halothane, cimetidine, nitroglycerin

• Decreased effects: sympathomimetics, lidocaine, indomethacin, theophylline, cimetidine

• Increased hypoglycemia: insulin

Lab test interferences:

False increase: Urinary catecholamines

NURSING CONSIDERATIONS

Assess:

• I&O, weight daily

• B/P during beginning treatment, periodically thereafter, pulse q4h; note rate, rhythm, quality

• Apical/radial pulse before administration; notify prescriber of any significant changes

• Baselines in renal, liver function tests before therapy begins

• Edema in feet, legs daily

• Skin turgor, dryness of mucous membranes for hydration status

Administer:

• PO ac, hs; tab may be crushed or swallowed whole

• Reduced dosage in renal dysfunction

IV

• Undiluted or diluted in LR, D₅W, D₅ in 0.2%, 0.9%, 0.33% NaCl or Ringer's inj; give undiluted 20 mg or less/2 min; infusion is titrated to patient response; 200 mg of drug/160 ml sol = 1 mg/ml; 300 mg of drug/240 ml sol = 1 mg/ml; 200 mg of drug/250 ml sol = 2 mg/3 ml; use infusion pump

• Keeping patient recumbent during and for 3 hr after administration

Solution compatibilities: D₅R, D₅LR, D₂ ½/0.45% NaCl, D₅/0.2% NaCl, D₅/0.33% NaCl, D₅0.9% NaCl, D₅W, Ringer's, LR

Y-site compatibilities: Amikacin, aminophylline, amiodarone, ampicillin, butorphanol, calcium gluconate, cefazolin, ceftazidime, ceftizoxime, chloramphenicol, cimetidine, clindamycin, diltiazem, dobutamine, dopamine, enalaprilat, epinephrine, erythromycin, esmolol, famotidine, fentanyl, gentamicin, hydromorphone, lidocaine, lorazepam, magnesium sulfate, meperidine, metronidazole, midazolam, milrinone, morphine, nicardipine, nitroglycerin, norepinephrine, nitroprusside, oxacillin, penicillin G potassium, piperacillin, potassium chloride, potassium phosphate, propofol, ranitidine, sodium acetate, tobramycin, trimethoprim-sulfamethoxazole, vancomycin, vecuronium

Perform/provide:

• Storage in dry area at room temp; do not freeze

Evaluate:

• Therapeutic response: decreased B/P after 1-2 wk

Teach patient/family:

• Not to discontinue drug abruptly; taper over 2 wk; may cause precipitate angina

• Not to use OTC products containing α-adrenergic stimulants (nasal decongestants, OTC cold preparations) unless directed by prescriber

• To report bradycardia, dizziness, confusion, depression, fever

• To take pulse at home, advise when to notify prescriber

• To avoid alcohol, smoking, Na intake

• To comply with weight control, dietary adjustments, modified exercise program

• To carry Medic Alert ID to identify drug, allergics

• To avoid hazardous activities if dizziness is present

• To report symptoms of CHF: difficulty breathing, especially on exertion or when lying down, night cough, swelling of extremities

• To take medication at bedtime to prevent effect of orthostatic hypotension

• To wear support hose to minimize effects of orthostatic hypotension

Treatment of overdose: Lavage, IV atropine for bradycardia, IV theophylline for bronchospasm, digitalis, O_2, diuretic for cardiac failure;

hemodialysis is useful for removal, hypotension; administer vasopressor (norepinephrine)

---

lactulose (℞)

(lak'tyoo-lose)
Cephulac, Cholac, Chronulac, Constilac, Constulose, Duphalac, Emulose, Enulose Lactulax*

Func. class.: Laxative; ammonia detoxicant (hyperosmotic)

Chem. class.: Lactose synthetic derivative

Action: Prevents absorption of ammonia in colon; increases water in stool

Uses: Chronic constipation, portal-systemic encephalopathy in patients with hepatic disease

Dosage and routes:

Constipation

• *Adult:* PO 15-60 ml qd

Encephalopathy

• *Adult:* PO 20-30 g tid or qid until stools are soft; RET ENEMA 30-45 ml in 100 ml of fluid

• *Infant:* 2.5-10 ml/day

• *Child:* 40-90 ml/day in divided doses given 2-4 ×/day

Available forms: Oral sol, rec sol 3.33 g/5 ml

Side effects/adverse reactions:

GI: Nausea, vomiting, anorexia, abdominal cramps, diarrhea, flatulence, distention, belching

Contraindications: Hypersensitivity, low-galactose diet

Precautions: Pregnancy (C), lactation, diabetes mellitus, elderly, debilitated patients

Pharmacokinetics: Metabolized in intestine, excreted by kidneys; onset 1-2 days, peak unknown, duration unknown

L

Interactions:
• Decreased effects of lactulose: neomycin, other oral antiinfectives

NURSING CONSIDERATIONS
Assess:
• Stool: amount, color, consistency
• Blood ammonia level (30-70 mg/100 ml); may decrease ammonia level by 25%-50%
• Blood, urine electrolytes if drug is used often; may cause diarrhea, hypokalemia, hyponatremia
• I&O ratio to identify fluid loss
• Cause of constipation; determine whether fluids, bulk, or exercise is missing from lifestyle
• Cramping, rectal bleeding, nausea, vomiting; if these symptoms occur, drug should be discontinued
• Clearing of confusion, lethargy, restlessness, irritability

Administer:
PO
• With 8 oz fruit juice, water, milk to increase palatability of oral form
RECT
• Retention enema by diluting 300 ml lactose/700 ml of water; administer by rectal balloon catheter
• Increased fluids to 2 L/day; do not give with other laxatives; if diarrhea occurs, reduce dosage

Evaluate:
• Therapeutic response: decreased constipation, decreased blood ammonia level, clearing of mental state

Teach patient/family:
• Not to use laxatives long-term
• To dilute with water or fruit juice to counteract sweet taste
• To store in cool environment; do not freeze
• To take on an empty stomach for rapid action
• To report diarrhea; may indicate overdose

lamivudine (℞)
(lam-i-voo′deen)
Epivir
Func. class.: Antiviral

Action: Inhibits replication of HIV virus by incorporating into cellular DNA by viral reverse transcriptase, thereby terminating cellular DNA chain

Uses: HIV infection in combination with zidovudine

Dosage and routes:
• Dosage reduction needed in renal disease (CrCl <50 ml/min)
• *Adult and adolescent (12-16 yr):* **PO** 150 mg bid with zidovudine; <50 kg (110 lbs): **PO** 2 mg/kg bid with zidovudine
• *Child 3 mo to 12 yr:* **PO** 4 mg/kg bid, may be given 150 mg bid with zidovudine

Available forms: Tabs 150 mg; oral sol 10 mg/ml

Side effects/adverse reactions:
HEMA: **Neutropenia, anemia, thrombocytopenia**
CNS: Fever, headache, malaise, dizziness, insomnia, depression, fatigue, chills
GI: Nausea, vomiting, diarrhea, anorexia, cramps, dyspepsia
RESP: Cough
EENT: Taste change, hearing loss, photophobia
INTEG: Rash
MS: Myalgia, arthralgia, pain

Contraindications: Hypersensitivity

Precautions: Granulocyte count <1000/mm^3 or Hgb <9.5 g/dl, pregnancy (C), lactation, child, renal disease, severe hepatic function, pancreatitis

Pharmacokinetics: Rapidly absorbed, distributed to extravascular space, excreted unchanged in urine

---

◆ = Nursing alert   ⫽ = Herb-drug interaction   ⊘ = Do not crush

Interactions:
- Increased level of zidovudine when given with lamivudine
- Increased level of lamivudine: trimethoprim/sulfamethoxazole

NURSING CONSIDERATIONS
Assess:
- Blood counts q2wk; watch for neutropenia, thrombocytopenia, Hgb; if low, therapy may have to be discontinued and restarted after hematologic recovery; blood transfusions may be required
- Liver studies: AST, ALT, bilirubin; amylase
- Children for pancreatitis

Administer:
- PO bid
- With zidovudine only

Perform/provide:
- Storage in cool environment; protect from light

Evaluate:
- Blood dyscrasias: bruising, fatigue, bleeding, poor healing

Teach patient/family:
- That GI complaints, insomnia resolve after 3-4 wk of treatment
- That drug is not a cure for AIDS, but will control symptoms
- To notify prescriber of sore throat, swollen lymph nodes, malaise, fever; other infections may occur
- That patient is still infective, may pass HIV virus on to others
- That follow-up visits must be continued since serious toxicity may occur; blood counts must be done q2wk
- That drug must be taken twice a day, even if patient feels better
- That other drugs may be necessary to prevent other infections
- That drug may cause fainting or dizziness

lamotrigine (℞)
(la-mot'ri-geen)
Lamictal
Func. class.: Anticonvulsant
Chem. class.: Phenyltriazine

Action: Unknown, may inhibit voltage-sensitive sodium channels
Uses: Adjunct in the treatment of partial seizures
Investigational uses: Generalized tonic-clonic, absence, atypical absence and myoclonic seizures; children with Lennox-Gastaut syndrome; refractory bipolar disorder
Dosage and routes:
No valproic acid
- *Adult:* 50 mg/day for wk 1-2, then increase to 100 mg divided bid for wk 3-4; maintenance, 300-500 mg/day
- *Child:* 2 mg/kg/day in 2 divided doses × 2 wks, then 10 mg/kg/day, max 15 mg/kg/day or 400 mg/day
With valproic acid
- *Adult:* 25 mg qod wk 1-4, then 150 mg/day in divided doses
- *Child:* 0.1-0.2 mg/kg/day initially, then increase q2wk as needed to 2 mg/kg/day or 150 mg/day
Available forms: Tabs 25, 100, 150, 200 mg; chew dispersible tabs
Side effects/adverse reactions:
CNS: Dizziness, ataxia, *headache,* fever, insomnia, tremor, depression, anxiety
EENT: Nystagmus, *diplopia, blurred vision*
GI: Nausea, vomiting, anorexia, abdominal pain, hepatotoxicity
GU: Dysmenorrhea
INTEG: **Rash (potentially life-threatening),** alopecia, photosensitivity
SYST: **Stevens-Johnson syndrome**
Contraindications: Hypersensitivity

Precautions: Pregnancy (C), lactation, child <16 yr, renal, hepatic disease

Pharmacokinetics: Half-life varies depending on dose

Interactions:

• Increased metabolic clearance: carbamazepine, phenobarbital, phenytoin

• Decreased metabolic clearance: valproic acid

NURSING CONSIDERATIONS
Assess:

• For seizure activity: duration, type, intensity, halo before seizure

⬥ For rash (Stevens-Johnson syndrome or toxic epidermal necrolysis) in pediatric patients, drug should be discontinued at first sign of rash

Evaluate:

• Therapeutic response: decrease in severity of seizures

Teach patient/family:

• To take PO doses divided with or after meals to decrease adverse effects, not to discontinue drug abruptly; seizures may occur

• To avoid hazardous activities until stabilized on drug

• To carry Medic Alert ID, to notify prescriber of skin rash or increased seizure activity, to use sunscreen and protective clothing if photosensitivity occurs

• To notify prescriber if pregnant or intend to become pregnant

---

lansoprazole (℞)

(lan-so-prey′zole)
Prevacid

Func. class.: Antisecretory compound-proton pump inhibitor

Chem. class.: Benzimidazole

Action: Suppresses gastric secretion by inhibiting hydrogen/potassium ATPase enzyme system in gastric parietal cell; characterized as gastric acid pump inhibitor, since it blocks final step of acid production

Uses: Gastroesophageal reflux disease (GERD), severe erosive esophagitis, poorly responsive systemic GERD, pathologic hypersecretory conditions (Zollinger-Ellison syndrome, systemic mastocytosis, multiple endocrine adenomas); possibly effective for treatment of duodenal ulcers, maintenance of healed duodenal ulcers

Dosage and routes:
NG tube

• *Adult:* Use intact granules mixed in 40 ml of apple juice and injected through **NG** tube, then flush with apple juice

Duodenal ulcer

• *Adult:* **PO** 15 mg qd before eating for 4 wk

Erosive esophagitis

• *Adult:* **PO** 30 mg qd before eating for up to 8 wk, may use another 8 wk course if needed

Pathologic hypersecretory conditions

• *Adult:* **PO** 60 mg qd, may give up to 90 mg bid

Available forms: Caps, delayed rel 15, 30 mg

Side effects/adverse reactions:

CNS: Headache, dizziness, confusion, agitation, amnesia, depression

GI: Diarrhea, abdominal pain, vomiting, nausea, constipation, flatulence, acid regurgitation, anorexia, irritable colon

RESP: Upper respiratory infections, cough, epistaxis, asthma, bronchitis, dyspnea

INTEG: Rash, urticaria, pruritus, alopecia

META: Weight gain/loss, gout

⬥ = Nursing alert   🖊 = Herb-drug interaction   🚫 = Do not crush

EENT: Tinnitus, taste perversion, deafness, eye pain, otitis media
CV: Chest pain, angina, tachycardia, bradycardia, palpitations, **CVA,** hypertension/hypotension, **MI, shock,** vasodilation
GU: **Hematuria,** glycosuria, impotence, kidney calculus, breast enlargement
HEMA: **Hemolysis,** anemia
Contraindications: Hypersensitivity
Precautions: Pregnancy (B), lactation, children
Pharmacokinetics: Absorption after granules leave stomach—rapid; plasma half-life 1½ hr, protein binding 97%, extensively metabolized in liver, excreted in urine, feces; clearance decreased in the elderly, renal and hepatic impairment
Interactions:
• Decreased clearance of theophylline when given with lansoprazole
• Delayed absorption of lansoprazole: sucralfate
• May be decreased absorption of ketoconazole, ampicillin, iron, digoxin

NURSING CONSIDERATIONS
Assess:
• GI system: bowel sounds q8h, abdomen for pain, swelling, anorexia
• Hepatic enzymes: AST (SGOT), ALT (SGPT), alk phosphatase during treatment
Administer:
🚫 Before eating; swallow capsule whole; do not break, crush, or chew caps
Evaluate:
• Therapeutic response: absence of epigastric pain, swelling, fullness
Teach patient/family:
• To report severe diarrhea; drug may have to be discontinued
• That diabetic patient should know that hypoglycemia may occur

• To avoid hazardous activities; dizziness may occur
• To avoid alcohol, salicylates, ibuprofen; may cause GI irritation

---

letrozole (℞)
(let′tro-zohl)
Femara
Func. class.: Antineoplastic nonsteroidal aromatase inhibitor

Action: Binds to the heme group of aromatase. Inhibits conversion of androgens to estrogens to reduce plasma estrogen levels. 30% of breast cancers decrease in size when deprived of estrogen
Uses: Metastatic breast cancer in postmenopausal women
Dosage and routes:
• *Adult:* **PO** 2.5 mg qd
Available forms: Tabs 2.5 mg
Side effects/adverse reactions:
RESP: Dyspnea, cough
*GI: Nausea, vomiting, anorexia, **hepatotoxicity,** constipation, heartburn, diarrhea
INTEG: Rash, pruritus, alopecia, sweating, hot flashes
CV: Hypertension
CNS: Headache, lethargy, somnolence, *dizziness, depression,* anxiety
Contraindications: Hypersensitivity, pregnancy (D)
Precautions: Hepatic disease, respiratory disease
Pharmacokinetics: Metabolized in liver, excreted in urine
Interactions: Unknown
NURSING CONSIDERATIONS
Assess:
• Renal function studies: BUN, serum uric acid, urine CrCl, electrolytes before, during therapy
• I&O ratio; report fall in urine output of 30 ml/hr

• Monitor temp q4h; may indicate beginning infection
• Liver function tests before, during therapy (bilirubin, AST, ALT, LDH) as needed or monthly
• RBC, Hct, Hgb, since these may be decreased, lymphocyte count, thyroid function tests
• Food preferences; list likes, dislikes
• Inflammation of mucosa, breaks in skin
• Yellowing of skin, sclera, dark urine, clay-colored stools, itchy skin, abdominal pain, fever, diarrhea

Perform/provide:
• Liquid diet, including cola, Jell-O; dry toast or crackers as ordered may be added if patient is not nauseated or vomiting
• Nutritious diet with iron and vitamin supplements as ordered

Evaluate:
• Therapeutic response: decrease in size of tumor

Teach patient/family:
• To report any complaints, side effects to nurse or prescriber
• That masculinization can occur, is reversible after discontinuing treatment
• To avoid self-administration of corticosteroids
• That drowsiness may occur and to avoid driving or operating heavy machinery

---

leucovorin (℞)

(loo-koe-vor'in)
leucovorin calcium, Wellcovorin
Func. class.: Vitamin, folic acid/ methotrexate antagonist antidote
Chem. class.: Tetrahydrofolic acid derivative

Action: Needed for normal growth patterns; prevents toxicity during antineoplastic therapy by protecting normal cells

Uses: Megaloblastic or macrocytic anemia caused by folic acid deficiency, overdose of folic acid antagonist, methotrexate toxicity, toxicity caused by pyrimethamine or trimethoprim, pneumocystosis, toxoplasmosis

Dosage and routes:
Megaloblastic anemia caused by enzyme deficiency
• *Adult and child:* PO/IV/IM up to 1 mg/day
Megaloblastic anemia caused by deficiency of folate
• *Adult and child:* IM 1 mg or less qd until adequate response
Methotrexate toxicity
• *Adult and child:* PO/IM/IV given 6-24 hr after dose of methotrexate 10 mg/m^2, then 10 mg/m^2 q6h × 72 hr
Pyrimethamine toxicity
• *Adult and child:* PO/IM 5 mg qd
Trimethoprim toxicity
• *Adult and child:* PO/IM 400 mg qd
Available forms: Tabs 5, 10, 15, 25 mg; inj 3, 5 mg/ml; powder for inj 10 mg/ml

Side effects/adverse reactions:
RESP: Wheezing
INTEG: Rash, pruritus, erythema, thrombocytosis, urticaria

Contraindications: Hypersensitivity, anemias other than megaloblastic not associated with vit B$_{12}$ deficiency

Precautions: Pregnancy (C)

Interactions:
• Decreased folate levels: chloramphenicol
• Increased metabolism of phenobarbital, hydantoins

NURSING CONSIDERATIONS
Assess:
• CrCl before leucovorin rescue and qd to detect nephrotoxicity

---

- I&O; watch for nausea and vomiting
- Nutritional status: bran, yeast, dried beans, nuts, fruits, fresh vegetables, asparagus, which have high folic acid levels
- Other drugs taken: alcohol, hydantoins, trimethoprim may cause increased folic acid use by body

Administer:
- Within 1 hr of folic acid antagonist

IV
- For IV reconstitute 50 mg/5 ml bacteriostatic or sterile H_2O for inj (10 mg/ml) or (100 mg/10 ml); use immediately if sterile H_2O is used
- Give by direct IV over 60 mg/min or less
- Give by intermittent inf after diluting in 100-500 ml of 0.9% NaCl, D_5W, $D_{10}W$, LR, Ringer's sol

Additive compatibilities: Cisplatin, cisplatin/floxuridine, floxuridine

Syringe compatibilities: Bleomycin, cisplatin, cyclophosphamide, doxorubicin, fluorouracil, furosemide, heparin, methotrexate, metoclopramide, mitomycin, vinblastine, vincristine

Y-site compatibilities: Amifostine, aztreonam, bleomycin, cefepime, cisplatin, cladribine, cyclophosphamide, doxorubicin, filgrastim, fluconazole, fluorouracil, furosemide, granisetron, heparin, methotrexate, metoclopramide, mitomycin, piperacillin/tazobactam, tacrolimus, teniposide, thiotepa, vinblastine, vincristine

Perform/provide:
- Increase fluid intake if used to treat folic acid inhibitor overdose
- Protection from light and heat

Evaluate:
- Therapeutic response: increased weight; improved orientation, well-being; absence of fatigue

Teach patient/family:
- For leucovorin rescue have patient drink 3 L fluid qd of rescue
- For folic acid deficiency eat folic acid rich foods: bran, yeast, dried beans, nuts, fresh, green leafy vegetables
- To take drug exactly as prescribed
- To notify prescriber of side effects
- To report signs of hyposensitivity reaction immediately

---

leuprolide (℞)

(loo-proe'lide)
Leupron Depo Ped, Lupron, Lupron Depot, Lupron Depot-3 month
Func. class.: Antineoplastic hormone
Chem. class.: Gonadotropin-releasing hormone

Action: Causes initial increase in circulating levels of LH, FSH; continuous administration results in decreased LH, FSH; in men, testosterone is reduced to castrate levels; in premenopausal women, estrogen is reduced to menopausal levels

Uses: Metastatic prostate cancer, management of endometriosis, central precocious puberty

Dosage and routes:
- *Adult:* SC 1 mg/day; **IM:** 7.5 mg/dose qmo

Available forms: Inj (depot) 3.75 mg, 7.5 mg single dose, multiple dose vials (5 mg/ml), single-use kit 11.25 mg vial, pediatric depot 7.5, 11.25, 15 mg

Side effects/adverse reactions:
GU: Edema, hot flashes, impotence, decreased libido, amenorrhea, vaginal dryness, gynecomastia

Contraindications: Hypersensitivity to GnRH or analogs, thromboembolic disorders, pregnancy (X), lactation, undiagnosed vaginal bleeding

Precautions: Edema, hepatic disease, CVA, MI, seizures, hypertension, diabetes mellitus

Pharmacokinetics:
SC: Onset 1-2 wk, peak 2-4 wk; absorbed rapidly (SC), slowly (IM depot); half-life 3 hr

NURSING CONSIDERATIONS
Assess:

• For symptoms of endometriosis (lower abdominal pain)

• Liver function tests before, during therapy (bilirubin, AST [SGOT], ALT [SGPT], LDH) as needed or monthly

• Pituitary gonadotropic and gonadal function during therapy and 4-8 wk after therapy is decreased

• Worsening of signs and symptoms; normal during beginning therapy

• Fatigue, increased pulse, pallor, lethargy

• Food preferences; list likes, dislikes

• Edema in feet, joints; stomach pain; shaking

◆ Symptoms indicating severe allergic reaction: rash, pruritus, urticaria, purpuric skin lesions, itching, flushing

• For central precocious puberty (CPP) if treatment is for this condition; secondary S4 characteristics to child <9 yr, estradiol/testosterone levels, GnRH test, tomography of head, adrenal steroids, chorionic gonadotropin, wrist x-ray, height, weight

Administer:

• IM/SC using syringe and drug packaged together, give deep in large muscle mass, rotate sites

• Use depot IM only

• Reconstitute vial (single dose)/1 ml of diluent, shake, use immediately

Perform/provide:

• Nutritious diet with iron, vitamin supplements as ordered

• Storage in tight container at room temp

Evaluate:

• Therapeutic response: decreased tumor size and spread of malignancy

Teach patient/family:

• To notify prescriber if menstruation continues; menstruation should stop

• To use a nonhormonal method of contraception during therapy

• That bone pain will disappear after 1 wk

• To report any complaints, side effects to nurse or prescriber

• How to prepare, give; to rotate sites for SC injections

• To keep accurate records of dose

• That tumor flare may occur: increase in size of tumor, increased bone pain, will subside rapidly; may take analgesics for pain; premenopausal women must use mechanical birth control; ovulation may be induced

---

levamisole (℞)
(leh-vam′ih-sole)
Ergamisol
Func. class.: Antineoplastic-immunomodulator

Action: May increase the action of macrophages, monocytes, T cells, which will restore immune function; complete action unknown

Uses: Treatment of Dukes' stage C colon cancer given with fluorouracil after surgical resection

Investigational uses: Malignant melanoma (advanced)

Dosage and routes:

• *Adult:* **PO** 50 mg q8h × 3d; begin treatment at least 1 wk but no more than 4 wk after resection; given with

---

◆ = Nursing alert   ▮ = Herb-drug interaction   ⊘ = Do not crush

fluorouracil 450 mg/m²/d; **IV** given daily × 5d beginning 21-34d after resection; maintenance is 50 mg q8h × 3d q2wk × 1 yr; given with fluorouracil 45 mg/m²/d by **IV** push qwk starting 28d after the initial 5-d course × 1 yr

Available forms: Tabs 50 mg (base), IV

Side effects/adverse reactions:

CNS: Dizziness, headache, paresthesia, somnolence, depression, anxiety, fatigue, fever, mental changes, ataxia, insomnia

GI: Nausea, vomiting, anorexia, diarrhea, stomatitis, constipation, flatulence, dyspepsia, abdominal pain

INTEG: Rash, pruritus, alopecia, dermatitis, urticaria

HEMA: Granulocytopenia, leukopenia, thrombocytopenia

CV: Chest pain, edema

META: Hyperbilirubinemia

EENT: Blurred vision, conjunctivitis

OTHER: Rigors, infection, altered sense of smell, arthralgia, myalgia

Contraindications: Hypersensitivity

Precautions: Pregnancy (C), lactation, children, blood dyscrasias

Pharmacokinetics: Peak 1½-2 hr, elimination half life 3-4 hr; metabolized by the liver

Interactions:

• Increased plasma levels: phenytoin

• Disulfiram-like reaction: alcohol

NURSING CONSIDERATIONS
Assess:

• Kidney, liver function studies: BUN, creatinine, AST (SGOT), ALT (SGPT), alk phosphatase, bilirubin

• Baseline blood counts with differential, platelets, electrolyte, repeat q3mo for 1 yr; if platelets are <100,000/mm³, therapy should be discontinued and restarted after recovery; fluorouracil should not be given if WBC is 2500-3500/mm³;

after WBC is >3500/mm³, dose should be reduced by 20%; if WBC <2500/mm³ for 10 days, discontinue levamisole

• Stomatitis or GI symptoms: drug may have to be discontinued; then start fluorouracil 28 days after the start of first course

⬧ Blood dyscrasias (anemia, granulocytopenia); bruising, fatigue, bleeding, poor healing

• Allergic reactions: dermatitis, exfoliative dermatitis, pruritus, urticaria

Administer:

• 7-20 days after surgery; start fluorouracil with second course of levamisole; begin no sooner than 21 days and no later than 35 days after surgery; if levamisole therapy begins 21-30 days after resection, fluorouracil should be given with first course; apply pressure to venipuncture sites for 10 min, especially if platelets are low

Evaluate:

• Therapeutic response: decrease in size and spread of tumor

Teach patient/family:

• To call prescriber if sore throat, swollen lymph nodes, malaise, fever occur, since other infections may occur

• To use contraception during therapy and 4 mo after

• To avoid alcohol; disulfiram reaction can occur; also to avoid tyramine-containing products

• To avoid use of products containing aspirin, ibuprofen; to report bleeding

• To report signs of anemia or CNS reactions

• That hair may be lost during treatment; a wig or hairpiece may be worn

levodopa (℞)

(lee′voe-doe-pa)
Dopar, Larodopa, L-Dopa
Func. class.: Antiparkinson agent
Chem. class.: Catecholamine

Action: Decarboxylation to dopamine, which increases dopamine levels in brain

Uses: Parkinsonism

Dosage and routes:
• *Adult:* PO 0.5-1 g qd divided bid-qid with meals; may increase by up to 0.75 g q3-7d not to exceed 8 g/day unless closely supervised
Available forms: Caps 100, 250, 500 mg; tabs 100, 250, 500 mg

Side effects/adverse reactions:
HEMA: **Hemolytic anemia, leukopenia, agranulocytosis**
CNS: Involuntary choreiform movements, hand tremors, fatigue, headache, anxiety, twitching, numbness, weakness, confusion, agitation, insomnia, nightmares, psychosis, hallucination, hypomania, severe depression, dizziness
GI: Nausea, vomiting, anorexia, abdominal distress, dry mouth, flatulence, dysphagia, bitter taste, diarrhea, constipation
INTEG: Rash, sweating, alopecia
CV: Orthostatic hypotension, tachycardia, hypertension, palpitation
EENT: Blurred vision, diplopia, dilated pupils
MISC: Urinary retention, incontinence, weight change, dark urine

Contraindications: Hypersensitivity, narrow-angle glaucoma, undiagnosed skin lesions

Precautions: Renal disease, cardiac disease, hepatic disease, respiratory disease, MI with dysrhythmias, convulsions, peptic ulcer, pregnancy (C), asthma, endocrine disease, affective disorders, psychosis, lactation, children <12 yr, peptic ulcer

Pharmacokinetics:
PO: Peak 1-3 hr, excreted in urine (metabolites)

Interactions:
• Hypertensive crisis: MAOIs, furazolidone
• Decreased effects of levodopa: anticholinergics, hydantoins, methionine, papaverine, pyridoxine, tricyclics, benzodiazepines
• Increased effects of levodopa: antacids, metoclopramide
Drug/food
• Increased pyridoxine will decrease levodopa effect
⚫ Decreased action of levodopa, increased EPS: Indian snakeroot

Lab test interferences:
False positive: Urine ketones, urine glucose, Coombs' test
False negative: Urine glucose (glucose oxidase)
False increase: Uric acid, urine protein
Decrease: VMA

NURSING CONSIDERATIONS

Assess:
• Liver function enzymes: AST (SGOT), ALT (SGPT), alk phosphatase, LDH, bilirubin, CBC
• Involuntary movements in parkinsonism: akinesia, tremors, staggering gait, muscle rigidity, drooling
◆ Levodopa toxicity: mental, personality changes, increased twitching, grimacing, tongue protrusion
• B/P, respiration during initial treatment; hypo/hypertension should be reported
• Mental status: affect, mood, behavioral changes, depression; complete suicide assessment

Administer:
• Drug until NPO before surgery
• Adjust dosage to patient response

• With meals; limit protein taken with drug

• Only after MAOIs have been discontinued for 2 wk

Perform/provide:

• Assistance with ambulation during beginning therapy

• Testing for diabetes mellitus, acromegaly if on long-term therapy

Evaluate:

• Therapeutic response: decrease in akathisia, increased mood

Teach patient/family:

• That therapeutic effects may take several wk to a few mo

• To change positions slowly to prevent orthostatic hypotension

• To report side effects: twitching, eye spasms; indicate overdose

• To use drug exactly as prescribed; if drug is discontinued abruptly, parkinsonian crisis may occur

• That urine, sweat may darken

• To avoid vit B_6 preparations, vitamin-fortified foods containing B_6; these foods can reverse effects of levodopa

---

levofloxacin (R)

(lee-voh-floks′a-sin)

Levaquin

Func. class.: Antiinfective

Chem. class.: Fluoroquinolone

Action: Interferes with conversion of intermediate DNA fragments into high-molecular-weight DNA in bacteria; DNA gyrase inhibitor

Uses: Acute sinusitis, acute chronic bronchitis, community-acquired pneumonia, uncomplicated skin infections, complicated UTI, acute pyelonephritis caused by *S. pneumoniae, H. influenzae, H. parainfluenzae, M. catarrhalis*

Dosage and routes:

• *Adult:* **IV INF** 500 mg by slow inf

over 1 hr q24h × 7-14 days depending on infection; **PO:** 500 mg q24h × 7-14 days depending on infection

Renal disease

• CrCl 20-49 ml/min initial 500 mg, then 250 mg, q24h; CrCl 10-19 ml/min 500 mg, then 750 mg q48h

Available forms: Single use vials (500 mg); 25 mg/ml 20 ml vials; premixed flexible containers; tabs 250, 500 mg

Side effects/adverse reactions:

CNS: Headache, dizziness, *insomnia,* anxiety

GI: Nausea, flatulence, *vomiting,* diarrhea, abdominal pain, ***pseudomembranous colitis***

GU: Vaginitis, crystalluria

INTEG: Rash, pruritus, photosensitivity

Contraindications: Hypersensitivity to quinolones, photosensitivity

Precautions: Pregnancy (C), lactation, children

Pharmacokinetics: Metabolized in liver, excreted in urine unchanged, half-life 6-8 hr

Interactions:

• Decreased absorption of levofloxacin: antacids, zinc, calcium, iron

• Increased toxicity: digoxin, caffeine, warfarin, cyclosporine

• Increased effect of levofloxacin: cimetidine, probenecid

• Do not use with magnesium in the same IV line

Lab test interferences:

Decrease: Glucose, lymphocytes

NURSING CONSIDERATIONS
Assess:

• For previous sensitivity reaction

• For signs and symptoms of infection: characteristics of sputum, WBC >10,000, fever; obtain baseline information before and during treatment

• C&S before beginning drug therapy to identify if correct treatment has been initiated

---

• For allergic reactions: rash, urticaria, pruritus, chills, fever, joint pain; may occur a few days after therapy begins; epinephrine and resuscitation equipment should be available for anaphylactic reaction

• Bowel pattern qd; if severe diarrhea occurs, drug should be discontinued

• For overgrowth of infection: perineal itching, fever, malaise, redness, pain, swelling, drainage, rash, diarrhea, change in cough, sputum

Administer:

• PO 4 hr before or 2 hr after antacids, iron, calcium, zinc

IV

• Only by slow IV infusion over 1 hr

• Discard any unused sol in the single-dose vial

• Using premix, tear outer wrap at notch and remove sol container, check for leaks, close control clamps; remove cover from port at bottom of container, insert pin into port with a twist; suspend container from hanger, squeeze and release drip chamber to proper fluid level, open flow control to expel air, close clamp; regulate rate with flow control clamps

Solution compatibilities: 0.9% NaCl, D_5W, $D_5/0.9\%$ NaCl, D_5LR, $D_5/0.45\%$ NaCl, sodium lactate

Evaluate:

• Therapeutic response: absence of signs/symptoms of infection (WBC <10,000/mm³, temp WNL)

Teach patient/family:

• To contact prescriber if vaginal itching, loose, foul-smelling stools, furry tongue occur; may indicate superinfection; report itching, rash, pruritus, urticaria

• To notify prescriber of diarrhea with blood or pus

• To take 4 hr before or 2 hr after antacids, iron, calcium, zinc products

• To complete full course of therapy

---

levomethadyl (R)

(lev-oh-meth'ah-dil)
ORLAMM
Func. class.: Narcotic agonist analgesic

Action: Depresses pain impulse transmission at the spinal cord level by interacting with opioid receptors

Uses: Management of opiate dependency

Dosage and routes:

Opiate withdrawal

• Usually given 3×/wk (Monday, Wednesday, Friday or Tuesday, Thursday, Saturday)

• *Initial dose:* 20-40 mg each dose at 48 or 72 hr; may be adjusted in increments of 5-10 mg until steady state occurs (1-2 wk); patients dependent on methadone may require larger doses

• *Maintenance:* 60-90 mg 3×/wk

• *Transfer to methadone:* Initial treatment given after 48 hr; may give increased or decreased (5-10 mg) in the daily methadone dose (symptoms of withdrawal)

Available forms: Oral sol 10 mg/ml

Side effects/adverse reactions:

CNS: Drowsiness, dizziness, confusion, headache, sedation, euphoria

CV: Palpitations, bradycardia, change in B/P

EENT: Tinnitus, blurred vision, miosis, diplopia

GI: Nausea, vomiting, anorexia, constipation, cramps, biliary tract spasm

GU: Increased urinary output, dysuria, urinary retention

INTEG: Rash, urticaria, bruising, flushing, diaphoresis, pruritus

*RESP: **Respiratory depression***

Contraindications: Hypersensitivity

Precautions: Addictive personality, pregnancy (B), lactation, increased intracranial pressure, MI (acute), severe heart disease, respiratory depression, hepatic disease, renal disease, child <18 yr

Pharmacokinetics:

PO: Onset 30-60 min, duration 6-8 hr, cumulative 22-48 hr

Metabolized by liver, excreted by kidneys, crosses placenta, excreted in breast milk

Interactions:

• Increased effects with other CNS depressants: alcohol, narcotics, sedative/hypnotics, antipsychotics, skeletal muscle relaxants, rifampin, phenytoin

NURSING CONSIDERATIONS

Assess:

• I&O ratio, check for decreasing output; may indicate urinary retention

Administer:

• With antiemetic for nausea, vomiting

Perform/provide:

• Storage in light-resistant container at room temp

Evaluate:

• Therapeutic response: decreased dependence on opiate

• CNS changes: dizziness, drowsiness, hallucinations, euphoria, LOC, pupil reaction

• Allergic reactions: rash, urticaria

• Respiratory dysfunction: depression, character, rate, rhythm

Teach patient/family:

• To report any symptoms of CNS changes, allergic reactions

• That physical dependency may result after extended period of use

• That withdrawal symptoms may occur: nausea, vomiting, cramps, fever, faintness, anorexia

---

levonorgestrel implant (R)

(lee-voe-nor-jess'trel)
Norplant System
Func. class.: Contraceptive system
Chem. class.: Synthetic progestin

Action: As a progestin, transforms proliferative endometrium into secretory endometrium; inhibits secretion of pituitary gonadotropins, which prevents follicular maturation and ovulation

Uses: Prevention of pregnancy for 5 yr

Dosage and routes:

• *Adult:* 6 caps subdermally implanted in the upper arm during first 7 days after onset of menses

Available forms: Kit of 6 caps, 36 mg/cap

Side effects/adverse reactions:

CNS: Dizziness, headache, nervousness

GU: Amenorrhea, cervical erosion, breakthrough bleeding, dysmenorrhea, vaginal candidiasis, breast changes, vaginitis

GI: Nausea, abdominal discomfort

INTEG: Alopecia, dermatitis, hirsutism, acne, hypertrichosis, infection at site, pain/itching at site

OTHER: Change in appetite, weight gain

Contraindications: Hypersensitivity, pregnancy (X), thrombophlebitis, undiagnosed genital bleeding, liver tumors, breast carcinoma, liver disease

Precautions: Depression, psychosis, lactation, fluid retention, contact lens wearers

Pharmacokinetics: Max concentration at 24 hr

Interactions:
• Decreased contraception: phenytoin, carbamazepine

NURSING CONSIDERATIONS
Assess:
• Blood studies: cholesterol, triglycerides; may be increased or decreased; sex hormone—binding globulin, thyroxine, T_3 uptake
• Menstrual irregularities: spotting, prolonged bleeding, amenorrhea; usually diminish
• For jaundice, thrombophlebitis; implants should be removed
• For acne, dermatitis, hirsutism, alopecia

Administer:
• 8 cm (3 in) above the crease of the elbow; implantation should be during first 7 days after onset of menses; implantation should be fanlike, 15 degrees apart

Evaluate:
• Therapeutic response: absence of pregnancy

Teach patient/family:
• That if vision problems occur, an ophthalmologist should be seen
• That physical examinations are necessary

---

levorphanol (R)

(lee-vor′fa-nole)
Levo-Dromoran
Func. class.: Narcotic analgesic (opioid analgesic agonist)
Chem. class.: Opiate, synthetic morphine derivative

Controlled Substance Schedule II
Action: Depresses pain impulse transmission at the spinal cord level by interacting with opioid receptors
Uses: Moderate to severe pain
Dosage and routes:
• *Adult:* PO/SC/IV 2-3 mg q4-5h prn; **PCA** 0.1 mg/ml

Available forms: Inj 2 mg/ml; tabs 2 mg
Side effects/adverse reactions:
CNS: Drowsiness, dizziness, confusion, headache, sedation, euphoria
GI: Nausea, vomiting, anorexia, constipation, cramps
GU: Urinary retention, dysuria
INTEG: Rash, urticaria, diaphoresis, pruritus
EENT: Tinnitus, blurred vision, miosis, diplopia
CV: Palpitations, bradycardia, change in B/P
*RESP: **Respiratory depression***
Contraindications: Hypersensitivity, addiction (narcotic)
Precautions: Addictive personality, pregnancy (B), lactation, increased intracranial pressure, MI (acute), severe heart disease, respiratory depression, hepatic disease, renal disease, child <18 yr
Pharmacokinetics:
PO: Onset up to ½-1½ hr, peak ½-1 hr, duration 6-8 hr
SC: Peak ½-1 hr, duration 6-8 hr
IV: Peak 20 min, duration 6-8 hr; metabolized by liver; excreted by kidneys; crosses placenta; excreted in breast milk; half-life 12-16 hr
Interactions:
• Effects may be increased with other CNS depressants: alcohol, narcotics, sedative/hypnotics, antipsychotics, skeletal muscle relaxants
🖊 Increased action: kava kava
Lab test interferences:
Increase: Amylase

NURSING CONSIDERATIONS
Assess:
• I&O ratio; check for decreasing output; may indicate urinary retention
• CNS changes: dizziness, drowsiness, hallucinations, euphoria, LOC, pupil reaction

---

◆ = Nursing alert   🖊 = Herb-drug interaction   🚫 = Do not crush

- Allergic reactions: rash, urticaria
- Respiratory dysfunction: respiratory depression, character, rate, rhythm; notify prescriber if respirations are <10/min
- Need for pain medication, physical dependence

Administer:
- With antiemetic if nausea, vomiting occur
- When pain is beginning to return; determine dosage interval by patient response

IV
- IV directly through Y-tube or 3-way stopcock over 5 min; do not give rapidly; circulatory collapse may occur

Syringe compatibilities: Glycopyrrolate, propofol

Perform/provide:
- Storage in light-resistant area at room temp
- Assistance with ambulation
- Safety measures: side rails, nightlight, call bell within easy reach

Evaluate:
- Therapeutic response: decrease in pain

Teach patient/family:
- To report any symptoms of CNS changes, allergic reactions
- That physical dependency may result from extended period of use
- That the following withdrawal symptoms may occur: nausea, vomiting, cramps, fever, faintness, anorexia

Treatment of overdose: Naloxone (Narcan) 0.2-0.8 mg IV, O$_2$, IV fluids, vasopressors

---

levothyroxine (T$_4$) (℞)

(lee-voe-thye-rox′een)
Eltroxin*, Levo-T, Levoxyl, Levothroid, levothyroxine sodium, Levoxine, PMS-Levothyroxine sodium*, Synthroid, T$_4$

Func. class.: Thyroid hormone
Chem. class.: Levoisomer of thyroxine

Action: Increases metabolic rate, controls protein synthesis, increases cardiac output, renal blood flow, O$_2$ consumption, body temp, blood volume, growth, development at cellular level

Uses: Hypothyroidism, myxedema coma, thyroid hormone replacement, congenital hypothyroidism, thyrotoxicosis, congenital hypothyroidism, some types of thyroid cancer

Dosage and routes:
Severe hypothyroidism
- *Adult:* **PO** 12.5-50 µg qd, increased by 50-100 µg q1-4 wk until desired response, maintenance dose 75-125 µg qd; **IM/IV** 50-100 µg/day as a single dose
- *Child >12 yr:* **PO** 2-3 µg/kg/day as a single dose AM
- *Child 6-12 yr:* **PO** 4-5 µg/kg/day as a single dose AM
- *Child 1-5 yr:* **PO** 5-6 µg/kg/day as a single dose AM
- *Child 6-12 mo:* **PO** 6-8 µg/kg/day as a single dose AM
- *Child to 6 mo:* **PO** 8-10 µg/kg/day as a single dose AM

Myxedema coma
- *Adult:* **IV** 200-500 µg, may increase by 100-300 µg after 24 hr; place on oral medication as soon as possible

Available forms: Inj 50, 200, 500 µg/vial; tabs 0.025, 0.05, 0.075, 0.088, 0.1, 0.112, 0.125, 0.15, 0.175, 0.2, 0.3 mg

---

Side effects/adverse reactions:

CNS: Anxiety, insomnia, tremors, headache, ***thyroid storm***

CV: Tachycardia, palpitations, angina, dysrhythmias, hypertension, ***cardiac arrest***

GI: Nausea, diarrhea, increased or decreased appetite, cramps

MISC: Menstrual irregularities, weight loss, sweating, heat intolerance, fever

Contraindications: Adrenal insufficiency, myocardial infarction, thyrotoxicosis, hypersensitivity to beef, alcohol intolerance (inj only)

Precautions: Elderly, angina pectoris, hypertension, ischemia, cardiac disease, pregnancy (A), lactation

Pharmacokinetics:

PO: Onset unknown, peak 1-3 wk, duration 1-3 wk

IV: Onset 6-8 hr, peak 24 hr, duration unknown

Half-life 6-7 days; distributed throughout body tissues

Interactions:

• Decreased absorption of levothyroxine: cholestyramine

• Increased effects of anticoagulants, sympathomimetics, tricyclic antidepressants

• Decreased effects of digitalis drugs, insulin, hypoglycemics

• Decreased effects of levothyroxine: estrogens

• Considered to be incompatible in syringe with all other drugs

🌿 Do not give with bugleweed

Lab test interferences:

Increase: CPK, LDH, AST (SGOT), PBI, blood glucose

Decrease: TSH, ¹³¹I uptake test, uric acid, triglycerides

NURSING CONSIDERATIONS
Assess:

• B/P, pulse before each dose
• I&O ratio

• Weight qd in same clothing, using same scale, at same time of day

• Height, growth rate of a child

• T₃, T₄, FTIs, which are decreased; radioimmunoassay of TSH, which is increased; radio uptake, which is increased if patient is on too low a dose of medication

• Pro-time may require decreased anticoagulant; check for bleeding, bruising

• Increased nervousness, excitability, irritability, which may indicate too high dose of medication, usually after 1-3 wk of treatment

• Cardiac status: angina, palpitation, chest pain, change in VS

Administer:

• IV after diluting with provided diluent 0.5 mg/5 ml; shake; give through Y-tube or 3-way stopcock; give 0.1 mg or less over 1 min; do not add to IV inf; 0.1 mg = 1 ml

• In AM if possible as a single dose to decrease sleeplessness

• At same time each day to maintain drug level

• Only for hormone imbalances; not to be used for obesity, male infertility, menstrual conditions, lethargy

• Lowest dose that relieves symptoms; lower dose to the elderly and in cardiac diseases

• Crushed and mixed with water, nonsoy formula, or breast milk for infants/children

Perform/provide:

• Storage in tight, light-resistant container; sol should be discarded if not used immediately

• Withdrawal of medication 4 wk before RAIU test

Evaluate:

• Therapeutic response: absence of depression; increased weight loss, diuresis, pulse, appetite; absence of constipation, peripheral edema, cold intolerance; pale, cool, dry skin;

◆ = Nursing alert   🌿 = Herb-drug interaction   🚫 = Do not crush

brittle nails, alopecia, coarse hair, menorrhagia, night blindness, paresthesias, syncope, stupor, coma, rosy cheeks

Teach patient/family:

• That hair loss will occur in child, is temporary

• To report excitability, irritability, anxiety, which indicate overdose

• Not to switch brands unless approved by prescriber

• That drug may be discontinued after giving birth, thyroid panel evaluated after 1-2 mo

• That hypothyroid child will show almost immediate behavior/personality change

• That drug is not to be taken to reduce weight

• To avoid OTC preparations with iodine; read labels

• To avoid iodine food, iodized salt, soybeans, tofu, turnips, some seafood, some bread

• That drug is not a cure but controls symptoms and treatment is lifelong

---

lidocaine (℞)

(lye'doe-kane)

Anestacon, Baylocaine, L-Caine, lidocaine HCl IV for Cardiac Arrhythmias, Lidopen Auto Injector, Xylocaine HCl IM for Cardiac Arrythmias, Xylocaine HCl IV for Cardiac Arrhythmias

Func. class.: Antidysrhythmic (Class Ib)

Chem. class.: Aminoacyl amide

Action: Increases electrical stimulation threshold of ventricle, His-Purkinje system, which stabilizes cardiac membrane, decreases automaticity

Uses: Ventricular tachycardia, ventricular dysrhythmias during cardiac surgery, myocardial infarction, digitalis toxicity, cardiac catheterization

Dosage and routes:

• *Adult:* **IV BOL** 50-100 mg (1 mg/kg) over 2-3 min, repeat q3-5min, not to exceed 300 mg in 1 hr; begin **IV INF; IV INF** 20-50 μg/kg/min; **IM** 200-300 mg (4.3 mg/kg) in deltoid muscle, may repeat in 1-1½ hr if needed

• *Elderly, CHF, reduced liver function:* **IV BOL** give ½ adult dose

• *Child:* **IV BOL** 1 mg/kg, then **IV INF** 30 μg/kg/min

Available forms: IV INF 0.2% (2 mg/ml), 0.4% (4 mg/ml), 0.8% (8 mg/ml); IV ad 4% (40 mg/ml), 10% (100 mg/ml), 20% (200 mg/ml); IV dir 1% (10 mg/ml), 2% (20 mg/ml); IM 300 mg/ml, 10%

Side effects/adverse reactions:

CNS: Headache, dizziness, involuntary movement, confusion, tremor, drowsiness, euphoria, ***convulsions***

EENT: Tinnitus, blurred vision

GI: Nausea, vomiting, anorexia

*CV: Hypotension, bradycardia, **heart block, cardiovascular collapse, arrest***

RESP: Dyspnea, ***respiratory depression***

INTEG: Rash, urticaria, edema, swelling

MISC: Febrile response, phlebitis at injection site

Contraindications: Hypersensitivity to amides, severe heart block, supraventricular dysrhythmias, Adams-Stokes syndrome, Wolff-Parkinson-White syndrome

Precautions: Pregnancy (B), lactation, children, renal disease, liver disease, CHF, respiratory depression, malignant hyperthermia

Pharmacokinetics:

IV: Onset 2 min, duration 20 min

IM: Onset 5-15 min, duration 1½

---

hr; half-life 8 min, 1-2 hr (terminal); metabolized in liver; excreted in urine; crosses placenta

Interactions:

• Increased neuromuscular blockade of neuromuscular blockers, tubocurarine

• Increased effects of lidocaine: cimetidine, phenytoin, propranolol, metoprolol

• Decreased effects of lidocaine: barbiturates

💉 Increased action of lidocaine: aloe, buckthorn bark/berry, cascara sagrada bark, senna pod/leaf

Lab test interferences:

Increase: CPK

NURSING CONSIDERATIONS
Assess:

• ECG continuously to determine increased PR or QRS segments; if these develop, discontinue or reduce rate; watch for increased ventricular ectopic beats; may have to rebolus

• IV infusion rate using infusion pump; run at less than 4 mg/min

• Blood levels (therapeutic level: 1.5-6 µg/ml)

• B/P continuously for fluctuations in cardiac rate

• I&O ratio, electrolytes (K, Na, Cl)

➡️ Malignant hyperthermia: tachypnea, tachycardia, changes in B/P, increased temp

• Respiratory status: rate, rhythm, lung fields for rales, watch for respiratory depression

• CNS effects: dizziness, confusion, psychosis, paresthesias, convulsions; drug should be discontinued

• Lung fields, bilateral rales may occur in CHF patient

• Increased respiration, increased pulse; drug should be discontinued

Administer:

• IM injection in deltoid; aspirate to avoid intravascular administration; check site daily for infiltration or extravasation

IV

• Bolus undiluted (1%, 2% only) give 50 mg or less over 1 min or dilute 1 g/250-500 ml of D_5W; titrate to patient response; use infusion pump; pediatric inf is 120 mg of lidocaine/100 ml D_5W; 1-2.5 ml/ kg/hr = 20-50 µg/kg/min; use only 1%, 2% sol for IV bol

Additive compatibilities: Alteplase, aminophylline, amiodarone, atracurium, bretylium, calcium chloride, calcium gluceptate, calcium gluconate, chloramphenicol, chlorothiazide, cimetidine, dexamethasone, digoxin, diphenhydramine, dobutamine, dopamine, ephedrine, erythromycin lactobionate, floxacillin, flumazenil, furosemide, heparin, hydrocortisone, hydroxyzine, insulin (regular), mephentermine, metaraminol, nafcillin, nitroglycerin, penicillin G potassium, pentobarbital, phenylephrine, potassium chloride, procainamide, prochlorperazine, promazine, ranitidine, sodium bicarbonate, sodium lactate, theophylline, verapamil, vit B/C

Solution compatibilities: D_5W, D_5/ 0.9% NaCl, D_5/0.45% NaCl, D_5/ LR, LR, 0.9% NaCl, 0.45% NaCl

Syringe compatibilities: Cloxacillin, glycopyrrolate, heparin, hydroxyzine, methicillin, metoclopramide, milrinone, moxalactam, nalbuphine

Y-site compatibilities: Alteplase, amiodarone, amrinone, cefazolin, ciprofloxacin, diltiazem, dobutamine, dopamine, enalaprilat, etomidate, famotidine, haloperidol, heparin, heparin/hydrocortisone, labetalol, meperidine, morphine, nitroglycerin, nitroprusside, potassium chloride, propofol, streptokinase, theophylline, vit B/C, warfarin

---

➡️ = Nursing alert   💉 = Herb-drug interaction   🚫 = Do not crush

Evaluate:
• Therapeutic response: decreased dysrhythmias
Teach patient/family:
• The use of automatic lidocaine injection device if ordered
Treatment of overdose: O_2, artificial ventilation, ECG; administer dopamine for circulatory depression, diazepam or thiopental for convulsions; decrease drug if needed

---

lindane (R)

(lin'dane)
GBH*, G-Well*, Kwell, Kwellada*, Kwildane, lindane, Scabene, Thionex
Func. class.: Scabicide, pediculicide
Chem. class.: Chlorinated hydrocarbon (synthetic)

Action: Stimulates nervous system of arthropods, resulting in seizures, death of organism
Uses: Scabies, lice (head/pubic/body), nits
Dosage and routes:
Lice
• *Adult and child:* CREAM/LOTION wash area with soap, water; remove visible crusts; apply to skin surfaces; remove with soap, water in 8-12 hr; may reapply in 1 wk if needed; shampoo using 30 ml: work into lather, rub for 5 min, rinse, dry with towel; comb with fine-toothed comb to remove nits
Scabies
• *Adult and child:* TOP apply 1% cream/lotion to skin, neck to bottom of feet, toes, repeat in 1 wk prn
Available forms: Lotion, shampoo, cream (1%)
Side effects/adverse reactions:
INTEG: Pruritus, rash, irritation, contact dermatitis

GI: Nausea, vomiting, diarrhea, liver damage (inhalation of vapors)
*HEMA: **Aplastic anemia** (chronic inhalation of vapors)
*CV: **Ventricular fibrillation** (chronic inhalation of vapors)
*GU: **Kidney damage** (chronic inhalation of vapors)
CNS: Tremors, ***convulsions,*** stimulation, dizziness (chronic inhalation of vapors)
Contraindications: Hypersensitivity; premature neonate; patients with known seizure disorders; inflammation of skin, abrasions, or breaks in skin
Precautions: Pregnancy (B); avoid contact with eyes; children <10 yr, infants, lactation
Interactions:
• Oils may enhance absorption; if an oil-based hair dressing is used, shampoo, rinse, dry hair before applying lindane shampoo
NURSING CONSIDERATIONS
Assess:
• Head, hair for lice and nits before and after treatment; if scabies are present check all skin surfaces
• Identify source of infection: school, family, sexual contacts
Administer:
• To body areas, scalp only; do not apply to face, lips, mouth, eyes, any mucous membrane, anus, or meatus
• Topical corticosteroids as ordered to decrease contact dermatitis
• Antihistamines
• Lotions of menthol or phenol to control itching
• Topical antibiotics for infection
Perform/provide:
• Isolation until areas on skin, scalp have cleared and treatment is completed
• Removal of nits by using a fine-toothed comb rinsed in vinegar after treatment; use gloves

Evaluate:

• Therapeutic response: decreased crusts, nits, brownish trails on skin, itching papules in skin folds, decreased itching after several wk

Teach patient/family:

• To wash all inhabitants' clothing, using insecticide; preventive treatment may be required of all persons living in same house, using lotion or shampoo to decrease spread of infection; use rubber gloves when applying drug

• That itching may continue for 4-6 wk

• That drug must be reapplied if accidently washed off, or treatment will be ineffective

• Not to apply to face; if accidental contact with eyes occurs, flush with water

• To treat sexual contacts simultaneously

Treatment of ingestion: Gastric lavage, saline laxatives, IV diazepam (Valium) for convulsions

---

liothyronine (T₃) (Rx)

(lye-oh-thye'roe-neen)

Cytomel, liothyronine sodium, Triostat

Func. class.: Thyroid hormone
Chem. class.: Synthetic T_3

Action: Increases metabolic rates, cardiac output, O_2 consumption, body temp, blood volume, growth, development at cellular level

Uses: Hypothyroidism, myxedema coma, thyroid hormone replacement, congenital hypothyroidism, nontoxic goiter, T_3 suppression test

Dosage and routes:

• *Adult:* **PO** 25 µg qd, increased by 12.5-25 µg q1-2wk until desired response, maintenance dose 25-75 µg qd

• *Geriatric:* **PO** 5 µg/day, increase by 5 µg/day q1-2wk

Congenital hypothyroidism

• *Child >3 yr:* **PO** 50-100 µg qd

• *Child <3 yr:* **PO** 5 µg qd, increased by 5 µg q3-4d titrated to response

Myxedema, severe hypothyroidism

• *Adult:* **PO** 5 µg qd; may increase by 5-10 µg q1-2wk; maintenance dose 50-100 µg qd

Nontoxic goiter

• *Adult:* **PO** 5 µg qd, increased by 12.5-25 µg q1-2wk; maintenance dose 75 µg qd

Suppression test

• *Adult:* **PO** 75-100 µg qd × 1 wk; radioactive ^{131}I is given before and after 1 wk dose

Available forms: Tabs 5, 25, 50 µg; inj 10 µg/ml

Side effects/adverse reactions:

CNS: Insomnia, tremors, headache, **thyroid storm**

CV: Tachycardia, palpitations, angina, dysrhythmias, hypertension, **cardiac arrest**

GI: Nausea, diarrhea, increased or decreased appetite, cramps

MISC: Menstrual irregularities, weight loss, sweating, heat intolerance, fever

Contraindications: Adrenal insufficiency, myocardial infarction, thyrotoxicosis

Precautions: Elderly, angina pectoris, hypertension, ischemia, cardiac disease, pregnancy (A), lactation

Pharmacokinetics:

PO/IV: Peak 12-48 hr, duration 72 hr, half-life 6-7 days

Interactions:

• Decreased absorption of liothyronine: cholestyramine

• Increased effects of anticoagulants, sympathomimetics, tricyclic antidepressants

---

◆ = Nursing alert   🌿 = Herb-drug interaction   🚫 = Do not crush

• Decreased effects of digitalis drugs, insulin, hypoglycemics
• Decreased effects of liothyronine: estrogens

🖋 Do not use with bugleweed

Lab test interferences:
Increase: CPK, LDH, AST (SGOT), PBI, blood glucose
Decrease: TSH, ^{131}I uptake test, uric acid, triglycerides

NURSING CONSIDERATIONS
Assess:
• B/P, pulse before each dose
• I&O ratio
• Weight qd in same clothing, using same scale, at same time of day
• Height, growth rate of child
• T_3, T_4, which are decreased; radioimmunoassay of TSH, which is increased; radio uptake, which is increased if patient is on too low a dose of medication
• Pro-time may require decreased anticoagulant; check for bleeding, bruising
• Increased nervousness, excitability, irritability, which may indicate too high dose of medication, usually after 1-3 wk of treatment
• Cardiac status: angina, palpitation, chest pain, change in VS

Administer:
• In AM if possible as a single dose to decrease sleeplessness
• At same time each day to maintain drug level
• Only for hormone imbalances; not to be used for obesity, male infertility, menstrual conditions, lethargy
• Lowest dose that relieves symptoms
• Liothyronine after discontinuing other thyroid preparation

Perform/provide:
• Removal of medication 4 wk before RAIU test

Evaluate:
• Therapeutic response: absence of depression; increased weight loss, diuresis, pulse, appetite; absence of constipation, peripheral edema, cold intolerance; pale, cool, dry skin; brittle nails, alopecia, coarse hair, menorrhagia, night blindness, paresthesia, syncope, stupor, coma, rosy cheeks

Teach patient/family:
• That hair loss will occur in child but is temporary
• To report excitability, irritability, anxiety, which indicates overdose
• Not to switch brands unless approved by prescriber
• That hypothyroid child will show almost immediate behavior/personality change
• That drug is not to be taken to reduce weight
• To avoid OTC preparations with iodine; read labels
• To avoid iodine food, iodized salt, soybeans, tofu, turnips, some seafood, some bread
• That drug controls symptoms but does not cure; treatment is lifelong

---

liotrix (℞)
(lye′oh-trix)
Euthroid, Thyrolar, T_3/T_4
Func. class.: Thyroid hormone
Chem. class.: Levothyroxine/liothyronine (synthetic T_4, T_3)

Action: Increases metabolic rates, cardiac output, O_2 consumption, body temp, blood volume, growth, development at cellular level

Uses: Hypothyroidism, thyroid hormone replacement

Dosage and routes:
• *Adult and child:* PO 15-30 mg qd, increased by 15-30 mg q1-2wk until desired response; may increase by 15-30 mg q2wk in child

---

• *Elderly:* **PO** 15 mg initially, increase q2-4wk by 15 mg until desired response

Available forms: Euthroid- ½, 1, 2, 3 gr; Thyrolar- ¼, ½, 1, 2, 3 gr; ½ gr = 30 mg

Side effects/adverse reactions:

CNS: Insomnia, tremors, headache, *thyroid storm*

CV: Tachycardia, palpitations, angina, dysrhythmias, hypertension, *cardiac arrest*

GI: Nausea, diarrhea, increased or decreased appetite, cramps

MISC: Menstrual irregularities, weight loss, sweating, heat intolerance, fever

Contraindications: Adrenal insufficiency, myocardial infarction, thyrotoxicosis

Precautions: Elderly, angina pectoris, hypertension, ischemia, cardiac disease, pregnancy (A), lactation

Pharmacokinetics:

PO (T₄): Onset unknown, peak 1-3 wk, duration 1-3 wk

PO (T₃): Onset unknown, peak 24-72 hr, duration 72 hr, half-life 1 wk

Interactions:

• Decreased absorption of liotrix: cholestyramine, colestipol

• Increased effects of anticoagulants, sympathomimetics, tricyclic antidepressants, catecholamines

• Decreased effects of digitalis, insulin, hypoglycemics

• Decreased effects of liotrix: estrogens

🍵 Do not use with bugleweed

Lab test interferences:

Increase: CPK, LDH, AST (SGOT), PBI, blood glucose

Decrease: TSH, ¹³¹I uptake test, uric acid, triglycerides

NURSING CONSIDERATIONS

Assess:

• B/P, pulse before each dose

• I&O ratio

• Weight qd in same clothing, using same scale, at same time of day

• Height, growth rate of child

• T₃, T₄, FTIs, which are decreased; radioimmunoassay of TSH, which is increased; radio uptake, which is increased if patient is on too low a dose of medication

• Pro-time may require decreased anticoagulant; check for bleeding, bruising

• Increased nervousness, excitability, irritability, which may indicate too high dose of medication, usually after 1-3 wk of treatment

• Cardiac status: angina, palpitation, chest pain, change in VS

Administer:

• In ᴀᴍ if possible as a single dose to decrease sleeplessness

• At same time each day to maintain drug level

• Only for hormone imbalances; not to be used for obesity, male infertility, menstrual conditions, lethargy

• Lowest dose that relieves symptoms

Perform/provide:

• Withdrawal of medication 4 wk before RAIU test

• Storage in airtight, light-resistant container

Evaluate:

• Therapeutic response: absence of depression; increased weight loss, diuresis, pulse, appetite; absence of constipation, peripheral edema, cold intolerance; pale, cool, dry skin; brittle nails, coarse hair, menorrhagia, night blindness, paresthesias, syncope, stupor, coma, rosy cheeks

Teach patient/family:

• That hair loss will occur in child, is temporary

• To report excitability, irritability, anxiety, which indicate overdose

- Not to switch brands unless approved by prescriber
- That hypothyroid child will show almost immediate behavior/personality change
- That drug is not to be taken to reduce weight
- To avoid OTC preparations with iodine; read labels
- To avoid iodine food, iodized salt, soybeans, tofu, turnips, some seafood, some bread
- That drug does not cure, but controls symptoms, treatment is lifelong

---

lisinopril (R)

(lyse-in'oh-pril)

Prinivil, Zestril

Func. class.: Antihypertensive, angiotensin converting enzyme inhibitor (ACE)

Chem. class.: Enalaprilat lysine analog

Action: Selectively suppresses renin-angiotensin-aldosterone system; inhibits ACE, preventing conversion of angiotensin I to angiotensin II

Uses: Mild to moderate hypertension, adjunctive therapy of systolic CHF

Dosage and routes:

Hypertension

- *Adult:* **PO** 10-40 mg qd; may increase to 80 mg qd if required
- *Geriatric:* **PO** 2.5-5 mg/day, increase q7 days

CHF

- *Adult:* **PO** 5 mg initially with diuretics/digitalis

Available forms: Tabs 2.5, 5, 10, 20, 40 mg

Side effects/adverse reactions:

GI: Nausea, vomiting, anorexia, constipation, flatulence, GI irritation

GU: **Proteinuria, renal insufficiency,** sexual dysfunction, impotence

INTEG: Rash, pruritus

CNS: Vertigo, depression, stroke, insomnia, paresthesias, headache, *fatigue,* asthenia

EENT: Blurred vision, nasal congestion

SYST: **Angioedema**

RESP: Dry cough, dyspnea

Contraindications: Hypersensitivity

Precautions: Pregnancy (C), lactation, renal disease, hyperkalemia, renal artery stenosis

Pharmacokinetics: Onset 1 hr, peak 6-8 hr, duration 24 hr, excreted unchanged in urine

Interactions:

- Increased hypotensive effect: diuretics, other hypertensives, probenecid
- Decreased effects of lisinopril: aspirin, indomethacin
- Increased K levels: K salt substitutes, K-sparing diuretics, K supplements
- Increased effects of antihypertensives, reserpine, diuretics
- Increased hypersensitivity reactions: allopurinol

Drug/food

- High-potassium diet (bananas, orange juice, avocados, nuts, spinach) should be avoided; hyperkalemia may occur

Lab test interferences:

Interference: Glucose/insulin tolerance tests

NURSING CONSIDERATIONS

Assess:

- B/P, pulse q4h; note rate, rhythm, quality
- Electrolytes: K, Na, Cl
- Apical/pedal pulse before administration; notify prescriber of any significant changes

- Baselines in renal, liver function tests before therapy begins
- Edema in feet, legs qd
- Skin turgor, dryness of mucous membranes for hydration status
- Symptoms of CHF: edema, dyspnea, wet rales

Evaluate:

- Therapeutic response: decreased B/P, CHF symptoms

Teach patient/family:

- Not to discontinue drug abruptly
- To rise slowly to sitting or standing position to minimize orthostatic hypotension
- To avoid increasing K in the diet

Treatment of overdose: Lavage, IV atropine for bradycardia, IV theophylline for bronchospasm, digitalis, O_2, diuretic for cardiac failure

---

lithium (℞)

(li'thee-um)

Carbolith*, Cibalith-S, Duralith*, Eskalith, Eskalith-CR, Lithane, lithium carbonate, Lithizine*, Lithonate, Lithotabs

Func. class.: Antimanic

Chem. class.: Alkali metal ion salt

Action: May alter sodium, potassium ion transport across cell membrane in nerve, muscle cells; may balance biogenic amines of norepinephrine, serotonin in CNS areas involved in emotional responses

Uses: Manic-depressive illness (manic phase), prevention of bipolar manic-depressive psychosis

Dosage and routes:

- *Adult:* **PO** 300-600 mg tid, maintenance 300 mg tid or qid; slow rel tabs 300 mg bid; dose should be individualized to maintain blood levels at 0.5-1.5 mEq/L

- *Geriatric:* **PO** 300 mg bid, increase q7 days by 300 mg to desired dose

Renal dose

- **PO** CrCl 10-50 ml/min 50%-75% of dose; CrCl <10 ml/min 25%-50% of dose

- *Child:* **PO** 15-20 mg (0.4-0.5 mEq)/kg/day in 2-3 divided doses, increase as needed, do not exceed adult doses

Available forms: Caps 300, 600 mg; tabs 300 mg; tabs cont rel 450 mg; syr 300 mg/5 ml (8 mEq/5 ml); cap slow rel 300 mg*

Side effects/adverse reactions:

CNS: Headache, drowsiness, dizziness, tremors, twitching, ataxia, *seizure,* slurred speech, restlessness, confusion, stupor, memory loss, clonic movements, fatigue

GI: Dry mouth, anorexia, nausea, vomiting, diarrhea, incontinence, abdominal pain, metallic taste

GU: Polyuria, glycosuria, proteinuria, albuminuria, urinary incontinence, polydipsia, edema

CV: Hypotension, ECG changes, dysrhythmias, *circulatory collapse,* edema

INTEG: Drying of hair, alopecia, rash, pruritus, hyperkeratosis, acneiform lesions, folliculitis

HEMA: Leukocytosis

EENT: Tinnitus, blurred vision

ENDO: Hyponatremia, hypothyroidism, goiter, hyperglycemia, hyperthyroidism

MS: Muscle weakness

Contraindications: Hepatic disease, renal disease, brain trauma, OBS, pregnancy (D), lactation, children <12 yr, schizophrenia, severe cardiac disease, severe renal disease, severe dehydration

Precautions: Elderly, thyroid disease, seizure disorders, diabetes mellitus, systemic infection, urinary retention

---

◆ = Nursing alert ⬤ = Herb-drug interaction ⊘ = Do not crush

Pharmacokinetics:
PO: Onset rapid, peak ½-4 hr, half-life 18-36 hr depending on age; crosses blood-brain barrier; 80% of filtered lithium is reabsorbed by the renal tubules, excreted in urine; crosses placenta; enters breast milk; well absorbed by oral method

Interactions:
• Increased hypothyroid effects: antithyroid agents, calcium iodide, potassium iodide, iodinated glycerol
• Brain damage: haloperidol, thioridazine
• Increased effects of neuromuscular blocking agents, phenothiazines
• Increased renal clearance: sodium bicarbonate, acetazolamide, mannitol, aminophylline
• Increased toxicity: indomethacin, diuretics, nonsteroidal antiinflammatories
• Decreased effects of lithium: theophyllines, urea, urinary alkalinizers

Drug/food
• Significant changes in sodium intake will alter lithium excretion

Lab test interferences:
Increase: K excretion, urine glucose, blood glucose, protein, BUN
Decrease: VMA, T_3, T_4, PBI, ^{131}I

NURSING CONSIDERATIONS
Assess:
• Weight qd; check for and report edema in legs, ankles, wrists
• Na intake; decreased Na intake with decreased fluid intake may lead to lithium retention; increased Na and fluids may decrease lithium retention
• Skin turgor at least qd
• Urine for albuminuria, glycosuria, uric acid during beginning treatment, q2mo thereafter
• Neuro status: LOC, gait, motor reflexes, hand tremors

• Serum lithium levels qwk initially, then q2mo (therapeutic level: 0.5-1.5 mEq/L)

Administer:
• Reduced dose to elderly
• With meals to avoid GI upset
• Adequate fluids (2-3 L/day) to prevent dehydration during initial treatment, 1-2 L/day during maintenance

Evaluate:
• Therapeutic response: decrease in excitement, manic phase

Teach patient/family:
• The symptoms of minor toxicity: vomiting, diarrhea, poor coordination, fine motor tremors, weakness, lassitude; major toxicity: coarse tremors, severe thirst, tinnitus, diluted urine
• To monitor urine specific gravity, emphasize need for follow-up care to determine lithium levels
• That contraception is necessary, since lithium may harm fetus
• Not to operate machinery until lithium levels are stable
• That beneficial effects may take 1-3 wk
• About drugs that interact with lithium (provide list) and discuss need for adequate stable intake of salt and fluids
Ⓝ Not to break, crush, or chew caps

Treatment of overdose: Induce emesis or lavage, maintain airway, respiratory function; dialysis for severe intoxication

---

lomefloxacin (℞)
(lo-meh-flox′a-sin)
Maxaquin
Func. class.: Antiinfective
Chem. class.: Fluoroquinolone

Action: Interferes with conversion of intermediate DNA fragments into high-molecular-weight DNA in bacteria; DNA gyrase inhibitor

Uses: Treatment of lower respiratory tract infections (pneumonia, bronchitis), genitourinary infections (prostatitis, UTIs), preoperatively to reduce UTIs in transurethral surgical procedures; gram-negative bacteria: *Aeromonas, Citrobacter, Enterobacter, Escherichia coli, Haemophilus influenzae, Klebsiella, Legionella, Moraxella catarrhalis, Morganella morganii, Proteus vulgaris, P. mirabilis, Providencia alcalifaciens, P. rettgeri, Pseudomonas aeruginosa, Serratia;* gram-positive bacteria: *Staphylococcus aureus, S. epidermidis, S. saprophyticus*

Dosage and routes:
• *Adult:* **PO** 400 mg/day for 7-14 days depending on type of infection
In renal impairment
• *Adult:* **PO** 200 mg/day
Surgical prophylaxis
• *Adult:* **PO** 400 mg 2-6 hr before surgery
Available forms: Tabs 400 mg
Side effects/adverse reactions:
CNS: Dizziness, headache, somnolence, depression, insomnia, nervousness, confusion, agitation
GI: Diarrhea, nausea, vomiting, anorexia, flatulence, heartburn, dry mouth; increased AST (SGOT), ALT (SGPT); constipation, abdominal pain, oral thrush, glossitis, stomatitis
INTEG: Rash, pruritus, urticaria, *photosensitivity*
EENT: Visual disturbances
Contraindications: Hypersensitivity to quinolones
Precautions: Pregnancy (C), lactation, children, elderly, renal disease, seizure disorders, excessive exposure to sunlight
Pharmacokinetics:
PO: Peak 1-2 hr, half-life 6-8 hr;

excreted in urine as active drug, metabolites

Interactions:
• Decreased effects of lomefloxacin: antacids, nitrofurantoin, sucralfate, iron salts, zinc salts, calcium
• Increased lomefloxacin levels: probenecid, cimetidine
• Increased levels of cyclosporine, warfarin, caffeine, theophylline

NURSING CONSIDERATIONS
Assess:
• Kidney, liver function studies: BUN, creatinine, AST (SGOT), ALT (SGPT)
• I&O ratio; urine pH, <5.5 is ideal
• CNS symptoms: insomnia, vertigo, headache, agitation, confusion
• Allergic reactions: rash, flushing, urticaria, pruritus
Administer:
• After clean-catch urine for C&S
• 2 hr before or 2 hrs after antacids, iron, calcium, zinc products
Evaluate:
• Therapeutic response: negative C&S, absence of signs/symptoms of infection
Teach patient/family:
• That fluids must be increased to 3 L/day to avoid crystallization in kidneys
• That if dizziness or light-headedness occurs, to ambulate, perform activities with assistance
• To complete full course of drug therapy
• To contact prescriber if adverse reactions occur
• To avoid iron- or mineral-containing supplements or antacids within 2 hr before and after dosing
• That photosensitivity may occur and sunscreen should be used

---

lomustine (℞)

(loe-mus'teen)
CCNU, CeeNU
Func. class.: Antineoplastic
alkylating agent
Chem. class.: Nitrosourea

Action: Responsible for crosslinking DNA strands, which leads to cell death; activity is not cell cycle phase specific

Uses: Hodgkin's disease, lymphomas, melanomas, multiple myeloma; brain, lung, bladder, kidney, colon cancer

Investigational uses: Brain, breast, renal, GI tract, bronchogenic carcinoma; melanomas

Dosage and routes:
• *Adult:* **PO** 130 mg/m² as a single dose q6wk; titrate dose to WBC; do not give repeat dose unless WBC >4000/mm³, platelet count >100,000/mm³

Available forms: Caps 10, 40, 100 mg

Side effects/adverse reactions:
*HEMA: **Thrombocytopenia, leukopenia, myelosuppression, anemia***
*GI: Nausea, vomiting, anorexia, stomatitis, **hepatotoxicity***
*GU: **Azotemia, renal failure***
INTEG: Burning at injection site
*RESP: **Fibrosis, pulmonary infiltrate***

Contraindications: Hypersensitivity, leukopenia, thrombocytopenia, pregnancy (D)

Precautions: Radiation therapy

Pharmacokinetics: Metabolized in liver, excreted in urine; half-life 16-48 hr; 50% protein bound; crosses blood-brain barrier; appears in breast milk

Interactions:
• Increased toxicity: barbiturates, phenytoin, chloral hydrate

• Increased metabolism of lomustine: phenobarbital
• Potentiation of lomustine: succinylcholine
• Increased bone marrow depression: allopurinol

NURSING CONSIDERATIONS
Assess:
• CBC, differential, platelet count qwk; withhold drug if WBC <4000 or platelet count <75,000; notify prescriber
• Pulmonary function tests, chest x-ray films before, during therapy; chest film should be obtained q2wk during treatment
• Renal function studies: BUN, serum uric acid, urine CrCl before, during therapy
• I&O ratio; report fall in urine output of 30 ml/hr
• Monitor temp q4h (may indicate beginning infection); no rectal temps
• Liver function tests before, during therapy (bilirubin, AST [SGOT], ALT [SGPT], LDH) as needed or monthly
• Bleeding: hematuria, guaiac, bruising or petechiae, mucosa or orifices q8h
• Dyspnea, rales, unproductive cough, chest pain, tachypnea
• Food preferences; list likes, dislikes
• Yellowing of skin and sclera, dark urine, clay-colored stools, itchy skin, abdominal pain, fever, diarrhea
• Inflammation of mucosa, breaks in skin
• Buccal cavity q8h for dryness, sores or ulceration, white patches, oral pain, bleeding, dysphagia
• Local irritation, pain, burning, discoloration at injection site
◆ Symptoms indicating severe allergic reaction: rash, pruritus, urticaria, purpuric skin lesions, itching, flushing

---

Side effects: *italics* = common; ***bold italics*** = life-threatening

Administer:
- Antiemetic 30-60 min before giving drug to prevent vomiting
- Antibiotics for prophylaxis of infection
- Topical or systemic analgesics for pain
- Local or systemic drugs for infection

Perform/provide:
- Storage in tight container at room temp
- Strict medical asepsis, protective isolation if WBC levels are low
- Special skin care
- Deep-breathing exercises with patient tid-qid; place in semi-Fowler's position
- Increase fluid intake to 2-3 L/day to prevent urate deposits, calculi formation
- Rinsing of mouth tid-qid with water, club soda; brushing of teeth bid-tid with soft brush or cotton-tipped applicators for stomatitis; use unwaxed dental floss

Evaluate:
- Therapeutic response: decreased tumor size, spread of malignancy

Teach patient/family:
- About protective isolation
- To report any changes in breathing or coughing
- To avoid foods with citric acid, hot or rough texture if buccal inflammation is present
- To report any bleeding, white spots, or ulcerations in mouth to prescriber; tell patient to examine mouth qd
- To report signs of infection: fever, sore throat, flu symptoms
- To report signs of anemia: fatigue, headache, faintness, shortness of breath, irritability
- To avoid use of razors, commercial mouthwash
- To avoid use of aspirin products or ibuprofen

---

loperamide (OTC, ℞)
(loe-per'a-mide)
A-D Kaopectate II Caplets, loperamide solution, Imodium, Imodium A-D, Imodium A-D Caplet, loperamide, Maalox Antidiarrheal Caplets, Pepto Diarrhea Control
Func. class.: Antidiarrheal
Chem. class.: Piperidine derivative

Action: Direct action on intestinal muscles to decrease GI peristalsis; reduces volume, increases bulk, electrolytes not lost

Uses: Diarrhea (cause undetermined), chronic diarrhea, ileostomy discharge

Dosage and routes:
- *Adult:* **PO** 4 mg, then 2 mg after each loose stool, not to exceed 16 mg/day
- *Child 2-5 yr:* **PO** 1 mg then 0.1 mg/kg after each loose stool
- *Child 5-8 yr:* **PO** 2 mg bid on day 1, then 0.1 mg/kg after each loose stool
- *Child 8-12 yr:* **PO** 2 mg tid on day 1, then 0.1 mg/kg after each loose stool

Available forms: Caps 2 mg; liq 1 mg/5 ml; tabs 2 mg

Side effects/adverse reactions:
CNS: Dizziness, drowsiness, fatigue, fever
GI: Nausea, dry mouth, vomiting, constipation, abdominal pain, anorexia, **toxic megacolon**
INTEG: Rash

Contraindications: Hypersensitivity, severe ulcerative colitis, pseudomembranous colitis, acute diarrhea associated with *E. coli*

Precautions: Pregnancy (B), lactation, children <2 yr, liver disease, dehydration, bacterial disease

---

Pharmacokinetics:
PO: Onset ½-1 hr, duration 4-5 hr, half-life 7-14 hr; metabolized in liver; excreted in feces as unchanged drug; small amount in urine

Interactions:
• Do not mix oral sol with other sols

NURSING CONSIDERATIONS
Assess:
• Stools: volume, color, characteristics
• Electrolytes (K, Na, Cl) if on long-term therapy
• Skin turgor q8h if dehydration is suspected
• Bowel pattern before; for rebound constipation
• Response after 48 hr; if no response, drug should be discontinued
• Dehydration in children
• Abdominal distention, toxic megacolon; may occur in ulcerative colitis

Administer:
• For 48 hr only

Perform/provide:
• Storage in tight container

Evaluate:
• Therapeutic response: decreased diarrhea

Teach patient/family:
• To avoid OTC products unless directed by prescriber
• That ostomy patient may take this drug for extended time
• That if drowsiness occurs, not to operate machinery
• To use hard candy, sips of water for dry mouth
🚫 Not to break, crush, or chew caps

loracarbef
See cephalosporins—2nd generation

---

loratadine (℞)
(lor-a′ti-deen)
Claritin, Claritin Reditabs
Func. class.: Antihistamine, 2nd generation
Chem. class.: Selective histamine (H_1)-receptor antagonist

Action: Binds to peripheral histamine receptors, providing antihistamine action without sedation

Uses: Seasonal rhinitis

Dosage and routes:
• *Adult and child ≥12 yr:* **PO** 10 mg qd
• *Child 6-12 yr:* **PO** 10 mg (10 ml) qd

Available forms: Tabs 10 mg; tabs rapid-disintegrating 10 mg; syr 1 mg/ml

Side effects/adverse reactions:
CNS: Sedation (more common with increased doses), headache

Contraindications: Hypersensitivity, acute asthma attacks, lower respiratory tract disease

Precautions: Pregnancy (B), increased intraocular pressure, bronchial asthma

Pharmacokinetics: Peak 1½ hr, elimination half-life 8½-28 hr; metabolized in liver to active metabolites, excreted in urine

Interactions:
• Additive CNS depressant effects: alcohol, other CNS depressants
• Increased CV effects: azole antifungals, macrolide antibiotics
• Increased loratadine levels: cimetidine
• Increased anticholinergic/sedative effects: MAOIs
🌿 Increased anticholinergic effect: henbane leaf

NURSING CONSIDERATIONS
Administer:
• Rapid-disintegrating tabs by plac-

ing on tongue, then swallow after disintegrated with or without water
• On empty stomach
Perform/provide:
• Storage in tight container at room temp
Evaluate:
• Therapeutic response: absence of running or congested nose
Teach patient/family:
• To avoid driving, other hazardous activities if drowsiness occurs

---

lorazepam (℞)

(lor-a′ze-pam)
Alzapam, Apo-Lorazepam*, Ativan, Loraz, lorazepam, Novolorazem*
Func. class.: Sedative, hypnotic; antianxiety
Chem. class.: Benzodiazepine

Controlled Substance Schedule IV
Action: Potentiates the actions of GABA, especially in system and reticular formation
Uses: Anxiety, irritability in psychiatric or organic disorders, preoperatively, insomnia, adjunct in endoscopic procedures
Dosage and routes:
Anxiety
• *Adult:* **PO** 2-6 mg/day in divided doses, not to exceed 10 mg/day
• *Geriatric:* **PO** 0.5-1 mg/day in divided doses; or 0.5-1 mg hs
• *Child:* **PO** 0.05 mg/kg/dose, q4-8h
Insomnia
• *Adult:* **PO** 2-4 mg hs; only minimally effective after 2 wk continuous therapy
Preoperatively
• *Adult:* **IM** 50 μg/kg 2 hr prior to surgery; **IV** 44 μg/kg 15-20 min prior to surgery
• *Child:* 0.05 mg/kg

Status epilepticus
• *Neonate:* 0.05 mg/kg
• *Child:* 0.1 mg/kg up to 4 mg/dose
Available forms: Tabs 0.5, 1, 2 mg; inj 2, 4 mg/ml; conc sol 2 mg/ml
Side effects/adverse reactions:
CNS: Dizziness, drowsiness, confusion, headache, anxiety, tremors, stimulation, fatigue, depression, insomnia, hallucinations, weakness, unsteadiness
INTEG: Rash, dermatitis, itching
CV: Orthostatic hypotension, **ECG changes, tachycardia,** hypotension
EENT: Blurred vision, tinnitus, mydriasis
Contraindications: Hypersensitivity to benzodiazepines, narrow-angle glaucoma, psychosis, pregnancy (D), lactation, child <12 yr, history of drug abuse, COPD
Precautions: Elderly, debilitated, hepatic disease, renal disease
Pharmacokinetics:
PO: Onset ½ hr, peak 1-6 hr, duration 24-48 hr
IM: Onset 15-30 min, peak 1-1 ½ hr, duration 24-48 hr
IV: Onset 5-15 min, peak unknown, duration 24-48 hr
Metabolized by liver; excreted by kidneys; crosses placenta, breast milk; half-life 14 hr
Interactions:
• Decreased effects of lorazepam: oral contraceptives, valproic acid
• Increased effects of lorazepam: CNS depressants, alcohol, disulfiram, oral contraceptives
🌿 Increased action: kava kava
Lab test interferences:
Increase: AST (SGOT), ALT (SGPT), serum bilirubin
Decrease: RAIU
False increase: 17-OHCS

◆ = Nursing alert   🌿 = Herb-drug interaction   🚫 = Do not crush

NURSING CONSIDERATIONS
Assess:
• B/P (lying, standing), pulse; if systolic B/P drops 20 mm Hg, hold drug, notify prescriber; respirations q5-15min if given IV
• Blood studies: CBC during long-term therapy; blood dyscrasias have occurred rarely
• Hepatic studies: AST (SGOT), ALT (SGPT), bilirubin, creatinine, LDH, alk phosphatase
• Mental status: mood, sensorium, affect, sleeping pattern, drowsiness, dizziness
• Physical dependency, withdrawal symptoms: headache, nausea, vomiting, muscle pain, weakness, tremors, convulsions, after long-term, excessive use
• Suicidal tendencies
Administer:
• With food or milk for GI symptoms
• Crushed if patient is unable to swallow medication whole
• Sugarless gum, hard candy, frequent sips of water for dry mouth
• Deep into large muscle mass (IM inj)
IV
• IV after diluting in equal vol sterile H₂O, 5% dextrose or 0.9% NaCl for inj; give through Y-tube or 3-way stopcock, give at 2 mg or less over 1 min
Syringe compatibilities: Cimetidine, hydromorphone
Y-site compatibilities: Acyclovir, albumin, allopurinol, amifostine, amikacin, amoxicillin, amoxicillin/clavulanate, amsacrine, atracurium, bumetanide, cefepime, cefmetazole, cefotaxime, ciprofloxacin, cisplatin, cladribine, clonidine, cyclophosphamide, cytarabine, dexamethasone, diltiazem, dobutamine, dopamine, doxorubicin, epinephrine, erythro-

mycin, etomidate, famotidine, fentanyl, filgrastim, fluconazole, fludarabine, furosemide, gentamicin, granisetron, haloperidol, heparin, hydrocortisone, hydromorphone, ketanserin, labetalol, melphalan, methotrexate, metronidazole, midazolam, milrinone, morphine, nicardipine, nitroglycerin, norepinephrine, paclitaxel, pancuronium, piperacillin, piperacillin/tazobactam, potassium chloride, propofol, ranitidine, tacrolimus, teniposide, thiotepa, trimethoprim-sulfamethoxazole, vancomycin, vecuronium, vinorelbine, zidovudine
Perform/provide:
• Assistance with ambulation during beginning therapy, since drowsiness/dizziness occurs
• Check to see if PO medication has been swallowed
• Refrigerate parenteral form
Evaluate:
• Therapeutic response: decreased anxiety, restlessness, insomnia
Teach patient/family:
• That drug may be taken with food
• Not to use drug for everyday stress or used longer than 4 mo unless directed by prescriber
• Not to take more than prescribed amount; may be habit forming
• To avoid OTC preparations (cough, cold, hay fever) unless approved by prescriber
• To avoid driving, activities that require alertness, since drowsiness may occur
• To avoid alcohol ingestion, other psychotropic medications, unless directed by prescriber
• Not to discontinue medication abruptly after long-term use
• To rise slowly or fainting may occur, especially elderly
• That drowsiness may worsen at beginning of treatment

• To use birth control if child-bearing age

Treatment of overdose: Lavage, VS, supportive care, flumazenil

---

losartan (R)

(lo-zar'tan)
Cozaar
Func. class.: Antihypertensive
Chem. class.: Angiotensin II receptor (Type AT₁)

Action: Blocks the vasoconstrictor and aldosterone-secreting effects of angiotensin II; selectively blocks the binding of angiotensin II to the AT₁ receptor found in tissues

Uses: Hypertension, alone or in combination

Dosage and routes:
• *Adult:* **PO** 50 mg qd alone or 25 mg qd when used in combination

Available forms: Tabs 25, 50 mg

Side effects/adverse reactions:

CNS: Dizziness, insomnia, anxiety, confusion, abnormal dreams, migraine, tremor, vertigo

CV: Angina pectoris, 2nd-degree AV block, *cerebrovascular accident,* hypotension, *myocardial infarction, dysrhythmias*

EENT: Blurred vision, burning eyes, conjunctivitis, task perversion

GI: Diarrhea, dyspepsia, anorexia, constipation, dry mouth, flatulence, gastritis, vomiting

GU: Impotence, nocturia, urinary frequency, UTI

HEMA: Anemia

INTEG: Alopecia, dermatitis, dry skin, flushing, photosensitivity, rash, pruritus, sweating

META: Gout

MS: Cramps, myalgia, pain, stiffness

RESP: Cough, upper respiratory infection, congestion, dyspnea, bronchitis

Contraindications: Hypersensitivity

Precautions: Hypersensitivity to ACE inhibitors; Pregnancy (C) 1st trimester, (D) 2nd and 3rd trimesters; lactation, children, elderly

Pharmacokinetics: Extensively metabolized, half-life 2 hr, metabolite 6-9 hr, highly bound to plasma proteins, excreted in urine and feces

NURSING CONSIDERATIONS

Assess:
• B/P, pulse q4h; note rate, rhythm, quality
• Electrolytes: K, Na, Cl
• Baselines in renal, liver function tests before therapy begins
• Edema in feet, legs qd
• Skin turgor, dryness of mucous membranes for hydration status

Administer:
• Without regard to meals

Evaluate:
• Therapeutic response: decreased B/P

Teach patient/family:
• To avoid sunlight or wear sunscreen if in sunlight; photosensitivity may occur
• To comply with dosage schedule, even if feeling better
• To notify prescriber of mouth sores, fever, swelling of hands or feet, irregular heartbeat, chest pain
• That excessive perspiration, dehydration, vomiting, diarrhea may lead to fall in blood pressure; consult prescriber if these occur
• That drug may cause dizziness, fainting; light-headedness may occur
• To rise slowly to sitting or standing position to minimize orthostatic hypotension

---

◆ = Nursing alert   ⫻ = Herb-drug interaction   ⊘ = Do not crush

lovastatin (℞)

(loh-vah-stat′in)

Mevacor

Func. class.: Antilipemic

Chem. class.: Aspergillus terreus strain derivative

Action: Inhibits HMG-CoA reductase enzyme, which reduces cholesterol synthesis

Uses: As an adjunct in primary hypercholesterolemia (types IIa, IIb), mixed hyperlipidemia, atherosclerosis

Dosage and routes:

(Patient should first be placed on a cholesterol-lowering diet)

• *Adult:* **PO** 20 mg qd with evening meal; may increase to 20-80 mg/day in single or divided doses, not to exceed 80 mg/day; dosage adjustments should be made qmo, reduce dose in renal disease

Available forms: Tabs 10, 20, 40 mg

Side effects/adverse reactions:

*GI: Flatus, nausea, constipation, diarrhea, dyspepsia, abdominal pain, heartburn, **liver dysfunction***

*MS: Muscle cramps, myalgia, **myositis, rhabdomyolysis***

CNS: Dizziness, headache, tremor

INTEG: Rash, pruritus, photosensitivity

EENT: Blurred vision, dysgeusia, lens opacities

Contraindications: Hypersensitivity, pregnancy (X), lactation, active liver disease

Precautions: Past liver disease, alcoholism, severe acute infections, trauma, hypotension, uncontrolled seizure disorders, severe metabolic disorders, electrolyte imbalances, visual disorder, children

Pharmacokinetics:

PO: Peak 2-4 hr, metabolized in liver (metabolites), highly protein bound; excreted in urine, feces; crosses placenta, excreted in breast milk; half-life 3-4 hr

Interactions:

• Increased effects: bile acid sequestrants, warfarin

• Increased myalgia, myositis: cyclosporine, gemfibrozil, niacin

• Decreased antihyperlipidemic effect: propranolol

• Increased bleeding: warfarin

Drug/food:

• Increased levels of lovastatin with food

Lab test interferences:

Increase: CPK, liver function tests

NURSING CONSIDERATIONS

Assess:

• Fasting cholesterol, LDL, HDL, triglycerides periodically during treatment

• Liver function studies q1-2mo during the first 1½ yr of treatment; AST (SGOT), ALT (SGPT), liver function tests may increase

• Renal function in patients with compromised renal system: BUN, creatinine, I&O ratio

• Eyes with slit lamp before, 1 mo after treatment begins, annually; lens opacities may occur

Administer:

• In evening with meal; if dose is increased, take with breakfast and evening meal

Perform/provide:

• Storage in cool environment in airtight, light-resistant container

Evaluate:

• Therapeutic response: cholesterol at desired level after 8 wk

Teach patient/family:

• That blood work and eye exam will be necessary during treatment

• To report blurred vision, severe GI symptoms, dizziness, headache, muscle pain, weakness

---

• That previously prescribed regimen will continue: low-cholesterol diet, exercise program

---

loxapine (℞)

(lox'a-peen)
Loxapac*, loxapine succinate*, Loxitane, Loxitane IM, Loxitane-C
Func. class.: Antipsychotic, neuroleptic
Chem. class.: Dibenzoxazepine

Action: Depresses cerebral cortex, hypothalamus, limbic system, which control activity and aggression; blocks neurotransmission produced by dopamine at synapse; exhibits strong α-adrenergic, anticholinergic blocking action; mechanism for antipsychotic effects is unclear

Uses: Psychotic disorders, nonpsychotic symptoms associated with dementia

Investigational uses: Depression, anxiety

Dosage and routes:
• *Adult:* PO 10 mg bid-qid initially, may be rapidly increased depending on severity of condition, maintenance 60-100 mg/day; **IM** 12.5-50 mg q4-6h or more until desired response, then start **PO** form
• *Geriatric:* PO 5-10 mg qd-bid, increase q4-7 days by 5-10 mg, max 125 mg

Available forms: Caps 5, 10, 25, 50 mg; conc 25 mg/ml; inj 50 mg/ml

Side effects/adverse reactions:
*RESP: **Laryngospasm,** dyspnea, **respiratory depression***
*CNS: EPS: pseudoparkinsonism, akathisia, dystonia, tardive dyskinesia, drowsiness, headache, **seizures,** confusion*
*HEMA: **Anemia, leukopenia, leukocytosis, agranulocytosis***

*INTEG: **Rash,** photosensitivity, dermatitis*
EENT: Blurred vision, glaucoma
*GI: **Dry mouth, nausea, vomiting, anorexia, constipation,** diarrhea, jaundice, weight gain*
GU: Urinary retention, urinary frequency, enuresis, impotence, amenorrhea, gynecomastia
*CV: Orthostatic hypotension, **cardiac arrest,** ECG changes, tachycardia*

Contraindications: Hypersensitivity, blood dyscrasias, coma, child <16 yr, brain damage, bone marrow depression, alcohol and barbiturate withdrawal states

Precautions: Pregnancy (C), lactation, seizure disorders, hepatic disease, cardiac disease, prostatic hypertrophy, cardiac conditions, child <16 yr, elderly

Pharmacokinetics:
PO: Onset 20-30 min, peak 2-4 hr, duration 12 hr
IM: Onset 15-30 min, peak 15-20 min, duration 12 hr
Metabolized by liver; excreted in urine; crosses placenta; enters breast milk; initial half-life 5 hr; terminal half-life 19 hr

Interactions:
• Toxicity: epinephrine
• Increased EPS: other antipsychotics
• Decreased effects: guanadrel, guanethidine
• Increased CNS depression: MAOIs, antidepressants
🌿 Increased action: kava kava

NURSING CONSIDERATIONS
Assess:
• Mental status before initial administration
• Swallowing of PO medication; check for hoarding or giving of medication to other patients
• I&O ratio; palpate bladder if low urinary output occurs

◆ = Nursing alert   🌿 = Herb-drug interaction   🚫 = Do not crush

• Bilirubin, CBC, liver function studies qmo
• Urinalysis is recommended before and during prolonged therapy
• Affect, orientation, LOC, reflexes, gait, coordination, sleep pattern disturbances
• B/P standing and lying; take pulse and respirations q4h during initial treatment; establish baseline before starting treatment; report drops of 30 mm Hg
• Dizziness, faintness, palpitations, tachycardia on rising
• EPS including akathisia (inability to sit still, no pattern to movements), tardive dyskinesia (bizarre movements of the jaw, mouth, tongue, extremities), pseudoparkinsonism (rigidity, tremors, pill rolling, shuffling gait)
• Skin turgor qd
⬥ For neuroleptic malignant syndrome: muscle rigidity, increased CPK, altered mental status, hyperthermia
• Constipation, urinary retention qd; if these occur, increase bulk, water in diet

Administer:
• Reduced dose to elderly
• Antiparkinsonian agent if EPS symptoms occur

IM
• IM injection into large muscle mass

PO
• Concentrate mixed in orange or grapefruit juice

Perform/provide:
• Decreased noise input by dimming lights, avoiding loud noises
• Supervised ambulation until stabilized on medication; do not involve in strenuous exercise program because fainting is possible; patient should not stand still for long periods
• Increased fluids to prevent constipation
• Sips of water, candy, gum for dry mouth
• Storage in air-tight, light-resistant container

Evaluate:
• Therapeutic response: decrease in emotional excitement, hallucinations, delusions, paranoia; reorganization of patterns of thought, speech

Teach patient/family:
• That orthostatic hypotension may occur and to rise from sitting or lying position gradually
• To remain lying down after IM injection for at least 30 min
• To avoid hot tubs, hot showers, tub baths, as hypotension may occur; that in hot weather heat stroke may occur; take extra precautions to stay cool
• To avoid abrupt withdrawal of this drug, or EPS may result; drug should be withdrawn slowly
• To avoid OTC preparations (cough, hay fever, cold) unless approved by prescriber; serious drug interactions may occur; avoid use with alcohol, CNS depressants; increased drowsiness may occur
• To avoid hazardous activities until stabilized on medication
• To use a sunscreen during sun exposure to prevent burns
• About necessity for meticulous oral hygiene, since oral candidiasis may occur
• To report impaired vision, jaundice, tremors, muscle twitching

Treatment of overdose: Lavage if orally ingested; provide an airway

---

Side effects: *italics* = common; ***bold italics*** = life-threatening

lypressin (℞)

(lye-press'in)
Diapid
Func. class.: Pituitary hormone
Chem. class.: Lysine vasopressin

Action: Promotes reabsorption of water by action on renal tubular epithelium

Uses: Nonnephrogenic diabetes insipidus

Dosage and routes:
• *Adult:* **INTRANASAL** 1-2 sprays in one or both nostrils qid, an extra dose hs if needed

Available forms: Intranasal 0.185 mg/ml

Side effects/adverse reactions:
EENT: Nasal irritation, congestion, rhinitis, conjunctivitis, rhinorrhea
CNS: Headache
GI: Nausea, heartburn, cramps
MISC: Chest tightness, cough, dyspnea

Precautions: CAD, pregnancy (B)

Pharmacokinetics:
Nasal: Onset 1 hr, duration 3-8 hr, half-life 15 min
Metabolized in liver, kidneys, excreted in urine

NURSING CONSIDERATIONS
Assess:
• Nares for irritation
• I&O ratio; weight qd; check for edema in extremities; if water retention is severe, diuretic may be prescribed
◆ Water intoxication: lethargy, behavioral changes, disorientation, neuromuscular excitability

Perform/provide:
• Storage at room temp

Evaluate:
• Therapeutic response: absence of severe thirst, decreased urine output, osmolality

Teach patient/family:
• To clear nasal passages before using drug, not to inhale spray
• To carry drug at all times

magaldrate (OTC)

(mag'al-drate)
Antiflux, Lowsium, Riopan, Riopan Extra Strength
Func. class.: Antacid
Chem. class.: Aluminum/magnesium hydroxide

Action: Neutralizes gastric acidity; drug is dissolved in gastric contents; combination of aluminum, magnesium

Uses: Antacid, peptic ulcer disease (adjunct), duodenal, gastric ulcers, reflux esophagitis, hyperacidity, indigestion, heartburn

Dosage and routes:
• *Adult:* **PO** 1-2 (480-1080 mg) between meals, hs, not to exceed 20 tabs/day; **CHEW TAB** 1-2 (480-960 mg) between meals, hs, not to exceed 20 tabs/day; **SUSP** 5-10 ml (400-800 mg) with H_2O between meals, hs, not to exceed 100 ml/day

Available forms: Tabs 480 mg; chew tabs 480 mg; susp 540 mg/5 ml, 480 mg/5 ml, 1080 mg/5 ml

Side effects/adverse reactions:
GI: Constipation, diarrhea
META: Hypermagnesemia, hypophosphatemia

Contraindications: Hypersensitivity to this drug or aluminum

Precautions: Elderly, fluid restriction, decreased GI motility, GI obstruction, dehydration, renal disease, Na-restricted diets, pregnancy (C)

Pharmacokinetics:
PO: Duration 60 min

Interactions:
• Decreased effectiveness of tetracyclines, ketoconazole

 = Nursing alert   = Herb-drug interaction   🚫 = Do not crush

• Decreased absorption of anticholinergics, chlordiazepoxide, cimetidine, corticosteroids, iron salts, phenothiazines, phenytoin, salicylates

NURSING CONSIDERATIONS

Assess:

• GI status: location of pain, intensity, characteristics, heartburn, hematemesis

• Serum Mg^{++} levels with impaired renal function

• Constipation: increase bulk in diet if needed

Administer:

• Laxatives or stool softeners if constipation occurs

• After shaking; give between meals and hs

Evaluate:

• Therapeutic response: absence of pain, decreased acidity

Teach patient/family:

• To separate enteric-coated drugs and antacid by 1 hr

• To notify prescriber immediately of coffee-ground emesis, emesis with frank blood, black tarry stools

---

magnesium oxide
Mag-Ox, Maox, Uro-Mag
Func. class.: Antacid
Chem. class.: Magnesium product

Action: Neutralizes gastric acidity
Uses: Constipation, hypomagnesemia, antacid

Dosage and routes:
• *Adult:* **PO** 250 mg-1 g pc, hs with 4-8 oz water
• *Child:* 10-20 mg/kg/dose (elemental magnesium)
Laxative
• *Adult:* **PO** 2-4 g with water hs
Hypomagnesemia
• *Adult:* **PO** 650-1.3 g qd
Available forms: Caps 140 mg; tabs 400, 420 mg

Side effects/adverse reactions:
GU: Renal stones
GI: Diarrhea, flatulence, cramps, belching, nausea, vomiting
META: Hypermagnesemia: *weakness, lethargy, depression, decreased B/P, increased pulse, **respiratory depression, coma***

Contraindications: Hypersensitivity

Precautions: Severe renal disease, GI bleeding, diarrhea, intestinal obstruction, pregnancy (C)

Pharmacokinetics:
PO: Excreted in urine

Interactions:
• Decreased effectiveness of tetracyclines, ketoconazole
• Decreased absorption of anticholinergics, chlordiazepoxide, cimetidine, corticosteroids, iron salts, phenothiazines, phenytoin

Lab test interferences:
Increase: Urinary pH, gastrin
Decrease: K$^+$

NURSING CONSIDERATIONS
Assess:
• Decreased constipation, characteristics of stools
Perform/provide:
• Storage in airtight container
Evaluate:
• Therapeutic response: absence of pain, decreased acidity
Teach patient/family:
• Not to change antacids unless directed by prescriber

---

magnesium salicylate (OTC, ℞)
Doan's pills, Magan, Mobidin
Func. class.: Nonnarcotic analgesic
Chem. class.: Salicylate

Action: Blocks pain impulses in CNS that occur in response to

---

inhibition of prostaglandin synthesis; antipyretic action results from inhibition of hypothalamic heat-regulating center to produce vasodilation to allow heat dissipation

Uses: Mild to moderate pain or fever including arthritis, juvenile rheumatoid arthritis

Dosage and routes:

Arthritis

• *Adult:* **PO** not to exceed 4.8 g/day in divided doses

Pain/fever

• *Adult:* **PO** 600 mg tid or qid

Available forms: Tabs 325, 545, 600 mg

Side effects/adverse reactions:

HEMA: ***Thrombocytopenia, agranulocytosis, leukopenia, neutropenia, hemolytic anemia,*** increased pro-time

CNS: Stimulation, drowsiness, dizziness, confusion, ***convulsion,*** headache, flushing, hallucinations, coma

GI: Nausea, vomiting, GI bleeding, diarrhea, heartburn, anorexia, ***hepatitis***

INTEG: Rash, urticaria, bruising

EENT: Tinnitus, hearing loss

CV: Rapid pulse, ***pulmonary edema***

RESP: Wheezing, hyperpnea

ENDO: Hypoglycemia, hyponatremia, hypokalemia

Contraindications: Hypersensitivity to salicylates, GI bleeding, bleeding disorders, children <12 yr, vit K deficiency

Precautions: Anemia, hepatic disease, renal disease, Hodgkin's disease, pregnancy (C), lactation

Pharmacokinetics:

PO: Onset 15-30 min, peak 1-2 hr, duration 4-6 hr; metabolized by liver; excreted by kidneys; crosses placenta; excreted in breast milk; half-life 1-3½ hr

Interactions:

• Decreased effects of magnesium-salicylate: antacids, steroids, urinary alkalizers

• Increased blood loss: alcohol, heparin

• Increased effects of anticoagulants, insulin, methotrexate

• Decreased effects of probenecid, spironolactone, sulfinpyrazone, sulfonylamides

• Toxic effects: PABA

• Decreased blood sugar levels: salicylates

Lab test interferences:

Increase: Coagulation studies, liver function studies, serum uric acid, amylase, CO_2, urinary protein

Decrease: Serum K, cholesterol, blood glucose

Interference: Urine catecholamines, pregnancy test

NURSING CONSIDERATIONS

Assess:

• Liver function studies: AST, ALT, bilirubin, creatinine (long-term therapy)

• Renal function studies: BUN, urine creatinine (long-term therapy)

• Blood studies: CBC, Hct, Hgb, pro-time (long-term therapy)

• I&O ratio; decreasing output may indicate renal failure (long-term therapy)

Hepatotoxicity: dark urine, clay-colored stools, yellow skin and sclera, itching, abdominal pain, fever, diarrhea (long-term therapy)

• Allergic reactions: rash, urticaria; if these occur, drug may have to be discontinued

• Renal dysfunction: decreased urine output

• Ototoxicity: tinnitus, ringing, roaring in ears; audiometric testing is needed before, after long-term therapy

---

Acetaminophen/Codeine

Tylenol with Codeine
300/15mg: McNeil

Vicodin
500/5mg: Knoll

Tylenol with Codeine
300/30mg: McNeil

Vicodin ES
750/7.5mg: Knoll

Tylenol with Codeine
300/60mg: McNeil

Anexsia
650/7.5mg: Monarch

Acetaminophen/ Hydrocodone

Lorcet Plus
650/7.5mg: Forest

Lortab
500/5mg: Whitby

Lorcet
650/10mg: Forest

Lortab
500/7.5mg: Whitby

Acetaminophen/ Propoxyphene HCl

Wygesic
650/65mg: Wyeth-Ayerst

Albuterol

Proventil
4mg: Schering

Proventil Repetabs
4mg: Schering

Amlodipine

Norvasc
2.5mg: Pfizer

Norvasc
5mg: Pfizer

Norvasc
10mg: Pfizer

Amoxicillin

Trimox
250mg: Bristol-Myers Squibb

Trimox
500mg: Bristol-Myers Squibb

Amoxil
125mg: SmithKline Beecham

Amoxil
250mg: SmithKline Beecham

Amoxil
250mg: SmithKline Beecham

Amoxil
500mg: SmithKline Beecham

Amoxicillin/Clavulanate

Augmentin
125/31.25mg: SmithKline Beecham

Augmentin
250/62.5mg: SmithKline Beecham

Augmentin
250/125mg: SmithKline Beecham

Augmentin
500/125mg: SmithKline Beecham

Augmentin
875/125mg: SmithKline Beecham

Azithromycin

Zithromax
250mg: Pfizer

Zithromax
250mg: Pfizer

Cephalexin

Keflex
250mg: Dista

Keflex
500mg: Dista

Ciprofloxacin HCl

Cipro
250mg: Miles

Cipro
500mg: Miles

Cipro
750mg: Miles

Clarithromycin

Biaxin
250mg: Abbott

Biaxin
500mg: Abbott

Digoxin

Lanoxicaps
0.1mg: Glaxo Wellcome

Diltiazem HCl

Cardizem
30mg: Hoechst Marion Roussel

Cardizem
60mg: Hoechst Marion Roussel

Cardizem
90mg: Hoechst Marion Roussel

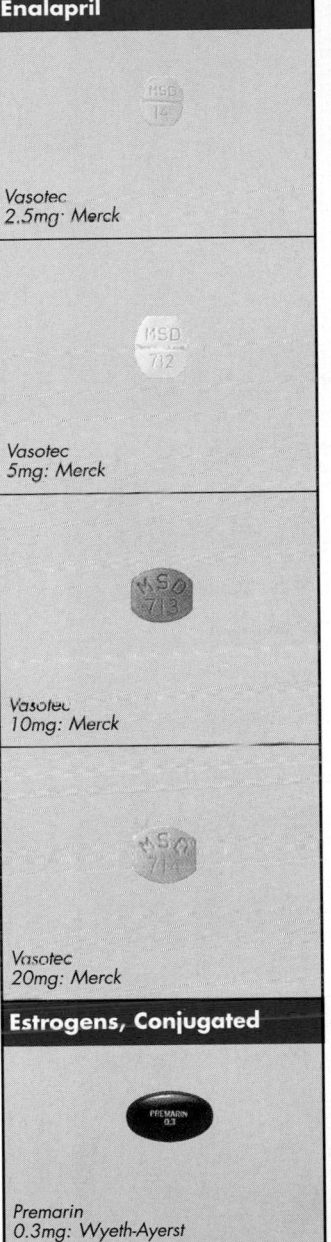

Cardizem CD
120mg: Hoechst Marion Roussel

Cardizem CD
180mg: Hoechst Marion Roussel

Cardizem CD
240mg: Hoechst Marion Roussel

Dilacor XR
180mg: Rhone-Poulenc Rorer

Dilacor XR
240mg: Rhone-Poulenc Rorer

Enalapril

Vasotec
2.5mg· Merck

Vasotec
5mg: Merck

Vasotec
10mg: Merck

Vasotec
20mg: Merck

Estrogens, Conjugated

Premarin
0.3mg: Wyeth-Ayerst

Premarin
0.625mg: Wyeth-Ayerst

Premphase
0.625/5mg: Wyeth-Ayerst

Premarin
0.9mg: Wyeth-Ayerst

Fluoxetine HCl

Prozac
10mg: Dista

Premarin
1.25mg: Wyeth-Ayerst

Prozac
20mg: Dista

Premarin
2.5mg: Wyeth-Ayerst

Furosemide

Lasix
20mg: Hoechst Marion Roussel

**Estrogens, Conjugated/
Medroxyprogesterone**

Prempro
0.625/2.5mg: Wyeth-Ayerst

Lasix
40mg: Hoechst Marion Roussel

Lasix
80mg: Hoechst Marion Roussel

Generic
20mg: Rugby

Generic
40mg: Rugby

Generic
80mg: Rugby

Levothyroxine

Levothroid
0.025mg: Forest

Levothroid
0.05mg: Forest

Levothroid
0.075mg: Forest

Levothroid
0.088mg: Forest

Levothroid
0.1mg: Forest

Levothroid
0.112mg: Forest

Levothroid
0.125mg: Forest

Synthroid
0.025mg: Knoll

Levothroid
0.137mg: Forest

Synthroid
0.05mg: Knoll

Levothroid
0.150mg: Forest

Synthroid
0.075mg: Knoll

Levothroid
0.2mg: Forest

Synthroid
0.1mg: Knoll

Levothroid
0.3mg: Forest

Synthroid
0.112mg: Knoll

Synthroid
0.125mg: Knoll

Synthroid
0.15mg: Knoll

Synthroid
0.2mg: Knoll

Synthroid
0.3mg: Knoll

Generic
0.1mg: Mova

Lisinopril

Prinivil
5mg: Merck

Prinivil
10mg: Merck

Prinivil
20mg: Merck

Prinivil
25mg: Merck

Prinivil
40mg: Merck

Drug identification guide

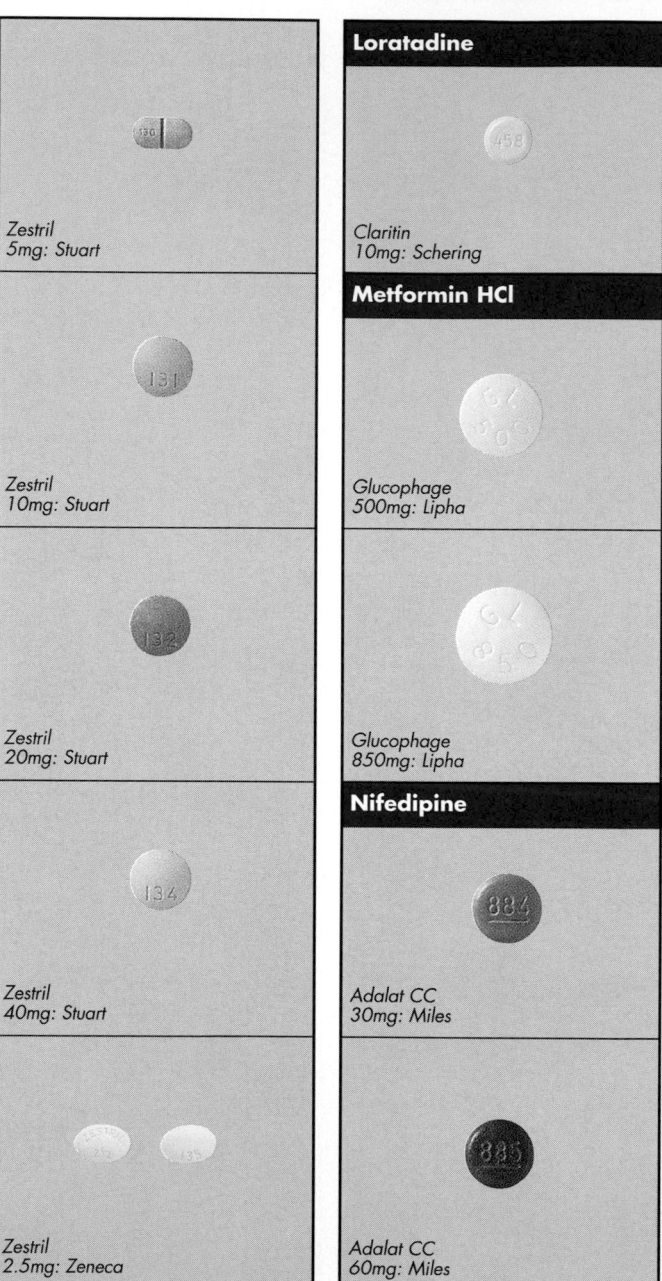

Zestril
5mg: Stuart

Zestril
10mg: Stuart

Zestril
20mg: Stuart

Zestril
40mg: Stuart

Zestril
2.5mg: Zeneca

Loratadine

Claritin
10mg: Schering

Metformin HCl

Glucophage
500mg: Lipha

Glucophage
850mg: Lipha

Nifedipine

Adalat CC
30mg: Miles

Adalat CC
60mg: Miles

Adalat CC
90mg: Miles

Procardia
10mg: Pfizer

Procardia
20mg: Pfizer

Procardia XL
30mg: Pfizer

Procardia XL
60mg: Pfizer

Procardia XL
90mg: Pfizer

Omeprazole

Prilosec
20mg: Merck

Paroxetine HCl

Paxil
10mg: SmithKline Beecham

Paxil
20mg: SmithKline Beecham

Paxil
30mg: SmithKline Beecham

Paxil
40mg: SmithKline Beecham

Penicillin V Potassium

Veetids
250mg: Bristol-Myers Squibb

Veetids
500mg: Bristol-Myers Squibb

V-Cillin K
250mg: Lilly

V-Cillin K
500mg: Lilly

Beepen-VK
250mg: SmithKline Beecham

Beepen-VK
500mg: SmithKline Beecham

Potassium Chloride

Micro-K
600mg: A. H. Robins

Micro-K
750mg: A. H. Robins

K-Dur
750mg: Schering

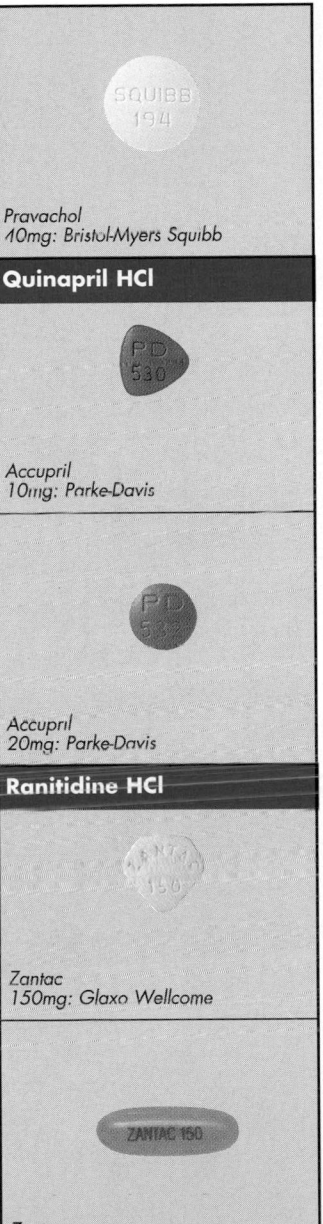

K-Dur
1500mg: Schering

Klor-Con
600mg: Upsher-Smith

Klor-Con
750mg: Upsher-Smith

Pravastatin

Pravachol
10mg: Bristol-Myers Squibb

Pravachol
20mg: Bristol-Myers Squibb

Pravachol
10mg: Bristol-Myers Squibb

Quinapril HCl

Accupril
10mg: Parke-Davis

Accupril
20mg: Parke-Davis

Ranitidine HCl

Zantac
150mg: Glaxo Wellcome

Zantac
150mg: Glaxo Wellcome

Zantac 150 Efferdose
150mg: Glaxo Wellcome

Zantac
300mg: Glaxo Wellcome

Zantac
300mg: Glaxo Wellcome

Sertraline HCl

Zoloft
50mg: Roerig

Zoloft
100mg: Roerig

Simvastatin

Zocor
5mg: Merck

Zocor
10mg: Merck

Zocor
20mg: Merck

Zocor
40mg: Merck

Sulfamethoxazole/ Trimethoprim

Septra
400/80mg: Glaxo Wellcome

Septra
800/160mg: Glaxo Wellcome

Cotrim
800/160mg: Lemmon

Generic
800/160mg: Mutual

Bactrim
400/80mg: Roche

Bactrim DS
800/160mg: Roche

Terazosin HCl

Hytrin
1mg: Abbott

Hytrin
2mg: Abbott

Hytrin
5mg: Abbott

Hytrin
10mg: Abbott

Tramadol HCl

Ultram
50mg: McNeil

Warfarin Sodium

Coumadin
1mg: DuPont

Coumadin
2mg: DuPont

Coumadin
2.5mg: DuPont

Coumadin
3mg: DuPont

Coumadin
4mg: DuPont

Coumadin
5mg: DuPont

Coumadin
7.5mg: DuPont

Coumadin
10mg: DuPont

Zolpidem

Ambien
5mg: Searle

Ambien
10mg: Searle

• Visual changes: blurring, halos, corneal and retinal damage
• Edema in feet, ankles, legs
• Prior drug history; there are many drug interactions

Administer:
• To patient crushed or whole; chewable tablets may be chewed
• With food or milk to decrease gastric symptoms; give 30 min before or 2 hr after antacids
• With full glass of water

Evaluate:
• Therapeutic response: decreased pain, fever

Teach patient/family:
• To report any symptoms of hepatotoxicity, renal toxicity, visual changes, ototoxicity, allergic reactions, bleeding (long-term therapy)
• Not to exceed recommended dosage; acute poisoning may result
• To read label on other OTC drugs; many contain aspirin
• That therapeutic response takes 2 wk (arthritis)
• To avoid alcohol ingestion; GI bleeding may occur
• That if anticoagulants are given with this drug, both should be discontinued 2 wk before surgery

Treatment of overdose: Lavage, activated charcoal, monitor electrolytes, VS

---

magnesium salts (OTC)

Concentrated Phillips Milk of Magnesia, Milk of Magnesia, Phillips Milk of Magnesia

Func. class.: Laxative, saline; antacid

Action: Increases osmotic pressure, draws fluid into colon, neutralizes HCl

Uses: Constipation, bowel preparation before surgery or exam

Dosage and routes:
Laxative
• *Adult:* PO 30-60 ml hs (Milk of Magnesia), 300 mg
• *Adult and child >6 yr:* PO 15 g in 8 oz H_2O (magnesium sulfate); PO 10-20 ml (Concentrated Milk of Magnesia); PO 5-10 oz hs (magnesium citrate)
• *Child 2-6 yr:* 5-15 ml (Milk of Magnesia)

Available forms: Liquid 395 mg/5 ml; tabs chew 300, 600 mg; conc. liquid 1.2 g/5 ml

Side effects/adverse reactions:
CNS: Muscle weakness, flushing, sweating, confusion, sedation, depressed reflexes, *flaccidity, paralysis,* hypothermia
GI: Nausea, vomiting, anorexia, cramps
CV: Hypotension, heart block, *circulatory collapse*
META: Electrolyte, fluid imbalances

Contraindications: Hypersensitivity, renal diseases, abdominal pain, nausea/vomiting, obstruction, acute surgical abdomen, rectal bleeding

Precautions: Pregnancy (B)

Pharmacokinetics:
PO: Peak 1-2 hr; excreted in feces

Interactions:
• Increased CNS depression: CNS depressants, barbiturates, narcotics, anesthetics

NURSING CONSIDERATIONS
Assess:
• I&O ratio; check for decrease in urinary output
• Cause of constipation; lack of fluids, bulk, exercise
• Cramping, rectal bleeding, nausea, vomiting; drug should be discontinued

◆ Mg toxicity: thirst, confusion, decrease in reflexes

Administer:
• With 8 oz H_2O

M

Evaluate:
• Therapeutic response: decreased constipation
Teach patient/family:
• Not to use laxatives for long-term therapy; bowel tone will be lost
• That chilling helps the taste of magnesium citrate
• To shake suspension well
• To not give at hs as a laxative; may interfere with sleep
• To give citrus fruit after administering to counteract unpleasant taste

---

magnesium sulfate (℞)
Func. class.: Anticonvulsant
Chem. class.: Magnesium product

Action: Decreases acetylcholine in motor nerve terminals, which is responsible for anticonvulsant properties; osmotically retains fluid, which increases amount of water in feces when used as laxative; reduces SA node impulse formation, prolongs conduction time in myocardium

Uses: Hypomagnesemic seizures, control of seizures in pregnancy-induced hypertension, seizures in acute nephritis

Dosage and routes:
Hypomagnesemic seizures
• *Adult:* **IV** 1-2 g over 15 min, then 1 g **IM** q4-6h, depending on response
Nephritis
• *Child:* **IM** 20-40 mg/kg in 20% sol, repeat as needed
Preeclampsia/eclampsia
• *Adult:* **IV** 4 g/250 ml D$_5$W and 4 g **IM,** then 4 g (50% sol) **IM** q4h prn; or 4 g (10-20% sol) **IV** loading dose, then 1-4 g (5% sol) **IV** inf qh, not to exceed 3 ml/min

Available forms: Inj 10%, 12.5%, 25%, 50%; granules
Side effects/adverse reactions:
CNS: Sweating, depressed deep tendon reflexes, flushing, drowsiness, flaccid paralysis, hypothermia, weakness, sedation
RESP: Paralysis
*CV: Hypotension, **circulatory collapse, heart block,*** decreased cardiac function
Contraindications: Hypersensitivity, 2 hr preceding delivery in PIH
Precautions: Pregnancy (A)
Pharmacokinetics:
IV: Onset 1-5 min, duration 30 min
IM: Onset 1 hr, duration 3-4 hr
Excreted by kidneys

Interactions:
• Increased CNS depression: barbiturates, general anesthetics, narcotics, antipsychotics
• Increased effects of neuromuscular blockers

NURSING CONSIDERATIONS
Assess:
• VS q15min after IV dose; do not exceed 150 mg/min
• Cardiac function: monitoring, Mg levels
• Blood levels: 2.5-7.5 mEq/L (therapeutic)
• Timing of contractions; determine intensity; monitor fetal heart rate, reactivity; may decrease with this drug during labor
• I&O: should remain at 30 ml/hr or more; if less than this, notify prescriber
• Urine output before each dose; should be >100 ml/4 hr
• Mental status: mood, sensorium, affect, memory (long, short)
• Respiratory dysfunction: respiratory depression, character, rate, rhythm; hold drug if respirations are <16/min

---

• Hypermagnesemia: depressed patellar reflex, flushing, polydipsia, confusion, weakness, flaccid paralysis, hypothermia, dyspnea begin to appear at blood levels of 4 mEq/L

• Respiratory rate, rhythm of newborn if drug was given 24 hr before delivery or less; check reflexes of newborn whose mother received this drug before delivery

◆ Reflexes: knee jerk, patellar; decrease signals Mg^{++} toxicity; mild depression will occur in therapeutic range

Administer:

IV

• Only when calcium gluconate available for magnesium toxicity

• IV undiluted 1.5 ml of 10% sol over 1 min; may dilute to 20% sol, infuse over 3 hr

• IV at less than 150 mg/min; circulatory collapse may occur

Additive compatibilities: Calcium gluconate, cephalothin, chloramphenicol, cisplatin, heparin, hydrocortisone, isoproterenol, meropenem, methyldopa, norepinephrine, penicillin G potassium, potassium phosphate, verapamil

Y-site compatibilities: Acyclovir, aldesleukin, amifostine, amikacin, ampicillin, aztreonam, cefamandole, cefazolin, cefmetazole, cefoperazone, cefotaxime, cefoxitin, cephalothin, cephapirin, chloramphenicol, clindamycin, dobutamine, doxycycline, enalaprilat, erythromycin, esmolol, famotidine, fludarabine, gallium, gentamicin, granisetron, heparin, hydrocortisone, hydromorphone, idarubicin, insulin, kanamycin, labetalol, meperidine, metronidazole, minocycline, morphine, moxalactam, nafcillin, ondansetron, oxacillin, paclitaxel, penicillin G potassium, piperacillin, piperacillin/tazobactam, potassium chloride, propofol, sargramostim, thiotepa, ticarcillin, tobramycin, trimethoprim/sulfamethoxazole, vancomycin, vit B complex/C

Perform/provide:

• Seizure precautions: dark room with decreased stimuli, padded side rails

Evaluate:

• Therapeutic response; absence of seizures

Teach patient/family:

• The symptoms of hypermagnesemia

Treatment of overdose: Stop drug; administer calcium gluconate; monitor reflexes, Mg levels; ECG monitoring if Ca is administered

---

mannitol (℞)

(man'i-tole)

mannitol, Osmitrol, Resectial

Func. class.: Osmotic diuretic

Chem. class.: Hexahydric alcohol

Action: Acts by increasing osmolarity of glomerular filtrate, which raises osmotic pressure of fluid in renal tubules; decrease in reabsorption of water, electrolytes; increase in urinary output, sodium, chloride excretion

Uses: Edema, promote systemic diuresis in cerebral edema, decrease intraocular pressure, improve renal function in acute renal failure, chemical poisoning

Dosage and routes:

Oliguria, prevention

• *Adult:* IV 50-100 g 5%-25% sol

Oliguria, treatment

• *Adult:* IV 300-400 mg/kg 20%-25% sol up to 100 g 15%-20% sol

• *Child:* IV 0.25-2 g/kg as 15%-20% sol run over 2-6 hr

Intraocular pressure/intracranial pressure
• *Adult:* **IV** 1½-2 g/kg 15%-25% sol over ½-1 hr
• *Child:* **IV** 1-2 g/kg (30-60 g/m²) as 15%-20% sol run over ½-1 hr
Renal failure
• *Adult:* **IV** 50-200 g/24 hr, adjusted to maintain output of 30-50 mg/hr
Diuresis in drug intoxication
• *Adult and child >12 yr:* 5%-10% sol continuously up to 200 g **IV**, while maintaining 100-500 ml urine output/hr
Available forms: Inj 5%, 10%, 15%, 20%
Side effects/adverse reactions:
GU: Marked diuresis, urinary retention, thirst
CNS: Dizziness, headache, *convulsions, rebound increased ICP,* confusion
GI: Nausea, vomiting, dry mouth, diarrhea
CV: Edema, thrombophlebitis, hypotension, hypertension, tachycardia, angina-like chest pains, fever, chills
RESP: Pulmonary congestion
ELECT: Fluid, electrolyte imbalances, *acidosis,* electrolyte loss, dehydration
EENT: Loss of hearing, blurred vision, nasal congestion, decreased intraocular pressure
Contraindications: Active intracranial bleeding, hypersensitivity, anuria, severe pulmonary congestion, edema, severe dehydration, progressive heart, renal failure
Precautions: Dehydration, pregnancy (C), severe renal disease, CHF, lactation
Pharmacokinetics:
IV: Onset 30-60 min for diuresis, ½-1 hr for intraocular pressure, 25 min for cerebrospinal fluid; duration 4-6 hr for intraocular pressure,

3-8 hr for cerebrospinal fluid; excreted in urine, half-life 100 min
Interactions:
• Decreased effect: lithium
• Increased effects of EDTA
• Drug/food: potassium foods: increased hyperkalemia
Lab test interferences:
Interference: Inorganic phosphorus, ethylene glycol

NURSING CONSIDERATIONS
Assess:
• Weight, I&O qd to determine fluid loss; effect of drug may be decreased if used qd; output qh prn
• Rate, depth, rhythm of respiration, effect of exertion
• B/P lying, standing; postural hypotension may occur
• Electrolytes: K, Na, Cl; include BUN, CBC, serum creatinine, blood pH, ABGs
• Signs of metabolic acidosis: drowsiness, restlessness
• Signs of hypokalemia: postural hypotension, malaise, fatigue, tachycardia, leg cramps, weakness
• Rashes, temp qd
• Confusion, especially in elderly; take safety precautions if needed
• Hydration including skin turgor, thirst, dry mucous membranes
Administer:
• In 15%-25% sol with filter; give over ½-1½ hr; rapid infusion may worsen CHF; warm in hot water and shake to dissolve crystals
• Test dose in severe oliguria, 0.2 g/kg over 3-5 min; if no urine increase, give second test dose; if no response, reassess patient
Additive compatibilities: Amikacin, bretylium, cefamandole, cefoxitin, cimetidine, cisplatin, dopamine, furosemide, gentamicin, metoclopramide, netilmicin, nizatidine, ofloxacin, ondansetron, sodium bicarbonate, tobramycin, verapamil

---

➡ = Nursing alert   ✍ = Herb-drug interaction   ◒ = Do not crush

Y-site compatibilities: Allopurinol, amifostine, aztreonam, cladribine, fludarabine, fluorouracil, gallium, idarubicin, melphalan, ondansetron, paclitaxel, piperacillin, propofol, sargramostim, teniposide, thiotepa, vinorelbine

Evaluate:
• Therapeutic response: improvement in edema of feet, legs, sacral area daily if medication is being used in CHF; decreased intraocular pressure, prevention of hypokalemia, increased excretion of toxic substances

Teach patient/family:
• To rise slowly from lying or sitting position
• The reason for and method of treatment

Treatment of overdose: Discontinue infusion; correct fluid, electrolyte imbalances; hemodialysis; monitor hydration, CV, renal function

---

maprotiline (Ŗ)

(n ia-proe′ti leen)
Ludiomil, maprotiline
Func. class.: Antidepressant
Chem. class.: Tetracyclic

Action: Blocks reuptake of norepinephrine, serotonin into nerve endings, increasing action of norepinephrine, serotonin in nerve cells

Uses: Depression, dysthymic disorder, bipolar disorder—depressed, agitated depression

Dosage and routes:
• *Adult:* **PO** 75 mg/day in moderate depression, may increase to 150 mg/day; not to exceed 225 mg in hospitalized patients; severely depressed hospitalized patients may be given 300 mg/day
• *Elderly:* initiate 25 mg q hs, increase by 25 mg q4-7 days as needed

Available forms: Tabs 25, 50, 75 mg

Side effects/adverse reactions:
HEMA: ***Agranulocytosis, thrombocytopenia, eosinophilia, leukopenia***
CNS: Dizziness, drowsiness, confusion, headache, anxiety, tremors, stimulation, weakness, insomnia, nightmares, EPS (elderly), increased psychiatric symptoms, ***seizures***
GI: Diarrhea, dry mouth, nausea, vomiting, ***paralytic ileus,*** increased appetite, cramps, epigastric distress, jaundice, ***hepatitis,*** stomatitis
GU: Retention, **acute renal failure**
INTEG: Rash, urticaria, sweating, pruritus, photosensitivity
CV: Orthostatic hypotension, ECG changes, tachycardia, ***hypertension,*** palpitations
EENT: Blurred vision, tinnitus, mydriasis

Contraindications: Hypersensitivity to tricyclic antidepressants, recovery phase of MI, convulsive disorders, prostatic hypertrophy

Precautions: Suicidal patients, severe depression, increased intraocular pressure, narrow-angle glaucoma, urinary retention, cardiac disease, hepatic disease, hypothyroidism, hyperthyroidism, elective surgery, elderly, pregnancy (B)

Pharmacokinetics:
PO: Onset 15-30 min, peak 12 hr, duration up to 3 wk, steady state 6-10 days; metabolized by liver; excreted in urine, feces; crosses placenta; half-life 51 hr

Interactions:
• Decreased effects of guanethidine, clonidine, indirect-acting sympathomimetics (ephedrine)
• Increased effects of direct-acting sympathomimetics (epinephrine), alcohol, barbiturates, benzodiazepines, CNS depressants
• Hyperpyretic crisis, convulsions,

M

---

hypertensive episode: MAOI (par-gyline [Eutonyl])

💉 Increased anticholinergic effects: belladonna leaf/root, henbane leaf

💉 Increased antidepressant effect: scopolia root

Lab test interferences:

Increase: Serum bilirubin, blood glucose, alk phosphatase

False increase: Urinary catecholamines

Decrease: VMA, 5-HIAA

NURSING CONSIDERATIONS
Assess:

• B/P (lying, standing), pulse q4h; if systolic B/P drops 20 mm Hg, hold drug, notify prescriber; take vital signs q4h in patients with cardiovascular disease

• Blood studies: CBC, leukocytes, differential, cardiac enzymes if patient is receiving long-term therapy

• Hepatic studies: AST (SGOT), ALT (SGPT), bilirubin, creatinine

• Weight qwk; appetite may increase with drug

• ECG for flattening of T wave, bundle branch block, AV block, dysrhythmias in cardiac patients

• EPS primarily in elderly: rigidity, dystonia, akathisia

• Mental status: mood, sensorium, affect, suicidal tendencies, increase in psychiatric symptoms: depression, panic

• Urinary retention, constipation; constipation is more likely to occur in children, elderly

⬥ Withdrawal symptoms: headache, nausea, vomiting, muscle pain, weakness; do not usually occur unless drug was discontinued abruptly

• Alcohol consumption; if alcohol is consumed, hold dose until morning

Administer:

• Increased fluids, bulk in diet for constipation, especially elderly

• With food, milk for GI symptoms

• Dosage hs if oversedation occurs during day; may take entire dose hs; elderly may not tolerate once/day dosing

• Gum, hard candy, or frequent sips of water for dry mouth

• Concentrate with fruit juice, water, or milk to disguise taste

Perform/provide:

• Storage in tight container at room temp; do not freeze

• Assistance with ambulation during beginning therapy, since drowsiness/dizziness occurs

• Safety measures, including side rails, primarily in elderly

• Checking to see if PO medication swallowed

Evaluate:

• Therapeutic response: decreased depression

Teach patient/family:

• That therapeutic effects may take 2-3 wk

• The use of caution in driving, other activities requiring alertness, because of drowsiness, dizziness, blurred vision

• To avoid alcohol ingestion, other CNS depressants

• Not to discontinue medication quickly after long-term use; may cause nausea, headache, malaise

• To wear sunscreen or large hat, since photosensitivity occurs

Treatment of overdose: ECG monitoring, induce emesis; lavage, activated charcoal; administer anticonvulsant

---

measles, mumps, and rubella vaccine (℞)

M-M-R-II

Func. class.: Vaccine

Action: Produces antibodies to measles, mumps, rubella

⬥ = Nursing alert   *💉* = Herb-drug interaction   🚫 = Do not crush

Uses: Prevention of measles, mumps, rubella

Dosage and routes:
• *Child >15 mo and adult:* **SC** 0.5 ml

Available forms: Inj SC measles 1000 TCID$_{50}$, mumps 20,000 TCID$_{50}$, rubella 1000 TCID$_{50}$ (0.5 ml)

Side effects/adverse reactions:

CNS: Fever, ***subacute sclerosing panencephalitis and blindness associated with optic neuritis,*** paresthesias

INTEG: Urticaria, erythema, burning, stinging at injection site

SYST: Lymphadenitis, ***anaphylaxis,*** malaise, sore throat, headache

MS: Osteomyelitis, arthralgia, arthritis

Contraindications: Hypersensitivity, blood dyscrasias, anemia, active infection, immunosuppression; egg, chicken allergy; pregnancy, febrile illness, neomycin allergy, neoplasms

Precautions: Elderly, lactation, children with TB

Interactions:
• Decreased response to TB skin test
• Other live virus vaccines

NURSING CONSIDERATIONS

Assess:
• For skin reactions. rash, induration, erythema
• For anaphylaxis. inability to breathe, bronchospasm

Administer:
• Only with epinephrine 1:1000 on unit to treat laryngospasm
• Only SC

Perform/provide:
• Storage at 39° F (4° C); protect from heat, light; do not give within 1 mo of other live virus vaccines
• Written record of immunization

Evaluate:
• For history of allergies, skin disorders (eczema, psoriasis, dermatitis), reactions to vaccinations

Teach patient/family:
• That fever may occur 5-12 days after vaccine given
• That joint pains, tingling in extremities may occur 5-12 days after vaccine given
• That pain and inflammation may occur
• To take acetaminophen for fever

---

mebendazole (℞)

(me-ben′da-zole)

Nemasole*, Vermox*

Func. class.: Anthelmintic

Chem. class.: Carbamate

Action: Inhibits glucose uptake, degeneration of cytoplasmic microtubules in the cell; interferes with absorption, secretory function

Uses: Pinworms, roundworms, hookworms, whipworms, threadworms, pork tapeworms, dwarf tapeworms, beef tapeworms, hydatid cyst

Dosage and routes:
• *Adult and child >2 yr:* **PO** 100 mg as a single dose or bid × 3 days, depending on type of infection; course may be repeated in 3 wk if needed

Available forms: Tabs, chewable 100 mg

Side effects/adverse reactions:

CNS: Dizziness, fever, headache

GI: Transient diarrhea, abdominal pain, nausea, vomiting

Contraindications: Hypersensitivity

Precautions: Child <2 yr, lactation, pregnancy (1st trimester) (C)

Pharmacokinetics:

PO: Peak ½-7 hr; excreted in feces primarily (metabolites), small amount in urine (unchanged); highly bound to plasma proteins

Interactions:
• Decreased effect of mebendazole: carbamazepine, hydantoins

NURSING CONSIDERATIONS
Assess:
• Stools during entire treatment; specimens must be sent to lab while still warm, also 1-3 wk after treatment is completed
• For allergic reaction: rash (rare)
• For diarrhea during expulsion of worms; avoid self-contamination with patient's feces
• For infection in other family members, since infection from person to person is common
• Blood studies: AST (SGOT), ALT (SGPT), alk phosphatase, BUN, CBC during treatment

Administer:
• May be crushed, chewed, swallowed whole
• PO after meals to avoid GI symptoms, since absorption is not altered by food
• Second course after 3 wk if needed; usually recommended

Perform/provide:
• Storage in tight container

Evaluate:
• Therapeutic response: expulsion of worms and 3 negative stool cultures after completion of treatment

Teach patient/family:
• Proper hygiene after BM, including hand-washing technique; tell patient to avoid putting fingers in mouth; clean fingernails
• That infected person should sleep alone; do not shake bed linen, change bed linen qd, wash in hot water, change and wash undergarments daily
• To clean toilet qd with disinfectant (green soap solution)
• The need for compliance with dosage schedule, duration of treatment
• To wear shoes, wash all fruits and vegetables well before eating; use commercial fruit/vegetable cleaner

---

mecamylamine (℞)
(mek-a-mill′a-meen)
Inversine
Func. class.: Antihypertensive
Chem. class.: Ganglionic blocker

Action: Occupies receptor site, prevents acetylcholine from attaching to postsynaptic nerve ending in sympathetic and parasympathetic ganglia

Uses: Moderate to severe hypertension, malignant hypertension

Dosage and routes:
• *Adult:* PO 2.5 mg bid, may increase in increments of 2.5 mg × 2 days until desired response; maintenance 25 mg/day in 3 divided doses

Available forms: Tabs 2.5 mg

Side effects/adverse reactions:
CV: Postural hypotension, irregular heart rate, ***CHF***
CNS: *Drowsiness, sedation,* headache, tremors, weakness, syncope, paresthesia, dizziness, ***convulsions***
EENT: *Blurred vision,* nasal congestion, dry mouth, dilated pupils
GU: Impotence, urinary retention, decreased libido
GI: Anorexia, glossitis, nausea, vomiting, constipation, ***paralytic ileus***

Contraindications: Hypersensitivity, MI, coronary insufficiency, renal disease, glaucoma, organic pyloric stenosis, uremia, uncooperative patients, mild/labile hypertension

Precautions: CVA, prostatic hypertrophy, bladder neck obstruction, urethral stricture, renal dysfunction (elevated BUN), cerebral dysfunction, pregnancy (C), lactation

Pharmacokinetics:
PO: Onset ½-2 hr, duration 6-12 hr; excreted in urine, feces, breast milk; crosses placenta

---

Interactions:
• Increased effects: thiazide diuretics, antihypertensives, CNS depressants (alcohol, anesthetics, MAOIs), bethanechol

NURSING CONSIDERATIONS
Assess:
• B/P lying and standing, other VS throughout treatment
• Weight qd, I&O
• Edema in feet, legs qd
• Skin turgor, dryness of mucous membranes for hydration status
• Tolerance to drug with prolonged use
• Constipation: number of stools, consistency; give stool softener as ordered or increase bulk in diet

Administer:
🚫 Whole; do not break, crush, or chew
• After meals for better absorption; give larger dose at noon and evening, smaller dose in AM
• Gum, frequent rinsing of mouth, hard candy for dry mouth

Evaluate:
• Therapeutic response: decreased B/P

Teach patient/family:
• To notify prescriber of tremor, seizure, signs of paralytic ileus
• To avoid OTC preparations unless directed by prescriber
• To rise slowly from sitting or lying position; orthostatic hypotension may occur
• That impotence may occur but is reversible after discontinuing drug

Treatment of overdose: Administer gastric lavage, discontinue drug, administer small doses of pressor amines for hypotension

---

mechlorethamine (℞)

(me-klor-eth′a-meen)
Mustargen, Nitrogen mustard
Func. class.: Antineoplastic alkylating agent
Chem. class.: Nitrogen mustard

Action: Responsible for cross-linking DNA strands leading to cell death; rapidly degraded, a vesicant; activity is not cell cycle phase-specific

Uses: Hodgkin's disease, leukemias, lymphomas, lymphosarcoma; ovarian, breast, lung carcinoma; neoplastic effusions

Dosage and routes:
• *Adult:* IV 0.4 mg/kg or 10 mg/m^2 as 1 dose or 2-4 divided doses over 2-4 days; second course after 3 wk depending on blood cell count

Neoplastic effusions
• *Adult:* **INTRACAVITARY** 10-20 mg, may be 200-400 μg/kg

Available forms: Inj 10 mg; powder for inj

Side effects/adverse reactions:
EENT: Tinnitus, hearing loss
HEMA: **Thrombocytopenia, leukopenia, agranulocytosis,** anemia
GI: *Nausea, vomiting, diarrhea, stomatitis, weight loss,* colitis, **hepatotoxicity**
CNS: *Headache, dizziness, drowsiness, paresthesia,* peripheral neuropathy, **coma**
INTEG: *Alopecia,* pruritus, herpes zoster, extravasation

Contraindications: Lactation, pregnancy (1st trimester) (D), myelosuppression, acute herpes zoster

Precautions: Radiation therapy, chronic lymphocytic leukopenia

Pharmacokinetics: Metabolized in liver, excreted in urine

Interactions:
• Increased toxicity: antineoplastics, radiation
• Blood dyscrasias: amphotericin B

NURSING CONSIDERATIONS
Assess:
• CBC, differential, platelet count qwk; withhold drug if WBC is <4000 or platelet count is <75,000; notify prescriber
• Renal function studies: BUN, serum uric acid, urine CrCl before, during therapy
• I&O ratio; report fall in urine output of 30 ml/hr
• Monitor temp q4h (may indicate beginning infection); no rectal temps
• Liver function tests before, during therapy (bilirubin, AST [SGOT], ALT [SGPT], LDH) as needed or monthly
• Bleeding: hematuria, guaiac, bruising or petechiae, mucosa or orifices q8h
• Food preferences; list likes, dislikes
• Yellow skin and sclera, dark urine, clay-colored stools, itchy skin, abdominal pain, fever, diarrhea
• Effects of alopecia on body image; discuss feelings about body changes
• Inflammation of mucosa, breaks in skin
• Buccal cavity q8h for dryness, sores, ulceration, white patches, oral pain, bleeding, dysphagia
• Local irritation, pain, burning, discoloration at injection site
⬥ Symptoms indicating severe allergic reaction: rash, pruritus, urticaria, purpuric skin lesions, itching, flushing

Administer:
• After using guidelines for preparation of cytotoxic drugs
• Antiemetic 30-60 min before giving drug and prn
• Antibiotics for prophylaxis of infection
• IV after diluting 10 mg/10 ml sterile H_2O or NaCl; leave needle in vial, shake, withdraw dose, give through Y-tube or 3-way stopcock or directly over 3-5 min
• Watch for infiltration; infiltrate area with isotonic sodium thiosulfate or 1% lidocaine; apply ice for 6-12 hr
• Topical or systemic analgesics for pain
• Local or systemic drugs for infection

Y-site compatibilities: Amifostine, aztreonam, filgrastim, fludarabine, granisetron, melphalan, ondansetron, sargramostim, teniposide, vinorelbine

Perform/provide:
• Storage at room temp in dry form
• Strict medical asepsis, protective isolation if WBC levels are low
• Special skin care
• Increase fluid intake to 2-3 L/day to prevent urate deposits, calculi formation
• Diet low in purines: organ meats (kidney, liver), dried beans, peas to maintain alkaline urine
• Preparation under hood using gloves and mask
• Rinsing of mouth tid-qid with water, club soda; brushing of teeth bid-tid with soft brush or cotton-tipped applicators for stomatitis; use unwaxed dental floss
• Warm compresses at injection site for inflammation

Evaluate:
• Therapeutic response: decreased tumor size, spread of malignancy

Teach patient/family:
• The rationale for and techniques of protective isolation
• That sterility, amenorrhea can occur; reversible after discontinuing treatment
• That hair may be lost during treat-

ment; a wig or hairpiece may make patient feel better; new hair may be different in color, texture

• To avoid foods with citric acid, hot or rough texture

• To report any bleeding, white spots, or ulcerations in mouth to prescriber; tell patient to examine mouth qd

• To report signs of infection: fever, sore throat, flu symptoms

• To report signs of anemia: fatigue, headache, faintness, shortness of breath, irritability

• To avoid use of razors, commercial mouthwash

• To avoid use of aspirin products, ibuprofen

---

meclizine (OTC, ℞)

(mek'li-zeen)
Antivert, Antivert/25, Antivert/25 Chewable, Antivert-50, Antrizine, Bonamine*, Bonine, Dizmiss, Dramamine II, meclizine HCl, Meni-D, Ru-Vert-M

Func. class.: Antiemetic, antihistamine, anticholinergic

Chem. class.: H₁-receptor antagonist, piperazine derivative

Action: Acts centrally by blocking chemoreceptor trigger zone, which in turn acts on vomiting center

Uses: Vertigo, motion sickness

Dosage and routes:
• *Adult:* PO 25-100 mg qd in divided doses or 1 hr before traveling

Available forms: Tabs 12.5, 25, 50 mg; chew tabs 25 mg; tabs film coated 25 mg

Side effects/adverse reactions:
CNS: Drowsiness, fatigue, restlessness, headache, insomnia
CV: Hypotension
GU: Retention
GI: Nausea, anorexia
EENT: Dry mouth, blurred vision

Contraindications: Hypersensitivity to cyclizines, shock, lactation

Precautions: Children, narrow-angle glaucoma, glaucoma, urinary retention, lactation, prostatic hypertrophy, elderly, pregnancy (B), CV disease, hypertension, seizure disease

Pharmacokinetics:
PO: Duration 8-24 hr, half-life 6 hr

Interactions:
• Increased effect of alcohol, tranquilizers, narcotics

Increased anticholinergic effect: henbane leaf

Lab test interferences:
False negative: Allergy skin testing

NURSING CONSIDERATIONS

Assess:
• VS, B/P

➡ Signs of toxicity of other drugs or masking of symptoms of disease: brain tumor, intestinal obstruction

• Observe for drowsiness, dizziness, LOC

Administer:
PO
• Tablets may be swallowed whole, chewed, or allowed to dissolve
• Lowest possible dose in elderly, anticholinergic effects

Evaluate:
• Therapeutic response: absence of dizziness, vomiting

Teach patient/family:
• That a false-negative result may occur with skin testing for allergies; these procedures should not be scheduled for 4 days after discontinuing use
• To avoid hazardous activities, activities requiring alertness; dizziness may occur; instruct patient to request assistance with ambulation
• To avoid alcohol, other depressants

---

meclofenamate (℞)

(me-kloe-fen'ah-mate)
meclofenamate,   meclofen,
Meclomen
Func. class.: Nonsteroidal anti-inflammatory
Chem. class.: Anthranilic acid derivative

Action: Inhibits prostaglandin synthesis by decreasing an enzyme needed for biosynthesis; analgesic, antiinflammatory, antipyretic

Uses: Mild to moderate pain, osteoarthritis, rheumatoid arthritis

Dosage and routes:
• *Adult:* **PO** 200-400 mg/day in divided doses tid-qid

Available forms: Caps 50, 100 mg

Side effects/adverse reactions:

GI: Nausea, anorexia, vomiting, diarrhea, jaundice, ***cholestatic hepatitis,*** constipation, flatulence, cramps, dry mouth, peptic ulcer, ***ulceration, perforation***

CNS: Dizziness, drowsiness, fatigue, tremors, confusion, insomnia, anxiety, depression

CV: Tachycardia, hypertension, peripheral edema, palpitations, dysrhythmias

INTEG: Purpura, rash, pruritus, sweating

*GU: **Nephrotoxicity: dysuria, hematuria, oliguria, azotemia***

*HEMA: **Blood dyscrasias***

EENT: Tinnitus, hearing loss, blurred vision

Contraindications: Hypersensitivity, asthma, severe renal disease, severe hepatic disease, ulcer disease

Precautions: Pregnancy (B), lactation, children, bleeding disorders, GI disorders, cardiac disorders, hypersensitivity to other antiinflammatory agents

Pharmacokinetics:
PO: Peak 2 hr, half-life 3-3 ½ hr; metabolized in liver, excreted in urine (metabolites), excreted in breast milk

Interactions:
• Increased action of coumadin, phenytoin, sulfonamides

NURSING CONSIDERATIONS
Assess:
• Pain: frequency, intensity, characteristics, relief after med
• Asthma, aspirin hypersensitivity, or nasal polyps are at increased risk for hypersensitive reactions
• Renal, liver, blood studies: BUN, creatinine, AST (SGOT), ALT (SGPT), Hgb, Hct before treatment, periodically thereafter
• Audiometric and ophthalmic exam before, during, after treatment
• For history of peptic ulcer disease
• For eye, ear problems: blurred vision, tinnitus (may indicate toxicity)

Administer:
• With food to decrease GI symptoms; best to take on empty stomach to facilitate absorption

Perform/provide:
• Storage at room temp

Evaluate:
• Therapeutic response: decreased pain, stiffness, swelling in joints, ability to move more easily

Teach patient/family:
• To report increased GI symptoms; dose may have to be reduced
• To report blurred vision, ringing, roaring in ears (may indicate toxicity)
• To avoid driving, other hazardous activities for dizziness, drowsiness
• To report change in urine pattern, weight increase, edema, pain increase in joints, fever, blood in urine (indicates nephrotoxicity)
• That therapeutic effects may take up to 1 mo

⬥ = Nursing alert   ▮▮ = Herb-drug interaction   🚫 = Do not crush

- To take with full glass of water
- To avoid other NSAIDs, alcohol, steroids
- 🚫 Not to break, crush, or chew caps

---

medroxyprogesterone (℞)

(me-drox'ee-proe-jess'te-rone)
Amen, Curretab, Cycrin, Depo-Provera, medroxyprogesterone acetate, Provera
Func. class.: Progestogen
Chem. class.: Progesterone derivative

Action: Inhibits secretion of pituitary gonadotropins, which prevents follicular maturation and ovulation; stimulates growth of mammary tissue; antineoplastic action against endometrial cancer

Uses: Uterine bleeding (abnormal), secondary amenorrhea, endometrial cancer, renal cancer, contraceptive, prevent endometrial changes associated with estrogen replacement therapy (ERT)

Investigational uses: Pickwickian syndrome, sleep apnea, hypersomnolence

Dosage and routes:
Secondary amenorrhea
- *Adult:* **PO** 5-10 mg qd × 5-10 days
Endometrial/renal cancer
- *Adult:* **IM** 400-1000 mg/wk
Uterine bleeding
- *Adult:* **PO** 5-10 mg qd × 5-10 days starting on 16th day of menstrual cycle
Contraceptive
- *Adult:* **INJ** q3mo
With ERT
- *Adult:* **PO** monophasic 2.5 mg qd; Biphasic 5 mg days 15-28 of cycle
Available forms: Tabs 2.5, 5, 10 mg; inj susp 100, 150, 400 mg/ml

Side effects/adverse reactions:
CNS: Dizziness, headache, migraines, depression, fatigue
CV: Hypotension, thrombophlebitis, edema, ***thromboembolism, stroke, pulmonary embolism, MI***
GI: Nausea, vomiting, anorexia, cramps, increased weight, ***cholestatic jaundice***
EENT: Diplopia
GU: Amenorrhea, cervical erosion, breakthrough bleeding, dysmenorrhea, vaginal candidiasis, breast changes, *gynecomastia, testicular atrophy, impotence,* endometriosis, ***spontaneous abortion***
INTEG: Rash, urticaria, acne, hirsutism, alopecia, oily skin, seborrhea, purpura, melasma, photosensitivity
META: Hyperglycemia

Contraindications: Breast cancer, hypersensitivity, thromboembolic disorders, reproductive cancer, genital bleeding (abnormal, undiagnosed), pregnancy (D)

Precautions: Lactation, hypertension, asthma, blood dyscrasias, gallbladder disease, CHF, diabetes mellitus, bone disease, depression, migraine headache, convulsive disorders, hepatic disease, renal disease, family history of cancer of breast or reproductive tract

Pharmacokinetics:
PO: Duration 24 hr, excreted in urine and feces, metabolized in liver

Lab test interferences:
Increase: Alk phosphatase, N (urine), pregnanediol, amino acids
Decrease: GTT, HDL

NURSING CONSIDERATIONS
Assess:
- Weight qd; notify prescriber of weekly weight gain >5 lb
- B/P at beginning of treatment and periodically
- I&O ratio; be alert for decreasing urinary output, increasing edema

M

- Liver function studies: ALT (SGPT), AST (SGOT), bilirubin, periodically during long-term therapy
- Edema, hypertension, cardiac symptoms, jaundice
- Mental status: affect, mood, behavioral changes, depression
- Hypercalcemia

Administer:
- Titrated dose; use lowest effective dose
- Oil solution deep in large muscle mass (IM), rotate sites
- After warming to dissolve crystals
- With food or milk to decrease GI symptoms (PO)

Perform/provide:
- Storage in dark area

Evaluate:
- Therapeutic response: decreased abnormal uterine bleeding, absence of amenorrhea

Teach patient/family:
- To avoid sunlight or use sunscreen; photosensitivity can occur
- About cushingoid symptoms
- To report breast lumps, vaginal bleeding, edema, jaundice, dark urine, clay-colored stools, dyspnea, headache, blurred vision, abdominal pain, numbness or stiffness in legs, chest pain; male to report impotence or gynecomastia
- To report suspected pregnancy

---

megestrol (℞)

(me-jess'trole)
Megace, megestrol acetate
Func. class.: Antineoplastic
Chem. class.: Hormone, progestin

Action: Affects endometrium by antiluteinizing effect; this is thought to bring about cell death

Uses: Breast, endometrial cancer, renal cell cancer, cachexia

Dosage and routes:
Endometrial/ovarian carcinoma
- *Adult:* PO 40-320 mg/day in divided doses

Breast carcinoma
- *Adult:* PO 40 mg qid

Anorexia (AIDS)
- *Adult:* PO 40 mg qid

Available forms: Tabs 20, 40 mg; oral susp 40 mg/ml

Side effects/adverse reactions:
GI: Nausea, vomiting, diarrhea, abdominal cramps, weight gain
GU: Gynecomastia, fluid retention, *hypercalcemia*, vaginal bleeding, discharge, impotence, decreased libido
CV: **Thrombophlebitis**
INTEG: Alopecia, rash, pruritus, purpura, itching
CNS: Mood swings

Contraindications: Hypersensitivity, pregnancy (X)

Pharmacokinetics:
PO: Duration 1-3 days, half-life 60 min; metabolized in liver; excreted in feces, breast milk

Lab test interferences:
Increase: Alk phosphatase, urinary N, urinary pregnanediol, plasma amino acids
False positive: Urine glucose
Decrease: HDL, glucose tolerance test

NURSING CONSIDERATIONS
Assess:
- I&O ratio; weights
- Serum Ca levels
- Homan's sign
- Food preferences; list likes, dislikes
- Effects of alopecia on body image; discuss feelings about body changes
- ⬥ Symptoms indicating severe allergic reaction: rash, pruritus, urti-

---

caria, purpuric skin lesions, itching, flushing
- Frequency of stools, characteristics: cramping, acidosis, signs of dehydration (rapid respirations, poor skin turgor, decreased urine output, dry skin, restlessness, weakness)
- Mood swings
- Anorexia, nausea, vomiting, constipation, weakness, loss of muscle tone

Administer:
- Diuretics for increased fluids
- Oral susp for AIDS patients

Perform/provide:
- Increase fluid intake to 2-3 L/day to prevent dehydration and maintain normal Ca
- Nutritious diet with iron, vitamin supplements as ordered
- Storage in tight container at room temp

Evaluate:
- Therapeutic response: decreased tumor size, spread of malignancy; weight gain in AIDS patients

Teach patient/family:
- To report vaginal bleeding
- That nonhormonal contraception should be used during and 4 mo after treatment
- That gynecomastia can occur; reversible after discontinuing treatment
- To recognize and report signs of fluid retention, thromboemboli, hepatotoxicity

---

melphalan (℞)

(mel'fa-lan)
Alkeran, Alkeran IV, L-PAM, L-Sarcolysin
Func. class.: Antineoplastic alkylating agent
Chem. class.: Nitrogen mustard

Action: Responsible for cross-linking DNA strands leading to cell death; activity is not cell cycle phase-specific

Uses: Multiple myeloma, breast cancer, reticulum cell sarcoma, testicular seminoma, malignant melanoma, advanced ovarian cancer

Investigational uses: Breast, testicular, prostate carcinoma; osteogenic sarcoma, chronic myelogenous leukemia

Dosage and routes:
Multiple myeloma
- *Adult:* PO 6 mg qd × 2-3 wk; stop drug for 4 wk or until WBC level begins to rise; do not administer if WBC <3000/mm^3 or platelets <100,000/mm^3; may be given 0.15 mg/kg/day × 7 days; wait until platelets and WBCs rise, then 0.05 mg/kg/day

Ovarian carcinoma
- *Adult:* IV INF 16 mg/m^2, reduce in renal insufficiency, give over 15-20 min, give at 2 wk intervals × 4 doses, then at 4 wk intervals

Available forms: Tabs 2 mg, powder for inj 50 mg

Side effects/adverse reactions:
HEMA: **Thrombocytopenia, neutropenia, leukopenia,** anemia
GI: Nausea, vomiting, stomatitis, diarrhea
GU: Amenorrhea, hyperuricemia, gonadal suppression
INTEG: Rash, urticaria, alopecia, pruritus
RESP: **Fibrosis, dysplasia**
SYST: **Anaphylaxis,** allergic reactions

Contraindications: Lactation, pregnancy (D), hypersensitivity to this drug or other nitrogen mustards

Precautions: Radiation therapy, bone marrow depression, infections, renal disease, children

Pharmacokinetics: Metabolized in liver, excreted in urine, half-life 1½ hr

M

Side effects: *italics* = common; ***bold italics*** = life-threatening

Interactions:
- Increased toxicity: antineoplastics, radiation

NURSING CONSIDERATIONS
Assess:
- CBC, differential, platelet count qwk; withhold drug if WBC is <4000 or platelet count is <75,000; notify prescriber
- Renal function studies: BUN, serum uric acid, urine CrCl before, during therapy
- I&O ratio; report fall in urine output to 30 ml/hr
- Monitor temp q4h (may indicate beginning infection); no rectal temps
- Liver function tests before, during therapy (bilirubin, AST [SGOT], ALT [SGPT], LDH) as needed or monthly
- Bleeding: hematuria, guaiac, bruising or petechiae, mucosa or orifices q8h
- Food preferences; list likes, dislikes
- Yellow skin and sclera, dark urine, clay-colored stools, itchy skin, abdominal pain, fever, diarrhea
- Inflammation of mucosa, breaks in skin
- Buccal cavity q8h for dryness, sores, ulceration, white patches, oral pain, bleeding, dysphagia
- Local irritation, pain, burning, discoloration at injection site
- Symptoms indicating severe allergic reaction: rash, pruritus, urticaria, purpuric skin lesions, itching, flushing

Administer:
- Antiemetic 30-60 min before giving drug to prevent vomiting
- Antibiotics for prophylaxis of infection
- Topical or systemic analgesics for pain
- Local or systemic drugs for infection

Y-site compatibilities: Acyclovir, amikacin, aminophylline, ampicillin, aztreonam, bleomycin, bumetanide, buprenorphine, butorphanol, calcium gluconate, carboplatin, carmustine, cefazolin, cefepime, cefoperazone, cefotaxime, cefotetan, ceftazidime, ceftizoxime, ceftriaxone, cefuroxime, cimetidine, cisplatin, clindamycin, cyclophosphamide, cytarabine, dacarbazine, dactinomycin, daunorubicin, dexamethasone, diphenhydramine, doxorubicin, doxycycline, droperidol, enalaprilat, etoposide, famotidine, floxuridine, fluconazole, fludarabine, fluorouracil, furosemide, gallium, ganciclovir, gentamicin, granisetron, haloperidol, heparin, hydrocortisone, hydrocortisone sodium phosphate, hydromorphone, hydroxyzine, idarubicin, ifosfamide, imipenem-cilastatin, lorazepam, mannitol, mechlorethamine, meperidine, mesna, methotrexate, methylprednisolone, metoclopramide, metronidazole, miconazole, minocycline, mitomycin, mitoxantrone, morphine, nalbuphine, netilmicin, ondansetron, pentostatin, piperacillin, plicamycin, potassium chloride, prochlorperazine, promethazine, ranitidine, sodium bicarbonate, streptozocin, teniposide, thiotepa, ticarcillin, ticarcillin/clavulanate, tobramycin, trimethoprim-sulfamethoxazole, vancomycin, vinblastine, vincristine, vinorelbine, zidovudine

Perform/provide:
- Storage in air-tight, light-resistant container
- Strict medical asepsis, protective isolation if WBC levels are low
- Special skin care
- Increase fluid intake to 2-3 L/day to prevent urate deposits, calculi formation

---

 = Nursing alert   ✏ = Herb-drug interaction   🚫 = Do not crush

• Diet low in purines: organ meats (kidney, liver), dried beans, peas to maintain alkaline urine

• Rinsing of mouth tid-qid with water, club soda; brushing of teeth bid-tid with soft brush or cotton-tipped applicators for stomatitis; use unwaxed dental floss

• Warm compresses at injection site for inflammation

Evaluate:

• Therapeutic response: decreased tumor size, spread of malignancy

Teach patient/family:

• About protective isolation

• That sterility, amenorrhea can occur; reversible after discontinuing treatment

• To avoid foods with citric acid, hot or rough texture

• To report any bleeding, white spots, or ulcerations in mouth to prescriber; tell patient to examine mouth qd

• To report signs of infection: fever, sore throat, flu symptoms

• To report signs of anemia: fatigue, headache, faintness, shortness of breath, irritability

• To avoid use of razors, commercial mouthwash

• To avoid use of aspirin products, ibuprofen

---

menadione/menadiol sodium diphosphate (vit K₃) (℞)

(men-a-dye'ohn)
Synkavite*, Synkayvite
Func. class.: Vitamin, fat soluble

Action: Needed for adequate blood clotting (factors II, VII, IX, X)

Uses: Vit K malabsorption, hypoprothrombinemia

Dosage and routes:

• *Adult:* PO 2-10 mg (menadione)

• *Adult:* PO/IM/IV 5-15 mg (menadiol sodium diphosphate)

Available forms: Tabs 5 mg; inj 5, 10, 37.5 mg/ml

Side effects/adverse reactions:

CNS: Headache, ***brain damage*** (large doses)

GI: Nausea, decreased liver function tests

HEMA: ***Hemolytic anemia, hemoglobinuria, hyperbilirubinemia***

INTEG: Rash, urticaria

Contraindications: Hypersensitivity, severe hepatic disease, last few weeks of pregnancy (X)

Precautions: Neonates

Pharmacokinetics: Metabolized, crosses placenta

Interactions:

• Decreased action of menadione: oral antibiotics, cholestyramine, mineral oil

• Decreased action of oral anticoagulants

• Incompatible with alkaloids, codeine, levorphanol, meperidine, methadone, procaine

NURSING CONSIDERATIONS

Assess:

• Pro-time during treatment (2 sec deviation from control time, bleeding time, and clotting time), monitor for bleeding, pulse, and B/P

• Nutritional status: liver (beef), spinach, tomatoes, coffee, asparagus, broccoli, cabbage, lettuce, greens

Administer:

• Deep IM, IV slowly over 7 min; may be given IV undiluted or added to infusions

Evaluate:

• Therapeutic response: decreased bleeding tendencies, decreased pro-time, decreased clotting time

Teach patient/family:

• Not to take other supplements unless directed by prescriber

• The necessary foods in diet

M

- To avoid use of mineral oil
- To avoid IM injections, activities leading to injury, use soft toothbrush, don't floss; use electric razor until coagulation defect corrected
- Not to take OTC drugs, especially containing aspirin or alcohol
- The importance of frequent lab tests to monitor coagulation factors

---

menotropins (℞)

(men-oh-troe′pins)
Humegon, Pergonal
Func. class.: Gonadotropin
Chem. class.: Exogenous gonadotropin

Action: In women, increases follicular growth, maturation; in men, when given with HCG, stimulates spermatogenesis

Uses: Infertility, anovulation in women, stimulates spermatogenesis in men

Dosage and routes:

Infertility

- *Men:* **IM** 1 ampule 3 × wk with HCG 2000 U 2 × wk × 4 mo
- *Women:* **IM** 75 IU FSH, LH qd × 9-12 days, then 10,000 U HCG 1 day after these drugs; repeat × 2 menstrual cycles, then increase to 150 IU FSH, LH qd × 9-12 days, then 10,000 U HCG 1 day after these drugs × 2 menstrual cycles

Anovulation

- *Women:* **IM** 75 IU FSH, LH qd × 9-12 days, then 10,000 U HCG 1 day after last dose of these drugs; repeat × 1-3 menstrual cycles

Available forms: Powder for inj lyophilized 75 IU FSH, LH activity 150 IU FSH, LH activity

Side effects/adverse reactions:

CNS: Fever

CV: Hypovolemia

GI: Nausea, vomiting, diarrhea, anorexia

GU: Ovarian enlargement, abdominal distention/pain, multiple births, ovarian hyperstimulation: sudden ovarian enlargement, ascites with or without pain, pleural effusion; gynecomastia in men

*HEMA: **Hemoperitoneum, arterial thromboembolism***

Contraindications: Primary ovarian failure, abnormal bleeding, thyroid/adrenal dysfunction, organic intracranial lesion, ovarian cysts, primary testicular failure

Precautions: Pregnancy (C)

NURSING CONSIDERATIONS

Assess:

- Weight qd; notify prescriber if weight increases rapidly
- Estrogen excretion level; if >100 µg/24 hr, drug is withheld; hyperstimulation syndrome may occur
- I&O ratio; be alert for decreasing urinary output
- Ovarian enlargement, abdominal distention/pain; report symptoms immediately

Administer:

IM

- After reconstituting with 1-2 ml sterile saline inj; use immediately

Evaluate:

- Therapeutic response: ovulation, pregnancy

Teach patient/family:

- That multiple births are possible; if pregnancy occurs, usually 4-6 wk after start of treatment
- To keep appointment during treatment qd × 2 wk
- That daily intercourse is necessary from day preceding administration of gonadotropin until ovulation occurs

---

meperidine (℞)

(me-per'i-deen)

Demerol, meperidine, Peth-adol, Pethidine

Func. class.: Narcotic analgesic

Chem. class.: Opiate, phenylpi-peridine derivative

Controlled Substance Schedule II

Action: Depresses pain impulse transmission at the spinal cord level by interacting with opioid receptors

Uses: Moderate to severe pain, pre-operatively, postoperatively

Dosage and routes:

Pain

• *Adult:* **PO/SC/IM** 50-150 mg q3-4h prn; dose should be decreased if given **IV**

• *Child:* **PO/SC/IM** 1 mg/kg q4-6h prn, not to exceed 100 mg q4h

Labor analgesia

• *Adult:* **SC/IM** 50-100 mg given when contractions are regularly spaced, repeat q1-3h prn

Preoperatively

• *Adult:* **IM/SC** 50-100 mg q30-90 min before surgery; dose should be reduced if given **IV**

• *Child:* **IM/SC** 1-2.2 mg/kg 30-90 min before surgery

Renal disease

• CrCl 10-50 ml/min 75% of dose; CrCl <10 ml/min 50% of dose

Available forms include: Inj 10, 50, 75, 100 mg/ml; tabs 50, 100 mg; syr 50 mg/5 ml

Side effects/adverse reactions:

CNS: Drowsiness, dizziness, confusion, headache, sedation, euphoria, increased intracranial pressure, seizures

CV: Palpitations, bradycardia, change in B/P, tachycardia (IV)

EENT: Tinnitus, blurred vision, miosis, diplopia, depressed corneal reflex

GI: Nausea, vomiting, anorexia, constipation, cramps

GU: Urinary retention, dysuria

INTEG: Rash, urticaria, bruising, flushing, diaphoresis, pruritus

*RESP: **Respiratory depression***

Contraindications: Hypersensitivity, addiction (narcotic)

Precautions: Addictive personality, pregnancy (B), lactation, increased intracranial pressure, MI (acute), severe heart disease, respiratory depression, hepatic disease, renal disease, child <18 yr, elderly

Pharmacokinetics:

Absorption 50% (PO), well absorbed IM, SC

PO: Onset 15 min, peak ½-1 hr, duration 2-4 hr

SC/IM: Onset 10 min, peak ½-1 hr, duration 2-4 hr

IV: Onset 5 min, duration 2 hr

Metabolized by liver (to active/inactive metabolites), excreted by kidneys; crosses placenta, excreted in breast milk; half-life 3-4 hr; toxic by-product can result from regular use

Interactions:

• Increased effects with other CNS depressants: alcohol, narcotics, sedative/hypnotics, antipsychotics, skeletal muscle relaxants, MAOIs, chlorpromazine

Lab test interferences:

Increase: Amylase, lipase

NURSING CONSIDERATIONS

Assess:

• Pain: location, type, character; give before pain becomes extreme

• Renal function prior to initiating therapy; poor renal function can lead to accumulation of toxic metabolite and seizures

• I&O ratio; check for decreasing output; may indicate urinary retention

• Need for drug

M

- For constipation; increase fluids, bulk in diet
- CNS changes: dizziness, drowsiness, hallucinations, euphoria, LOC, pupil reactions
- Allergic reactions: rash, urticaria
- Respiratory dysfunction: depression, character, rate, rhythm; notify prescriber if respirations are <12/min

Administer:
- Patient should remain recumbent for 1 hr after IM/SC route
- With antiemetic for nausea, vomiting
- When pain is beginning to return; determine dosage interval by patient response
- In gradually decreasing dose after long-term use; withdrawal symptoms may occur

IV
- After diluting with 5 ml or more sterile H_2O or NS; give directly over 4-5 min; may be further diluted in sol to 1 mg/ml during anesthesia in D_5W or NS; if diluted in NS, may be given through patient-controlled inf device

Additive compatibilities: Cefazolin, dobutamine, ondansetron, scopolamine, succinylcholine, triflupromazine, verapamil

Syringe compatibilities: Atropine, benzquinamide, butorphanol, chlorpromazine, cimetidine, dimenhydrinate, diphenhydramine, droperidol, fentanyl, glycopyrrolate, hydroxyzine, ketamine, metoclopramide, midazolam, pentazocine, perphenazine, prochlorperazine, promazine, promethazine, ranitidine, scopolamine

Y-site compatibilities: Amifostine, amikacin, ampicillin, atenolol, aztreonam, bumetanide, cefamandole, cefazolin, cefmetazole, cefotaxime, cefotetan, cefoxitin, ceftazidime, ceftizoxime, ceftriaxone, cefurox-ime, cephalothin, cephapirin, chloramphenicol, cladribine, clindamycin, dexamethasone, diltiazem, diphenhydramine, dobutamine, dopamine, doxycycline, droperidol, erythromycin, famotidine, filgrastim, fluconazole, fludarabine, gallium, gentamicin, granisetron, heparin, hydrocortisone, insulin (regular), kanamycin, labetalol, lidocaine, methyldopa, magnesium sulfate, melphalan, methylprednisolone, metoclopramide, metoprolol, metronidazole, moxalactum, ondansetron, oxacillin, oxytocin, paclitaxel, penicillin G potassium, piperacillin, potassium chloride, propofol, propranolol, ranitidine, sargramostim, teniposide, thiotepa, ticarcillin, ticarcillin/clavulanate, tobramycin, trimethoprim/sulfamethoxazole, vancomycin, verapamil, vinorelbine

Perform/provide:
- Storage in light-resistant container at room temp
- Assistance with ambulation
- Safety measures: side rails, nightlight, call bell within easy reach

Evaluate:
- Therapeutic response: decrease in pain

Teach patient/family:
- To report any symptoms of CNS changes, allergic reactions
- That physical dependency may result from extended use
- That drowsiness, dizziness may occur; to call for assistance
- That withdrawal symptoms may occur: nausea, vomiting, cramps, fever, faintness, anorexia
- To make position changes slowly; orthostatic hypotension can occur
- To avoid OTC medications, alcohol unless directed by prescriber

Treatment of overdose: Naloxone (Narcan) 0.2-0.8 mg IV, O_2, IV fluids, vasopressors

mephentermine (℞)

(me-fen'ter-meen)

Wyamine

Func. class.: Adrenergic, direct and indirect acting

Chem. class.: Substituted phenylethylamine

Action: Causes increased contractility and heart rate by acting on β-receptors in heart; also acts on α-receptors, causing vasoconstriction in blood vessels; cardiac output is elevated and systolic and diastolic pressures are increased

Uses: Shock and hypotension following variety of procedures

Dosage and routes:

Hypotension

• *Adult:* IV 15-45 mg depending on procedure

Hypotension/shock

• *Adult:* IV 0.5 mg/kg

• *Child:* IV 0.4 mg/kg

Available forms: Inj 15, 30 mg/ml

Side effects/adverse reactions:

CV: Palpitations, tachycardia, hypertension

CNS: Tremors, drowsiness, confusion, incoherence

Contraindications: Hypersensitivity to sympathomimetics

Precautions: Pregnancy (B), cardiac disorders, hyperthyroidism, diabetes mellitus, prostatic hypertrophy

Pharmacokinetics:

IV: Onset immediate, duration ½-1 hr; metabolized in liver, excreted in urine

Interactions:

• Severe hypertension: oxytocics

• Do not use with MAOIs or tricyclic antidepressants; hypertensive crisis may occur

• Decreased effect of mephentermine: methyldopa, urinary acidifiers, rauwolfia alkaloids

• Increased effect of mephentermine: urinary alkalizers

• Dysrhythmias: halothane, digitalis

• Incompatible with epinephrine, hydralazine

NURSING CONSIDERATIONS

Assess:

• I&O ratio; notify prescriber if output is <30 ml/hr

• ECG during administration continuously; if B/P increases, drug is decreased

• B/P, pulse q5min after parenteral route

• CVP or PWP during infusion if possible

Administer:

IV

• Plasma expanders for hypovolemia

• IV undiluted 30 mg or less/1 min, or diluted 600 mg/500 ml D_5W, titrate to patient response, check site for extravasation; use an infusion pump

Perform/provide:

• Refrigerated storage of reconstituted sol no longer than 24 hr

• Do not use discolored sol

Evaluate:

• Therapeutic response: increased B/P with stabilization

Teach patient/family:

• The reason for drug administration

Treatment of overdose: Symptomatic treatment, may use a β-blocker

mephenytoin (℞)

(me-fen'i-toyn)

Mesantoin

Func. class.: Anticonvulsant

Chem. class.: Hydantoin derivative

Action: Reduces electrical discharges in motor cortex, reducing seizures

Uses: Generalized tonic-clonic, complex-partial seizures

Dosage and routes:

• *Adult:* **PO** 50-100 mg/day, may increase by 50-100 mg q7d, up to 200 mg tid

• *Child:* **PO** 50-100 mg/day or 100-450 mg/m^2/day in 3 divided doses, initially; then increase 50-100 mg q7d, up to 200 mg tid in divided doses q8h

Available forms: Tabs 100 mg

Side effects/adverse reactions:

HEMA: Agranulocytosis, neutropenia, leukopenia, pancytopenia, eosinophilia, lymphadenopathy

CNS: Drowsiness, dizziness, fatigue, irritability, tremors, insomnia, depression

GI: Nausea, vomiting

INTEG: Rash, *exfoliative dermatitis*

EENT: Photophobia, conjunctivitis, nystagmus, diplopia

RESP: Pulmonary fibrosis

Contraindications: Hypersensitivity to hydantoins, sinus bradycardia, heart block, Adams-Stokes syndrome

Precautions: Alcoholism, hepatic disease, renal disease, blood dyscrasias, CHF, elderly, pregnancy (C), respiratory depression, diabetes mellitus

Pharmacokinetics:

PO: Onset 30 min, duration 24-48 hr, metabolized by liver, excreted by kidneys, half-life 144 hr

Interactions:

• Decreased effects: rifampin, chronic alcohol use, barbiturates, antihistamines, antacids, other anticonvulsants, antineoplastics, Ca products, folic acid, oxacillin

• Increased effects: benzodiazepines, cimetidine, salicylates, sulfonamide, pyrazolones, phenothiazines, estrogens, disulfiram, chloramphenicol, anticoagulants

• Seizures: valproic acid

• Myocardial depression: lidocaine, propranolol, sympathomimetics

NURSING CONSIDERATIONS

Assess:

• Blood studies: CBC, platelets q2 wk until stabilized, then qmo × 12, then q3mo; discontinue drug if neutrophils are <1600/mm^3; liver function tests with long-term use

• Blood glucose may be increased

• Mental status: mood, sensorium, affect, behavioral changes; if mental status changes, notify prescriber

• Eye problems: need for ophthalmic examinations before, during, after treatment (slit lamp, fundoscopy, tonometry)

• Allergic reaction: red raised rash; drug should be discontinued

• Blood dyscrasias: fever, sore throat, bruising, rash, jaundice

 Toxicity: bone marrow depression, nausea, vomiting, ataxia, diplopia, cardiovascular collapse, Stevens-Johnson syndrome

Evaluate:

• Therapeutic response: decreased seizure activity

Teach patient/family:

• Not to discontinue drug quickly; should be tapered

• To avoid activities that require alertness if drowsiness, dizziness occurs

---

• That use of alcohol may decrease effects of drug
• To inform dentist; use good oral hygiene

---

mephobarbital (℞)

(me-foe-bar'bi-tal)
Mebaral
Func. class.: Anticonvulsant
Chem. class.: Barbiturate

Controlled Substance Schedule IV
Action: Depresses sensory cortex, motor activity; inhibits ascending conduction in reticular formation of thalamus
Uses: Generalized tonic-clonic (grand mal), absence (petit mal) seizures
Dosage and routes:
• *Adult:* **PO** 400-600 mg/day or in divided doses
• *Child:* **PO** <5 yr: 16-32 mg tid or qid, >5 yr: 32-64 mg tid or qid
Available forms: Tabs 32, 50, 100, 200* mg
Side effects/adverse reactions:
*HEMA: **Thrombocytopenia, agranulocytosis, megaloblastic anemia***
CNS: Dizziness, headache, hangover, paradoxic stimulation, drowsiness, increased pain
GI: Nausea, vomiting, epigastric pain
INTEG: Rash, urticaria, purpura, erythema multiforme, facial edema
EENT: Tinnitus, hearing loss
CV: Hypotension, bradycardia
RESP: Wheezing, hyperpnea
ENDO: Hypoglycemia, hyponatremia, hypokalemia
Contraindications: Hypersensitivity to barbiturates, pregnancy (D)
Precautions: Hepatic disease, renal disease, lactation, alcoholism, drug abuse, hyperthyroidism
Pharmacokinetics:
PO: Onset 20-60 min, duration 10-16 hr

Interactions:
• Increased effects: CNS depressants, chloramphenicol, valproic acid, sulfonamides
NURSING CONSIDERATIONS
Assess:
• Drug level, CBC, BUN, creatinine
• Mental status: mood, sensorium, affect, memory (long, short)
• Respiratory depression: respiration <10/min, shallow
◆ Blood dyscrasias: fever, sore throat, bruising, rash, jaundice
Perform/provide:
• Storage in light-resistant container
Evaluate:
• Therapeutic response: decreased seizure activity
Teach patient/family:
• Never to withdraw drug abruptly; notify prescriber of side effects
• To avoid hazardous activities until stabilized on drug
• That dreaming may increase when drug is discontinued
Treatment of overdose: Administer calcium gluconate IV

---

mepivacaine (℞)

(meh-piv'ah-kane)
Carbocaine, Carbocaine with Neo Cobefrin, Isocaine HCl, mepivicaine HCl, Polocaine
Func. class.: Local anesthetic
Chem. class.: Amide

Action: Competes with calcium for sites in nerve membrane that control sodium transport across cell membrane; decreases rise of depolarization phase of action potential
Uses: Nerve block, caudal anesthesia, epidural, pain relief, paracervical block, transvaginal block or infiltration
Dosage and routes:
Varies with route of anesthesia

Side effects: *italics* = common; ***bold italics*** = life-threatening

Available forms: Inj 1%, 1.5%, 2%, 3%

Side effects/adverse reactions:

CNS: Anxiety, restlessness, *convulsions, loss of consciousness,* drowsiness, disorientation, tremors, shivering

CV: Myocardial depression, cardiac arrest, dysrhythmias, bradycardia, hypotension, hypertension, *fetal bradycardia*

GI: Nausea, vomiting

EENT: Blurred vision, tinnitus, pupil constriction

INTEG: Rash, urticaria, allergic reactions, edema, burning, skin discoloration at injection site, tissue necrosis

RESP: Status asthmaticus, respiratory arrest, anaphylaxis

Contraindications: Hypersensitivity, child <12 yr, elderly, severe liver disease

Precautions: Elderly, severe drug allergies, pregnancy (C)

Pharmacokinetics: Onset 15 min, duration 3 hr; metabolized by liver, excreted in urine (metabolites)

Interactions:

• Dysrhythmias: epinephrine, halothane, enflurane

• Hypertension: MAOIs, tricyclic antidepressants, phenothiazines

• Decreased action of mepivacaine: chloroprocaine

NURSING CONSIDERATIONS

Assess:

• B/P, pulse, respiration during treatment

• Fetal heart tones during labor

• Allergic reactions: rash, urticaria, itching

• Cardiac status: ECG for dysrhythmias, pulse, B/P during anesthesia

Administer:

• Only with crash cart, resuscitative equipment nearby

• Only drugs without preservatives for epidural or caudal anesthesia

Perform/provide:

• Use of new sol; discard unused portion

Evaluate:

• Therapeutic response: anesthesia necessary for procedure

Treatment of overdose: Airway, O_2, vasopressor, IV fluids, anticonvulsants for seizures

---

meprobamate (℞)

(me-proe-ba′mate)

Equanil, Meditran*, meprobamate, Meprospan, Miltown, Miltown 600, Neo-Tran*, Novomepro*, Saronil, Sedabamate, Tranhep

Func. class.: Antianxiety/sedative, hypnotic

Chem. class.: Propanediol carbamate derivative

Controlled Substance Schedule IV

Action: Produces widespread depression of the CNS

Uses: Anxiety

• *Adult:* **PO** 1.2-1.6 g/day in 2-3 divided doses, not to exceed 2.4 g/day or 800-1600 mg/day in 2 divided doses (SUS REL); max 2.4 g/day

• *Geriatric:* **PO** 200 mg bid-tid, adjust to lowest possible dose

• *Child 6-12 yr:* **PO** 100-200 mg bid-tid or 200 mg (SUS REL) bid

Available forms: Tabs 200, 400, 600 mg; caps 400 mg; sus rel caps 200, 400 mg

Side effects/adverse reactions:

HEMA: Thrombocytopenia, leukopenia, eosinophilia

CNS: Dizziness, drowsiness, headache, *convulsions,* ataxia

GI: Nausea, vomiting, anorexia, diarrhea, stomatitis

INTEG: Urticaria, pruritus, maculopapular rash

◆ = Nursing alert   ⫸ = Herb-drug interaction   ⊘ = Do not crush

CV: Hypotension, tachycardia, palpitations, *hyperthermia*

EENT: Blurred vision, tinnitus, mydriasis, slurred speech

Contraindications: Hypersensitivity, renal failure, porphyria, pregnancy (D), history of drug abuse or dependence

Precautions: Suicidal patients, severe depression, renal disease, hepatic disease, elderly

Pharmacokinetics:

PO: Onset 1 hr; metabolized by liver; excreted in urine, in feces, breast milk; crosses placenta; half-life 6-16 hr

Interactions:

• Increased effects of meprobamate: CNS depressants, alcohol, tricyclic antidepressants

Lab test interferences:

False increase: 17-OHCS

False positive: Phentolamine test

NURSING CONSIDERATIONS

Assess:

• Sleep pattern; note sleep apnea, obstructed airway, pain/discomfort, urinary, frequency other circumstances that interrupt sleep

• B/P (lying, standing), pulse; if systolic B/P drops 20 mm Hg, hold drug, notify prescriber

• Blood studies: CBC during longterm therapy; blood dyscrasias have occurred rarely

• Therapeutic blood levels 0.5-2 mg/ 100 ml

• Hepatic studies: AST (SGOT), ALT (SGPT), bilirubin, creatinine, LDH, alk phosphatase

• Mental status: mood, sensorium, affect, drowsiness, dizziness; suicidal tendencies

➜ Tolerance, withdrawal symptoms: headache, nausea, vomiting, muscle pain, weakness, hyperthermia, death, convulsions after longterm use

Administer:

PO

• With food, milk for GI symptoms

• Crushed tabs if patient is unable to swallow medication whole

🚫 Do not break, crush, or chew sus rel cap

• Sugarless gum, hard candy, frequent sips of water for dry mouth

Perform/provide:

• Assistance with ambulation during beginning therapy, since drowsiness/dizziness occurs

• Safety measures, side rails

• Check to see if PO medication has been swallowed

Evaluate:

• Therapeutic response: decreased anxiety, restlessness, insomnia

Teach patient/family:

• That drug may be taken with food

• Not to be used for everyday stress or used longer than 4 mo unless directed by prescriber; not to take more than prescribed amount; may be habit forming

• To avoid OTC preparations (alcohol, cold, hay fever) unless approved by prescriber

• To avoid driving, activities that require alertness, since drowsiness may occur

• To avoid alcohol ingestion, other psychotropic medications unless directed by prescriber

• Not to discontinue medication abruptly after long-term use

• To rise slowly or fainting may occur, especially elderly

• That drowsiness may worsen at beginning of treatment

Treatment of overdose: Lavage, VS, supportive care

M

mercaptopurine (℞)

(mer-kap-toe-pyoor'een)
Purinethol, 6-MP
Func. class.: Antineoplastic-antimetabolite
Chem. class.: Purine analog

Action: Inhibits purine metabolism at multiple sites, which inhibits DNA and RNA synthesis, S phase of cell cycle specific

Uses: Chronic myelocytic leukemia, acute lymphoblastic leukemia in children, acute myelogenous leukemia

Investigational uses: Polycythemia vera, psoriatic arthritis, colitis, lymphoma

Dosage and routes:
• *Adult and child:* PO 2.5 mg/kg/day, not to exceed 5 mg/kg/day; maintenance 1.5-2.5 mg/kg/day
• *Child:* 70 mg/m²/day
Available forms: Tabs 50 mg

Side effects/adverse reactions:
CNS: Fever, headache, weakness
HEMA: ***Thrombocytopenia, leukopenia, myelosuppression, anemia***
GI: *Nausea, vomiting, anorexia, diarrhea, stomatitis,* **hepatotoxicity** (high doses), jaundice, gastritis
GU: **Renal failure,** hyperuricemia, *oliguria,* crystalluria, **hematuria**
INTEG: *Rash,* dry skin, urticaria

Contraindications: Patients with prior drug resistance, leukopenia (<2500/mm³), thrombocytopenia (<100,000/mm³), anemia, pregnancy (D)

Precautions: Renal disease

Pharmacokinetics: Incompletely absorbed when taken orally; metabolized in liver, excreted in urine

Interactions:
• Increased toxicity: radiation or other antineoplastics
• Increased bone marrow depression: allopurinol
• Reversal of neuromuscular blockade: nondepolarizing muscle relaxants

NURSING CONSIDERATIONS
Assess:
• CBC, differential, platelet count qwk; withhold drug if WBC is <3500 or platelet count is <100,000; notify prescriber; drug should be discontinued
• Renal function studies: BUN, serum uric acid, urine CrCl, electrolytes before, during therapy
• I&O ratio; report fall in urine output to <30 ml/hr
• Monitor temp q4h; fever may indicate beginning infection; no rectal temps
• Liver function tests before, during therapy: bilirubin, alk phosphatase, AST (SGOT), ALT (SGPT), qwk during beginning therapy
• Bleeding: hematuria, guaiac, bruising, petechiae; mucosa or orifices q8h
• Food preferences; list likes, dislikes
• Inflammation of mucosa, breaks in skin
• Buccal cavity q8h for dryness, sores, ulceration, white patches, oral pain, bleeding, dysphagia
◆ Symptoms indicating severe allergic reaction: rash, urticaria, itching, flushing

Administer:
• Antacid before oral agent; give drug after evening meal before bedtime
• Allopurinol or sodium bicarbonate to maintain uric acid levels, alkalinization of urine
• Antibiotics for prophylaxis of infection
• Topical or systemic analgesics for pain
• Transfusion for anemia

◆ = Nursing alert   🌿 = Herb-drug interaction   ⊘ = Do not crush

Perform/provide:
• Strict medical asepsis, protective isolation if WBC levels are low
• Increase fluid intake to 2-3 L/day to prevent urate deposits, calculi formation, unless contraindicated
• Diet low in purines: absence of organ meats (kidney, liver), dried beans, peas to maintain alkaline urine
• Rinsing of mouth tid-qid with water, club soda; brushing of teeth bid-tid with soft brush or cotton-tipped applicators for stomatitis; use unwaxed dental floss
• Nutritious diet with iron, vitamin supplements as ordered
• Storage in tightly closed container in cool environment
Evaluate:
• Therapeutic response: decreased size of tumor, spread of malignancy
Teach patient/family:
• To avoid foods with citric acid, hot or rough texture for stomatitis
• To report stomatitis: any bleeding, white spots, ulcerations in mouth; tell patient to examine mouth qd, report symptoms
• That contraceptive measures are recommended during therapy
• To drink 10-12 (8 oz) glasses of fluid/day
• To notify prescriber of fever, chills, sore throat, nausea, vomiting, anorexia, diarrhea, bleeding, bruising, which may indicate blood dyscrasias
• To report signs of infection: fever, sore throat, flu symptoms
• To report signs of anemia: fatigue, headache, faintness, shortness of breath, irritability
• To report bleeding: avoid use of razors, commercial mouthwash
• To avoid use of aspirin products, ibuprofen

meropenem (R̥)
(mer-oh-pen′em)
Merrem IV
Func. class.: Antiinfective-misc.
Chem. class.: Carbapenem

Action: Interferes with cell wall replication of susceptible organisms; osmotically unstable cell wall swells, bursts from osmotic pressure
Uses: Serious infections caused by gram-positive: *S. pneumoniae,* group A β-hemolytic streptococci, enterococcus; gram-negative: *Klebsiella, Proteus, E. coli, P. aeruginosa;* appendicitis, peritonitis caused by *viridans* group streptococci; *B. fragilis, B. thetaiotamicron,* bacterial meningitis (≥3 mo)
Dosage and routes:
Renal disease
• CrCl 26-50 ml/min 1 g q12h; CrCl 10-25 ml/min 500 mg q12h; CrCl <10 ml/min 500 mg q24h
• *Adult:* IV 1 g q8h, given over 15-30 min or as an **IV BOL** 5-20 ml given over 3-5 min
• *Child ≥3 mo:* IV 20-40 mg/kg q8h (max 2g q8h meningitis)
• *Child >50 kg:* IV 1 g q8h (intraabdominal infection) or 2 g q8h (meningitis) given over 15-30 min or as an **IV BOL** 5-20 ml over 3-5 min
Available forms: Inj 500 mg, 1 g
Side effects/adverse reactions:
CNS: Fever, somnolence, *seizures,* dizziness, weakness, myoclonia, *headache*
GI: Diarrhea, nausea, vomiting, ***pseudomembranous colitis, hepatitis,*** glossitis
CV: Hypotension, palpitations
HEMA: ***Eosinophilia, neutropenia,*** decreased Hgb, Hct
INTEG: Rash, urticaria, *pruritus,* pain

at injection site, phlebitis, erythema at injection site
*SYST: **Anaphylaxis***
RESP: Chest discomfort, dyspnea, hyperventilation
Contraindications: Hypersensitivity to meropenem or imipenem
Precautions: Pregnancy (B), lactation, elderly, renal disease
Pharmacokinetics:
IV: Onset immediate, peak dose dependent, half-life 1 hr, hepatic metabolism
Interactions:
• Increased meropenem plasma levels: probenecid
Lab test interferences:
Increase: AST (SGOT), ALT (SGPT), LDH, BUN, alk phosphatase, bilirubin, creatinine
False positive: Direct Coombs' test
NURSING CONSIDERATIONS
Assess:
• Sensitivity to carbapenem antibiotics
• Renal disease: lower dose may be required
• Bowel pattern qd; if severe diarrhea occurs, drug should be discontinued; may indicate pseudomembranous colitis
• Allergic reactions: rash, urticaria, pruritus; may occur few days after therapy begins
• Overgrowth of infection: perineal itching, fever, malaise, redness, pain, swelling, drainage, rash, diarrhea, change in cough, sputum
Administer:
• By IV INF or IV BOL
• After C&S is taken
Additive compatibilities: Aminophylline, atropine, cimetidine, dexamethasone, dobutamine, dopamine, enalaprilat, fluconazole, furosemide, gentamicin, heparin, insulin (regular), magnesium sulfate, metoclopramide, morphine, norepi-

nephrine, phenobarbital, ranitidine, vancomycin
Y-site compatibilities: Aminophylline, atenolol, atropine, cimetidine, dexamethasone, digoxin, diphenhydramine, enalaprilat, fluconazole, furosemide, gentamicin, heparin, insulin (regular), metoclopramide, morphine, norepinephrine, phenobarbital, vancomycin
Evaluate:
• Therapeutic response: negative C&S; absence of symptoms and signs of infection
Teach patient/family:
• To report severe diarrhea; may indicate pseudomembranous colitis
• To report sore throat, bruising, bleeding, joint pain; may indicate blood dyscrasias (rare)
Treatment of overdose: Epinephrine, antihistamines; resuscitate if needed (anaphylaxis)

---

mesalamine (R_x)
(mez-al′a-meen)
Asacol, Pentasa, Rowasa
Salofalk*
Func. class.: GI antiinflammatory
Chem. class.: 5-aminosalicylic acid

Action: May diminish inflammation by blocking cyclooxygenase, inhibiting prostaglandin production in colon; local action only
Uses: Mild to moderate active distal ulcerative colitis, proctosigmoiditis, proctitis
Dosage and routes:
• *Adult:* **RECT** 60 ml (4 g) hs, retained for 8 hr × 3-6 wk; **PO** 800 mg tid for 6 wk; **SUPP** 500 mg bid for 3-6 wk
Available forms: Rect susp 4 g/60 ml; supp 500 mg; tab del rel 400 mg; cap con rel 250 mg (Pentasa)

◆ = Nursing alert   ▰ = Herb-drug interaction   ⊘ = Do not crush

Side effects/adverse reactions:

CV: Pericarditis, myocarditis

GI: Cramps, gas, nausea, diarrhea, rectal pain, constipation

CNS: Headache, fever, dizziness, insomnia, asthenia, weakness, fatigue

INTEG: Rash, itching, acne

SYST: Flu, malaise, back pain, peripheral edema, leg and joint pain, arthralgia, dysmenorrhea

EENT: Sore throat, cough, pharyngitis, rhinitis

Contraindications: Hypersensitivity to this drug or salicylates

Precautions: Renal disease, pregnancy (B), lactation, children, sulfite sensitivity

Pharmacokinetics:

RECT: Primarily excreted in feces but some in urine as metabolite; half-life 1 hr, metabolite half-life 5-10 hr

NURSING CONSIDERATIONS

Assess:

• GI symptoms: cramps, gas, nausea, diarrhea, rectal pain; if severe, drug should be discontinued

• Renal function prior to treatment

Administer:

• May give orally; tabs should be swallowed whole

• Rectally; drug should be given hs, retained until morning

Perform/provide:

• Storage at room temp

Evaluate:

• Therapeutic response: absence of pain, bleeding from GI tract, decrease in number of diarrhea stools

Teach patient/family:

• That usual course of therapy is 3-6 wk

• To shake bottle well

• Method of rectal administration

• To inform prescriber of GI symptoms

🚫 Not to break, crush, or chew tabs

• To report abdominal cramping, pain, diarrhea with blood, headache, fever, rash, chest pain; drug should be discontinued

---

mesoridazine (R)

(mez-oh-rid'a-zeen)

Serentil

Func. class.: Antipsychotic, neuroleptic

Chem. class.: Phenothiazine, piperidine

Action: Depresses cerebral cortex, hypothalamus, limbic system, which control activity, aggression; blocks neurotransmission produced by dopamine at synapse; exhibits strong α-adrenergic, anticholinergic blocking action; mechanism for antipsychotic effects is unclear

Uses: Psychotic disorders, schizophrenia, anxiety, alcoholism, behavioral problems in mental deficiency, chronic brain syndrome

Dosage and routes:

Schizophrenia

• *Adult:* **PO** 50 mg tid; optimum dose 100-400 mg/day; **IM** 25 mg may repeat ½-1 hr; dosage range 25-200 mg/day

Behavior problems

• *Adult:* **PO** 25 mg tid; optimum dose 75-300 mg/day

• *Geriatric:* **PO** 10 mg qd-bid, increase q3-7 days by 10-25 mg to desired dose

Alcoholism

• *Adult:* **PO** 25 mg bid; optimum dose 50-200 mg/day

Schizoaffective disorders

• *Adult:* **PO** 10 mg tid; optimum dose 30-150 mg/day

Available forms: Tabs 10, 25, 50, 100 mg; conc 25 mg/ml; inj 25 mg/ml

Side effects/adverse reactions:

RESP: Laryngospasm, dyspnea, *respiratory depression*

M

CNS: EPS: pseudoparkinsonism, akathisia, dystonia, tardive dyskinesia, drowsiness, headache
HEMA: **Anemia, leukopenia, leukocytosis, agranulocytosis**
INTEG: Rash, photosensitivity, dermatitis
EENT: Blurred vision, glaucoma
GI: Dry mouth, nausea, vomiting, anorexia, constipation, diarrhea, jaundice, weight gain
GU: Urinary retention, urinary frequency, enuresis, impotence, amenorrhea, gynecomastia
CV: Orthostatic hypotension, hypertension, **cardiac arrest,** ECG changes, tachycardia
Contraindications: Hypersensitivity, circulatory collapse, liver damage, cerebral arteriosclerosis, coronary disease, severe hypertension/hypotension, blood dyscrasias, coma, brain damage, bone marrow depression, narrow-angle glaucoma
Precautions: Pregnancy (C), lactation, seizure disorders, hypertension, hepatic disease, cardiac disease, prostatic hypertrophy, intestinal obstruction, respiratory conditions
Pharmacokinetics:
PO: Onset erratic, peak 2 hr, duration 4-6 hr
IM: Onset 15-30 min, peak 30 min, duration 6-8 hr
Metabolized by liver, excreted in urine, crosses placenta, enters breast milk
Interactions:
• Oversedation: other CNS depressants, alcohol, barbiturate anesthetics
• Toxicity: epinephrine
• Decreased absorption: aluminum hydroxide, magnesium hydroxide antacids
• Decreased effects of lithium, levodopa
• Increased effects of both drugs: β-adrenergic blockers, alcohol
• Increased anticholinergic effects: anticholinergics
🌿 Increased anticholinergic effect: henbane leaf
Lab test interferences:
Increase: Liver function tests, cardiac enzymes, cholesterol, blood glucose, prolactin, bilirubin, PBI, cholinesterase, ^{131}I
Decrease: Hormones (blood, urine)
False positive: Pregnancy tests, PKU
False negative: Urinary steroids, 17-OHCS

NURSING CONSIDERATIONS
Assess:
• Mental status before initial administration
• Swallowing of PO medication; check for hoarding or giving to other patients
• I&O ratio; palpate bladder if low urinary output occurs
• Bilirubin, CBC, liver function studies monthly
• Urinalysis is recommended before, during prolonged therapy
• Affect, orientation, LOC, reflexes, gait, coordination, sleep pattern disturbances
• B/P standing and lying, pulse, respirations q4h during initial treatment; establish baseline before starting treatment; report drops of 30 mm Hg
• Dizziness, faintness, palpitations, tachycardia on rising
• EPS including akathisia (inability to sit still, no pattern to movements), tardive dyskinesia (bizarre movements of jaw, mouth, tongue, extremities), pseudoparkinsonism (rigidity, tremors, pill rolling, shuffling gait)
➡ For neuroleptic malignant syndrome: hyperthermia, altered mental status, muscle rigidity, increased CPK

➡ = Nursing alert   🌿 = Herb-drug interaction   🚫 = Do not crush

• Skin turgor daily
• Constipation, urinary retention daily; if these occur, increase bulk, water in diet

Administer:
• Antiparkinsonian agent after securing order from prescriber for EPS
• Concentrate mixed in distilled water, orange, grape juice; do not prepare, store bulk dilutions
• IM inj into large muscle mass; do not use if precipitate present
• Lowest possible dose to elderly to minimize side effects

Perform/provide:
• Decreased noise input by dimming lights, avoiding loud noises
• Supervised ambulation until stabilized on medication; do not involve in strenuous exercise program because fainting is possible; patient should not stand still for long periods
• Dose reduction in patients treated for behavior problems
• Increased fluids to prevent constipation
• Sips of water, candy, gum for dry mouth
• Storage in air tight, light-resistant container

Evaluate:
• Therapeutic response: decrease in emotional excitement, hallucinations, delusions, paranoia, and reorganization of patterns of thought, speech

Teach patient/family:
• That orthostatic hypotension is common and to rise from sitting or lying position gradually; to avoid hazardous activities until stabilized on medication
• To remain lying down for at least 30 min after IM injection
• To avoid hot tubs, hot showers, tub baths; hypotension may occur
• To avoid abrupt withdrawal of

mesoridazine, or EPS may result; drug should be withdrawn slowly
• To avoid OTC preparations (cough, hay fever, cold) unless approved by prescriber; serious drug interactions may occur; to avoid use with alcohol, CNS depressants; increased drowsiness may occur
• To use sunscreen during sun exposure to prevent burns
• Regarding compliance with drug regimen
• About necessity for meticulous oral hygiene, since oral candidiasis may occur
• To report sore throat, malaise, fever, bleeding, mouth sores; if these occur, a CBC should be drawn and drug discontinued
• That in hot weather heat stroke may occur; take extra precautions to stay cool

Treatment of overdose: Lavage if orally ingested; provide an airway; *do not induce vomiting*

---

metaproterenol (R)

(met-a-proe-ter'e-nole)
Alupent, Arm-A-Med Metaproterenol Sulfate, Metaprel
Func. class.: Bronchodilator-selective β₂-agonist

Action: Relaxes bronchial smooth muscle by direct action on β₂-adrenergic receptors with increased levels of cAMP with increased bronchodilation, diuresis, cardiac CNS stimulation

Uses: Bronchial asthma, bronchospasm

Dosage and routes:
• *Adult and child >12 yr:* **INH** 2-3 puffs; may repeat q3-4h, not to exceed 12 puffs/day
• *Adult:* **PO** 20 mg q6-8h
• *Geriatric:* **PO** 10 mg tid-qid, initially

• *Child >9 yr or >27 kg:* **PO** 20 mg q6-8h or 0.4-0.9 mg/kg tid
• *Child 6-9 yr or <27 kg:* **PO** 10 mg q6-8h or 0.4-0.9 mg/kg tid
• *Child 2-6 yr:* **PO** 1.3-2.6 mg/kg divided q6-8h

Available forms: Tabs 10, 20 mg; aerosol 0.65 mg/dose; syrup 10 mg/5 ml; sol nebulizer 0.4%, 0.6%, 5%

Side effects/adverse reactions:
CNS: Tremors, anxiety, insomnia, headache, dizziness, stimulation
CV: Palpitations, tachycardia, hypertension, dysrhythmias, *cardiac arrest*
GI: Nausea, vomiting

Contraindications: Hypersensitivity to sympathomimetics, narrow-angle glaucoma

Precautions: Pregnancy (C), cardiac disorders, hyperthyroidism, diabetes mellitus, prostatic hypertrophy

Pharmacokinetics: Well absorbed (PO)
PO: Onset 15-30 min, peak 1 hr, duration 4 hr, excreted in urine as metabolites
INH: Onset 5 min, peak 1 hr, duration 4 hr

Interactions:
• Increased effects of both drugs: other sympathomimetics
• Decreased action of β-blockers, oral hypoglycemics
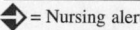 Increased effect: ephedra

Lab test interferences:
Decrease: K

NURSING CONSIDERATIONS
Assess:
• Respiratory function: vital capacity, forced expiratory volume, ABGs; also B/P; lung sounds, secretion before and after treatment
• Tolerance over long-term therapy; dose may have to be changed; check for rebound bronchospasm

Administer:
• 2 hr before hs to avoid sleeplessness
• PO with food for GI upset

Perform/provide:
• Storage at room temp; do not use discolored sol
• Spacer device for elderly

Evaluate:
• Therapeutic response: absence of dyspnea, wheezing; improved ABGs

Teach patient/family:
• To increase fluid intake to liquefy secretions
• Not to use OTC medications; excess stimulation may occur
• To notify prescriber of headaches, chest pain, weakness, dizziness, anxiety
• Use of inhaler; review package insert with patient
• To avoid getting aerosol in eyes
• To wash inhaler in warm water and dry qd
• All aspects of drug; avoid smoking, smoke-filled rooms, persons with respiratory infections

---

metformin (R_x)
(met-for'min)
Glucophage
Func. class.: Antidiabetic, oral
Chem. class.: Biguanide

Action: Inhibits hepatic glucose production and increases sensitivity of peripheral tissue to insulin
Uses: Stable adult-onset diabetes mellitus (type II) NIDDM
Dosage and routes:
• *Adult:* **PO** 500 mg bid initially, then increase to desired response 1-3 g; dosage adjustment q2-3wk or 850 mg qd with morning meal with dosage increased every other wk, max 2550 mg/day
Available forms: Tabs 500, 850 mg

Side effects/adverse reactions:

CNS: Headache, weakness, dizziness, drowsiness, tinnitus, fatigue, vertigo, *agitation*

GI: Nausea, vomiting, diarrhea, heartburn, anorexia, metallic taste

HEMA: **Thrombocytopenia,** decreased vit B_{12} concentration

INTEG: Rash

ENDO: **Lactic acidosis,** hypoglycemia

Contraindications: Hypersensitivity, hepatic, renal disease, alcoholism, cardiopulmonary disease, history of lactic acidosis

Precautions: Previous hypersensitivity to phenformin or buformin, pregnancy (B), elderly, thyroid disease, CHF, renal disease

Pharmacokinetics: Excreted by the kidneys unchanged 35%-50%, half-life 1½-5 hr, terminal 9-17 hr, peak 1-3 hr

Interactions:

• Increased risk of lactic acidosis, ethanol, glucocorticoids

• Increased blood glucose levels: acetazolamide

• Increased hypoglycemia: cimetidine

• Do not give with iodinated contrast media; may cause renal failure

NURSING CONSIDERATIONS

Assess:

• For hypoglycemic reactions (sweating, weakness, dizziness, anxiety, tremors, hunger), hyperglycemic reactions soon after meals

• CBC (baseline, q3mo) during treatment; check liver function tests periodically AST (SGOT), LDH, renal studies: BUN, creatinine during treatment

• For lactic acidosis: malaise, myalgia, abdominal distress; risk increases with age, poor renal function

Administer:

PO

• Twice a day given with meals to decrease GI upset and provide best absorption

• Tabs crushed and mixed with meal or fluids for patients with difficulty swallowing

Perform/provide:

• Conversion from other oral hypoglycemic agents; change may be made without gradual dosage change; monitor serum or urine glucose and ketones tid during conversion

• Storage in tight container in cool environment

Evaluate:

• Therapeutic response: decrease in polyuria, polydipsia, polyphagia; clear sensorium; absence of dizziness; stable gait, blood glucose at normal level

Teach patient/family:

• To use capillary blood glucose test or Chemstrip tid

• The symptoms of hypo/hypergly cemia, what to do about each

• That drug must be continued on daily basis; explain consequence of discontinuing drug abruptly

• To take drug in morning to prevent hypoglycemic reactions at night

• To avoid OTC medications unless approved by prescriber

• That diabetes is a lifelong illness; that this drug is not a cure; only controls symptoms

• That all food included in diet plan must be eaten to prevent hypoglycemia

• To carry Medic Alert ID and glucagon emergency kit for emergencies

Treatment of overdose: Glucose 25 g IV via dextrose 50% sol, 50 ml or 1 mg glucagon

M

---

methadone (℞)

(meth'a-done)
Dolophine HCl, methadone, methadone HCl Diskets, methadone HCl Intensol
Func. class.: Narcotic analgesic
Chem. class.: Opiate, synthetic diphenylheptane derivative

Controlled Substance Schedule II

Action: Depresses pain impulse transmission at the spinal cord level by interacting with opioid receptors, produce CNS depression

Uses: Severe pain, narcotic withdrawal

Dosage and routes:

Pain
• *Adult:* **PO/SC/IM** 2.5-10 mg q4-12h prn

Narcotic withdrawal
• *Adult:* **PO** 15-40 mg/day individualized initially, then 20-120 mg/day titrated to patient response
• *Child:* 0.05-0.1 mg/kg/dose q6-12h

Renal disease
• CrCl 10-50 ml/min dose q8h; CrCl <10 ml/min dose q8-12h

Available forms: Inj 10 mg/ml; tabs 5, 10 mg; oral sol 5, 10 mg/5 ml; dispersible tabs 40 mg; oral conc 10 mg/ml

Side effects/adverse reactions:

CNS: Drowsiness, dizziness, confusion, headache, sedation, euphoria
GI: Nausea, vomiting, anorexia, constipation, cramps, biliary tract spasm
GU: Increased urinary output, dysuria, urinary retention
INTEG: Rash, urticaria, bruising, flushing, diaphoresis, pruritus
EENT: Tinnitus, blurred vision, miosis, diplopia
CV: Palpitations, bradycardia, change in B/P

*RESP: **Respiratory depression***

Contraindications: Hypersensitivity to this drug or chlorobutanol (inj), addiction (narcotic)

Precautions: Addictive personality, pregnancy (B), lactation, increased intracranial pressure, MI (acute), severe heart disease, respiratory depression, hepatic disease, renal disease, child <18 yr, elderly

Pharmacokinetics:

PO: Onset 30-60 min, peak ½-1 hr, duration 6-8 hr, cumulative 22-48 hr
SC/IM: Onset 10-20 min, peak ½-1 hr, duration 6-8 hr, cumulative 22-48 hr

Metabolized by liver; excreted by kidneys; crosses placenta; excreted in breast milk; half-life 15-30 hr, extended interval with continued dosing; 90% bound to plasma proteins

Interactions:
• Increased effects with other CNS depressants: alcohol, narcotics, sedative/hypnotics, antipsychotics, skeletal muscle relaxants, rifampin, phenytoin

Lab test interferences:
Increase: Amylase

NURSING CONSIDERATIONS
Assess:
• I&O ratio; check for decreasing output; may indicate urinary retention
• CNS changes: dizziness, drowsiness, hallucinations, euphoria, LOC, pupil reaction
• Allergic reactions: rash, urticaria
• Respiratory dysfunction: respiratory depression, character, rate, rhythm; notify prescriber if respirations are <10/min
• Need for pain medication; possible physical dependence

Administer:
• With antiemetic if nausea/vomiting occurs

 = Nursing alert   = Herb-drug interaction   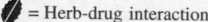 = Do not crush

• When pain is beginning to return; determine dosage interval by patient response
• Rotating inj sites, give deep in large muscle mass (IM)

Perform/provide:
• Storage in light-resistant container at room temp
• Assistance with ambulation
• Safety measures: side rails, night-light, call bell within easy reach

Evaluate:
• Therapeutic response: decrease in pain, successful narcotic withdrawal

Teach patient/family:
• To report any symptoms of CNS changes, allergic reactions
• That physical dependency may result from extended use
➡ Withdrawal symptoms may occur: nausea, vomiting, cramps, fever, faintness, anorexia

Treatment of overdose: Naloxone (Narcan) 0.2-0.8 mg IV, O$_2$, IV fluids, vasopressors

---

methamphetamine (℞)

(meth-am-fet′a-meen)
Desoxyn, Desoxyn Gradumet
Func. class.: Cerebral stimulant
Chem. class.: Amphetamine

Controlled Substance Schedule II
Action: Increases release of norepinephrine and dopamine in cerebral cortex to reticular activating system

Uses: Exogenous obesity, minimal brain dysfunction, attention deficit disorder with hyperactivity

Dosage and routes:
Attention deficit disorder
• *Child >6 yr:* **PO** 2.5-5 mg qd or bid increasing by 5 mg/wk
Obesity
• *Adult:* **PO** 2.5-5 mg, 30 min ac or 10-15 mg long-acting tab qd in AM

Available forms: Tabs 5 mg; tabs long-acting 5, 10, 15 mg

Side effects/adverse reactions:
CNS: Hyperactivity, insomnia, restlessness, talkativeness, dizziness, headache, chills, stimulation, dysphoria, irritability, aggressiveness, tremor
GI: Anorexia, dry mouth, diarrhea, constipation, weight loss, metallic taste, cramps
GU: Impotence, change in libido
CV: Palpitations, tachycardia, hypertension, decreased heart rate, dysrhythmia
INTEG: Urticaria

Contraindications: Hypersensitivity to sympathomimetic amines, hyperthyroidism, hypertension, glaucoma hypertrophy, severe arteriosclerosis, drug abuse, cardiovascular disease, anxiety

Precautions: Gilles de la Tourette's disorder, pregnancy (C), lactation, child <3 yr

Pharmacokinetics:
PO: Duration 3-6 hr, metabolized by liver, excreted by kidneys, crosses blood-brain barrier

Interactions:
• Hypertensive crisis: MAOIs or within 14 days of MAOIs
• Increased effect of methamphetamine: acetazolamide, antacids, sodium bicarbonate
• Decreased effects of methamphetamine: barbiturates, tricyclics, ascorbic acid, ammonium chloride
• Decreased effect of guanethidine

NURSING CONSIDERATIONS
Assess:
• VS, B/P; may reverse antihypertensives; check patients with cardiac disease more often
• CBC, urinalysis, in diabetes: blood sugar, urine sugar; insulin changes may have to be made, since eating will decrease

M

• Height, growth rate in children; growth rate may be decreased
• Mental status: mood, sensorium, affect, stimulation, insomnia, aggressiveness
• Physical dependency: should not be used for extended time; dose should be discontinued gradually; tolerance will occur (long-term use)

◆ Withdrawal symptoms: headache, nausea, vomiting, muscle pain, weakness
• Weight per regimen protocol

Administer:
• At least 6 hr before hs to avoid sleeplessness
• For obesity only if patient is on program including dietary changes, exercise; patient will develop tolerance; loss of weight won't occur without additional methods; give 2 hr before meals
• Gum, hard candy, or frequent sips of water for dry mouth

Evaluate:
• Therapeutic response: decreased weight, decreased hyperactivity

Teach patient/family:
• To decrease caffeine consumption (coffee, tea, cola, chocolate), which may increase irritability, stimulation
• To avoid OTC preparations unless approved by prescriber
• To taper off drug over several wk, or depression, increased sleeping, lethargy may ensue
• To avoid alcohol ingestion
• To avoid hazardous activities until patient is stabilized on medication
• To get needed rest; patients will feel more tired at end of day

🚫 Not to break, crush, or chew sus rel forms

Treatment of overdose: Administer fluids, hemodialysis or peritoneal dialysis; antihypertensive for increased B/P; ammonium Cl for increased excretion

---

methantheline (℞)

(meth-an'tha-leen)
Banthine
Func. class.: GI anticholinergic
Chem. class.: Synthetic quaternary ammonium antimuscarinic

Action: Inhibits muscarinic actions of acetylcholine at postganglionic parasympathetic neuroeffector sites

Uses: Treatment of peptic ulcer disease, irritable bowel syndrome, pancreatitis, gastritis, biliary dyskinesia, pylorospasm, reflex neurogenic bladder in children

Dosage and routes:
• *Adult:* PO 50-100 mg q6h
• *Child >1 yr:* PO 12.5-50 mg qid
• *Child <1 yr:* PO 12.5-25 mg qid
• *Neonate:* PO 12.5 mg bid-tid
Available forms: Tabs 50 mg

Side effects/adverse reactions:
CNS: Confusion, stimulation in elderly, headache, insomnia, dizziness, drowsiness, anxiety, weakness, hallucination
GI: Dry mouth, constipation, paralytic ileus, heartburn, nausea, vomiting, dysphagia, absence of taste
GU: Hesitancy, retention, impotence
CV: Palpitations, tachycardia
EENT: Blurred vision, photophobia, mydriasis, cycloplegia, increased ocular tension
INTEG: Urticaria, rash, pruritus, anhidrosis, fever, allergic reactions

Contraindications: Hypersensitivity to anticholinergics, narrow-angle glaucoma, GI obstruction, myasthenia gravis, paralytic ileus, GI atony, toxic megacolon

---

Precautions: Hyperthyroidism, coronary artery disease, dysrhythmias, CHF, ulcerative colitis, hypertension, hiatal hernia, hepatic disease, renal disease, pregnancy (C), urinary retention, prostatic hypertrophy, elderly

Pharmacokinetics:

PO: Onsct 30-45 min, duration 4-6 hr; metabolized by liver, excreted in urine, bile

Interactions:

• Increased anticholinergic effect: amantadine, tricyclic antidepressants, MAOIs, H₁-antihistamines
• Increased effect of nitrofurantoin
• Decreased effect of phenothiazines, levodopa

NURSING CONSIDERATIONS

Assess:

• VS, cardiac status: check for dysrhythmias, increased rate, palpitations
• I&O ratio; check for urinary retention, hesitancy
• GI complaints: pain, bleeding (frank or occult), nausea, vomiting, anorexia

Administer:

• ½-1 hr ac for better absorption
• Decreased dose to elderly patients; metabolism may be slowed
• Gum, hard candy, frequent rinsing of mouth for dryness of oral cavity

Perform/provide:

• Storage in tight container protected from light
• Increased fluids, bulk, exercise to decrease constipation

Evaluate:

• Therapeutic response: absence of epigastric pain, bleeding, nausea, vomiting

Teach patient/family:

• To avoid driving, other hazardous activities until stabilized on medication
• To avoid alcohol, other CNS depressants; will enhance sedating properties of this drug
• That drug may cause blurred vision

---

methazolamide (℞)

(meth-a-zoe'la-mide)
GlaucTabs, MZM, Neptazane
Func. class.: Carbonic anhydrase inhibitor diuretic
Chem. class.: Sulfonamide derivative

Action: Decreases production of aqueous humor in eye, which lowers intraocular pressure

Uses: Open-angle glaucoma or preoperatively in narrow-angle glaucoma; can be used with miotic, osmotic agents

Dosage and routes:

• *Adult:* **PO** 50-100 mg bid or tid
Available forms: Tabs 25, 50 mg

Side effects/adverse reactions:

GU: Frequency, hypokalemia, polyuria, uremia, *glucosuria, hematuria,* dysuria, renal calculi

CNS: Drowsiness, paresthesia, anxiety, depression, headache, dizziness, confusion, stimulation, fatigue, *convulsions,* sedation, nervousness

GI: Nausea, vomiting, anorexia, constipation, diarrhea, melena, weight loss, *hepatic insufficiency,* metallic taste in mouth

EENT: Myopia

INTEG: Rash, pruritus, urticaria, fever, photosensitivity, *Stevens-Johnson syndrome*

ENDO: Hyperglycemia

HEMA: Aplastic anemia, hemolytic anemia, leukopenia, agranulocytosis, thrombocytopenia, purpura, pancytopenia

Contraindications: Hypersensitivity to sulfonamides, severe renal disease, severe hepatic disease, elec-

trolyte imbalances (hyponatremia, hypokalemia), hyperchloremic acidosis, Addison's disease, COPD
Precautions: Hypercalciuria, pregnancy (C), diabetes mellitus
Pharmacokinetics:
PO: Onset 2-4 hr, peak 6-8 hr, duration 10-18 hr; excreted in urine, crosses placenta
Interactions:
• Decreased effectiveness of lithium, barbiturates
• Hypokalemia: with other diuretics, corticosteroids, amphotericin B
• Increased toxicity: salicylates, methazolamide
Lab test interferences:
False positive: Urinary protein
NURSING CONSIDERATIONS
Assess:
• Weight, I&O daily to determine fluid loss; effect of drug may be decreased if used qd
• Rate, depth, rhythm of respiration, effect of exertion
• B/P lying, standing; postural hypotension may occur
• Electrolytes: K, Na, Cl; include BUN, blood sugar, CBC, serum creatinine, blood pH, ABGs, liver function tests
• Signs of metabolic acidosis: drowsiness, restlessness
• Signs of hypokalemia: postural hypotension, malaise, fatigue, tachycardia, leg cramps, weakness
• Rashes, temp qd
• Confusion, especially in elderly; take safety precautions if needed
Administer:
• In AM to avoid sleeplessness
• K replacement if <3 mg/dl
• With food if nausea occurs; absorption may be decreased slightly
Evaluate:
• Therapeutic response: decrease in aqueous humor
Teach patient/family:
• To increase fluid intake to 2-3

L/day unless contraindicated; to rise slowly from lying or sitting position
• To use sunscreen for photosensitivity
• To notify prescriber of sore throat, unusual bleeding, bruising, paresthesias, tremors, flank pain, or skin rash
• To avoid hazardous activities if drowsiness occurs
Treatment of overdose: Lavage if taken orally; monitor electrolytes; administer dextrose in saline; monitor hydration, CV, renal status

---

methenamine (Ŗ)

(meth-en'a-meen)
Hiprex, Hip-Rex*, Urex, Mandameth, Mandelamine, methenamine mandelate
Func. class.: Urinary antiinfective
Chem. class.: Methenamine, mandelic acid

Action: In acid urine, hydrolyzed to ammonia, formaldehyde, which are bactericidal
Uses: UTIs caused by *E. coli, Klebsiella, Enterobacter, P. mirabilis, P. morganii, Serratia, Citrobacter*
Dosage and routes:
• *Adult and child >12 yr:* **PO** 1 g q12h (as hippurate) or 1 g q6h (as mandelate)
• *Child 6-12 yr:* **PO** 500 mg-1 g q12h (hippurate) or 500 mg q6h (mandelate)
Neurogenic bladder
• *Adult:* **PO** 1 g qid pc
• *Child 6-12 yr:* **PO** 500 mg qid pc
• *Child <6 yr:* **PO** 50 mg/kg in 4 divided doses pc
Available forms: Hippurate: tabs 1 g; Mandelate: tabs 500 mg, 1 g; tabs enteric-coated 500 mg, 1 g; tab film-coated 500 mg, 1 g; oral susp 250, 500 mg/5 ml

---

Side effects/adverse reactions:

CNS: Headache

INTEG: Pruritus, rash, urticaria

GI: Nausea, vomiting, anorexia, abdominal pain, increased AST (SGOT), ALT (SGPT)

GU: Dysuria, bladder irritation, *albuminuria, hematuria,* crystalluria

EENT: Tinnitus, stomatitis

Contraindications: Hypersensitivity, severe dehydration, renal insufficiency, sulfonamide therapy, hepatic disease (hippurate)

Precautions: Renal disease, pregnancy (C), lactation

Pharmacokinetics:

PO: Excreted in urine, half-life 4 hr

Interactions:

• Insoluble precipitate in urine: sulfonamides

• Do not use with silver, iron, mercury salts

Lab test interferences:

Interference: VMA, urinary catecholamines

False decrease: Urine estriol, 5-HIAA

False increase: 17-OHCS

NURSING CONSIDERATIONS

Assess:

• I&O ratio; urine pH <5.5 is ideal; monitor for hematuria indicating crystalluria

• Periodic liver function tests: AST (SGOT), ALT (SGPT), alk phosphatase

• C&S before treatment, after completion

• Allergy: fever, flushing, rash, urticaria, pruritus

Administer:

• After clean-catch urine for C&S

• Two daily doses if urine output is high or if patient has diabetes

• Up to 12 g of vit C if needed to acidify urine; cranberry, prune juice may be used; give with food

Perform/provide:

• Storage protected from heat

• Limited intake of alkaline foods or drugs: milk, dairy products, peanuts, vegetables, alkaline antacids, sodium bicarbonate

Evaluate:

• Therapeutic response: decreased pain, frequency, urgency, negative C&S, absence of infection

Teach patient/family:

• To keep urine acidic by eating meats, eggs, fish, gelatin products, prunes, plums, cranberries

• That fluids must be increased to 3 L/day to avoid crystallization in kidneys

• To complete full course of drug therapy; to take drug at evenly spaced intervals around clock for best results

---

methicillin (℞)

(meth-i-sill′in)

Staphcillin

Func. class.: Broad-spectrum antiinfective

Chem. class.: Penicillinase-resistant penicillin

Action: Interferes with cell wall replication of susceptible organisms; osmotically unstable cell wall swells, bursts from osmotic pressure

Uses: Effective for gram-positive cocci (*S. aureus, S. pyogenes, S. viridans, S. faecalis, S. bovis, S. pneumoniae*), infections caused by penicillinase-producing *Staphylococcus*

Dosage and routes:

Renal disease

• CrCl <10 ml/min no more than 2 g q12h

• *Adult:* **IM/IV** 4-12 g/day in divided doses q4-6h

• *Child:* **IM/IV** 50-300 mg/kg/day in divided doses q4-12h

Available forms: Powder for inj 1, 4, 6, 10 g; inf only 1 g

Side effects/adverse reactions:

HEMA: Anemia, increased bleeding time, **bone marrow depression, granulocytopenia**

GI: Nausea, vomiting, diarrhea; increased AST (SGOT), ALT (SGPT); abdominal pain, glossitis, colitis, interstitial nephritis

GU: Oliguria, **proteinuria, hematuria,** vaginitis, moniliasis, **glomerulonephritis**

CNS: Lethargy, hallucinations, anxiety, depression, twitching, **coma, convulsions**

Contraindications: Hypersensitivity to penicillins

Precautions: Pregnancy (B), hypersensitivity to cephalosporins, neonates

Pharmacokinetics:

IM: Peak ½-1 hr, duration 4 hr

IV: Peak 15 min, duration 2 hr

Metabolized in liver; excreted in urine, bile, breast milk; crosses placenta

Interactions:

• Decreased antimicrobial effectiveness of methicillin: tetracyclines, erythromycins

• Increased methicillin concentrations: aspirin, probenecid

• Drug/food: decreased absorption: food, carbonated drinks, citrus fruit juices

Lab test interferences:

False positive: Urine glucose, urine protein

NURSING CONSIDERATIONS

Assess:

• I&O ratio; report hematuria, oliguria, since penicillin in high doses is nephrotoxic

• Any patient with compromised renal system; drug is excreted slowly in poor renal system function; toxicity may occur rapidly

• Liver studies: AST (SGOT), ALT (SGPT)

• Blood studies: WBC, RBC, H&H, bleeding time

• Renal studies: urinalysis, protein, blood

• C&S before therapy; drug may be given as soon as culture is taken

• Bowel pattern before, during treatment

• Skin eruptions after administration of penicillin to 1 wk after discontinuing drug

• For thrombophlebitis at IV site, change IV site q48h

• Respiratory status: rate, character, wheezing, tightness in chest

• Allergies before initiation of treatment, reaction of each medication; highlight allergies on chart

Administer:

Drug after C&S completed

IV

• After diluting 1 g/1.8 ml sterile H_2O; further dilute each 500 mg/25 ml or more NaCl; give directly at 10 ml/min, added to D_5W, NS, LR, or by inf over ½ hr

Additive compatibilities: Aminophylline, ascorbic acid, calcium chloride or gluconate, cephalothin, chloramphenicol, colistimethate, corticotropin, dimenhydrinate, diphenhydramine, erythromycin, gentamicin, penicillin G potassium, penicillin G sodium, polymyxin B, potassium chloride, prednisolone, procaine, verapamil

Syringe compatibilities: Chloramphenicol, colistimethate, erythromycin, gentamicin, lidocaine, polymyxin B, procaine, streptomycin

Y-site compatibilities: Heparin, hydrocortisone sodium succinate, potassium chloride, verapamil, vit B/C

Perform/provide:

• Adrenalin, suction, tracheostomy set, endotracheal intubation equipment

---

◆ = Nursing alert   ✏ = Herb-drug interaction   ⊘ = Do not crush

- Adequate fluid intake (2 L) during diarrhea episodes
- Scratch test to assess allergy after securing order from prescriber; usually done when penicillin is only drug of choice
- Storage at room temp; reconstituted sol stable for 8 hr

Evaluate:
- Therapeutic response: absence of fever, draining wounds

Teach patient/family:
- That culture may be taken after completed course of medication
- To report sore throat, fever, fatigue (may indicate superinfection)
- To wear or carry Medic Alert ID if allergic to penicillins
- To notify nurse of diarrhea

Treatment of anaphylaxis: Withdraw drug; maintain airway; administer epinephrine, aminophylline, O_2, IV corticosteroids

---

methimazole (℞)

(meth-im′a-zole)
Tapazole
Func. class.: Thyroid hormone antagonist (antithyroid)
Chem. class.: Thioamide

Action: Inhibits synthesis of thyroid hormones by decreasing iodine use in manufacture of thyroglobin and iodothyronine; does not affect already formed hormones

Uses: Hyperthyroidism, preparation for thyroidectomy, thyrotoxic crisis, thyroid storm

Dosage and routes:
Hyperthyroidism
- *Adult:* **PO** 5-20 mg tid depending on severity of condition; continue until euthyroid; maintenance dose 5-10 mg qd-tid, maximal dose 150 mg qd

- *Child:* **PO** 0.4 mg/kg/day in divided doses q8h; continue until euthyroid; maintenance dose 0.2 mg/kg/day in divided doses q8h
Preparation for thyroidectomy
- *Adult and child:* **PO** same as above; iodine may be added × 10 days before surgery
Thyrotoxic crisis
- *Adult and child:* **PO** same as hyperthyroidism with iodine and propranolol

Available forms: Tabs 5, 10 mg
Side effects/adverse reactions:
ENDO: Enlarged thyroid
INTEG: Rash, urticaria, pruritus, alopecia, hyperpigmentation, lupus-like syndrome
GU: **Nephritis**
CNS: Drowsiness, headache, vertigo, fever, paresthesias, neuritis
HEMA: **Agranulocytosis, leukopenia, thrombocytopenia, hypothrombinemia, lymphadenopathy,** bleeding, vasculitis
GI: Nausea, diarrhea, vomiting, **jaundice, hepatitis,** loss of taste
MS: Myalgia, arthralgia, nocturnal muscle cramps

Contraindications: Hypersensitivity, pregnancy (D), 3rd trimester, lactation
Precautions: Infection, bone marrow depression, hepatic disease, pregnancy (D), 1st, 2nd trimester
Pharmacokinetics:
PO: Onset 1 wk, duration is up to 10 wk, half-life 1-2 hr; excreted in urine, breast milk; crosses placenta
Interactions:
- Increased bone marrow depression: radiation, antineoplastic agents
- Decreased effectiveness: amiodarone, potassium iodide
- Agranulocytosis: phenothiazines
- Altered response to digitalis, warfarin

Lab test interferences:
Increase: Pro-time, AST (SGOT)/ALT (SGPT), alk phosphatase

NURSING CONSIDERATIONS
Assess:
• Pulse, B/P, temp
• I&O ratio; check for edema: puffy hands, feet, periorbits; indicate hypothyroidism
• Weight qd; same clothing, scale, time of day
• T_3, T_4, which are increased; serum TSH, which is decreased; free thyroxine index, which is increased if dosage is too low; discontinue drug 3-4 wk before RAIU
• Blood work: CBC for blood dyscrasias: leukopenia, thrombocytopenia, agranulocytosis; LFTs
⬧ Overdose: peripheral edema, heat intolerance, diaphoresis, palpitations, dysrhythmias, severe tachycardia, fever, delirium, CNS irritability
• Hypersensitivity: rash, enlarged cervical lymph nodes; drug may have to be discontinued
• Hypoprothrombinemia: bleeding, petechiae, ecchymosis
• Clinical response: after 3 wk should include increased weight, pulse; decreased T_4
• Bone marrow depression: sore throat, fever, fatigue

Administer:
• With meals to decrease GI upset
• At same time each day to maintain drug level
• Lowest dose that relieves symptoms; discontinue before RAIU

Perform/provide:
• Storage in light-resistant container
• Fluids to 3-4 L/day, unless contraindicated

Evaluate:
• Therapeutic response: weight gain, decreased pulse, decreased T_4, B/P

Teach patient/family:
• Not to breastfeed
• To take pulse daily
• To report redness, swelling, sore throat, mouth lesions, fever, which indicate blood dyscrasias
• To keep graph of weight, pulse, mood
• To avoid OTC products that contain iodine
• That seafood, other iodine products may be restricted
• Not to discontinue this medication abruptly; thyroid crisis may occur; stress patient response
• That response may take several mo if thyroid is large
• The symptoms and signs of overdose: periorbital edema, cold intolerance, mental depression
• The symptoms of inadequate dose: tachycardia, diarrhea, fever, irritability

---

methocarbamol (℞)

(meth-oh-kar′ba-mole)
Delaxin, Marbaxin 750, methocarbamol, Robaxin, Robaxin-750, Robomol-500, Robomol-750, Tresortil*

Func. class.: Skeletal muscle relaxant, central acting
Chem. class.: Carbamate derivative

Action: Depresses multisynaptic pathways in the spinal cord, causing skeletal muscle relaxation
Uses: Adjunct for relief of spasm and pain in musculoskeletal conditions, tetanus management
Dosage and routes:
Pain
• *Adult:* **PO** 1.5 g × 2-3 days, then 1 g qid; **IM** 500 mg in each gluteal region, may repeat q8h; **IV BOL** 1-3 g/day at 3 ml/min; **IV INF** 1 g/250 ml D_5W or NS, not to exceed 3 g/day

---

• *Geriatric:* **PO** 500 mg qid, titrate to needed dose

Tetanus

• *Adult:* **IV INF** 1-3 g/L of solution q6h; **IV BOL** 1-2 g injected into running **IV**

• *Child:* **IV** 15 mg/kg q6h

Available forms: Tabs 500, 750 mg; inj 100 mg/ml

Side effects/adverse reactions:

CNS: Dizziness, weakness, drowsiness, headache, tremor, depression, insomnia, *seizures*

HEMA: Hemolysis, increased hemoglobin (IV only)

EENT: Diplopia, temporary loss of vision, blurred vision, nystagmus

CV: Postural hypotension, bradycardia

GI: Nausea, vomiting, hiccups, anorexia, metallic taste

GU: Brown, black, green urine

INTEG: Rash, pruritus, fever, facial flushing, urticaria

Contraindications: Hypersensitivity, child <12 yr, intermittent porphyria

Precautions: Renal disease, hepatic disease, addictive personalities, pregnancy (C), myasthenia gravis, epilepsy

Pharmacokinetics:

IM/IV: Onset rapid

PO: Onset ½ hr, peak 1-2 hr, half-life 1-2 hr

Metabolized in liver, excreted in urine unchanged, crosses placenta

Interactions:

• Increased CNS depression: alcohol, tricyclic antidepressants, narcotics, barbiturates, sedatives, hypnotics

• Considered incompatible with any drug in sol or syringe

Lab test interferences:

False increase: VMA, urinary 5-HIAA

NURSING CONSIDERATIONS

Assess:

• Blood studies: CBC, WBC, differential; blood dyscrasias may occur

• During and after injection: CNS effects, rash, conjunctivitis, nasal congestion may occur

• Liver function studies: AST (SGOT), ALT (SGPT), alk phosphatase; hepatitis may occur

• ECG in epileptic patients; poor seizure control has occurred

• Allergic reactions: rash, fever, respiratory distress

• Severe weakness, numbness in extremities

• Tolerance: increased need for medication, more frequent requests for medication, increased pain

• CNS depression: dizziness, drowsiness, psychiatric symptoms

Administer:

• With meals for GI symptoms

• IV undiluted over 1 min or more, give 300 mg or less/1 min or longer; may be diluted in 250 ml or less D_5 or isotonic NaCl sol

• By slow IV to prevent phlebitis; keep recumbent for 15 min to prevent orthostatic hypotension; check for extravasation

• IM deep in large muscle mass; rotate sites

Perform/provide:

• Storage in tight container at room temp

• Assistance with ambulation if dizziness/drowsiness occurs

• Recumbent position after IV administration

Evaluate:

• Therapeutic response: decreased pain, spasticity

Teach patient/family:

• Not to discontinue medication quickly; insomnia, nausea, headache, spasticity, tachycardia will oc-

M

cur; drug should be tapered off over 1-2 wk

• That urine may turn green, black, or brown

• Not to take with alcohol, other CNS depressants

• To avoid altering activities while taking this drug

• To avoid hazardous activities if drowsiness, dizziness occurs

• To avoid using OTC medication: cough preparations, antihistamines, unless directed by prescriber

Treatment of overdose: Induce emesis of conscious patient, lavage, dialysis; have epinephrine, antihistamines, and corticosteroids available

---

methohexital (℞)
(meth-oh-hex′i-tal)
Brevital Sodium, Brietal Sodium*
Func. class.: General anesthetic
Chem. class.: Barbiturate

Controlled Substance Schedule IV

Action: Acts in reticular-activating system to produce anesthesia; may be potentiated by GABA

Uses: General anesthesia for electroshock therapy, reduction of fractures, adjunct with other anesthetics, balanced anesthesia

Dosage and routes:

• *Adult and child:* **IV** 50-120 mg given 1 ml/5 sec

Maintenance

• *Adult and child:* **IV** 20-40 mg q4-7min 0.1% sol; **CONT IV** 3 ml/min (6 mg/min) 0.2% sol

Available forms: Powder for inj 500 mg, 2.5, 5 g; powder for inj 10 mg/ml*

Side effects/adverse reactions:

*RESP: **Respiratory depression, bronchospasm***

CNS: Retrograde amnesia, prolonged somnolence

CV: Tachycardia, hypotension, ***myocardial depression, dysrhythmias***

EENT: Sneezing, coughing

INTEG: Chills, *shivering,* necrosis, pain at injection site

MS: Muscle irritability

Contraindications: Hypersensitivity, status asthmaticus, hepatic/intermittent porphyrias, pregnancy (D)

Precautions: Severe cardiovascular disease, renal disease, hypotension, liver disease, myxedema, myasthenia gravis, asthma, increased intracranial pressure

Pharmacokinetics:

IV: Onset 30-40 sec; half-life 11.5 hr; crosses placenta

Interactions:

• Increased action: CNS depressants

• Do not mix with other drugs in sol or syringe

NURSING CONSIDERATIONS

Assess:

• VS q3-5min during IV administration, after dose, q4h postoperatively

• Extravasation; use chloroprocaine to decrease pain, increase circulation

• Dysrhythmias, myocardial depression

Administer:

IV

• After preparation with sterile water, 0.9% NaCl, or 5% dextrose

• Only with crash cart, resuscitative equipment nearby

• IV slowly only by qualified persons

Evaluate:

• Therapeutic response: induction of anesthesia

---

methotrexate (amethopterin, MTX) (℞)

(meth-oh-trex'ate)

Folex PFS, methotrexate, Methotrexate LPF, Rheumatrex Dose Pack

Func. class.: Antineoplastic-antimetabolite

Chem. class.: Folic acid antagonist

Action: Inhibits an enzyme that reduces folic acid, which is needed for nucleic acid synthesis in all cells; S phase of cell cycle specific; immunosuppressive

Uses: Acute lymphocytic leukemia, in combination for breast, lung, head, neck carcinoma; lymphosarcoma, gestational choriocarcinoma, hydatidiform mole psoriasis, rheumatoid arthritis, mycosis fungoides

Investigational uses: Used investigationally to produce abortion

Dosage and routes:

Leukemia

• *Adult and child:* **PO** 3.3 mg/m²/day with prednisone **IT** 12 mg/m², maintenance 30 mg/m²/day 2 x/wk; **IV** 2.5 mg/kg q2wk

Choriocarcinoma

• *Adult and child:* **PO** 15-30 mg/m² qd × 5 days, then off 1 wk; may repeat

Osteosarcoma

• *Adult and child:* **IV** 12 g/m² given over 4 hr, then leucovorin rescue

Mycosis fungoides

• *Adult:* **PO** 2.5-10 mg/day until cleared (may be many months); **IM** 50 mg qwk or 25 mg 2 x /wk

Psoriasis

• *Adult:* **PO/IM/IV** 10 mg qwk, may increase to 25 mg qwk

Available forms: Tabs 2.5 mg; inj 25 mg/ml; powder for inj 20, 25, 50, 100, 250 mg, 1 g; sodium inj 2.5, 25 mg/ml

Side effects/adverse reactions:

HEMA: **Leukopenia, thrombocytopenia, myelosuppression, anemia**

GI: Nausea, vomiting, anorexia, diarrhea, stomatitis, **hepatotoxicity,** cramps, ulcer, gastritis, **GI hemorrhage,** abdominal pain, hematemesis

GU: Urinary retention, **renal failure,** menstrual irregularities, defective spermatogenesis, **hematuria, azotemia, uric acid nephropathy**

INTEG: Rash, alopecia, dry skin, urticaria, photosensitivity, folliculitis, vasculitis, petechiae, ecchymosis, acne, alopecia

CNS: Dizziness, **convulsions,** headache, confusion, hemiparesis, malaise, fatigue, chills, fever

Contraindications: Hypersensitivity, leukopenia (<2500/mm³), thrombocytopenia (<100,000/mm³), anemia, psoriatic patients with severe renal/hepatic disease, pregnancy (D), alcoholism, HIV

Precautions: Renal disease, lactation

Pharmacokinetics:

PO: Readily absorbed

PO/IM/IV: Onset 4-7 days; peak 1-2 wk; duration 3 wk

IT: Onset, peak, duration unknown

Not metabolized; excreted in urine (unchanged); crosses placenta, blood-brain barrier; 50% plasma protein bound

Interactions:

• Increased toxicity: aspirin, sulfa drugs, other antineoplastics, radiation, alcohol, probenecid, phenytoin, phenylbutazone, pyrimethamine, penicillins

• Decreased effect of oral digoxin

• Increased hypoprothrombinemia: oral anticoagulants

• Decreased effect of methotrexate: folic acid supplements

M

- Possible fatal interactions: non-steroidal antiinflammatory drugs

NURSING CONSIDERATIONS
Assess:

- CBC, differential, platelet count weekly; withhold drug if WBC is <3500/mm³ or platelet count is <100,000/mm³; notify prescriber; drug should be discontinued
- Renal function studies: BUN, serum uric acid, urine CrCl, electrolytes before, during therapy
- I&O ratio; report fall in urine output to <30 ml/hr
- Monitor temp q4h; fever may indicate beginning infection; no rectal temps
- Liver function tests before and during therapy: bilirubin, alk phosphatase, AST (SGOT), ALT (SGPT); liver biopsy should be done before start of therapy (psoriasis patients)
- Bleeding time, coagulation time during treatment
- Bleeding: hematuria, guaiac, bruising or petechiae, mucosa or orifices q8h
- Food preferences; list likes, dislikes
- Effects of alopecia on body image; discuss feelings about body changes
- ◆ Hepatotoxicity: yellow skin and sclera, dark urine, clay-colored stools, pruritus, abdominal pain, fever, diarrhea
- Buccal cavity q8h for dryness, sores, ulceration, white patches, oral pain, bleeding, dysphagia
- Symptoms indicating severe allergic reaction: rash, urticaria, itching, flushing

Administer:

- Antacid before oral agent; give drug after evening meal before bedtime
- Antiemetic 30-60 min before giving drug
- Allopurinol or sodium bicarbonate to maintain uric acid levels, alkalinization of urine, adequate fluids
- Antibiotics for prophylaxis of infection
- Topical or systemic analgesics for pain
- Transfusion for anemia

IV

- After diluting 5 mg/2 ml of sterile H₂O for inj; give through Y-tube or 3-way stopcock at 10 mg or less/min
- ◆ Leucovorin Ca within 12 hr of this drug to prevent tissue damage; check agency policy

Additive compatibilities: Cephalothin, cyclophosphamide, cytarabine, fluorouracil, hydroxyzine, mercaptopurine, ondansetron, sodium bicarbonate, vincristine

Solution compatibilities: Amino acids, 4.25%/D₂₅, D₅W, sodium bicarbonate 0.05 mol/L, sodium chloride 0.9%

Syringe compatibilities: Bleomycin, cisplatin, cyclophosphamide, doxapram, doxorubicin, fluorouracil, furosemide, heparin, leucovorin, mitomycin, vinblastine, vincristine

Y-site compatibilities: Allopurinol, amifostine, asparaginase, aztreonam, bleomycin, cefepime, ceftriaxone, cimetidine, cisplatin, cyclophosphamide, cytarabine, daunorubicin, dexchlorpheniramine, diphenhydramine, doxorubicin, etoposide, famotidine, filgrastim, fludarabine, fluorouracil, furosemide, gallium, ganciclovir, granisetron, heparin, hydromorphone, imipenem-cilastatin, leucovorin, lorazepam, melphalan, mesna, methylprednisolone, metoclopramide, mitomycin, morphine, ondansetron, oxacillin, paclitaxel, piperacillin/tazobactam, prochlorperazine, ranitidine, sargramostim,

---

◆ = Nursing alert   ⧸⧸ = Herb-drug interaction   ⊘ = Do not crush

teniposide, thiotepa, vinblastine, vincristine, vinorelbine
Perform/provide:
• Strict medical asepsis and protective isolation if WBC levels are low
• Liquid diet: carbonated beverage, Jell-O; dry toast, crackers may be added when patient is not nauseated or vomiting
• Increased fluid intake to 2-3 L/day to prevent urate deposits, calculi formation, unless contraindicated
• Diet low in purines: absence of organ meats (kidney, liver), dried beans, peas to maintain alkaline urine
• Rinsing of mouth tid-qid with water, club soda; brushing of teeth bid-tid with soft brush or cotton-tipped applicators for stomatitis; use unwaxed dental floss
• Nutritious diet with iron, vitamin supplements
• Storage in tightly closed container in cool environment; store injection, powder for injection in dark, dry area
Evaluate:
• Therapeutic response: decreased tumor size, spread of malignancy
Teach patient/family:
• To report any complaints, side effects to nurse or prescriber: black tarry stools, chills, fever, sore throat, bleeding, bruising, cough, shortness of breath, dark or bloody urine
• That hair may be lost during treatment; wig or hairpiece may make patient feel better; tell patient that new hair may be different in color, texture (alopecia is rare)
• To avoid foods with citric acid, hot or rough texture if stomatitis is present
• To report stomatitis: any bleeding, white spots, ulcerations in mouth to prescriber; tell patient to examine mouth qd, report symptoms to nurse
• That contraceptive measures are recommended during therapy for at least 8 wk following cessation of therapy
• To drink 10-12 glasses of fluid/day
• To avoid alcohol, salicylates, live vaccines
• To avoid use of razors, commercial mouthwash

---

methotrimeprazine (℞)

(meth-oh-trye-mep'ra-zeen)
Levoprome, Nozinan*
Func. class.: Nonopiate analgesic
Chem. class.: Aliphatic (propylamine-phenothiazine derivative)

Action: Depresses cerebral cortex, hypothalamus, limbic system; blocks neurotransmission produced by dopamine at synapse; exhibits strong α-adrenergic, anticholinergic blocking action, antihistamine
Uses: Sedation, analgesia, preoperative and postoperative analgesia, obstetric analgesia in nonambulatory patients
Dosage and routes:
Analgesia/sedation
• *Adult and child >12 yr:* IM 10-20 mg q4-6h prn
• *Elderly:* IM 5-10 mg q4-6h
Preoperative medication
• *Adult and child >12 yr:* IM 2-20 mg 45 min to 3 hr before surgery
Postoperative medication
• *Adult and child >12 yr:* IM 2.5-7.5 mg q4-6h titrated to patient's needs
Obstetric analgesia
• *Adult:* 15-20 mg, may be repeated
Available forms: Inj 20 mg/ml
Side effects/adverse reactions:
*HEMA: **Thrombocytopenia, agranulocytosis, leukopenia, neutropenia, hemolytic anemia*** (long-term, high dose)
CNS: Weakness, dizziness, drowsi-

ness, confusion, delirium, euphoria, headache, sedation, EPS

GI: Nausea, vomiting, abdominal pain, dry mouth, jaundice (long-term use)

*GU: **Hematuria**,* dysuria, hesitancy, retention, uterine inertia (rare)

INTEG: Pain, edema at injection site, fever, chills

EENT: Nasal congestion, blurred vision, slurred speech

CV: Orthostatic hypotension, palpitations, tachycardia, bradycardia

Contraindications: Hypersensitivity to this drug, phenothiazines, bisulfite; seizures; severe hepatic disease; severe renal disease; severe cardiac disease; coma

Precautions: Elderly, pregnancy (C)

Pharmacokinetics:

IM: Onset 20-30 min, peak 1-2 hr, duration 4 hr; metabolized by liver, excreted by kidneys and in feces, crosses placenta, excreted in breast milk

Interactions:

• Increased sedation: CNS depressants, alcohol, barbiturates, reserpine, narcotics, general anesthetics, meprobamate

NURSING CONSIDERATIONS

Assess:

• Blood studies: CBC, ALT (SGPT), AST (SGOT), bilirubin

• VS q10min for 30 min; watch for decreasing B/P with increased pulse that may occur 10-30 min after injection; continue to monitor closely for 6-12 hr after several injections

• Effect on uterine contractions, fetal heart tones if using for labor

Administer:

• After removal of cigarettes to prevent fires

• IM inj deep in large muscle mass to prevent tissue sloughing; rotate sites

• Lowest dose, then gradually increase; lower doses are required after general anesthesia

Syringe compatibilities: Butorphanol, hydroxyzine, metoclopramide, perphenazine, sufentanil

Y-site compatibilities: Sufentanil

Perform/provide:

• Bed rest for several hr after injection if orthostatic hypotension occurs

• Safety measures: side rails, nightlight, call bell within easy reach

• Storage in darkness; expires after 5 yr

• Assistance with ambulation for 6 hr after injection

Evaluate:

• Therapeutic response: decrease in pain, grimacing, absence of change in VS, ability to cough and breathe deep after surgery

Teach patient/family:

• To avoid ambulation without assistance for 6 hr after drug is given

Treatment of overdose: Monitor electrolytes, vital signs

---

methylcellulose (OTC)

(meth-ill-sell'yoo-lose)

Citrucel

Func. class.: Laxative, bulk

Chem. class.: Hydrophilic semi-synthetic cellulose derivative

Action: Attracts water, expands in intestine to increase peristalsis; also absorbs excess water in stool; decreases diarrhea

Uses: Constipation

Dosage and routes:

• *Adult:* **PO** 5-20 ml tid with 8 oz H_2O

• *Child:* **PO** 5-10 ml qd or bid with H_2O or 500 mg tid with 8 oz H_2O

Available forms: Powder 105 mg/g; sol 450 mg/5 ml; tab 500 mg

---

⬧ = Nursing alert   🌿 = Herb-drug interaction   ⊘ = Do not crush

Side effects/adverse reactions:
GI: Obstruction, abdominal distention .

Contraindications: Hypersensitivity, GI obstruction, hepatitis

Pharmacokinetics:
PO: Onset 12-24 hr, peak 1-3 days

Interactions:
• Decreased absorption: antibiotics, digitalis, nitrofurantoin, salicylates, tetracyclines, oral anticoagulants

NURSING CONSIDERATIONS
Assess:
• Blood, urine electrolytes if used often
• I&O ratio to identify fluid loss
• Cause of constipation; lack of fluids, bulk, exercise
• Cramping, rectal bleeding, nausea, vomiting; drug should be discontinued

Administer:
PO
• Alone for better absorption; do not take within 1 hr of other drugs
• In morning or evening (oral dose)

Evaluate:
• Therapeutic response: decrease in constipation

Teach patient/family:
🚫 To swallow tabs whole; do not break, crush, or chew
• To increase fluid intake
• That normal bowel movements do not always occur daily
• Not to use in presence of abdominal pain, nausea, vomiting
• To notify prescriber if constipation unrelieved or if symptoms of electrolyte imbalance occur: muscle cramps, pain, weakness, dizziness, excessive thirst

---

methyldopa/methyldopate (℞)

(meth-ill-doe′pa)
Aldomet, methyldopa/methyldopate

Func. class.: Antihypertensive
Chem. class.: Centrally acting α-adrenergic inhibitor

Action: Stimulates central inhibitory α-adrenergic receptors or acts as false transmitter, resulting in reduction of arterial pressure

Uses: Hypertension

Dosage and routes:
• *Adult:* **PO** 250-500 mg bid or tid, then adjusted q2d as needed, 0.5-2 g qd in 2-4 divided doses (maintenance), not to exceed 3 g/day; **IV** 250-500 mg in 100 ml D_5W q6h, run over 30-60 min, not to exceed 1 g q6h
• *Geriatric:* **PO** 125 mg bid-tid, increase q2d as needed, max 3 g/day
• *Child:* **PO** 10 mg/kg/day in 2-4 divided doses, not to exceed 65 mg/kg or 3 g/day, whichever is less; **IV** 20-40 mg/kg/day in 4 divided doses, not to exceed 65 mg/kg or 3 g, whichever is less

Available forms: Methyldopa: Tabs 125, 250, 500 mg; oral susp 50 mg/ml; Methyldopate: Inj 50 mg/ml

Side effects/adverse reactions:
ENDO: Breast enlargement, gynecomastia, lactation, amenorrhea
GI: Nausea, vomiting, diarrhea, constipation, hepatic dysfunction, sore or "black" tongue, pancreatitis
CV: Bradycardia, myocarditis, orthostatic hypotension, angina, edema, weight gain, *CHF*
CNS: Drowsiness, weakness, dizziness, sedation, headache, depression, psychosis paresthesias, parkinsonism, Bell's palsy, nightmares

EENT: Nasal congestion, eczema
HEMA: ***Leukopenia, thrombocyto-***
penia, hemolytic anemia, granulo-
cytopenia, positive Coombs' test
INTEG: Rash, toxic epidermal
necrolysis, lupuslike syndrome
GU: Impotence, failure to ejaculate
Contraindications: Active hepatic
disease, hypersensitivity, blood dys-
crasias
Precautions: Pregnancy (C), liver
disease, eclampsia, severe cardiac
disease
Pharmacokinetics:
PO: Peak 2-4 hr, duration 12-24 hr
IV: Peak 2 hr, duration 10-16 hr
Metabolized by liver, excreted in
urine
Interactions:
• Increased pressor effect: sympa-
thomimetic amines (norepinephrine,
phenylpropanolamine)
• Increased hypotension: levodopa
• Increased psychosis: haloperidol
• Increased action of anesthetics
• Lithium toxicity: lithium
• Increased B/P: phenothiazines,
beta blockers
• Increased hypoglycemia: tolbuta-
mide
• Decreased effects of methyldopa:
barbiturates, tricyclic antidepres-
sants
🌿 Decreased effect, increased EPS:
Indian snakeroot
Lab test interferences:
Interference: Urinary uric acid, se-
rum creatinine, AST
False increase: Urinary catechol-
amines

NURSING CONSIDERATIONS
Assess:
• Blood studies: neutrophils, de-
creased platelets
• Baselines in renal, liver function
tests before therapy begins
• B/P during beginning treatment,
periodically thereafter

• Allergic reaction: rash, fever, pruritus, urticaria; drug should be discontinued if antihistamines fail to
help
• CNS symptoms especially in the
elderly
• Symptoms of CHF: edema, dyspnea, wet rales, B/P
• Renal symptoms: polyuria, oliguria, frequency
Administer:
IV
• After diluting with 100-200 ml
D_5W; run over ½-1 hr
Additive compatibilities: Aminophylline, ascorbic acid, chloramphenicol, diphenhydramine, heparin, magnesium sulfate, multivitamins, netilmicin, potassium chloride,
promazine, sodium bicarbonate, suc-
cinylcholine, verapamil, vit B/C
Solution compatibilities: D_5W, D_5/
0.9% NaCl, Ringer's, sodium bicar-
bonate 5%, 0.9% NaCl, amino acids
4.25%/D_{25}, Dextran$_6$/0.9% NaCl,
Normosol R, Normosol M/D_5W
Y-site compatibilities: Esmolol,
heparin, meperidine, morphine, theophylline
Perform/provide:
• Storage of tabs in tight container
Evaluate:
• Therapeutic response: decrease in
B/P in hypertension
Teach patient/family:
• To avoid hazardous activities
• To administer 1 hr before meals
• Not to discontinue drug abruptly,
or withdrawal symptoms may oc-
cur: anxiety, increased B/P, head-
ache, insomnia, increased pulse,
tremors, nausea, sweating
• Not to use OTC (cough, cold, al-
lergy) products unless directed by
prescriber
• To avoid sunlight or wear sun-
screen; photosensitivity may occur

➤ = Nursing alert   🌿 = Herb-drug interaction   🚫 = Do not crush

• To comply with dosage schedule even if feeling better
• To rise slowly to sitting or standing position to minimize orthostatic hypotension
• To notify prescriber of mouth sores, sore throat, fever, swelling of hands or feet, irregular heartbeat, chest pain, signs of angioedema
• That excessive perspiration, dehydration, vomiting, diarrhea may lead to fall in blood pressure; consult prescriber
• That dizziness, fainting, lightheadedness may occur during first few days of therapy
• That compliance is necessary; not to skip or stop drug unless directed by prescriber
• That drug may cause skin rash or impaired perspiration

Treatment of overdose: Gastric evacuation, sympathomimetics may be indicated; if severe, hemodialysis

---

methylene blue (℞)

(meth'i-leen)
methylene blue, Urolene Blue
Func. class.: Urinary tract antiseptic
Chem. class.: Antiseptic dye

Action: Oxidation-reduction; has opposite action on hemoglobin depending on concentration; with increased concentration, converts ferrous ion of reduced hemoglobin to ferric form; methemoglobin is thus produced; prolonged administration accelerates destruction of erythrocytes

Uses: Oxalate urinary tract calculi; UTIs caused by *E. coli, Klebsiella, Enterobacter, P. mirabilis, P. vulgaris, P. morganii, Serratia, Citro-*

bacter, cyanide poisoning, methemoglobinemia

Dosage and routes:
• *Adult:* **PO** 65-130 mg pc with full glass of water

Cyanide poisoning/methemoglobinemia
• *Adult and child:* **IV** 1-2 mg/kg of 1% sol; inject slowly over 5 min or more

Available forms: Tabs 65 mg; inj 10 mg/ml

Side effects/adverse reactions:
CV: Cyanosis, CV abnormalities
INTEG: Pruritus, rash, urticaria, photosensitivity, profuse sweating
CNS: Dizziness, headache, drowsiness, mental confusion, fever with large doses
GI: Nausea, vomiting, abdominal pain, diarrhea
GU: Bladder irritation

Contraindications: Hypersensitivity to this drug, renal insufficiency

Precautions: Anemia, renal disease, hepatic disease, G6PD deficiency, pregnancy (C)

Pharmacokinetics:
PO/IV: Excreted in urine, bile, feces

NURSING CONSIDERATIONS
Assess:
• For cyanosis
• I&O ratio; urine pH <5.5 is ideal
• Hct, Hgb
• CNS symptoms: insomnia, headache, drowsiness, confusion
• Allergic reactions: fever, flushing, rash, urticaria, pruritus

Administer:
• After clean-catch urine is obtained for C&S
• Two daily doses if urine output is high or if patient has diabetes

Perform/provide:
• Limited intake of alkaline foods, drugs: milk, dairy products, peanuts, vegetables, alkaline antacids, sodium bicarbonate

---

Evaluate:
• Therapeutic response: decreased pain, frequency, urgency, C&S absence of infection

Teach patient/family:
• That anemia may result with continued administration
• That drug turns urine, sometimes stool, blue-green
• To notify prescriber if symptoms do not improve
• To notify prescriber of any sign/symptoms of side effects or adverse reactions

---

methylergonovine (℞)

(meth-ill-er-goe-noe'veen)
Methergine, Methylergobasine*, methylergonovine
Func. class.: Oxytocic
Chem. class.: Ergot alkaloid

Action: Stimulates uterine, vascular, smooth muscle, causing contractions; decreases bleeding

Uses: Treatment of hemorrhage postpartum or postabortion, uterine contractions

Dosage and routes:
• *Adult:* **IM** 0.2 mg q2-5h, not to exceed 5 doses; **IV** 0.2 mg given over 1 min; **PO** 0.2-0.4 mg q6-12h × 2-7 days after initial **IM** or **IV** dose

Available forms: Inj 0.2 mg/ml; tabs 0.2 mg

Side effects/adverse reactions:
RESP: Dyspnea
GU: Cramping
CNS: Headache, dizziness
GI: Nausea, vomiting
CV: Chest pain, palpitation, *hypertension,* dysrhythmias
EENT: Tinnitus
INTEG: Sweating, rash, allergic reactions

Contraindications: Hypersensitivity to ergot preparations, indication of labor, before delivery of placenta, hypertension, pelvic inflammatory disease, respiratory disease, cardiac disease, peripheral vascular disease

Precautions: Pregnancy (C), severe hepatic disease, severe renal disease, jaundice, diabetes mellitus, convulsive disorders, sepsis

Pharmacokinetics:
PO: Onset 5-25 min, duration 3 hr
IM: Onset 2-5 min, duration 3 hr
IV: Onset immediate, duration 45 min
Metabolized in liver, excreted in urine

Interactions:
• Exercise caution: vasoconstrictors

NURSING CONSIDERATIONS
Assess:
• B/P, pulse, character and amount of vaginal bleeding; watch for indications of hemorrhage
• Respiratory rate, rhythm, depth; notify prescriber of abnormalities
• For uterine relaxation; observe for severe cramping
◆ Ergot toxicity: tinnitus, hypertension, palpitations, chest pain

Administer:
• Only during fourth stage of labor; not to be used to augment labor
• IM in deep muscle mass; rotate injection sites of additional doses

IV
• Undiluted through Y-tube or 3-way stopcock; give 0.2 mg or less/min
• With crash cart available on unit; IV route used only in emergencies

Y-site compatibilities: Heparin, hydrocortisone sodium succinate, potassium chloride, vit B/C

Evaluate:
• Therapeutic response: absence of hemorrhage

◆ = Nursing alert   ⬳ = Herb-drug interaction   ⃠ = Do not crush

Teach patient/family:
• To report increased blood loss, severe abdominal cramps, fever or foul-smelling lochia

---

methylphenidate (℞)

(meth-ill-fen'i-date)
Methidate, Ritalin, Ritalin SR
Func. class.: Cerebral stimulant
Chem. class.: Piperidine derivative

Controlled Substance Schedule II
Action: Increases release of norepinephrine, dopamine in cerebral cortex to reticular activating system; exact action not known
Uses: Attention deficit hyperactivity disorder, narcolepsy
Investigational uses: Depression in the elderly; cancer, stroke patients
Dosage and routes:
Attention deficit hyperactivity disorder
• *Child >6 yr:* 5 mg before breakfast and lunch, increasing by 5-10 mg/wk, not to exceed 60 mg/day
Narcolepsy
• *Adult:* PO 10 mg bid-tid, 30-45 min before meals, may increase up to 40-60 mg/day
Depression (elderly)
• *Geriatric:* PO 2.5 mg qAM, increase q 3rd day by 2.5 mg to desired dose, max 20 mg/day
Available forms: Tabs 5, 10, 20 mg; tabs sus rel 20 mg
Side effects/adverse reactions:
MISC: Fever, arthralgia, scalp hair loss
CNS: Hyperactivity, insomnia, restlessness, talkativeness, dizziness, headache, akathisia, dyskinesia, Gilles de la Tourette's syndrome
GI: Nausea, anorexia, dry mouth, weight loss, abdominal pain

CV: Palpitations, tachycardia, B/P changes, angina, dysrhythmias, ***thrombocytopenic purpura***
*INTEG: **Exfoliative dermatitis,*** urticaria, rash, erythema multiforme
ENDO: Growth retardation
*GU: **Uremia***
*HEMA: **Leukopenia, anemia***
Contraindications: Hypersensitivity, anxiety, history of Gilles de la Tourette's syndrome; children <6 yr, glaucoma
Precautions: Hypertension, depression, pregnancy (C), seizures, lactation, drug abuse
Pharmacokinetics:
PO: Onset ½-1 hr, duration 4-6 hr, metabolized by liver, excreted by kidneys
Interactions:
• Hypertensive crisis: MAOIs or within 14 days of MAOIs, vasopressors
• Decreased effect of guanethidine
NURSING CONSIDERATIONS
Assess:
• VS, B/P; may reverse antihypertensives; check patients with cardiac disease more often for increased B/P
• CBC, urinalysis, in diabetes: blood sugar, urine sugar; insulin changes may have to be made, since eating will decrease
• Height, growth rate q3mo in children; growth rate may be decreased
• Mental status: mood, sensorium, affect, stimulation, insomnia, aggressiveness
◆ Withdrawal symptoms: headache, nausea, vomiting, muscle pain, weakness
• Appetite, sleep, speech patterns
Administer:
• At least 6 hr before hs to avoid sleeplessness
• Gum, hard candy, frequent sips of water for dry mouth

M

Evaluate:
• Therapeutic response: decreased hyperactivity or ability to stay awake
Teach patient/family:
• To decrease caffeine consumption (coffee, tea, cola, chocolate); may increase irritability, stimulation
🚫 Not to break, crush, or chew time-released medication
• To avoid OTC preparations unless approved by prescriber
• To taper off drug over several wk, or depression, increased sleeping, lethargy will occur
• To avoid alcohol ingestion
• To avoid hazardous activities until stabilized on medication
• To get needed rest; patients will feel more tired at end of day
Treatment of overdose: Administer fluids; hemodialysis or peritoneal dialysis; antihypertensive for increased B/P; administer short-acting barbiturate before lavage

---

methylprednisolone/ methylprednisolone acetate/methylpred-nisolone sodium succinate (℞)

(meth-il-pred-niss'oh-lone)
Medrol/Depo-Medrol, Dura-lone, Medralone, Rep-Pred/A-Methapred, Solu-Medrol
Func. class.: Corticosteroid
Chem. class.: Glucocorticoid, immediate acting

Action: Decreases inflammation by suppression of migration of polymorphonuclear leukocytes, fibroblasts; reversal of increased capillary permeability and lysosomal stabilization
Uses: Severe inflammation, shock, adrenal insufficiency, collagen disorders

Dosage and routes:
Adrenal insufficiency/inflammation
• *Adult:* PO 2-60 mg in 4 divided doses; IM 40-80 mg (acetate); IM/IV 10-250 mg (succinate); intraarticular 4-30 mg (acetate)
• *Child:* IV 117 μg-1.66 mg/kg in 3-4 divided doses (succinate)
Shock
• *Adult:* IV 100-250 mg q2-6h (succinate)
Available forms: Tabs 2, 4, 6, 8, 16, 24, 32 mg; inj 20, 40, 80 mg/ml acetate; inj 40, 125, 500, 1000 mg/vial succinate; dose pack 4 mg tabs
Side effects/adverse reactions:
CNS: Depression, flushing, sweating, headache, mood changes
CV: Hypertension, *circulatory collapse, thrombophlebitis, embolism,* tachycardia
EENT: Fungal infections, increased intraocular pressure, blurred vision, cataracts
GI: Diarrhea, nausea, abdominal distention, GI hemorrhage, increased appetite, pancreatitis
HEMA: Thrombocytopenia
INTEG: Acne, poor wound healing, ecchymosis, petechiae
MS: Fractures, osteoporosis, weakness
Contraindications: Psychosis, hypersensitivity, idiopathic thrombocytopenia, acute glomerulonephritis, amebiasis, fungal infections, nonasthmatic bronchial disease, child <2 yr, AIDS, TB
Precautions: Pregnancy (C), lactation, diabetes mellitus, glaucoma, osteoporosis, seizure disorders, ulcerative colitis, CHF, myasthenia gravis, renal disease, esophagitis, peptic ulcer
Pharmacokinetics: Well absorbed PO, IM
PO: Peak 1-2 hr, duration 1½ days

🔷 = Nursing alert   ⚗ = Herb-drug interaction   🚫 = Do not crush

IM: Peak 4-8 days, duration 1-4 wk
Intraarticular: Peak 1 wk
Half-life >3½ hr; crosses placenta, enters breast milk in small amounts; metabolized in liver, excreted by kidneys (unchanged)

Interactions:

• Decreased action of methylprednisolone: cholestyramine, colestipol, barbiturates, rifampin, ephedrine, phenytoin, theophylline
• Decreased effects of anticoagulants, anticonvulsants, antidiabetics, ambenonium, neostigmine, isoniazid, toxoids, vaccines, anticholinesterases, salicylates, somatrem
• Increased side effects: alcohol, salicylates, indomethacin, amphotericin B, digitalis, cyclosporine, diuretics
• Increased action of methylprednisolone: salicylates, estrogens, indomethacin, oral contraceptives, ketoconazole, macrolide antibiotics
🖉 Potassium deficiency: aloe, cascara sagrada bark, buckthorn bark/berry, rhubarb root, senna leaf/fruits

Lab test interferences:
Increase: Cholesterol, Na, blood glucose, uric acid, Ca, urine glucose
Decrease: Ca, K, T_4, T_3, thyroid ^{131}I uptake test, urine 17-OHCS, 17-KS
False negative: Skin allergy tests

NURSING CONSIDERATIONS
Assess:
• K depletion: parethesias, fatigue, nausea, vomiting, depression, polyuria, dysrhythmias, weakness
• Edema, hypertension, cardiac symptoms
• Mental status: affect, mood, behavioral changes, aggression
• K, blood sugar, urine glucose while on long-term therapy; hypokalemia and hyperglycemia
• Joint mobility, pain, edema if given intraarticularly

• Weight daily; notify prescriber of weekly gain >5 lb
• B/P q4h, pulse; notify prescriber of chest pain, rales
• I&O ratio; be alert for decreasing urinary output, increasing edema
• Adrenal insufficiency: weight loss, nausea, vomiting, confusion, anxiety, hypotension, weakness
• Plasma cortisol levels during long-term therapy (normal level: 138-635 nmol/L SI units when drawn at 8 AM)
• Growth in children on long-term treatment

Administer:
• Titrated dose; use lowest effective dose
• IM inj deep in large muscle mass; rotate sites; avoid deltoid; use 21G needle; after shaking suspension (parenteral)
• In one dose in AM to prevent adrenal suppression; avoid SC administration; may damage tissue
• With food or milk to decrease GI symptoms (PO)

IV
• After diluting with diluent provided; agitate slowly; give 500 mg or less/1 min or longer; may be given as IV infusion in its own diluent over 10-20 min

Additive compatibilities: Chloramphenicol, cimetidine, clindamycin, dopamine, granisetron, heparin, norepinephrine, penicillin G potassium, ranitidine, theophylline, verapamil
Syringe compatibilities: Granisetron, metoclopramide
Y-site compatibilities: Acyclovir, amifostine, amrinone, aztreonam, cefepime, cisplatin, cladribine, cyclophosphamide, cytarabine, dopamine, doxorubicin, enalaprilat, famotidine, fludarabine, granisetron, heparin, melphalan, meperidine, methotrexate, metronidazole, midazolam, morphine, piperacillin/

M

  Side effects: *italics* = common; **bold italics** = life-threatening

tazobactam, sodium bicarbonate, tacrolimus, teniposide, theophylline, thiotepa

Perform/provide:

• Assistance with ambulation in patient with bone tissue disease to prevent fractures

Evaluate:

• Therapeutic response: ease of respirations, decreased inflammation; decreased symptoms of adrenal insufficiency

• Infection: increased temp, WBC, even after withdrawal of medication; drug masks infection

Teach patient/family:

• To increase intake of K, Ca, protein

• That ID as steroid user should be carried

• To notify prescriber if therapeutic response decreases; dosage adjustment may be needed

• Not to discontinue abruptly, or adrenal crisis can result

• To avoid OTC products: salicylates, alcohol in cough products, cold preparations unless directed by prescriber; to avoid vaccinations, since immunosuppression occurs

• About cushingoid symptoms

• To recognize the symptoms of adrenal insufficiency: nausea, anorexia, fatigue, dizziness, dyspnea, weakness, joint pain

---

methysergide (℞)

(meth-i-ser′jide)

Sansert

Func. class.: Adrenergic blocker, serotonin antagonist

Chem. class.: Ergot derivative

Action: Competitively blocks serotonin HT receptors in CNS and periphery; potent vasoconstrictor

Uses: Prophylaxis for migraine and other vascular headaches. If no improvement is noted in 3 wk, drug is unlikely to be beneficial

Dosage and routes:

• *Adult:* **PO** 2 mg bid with meals

Available forms: Tabs 2 mg

Side effects/adverse reactions:

CNS: Tremors, anxiety, insomnia, headache, dizziness, euphoria, confusion, depersonalization, hallucination, paresthesias, drowsiness

CV: Retroperitoneal fibrosis, valvular thickening, palpitations, tachycardia, postural hypertension, angina, *thrombophlebitis,* ECG changes, *cardiac fibrosis*

GI: Nausea, vomiting, weight gain

MS: Arthralgia, myalgia

INTEG: Flushing, rash, alopecia

HEMA: Blood dyscrasias

Contraindications: Hypersensitivity to ergot, tartrazine, occlusion (peripheral, vascular), CAD, hepatic disease, renal disease, peptic ulcer, hypertension, connective tissue disease, fibrotic pulmonary disease

Precautions: Pregnancy (C), lactation, children

Pharmacokinetics:

PO: Half-life 10 hr, metabolized by liver, excreted in urine (metabolites/unchanged drug)

Interactions:

• Increased vasoconstriction: β-blockers

• Decreased effect of narcotic analgesics

NURSING CONSIDERATIONS

Assess:

• Weight daily; check for peripheral edema in feet, legs; B/P

• For stress, activity, recreation, coping mechanisms

• Neurologic status: LOC, blurring vision, nausea, vomiting, tingling in extremities that precede headache

• Ingestion of tyramine foods (pickled products, beer, wine, aged cheese), food additives, preserva-

---

tives, colorings, artificial sweeteners, chocolate, caffeine may precipitate these types of headaches

Administer:

PO

• Give with or after meals to avoid GI symptoms

• Only to women who are not pregnant; harm to fetus may occur

• For less than 6 mo continuously a 3-4 wk drug-free period must follow each 6 mo period

Perform/provide:

• Storage in dark area

• Quiet, calm environment with decreased stimulation for noise, bright light, or excessive talking

Evaluate:

• Therapeutic response: decrease in frequency, severity of headache

Teach patient/family:

• Not to use OTC medications; serious drug interactions may occur

• To maintain dose at approved level, not to increase even if drug does not relieve headache

• To report side effects: increased vasoconstriction starting with cold extremities, then paresthesia, weakness

• That headaches may increase when drug discontinued after long-term use

• To keep drug out of reach of children; death may occur

• To report at once: dyspnea, paresthesias, urinary problems, pain in abdomen, chest, back, legs

• To use drug for less than 6 mo unless a 3-4 wk rest period has been taken

• That drug may cause drowsiness

---

metipranolol (R)

(met-ee-pran'oh-lole)
Optipranolol

Func. class.: β-adrenergic blocker

Chem. class.: I-isomer

Action: Reduces production of aqueous humor by unknown mechanism

Uses: Ocular hypertension, chronic open-angle glaucoma

Dosage and routes:

• *Adult:* **INSTILL** 1 gtt bid

Available forms: Sol 0.3%

Side effects/adverse reactions:

CNS: Weakness, fatigue, depression, anxiety, headache, confusion

GI: Nausea, anorexia, dyspepsia

EENT: Eye irritation, conjunctivitis, keratitis

INTEG: Rash, urticaria

CV: **Bradycardia,** hypertension

RESP: **Bronchospasm,** dyspnea, bronchitis, coughing, rhinitis

Contraindications: Hypersensitivity, asthma, 2nd or 3rd degree heart block, right ventricular failure, congenital glaucoma (infants)

Precautions: Pregnancy (C), uncompensated CHF

Pharmacokinetics: Onset 15-30 min, peak 1-2 hr, duration 24 hr

Interactions:

• Increased effect: propranolol, metoprolol

NURSING CONSIDERATIONS

Assess:

• B/P, heart rate throughout treatment

• For increased intraocular pressure

• For eye irritation, conjunctivitis

Evaluate:

• Therapeutic response: decreased intraocular pressure

Teach patient/family:

• To report change in vision (blur-

M

ring or loss of sight), trouble breathing, sweating, flushing
• The proper method of instillation, including pressure on lacrimal sac for 1 min, and not to touch dropper to eye
• That long-term therapy may be required
• That blurred vision will decrease with continued use of drug

---

metoclopramide (R)

(met-oh-kloe-pra'mide)
Clopra, Emex*, Maxeran*, Maxolon, metoclopramide HCl, Octamide PFS, Reclomide, Reglan

Func. class.: Cholinergic
Chem. class.: Central dopamine receptor antagonist

Action: Enhances response to acetylcholine of tissue in upper GI tract, which causes contraction of gastric muscle; relaxes pyloric, duodenal segments; increases peristalsis without stimulating secretions, blocks dopamine in chemoreceptor trigger zone of CNS

Uses: Prevention of nausea, vomiting induced by chemotherapy, radiation, delayed gastric emptying, gastroesophageal reflux

Dosage and routes:
Renal dose
• CrCl <40 ml/min 50% of dose
Nausea/vomiting
• *Adult:* IV 2 mg/kg q2h × 5 doses 30 min before administration of chemotherapy
• *Child:* IV 0.1-0.2 mg/kg/dose
Delayed gastric emptying
• *Adult:* PO 10 mg 30 min ac, hs × 2-8 wk
• *Geriatric:* PO 5 mg ½ hr ac hs, increase to 10 mg if needed

Gastroesophageal reflux
• *Adult:* PO 10-15 mg qid 30 min ac
• *Child:* 0.4-0.8 mg/kg/day divided in 4 doses
Available forms: Tabs 5, 10 mg; syr 5 mg/5 ml; inj 5 mg/ml
Side effects/adverse reactions:
CNS: Sedation, fatigue, restlessness, headache, sleeplessness, dystonia, dizziness, drowsiness
GI: Dry mouth, constipation, nausea, anorexia, vomiting, diarrhea
GU: Decreased libido, prolactin secretion, amenorrhea, galactorrhea
CV: Hypotension, supraventricular tachycardia
INTEG: Urticaria, rash
HEMA: Neutropenia, leukopenia
Contraindications: Hypersensitivity to this drug or procaine or procainamide, seizure disorder, pheochromocytoma, breast cancer (prolactin dependent), GI obstruction
Precautions: Pregnancy (B), lactation, GI hemorrhage, CHF, Parkinson's disease
Pharmacokinetics:
IV: Onset 1-3 min, duration 1-2 hr
PO: Onset ½-1 hr, duration 1-2 hr
IM: Onset 10-15 min, duration 1-2 hr
Metabolized by liver, excreted in urine, half-life 4 hr
Interactions:
• Decreased action of digoxin
• Decreased action of metoclopramide: anticholinergics, opiates
• Increased sedation: alcohol, other CNS depressants
Lab test interferences:
Increase: Prolactin, aldosterone, thyrotropin
NURSING CONSIDERATIONS
Assess:
• For EPS and tardive dyskinesia, more likely to occur in elderly patient
• Mental status: depression, anxiety, irritability

◆ = Nursing alert   ⫽ = Herb-drug interaction   ⊘ = Do not crush

• GI complaints: nausea, vomiting, anorexia, constipation

Administer:

• ½-1 hr before meals for better absorption

• Gum, hard candy, frequent rinsing of mouth for dry oral cavity

IV

• Undiluted if dose is <10 mg; give over 2 min; 10 mg or more may be diluted in 50 ml or more D_5W, NaCl, Ringer's, LR and given over 15 min or more

Additive compatibilities: Clindamycin, meropenem, morphine, multivitamins, potassium acetate, potassium chloride, potassium phosphate, verapamil

Syringe compatibilities: Aminophylline, ascorbic acid, atropine, benztropine, bleomycin, butorphanol, chlorpromazine, cisplatin, cyclophosphamide, cytarabine, dexamethasone, dimenhydrinate, diphenhydramine, doxorubicin, droperidol, fentanyl, fluorouracil, heparin, hydrocortisone, hydroxyzine, insulin (regular), leucovorin, lidocaine, magnesium sulfate, meperidine, methotrimeprazine, methylprednisolone, midazolam, mitomycin, morphine, pentazocine, perphenazine, prochlorperazine, promazine, promethazine, ranitidine, scopolamine, sufentanil, vinblastine, vincristine, vit B/C

Y-site compatibilities: Acyclovir, aldesleukin, amifostine, aztreonam, bleomycin, ciprofloxacin, cisplatin, cladribine, cyclophosphamide, cytarabine, diltiazem, doxorubicin, droperidol, famotidine, filgrastim, fluconazole, fludarabine, fluorouracil, foscarnet, gallium, granisetron, heparin, idarubicin, leucovorin, melphalan, meperidine, meropenum, methotrexate, mitomycin, morphine, ondansetron, paclitaxel, piperacillin/tazobactam, propofol, sargramostim, sufentanil, tacrolimus, teniposide, thiotepa, vinblastine, vincristine, vinorelbine, zidovudine

Perform/provide:

• Protect from light with aluminum foil during infusion

• Discard open ampules

Evaluate:

• Therapeutic response: absence of nausea, vomiting, anorexia, fullness

Teach patient/family:

• To avoid driving, other hazardous activities until patient is stabilized on this medication

• To avoid alcohol, other CNS depressants that will enhance sedating properties of this drug

---

metocurine (R)

(met-oh-kyoor′een)
Metubine
Func. class.: Neuromuscular blocker (nondepolarizing)
Chem. class.: Methyl analog of tubocurarine

Action: Inhibits transmission of nerve impulses by binding with cholinergic receptor sites, antagonizing action of acetylcholine

Uses: Facilitation of endotracheal intubation, skeletal muscle relaxation during mechanical ventilation, surgery, or general anesthesia, reduction of fractures/dislocations

Dosage and routes:

Surgery

• *Adult:* IV 150-400 µg/kg, may give 0.5-1 mg q½-1½h

ECT (electroconvulsive therapy) adjunct

• *Adult:* IV 2-3 mg

Available forms: Inj 2 mg/ml

M

Side effects: *italics* = common; **bold italics** = life-threatening

Side effects/adverse reactions:

CV: Bradycardia, tachycardia, increased B/P

*RESP: **Prolonged apnea, bronchospasm, cyanosis, respiratory depression***

EENT: Increased secretions

INTEG: Rash, flushing, pruritus, urticaria

Contraindications: Hypersensitivity to iodides

Precautions: Pregnancy (C), cardiac disease, hepatic disease, renal disease, lactation, children <2 yr, electrolyte imbalances, dehydration, neuromuscular disease (myasthenia gravis), respiratory disease, or when histamine release is a definite hazard (e.g., asthma)

Pharmacokinetics:

IV: Peak 3-5 min, duration 35-90 min, half-life 3½ hr; excreted in urine, bile (½ unchanged); crosses placenta

Interactions:

• Increased neuromuscular blockade: aminoglycosides, clindamycin, lincomycin, quinidine, local anesthetics, polymyxin antibiotics, lithium, narcotic analgesics, thiazides, enflurane, isoflurane, magnesium sulfate

• Dysrhythmias: theophylline

• Do not mix with barbiturates in sol or syringe; unstable in alkaline sol

NURSING CONSIDERATIONS
Assess:

• For electrolyte imbalances (K, Mg); may lead to increased action of this drug

• Vital signs (B/P, pulse, respirations, airway) until fully recovered; rate, depth, pattern of respirations (keep airway clear), strength of hand grip

• I&O ratio; check for urinary retention, frequency, hesitancy

• Recovery: decreased paralysis of face, diaphragm, leg, arm, rest of body

• Allergic reactions: rash, fever, respiratory distress, pruritus; drug should be discontinued

Administer:

• Using nerve stimulator by anesthesiologist to determine neuromuscular blockade

• Anticholinesterase to reverse neuromuscular blockade

• By slow IV over 1-2 min (only by qualified person, usually an anesthesiologist)

• Only slightly discolored sol

Perform/provide:

• Storage in light-resistant, cool area

• Reassurance if communication is difficult during recovery from neuromuscular blockade

Evaluate:

• Therapeutic response: paralysis of jaw, eyelid, head, neck, rest of body

Teach patient/family:

• That postoperative stiffness is normal and will subside

Treatment of overdose: Edrophonium or neostigmine, atropine; monitor VS; may require mechanical ventilation

---

metolazone (Ŗ)

(me-tole'a-zone)
Diulo, Mykrox, Zaroxolyn
Func. class.: Diuretic
Chem. class.: Thiazide-like quinazoline derivative

Action: Acts on distal tubule and cortical thick ascending limb of the loop of Henle by increasing excretion of water, sodium, chloride, potassium, magnesium, bicarbonate

Uses: Edema, hypertension, CHF

Dosage and routes:

Edema

• *Adult:* **PO** 5-20 mg/day

 = Nursing alert   = Herb-drug interaction   = Do not crush

Hypertension
- *Adult:* **PO** 2.5-5 mg/day (Diulo, Zaroxolyn)
- *Child:* **PO** 0.2-0.4 mg/kg/day divided q12-24h
- *Adult:* **PO** 0.5 mg (Mykrox) qd in AM, may increase to 1 mg

Available forms: Tabs 0.5 (Mykrox), 2.5, 5, 10 mg

Side effects/adverse reactions:

GU: Frequency, polyuria, ***uremia, glucosuria***

CNS: Drowsiness, paresthesia, anxiety, depression, headache, *dizziness, fatigue, weakness*

GI: Nausea, vomiting, anorexia, constipation, diarrhea, cramps, pancreatitis, GI irritation, ***hepatitis***

EENT: Blurred vision

INTEG: Rash, urticaria, purpura, photosensitivity, fever

META: Hyperglycemia, increased creatinine, BUN

*HEMA: **Aplastic anemia, hemolytic anemia, leukopenia, agranulocytosis, neutropenia***

CV: Irregular pulse, orthostatic hypotension, palpitations, volume depletion

ELECT: Hypokalemia, hypomagnesemia, hypercalcemia, hyponatremia, hypochloremia, hypophosphatemia

Contraindications: Hypersensitivity to thiazides or sulfonamides, anuria, lactation

Precautions: Hypokalemia, renal disease, hepatic disease, gout, COPD, lupus erythematosus, diabetes mellitus, pregnancy (B)

Pharmacokinetics:

PO: Onset 1 hr, peak 2 hr, duration 12-24 hr; excreted unchanged by kidneys; crosses placenta; enters breast milk; half-life 8 hr

Interactions:
- Synergism: furosemide
- Increased toxicity of lithium, nondepolarizing skeletal muscle relaxants
- Decreased effects of antidiabetics, methenamine
- Decreased absorption of thiazides, cholestyramine, colestipol
- Decreased hypotensive response: indomethacin
- Hyperglycemia, hyperuricemia, hypotension: diazoxide
- Potassium deficiency: aloe, cascara sagrada bark, buckthorn bark/berry, rhubarb root, senna leaf/fruits

Lab test interferences:

Increase: BSP retention, Ca, amylase, parathyroid test

Decrease: PBI, PSP

NURSING CONSIDERATIONS

Assess:
- Weight, I&O daily to determine fluid loss; effect of drug may be decreased if used qd
- Rate, depth, rhythm of respiration, effect of exertion
- B/P lying, standing; postural hypotension may occur
- Electrolytes: K, Mg, Na, Cl; include BUN, blood sugar, CBC, serum creatinine, blood pH, ABGs, uric acid, Ca
- Glucose in urine of diabetic
- Improvement in edema of feet, legs, sacral area daily if medication is being used in CHF
- Improvement in CVP q8h
- Signs of metabolic alkalosis: drowsiness, restlessness
- Signs of hypokalemia: postural hypotension, malaise, fatigue, tachycardia, leg cramps, weakness
- Rashes, fever qd
- Confusion, especially in elderly; take safety precautions if needed

Administer:
- In AM to avoid interference with sleep if using drug as a diuretic
- K replacement if K <3 mg/dl

• With food; if nausea occurs, absorption may be decreased slightly
• Extended products are Diulo, Zaroxalyn; prompt product is Mykrox

Evaluate:
• Therapeutic response: decreased edema, B/P

Teach patient/family:
• To increase fluid intake to 2-3 L/day unless contraindicated, to rise slowly from lying or sitting position
• To notify prescriber of muscle weakness, cramps, nausea, dizziness
• That drug may be taken with food or milk
• To use sunscreen for photosensitivity
• That blood sugar may be increased in diabetics
• To take early in day to avoid nocturia

Treatment of overdose: Lavage if taken orally; monitor electrolytes; administer dextrose in saline; monitor hydration, CV, renal status

---

metoprolol (℞)

(meh-toe′proe-lole)
Apo-Metoprolol*, Betaloc*, Betaloc Durules*, Lopresor*, Lopressor, Lopressor SR*, Novometoprol*, Toprol XL
Func. class.: Antihypertensive, antianginal
Chem. class.: β₁-blocker

Action: Lowers B/P by β-blocking effects; elevated plasma renins are reduced; blocks β₂-adrenergic receptors in bronchial, vascular smooth muscle only at high doses

Uses: Mild to moderate hypertension, acute MI to reduce cardiovascular mortality, angina pectoris

Investigational uses: Dysrhythmias, hypertrophic cardiomyopathy, mitral valve prolapse, pheochromocytoma, tremors, prevention of vascular headaches, aggression

Dosage and routes:
Hypertension
• *Adult:* **PO** 50 mg bid, or 100 mg qd; may give up to 200-450 mg in divided doses; **SUS REL** give qd
• *Geriatric:* **PO** 25 mg/day initially, increase weekly as needed

Myocardial infarction
• *Adult:* (early treatment) **IV BOL** 5 mg q2min × 3, then 50 mg **PO** 15 min after last dose and q6h × 48 hr; (late treatment) **PO** maintenance 100 mg bid for 3 mo

Available forms: Tabs 50, 100 mg; inj 1 mg/ml; sus rel tab 50, 100, 200 mg

Side effects/adverse reactions:
CV: Hypotension, *bradycardia*
CHF: Palpitations, dysrhythmias, *cardiac arrest, AV block*
CNS: Insomnia, dizziness, mental changes, hallucinations, *depression,* anxiety, headaches, nightmares, confusion, fatigue
GI: Nausea, vomiting, colitis, cramps, *diarrhea,* constipation, flatulence, dry mouth, *hiccups*
INTEG: Rash, purpura, alopecia, dry skin, urticaria, pruritus
HEMA: Agranulocytosis, eosinophilia, thrombocytopenia, purpura
EENT: Sore throat; dry, burning eyes
GU: Impotence
RESP: Bronchospasm, dyspnea, wheezing

Contraindications: Hypersensitivity to β-blockers, cardiogenic shock, heart block (2nd, 3rd degree), sinus bradycardia, bronchial asthma

Precautions: Major surgery, pregnancy (C), lactation, diabetes mellitus, renal disease, thyroid disease, COPD, heart failure, CAD, nonallergic bronchospasm, hepatic disease, CHF

Pharmacokinetics:

PO: Peak 2-4 hr, duration 13-19 hr; half-life 3-4 hr; metabolized in liver (metabolites); excreted in urine; crosses placenta; enters breast milk

Interactions:

• Increased hypotension, bradycardia: reserpine, hydralazine, methyldopa, prazosin

• Decreased antihypertensive effects: indomethacin, sympathomimetics

• Increased hypoglycemic effects: insulin

• Decreased bronchodilation: theophyllines, β-agonists

• Decreased hypoglycemic effect: sulfonylureas

Lab test interferences:

Increase: Liver function tests, renal function tests

NURSING CONSIDERATIONS

Assess:

• ECG directly when giving IV during initial treatment

• I&O, weight daily

• B/P during initial treatment, periodically thereafter; pulse q4h; note rate, rhythm, quality

• Apical/radial pulse before administration; notify prescriber of any significant changes or pulse <50 bpm

• Baselines in renal, liver function tests before therapy begins

• Edema in feet, legs daily

• Skin turgor, dryness of mucous membranes for hydration status

Administer:

• PO ac, hs, tab may be crushed or swallowed whole

IV

• IV, undiluted, give over 1 min, keep patient recumbent for 3 hr

Y-site compatibilities: Alteplase, meperidine, morphine

Perform/provide:

• Storage in dry area at room temp, do not freeze

Evaluate:

• Therapeutic response: decreased B/P after 1-2 wk

Teach patient/family:

• To take with or immediately after meals

• Not to discontinue drug abruptly; taper over 2 wk; may cause precipitate angina

• Not to use OTC products containing α-adrenergic stimulants (nasal decongestants, OTC cold preparations) unless directed by prescriber

• To report bradycardia, dizziness, confusion, depression, fever, sore throat, shortness of breath to prescriber

• To take pulse at home; advise when to notify prescriber

• To avoid alcohol, smoking, Na intake

• To comply with weight control, dietary adjustments, modified exercise program

• To carry Medic Alert ID to identify drug, allergies

• To avoid hazardous activities if dizziness is present

• To report symptoms of CHF: difficult breathing, especially on exertion or when lying down, night cough, swelling of extremities

• To take medication hs to prevent effect of orthostatic hypotension

• To wear support hose to minimize effects of orthostatic hypotension

Treatment of overdose: Lavage, IV atropine for bradycardia, IV theophylline for bronchospasm, digitalis, O_2, diuretic for cardiac failure, hemodialysis, hypotension administer vasopressor (norepinephrine)

M

metronidazole (R)

(me-troe-ni′da-zole)
Apo-Metronidazole*, Fema-zole, Flagyl, Flagyl IV, Flagyl IV RTU, Metro IV, metronidazole, metronidazole Redi-Infusion, Metryl, Neo-Metric*, Novoni-dazole*, PMS-Metronidazole*, Protostat, Satric, Trikacide*

Func. class.: Trichomonacide, amebicide; antiinfective

Chem. class.: Nitroimidazole de-rivative

Action: Direct-acting amebicide/trichomonacide binds, degrades DNA in organism

Uses: Intestinal amebiasis, amebic abscess, trichomoniasis, refractory trichomoniasis, bacterial anaerobic infections, giardiasis, septicemia, en-docarditis, bone, joint infections, lower respiratory tract infections

Dosage and routes:

Trichomoniasis
• *Adult:* **PO** 250 mg tid × 7 days or 2 g in single dose; do not repeat treatment for 4-6 wk

Refractory trichomoniasis
• *Adult:* **PO** 250 mg bid × 10 days

Amebic abscess
• *Adult:* **PO** 500-750 mg tid × 5-10 days
• *Child:* **PO** 35-50 mg/kg/day in 3 divided doses × 10 days

Intestinal amebiasis
• *Adult:* **PO** 750 mg tid × 5-10 days
• *Child:* **PO** 35-50 mg/kg/day in 3 divided doses × 10 days; then oral iodoquinol

Anaerobic bacterial infections
• *Adult:* **IV INF** 15 mg/kg over 1 hr, then 7.5 mg/kg **IV** or **PO** q6h, not to exceed 4 g/day; first maintenance dose should be administered 6 hr following loading dose

Giardiasis
• *Adult:* **PO** 250 mg tid × 5 days
• *Child:* **PO** 5 mg/kg tid × 5 days

Antibiotic-associated pseudomem-branous colitis
• *Adult:* **PO** 250-500 mg 3-4 ×/day × 10-14 days
• *Child:* **PO** 20 mg/kg/day (max 2 g) divided q6h

Available forms: Tabs 250, 500 mg; film-coated tabs 250, 1500 mg; inj 5 mg/vial; HCl inj 500 mg

Side effects/adverse reactions:

CV: Flat T waves

CNS: Headache, dizziness, confu-sion, irritability, restlessness, ataxia, depression, fatigue, drowsiness, in-somnia, paresthesia, peripheral neu-ropathy, *convulsions,* incoordina-tion, depression

EENT: Blurred vision, sore throat, retinal edema, dry mouth, metallic taste, furry tongue, glossitis, stoma-titis

GI: Nausea, vomiting, diarrhea, epi-gastric distress, *anorexia,* constipa-tion, *abdominal cramps,* metallic taste, *pseudomembranous colitis*

GU: Darkened urine, vaginal dry-ness, polyuria, *albuminuria,* dys-uria, cystitis, decreased libido, *neu-rotoxicity,* incontinence, dyspareu-nia

HEMA: Leukopenia, bone marrow, depression, aplasia

INTEG: Rash, pruritus, urticaria, flushing

Contraindications: Hypersensitiv-ity to this drug, renal disease, he-patic disease, contracted visual or color fields, blood dyscrasias, preg-nancy (1st trimester), lactation, CNS disorders

Precautions: *Candida* infections, pregnancy (2nd, 3rd trimesters) (B)

Pharmacokinetics:

IV: Onset immediate, peak end of inf

 = Nursing alert   = Herb-drug interaction   = Do not crush

PO: Peak 1-2 hr, half-life 6-11 hr Crosses placenta, enters breast milk, excreted in feces; absorbed PO (80%-85%)

Interactions:
- Disulfiram reaction: alcohol
- May increase action of warfarin
- Decreased action of metronidazole: phenobarbital, phenytoin

Lab test interferences:
Decrease: AST (SGOT), ALT (SGPT)

NURSING CONSIDERATIONS
Assess:
- For infection: WBC, wound symptoms, fever, skin or vaginal secretions; start treatment after C&S
- Stools during entire treatment; should be clear at end of therapy; stools should be free of parasites for 1 yr before patient is considered cured (amebiasis)
- Vision by ophthalmic exam during, after therapy; vision problems frequent
- I&O; weight daily; stools for number, frequency, character

◆ Neurotoxicity: peripheral neuropathy, seizures, dizziness, uncoordination, pruritus, joint pains; may be discontinued
- Allergic reaction: fever, rash, itching, chills; drug should be discontinued if these symptoms occur
- Superinfection: fever, monilial growth, fatigue, malaise
- Renal and reproductive dysfunction: dysuria, polyuria, impotence, dyspareunia, decreased libido

Administer:
- PO with or after meals to avoid GI symptoms, metallic taste; crush tabs if needed

IV
- Prediluted; Flagyl IV, dilute with 4.4 ml sterile H_2O or 0.9% NaCl; must be diluted further with 8 mg/ml or more 0.9% NaCl, D_5W, or LR; must neutralize with 5 mEq Na_2CO_3/ 500 mg; CO_2 gas will be generated and may require venting; run over 1 hr; primary IV must be discontinued; may be given as continuous infusion; do not use aluminum products; IV may require venting

Additive compatibilities: Amikacin, aminophylline, cefazolin, cefotaxime, cefotiam, ceftazidime, ceftizoxime, ceftriaxone, cefuroxime, chloramphenicol, ciprofloxacin, clindamycin, disopyramide, floxacillin, fluconazole, gentamicin, heparin, moxalactam, multielectrolyte concentrate, multivitamins, netilmicin, penicillin G potassium, tobramycin

Y-site compatibilities: Acyclovir, allopurinol, amifostine, amiodarone, cefepime, cyclophosphamide, diltiazem, dopamine, enalaprilat, esmolol, fluconazole, foscarnet, granisetron, heparin, hydromorphone, labetalol, lorazepam, magnesium sulfate, melphalan, meperidine, methylprednisolone, midazolam, morphine, perphanazine, piperacillin/tazobactam, sargramostim, tacrolimus, teniposide, theophylline, thiotepa, vinorelbine

Perform/provide:
- Storage in light-resistant container; do not refrigerate

Evaluate:
- Therapeutic response: decreased symptoms of infection

Teach patient/family:
- That urine may turn dark-reddish brown, may cause metallic taste
- Proper hygiene after BM; handwashing technique
- To notify physician for numbness or tingling of extremities
- To avoid hazardous activities, since dizziness can occur
- Need for compliance with dosage schedule, duration of treatment

---

• To use condoms if treatment for trichomoniasis, or cross-contamination may occur
• To use frequent sips of water, sugarless gum for dry mouth
• That treatment of both partners is necessary in trichomoniasis
• Not to drink alcohol or use preparations containing alcohol; disulfiram reaction can occur

---

metyrosine (℞)

(me-tye′roe-seen)
Demser
Func. class.: Antihypertensive
Chem. class.: Adrenergic blocker

Action: Inhibits enzyme tyrosine hydroxylase, resulting in decreased levels of catecholamines

Uses: Pheochromocytoma

Dosage and routes:
• *Adult and child >12 yr:* **PO** 250 mg qid, may increase by 250-500 mg qd to a max of 4 g/day in divided doses

Available forms: Caps 250 mg

Side effects/adverse reactions:
CNS: Sedation, drowsiness, dizziness, headache, depression, EPS, hallucinations, psychosis, agitation
INTEG: Rash, urticaria
EENT: Dry mouth, nasal stuffiness
GU: Dysuria, *oliguria, hematuria,* enuresis, impotence
GI: Nausea, vomiting, anorexia, diarrhea, abdominal pain
MISC: Breast swelling

Contraindications: Hypersensitivity, essential hypertension, children <12 yr

Precautions: Pregnancy (C), lactation, hepatic disease, renal disease

Pharmacokinetics:
PO: Onset 2 days, duration 3-4 days; half-life 3.4-3.7 hr, excreted in urine

Interactions:
• Increased sedation: CNS depressants: alcohol, barbiturates, antipsychotics
• Decreased effects of levodopa
• EPS: phenothiazines, haloperidol

Lab test interferences:
False increase: Urinary catecholamines

NURSING CONSIDERATIONS
Assess:
• Electrolytes: K, Na, Cl, CO_2
• Renal function studies: catecholamines, BUN, creatinine
• Hepatic function studies: AST (SGOT), ALT (SGPT), alk phosphatase
• B/P, ECG, other VS throughout treatment
• Weight daily, I&O
• Change in behavior or personality: psychosis, anxiety, hallucinations, EPS
• Nausea, vomiting, diarrhea
• Edema in feet, legs daily
• Skin turgor, dryness of mucous membranes for hydration status

Administer:
• Antiemetic or antidiarrheals for vomiting, diarrhea

Perform/provide:
• Fluids to 2 L/day to prevent crystallization by kidneys

Evaluate:
• Therapeutic response: decreased B/P, decreased levels of catecholamines

Teach patient/family:
• To take each dose with a full glass of water; maintain sufficient daily intake
• Not to drive or perform hazardous tasks if behavioral changes, dizziness, or drowsiness occurs
• To avoid alcohol, other CNS depressants
• To notify prescriber of any of following: jaw stiffness, drooling,

speech difficulty, tremors, disorientation, diarrhea, painful urination
Treatment of overdose: Administer vasopressors, discontinue drug

---

mexiletine (R)
(mex-il'e-teen)
Mexitil
Func. class.: Antidysrhythmic (Class IB)
Chem. class.: Lidocaine analog

Action: Increases electrical stimulation threshold of ventricle, His-Purkinje system, which stabilizes cardiac membrane

Uses: Ventricular tachycardia, ventricular dysrhythmias during cardiac surgery, MI

Dosage and routes:
• *Adult:* PO 400 mg (loading dose), then 200 mg q8h, then 200-400 mg q8h

Available forms: Caps 150, 200, 250 mg

Side effects/adverse reactions:
CNS: Headache, dizziness, confusion, *convulsions,* tremors, psychosis, nervousness, paresthesias, weakness, fatigue, coordination difficulties, change in sleep habits
EENT: Blurred vision, hearing loss, tinnitus
GI: Nausea, vomiting, anorexia, diarrhea, abdominal pain, *hepatitis,* dry mouth, peptic ulcer, altered taste, GI bleeding
CV: Hypotension, bradycardia, angina, PVCs, *heart block, cardiovascular collapse or arrest,* sinus node slowing, *left ventricular failure,* syncope, *cardiogenic shock*
RESP: Dyspnea, *fibrosis, embolism,* pneumonia
INTEG: Rash, alopecia, dry skin
HEMA: **Thrombocytopenia, leukopenia, agranulocytosis, hypoplas-**

tic anemia, systemic lupus erythematosus syndrome
GU: Urinary hesitancy, decreased libido
MISC: Edema, arthralgia, fever

Contraindications: Hypersensitivity to amides, cardiogenic shock, blood dyscrasias, severe heart block

Precautions: Pregnancy (C), lactation, children, renal disease, liver disease, CHF, respiratory depression, myasthenia gravis

Pharmacokinetics:
PO: Peak 2-3 hr; half-life 12 hr, metabolized by liver, excreted unchanged by kidneys (10%), excreted in breast milk

Interactions:
• Decreased effects of mexiletine: cimetidine
• Decreased levels of mexiletine: phenytoin, phenobarbital, rifampin
• Increased effects of mexiletine: metoclopramide
Drug/smoking: Decreased drug effect
🌿 Increased potassium loss, increased antidysrhythmic action: aloe, cascara sagrada bark, buckthorn bark/berry, rhubarb root, senna leaf/fruits

Lab test interferences:
Increase: CPK

NURSING CONSIDERATIONS
Assess:
• ECG continuously for increased PR or QRS segments; discontinue or reduce rate; watch for increased ventricular ectopic beats; may have to rebolus
• Blood levels (therapeutic level 0.5-2 µg/ml)
• B/P continuously for fluctuations in cardiac rate
• I&O ratio, electrolytes (K, Na, Cl), liver enzymes
◆ Malignant hyperthermia: tachypnea, tachycardia, changes in B/P, fever

• Respiratory status: rate, rhythm, lung fields for rales, watch for respiratory depression
• CNS effects: dizziness, confusion, psychosis, paresthesias, convulsions; drug should be discontinued
• Lung fields, bilateral rales may occur in CHF patient
• Increased respiration, increased pulse; drug should be discontinued

Administer:
• With food for GI upset

Evaluate:
• Therapeutic response: decreased dysrhythmias

Treatment of overdose: O₂, artificial ventilation, ECG; administer dopamine for circulatory depression, diazepam or thiopental for convulsions, to acidify urine

---

mezlocillin (R)
(mez-loe-sill'in)
Mezlin
Func. class.: Antiinfective, broad-spectrum
Chem. class.: Extended-spectrum penicillin

Action: Interferes with cell wall replication of susceptible organisms; osmotically unstable cell wall swells, bursts from osmotic pressure

Uses: Effective for gram-positive cocci *(S. aureus, S. viridans, S. faecalis, S. pneumoniae),* gram-negative cocci *(N. gonorrhoeae),* gram-positive bacilli *(C. perfringens, C. tetani),* gram-negative bacilli *(Bacteroides, E. coli, H. influenzae, Klebsiella, P. mirabilis, Peptococcus, Peptostreptococcus, M. morganii, Enterobacter, Serratia, Pseudomonas, P. vulgaris, P. rettgeri, Shigella, Citrobacter, Veillonella)*

Dosage and routes:
• Dose reduction indicated in renal impairment (CrCl <30 ml/min)
• Hepatic dose give 50% of dose
• *Adult:* **IM/IV** 3-4 g q4-6h or **IV** 500 mg q8h, may give up to 24 g/day for severe infections
• *Child:* **IM/IV** 50 mg/kg q4-6h
• *Infant >8 days:* >2000 g: 75 mg/kg q6h; <2000 g: 75 mg/kg q8h
• *Infant <8 days:* 75 mg/kg q12h
Available forms: Powder for inj 1, 2, 3, 4, 20 g

Side effects/adverse reactions:
HEMA: Anemia, increased bleeding time, ***bone marrow depression, granulocytopenia***
GI: Nausea, vomiting, diarrhea; increased AST (SGOT), ALT (SGPT); abdominal pain, glossitis, colitis, abnormal taste
GU: Oliguria, proteinuria, hematuria, (vaginitis, moniliasis), ***glomerulonephritis,*** increased BUN, creatinine
CNS: Lethargy, hallucinations, anxiety, depression, twitching, ***coma, convulsions***
META: Hyperkalemia, hypokalemia, alkalosis, hypernatremia

Contraindications: Hypersensitivity to penicillins

Precautions: Pregnancy (B), lactation, hypersensitivity to cephalosporins, neonates, renal disease

Pharmacokinetics:
IM: Peak 45 min
IV: Peak 5 min
Half-life 50-55 min; partially metabolized in liver; excreted in urine, bile, breast milk (small amount); crosses placenta

Interactions:
• Decreased effectiveness of aminoglycosides if mixed together
• Decreased antimicrobial effectiveness of mezlocillin: tetracyclines, erythromycins

---

◆ = Nursing alert 　　 🌿 = Herb-drug interaction 　　 🚫 = Do not crush

• Increased mezlocillin concentrations: aspirin, probenecid

• Increased effect of heparin, vecuronium

Lab test interferences:

False positive: Urine glucose, urine protein

NURSING CONSIDERATIONS
Assess:

• I&O ratio; report hematuria, oliguria, since penicillin in high doses is nephrotoxic

• Any patient with compromised renal system, since drug is excreted slowly in poor renal system function; toxicity may occur rapidly

• Liver studies: AST (SGOT), ALT (SGPT)

• Blood studies: WBC, RBC, Hct, Hgb, bleeding time

• Renal studies: urinalysis, protein, blood, BUN, creatinine

• C&S before drug therapy; drug may be given as soon as culture is taken

• Bowel pattern before and during treatment

• Skin eruptions after administration of penicillin to 1 wk after discontinuing drug

• Respiratory status: rate, character, wheezing, and tightness in chest

• Check IV site for thrombophlebitis

• WBC, differential, liver, renal studies periodically for patients on long-term therapy

• Allergies before initiation of treatment, and reaction of each medication; highlight allergies on chart

Administer:

• Drug after C&S completed

IV

• After diluting 1 g or less/10 ml of sterile H_2O, D_5, or 0.9% NaCl for inj; shake, dilute further with D_5W or 0.45 NaCl, and give over 3-5 min; may be given by intermittent inf over ½ hr

Solution compatibilities: $D_{10}W$, F_5W, 0.9% NaCl

Syringe compatibilities: Heparin

Y-site compatibilities: Amifostine, aztreonam, cyclophosphamide, famotidine, fludarabine, granisetron, hydromorphone, morphine, perphenazine, propofol, sargramostim, tacrolimus, teniposide, thiotepa

Perform/provide:

• Adrenaline, suction, tracheostomy set, endotracheal intubation equipment

• Adequate fluid intake (2 L) during diarrhea episodes

• Scratch test to assess allergy after securing order from prescriber; usually done when penicillin is only drug of choice

• Storage at room temp; reconstituted sol is stable for 24 hr refrigerated

Evaluate:

• Therapeutic response: absence of fever, draining wounds

Teach patient/family:

• That culture may be taken after completed course of medication

• To report sore throat, fever, fatigue (may indicate superinfection)

• To wear or carry Medic Alert ID if allergic to penicillins

• To report diarrhea, symptoms of *Candida* vaginitis

Treatment of anaphylaxis: Withdraw drug, maintain airway, administer epinephrine, aminophylline, O_2, IV corticosteroids

---

miconazole (℞)

(mi-kon′a-zole)

Monistat, Monistat I.V.

Func. class.: Antifungal

Chem. class.: Imidazole

Action: Alters cell membranes, inhibits fungal enzymes

Uses: Coccidioidomycosis, candidiasis, cryptococcoses, paracoccidioidomycosis, chronic mucocutaneous candidiasis, fungal meningitis; IV for severe infections only

Dosage and routes:
• *Adult:* **IV INF** 200-3600 mg/day; may be divided in 3 infusions 200-1200 mg/infusion; may have to repeat course; **INTRATHECAL** 20 mg given simultaneously with **IV** for fungal meningitis q1-2d
• *Child:* **IV** 20-40 mg/kg/day, not to exceed 15 mg/kg/dose

Available forms: Inj 10 mg/ml; aerosol 2%

Side effects/adverse reactions:
CV: Tachycardia, dysrhythmias (rapid IV)
CNS: Drowsiness, headache, laziness
GI: Nausea, vomiting, anorexia, diarrhea, cramps
GU: Vulvovaginal burning, itching, hyponatremia, pelvic cramps (topical forms)
HEMA: **Decreased Hct, thrombocytopenia, hyperlipidemia**
INTEG: Pruritus, rash, fever, flushing, **anaphylaxis,** hives

Contraindications: Hypersensitivity

Precautions: Renal disease, hepatic disease, pregnancy (B)

Pharmacokinetics:
IV: Onset immediate; peak end of inf; half-life triphasic 0.4, 2.1, 24.1 hr; metabolized in liver; excreted in feces, urine (inactive metabolites); >90% protein binding

Interactions:
• Increased effect: warfarin, sulfonylureas, phenytoin
• Increased risk of cardiotoxicity: terfenadine, astemizole, cisapride
• Decreased action of both drugs: amphotericin

Lab test interferences:
False positive: Urine glucose, urine protein

NURSING CONSIDERATIONS
Assess:
• Cardiac system: B/P, pulse, ECG; watch for increasing pulse, cardiac dysrhythmias; drug should be discontinued
• Blood studies: WBC, RBC, Hct, Hgb, bleeding time
• Renal studies: urinalysis, protein, blood
• C&S before drug therapy; drug may be given as soon as culture is taken; monitor signs of infection prior to and throughout treatment
• Bowel pattern before and during treatment; diarrhea is common
• Skin eruptions after administration of drug to 1 wk after discontinuing drug
• Respiratory status: rate, character, wheezing, tightness in chest
• IV site for thrombophlebitis
• WBC and differential liver and renal studies periodically for patients on long-term therapy
• Allergies before initiation of treatment, and reaction of each medication; highlight allergies on chart

Administer:
• Drug after C&S completed
IV
• 200 mg initially to prevent severe hypersensitive reaction
• IV after diluting 1 g or less/10 ml of sterile H_2O, D_5W, or 0.45% NaCl; give over 3-5 min; may be given by intermittent INF over 2 hr

Y-site compatibilities: Allopurinol, filgrastim, foscarnet, granisetron, melphalan, ondansetron, propofol, sargramostim, teniposide, thiotepa, vinorelbine

Perform/provide:
• Adrenaline, suction, tracheostomy set, endotracheal intubation equipment
• Adequate fluid intake (2 L) during diarrhea episodes
• Scratch test to assess allergy after

= Nursing alert   = Herb-drug interaction   = Do not crush

securing order from prescriber; usually done when penicillin is only drug of choice

• Storage at room temp; reconstituted sol stable for 24 hr refrigerated

Evaluate:

• Therapeutic response: absence of fever, draining wounds

Teach patient/family:

• That culture may be taken after completed course of medication

• To report sore throat, fever, fatigue (may indicate superinfection)

• To wear or carry Medic Alert ID if allergic to drug

• To report diarrhea, symptoms of *Candida* vaginitis

Treatment of overdose: Withdraw drug; maintain airway; administer epinephrine, aminophylline, O_2, IV corticosteroids for anaphylaxis

---

microfibrillar collagen hemostat (℞)
Avitene
Func. class.: Hemostatic
Chem. class.: Purified cattle collagen

Action: Platelets adhere to hemostat, cause aggregation to and formation of thrombi

Uses: For hemostasis in surgery when ligature is ineffective/impractical

Dosage and routes:

• *Adult and child:* **TOP** apply to bleeding area after drying with sponge; compress for 1-5 min; may reapply if needed

Available forms: Fibrous form, nonwoven web form

Side effects/adverse reactions:
INTEG: Rash, abscess, allergic reactions, infection, wound dehiscence
HEMA: Hematoma

Contraindications: Hypersensitivity, closure of skin incision
Precautions: Pregnancy (C)
NURSING CONSIDERATIONS
Assess:

• Possible infection: hematoma, abscess

• Allergy: rash, itching

Administer:

• Dry, do not moisten

• Using gloves with forceps; area must be dry for drug to work

• Only new product; do not resterilize

Evaluate:

• Therapeutic response: decreased bleeding in surgery

---

midazolam (℞)
(mid'ay-zoe-lam)
Versed
Func. class.: Sedative, hypnotic
Chem. class.: Benzodiazepine, short-acting

Controlled Substance Schedule IV
Action: Depresses subcortical levels in CNS; may act on limbic system, reticular formation; may potentiate γ aminobutyric acid (GABA) by binding to specific benzodiazepine receptors

Uses: Preoperative sedation, general anesthesia induction, sedation for diagnostic endoscopic procedures, intubation

Investigational uses: Epileptic seizures, refractory status epilepticus

Dosage and routes:
Preoperative sedation

• *Adult:* **IM** 0.07-0.08 mg/kg ½-1 hr before general anesthesia

• *Child:* **IM** 0.1-0.15 mg/kg, may give up to 0.5 mg/kg if needed

Induction of general anesthesia

• *Adult and child 12-16 yr:* **IV** (unpremedicated patients) 0.3-0.35 mg/kg over 30 sec, wait 2 min, fol-

low with 25% of initial dose if needed; (premedicated patients) 0.15-0.35 mg/kg over 20-30 sec, allow 2 min for effect
- *Child 6-12 yr:* **IV** 0.025-0.05 mg/kg, total dose up to 0.4 mg/kg may be needed
- *Child 6 mo-5 yr:* **IV** 0.05-0.1 mg/kg, total dose up to 0.6 mg/kg may be needed
- *Child <6 mo:* Titrate with small increments

Available forms: Inj 1, 5 mg/ml

Side effects/adverse reactions:

CNS: Retrograde amnesia, euphoria, confusion, headache, anxiety, insomnia, slurred speech, paresthesia, tremors, weakness, chills

RESP: Coughing, ***apnea, bronchospasm, laryngospasm,*** dyspnea

CV: Hypotension, PVCs, tachycardia, bigeminy, nodal rhythm

EENT: Blurred vision, nystagmus, diplopia, blocked ears, loss of balance

GI: Nausea, vomiting, increased salivation, hiccups

INTEG: Urticaria, pain, swelling at injection site, rash, pruritus

Contraindications: Pregnancy (D), hypersensitivity to benzodiazepines, shock, coma, alcohol intoxication, acute narrow-angle glaucoma

Precautions: COPD, CHF, chronic renal failure, chills, elderly, debilitated, children, lactation

Pharmacokinetics:

IM: Onset 15 min, peak ½-1 hr
IV: Onset 3-5 min, onset of anesthesia 1½-2½ min; protein binding 97%; half-life 1.2-12.3 hr
Metabolized in liver; metabolites excreted in urine; crosses placenta, blood-brain barrier

Interactions:
- Prolonged respiratory depression: other CNS depressants, alcohol, barbiturates, narcotic analgesics, verapamil, ritonavir, indinavir, fluvoxamine
- Increased hypnotic effect: fentanyl, narcotic agonists, analgesics, droperidol
- Increased clearance and decreased half-life of midazolam: rifamycins
- Decreased metabolism of midazolam: valproic acid
- Decreased effect of midazolam: theophyllines
- Increased half-life of midazolam: oral contraceptives
- Increased levels of midazolam: cimetidine, azole antifungals
- Increased effect of midazolam: propofol

NURSING CONSIDERATIONS
Assess:
- Injection site for redness, pain, swelling
- Degree of amnesia in elderly; may be increased
- Anterograde amnesia
- Vital signs for recovery period in obese patient, since half-life may be extended
- Apnea, respiratory depression that may be increased in the elderly

Administer:
- IM deep into large muscle mass
IV
- After diluting with D₅W or 0.9% NaCl to 0.25 mg/ml; give over 2 min (conscious sedation) or over 30 sec (anesthesia induction)

Syringe compatibilities: Atracurium, atropine, benzquinamide, buprenorphine, butorphanol, chlorpromazine, cimetidine, diphenhydramine, droperidol, fentanyl, glycopyrrolate, hydromorphone, hydroxyzine, meperidine, metoclopramide, morphine, nalbuphine, promazine, promethazine, scopolamine, sufentanil, thiethylperazine, trimethobenzamide

Y-site compatibilities: Amikacin,

 = Nursing alert   = Herb-drug interaction   = Do not crush

amiodarone, atracurium, calcium gluconate, cefazolin, cefmetazole, cefotaxime, cimetidine, ciprofloxacin, clindamycin, digoxin, diltiazem, dopamine, epinephrine, erythromycin, esmolol, etomidate, famotidine, fentanyl, fluconazole, gentamicin, haloperidol, heparin, hydromorphone, insulin (regular), labetalol, lorazepam, methylprednisolone, metronidazole, milrinone, morphine, nicardipine, nitroglycerin, norepinephrine, pancuronium, piperacillin, potassium chloride, ranitidine, sodium nitroprusside, sufentanil, theophylline, tobramycin, vancomycin, vecuronium

Perform/provide:

• Assistance with ambulation until drowsy period relieved
• Storage at room temp
• Immediate availability of resuscitation equipment, O_2 to support airway, do not give by rapid bolus

Evaluate:

• Therapeutic response: induction of sedation, general anesthesia

Teach patient/family:

• That amnesia occurs; events may not be remembered

Treatment of overdose: O_2, vasopressors, physostigmine, resuscitation

---

midodrine (℞)

(mye'doh-dreen)
ProAmatine
Func. class.: Vasopressor

Action: Activates α-adrenergic receptors of arteriolar venous vasculature

Uses: Orthostatic hypotension

Dosage and routes:

• *Adult:* PO 10 mg tid

Renal dose

• *Adult:* PO 2.5 mg tid

Available forms: Tabs 2.5, 5 mg

Side effects/adverse reactions:

CNS: Drowsiness, restlessness, headache, *paresthesia, pain,* chills
GI: Nausea, anorexia
EENT: Dry mouth, blurred vision
INTEG: Pruritus, piloerection, rash
GU: Urinary urgency
CV: Supine hypertension

Contraindications: Hypersensitivity, severe organic heart disease, acute renal disease, urinary retention, pheochromocytoma, thyrotoxicosis, persistent/excessive supine hypertension

Precautions: Children, urinary retention, lactation, prostatic hypertrophy, pregnancy (C)

Pharmacokinetics:

PO: Peak 1-2 hr, half-life 3-4 hr

Interactions:

• Increased bradycardia: β-blockers, psychopharmacologics, cardiac glycosides
• Increased pressor effects: α-agonist
• Increased intraocular pressure: steroids

NURSING CONSIDERATIONS

Assess:

• VS, B/P (standing, supine)
• Observe for drowsiness, dizziness, LOC

Administer:

• Tablets may be swallowed whole, chewed, or allowed to dissolve
• Upon arising, midday, and late afternoon (no later than 6 PM)
• Avoid administering if patient is to be supine during day

Evaluate:

• Therapeutic response: decreased orthostatic hypotension

Teach patient/family:

• To avoid hazardous activities, activities requiring alertness; dizziness may occur; instruct patient to request assistance with ambulation
• To avoid alcohol, other depressants

miglitol (℞)

(mig'lih-tol)
Glyset
Func. class.: Oral hypoglycemic
Chem. class.: α-glucosidase inhibitor

Action: Delays digestion of ingested carbohydrates, results in smaller rise in blood glucose after meals; does not increase insulin production

Uses: Non–insulin-dependent diabetes mellitus (NIDDM) Type II

Dosage and routes:
• *Adult:* **PO** 25 mg tid initially, with first bite of meal; maintenance dose may be increased to 50 mg tid; may be increased to 100 mg tid if needed (only in patients >60 kg) with dosage adjustment at 4-8 wk intervals

Available forms: Tabs 25, 50, 100 mg

Side effects/adverse reactions:
*GI: Abdominal pain, diarrhea, flatulence, **hepatotoxicity***
HEMA: Low iron
INTEG: Rash

Contraindications: Hypersensitivity, diabetic ketoacidosis, cirrhosis, inflammatory bowel disease, colonic ulceration, partial intestinal obstruction, chronic intestinal disease

Precautions: Pregnancy (B), renal disease, lactation, children, hepatic disease

Pharmacokinetics: Not metabolized, excreted in urine as unchanged drug, half-life 2 hr

Interactions:
• Increased hypoglycemia: sulfonylureas, insulin
• Decreased levels of: digoxin, propranolol, ranitidine
• Decreased levels of miglitol: digestive enzymes, intestinal adsorbents; do not use together

NURSING CONSIDERATIONS

Assess:
• Hypoglycemia, hyperglycemia; even though drug does not cause hypoglycemia, if patient is on sulfonylureas or insulin, hypoglycemia may be additive
• Blood glucose levels, glycosylated hemoglobin, LFTs

Administer:
• tid with first bite of each meal

Perform/provide:
• Storage in tight container in cool environment

Evaluate:
• Therapeutic response: decreased signs/symptoms of diabetes mellitus (polyuria, polydipsia, polyphagia, clear sensorium, absence of dizziness, stable gait)

Teach patient/family:
• The symptoms of hypo/hyperglycemia, what to do about each
• That medication must be taken as prescribed; explain consequences of discontinuing medication abruptly
• To avoid OTC medications unless approved by health-care provider
• That diabetes is life-long illness; that this drug is not a cure
• To carry a Medic Alert ID for emergency purposes
• That diet and exercise regimen must be followed

milrinone (℞)

(mill'rih-nohn)
Primacor
Func. class.: Inotropic/vasodilator agent with phosphodiesterase activity
Chem. class.: Bipyridine derivative

Action: Positive inotropic agent with vasodilator properties; reduces pre-load and afterload by direct relaxation on vascular smooth muscle

Uses: Short-term management of CHF that has not responded to other medication; can be used with digitalis

Dosage and routes:

• *Adult:* IV BOL 50 µg/kg given over 10 min; start infusion of 0.375-0.75 µg/kg/min; reduce dose in renal impairment

Available forms: Inj 1 mg/ml

Side effects/adverse reactions:

HEMA: **Thrombocytopenia**

MISC: Headache, hypokalemia, tremor

CV: Dysrhythmias, hypotension, chest pain

GI: Nausea, vomiting, anorexia, abdominal pain, **hepatotoxicity,** jaundice

Contraindications: Hypersensitivity to this drug, severe aortic disease, severe pulmonic valvular disease, acute myocardial infarction

Precautions: Lactation, pregnancy (C), children, renal disease, hepatic disease, atrial flutter/fibrillation, elderly

Pharmacokinetics:

IV: Onset 2-5 min, peak 10 min, duration variable; half-life 4-6 hr; metabolized in liver; excreted in urine as drug and metabolites 60%-90%

Interactions:

• Excessive hypotension: antihypertensives

NURSING CONSIDERATIONS

Assess:

• B/P and pulse q5min during infusion; if B/P drops 30 mm Hg, stop infusion and call prescriber

• Electrolytes: K, Na, Cl, Ca; renal function studies: BUN, creatinine; blood studies: platelet count

• ALT (SGPT), AST (SGOT), bilirubin qd

• I&O ratio and weight qd; diuresis should increase with continuing therapy

• If platelets are <150,000/mm^3, drug is usually discontinued and another drug started

• Extravasation; change site q48h

Administer:

• K supplements if ordered for K levels <3 mg/dl

IV

• Into running dextrose infusion through Y-connector or directly into tubing; dilute with NS to 1-3 mg/ml; do not mix with glucose for long-term infusion

• By infusion pump for doses other than bolus

Additive compatibilities: Quinidine

Syringe compatibilities: Atropine, calcium chloride, digoxin, epinephrine, lidocaine, morphine, propranolol, sodium bicarbonate, verapamil

Y-site compatibilities: Digoxin, diltiazem, dobutamine, dopamine, epinephrine, fentanyl, heparin, hydromorphone, labetalol, lorazepam, midazolam, morphine, nicardipine, nitroglycerin, norepinephrine, propranolol, quinidine, ranitidine, thiopental, vecuronium

Evaluate:

• Therapeutic response: increased cardiac output, decreased PCWP, adequate CVP, decreased dyspnea, fatigue, edema, ECG

Treatment of overdose: Discontinue drug, support circulation

M

mineral oil

Agoral Plain, Fleet Mineral Oil Enema, Kondremul*, Kondremul Plain, Liqui-doss, Lansoyl*, Milkinol, Neo-Cultol, Nujol, Petrogalar Plain, Zymenol

Func. class.: Laxative-lubricant
Chem. class.: Petroleum hydrocarbon

Action: Eases passage of stool by increasing water retention in feces; acts as lubricant

Uses: Constipation, preparation for bowel surgery or exam

Dosage and routes:

• *Adult:* **PO** 15-30 ml hs; enema 4 oz

• *Child 6-12 yr:* **PO** 5-15 ml hs; enema 1-2 oz

• *Child 2-11 yr:* Enema 1-2 oz

Available forms: Oil, enema; jelly 55%; susp 1.4, 2.5, 2.75 mg/5 ml

Side effects/adverse reactions:

CNS: Muscle weakness

GI: Nausea, vomiting, anorexia, diarrhea, pruritus ani, hepatic infiltration

META: **Hypoprothrombinemia**

RESP: Lipid pneumonia

Contraindications: Hypersensitivity, intestinal obstruction, abdominal pain, nausea/vomiting

Precautions: Pregnancy (C), swallowing difficulty

Pharmacokinetics: Excreted in feces

Interactions:

• Increased effect of oral anticoagulants

• Decreased absorption: fat-soluble vitamins (A, D, E, K) if used for prolonged time

NURSING CONSIDERATIONS

Assess:

• Stool for color, consistency, amount

• Blood, urine electrolytes if drug is used often by patient

• I&O ratio to identify fluid loss

• Cause of constipation; lack of fluids, bulk, exercise

• Cramping, rectal bleeding, nausea, vomiting; drug should be discontinued

Administer:

• Alone for better absorption

• In morning or evening (oral dose)

• Cautiously in elderly to prevent aspiration

Evaluate:

• Therapeutic response: decrease in constipation

Teach patient/family:

• Not to use laxatives for long-term therapy; bowel tone will be lost

• That normal bowel movements do not always occur daily

• Not to use in presence of abdominal pain, nausea, vomiting

• To notify prescriber if constipation unrelieved or if symptoms of electrolyte imbalance occur: muscle cramps, pain, weakness, dizziness, excessive thirst

• Not to use with food or vitamin preparations; delays digestion and absorption of fat-soluble vitamins

minocycline (℞)

(min-oh-sye′kleen)
Minocin, Minocin IV

Func. class.: Broad-spectrum antiinfective
Chem. class.: Tetracycline

Action: Inhibits protein synthesis, phosphorylation in microorganisms by binding to 30S ribosomal subunits, reversibly binding to 50S ribosomal subunits; bacteriostatic

Uses: Syphilis, chlamydia trachomatis, gonorrhea, lymphogranuloma venereum, rickettsial infections, in-

 = Nursing alert   = Herb-drug interaction   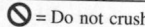 = Do not crush flammatory acne, *Neisseria meningitidis, N. gonorrheae, Treponema pallidum, Chlamydia trachomatis, Ureaplasma urealyticum, Mycoplasma pneumoniae, Nocardia*

Dosage and routes:
• *Adult:* **PO/IV** 200 mg, then 100 mg q12h or 50 mg q6h, not to exceed 400 mg/24 hr **IV**
• *Child >8 yr:* **PO/IV** 4 mg/kg then 4 mg/kg/day **PO** in divided doses q12h

Gonorrhea
• *Adult:* **PO** 200 mg, then 100 mg q12h × 4 days

Chlamydia trachomatis
• *Adult:* **PO** 100 mg bid × 7 days

Syphilis
• *Adult:* **PO** 200 mg, then 100 mg q12h × 10-15 days

Available forms: Tabs 50, 100 mg; caps 50, 100 mg; oral susp 50 mg/5 ml; powder for inj 100 mg/vial

Side effects/adverse reactions:
CNS: Dizziness, fever, light-headedness, vertigo
*HEMA: **Eosinophilia, neutropenia, thrombocytopenia, hemolytic anemia***
EENT: Dysphagia, glossitis, decreased calcification of deciduous teeth, permanent discoloration of teeth, oral candidiasis
GI: Nausea, abdominal pain, vomiting, diarrhea, anorexia, enterocolitis, ***hepatotoxicity,*** flatulence, abdominal cramps, epigastric burning, stomatitis
CV: Pericarditis
GU: Increased BUN, polyuria, polydipsia, ***renal failure, nephrotoxicity***
INTEG: Rash, urticaria, photosensitivity, increased pigmentation, ***exfoliative dermatitis,*** pruritus, angioedema, blue-gray color of skin, mucous membranes

Contraindications: Hypersensitivity to tetracyclines, children <8 yr, pregnancy (D)
Precautions: Hepatic disease, lactation

Pharmacokinetics:
PO: Peak 2-3 hr, half-life 11-17 hr; excreted in urine, feces, breast milk; crosses placenta; 70%-75% protein bound

Interactions:
• Decreased effect of minocycline: antacids, $NaHCO_3$, alkali products, iron, kaolin/pectin, cimetidine
• Increased effect: warfarin
• Decreased effect of barbiturates, carbamazepine, phenytoin, penicillins, oral contraceptives
• Nephrotoxicity: methoxyflurane

Lab test interferences:
False negative: Urine glucose with Clinistix or Tes-Tape

NURSING CONSIDERATIONS
Assess:
• I&O ratio
• Blood studies: PT, CBC, AST (SGOT), ALT (SGPT), BUN, creatinine
• Signs of anemia: Hct, Hgb, fatigue
• Allergic reactions: rash, itching, pruritus, angioedema
• Nausea, vomiting, diarrhea; administer antiemetic, antacids as ordered
• Overgrowth of infection: fever, malaise, redness, pain, swelling, drainage, perineal itching, diarrhea, changes in cough or sputum, black, furry tongue

Administer:
• After C&S obtained
• 2 hr before or after laxative or ferrous products; 3 hr after antacid or kaolin-pectin product (PO)
IV
• After diluting 100 mg/5 ml sterile H_2O for inj; further dilute in 500-

M

1000 ml of NaCl, dextrose sol, LR, Ringer's sol; run 100 mg/6 hr

Y-site compatibilities: Aztreonam, cyclophosphamide, filgrastim, fludarabine, granisetron, heparin, hydrocortisone, magnesium sulfate, melphalan, perphenazine, potassium chloride, sargramostim, teniposide, vinorelbine, vit B/C

Perform/provide:

• Storage in air-tight, light-resistant container at room temp

Evaluate:

• Therapeutic response: decreased temp, absence of lesions, negative C&S

Teach patient/family:

• To avoid sunlight; sunscreen does not seem to decrease photosensitivity

• That all prescribed medication must be taken to prevent superinfection

• To take with a full glass of water; may take with food for GI symptoms

---

minoxidil (℞)

(mi-nox'i-dill)

Loniten, Minodyl, minoxidil, Rogaine

Func. class.: Antihypertensive

Chem. class.: Vasodilator—peripheral

Action: Directly relaxes arteriolar smooth muscle, causing vasodilation

Uses: Severe hypertension unresponsive to other therapy (use with diuretic); topically to treat alopecia

Dosage and routes:

Severe hypertension

• *Adult:* PO 5 mg/day not to exceed 100 mg daily, usual range 10-40 mg/day in single doses

• *Geriatric:* PO 2.5 mg qd, may be increased gradually

• *Child <12 yr:* (initial) 0.2 mg/kg/day; (effective range) 0.25-1 mg/kg/day; (max) 50 mg/day

Alopecia

• *Adult:* Apply topically, rub into scalp daily

Available forms: Tabs 2.5, 10 mg; top 20, 50 mg/ml

Side effects/adverse reactions:

CV: Severe rebound hypertension, tachycardia, angina, increased T wave, **CHF, pulmonary edema, pericardial effusion,** edema, sodium, water retention

CNS: Drowsiness, dizziness, sedation, headache, depression, fatigue

GI: Nausea, vomiting

GU: Gynecomastia, breast tenderness

INTEG: Pruritus, **Stevens-Johnson syndrome,** rash, hirsutism

HEMA: Hct, Hgb, erythrocyte count may decrease initially

Contraindications: Acute MI, dissecting aortic aneurysm, hypersensitivity, pheochromocytoma

Precautions: Pregnancy (C), lactation, children, renal disease, CAD, CHF

Pharmacokinetics:

PO: Onset 30 min, peak 2-3 hr, duration 75 hr; half-life 4.2 hr; metabolized in liver; metabolites excreted in urine, feces

Interactions:

• Orthostatic hypotension: guanethidine

Lab test interferences:

Increase: Renal function studies

Decrease: Hgb/Hct/RBC

NURSING CONSIDERATIONS

Assess:

• Nausea, edema in feet, legs daily

• Skin turgor, dryness of mucous membranes for hydration status

---

- Rales, dyspnea, orthopnea
- Electrolytes: K, Na, Cl, CO_2
- Renal function studies: catecholamines, BUN, creatinine
- Hepatic function studies: AST (SGOT), ALT (SGPT), alk phosphatase
- B/P, pulse
- Weight daily, I&O

Administer:

TOP

- 1 ml no matter how much balding has occurred; increasing dosage does not speed growth

PO

- With meals for better absorption, to decrease GI symptoms
- With β-blocker and/or diuretic for hypertension

Perform/provide:

- Storage protected from light and heat

Evaluate:

- Therapeutic response: decreased B/P or increased hair growth

Teach patient/family:

- That body hair will increase but is reversible after discontinuing treatment
- Not to discontinue drug abruptly
- To report pitting edema, dizziness, weight gain >5 lb, shortness of breath, bruising or bleeding, heart rate >20 beats/min over normal, severe indigestion, dizziness, lightheadedness, panting, new or aggravated symptoms of angina
- To take drug exactly as prescribed, or serious side effects may occur
- That for topical use: treatment must continue long-term or new hair will be lost
- Not to use except on scalp

Treatment of overdose: Administer normal saline IV, vasopressors

mirtazapine (R)

(mer-ta′za-peen)
Remeron
Func. class.: Antidepressant
Chem. class.: Tetracyclic

Action: Blocks reuptake of norepinephrine, serotonin into nerve endings, increasing action of norepinephrine, serotonin in nerve cells

Uses: Depression, dysthymic disorder, bipolar disorder—depressed, agitated depression

Dosage and routes:

- *Adult:* **PO** 15 mg/day at hs, maintenance to continue for 6 mo
- *Geriatric:* **PO** 7.5 mg q hs, increase by 7.5 mg q1-2wk to desired dose, max 45 mg/day

Available forms: Tabs 15, 30 mg

Side effects/adverse reactions:

HEMA: Agranulocytosis, thrombocytopenia, eosinophilia, leukopenia

CNS: Dizziness, drowsiness, confusion, headache, anxiety, tremors, stimulation, weakness, insomnia, nightmares, EPS (elderly), increased psychiatric symptoms, *seizures*

GI: Diarrhea, dry mouth, nausea, vomiting, *paralytic ileus,* increased appetite, cramps, epigastric distress, jaundice, *hepatitis,* stomatitis

GU: Retention, acute renal failure

INTEG: Rash, urticaria, sweating, pruritus, photosensitivity

CV: Orthostatic hypotension, ECG changes, tachycardia, **hypertension,** palpitations

EENT: Blurred vision, tinnitus, mydriasis

Contraindications: Hypersensitivity to tricyclic antidepressants, recovery phase of MI, convulsive disorders, prostatic hypertrophy

Precautions: Suicidal patients, severe depression, increased intraocu-

M

lar pressure, narrow-angle glaucoma, urinary retention, cardiac disease, hepatic disease, hypothyroidism, hyperthyroidism, electroshock therapy, elective surgery, elderly, pregnancy (B)

Pharmacokinetics:

PO: Peak 12 hr, metabolized by liver; excreted in urine, feces; crosses placenta; half-life 20-40 hr

Interactions:

• Decreased effects of guanethidine, clonidine, indirect-acting sympathomimetics (ephedrine)

• Increased effects of direct-acting sympathomimetics (epinephrine), alcohol, barbiturates, benzodiazepines, CNS depressants

• Hyperpyretic crisis, convulsions, hypertensive episode: MAOI (pargyline [Eutonyl])

🍃 Increased anticholinergic effect: belladonna leaf/root, henbane leaf

🍃 Increased antidepressant action: scopolia root

Lab test interferences:

Increase: Serum bilirubin, blood glucose, alk phosphatase

False increase: Urinary catecholamines

Decrease: VMA, 5-HIAA

NURSING CONSIDERATIONS

Assess:

• B/P (lying, standing), pulse q4h; if systolic B/P drops 20 mm Hg, hold drug, notify prescriber; take vital signs q4h in patients with cardiovascular disease

• Blood studies: CBC, leukocytes, differential, cardiac enzymes if patient is receiving long-term therapy

• Hepatic studies: AST (SGOT), ALT (SGPT), bilirubin, creatinine

• Weight qwk; appetite may increase with drug

• ECG for flattening of T wave, bundle branch block, AV block, dysrhythmias in cardiac patients

• EPS primarily in elderly: rigidity, dystonia, akathisia

• Mental status: mood, sensorium, affect, suicidal tendencies, increase in psychiatric symptoms: depression, panic

• Urinary retention, constipation; constipation is more likely to occur in children

• Withdrawal symptoms: headache, nausea, vomiting, muscle pain, weakness; do not usually occur unless drug was discontinued abruptly

• Alcohol consumption; if alcohol is consumed, hold dose until morning

Administer:

• Increased fluids, bulk in diet for constipation, especially elderly

• With food, milk for GI symptoms

• Dosage hs if oversedation occurs during day; may take entire dose hs; elderly may not tolerate once/day dosing

• Gum, hard candy, or frequent sips of water for dry mouth

• Concentrate with fruit juice, water, or milk to disguise taste

Perform/provide:

• Storage in tight container at room temp; do not freeze

• Assistance with ambulation during beginning therapy, since drowsiness/dizziness occurs

• Safety measures, including side rails, primarily in elderly

• Checking to see PO medication swallowed

Evaluate:

• Therapeutic response: decreased depression

Teach patient/family:

• That therapeutic effects may take 2-3 wk

• To use caution in driving, other activities requiring alertness, because of drowsiness, dizziness, blurred vision

---

⬦ = Nursing alert   🍃 = Herb-drug interaction   🚫 = Do not crush

• Antiemetic 30-60 min before giving drug to prevent vomiting
• IV after diluting 5 mg/10 ml sterile H_2O for inj; allow to stand, give through Y-tube or 3-way stopcock; give over 5-10 min
• Transfusion for anemia
• Antispasmodic for GI symptoms

Additive compatibilities: Dexamethasone, hydrocortisone
Solution compatibilities: LR, 0.3% NaCl, 0.5% NaCl
Syringe compatibilities: Bleomycin, cisplatin, cyclophosphamide, doxorubicin, droperidol, fluorouracil, furosemide, heparin, leucovorin, methotrexate, metoclopramide, vinblastine, vincristine
Y-site compatibilities: Allopurinol, amifostine, bleomycin, cisplatin, cyclophosphamide, doxorubicin, droperidol, fluorouracil, furosemide, granisetron, heparin, leucovorin, melphalan, methotrexate, metoclopramide, ondansetron, teniposide, thiotepa, vinblastine, vincristine
Perform/provide:
• Liquid diet: carbonated beverages, gelatin may be added if patient is not nauseated or vomiting
• Rinsing of mouth tid-qid with water; brushing of teeth with soft brush or baking soda bid-tid with soft brush or cotton-tipped applicators for stomatitis; use unwaxed dental floss
• Storage at room temp 1 wk after reconstituting or 2 wk refrigerated
Evaluate:
• Therapeutic response: decreased tumor size, spread of malignancy
Teach patient/family:
• To report any complaints, side effects to nurse or prescriber
• That hair may be lost during treatment and wig or hairpiece may make the patient feel better; tell patient that new hair may be different in color, texture

• To avoid foods with citric acid, hot or rough texture
• To report any bleeding, white spots, ulcerations in mouth; tell patient to examine mouth qd
• To avoid crowds, people with infections if granulocyte count is low

---

mitoxantrone (℞)
(mye-toe-zan'trone)
Novantrone
Func. class.: Antineoplastic, antibiotic
Chem. class.: Synthetic anthraquinone

Action: DNA reactive agent, cytocidal effect on both proliferating and nonproliferating cells, suggesting lack of cell cycle phase specificity (vesicant)
Uses: Acute nonlymphocytic leukemia (adult), relapsed leukemia, breast cancer; used with steroids to treat bone pain (advanced prostate cancer)
Investigational uses: Breast and liver malignancies, non-Hodgkin's lymphoma
Dosage and routes:
• *Adult:* **IV INF** 12 mg/m^2/day on days 1-3, and 100 mg/m^2 cytosine arabinoside × 7 days as a continuous 24 hr infusion
Available forms: Inj 2 mg/ml
Side effects/adverse reactions:
*GI: Nausea, vomiting, diarrhea, anorexia, mucositis, **hepatotoxicity***
*HEMA: **Thrombocytopenia, leukopenia, myelosuppression, anemia***
INTEG: Rash, necrosis at injection site, dermatitis, thrombophlebitis at injection site, alopecia
*CV: **CHF, cardiopathy, dysrhythmias***
MISC: Fever
RESP: Cough, dyspnea

Contraindications: Hypersensitivity, pregnancy (D)

Precautions: Myelosuppression, lactation, cardiac disease, children; renal, hepatic disease; gout

Pharmacokinetics: Highly bound to plasma proteins, metabolized in liver, excreted via renal, hepatobiliary systems; half-life 24-72 hr

Interactions:

• Do not mix with heparin; precipitate will form

NURSING CONSIDERATIONS
Assess:

• CBC, differential, platelet count qwk; withhold drug if WBC is <4000/mm³ or platelet count is <75,000/mm³; notify prescriber of these results

• Liver function tests before, during therapy: bilirubin, AST (SGOT), ALT (SGPT), alk phosphatase prn or qmo

• Renal function studies: BUN, serum uric acid, urine CrCl, electrolytes before, during therapy

• Bleeding, hematuria, guaiac, bruising or petechiae, mucosa or orifices q8h

• Food preferences: list likes, dislikes

• Yellow skin and sclera, dark urine, clay-colored stools, itchy skin, abdominal pain, fever, diarrhea

• Acidosis, signs of dehydration: rapid respirations, poor skin turgor, decreased urine output, dry skin, restlessness, weakness

Administer:

• Medications by oral route if possible; avoid IM, SC, IV routes to prevent infections

• Antiemetic 30-60 min before giving drug to prevent vomiting

• IV after diluting with 50 ml or more normal saline or D₅W; give over 3-5 min, running IV of D₅W or NS; may be diluted further in D₅W, NS and run over 15-30 min; check for extravasation

Additive compatibilities: Cyclophosphamide, cytarabine, fluorouracil, hydrocortisone, potassium chloride

Solution compatibilities: D₅/0.9 NaCl, D₅W, 0.9% NaCl

Y-site compatibilities: Allopurinol, amifostine, cladribine, filgrastim, fludarabine, granisetron, melphalan, ondansetron, sargramostim, teniposide, thiotepa, vinorelbine

Perform/provide:

• Liquid diet: carbonated beverages, Jell-O; dry toast, crackers may be added if patient is not nauseated or vomiting

• Rinsing of mouth tid-qid with water, club soda; brushing of teeth bid-qid with soft brush or cotton-tipped applicators for stomatitis; use unwaxed dental floss

Evaluate:

• Therapeutic response: decreased tumor size, spread of malignancy

Teach patient/family:

• To report side effects to nurse or physician

• To avoid foods with citric acid, rough texture, or hot

• To report any bleeding, white spots, ulcerations in mouth; tell patient to examine mouth qd

---

mivacurium (℞)
(miv-a-kure'ee-um)
Mivacron
Func. class.: Nondepolarizing neuromuscular blocker

Action: Inhibits transmission of nerve impulses by binding competitively with cholinergic receptor sites, antagonizing action of acetylcholine

Uses: Facilitation of endotracheal

intubation, skeletal muscle relaxation during mechanical ventilation, surgery, or general anesthesia

Dosage and routes:
• *Adult:* IV 0.15 mg/kg; maintenance q15min
• *Child 2-12 yr:* IV 0.2 mg/kg for a 10 min block

Available forms: 5, 10 ml single-use vial (2 mg/ml); premixed infusion in D$_5$W 50-ml flex container

Side effects/adverse reactions:
CV: Decreased B/P, bradycardia, tachycardia
*RESP: **Prolonged apnea, bronchospasm, wheezing, respiratory depression***
EENT: Diplopia
MS: Weakness, prolonged skeletal muscle relaxation, *paralysis*
INTEG: Rash, urticaria

Contraindications: Hypersensitivity

Precautions: Pregnancy (C), renal or hepatic disease, lactation, children <3 mo, fluid and electrolyte imbalances, neuromuscular disease, respiratory disease, obesity, elderly

Pharmacokinetics: Rapidly hydrolyzed by plasma cholinesterases, peak 2-3 min, reversal within 15-30 min

Interactions:
• Increased neuromuscular blockade: aminoglycosides, quinidine, local anesthetics, polymyxin antibiotics, enflurane, isoflurane, tetracyclines, halothane, Mg, colistin, procainamide, bacitracin, lincomycin, clindamycin, lithium

NURSING CONSIDERATIONS
Assess:
• For electrolyte imbalances (K, Mg); may lead to increased action of this drug
• Vital signs (B/P, pulse, respirations, airway) until fully recovered; rate, depth, pattern of respirations, strength of hand grip

• I&O ratio; check for urinary retention, frequency, hesitancy
• Recovery: decreased paralysis of face, diaphragm, leg, arm, rest of body
• Allergic reactions: rash, fever, respiratory distress, pruritus; drug should be discontinued

Administer:
• Using nerve stimulator by anesthesiologist to determine neuromuscular blockade
• Anticholinesterase to reverse neuromuscular blockade
• By slow IV over 1-2 min (only by qualified persons, usually an anesthesiologist)
• Only fresh sol

Y-site compatibilities: Etomidate, thiopental

Perform/provide:
• Storage at room temp; do not freeze
• Reassurance if communication is difficult during recovery from neuromuscular blockade
• Frequent (q2h) instillation of artificial tears and covering eyes to prevent drying of cornea

Evaluate:
• Therapeutic response: paralysis of jaw, eyelid, head, neck, rest of body

Treatment of overdose: Neostigmine, monitor VS; may require mechanical ventilation

---

moexipril (℞)

(moe-ex'ih-prill)
Univasc
Func. class.: Antihypertensive
Chem. class.: Angiotensin-converting enzyme inhibitor

Action: Selectively suppresses renin-angiotensin-aldosterone system; inhibits ACE; prevents conversion of angiotensin I to angiotensin II; results in dilation of arterial, venous vessels

Uses: Hypertension, alone or in combination with thiazide diuretics

Dosage and routes:

Renal dose

• CrCl <40 ml/min 3.75 mg/day titrate to desired dose

• *Adult:* **PO** 7.5 mg 1 hr ac initially, may be increased or divided depending on B/P response; maintenance dosage; 7.5-30 mg qd in 1-2 divided doses 1 hr ac

Available forms: Tabs 7.5, 15 mg

Side effects/adverse reactions:

CV: Hypotension, postural hypotension

GU: Impotence, dysuria, nocturia, proteinuria, nephrotic syndrome, acute reversible renal failure, polyuria, oliguria, frequency

HEMA: **Neutropenia**

INTEG: Rash

RESP: **Bronchospasm,** dyspnea, dry cough

META: Hypokalemia

GI: Loss of taste

CNS: Fever, chills

SYST: **Angioedema**

Contraindications: Hypersensitivity, children, lactation, heart block, bilateral renal stenosis, K-sparing diuretics

Precautions: Dialysis patients, hypovolemia, leukemia, scleroderma, lupus erythematosus, blood dyscrasias, CHF, diabetes mellitus, renal disease, thyroid disease, COPD, asthma, pregnancy (C)

Pharmacokinetics: Metabolized by liver (metabolites), excreted in urine; crosses placenta; excreted in breast milk

Interactions:

• Increased hypotension: diuretics, other antihypertensives, ganglionic blockers, adrenergic blockers

• Do not use with potassium-sparing diuretics, sympathomimetics, potassium supplements

Lab test interferences:

False positive: Urine acetone

NURSING CONSIDERATIONS

Assess:

• Blood studies: neutrophils, decreased platelets

• B/P

• Renal studies: protein, BUN, creatinine; watch for increased levels that may indicate nephrotic syndrome

• Baselines in renal, liver function tests before therapy begins

• K levels, although hyperkalemia rarely occurs

• Edema in feet, legs daily

• Allergic reaction: rash, fever, pruritus, urticaria; drug should be discontinued if antihistamines fail to help

• Symptoms of CHF; edema, dyspnea, wet rales, B/P

• Renal symptoms: polyuria, oliguria, frequency

Administer:

• PO 1 hr before meals

Perform/provide:

• Storage in tight container at 86° F or less

Evaluate:

• Therapeutic response: decrease in B/P in hypertension

Teach patient/family:

• To take 1 hr ac

• Not to discontinue drug abruptly

• Not to use OTC (cough, cold, or allergy) products unless directed by prescriber

• To comply with dosage schedule, even if feeling better

• To rise slowly to sitting or standing position to minimize orthostatic hypotension

• To notify prescriber of mouth

 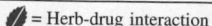

sores, sore throat, fever, swelling of hands or feet, irregular heartbeat, chest pain, signs of angioedema
• That excessive perspiration, dehydration, vomiting, diarrhea may lead to fall in blood pressure; consult prescriber if these occur
• That dizziness, fainting, lightheadedness may occur during first few days of therapy
• That skin rash or impaired perspiration may occur
• How to take B/P
Treatment of overdose: 0.9% NaCl IV inf, hemodialysis

---

moricizine (℞)

(more-i'siz-een)

Ethmozine

Func. class.: Antidysrhythmic, group I

Chem. class.: Phenothiazine

Action: Decreased rate of rise of action potential, prolonging refractory period and shortening the action potential duration; depression of inward influx if sodium mediates the effects; drug may slow atrial and AV nodal conduction

Uses: Life-threatening dysrhythmias

Dosage and routes:
• *Adult:* **PO** 10-15 mg/kg/day or 600-900 mg/day in 2-3 divided doses

Available forms: Film-coated tabs 200, 250, 300 mg

Side effects/adverse reactions:

GI: Nausea, abdominal pain, vomiting, diarrhea

CNS: Dizziness, headache, fatigue, perioral numbness, euphoria, nervousness, sleep disorders, depression, tinnitus, fatigue

RESP: Dyspnea, hyperventilation, ***apnea,*** asthma, pharyngitis, cough

GU: Sexual dysfunction, difficult urination, dysuria, incontinence

CV: Palpitations, chest pain, ***CHF,*** hypertension, syncope, dysrhythmias, bradycardia, ***MI, thrombophlebitis***

MISC: Sweating, musculoskeletal pain

Contraindications: 2nd or 3rd degree AV block, right bundle branch block, cardiogenic shock, hypersensitivity

Precautions: CHF, hypokalemia, hyperkalemia, sick sinus syndrome, pregnancy (B), lactation, children, impaired hepatic and renal function, cardiac dysfunction

Pharmacokinetics: Half-life 1.5-3.5 hr; peak 0.5-2.2 hr; metabolized by the liver; metabolites excreted in feces and urine, protein binding >90%

Interactions:
• Increased plasma levels of moricizine: amantadine, cimetidine
• Digoxin or propranolol may enhance some cardiac effects of moricizine; moricizine may decrease effects of theophylline
• Increased anticholinergic effect: henbane leaf
• Increased potassium loss, increased antidysrhythmic action: aloe, cascara sagrada bark, buckthorn bark/berry, rhubarb root, senna leaf/fruits

Lab test interferences:

Increase: CPK

NURSING CONSIDERATIONS

Assess:
• GI status: bowel pattern, number of stools
• Cardiac status: rate, rhythm, quality
• Chest x-ray, pulmonary function test during treatment
• I&O ratio; check for decreasing output
• B/P for fluctuations
• Lung fields: bilateral rales may occur in CHF patient

• Increased respiration, increased pulse; drug should be discontinued

◆ Toxicity: fine tremors, dizziness

• Cardiac status: respiration, rate, rhythm, character continuously

Evaluate:

• Therapeutic response: absence of dysrhythmias

Teach patient/family:

• To report side effects to prescriber

Treatment of overdose: O_2 artificial ventilation, ECG; administer dopamine for circulatory depression, diazepam or thiopental for convulsions

---

morphine (℞)

(mor′feen)

Astramorph PF, Duramorph, Epimorph*, Kadian, Infumorph 200, Infumorph 500, morphine sulfate, Morphitec*, M.O.S.*, M.O.S.-S.R.*, MS Contin, MSIR, OMS Concentrate, Oramorph SR, RMS, Roxanol, Roxanol 100, Roxanol Rescudose, Roxanol SR, UltraJect

Func. class.: Narcotic analgesic

Chem. class.: Opiate

Controlled Substance Schedule II

Action: Depresses pain impulse transmission at the spinal cord level by interacting with opioid receptors

Uses: Severe pain

Dosage and routes:

• *Adult:* **SC/IM** 4-15 mg q4h prn; **PO** 10-30 mg q4h prn; **EXT REL** q8-12h; **RECT** 10-20 mg q4h prn; **IV** 4-10 mg diluted in 4-5 ml H_2O for injection, over 5 min

• *Child:* **SC/IV** 0.1-0.2 mg/kg, not to exceed 15 mg; **PO** 0.2-0.5 mg/kg q4-6h (reg rel), q12h (sus rel)

Available forms: Inj 2, 4, 5, 8, 10, 15 mg/ml; sol tabs 10, 15, 30 mg; oral sol 10, 20 mg/5 ml, 20 mg/10 ml, 20 mg/ml; oral tabs 15, 30 mg; rect supp 5, 10, 20, 30 mg; ext rel tabs 15, 30, 60, 100, 200 mg; caps 15, 30 mg

Side effects/adverse reactions:

CNS: Drowsiness, dizziness, confusion, headache, sedation, euphoria

CV: Palpitations, bradycardia, change in B/P

EENT: Tinnitus, blurred vision, miosis, diplopia

GI: Nausea, vomiting, anorexia, constipation, cramps, biliary tract pressure

GU: Urinary retention

INTEG: Rash, urticaria, bruising, flushing, diaphoresis, pruritus

*RESP: **Respiratory depression***

Contraindications: Hypersensitivity, addiction (narcotic), hemorrhage, bronchial asthma, increased intracranial pressure

Precautions: Addictive personality, pregnancy (B), lactation, acute MI, severe heart disease, elderly, respiratory depression, hepatic disease, renal disease, child <18 yr

Pharmacokinetics:

PO: Onset variable, peak variable, duration variable

IM: Onset ½ hr, peak ½-1 hr, duration 3-7 hr

SC: Onset 15-20 min, peak 50-90 min, duration 3-5 hr

IV: Peak 20 min

RECT: Peak ½-1 hr, duration 4-5 hr

Intrathecal: Onset rapid, duration up to 24 hr

Metabolized by liver, crosses placenta; excreted in urine, breast milk; half-life 1½-2 hr

Interactions:

• Increased effects with other CNS depressants: alcohol, narcotics, sedative/hypnotics, antipsychotics, skeletal muscle relaxants

Lab test interferences:

Increase: Amylase

◆ = Nursing alert   🖋 = Herb-drug interaction   🚫 = Do not crush

NURSING CONSIDERATIONS
Assess:
• Pain: location, type, character; give dose before pain becomes severe
• Bowel status; constipation frequent
• I&O ratio; check for decreasing output; may indicate urinary retention
• B/P, pulse, respirations (character, depth, rate)
• CNS changes: dizziness, drowsiness, hallucinations, euphoria, LOC, pupil reaction
• Allergic reactions: *rash, urticaria*
• Respiratory dysfunction: depression, character, rate, rhythm; notify prescriber if respirations are <12/min

Administer:
• With antiemetic for nausea, vomiting
• When pain is beginning to return; determine dosage interval by response; continuous dosing is more effective than prn
• May be given by patient-controlled analgesia
• Epidurally cautiously in the elderly

IV
• After diluting with 5 ml or more sterile H$_2$O or NS; give 15 mg or less over 4-5 min; give through Y-tube or 3-way stopcock; may be added to IV sol, each 0.1-1 mg diluted in 1 ml D$_5$W, D$_{10}$W, 0.9% NaCl, 0.45% NaCl, Ringer's, LR, given with inf pump titrated to patient response

Additive compatibilities: Alteplase, atracurium, baclofen, bupivacaine, dobutamine, fluconazole, furosemide, meropenem, metoclopramide, ondansetron, succinylcholine, verapamil

Syringe compatibilities: Atropine, benzquinamide, bupivacaine, butorphanol, cimetidine, dimenhydrinate, diphenhydramine, droperidol, fentanyl, glycopyrrolate, hydroxyzine, ketamine, metoclopramide, midazolam, milrinone, pentazocine, perphenazine, promazine, ranitidine, scopolamine

Y-site compatibilities: Allopurinol, amifostine, amikacin, aminophylline, amiodarone, ampicillin, ampicillin/sulbactam, amsacrine, atenolol, atracurium, aztreonam, bumetanide, calcium chloride, cefamandole, cefazolin, cefmetazole, cefoperazone, cefotaxime, cefotetan, cefoxitin, ceftazidime, ceftizoxime, ceftriaxone, cefuroxime, cephalothin, cephapirin, chloramphenicol, cisplatin, cladribine, clindamycin, cyclophosphamide, cytarabine, dexamethasone, digoxin, diltiazem, dobutamine, dopamine, doxycycline, enalaprilat, epinephrine, erythromycin, esmolol, etomidate, famotidine, fentanyl, filgrastim, fluconazole, fludarabine, foscarnet, gentamicin, granisetron, heparin, hydrocortisone, hydromorphone, IL-2, insulin (regular), kanamycin, labetalol, lidocaine, lorazepam, magnesium sulfate, melphalan, meropenem, methotrexate, methyldopate, methylprednisolone, metoclopramide, metoprolol, metronidazole, mezlocillin, midazolam, milrinone, moxalactam, nafcillin, nicardipine, nitroglycerin, norepinephrine, ondansetron, oxacillin, oxytocin, paclitaxel, pancuronium, penicillin G potassium, piperacillin, piperacillin/tazobactam, potassium chloride, propofol, propranolol, ranitidine, sodium bicarbonate, sodium nitroprusside, teniposide, thiotepa, ticarcillin, ticarcillin/clavulanate, tobramycin, trimethoprim-sulfamethoxazole, vancomycin, vecuronium, vinorelbine, vit B/C, warfarin, zidovudine

M

Perform/provide:
• Storage in light-resistant container at room temp
• Assistance with ambulation
• Safety measures: side rails, night-light, call bell within easy reach
• Gradual withdrawal after long-term use

Evaluate:
• Therapeutic response; decrease in pain intensity

Teach patient/family:
• To change position slowly; orthostatic hypotension may occur
• To report any symptoms of CNS changes, allergic reactions
• That physical dependency may result from long-term use
• To avoid use of alcohol, CNS depressants
• That withdrawal symptoms may occur: nausea, vomiting, cramps, fever, faintness, anorexia

Treatment of overdose: Naloxone (Narcan) 0.2-0.8 mg IV, O_2, IV fluids, vasopressors

---

moxalactam
See cephalosporins—3rd generation

---

multivitamins (OTC, ℞)
Adavite, Dayalets, LKV Drops, Multi-75, Multiday, One-A-Day, Optilets, Poly-Vi-sol, Quin tabs, Ru-Lets, Sesame Street Vitamins, Tab-A-Vite, Therabid, Theragram, Unicaps, Vita-Bob, Vita-Kid, many other brands
Func. class.: Vitamins, multiple

Action: Needed for adequate metabolism

Uses: Prevention and treatment of vitamin deficiencies

Dosage and routes:
• *Adult and child:* **PO/IV**—depends on brand
Available forms: Many

Side effects/adverse reactions:
None known at recommended dosage

Precautions: Pregnancy (A)

NURSING CONSIDERATIONS
Assess:
• Vitamin deficiency: usually more than one vitamin is deficient

Administer:
• Liquid multivitamins diluted or dropped into patient's mouth using dropper provided with some brands
• Chew tabs should be chewed, not swallowed whole
• Give by cont IV inf only after diluting 5-10 ml multivitamins/500-1000 ml of D_5W, $D_{10}W$, $D_{20}W$, LR, D_5/LR, D_5/0.9% NaCl, 0.9% NaCl, 3% NaCl
• Do not use sol with crystals, precipate, or color other than bright yellow

Additive compatibilities: Cefoxitin, isoproterenol, methyldopa, metoclopramide, metronidazole, netilmicin, norepinephrine, sodium bicarbonate, verapamil

Y-site compatibilities: Acyclovir, ampicillin, cefazolin, cephalothin, cephapirin, diltiazem, erythromycin, fludarabine, gentamicin, tacrolimus

Evaluate:
• Therapeutic response: check each individual vitamin for guidelines

Teach patient/family:
• That adequate nutrition must be maintained to prevent further deficiencies
• The drug interactions that should be avoided
• To comply with regimen
• To avoid presenting flavored mul-

 = Nursing alert   = Herb-drug interaction   = Do not crush

tivitamins as candy; child may overdose
• To store out of children's reach

---

muromonab-CD3 (℞)

(mur-oo-mone'ab)
Orthoclone OKT3
Func. class.: Immunosuppres-
sant
Chem. class.: Murine monoclo-
nal antibody

Action: Reverses graft rejection by
blocking T-cell function
Uses: Acute allograft rejection in
renal, cardiac/hepatic transplant pa-
tients
Dosage and routes:
• *Adult:* **IV BOL** 5 mg/day × 10-14
days
• *Child:* **IV** 100 μg/kg/day × 10-14
days
*Cardiac/hepatic allograft rejection,
steroid resistant*
• *Adult:* **IV BOL** 5 mg/day × 10-14
days; begin when it is known that
rejection has not been reversed by
steroids
Available forms: Inj 5 mg/5 ml
Side effects/adverse reactions:
CNS: Pyrexia, chills, tremors
*RESP: Dyspnea, wheezing, **pulmo-
nary edema***
CV: Chest pain
GI: Vomiting, nausea, diarrhea
MISC: Infection
Contraindications: Hypersensitiv-
ity to murine origin, fluid overload
Precautions: Pregnancy (C), child
<2 yr, fever
Pharmacokinetics: Trough level
steady state 3-14 days
Interactions:
• Incompatible with any drug in sy-
ringe or sol
NURSING CONSIDERATIONS
Assess:
◆ For cytokine release syndrome

(CRS): nausea, vomiting, chills, fever, joint pain, weakness, dizziness,
diarrhea, tremors, abdominal pain
• For hypersensitivity: dyspnea,
bronchospasm, urticaria, tachycardia, angioedema; emergency equipment must be available
• Blood studies: Hgb, WBC, platelets during treatment qmo; if leukocytes are <3000/mm³, drug should
be discontinued
• Liver function studies: alk phosphatase, AST (SGOT), ALT (SGPT),
bilirubin
• Hepatotoxicity: dark urine, jaundice, itching, light-colored stools;
drug should be discontinued
Administer:
• For several days before transplant
surgery
• All medications PO if possible;
avoid IM injection, since infection
may occur
IV
• IV undiluted; withdraw with a 0.2-
0.22 low protein-binding μm filter,
discard and use new needle for administration; give over 1 min
Evaluate:
• Therapeutic response: absence of
graft rejection
Teach patient/family:
• To report fever, chills, sore throat,
fatigue, since serious infection may
occur
• To use contraceptive measures during treatment, for 12 wk after ending therapy; possible mutagenic effects

M

---

mycophenolate mofetil (R̲)

(mye-koe-phen'oh-late)
CellCept
Func. class.: Immunosuppressant

Action: Inhibits inflammatory responses that are mediated by the immune system; prolongs the survival of allogenic transplants

Uses: Organ transplants (to prevent rejection)

Dosage and routes:
• *Adult:* **PO** give initial dose 72 hr prior to transplantation; 1 g bid given to renal transplant patients in combination with corticosteroids, cyclosporine

Available forms: Caps 250 mg; tabs 500 mg

Side effects/adverse reactions:
GI: Nausea, vomiting, stomatitis
*HEMA: **Leukopenia, thrombocytopenia, anemia, pancytopenia***
INTEG: Rash
MS: Arthralgia, muscle wasting
RESP: Dyspnea, respiratory infection, increased cough, pharyngitis, bronchitis, pneumonia
CNS: Tremor, dizziness, insomnia, headache, fever
META: Peripheral edema, hypercholesterolemia, hypophosphatemia, edema, hyperkalemia, hypokalemia, hyperglycemia
GU: UTI, hematuria, ***renal tubular necrosis***

Contraindications: Hypersensitivity to this drug or mycophenolic acid

Precautions: Lymphomas, malignancies, neutropenia, renal disease, pregnancy (C), lactation

Pharmacokinetics: Rapidly and completely absorbed, metabolized to active metabolite (MPA), excreted in urine, feces

Interactions:
• Increased concentration of both drugs: acyclovir, ganciclovir
• Increased levels of mycophenolate: probenecid, salicylate
• Decreased levels of mycophenolate: antacids, cholestyramine
• Decreased binding of phenytoin, theophylline

NURSING CONSIDERATIONS
Assess:
• Blood studies: CBC during treatment monthly
• Liver function studies: alk phosphatase, AST (SGOT), ALT (SGPT), bilirubin

Administer:
• 72 hr prior to transplantation; may be given in combination with corticosteroids, cyclosporine
• Give alone for better absorption

Evaluate:
• Therapeutic response: absence of graft rejection

Teach patient/family:
• To report fever, rash, severe diarrhea, chills, sore throat, fatigue, since serious infections may occur
• To reduce risk of infection by avoiding crowds
🚫 Not to break, crush, or chew caps

nabumetone (R̲)

(na-byoo'me-tone)
Relafen
Func. class.: Nonsteroidal antiinflammatory
Chem. class.: Acetic acid derivative

Action: Inhibits prostaglandin synthesis by decreasing enzyme needed for biosynthesis; analgesic, antiinflammatory

Uses: Osteoarthritis, rheumatoid arthritis, acute or chronic treatment

---

 = Nursing alert   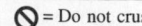 = Herb-drug interaction   🚫 = Do not crush

Dosage and routes:
• *Adult:* **PO** 1 g as a single dose; may increase to 1.5-2 g/day if needed; may give qd or bid as a divided dose
Available forms: Tabs 500, 750 mg
Side effects/adverse reactions:
CNS: Dizziness, headache, drowsiness, fatigue, tremors, confusion, insomnia, anxiety, depression, nervousness
*GU: **Nephrotoxicity, dysuria, hematuria, oliguria, azotemia,** cystitis*
GI: Nausea, anorexia, vomiting, diarrhea, jaundice, ***cholestatic hepatitis,*** constipation, flatulence, cramps, dry mouth, peptic ulcer, gastritis, ***ulceration, perforation***
CV: Tachycardia, peripheral edema, palpitations, dysrhythmias, ***CHF***
INTEG: Purpura, rash, pruritus, sweating, photosensitivity
*HEMA: **Blood dyscrasias***
EENT: Tinnitus, hearing loss, blurred vision
RESP: Dyspnea, pharyngitis, ***bronchospasm***
Contraindications: Hypersensitivity to this drug or aspirin, iodides, NSAIDs, asthma, severe renal disease, severe hepatic disease
Precautions: Pregnancy (B) 1st and 2nd trimester, lactation, children, bleeding disorders, GI disorders, cardiac disorders, renal disorders, hepatic dysfunction, elderly
Pharmacokinetics:
PO: Peak 2½-4 hr, plasma protein binding >90%, half-life 22-30 hr; metabolized in liver to active metabolite; excreted in urine (metabolites), breast milk
Interactions:
• May increase action or toxicity of warfarin, cyclosporine, phenytoin, methotrexate, probenecid, salicylates

• Decreased effect of diuretics, antihypertensives
• Increased risk of bleeding: cefamandole, cefotetan, cefoperazone, valproic acid, plicamycin, thrombolytics, anticoagulants

NURSING CONSIDERATIONS
Assess:
• Pain: frequency, intensity, characteristics; relief of pain after med
• Asthma, aspirin sensitivity or nasal polyps; increased hypersensitive reactions
• Renal, liver, blood studies: BUN, creatinine, AST (SGOT), ALT (SGPT), Hgb, before treatment, periodically thereafter
• Audiometric, ophthalmic exam before, during, after treatment
• For eye, ear problems: blurred vision, tinnitus; may indicate toxicity
Administer:
• With food for GI symptoms
Perform/provide:
• Storage at room temp
Evaluate:
• Therapeutic response: decreased pain and stiffness in joints
Teach patient/family:
• To avoid alcoholic beverages and aspirin
• To report blurred vision, ringing, roaring in ears; may indicate toxicity
• To avoid driving, other hazardous activities if dizziness, drowsiness occur
• To report change in urine pattern, increased weight, edema, increased pain in joints, fever, blood in urine; indicates nephrotoxicity
• That therapeutic effects may take up to 1 mo
• To take with a full glass of water to enhance absorption
• To report dark stools; may indicate GI bleeding

N

nadolol (℞)

(nay-doe'lole)
Corgard
Func. class.: Antihypertensive,
antianginal
Chem. class.: β-adrenergic receptor blocker

Action: Long-acting, nonselective β-adrenergic receptor blocking agent; mechanism is similar to that of propranolol

Uses: Chronic stable angina pectoris, mild to moderate hypertension, prophylaxis of migraine headaches

Investigational uses: Tachydysrhythmias, aggression, anxiety, tremors, esophageal varices (rebleeding only)

Dosage and routes:
Renal dose
• CrCl 31-50 ml/min give q24-36h; CrCl 10-30 ml/min give q24-48h
• *Adult:* **PO** 40 mg qd, increase by 40-80 mg q3-7d; maintenance 40-240 mg/day for angina, 40-320 mg/day for hypertension
• *Geriatric:* **PO** 20 mg/day, may increase by 20 mg until desired dose

Available forms: Tabs 20, 40, 80, 120, 160 mg

Side effects/adverse reactions:
RESP: Dyspnea, respiratory dysfunction, *bronchospasm,* cough, wheezing, nasal stuffiness, pharyngitis, *laryngospasm*
CV: Bradycardia, hypotension, CHF, palpitations, *AV block,* chest pain, peripheral ischemia, flushing, edema, vasodilation, conduction disturbances
HEMA: Agranulocytosis, thrombocytopenia
GI: Nausea, vomiting, diarrhea, colitis, constipation, cramps, dry mouth, flatulence, hepatomegaly, *pancreatitis,* taste distortion

INTEG: Rash, pruritus, fever
CNS: Depression, hallucinations, dizziness, fatigue, lethargy, paresthesias, headache
EENT: Sore throat

Contraindications: Hypersensitivity to this drug, cardiac failure, cardiogenic shock, 2nd or 3rd degree heart block, bronchospastic disease, sinus bradycardia, CHF, COPD

Precautions: Diabetes mellitus, pregnancy (C), renal disease, lactation, hyperthyroidism, peripheral vascular disease, myasthenia gravis

Pharmacokinetics:
PO: Onset variable, peak 3-4 hr, duration 17-24 hr; half-life 16-20 hr; not metabolized; excreted in urine (unchanged), bile, breast milk

Interactions:
• Increased effects of reserpine, digitalis, ergots, neuromuscular blocking agents, calcium channel blockers
• Increased hypotensive effects: other hypotensive agents, diuretics, phenothiazines
• Decreased effects of norepinephrine, xanthines, isoproterenol, thyroid

Lab test interferences:
Increase: Serum K, serum uric acid, ALT (SGPT), AST (SGOT), alk phosphatase, LDH, blood glucose, cholesterol

NURSING CONSIDERATIONS
Assess:
• B/P, pulse, respirations during beginning therapy
• Weight qd; report gain of 5 lb
• I&O ratio, CrCl if kidney damage is diagnosed
• qd, note need to be administered more often
• Pain: duration, time started, activity being performed, character
• Headache, light-headedness, decreased B/P; may indicate a need for decreased dosage

---

◆ = Nursing alert   ∥ = Herb-drug interaction   Ⓢ = Do not crush

Administer:
PO
• With 8 oz water
Evaluate:
• Therapeutic response: decreased B/P, symptoms of angina
Teach patient/family:
• That drug may mask signs of hypoglycemia or alter blood glucose in diabetics
• Not to discontinue abruptly
• To avoid OTC drugs unless prescriber approves
• To avoid hazardous activities if dizziness occurs
• To comply with complete medical regimen

---

nafarelin (R)
(naf-ah-rell'in)
Synarel
Func. class.: Gonadotropin
Chem. class.: Analog of gonadotropin-releasing hormone

Action: Stimulates the release of LH and FSH, which increases ovarian steroid production; repeated dosing prevents stimulation of the pituitary gland
Uses: Endometriosis, gonadotropin-dependent precocious puberty
Dosage and routes:
• *Adult:* NASAL 400 µg/day as one spray (200 µg) into one nostril in morning and one spray into other nostril in evening; start treatment between days 2 and 4 of menstrual cycle; may increase to 800 µg/day (one spray into each nostril twice a day); recommended duration of treatment is 6 mo
Available forms: Nasal sol 2 mg/ml
Side effects/adverse reactions:
GU: Decreased libido, vaginal dryness, breast tenderness, increased pubic hair

CNS: Headache, flushing, depression, insomnia, emotional lability, hot flashes
INTEG: Nasal irritation, acne
MISC: Body odor, seborrhea, rhinitis
SENSITIVITY: Shortness of breath, chest pain, urticaria, pruritus
Contraindications: Hypersensitivity, pregnancy (X), lactation, undiagnosed abnormal vaginal bleeding
Precautions: Children
Pharmacokinetics: Rapidly absorbed, peak 10-40 min, half-life 3 hr; 80% bound to plasma proteins
NURSING CONSIDERATIONS
Assess:
• Test results: pituitary/hypothalamus dysfunction (decreased LH); postmenopausal (increased LH)
Administer:
NASAL
• Repeated doses may be necessary to elevate pituitary gonadotropin reserve
Perform/provide:
• Storage at room temp; protect from light
Evaluate:
• Therapeutic response: decreased symptoms of endometriosis
Teach patient/family:
• To use nonhormonal contraception
• About correct nasal use, one spray in right nostril AM, one in left nostril PM
• That medication may cause hot flashes, decreased libido, vaginal dryness

N

Side effects: *italics* = common; ***bold italics*** = life-threatening

nafcillin (R)

(naf-sill'in)
Nafcil, nafcillin sodium, Nallpen, Unipen
Func. class.: Antiinfective, broad-spectrum
Chem. class.: Penicillinase-resistant penicillin

Action: Interferes with cell wall replication of susceptible organisms; osmotically unstable cell wall swells, bursts from osmotic pressure

Uses: Effective for gram-positive cocci *(S. aureus, S. viridans, S. pneumoniae),* infections caused by penicillinase-producing *Staphylococcus*

Dosage and routes:
• *Adult:* **PO** 250-1000 mg q4-6h; **IM** 500 mg q4-6h; **IV** 500-1500 mg q4-6h
• *Child and infants most infections:* **PO** 6.25-12.5 mg/kg q6h; pharyngitis **PO** 250 mg q8h; **IM** 25 mg/kg q12h; **IV** most infections 10-20 mg/kg q4h or 20-40 mg/kg q8h, max 200 mg/kg/day
• *Neonates:* **PO** 10 mg/kg q6-8h; **IM** 10 mg/kg q12h; **IV:** most infections 10-20 mg/kg q4h or 20-40 mg/kg q8h, max 200 mg/kg/day
Meningitis
• *Neonates* ≥2 *kg:* 50 mg/kg q8h × 1 wk of life, then 50 mg/kg q6h
• *Neonates* <2 *kg:* 25-50 mg/kg q12h × 1 wk of life, then 50 mg/kg q8h
Available forms: Caps 250 mg; tabs 500 mg; powder for oral susp 250 mg/5 ml; powder for inj 500 mg, 1, 2, 10 g; inj 1, 1.5, 2, 4 g

Side effects/adverse reactions:
HEMA: Anemia, increased bleeding time, *bone marrow depression, granulocytopenia*
GI: Nausea, vomiting, diarrhea, increased AST (SGOT), ALT (SGPT), abdominal pain, glossitis, *pseudomembranous colitis*
GU: Oliguria, *proteinuria, hematuria,* vaginitis, moniliasis, *glomerulonephritis,* interstitial nephritis
CNS: Lethargy, hallucinations, anxiety, depression, twitching, *coma, convulsions*

Contraindications: Hypersensitivity to penicillins
Precautions: Pregnancy (B), hypersensitivity to cephalosporins, neonates

Pharmacokinetics:
IM/PO: Peak 30-60 min, duration 4-6 hr, half-life 1 hr, metabolized by liver, excreted in bile, urine
Interactions:
• Decreased effect of oral contraceptives
• Increased nafcillin concentrations: aspirin, probenecid, disulfiram
Lab test interferences:
False positive: Urine glucose, urine protein

NURSING CONSIDERATIONS
Assess:
• I&O ratio; report hematuria, oliguria, since penicillin in high doses is nephrotoxic
 Any patient with compromised renal system, since drug is excreted slowly in poor renal system function; toxicity may occur rapidly
• Liver studies: AST (SGOT), ALT (SGPT)
• Blood studies: WBC, RBC, H&H, bleeding time
• Renal studies: urinalysis, protein, blood, BUN, creatinine
• C&S before drug therapy; drug may be given as soon as culture is taken
• Bowel pattern before and during treatment
• Skin eruptions after administration of penicillin to 1 wk after discontinuing drug

---

 = Nursing alert   ⚟ = Herb-drug interaction   ⛒ = Do not crush

• Respiratory status: rate, character, wheezing, and tightness in chest
• Allergies before initiation of treatment and reaction of each medication; highlight allergies on chart, Kardex
• Differential WBC in patients on long-term therapy

Administer:
• IM deep in gluteal muscle
• Drug after C&S has been completed
• Divided oral doses on empty stomach before meals; oral absorption is erratic

IV
• After diluting 500 mg/1.7 ml of sterile H_2O for inj; further dilute each 500 mg/15-30 ml sterile H_2O or NS sol; give through Y-tube or 3-way stopcock; 500 mg or less/5-10 min; may be further diluted and run over 24 hr

Additive compatibilities: Chloramphenicol, chlorothiazide, dexamethasone, diphenhydramine, ephedrine, heparin, hydroxyzine, lidocaine, potassium chloride, prochlorperazine, sodium bicarbonate, sodium lactate
Syringe compatibilities: Cimetidine, heparin
Y-site compatibilities: Acyclovir, atropine, cyclophosphamide, diazepam, enalaprilat, esmolol, famotidine, fentanyl, fluconazole, foscarnet, hydromorphone, magnesium sulfate, morphine, perphenazine, propofol, theophylline, zidovudine

Perform/provide:
• Adrenalin, suction, tracheostomy set, endotracheal intubation equipment
• Adequate fluid intake (2 L) during diarrhea episodes
• Scratch test to assess allergy after securing order from prescriber; usually done when penicillin is only drug of choice

• Storage in tight container; refrigerate reconstituted sol

Evaluate:
• Therapeutic response: absence of fever, draining wounds

Teach patient/family:
• All aspects of drug therapy, including need to complete course of medication to ensure organism death (10-14 days); culture may be taken after completed course
• To report sore throat, fever, fatigue (may indicate superinfection)
• To wear or carry Medic Alert ID if allergic to penicillins
• To notify nurse of diarrhea
🚫 Not to break, crush, or chew caps

Treatment of anaphylaxis: Withdraw drug; maintain airway; administer epinephrine, aminophylline, O_2, IV corticosteroids

---

nalbuphine (℞)

(nal′byoo-feen)
Nubain, nalbuphine HCl
Func. class.: Narcotic analgesic
Chem. class.: Synthetic narcotic agonist, antagonist

Controlled Substance Schedule II
Action: Depresses pain impulse transmission at the spinal cord level by interacting with opioid receptors
Uses: Moderate to severe pain
Dosage and routes:
Analgesic
• *Adult:* **SC/IM/IV** 10-20 mg q3-6h prn, not to exceed 160 mg/day
Balanced anesthesia supplement
• *Adult:* **IV** 0.3-3 mg/kg given over 10-15 min, may give 0.25-0.5 mg/kg as needed for maintenance
Available forms: Inj 10, 20 mg/ml
Side effects/adverse reactions:
CNS: Drowsiness, dizziness, confusion, headache, sedation, euphoria,

dysphoria (high doses), hallucinations, dreaming, tolerance, physical, psychological dependency
GI: Nausea, vomiting, anorexia, constipation, cramps
GU: Increased urinary output, dysuria, urinary retention, urgency
INTEG: Rash, urticaria, bruising, flushing, diaphoresis, pruritus
EENT: Tinnitus, blurred vision, miosis, diplopia
CV: Palpitations, bradycardia, change in B/P, orthostatic hypotension
RESP: Respiratory depression
Contraindications: Hypersensitivity, addiction (narcotic)
Precautions: Addictive personality, pregnancy (C), lactation, increased intracranial pressure, MI (acute), severe heart disease, respiratory depression, hepatic disease, renal disease
Pharmacokinetics:
SC/IM/IV: Duration 3-6 hr; metabolized by liver, excreted by kidneys, half-life 5 hr
Interactions:
• Increased effects with other CNS depressants: alcohol, narcotics, sedative/hypnotics, antipsychotics, skeletal muscle relaxants
Lab test interferences:
Increase: Amylase
NURSING CONSIDERATIONS
Assess:
• I&O ratio; check for decreasing output; may indicate urinary retention
 For withdrawal reactions in narcotic-dependent individuals: pulmonary embolus, vascular occlusion; abscesses, ulcerations, nausea, vomiting, convulsions
• CNS changes: dizziness, drowsiness, hallucinations, euphoria, LOC, pupil reaction
• Allergic reactions: rash, urticaria
• Respiratory dysfunction: respiratory depression, character, rate,

rhythm; notify prescriber if respirations are <10/min
• Need for pain medication by pain sedation scoring, physical dependency
Administer:
• With antiemetic if nausea, vomiting occur
• When pain is beginning to return; determine dosage interval by response
• IM deep in large muscle mass, rotate injection sites
IV
• Undiluted 10 mg or less over 3-5 min
Syringe compatibilities: Atropine, cimetidine, diphenhydramine, droperidol, glycopyrrolate, hydroxyzine, lidocaine, midazolam, prochlorperazine, ranitidine, scopolamine, trimethobenzamide
Y-site compatibilities: Amifostine, aztreonam, cefmetazole, cladribine, filgrastim, fludarabine, granisetron, melphalan, paclitaxel, propofol, teniposide, thiotepa, vinorelbine
Perform/provide:
• Storage in light-resistant area at room temp
• Assistance with ambulation
• Safety measures: night-light, call bell within easy reach
Evaluate:
• Therapeutic response: decrease in pain
Teach patient/family:
• To report any symptoms of CNS changes, allergic reactions
• That physical dependency may result from long-term use
• That withdrawal symptoms may occur: nausea, vomiting, cramps, fever, faintness, anorexia
Treatment of overdose: Naloxone (Narcan) 0.2-0.8 mg IV, O_2, IV fluids, vasopressors

nalidixic acid (℞)

(nal-i-dix'ik)

NegGram, NegGram Caplets

Func. class.: Urinary tract anti-infective

Chem. class.: Fluoroquinolone

Action: Appears to inhibit DNA polymerization, primary target being single-stranded DNA precursors in late stages of chromosomal replication

Uses: UTIs (acute/chronic) caused by *E. coli, Klebsiella, Enterobacter, P. mirabilis, P. vulgaris, P. morganii*

Dosage and routes:

Renal dose

• CrCl <50 ml/min avoid use

• *Adult:* **PO** 1 g qid × 1-2 wk, 2 g/day for long-term treatment

• *Child >3 mo:* **PO** 55 mg/kg/day in 4 divided doses for 1-2 wk; 33 mg/kg/day in 4 divided doses for long-term treatment

Available forms: Tabs 250, 500 mg, 1 g; susp 250 mg/5 ml

Side effects/adverse reactions:

INTEG: Pruritus, rash, urticaria, photosensitivity

CNS: Dizziness, headache, drowsiness, insomnia, ***convulsions***

GI: Nausea, vomiting, abdominal pain, diarrhea

EENT: Sensitivity to light, blurred vision, change in color perception

Contraindications: Hypersensitivity, CNS damage, liver disease, liver failure, infants <3 mo

Precautions: Elderly, renal disease, hepatic disease, pregnancy (B), lactation

Pharmacokinetics:

PO: Peak 1-2 hr, metabolized in liver, excreted in urine (unchanged/conjugates), crosses placenta, enters breast milk

Interactions:

• Increased effects of oral coagulants

• Decreased effects with antacids

Lab test interferences:

False positive: Urinary glucose

False increase: 17-OHCS, VMA

NURSING CONSIDERATIONS

Assess:

• Blood count for patients on chronic therapy

• I&O ratio; urine pH <5.5 is ideal

• Renal, hepatic function

• Photosensitivity: drug should be discontinued

• CNS symptoms: insomnia, vertigo, headache, drowsiness, convulsions

• Allergy: fever, flushing, rash, urticaria, pruritus

Administer:

PO

• After clean-catch urine for C&S

• Two daily doses if urine output is high or if patient has diabetes

• 2 hr before or 2 hr after antacids

Perform/provide:

• Protection from freezing

Evaluate:

• Therapeutic response: decreased dysuria, negative culture

Teach patient/family:

• That photosensitivity occurs; that patient should avoid sunlight or use sunscreen to prevent burns

• To take medication with food or milk to decrease GI irritation; take 2 hr before or 2 hr after antacids

• To protect suspension from freezing, shake well before taking

• That drug may cause drowsiness; instruct client to seek aid in walking, other activities; advise client not to drive or operate machinery while on medication

• That diabetics should monitor blood glucose

nalmefene
(nal'meh-feen)
Revex
Func. class.: Opioid antagonist
Chem. class.: Analog of nal-trexone

Action: Competes with opioids at opioid receptor sites; prevents or reverses the effects of opioids

Uses: Reversal of opioid effects, management of known or suspected opioid overdose

Dosage and routes:
Opioid overdose
• *Adult (green label):* Titrate to reverse effects of opioids; 0.5 mg/70 kg, may give 1 mg/70 kg at 2-5 min intervals; since this drug is longer acting, use incremental dosing to avoid over-reversal

Postoperative opioid depression
• *Adult (blue label):* 0.25 μg/kg, then 0.25 μg/kg at 2-5 min intervals

Available forms: Inj 1 mg/ml

Side effects/adverse reactions:
CNS: Drowsiness, nervousness, dizziness, headache, chills, fever
CV: Tachycardia, hypertension, hypotension, vasodilation, bradycardia
GI: Nausea, vomiting, diarrhea

Contraindications: Hypersensitivity

Precautions: Pregnancy (B), children, opioid dependency, lactation, respiratory depression, renal or hepatic disease, elderly

Pharmacokinetics: Complete bioavailability, rapidly distributed, metabolized by liver, excreted in urine, terminal half-life approx 40 min, 10-15 hr

Interactions:
• Seizures: flumazenil

NURSING CONSIDERATIONS
Assess:
• Withdrawal: cramping, hypertension, anxiety, vomiting
• VS q3-5min
• ABGs, including Po_2, Pco_2
• Cardiac status: tachycardia, hypertension; monitor ECG
• Respiratory dysfunction: respiratory depression, character, rate, rhythm; if respirations are <10/min, administer this drug; probably due to opioid overdose; monitor LOC

Administer:
• Only with resuscitative equipment, O_2 nearby

Perform/provide:
• Storage at room temp

Evaluate:
• Therapeutic response: reversal of respiratory depression; LOC-alert

naloxone (℞)
(nal-oks'one)
naloxone HCl, Narcan
Func. class.: Opioid antagonist
Chem. class.: Thebaine derivative

Action: Competes with narcotics at narcotic receptor sites

Uses: Respiratory depression induced by narcotics, pentazocine, propoxyphene; refractory circulatory shock

Dosage and routes:
Opioid-induced respiratory depression
• *Adult:* **IV/SC/IM** 0.4-2 mg; repeat q2-3min if needed
• *Child:* **IV/SC/IM** 0.5-2 μg/kg as small frequent, q/min **BOL** or as **INF** titrated to response

Postoperative respiratory depression
• *Adult:* **IV** 0.1-0.2 mg q2-3min prn
• *Child:* **IV/IM/SC** 0.01 mg/kg q2-3min prn

 = Nursing alert   = Herb-drug interaction   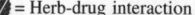 = Do not crush

Asphyxia neonatorum

• *Neonate:* **IV** 0.01 mg/kg given into umbilical vein after delivery; may repeat q2-3min × 3 doses

Available forms: Inj 0.02, 0.4, 1 mg/ml

Side effects/adverse reactions:

CNS: Drowsiness, nervousness

CV: Rapid pulse, increased systolic B/P (high doses), ventricular tachycardia, fibrillation

GI: Nausea, vomiting

RESP: Hyperpnea

Contraindications: Hypersensitivity, respiratory depression

Precautions: Pregnancy (B), children, cardiovascular disease, opioid dependency, lactation

Pharmacokinetics: Well absorbed IM, SC; metabolized by liver, crosses placenta; excreted in urine, breast milk; half-life 1 hr

IV: Onset 1 min, duration 45 min

IM/SC: Onset 2-5 min, duration 45-60 min

Interactions:

• Decreased effect of opioid analgesics

Lab test interferences:

Interference: Urine VMA, 5-HIAA, urine glucose

NURSING CONSIDERATIONS

Assess:

• Withdrawal: cramping, hypertension, anxiety, vomiting, signs of withdrawal in drug-dependent individuals

• VS q3-5min

• ABGs including Po_2, Pco_2

• Cardiac status: tachycardia, hypertension; monitor ECG

• Respiratory dysfunction: respiratory depression, character, rate, rhythm; if respirations are <10/min, administer naloxone; probably due to opioid overdose; monitor LOC

Administer:

• Only with resuscitative equipment, O_2 nearby

• Only sol prepared within 24 hr

IV

• Undiluted with sterile H_2O for inj; may be further diluted with NS or D_5 and given as an inf; give 0.4 mg or less over 15 sec or titrate inf to response

Additive compatibilities: Verapamil

Syringe compatibilities: Benzquinamide, heparin

Y-site compatibilities: Propofol

Perform/provide:

• Dark storage at room temp

Evaluate:

• Therapeutic response: reversal of respiratory depression; LOC-alert

---

naltrexone (Ŗ)

(nal-trex′one)

Trexan

Func. class.: Opioid antagonist

Chem. class.: Thebaine derivative

N

Action: Competes with narcotics at narcotic receptor sites

Uses: Blockage of opioid analgesics, used in treatment of opiate addiction

Dosage and routes:

• *Adult:* **PO** 25 mg, may give 25 mg after 1 hr if no withdrawal symptoms; 50-150 mg may be given qd depending on need, maintenance 50 mg q24h; 100-150 mg may be given on alternate days or 3 days per wk

Available forms: Tabs 50 mg

Side effects/adverse reactions:

MISC: Increased thirst, chills, fever

MS: Joint and muscle pain

GU: Delayed ejaculation, decreased potency

CNS: Stimulation, drowsiness, dizziness, confusion, ***convulsion,*** headache, flushing, hallucinations, nervousness, irritability

GI: Nausea, vomiting, diarrhea,

heartburn, anorexia, ***hepatitis,*** constipation

INTEG: Rash, urticaria, bruising, oily skin, acne, pruritus

EENT: Tinnitus, hearing loss, blurred vision

CV: Rapid pulse, ***pulmonary edema,*** hypertension

RESP: Wheezing, hyperpnea, nasal congestion, rhinorrhea, sneezing, sore throat

Contraindications: Hypersensitivity, opioid dependence, hepatic failure, hepatitis

Precautions: Pregnancy (C), hepatic disease, lactation, child

Pharmacokinetics:

PO: Onset 15-30 min, peak 1-2 hr, duration is dose dependent

Metabolized by liver, excreted by kidneys; crosses placenta, excreted in breast milk; half-life 4 hr; extensive first-pass metabolism

NURSING CONSIDERATIONS
Assess:

• VS q3-5min

• ABGs including Po_2, Pco_2

• Signs of withdrawal in drug-dependent individuals

• Cardiac status: tachycardia, hypertension

• Respiratory dysfunction: respiratory depression, character, rate, rhythm; if respirations are <10/min, respiratory stimulant should be administered

Administer:

• Only if resuscitative equipment is nearby

Perform/provide:

• Storage in tight container

Evaluate:

• Therapeutic response: blocking narcotic ingestion

Teach patient/family:

• That they must be drug-free to start treatment

• That using opioid while taking this drug could prove fatal because high dose is needed to overcome this antagonist

• To carry MedicAlert ID stating med used

• If surgery is needed, all involved should be aware of this drug

---

nandrolone decanoate/ nandrolone phenpropionate (℞)

(nan'droe-lone)

Androlone-D 200, Deca-Durabolin, Durabolin, Hybolin Decanoate-50, Hybolin Decanoate-100, Hybolin Improved, Nandrobolic, nandrolone decanoate, nandrolone phenpropionate, Neo-Durabolic

Func. class.: Androgenic anabolic steroid

Chem. class.: Halogenated testosterone derivative

Action: Increases weight by building body tissue, increases potassium, phosphorus, chloride, nitrogen levels, increases bone development

Uses: Tissue building, severe disease, refractory anemias, metastatic breast cancer

Dosage and routes:

Tissue building (possibly effective)

• *Adult:* **IM** 50-100 mg q3-4wk (decanoate)

• *Child 2-13 yr:* **IM** 25-50 mg q3-4wk (decanoate)

Severe disease/refractory anemias

• *Adult:* **IM** 100-200 mg qwk (decanoate)

Breast cancer

• *Adult:* **IM** 50-100 mg qwk (phenpropionate)

Available forms: Phenpropionate inj

 = Nursing alert   = Herb-drug interaction   = Do not crush

25, 50 mg/ml; decanoate inj 50, 100, 200 mg/ml

Side effects/adverse reactions:

INTEG: Rash, acneiform lesions, oily hair, skin, flushing, sweating, acne vulgaris, alopecia, hirsutism

CNS: Dizziness, headache, fatigue, tremors, paresthesias, flushing, sweating, anxiety, lability, insomnia, carpal tunnel syndrome

MS: Cramps, spasms

CV: Increased B/P

GU: **Hematuria,** amenorrhea, vaginitis, decreased libido, decreased breast size, clitoral hypertrophy, testicular atrophy

GI: Nausea, vomiting, constipation, weight gain, ***cholestatic jaundice***

EENT: Conjunctival edema, nasal congestion

ENDO: Abnormal GTT

Contraindications: Severe renal, severe cardiac, severe hepatic disease, hypersensitivity, pregnancy (X), lactation, abnormal genital bleeding, males with cancer of breast, prostate

Precautions: Diabetes mellitus, CV disease, MI

Pharmacokinetics:

IM: Metabolized in liver, crosses placenta, excreted in breast milk, urine

Interactions:

• Increased effects of oral antidiabetics, oxyphenbutazone
• Increased PT: anticoagulants
• Edema: ACTH, adrenal steroids
• Decreased effects of insulin

Lab test interferences:

Increase: Serum cholesterol, blood glucose, urine glucose

Decrease: Serum Ca, serum K, T_4, T_3, thyroid ^{131}I uptake test, urine 17-OHCS, 17-KS, PBI, BSP

NURSING CONSIDERATIONS

Assess:

• Weight daily; notify prescriber if weekly weight gain is >5 lb
• B/P q4h

• I&O ratio; be alert for decreasing urinary output, increasing edema
• Growth rate in children, since growth rate may be uneven (linear/bone growth) with extended use
• Electrolytes: K, Na, Cl, Ca; cholesterol
• Liver function studies: ALT (SGPT), AST (SGOT), bilirubin
• Edema, hypertension, cardiac symptoms, jaundice
• Mental status: affect, mood, behavioral changes, aggression
• Signs of masculinization in female: increased libido, deepening of voice, decreased breast tissue, enlarged clitoris, menstrual irregularities; male: gynecomastia, impotence, testicular atrophy
• Hypercalcemia: lethargy, polyuria, polydipsia, nausea, vomiting, constipation; drug may have to be decreased
• Hypoglycemia in diabetics, since oral antidiabetic action is increased

Administer:

• Titrated dose; use lowest effective dose

Perform/provide:

• Diet with increased calories, protein; decrease Na if edema occurs

Evaluate:

• Therapeutic response: increased appetite, increased stamina

Teach patient/family:

• That drug must be combined with complete health plan: diet, rest, exercise
• To notify prescriber if therapeutic response decreases
• Not to discontinue abruptly
• About changes in sex characteristics
• That females should report menstrual irregularities
• That 1-3 mo course is necessary for response in breast cancer

N

naproxen (OTC, ℞)

(na-prox'en)

Apo-Naproxen*, EC-Naprosyn, Naprelan, Napron X, Naprosyn, Naprosyn-E*, Naprosyn-SR*, Naxen*, Novo-Naprox*, Nu-Naprox*

naproxen sodium

Aleve, Anaprox, Anaprox DS, Apo-Napro-Na*, Apo-Napro-Na DS, Naprelan, Novo-Naprox Sodium*, Novo-Naprox Sodium DS*, Synflex*, Synflex DS*

Func. class.: Nonsteroidal antiinflammatory, nonopioid analgesic

Chem. class.: Propionic acid derivative

Action: Inhibits prostaglandin synthesis by decreasing an enzyme needed for biosynthesis; analgesic, antiinflammatory, antipyretic

Uses: Mild to moderate pain, osteoarthritis, rheumatoid, gouty arthritis, juvenile arthritis, primary dysmenorrhea

Dosage and routes:
• *Adult:* **PO** 250-500 mg bid, not to exceed 1 g/day (base); 525 mg, then 275 mg q6-8h prn, not to exceed 1475 mg (sodium)
• *Child:* **PO** 10 mg/kg in 2 divided doses

Available forms: Tabs, naproxen: 250, 375, 500 mg; oral susp 125 mg/5 ml; naproxen sodium tabs 220, 275, 550 mg

Side effects/adverse reactions:
GI: Nausea, anorexia, vomiting, diarrhea, jaundice, ***cholestatic hepatitis,*** constipation, flatulence, cramps, dry mouth, peptic ulcer, ***GI ulceration, bleeding, perforation***
CNS: Dizziness, drowsiness, fatigue, tremors, confusion, insomnia, anxiety, depression
CV: Tachycardia, peripheral edema, palpitations, dysrhythmias
INTEG: Purpura, rash, pruritus, sweating
GU: ***Nephrotoxicity: dysuria, hematuria, oliguria, azotemia***
HEMA: ***Blood dyscrasias***
EENT: Tinnitus, hearing loss, blurred vision

Contraindications: Hypersensitivity, asthma, severe renal disease, severe hepatic disease, ulcer disease

Precautions: Pregnancy (B), lactation, children <2 yr, bleeding disorders, GI disorders, cardiac disorders, hypersensitivity to other antiinflammatory agents, elderly, CrCl <25 ml/min

Pharmacokinetics:
PO: Peak 2-4 hr, half-life 3-3½ hr; metabolized in liver; excreted in urine (metabolites), breast milk; 99% protein binding

Interactions:
• May increase action of heparin
• Increased lithium toxicity: lithium

Lab test interferences:
Increase: BUN, alk phosphatase
False increase: 5-HIAA, 17KGS

NURSING CONSIDERATIONS

Assess:
• Pain: frequency, characteristics, intensity; relief after med
• Asthma, aspirin hypersensitivity or nasal polyps, increased risk of hypersensitivity
• Renal, liver, blood studies: BUN, creatinine, AST (SGOT), ALT (SGPT), Hgb before treatment, periodically thereafter
• Audiometric, ophthalmic exam before, during, after treatment
• For eye, ear problems: blurred vision, tinnitus (may indicate toxicity)

 = Nursing alert   🖋 = Herb-drug interaction   = Do not crush

Administer:
• With food to decrease GI symptoms; best to take on empty stomach to facilitate absorption
Perform/provide:
• Storage at room temp
Evaluate:
• Therapeutic response: decreased pain, stiffness, swelling in joints, ability to move more easily
Teach patient/family:
• To report blurred vision, ringing, roaring in ears (may indicate toxicity)
• To avoid driving, other hazardous activities if dizziness or drowsiness occurs
• To report change in urine pattern, weight increase, edema (face, lower extremities), pain increase in joints, fever, blood in urine (indicates nephrotoxicity)
• That therapeutic effects may take up to 1 mo
• To avoid ASA, alcohol, steroids

**nedocromil
inhaler** (℞)
(ned-o-kroe'mill)
Tilade
Func. class.: Antiasthmatic
Chem. class.: Mast cell stabilizer

Action: Stabilizes the membrane of the sensitized mast cell, preventing release of chemical mediators after an antigen-IgE interaction
Uses: Severe perennial bronchial asthma, exercise-induced bronchospasm (prevention), prevention of acute bronchospasm induced by environmental pollutants; *not* for treatment of acute asthma attacks
Dosage and routes:
Bronchospasm, bronchial asthma
Adult and child >12 yr: **INH** 2 inhalations 2-4 ×/day at regular intervals to provide 14 g/day
Available forms: 1.75 mg nedocromil Na per activation in 16.2 g canisters providing at least 112 metered inhalations
Side effects/adverse reactions:
EENT: Throat irritation, cough, nasal congestion, burning eyes, rhinitis
CNS: Headache, dizziness, neuritis, dysphonia
GI: Nausea, vomiting, anorexia, dry mouth, bitter taste
Contraindications: Hypersensitivity to this drug or lactose, status asthmaticus
Precautions: Pregnancy (B), lactation, children
Pharmacokinetics:
INH: Peak 15 min, duration 4-6 hr; excreted unchanged in urine; half-life 80 min
NURSING CONSIDERATIONS
Assess:
• Pulmonary function testing baseline
• Respiratory status: rate, rhythm, characteristics, cough, wheezing, dyspnea
Administer:
• By inhalation only, with spacer device if needed
• Gargle, sip of water to decrease irritation in throat
Evaluate:
• Therapeutic response: decrease in asthmatic symptoms, congested, runny nose
Teach patient/family:
• To clear mucus before using
• The proper technique: exhale; using inhaler, inhale deeply with head tipped back to open airway; remove, hold breath, exhale
• That therapeutic effect may take up to 4 wk
• That drug is preventive only, not restorative

---

nefazodone (℞)

(ne-faz'o-done)
Serzone
Func. class.: Antidepressant
Chem. class.: Phenylpiperazine

Action: Selectively inhibits serotonin uptake by brain, potentiates behavioral changes, occupies central S-H$_2$ receptors

Uses: Major depression

Dosage and routes:
• *Adult:* **PO** 200 mg/day (100 mg bid); dose may be increased to 300 mg/day (150 mg bid), max 600 mg/day
• *Elderly:* 100 mg/day (50 mg bid); increase to 100 mg bid after 2 wk to desired dose

Available forms: Tabs 100, 150, 200, 250 mg

Side effects/adverse reactions:
CNS: Somnolence, dizziness, *headache, insomnia*
GI: Nausea, constipation, dry mouth
GU: Urinary frequency, retention, UTI
CV: Postural hypotension
RESP: Pharyngitis, cough
EENT: Blurred vision, abnormal vision

Contraindications: Hypersensitivity to this drug or phenylpiperazines

Precautions: Pregnancy (C), lactation, children, elderly, cardiovascular disease, seizure disorder

Pharmacokinetics: Metabolized in liver extensively to metabolites; excreted in urine, breast milk; peak 1-3 hr; half-life triphasic 2-4 hr

Interactions:
• Increased effect: CNS depressants
• *Fatal reaction:* antihistamines, nonsedating (astemizole, terfenidine, cisapride)
• Increased plasma concentrations: benzodiazepines

• Hypertension crisis: MAOIs
• Increased toxicity: triazolam, alprazolam, midazolam, phenytoin, MAOI

Drug/smoking: Increases metabolism, decreases effects

NURSING CONSIDERATIONS
Assess:
• B/P (lying, standing), pulse q4h; if systolic B/P drops 20 mm Hg, hold drug, notify prescriber; take vital signs q4h in patients with cardiovascular disease
• Blood studies: CBC, leukocytes, differential, cardiac enzymes (long-term therapy)
• Hepatic studies: AST (SGOT), ALT (SGPT), bilirubin
• Mental status: mood, sensorium, affect, suicidal tendencies; increase in psychiatric symptoms: depression, panic
• Urinary retention, constipation; constipation is more likely in children, elderly
⬥ For withdrawal symptoms: headache, nausea, vomiting, muscle pain, weakness; unusual unless drug discontinued abruptly
• Alcohol consumption; hold dose until morning

Administer:
• With food, milk for GI symptoms
• Crushed if patient cannot swallow whole

Perform/provide:
• Storage at room temp; do not freeze

Evaluate:
• Therapeutic response: decrease in depression; absence of suicidal thoughts

Teach patient/family:
• That therapeutic effects may take 3-4 wk
• To use caution in driving, other activities requiring alertness because of drowsiness, dizziness; to avoid rising quickly from sitting to standing, especially elderly

---

⬥ = Nursing alert   ⬊ = Herb-drug interaction   ⊘ = Do not crush

• To avoid alcohol ingestion, other CNS depressants, benzodiazepines
• Not to discontinue medication quickly after long-term use; may cause nausea, headache, malaise
• To increase bulk in diet for constipation, especially elderly
• To take gum, hard sugarless candy, frequents sips of water for dry mouth
Treatment of overdose: ECG monitoring; induce emesis; lavage, activated charcoal; administer anticonvulsant

---

nelfinavir (℞)

(nell-fin'a-ver)
Viracept
Func. class.: Antiviral
Chem. class.: HIV protease inhibitor

Action: Inhibits human immunodeficiency virus (HIV) protease, which prevents maturation of the infectious virus

Uses: HIV alone or in combination

Dosage and routes:
• *Adult:* PO 750 mg tid
• *Child:* PO 20-30 mg/kg tid
Available forms: Tabs 250 mg; powder, oral 50 mg/g

Side effects/adverse reactions:
HEMA: **Anemia, leukopenia, thrombocytopenia, Hgb abnormalities**
GI: *Diarrhea,* anorexia, dyspepsia, nausea, flatulence
CNS: Headache, asthenia, poor concentration
INTEG: *Rash,* dermatitis
MS: Pain
CV: Bleeding
ENDO: Hypoglycemia, hyperlipidemia

Contraindications: Hypersensitivity to protease inhibitors
Precautions: Liver disease, pregnancy (B), lactation, renal disease, hemophilia, PKU
Pharmacokinetics: Half-life 3½-5 hr
Interactions:
• Increased effect: terfenadine, astemizole, cisapride, rifabutin, midazolam, triazolam
• Increased nelfinavir levels: ketoconazole, indinavir, ritonavir
• Decreased nelfinavir levels: rifamycins, nevirapine, phenobarbital, phenytoin, carbamazepine

NURSING CONSIDERATIONS
Assess:
• Signs of infection, anemia
• Liver function studies: ALT, AST
• C&S before drug therapy; drug may be taken as soon as culture is taken; repeat C&S after treatment; determine the presence of other sexually transmitted diseases
• Bowel pattern before, during treatment; if severe abdominal pain with bleeding occurs, drug should be discontinued; monitor hydration
• Skin eruptions, rash, urticaria, itching
• Allergies before treatment, reaction of each medication; place allergies on chart
Teach patient/family:
• If dose is missed, to take as soon as remembered up to 1 hr before next dose; do not double dose
• To take with food

---

neomycin (℞)

(nee-oh-mye'sin)
Mycifradin Sulfate
Func. class.: Antiinfective
Chem. class.: Aminoglycoside

Action: Interferes with protein synthesis in bacterial cell by binding to 30S ribosomal subunit, causing in-

---

accurate peptide sequence to form in protein chain, causing bacterial death

Uses: Severe systemic infections of CNS, respiratory, GI, urinary tract, eye, bone, skin, soft tissues caused by *P. aeruginosa, E. coli, Enterobacter, K. pneumoniae, P. vulgaris;* also used for hepatic coma, preoperatively to sterilize bowel, infectious diarrhea caused by enteropathogenic *E. coli*

Dosage and routes:
Severe systemic infections
• *Adult:* **IM** 15 mg/kg/day in 4 divided doses, not to exceed 1 g/day
Hepatic coma
• *Adult:* **PO** 4-12 g/day in divided doses × 5-6 days
• *Child:* 50-100 mg/kg/day in divided doses
Preoperative bowel sterilization
• *Adult:* **PO** on 3rd day of a 3-day regimen, give 1 g early PM, repeat in 1 hr, repeat at hs (given with erythromycin); give saline cathartic before giving this drug

Available forms: Tabs 500 mg; inj 500 mg; oral sol 125 mg/5 ml

Side effects/adverse reactions:
GU: Oliguria, hematuria, renal damage, azotemia, renal failure, nephrotoxicity
CNS: Confusion, depression, numbness, tremors, *convulsions,* muscle twitching, *neurotoxicity,* dizziness, vertigo
EENT: Ototoxicity, deafness, visual disturbances, tinnitus
HEMA: Agranulocytosis, thrombocytopenia, leukopenia, eosinophilia, anemia
GI: Nausea, vomiting, anorexia; increased ALT (SGPT), AST (SGOT), bilirubin; hepatomegaly, *hepatic necrosis,* splenomegaly
CV: Hypotension, hypertension, palpitation

INTEG: Rash, burning, urticaria, photosensitivity, dermatitis, alopecia

Contraindications: Bowel obstruction (oral use), severe renal disease, hypersensitivity, infants, children

Precautions: Mild renal disease, pregnancy (C), hearing deficits, lactation, myasthenia gravis, Parkinson's disease

Pharmacokinetics:
PO: Onset rapid, peak 1-2 hr
Plasma half-life 2-3 hr; not metabolized, excreted unchanged in feces, crosses placenta

Interactions:
• Increased ototoxicity, neurotoxicity, nephrotoxicity: other aminoglycosides, amphotericin B, polymyxin, vancomycin, ethacrynic acid, furosemide, mannitol, methoxyflurane, cisplatin, cephalosporins, bacitracin
• Do not mix in sol or syringe: carbenicillin, ticarcillin, amphotericin B, cephalothin, erythromycin, heparin
• Increased effects: nondepolarizing muscle relaxants, succinylcholine, oral anticoagulants when given with oral neomycin
• Decreased effects of digoxin, penicillin V when given with oral neomycin

NURSING CONSIDERATIONS
Assess:
• Weight before treatment; calculation of dosage is usually based on ideal body weight, but may be calculated on actual body weight
• I&O ratio, urinalysis qd for proteinuria, cells, casts; report sudden change in urine output
• Urine pH if drug is used for UTI; urine should be kept alkaline
• Renal impairment by securing urine for CrCl testing, BUN, serum creatinine; lower dosage should be

given in renal impairment (CrCl <80 ml/min)

• Deafness by audiometric testing, ringing, roaring in ears, vertigo; assess hearing before, during, after treatment

• Dehydration: high specific gravity, decrease in skin turgor, dry mucous membranes, dark urine

• Overgrowth of infection: fever, malaise, redness, pain, swelling, perineal itching, diarrhea, stomatitis, change in cough, sputum

• C&S before starting treatment to identify infecting organism

• Vestibular dysfunction: nausea, vomiting, dizziness, headache; drug should be discontinued if severe

• Injection sites for redness, swelling, abscesses; use warm compresses at site

Administer:

• IM inj deep in large muscle mass; rotate injection sites

• Drug in evenly spaced doses to maintain blood level

• Bicarbonate to alkalinize urine if ordered in treating UTI, as drug is most active in alkaline environment

Perform/provide:

• Adequate fluids of 2-3 L/day unless contraindicated to prevent irritation of tubules

• Supervised ambulation, other safety measures, with vestibular dysfunction

Evaluate:

• Therapeutic response: absence of fever, draining wounds, negative C&S after treatment

Teach patient/family:

• To report headache, dizziness, symptoms of overgrowth of infection, renal impairment

• To report loss of hearing, ringing, roaring in ears or a feeling of fullness in head

Treatment of overdose: Hemodialysis; monitor serum levels of drug

---

neostigmine (℞)

(nee-oh-stig′meen)
neostigmine methylsulfate, Prostigmin
Func. class.: Cholinergic stimulant; anticholinesterase
Chem. class.: Quaternary compound

Action: Inhibits destruction of acetylcholine, which increases concentration at sites where acetylcholine is released; this facilitates transmission of impulses across myoneural junction

Uses: Myasthenia gravis, nondepolarizing neuromuscular blocker antagonist, bladder distention, postoperative ileus

Dosage and routes:

Renal dose

• CrCl 10-50 ml/min 50% of dose; CrCl <10 ml/min 25% of dose

Myasthenia gravis

• *Adult:* **PO** 15-375 mg/day; **IM/IV** 0.5-2 mg q1-3h

• *Child:* **PO** 2 mg/kg/day q3-4h

Nondepolarizing neuromuscular blocker antagonist

• *Adult:* **IV** 0.5-2 mg slowly, may repeat if needed (give 0.6-1.2 mg atropine before this drug)

• *Infant/child:* **IV** 0.025-0.1 mg/kg/dose

Abdominal distention/postoperative ileus

• *Adult:* **IM/SC** 0.25-1 mg (1:4000) q4-6h depending on condition × 2-3 days

Available forms: Tabs 15 mg; inj 1:400*, 1:1000, 1:2000, 1:4000

Side effects/adverse reactions:

INTEG: Rash, urticaria, flushing

CNS: Dizziness, headache, sweating, weakness, *convulsions,* incoordination, *paralysis,* drowsiness, loss of consciousness

GI: Nausea, diarrhea, vomiting, cramps, increased peristalsis, salivary and gastric secretions

CV: Tachycardia, dysrhythmias, bradycardia, hypotension, AV block, ECG changes, *cardiac arrest,* syncope

GU: Frequency, incontinence, urgency

RESP: Respiratory depression, bronchospasm, constriction, laryngospasm, respiratory arrest, dyspnea

EENT: Miosis, blurred vision, lacrimation, visual changes

Contraindications: Obstruction of intestine, renal system, bromide sensitivity, peritonitis

Precautions: Bradycardia, pregnancy (C), hypotension, seizure disorders, bronchial asthma, coronary occlusion, hyperthyroidism, dysrhythmias, peptic ulcer, megacolon, poor GI motility, lactation, children

Pharmacokinetics:

PO: Onset 45-75 min, duration 2½-4 hr

IM/SC: Onset 10-30 min, duration 2½-4 hr

IV: Onset 4-8 min; duration 2-4 hr; metabolized in liver, excreted in urine

Interactions:

• Decreased action of gallamine, metocurine, pancuronium, tubocurarine, atropine

• Increased action of decamethonium, succinylcholine

• Decreased action of neostigmine: aminoglycosides, anesthetics, procainamide, quinidine, mecamylamine, polymyxin, magnesium

NURSING CONSIDERATIONS
Assess:

• VS, respiration q8h

• I&O ratio; check for urinary retention or incontinence

◆ For bradycardia, hypotension, bronchospasm, headache, dizziness, convulsions, respiratory depression; drug should be discontinued if toxicity occurs

Administer:

• Only with atropine sulfate available for cholinergic crisis

• Only after all other cholinergics have been discontinued

• Increased doses if tolerance occurs

• Larger doses after exercise or fatigue

PO

• On empty stomach for better absorption

IV

• Undiluted, give through Y-tube or 3-way stopcock; give 0.5 mg or less over 1 min

Additive compatibilities: Netilmicin

Syringe compatibilities: Glycopyrrolate, heparin, pentobarbital, thiopental

Y-site compatibilities: Heparin, hydrocortisone, potassium chloride, vit B/C

Perform/provide:

• Storage at room temp

Evaluate:

• Therapeutic response: increased muscle strength, hand grasp, improved gait, absence of labored breathing (if severe)

Teach patient/family:

• That drug is not a cure; it only relieves symptoms

• To wear Medic Alert ID specifying myasthenia gravis, drugs taken

Treatment of overdose: Respiratory support, atropine 1-4 mg (IV)

netilmicin (Ŗ)

(ne-til-mye′sin)
Netromycin
Func. class.: Antiinfective
Chem. class.: Aminoglycoside

Action: Interferes with protein synthesis in bacterial cell by binding to 30S ribosomal subunit, causing inaccurate peptide sequence to form in protein chain, causing bacterial death

Uses: Severe systemic infections of CNS, respiratory, GI, urinary tract, bone, skin, soft tissues caused by *P. aeruginosa, E. coli, Enterobacter, Citrobacter, Staphylococcus, K. pneumoniae, P. mirabilis, Serratia, Shigella, Salmonella, Acinetobacter, Neisseria*

Dosage and routes:
Renal dose
• CrCl 40-59 ml/min give q36h; CrCl 20-39 ml/min give q48h; CrCl <20 ml/min individualize dose
Normal renal function
• *Adult and child >12 yr:* **IM/IV** 3-6.5 mg/kg/day; may give q8-12h for severe infections
• *Child and infant 6 wk-12 yr:* **IM/IV** 5.5-8 mg/kg/day in divided doses q8-12h
• *Neonate <6 wk:* **IM/IV** 4-6.5 mg/kg/day in divided doses q12h
Available forms: Inj 100 mg/ml
Side effects/adverse reactions:
GU: Oliguria, hematuria, renal damage, azotemia, renal failure, nephrotoxicity
CNS: Confusion, depression, numbness, tremors, *convulsions,* muscle twitching, *neurotoxicity,* dizziness, vertigo
EENT: Ototoxicity, deafness, visual disturbances, tinnitus
HEMA: Agranulocytosis, thrombo-
cytopenia, leukopenia, eosinophilia, anemia
GI: Nausea, vomiting, anorexia; increased ALT (SGPT), AST (SGOT), bilirubin; hepatomegaly, *hepatic necrosis,* splenomegaly
CV: Hypotension, hypertension, palpitations
INTEG: Rash, burning, urticaria, dermatitis
Contraindications: Severe renal disease, hypersensitivity
Precautions: Neonates, pregnancy (C), mild renal disease, children <12 yr, lactation, myasthenia gravis, hearing deficit, Parkinson's disease, severe burns, cystic fibrosis
Pharmacokinetics:
IM: Onset rapid, peak 1-2 hr
IV: Onset immediate, peak 1-2 hr
Plasma half-life 2-3 hr, not metabolized, excreted unchanged in urine, crosses placental barrier, poor CSF penetration
Interactions:
• Increased ototoxicity, neurotoxicity, nephrotoxicity: other aminoglycosides, amphotericin B, polymyxin, vancomycin, ethacrynic acid, furosemide, mannitol, methoxyflurane, cisplatin, cephalosporins, bacitracin
• Increased effects: nondepolarizing muscle relaxants, succinylcholine

NURSING CONSIDERATIONS
Assess:
• Weight before treatment; calculation of dosage is usually based on ideal body weight, but may be calculated on actual body weight
• Daily I&O ratio, urinalysis for proteinuria, cells, casts; report sudden change in urine output
• IV site for thrombophlebitis, including pain, redness, swelling q30 min; change site if needed; apply warm compresses to discontinued

N

site; VS during infusion, watch for hypotension, change in pulse

• Serum peak, drawn at 30-60 min after IV inf or 60 min after IM inj; trough level drawn just before next dose; blood level should be 2-4 times bacteriostatic level; trough = 0.5-2 mEq/ml, peak = 6-10 mEq/ml

• Urine pH if drug is used for UTI; urine should be kept alkaline

• Renal impairment by securing urine for CrCl testing, BUN, serum creatinine; a lower dosage should be given in renal impairment (CrCl <80 ml/min)

• Deafness by audiometric testing, ringing, roaring in ears, vertigo; assess hearing before, during, after treatment

• Dehydration: high specific gravity, decrease in skin turgor, dry mucous membranes, dark urine

• Electrolytes: K, Na, Cl, Mg monthly if on long-term therapy

• Overgrowth of infection: fever, malaise, redness, pain, swelling, perineal itching, diarrhea, stomatitis, change in cough or sputum

• C&S before starting treatment to identify infecting organism

• Vestibular dysfunction: nausea, vomiting, dizziness, headache; drug should be discontinued if severe

• Inj sites for redness, swelling, abscesses; use warm compresses at site

Administer:

• Drug in evenly spaced doses to maintain blood level

• Bicarbonate to alkalinize urine if ordered in treating UTI, as drug is most active in alkaline environment

IM

• IM inj deep in large muscle mass; rotate inj sites

IV

• IV diluted in 50-200 ml D_5W, 0.9% NaCl; saline infuse over ½-2 hr; separate aminoglycosides and penicillins by ≥1 hr

Additive compatibilities: Aminocaproic acid, atropine, cefuroxime, chlorpromazine, ciprofloxacin, clindamycin, dexamethasone, diazepam, diphenhydramine, hydrocortisone, iron dextran, isoproterenol, methyldopate, metronidazole, multivitamins, neostigmine, norepinephrine, oxytocin, phytonadione, potassium chloride, procainamide, promethazine, triflupromazine, vit B/C

Syringe compatibilities: Doxapram

Y-site compatibilities: Amifostine, aminophylline, aztreonam, calcium gluconate, filgrastim, fludarabine, granisetron, melphalan, sargramostim, teniposide, thiotepa, vinorelbine

Perform/provide:

• Adequate fluids of 2-3 L/day unless contraindicated to prevent irritation of tubules

• Flush of IV line with NS or D_5W after inf

• Supervised ambulation, other safety measures, with vestibular dysfunction

Evaluate:

• Therapeutic response: absence of fever, draining wounds, negative C&S after treatment

Teach patient/family:

• To report headache, dizziness, symptoms of overgrowth of infection, renal impairment

• To report loss of hearing, ringing, roaring in ears or feeling of fullness in head

Treatment of overdose: Hemodialysis; monitor serum levels of drug

---

◆ = Nursing alert   ▮ = Herb-drug interaction   ⊘ = Do not crush

row in; aids in explusion of worms (dwarf tapeworms only)

Treatment of overdose: Enemas, laxatives; do not induce vomiting

---

nicotine resin complex (OTC, ℞)

(nik'o-teen)

Nicorette, Nicorette DS

Func. class.: Smoking deterrent

Chem. class.: Ganglionic cholinergic agonist

Action: Agonist at nicotinic receptors in peripheral, central nervous systems; acts at sympathetic ganglia, on chemoreceptors of aorta, carotid bodies; also affects adrenalin-releasing catecholamines

Uses: Deter cigarette smoking

Dosage and routes:

• *Adult:* Gum 1 piece chewed × ½ hr as needed to abstain from smoking, not to exceed 30/day

Available forms: Gum 2 mg/piece

Side effects/adverse reactions:

RESP: Breathing difficulty, cough, hoarseness, sneezing, wheezing

EENT: Jaw ache, irritation in buccal cavity

CNS: Dizziness, vertigo, insomnia, headache, confusion, convulsions, depression, euphoria, numbness, tinnitus

GI: Nausea, vomiting, anorexia, indigestion, diarrhea, abdominal pain, constipation, eructation

CV: Dysrhythmias, tachycardia, palpitations, edema, flushing, hypertension

Contraindications: Hypersensitivity, immediate post MI recovery period, severe angina pectoris, pregnancy (X)

Precautions: Vasospastic disease, dysrhythmias, diabetes mellitus, hyperthyroidism, pheochromocytoma, coronary disease, esophagitis, peptic ulcer, lactation, hepatic/renal disease

Pharmacokinetics: Onset 15-30 min, metabolized in liver, excreted in urine, half-life 2-3 hr, 30-120 hr (terminal)

Interactions:

• Decreased absorption: glutethimide

• Increased absorption: SC insulin

• Decreased metabolism of propoxyphene

• Smoking cessation increases diuretic effects of furosemide

• Increased blood levels with cessation of smoking: caffeine, theophylline, pentazocine, imipramine, oxazepam, propranolol, acetaminophen

NURSING CONSIDERATIONS

Assess:

• Adverse reaction: irritation of buccal cavity, dislike of taste, jaw ache

Evaluate:

• Therapeutic response: decrease in urge to smoke, decreased need for gum after 3-6 mo

Teach patient/family:

• To chew gum slowly for 30 min to promote buccal absorption of the drug; do not chew over 45 min

• To begin drug withdrawal after 3 mo use; not to exceed 6 mo

• All aspects of drug use; give package insert to patient and explain

• That gum will not stick to dentures, dental appliances

• That gum is as toxic as cigarette; to be used only to deter smoking

• Not to use during pregnancy; birth defects may occur

N

nicotine transdermal system (OTC, ℞)

Habitrol, Nicoderm, Nicotrol, Prostep

Func. class.: Smoking deterrent
Chem. class.: Ganglionic cholinergic agonist

Action: Binds to acetylcholine receptors at autonomic ganglia in the adrenal medulla, at neuromuscular junctions, in brain

Uses: Deter cigarette smoking

Dosage and routes:
• *Habitrol, Nicoderm:* 21 mg/day × 4-8 wk; 14 mg/day × 2-4 wk; 7 mg/day × 2-4 wk
• *Nicotrol:* 15 mg/day × 12 wk; 10 mg/day × 2 wk; 5 mg/day × 2 wk
• *Prostep:* 22 mg/day × 4-8 wk; 11 mg/day × 2-4 wk

Available forms: Transdermal patch delivering 7, 14, 21 mg/day (Habitrol, Nicoderm); 5, 10, 15 mg/day (Nicoderm); 11, 22 mg/day (Prostep)

Side effects/adverse reactions:
RESP: Cough, pharyngitis, sinusitis
MISC: Back pain, chest pain
INTEG: Erythema, pruritus, burning at application site, cutaneous hypersensitivity, sweating, rash
GI: Diarrhea, dyspepsia, constipation, nausea, abdominal pain, vomiting
MS: Arthralgia, myalgia
EENT: Dry mouth, abnormal taste
CNS: Abnormal dreams, insomnia, nervousness, headache, dizziness, paresthesia

Contraindications: Hypersensitivity, children, pregnancy (D), nonsmokers, immediate post MI period, life-threatening dysrhythmias, severe or worsening angina pectoris

Precautions: Skin disease, angina pectoris, MI, renal or hepatic insufficiency, peptic ulcer, accelerated hypertension, serious cardiac dysrhythmias, hyperthyroidism, pheochromocytoma, insulin-dependent diabetes, elderly

Pharmacokinetics: Half-life 3-4 hr, protein binding <5%, 30% is excreted unchanged in urine

Interactions:
• Decreased absorption: glutethimide
• Decreased dose at cessation of smoking: acetaminophen, caffeine, imipramine, oxazepam, pentazocine, propranolol, theophylline, insulin, adrenergic antagonists
• Increased dose at cessation of smoking: adrenergic agonists
• Decreased metabolism of propoxyphene
• Increased diuretic effects of furosemide
• Increased absorption: SC insulin

NURSING CONSIDERATIONS
Assess:
• Adverse reactions: irritation, pruritus, burning at patch site

Perform/provide:
• Storage below 86° F (30° C)

Evaluate:
• Therapeutic response: decrease in urge to smoke, absence of nicotine withdrawal symptoms

Teach patient/family:
• All aspects of drug use; give package insert to patient and explain
• That patch is as toxic as cigarettes; to be used only to deter smoking
• Not to use during pregnancy; birth defects may occur
• To keep used and unused system out of reach of children and pets
• To apply once a day to a nonhairy, clean, dry area of skin on upper body or upper outer arm; to rotate sites to prevent skin irritation
• To stop smoking immediately when beginning patch treatment

• To apply promptly after removing from protective patch; system may lose strength

---

nifedipine (R)

(nye-fed'i-peen)
Adalat, Adalat CC, Adalat P.A.*, Apo-Nifed*, nifedipine, Novo-Nifedin*, Nu N Sed*, Procardia, Procardia XL
Func. class.: Calcium-channel blocker, antianginal
Chem. class.: Dihydropyridine

Action: Inhibits calcium ion influx across cell membrane during cardiac depolarization; relaxes coronary vascular smooth muscle; dilates coronary arteries; increases myocardial oxygen delivery in patients with vasospastic angina; dilates peripheral arteries

Uses: Chronic stable angina pectoris, vasospastic angina, hypertension

Investigational uses: Hypertension (acute), migraines, CHF, Raynaud's disease

Dosage and routes:
• *Adult:* PO immediate release 10 mg tid, increase in 10 mg increments q4-6h, not to exceed 180 mg/24 hr or single dose of 30 mg
• *Child:* PO 0.25-0.5 mg/kg/dose q4-6h, max 1-2 mg/kg/day
• *Adult:* PO sus rel 30-60 mg/qd, may increase q7-14d, doses >120 mg not recommended
Available forms: Caps 5*, 10, 20 mg; tabs, sus rel 30, 60, 90 mg
Side effects/adverse reactions:
CNS: Headache, fatigue, drowsiness, dizziness, anxiety, depression, weakness, insomnia, light-headedness, paresthesia, tinnitus, blurred vision, nervousness

CV: Dysrhythmias, edema, ***CHF,*** hypotension, palpitations, ***MI, pulmonary edema,*** tachycardia
GI: Nausea, vomiting, diarrhea, gastric upset, constipation, increased liver function studies, dry mouth
GU: Nocturia, polyuria
INTEG: Rash, pruritus, flushing, photosensitivity, hair loss
MISC: Flushing, sexual difficulties, cough, fever, chills
Contraindications: Hypersensitivity
Precautions: CHF, hypotension, sick sinus syndrome, 2nd or 3rd degree heart block, hypotension less than 90 mm Hg systolic, hepatic injury, pregnancy (C), lactation, children, renal disease
Pharmacokinetics:
Well absorbed PO
PO-SR: Duration 24 hr
PO: Onset 20 min, peak 0.5-6 hr, duration 6-8 hr, half-life 2-5 hr
Metabolized by liver, excreted in urine (98% as metabolites)
Interactions:
• Increased effects of theophylline, β-blockers, antihypertensives, digitalis
• Increased nifedipine level: cimetidine, grapefruit juice
• Decreased effects: quinidine
NURSING CONSIDERATIONS
Assess:
• Cardiac status: B/P, pulse, respiration, ECG
Administer:
• Before meals, hs
Evaluate:
• Therapeutic response: decreased anginal pain, B/P, activity tolerance
Teach patient/family:
• To avoid hazardous activities until stabilized on drug, dizziness is no longer a problem
• To limit caffeine consumption; no alcohol products

N

- To avoid OTC drugs unless directed by a prescriber
- That sus rel nonabsorbable shell, may appear in stools
- To comply with all areas of medical regimen: diet, exercise, stress reduction, drug therapy
- To change position slowly; orthostatic hypotension is common

🚫 Not to break, crush, or chew sus rel tabs

- To notify prescriber of dyspnea, edema of extremities, nausea, vomiting, severe ataxia

Treatment of overdose: Defibrillation, atropine for AV block, vasopressor for hypotension

---

nilutamide
(nye-loo′ta-mide)
Nilandron, Anandron*
Func. class.: Antineoplastic-hormone
Chem. class.: Antiandrogen

Action: Interferes with testosterone uptake in the nucleus or testosterone activity in target tissues; arrests tumor growth in androgen-sensitive tissue, i.e., prostate gland, prostatic carcinoma is androgen-sensitive, so tumor growth is arrested

Uses: Metastatic prostatic carcinoma, stage D2 in combination with surgical castration

Dosage and routes:
- *Adult:* **PO** 300 mg qd × 30 days, then 150 mg qd

Available forms: Tabs 50, 100 mg*

Side effects/adverse reactions:

CNS: Hot flashes, drowsiness, insomnia, dizziness, hyperthesia, depression

GU: Decreased libido, impotence, testicular atrophy, UTI, hematuria, nocturia, gynecomastia

GI: Diarrhea, nausea, vomiting, increased liver function studies, constipation, dyspepsia

INTEG: Rash, sweating, alopecia, dry skin

RESP: Dyspnea, URI, pneumonia, *interstitial pneumonitis*

HEMA: Anemia

EENT: Delay in adaptation to dark

MISC: Edema

Contraindications: Hypersensitivity, severe hepatic impairment, severe respiratory disease

Precautions: Pregnancy (C)

Pharmacokinetics: Rapidly and completely absorbed; excreted in urine and feces as metabolites

Interactions:
- Increased toxicity of vit K, phenytoin, theophylline

NURSING CONSIDERATIONS
Assess:
- Liver function studies: AST (SGOT), ALT (SGPT), alk phosphatase, which may be elevated
- For CNS symptoms: drowsiness, insomnia, dizziness
- Chest x-rays, routinely; dyspnea, cough, which may indicate interstitial pneumonitis; discontinue treatment if this condition is suspected

Evaluate:
- Therapeutic response: decrease in prostatic tumor size, decrease in spread of cancer

Teach patient/family:
- To report side effects: decreased libido, impotence, breast enlargement, hot flashes, diarrhea, dyspnea, cough
- To wear tinted lens to alleviate delay in adapting to the dark

Treatment of overdose: Induce vomiting, provide supportive care

---

◆ = Nursing alert   🖋 = Herb-drug interaction   🚫 = Do not crush

nisoldipine
(nye-sole'dih-peen)
Sular
Func. class.: Antihypertensive,
calcium channel blocker
Chem. class.: Dihydropyridine

Action: Inhibits calcium ion influx
across cell membrane, resulting in
dilation of peripheral arteries
Uses: Essential hypertension, alone
or with other antihypertensives
Dosage and routes:
• *Adult:* **PO** 20 mg qd initially, may
increase by 10 mg/wk, usual dose
20-40 mg qd
• *Geriatric:* **PO** 10 mg/day, increase
by 10 mg/wk
Available forms: Tabs, ext rel 10,
20, 30, 40 mg
Side effects/adverse reactions:
CV: Dysrhythmia, edema, CHF, hypotension, palpitations, *MI, pulmonary edema,* tachycardia, syncope,
AV block, angina
GI: Nausea, vomiting, diarrhea, gastric upset, constipation, increased
liver function studies, dry mouth
GU: Nocturia, polyuria
INTEG: Rash, pruritus
MISC: Flushing, sexual difficulties,
cough, nasal congestion, shortness
of breath, wheezing, epistaxis, respiratory infection, chest pain
CNS: Headache, fatigue, drowsiness, dizziness, anxiety, depression,
nervousness, insomnia, light-
headedness, paresthesia, tinnitus,
psychosis, somnolence
HEMA: Anemia
Contraindications: Hypersensitivity, sick sinus syndrome, 2nd or 3rd
degree heart block
Precautions: CHF, hypotension <90
mm Hg systolic, hepatic injury, pregnancy (C), lactation, children, renal
disease, elderly

Pharmacokinetics: Metabolized by
liver, excreted in urine
Interactions:
• Increased effects of β-blockers, an-
tihypertensives, digitalis
• Increased felodipine level: cimet-
idine, ranitidine
NURSING CONSIDERATIONS
Assess:
• Cardiac status: B/P, pulse, respi-
ration, ECG
Administer:
• Once daily as whole tablet; avoid
high fat foods, grapefruit
Evaluate:
• Therapeutic response: decreased
B/P
Teach patient/family:
🚫 To swallow whole; not to break,
crush, or chew
• To avoid hazardous activities un-
til stabilized on drug, dizziness is no
longer a problem
• To limit caffeine consumption
• To avoid OTC drugs unless di-
rected by a prescriber
• The importance of complying with
all areas of medical regimen: diet,
exercise, stress reduction, drug
therapy
Treatment of overdose: Defibrillation, atropine for AV block, vaso-
pressor for hypotension

N

nitrofurantoin (R)

(nye-troe-fyoor'an-toyn)
Apo-Nitrofurantoin*, Furadantin*, Furalan, Macpac, Macrobid, Macrodantin, Nephronex*, Nitrofuracot, Nitrofurantoin, Novofuran*

Func. class.: Urinary tract antiinfective

Chem. class.: Synthetic nitrofuran derivative

Action: Appears to inhibit bacterial enzymes

Uses: Urinary tract infections caused by *E. coli, Klebsiella, Pseudomonas, P. vulgaris, P. morganii, Serratia, Citrobacter, S. aureus, S. epidermidis, Enterococcus, Salmonella, Shigella*

Dosage and routes:
• *Adult and child >12 yr:* **PO** 50-100 mg qid pc or 50-100 mg hs for long-term treatment
• *Child 1 mo-3 yr:* **PO** 5-7 mg/kg/day in 4 divided doses; 1-3 mg/kg/day for long-term treatment

Available forms: Caps 25, 50, 100 mg; tabs 50, 100 mg; susp 25 mg/5 ml; ext rel caps 100 mg; macrocrystal caps (Macrodantin) 25, 50, 100 mg

Side effects/adverse reactions:
INTEG: Pruritus, rash, urticaria, angioedema, alopecia, tooth staining
CNS: Dizziness, headache, drowsiness, peripheral neuropathy
*GI: Nausea, vomiting, abdominal pain, diarrhea, **cholestatic jaundice***

Contraindications: Hypersensitivity, anuria, severe renal disease, infants <1 mo

Precautions: Pregnancy (B), lactation, G-6-PD deficiency, elderly

Pharmacokinetics:
PO: Half-life 20-60 min; crosses blood-brain barrier, placenta; enters breast milk; excreted as inactive metabolites in liver, unchanged in urine

Interactions:
• Increased levels of nitrofurantoin: probenecid
• Antagonistic effect: nalidixic acid
• Decreased absorption of Mg trisilicate antacid

NURSING CONSIDERATIONS
Assess:
• Blood count during chronic therapy
• I&O ratio; urine pH <5.5 is ideal; C&S before treatment, after completion
• Renal and hepatic function
• CNS symptoms: insomnia, vertigo, headache, drowsiness, convulsions
• Allergy: fever, flushing, rash, urticaria, pruritus
• Liver function tests periodically: AST, ALT, alk phosphatase

Administer:
PO
• After clean-catch urine for C&S
• Two daily doses if urine output is high or if patient has diabetes

Evaluate:
• Therapeutic response: decreased dysuria, fever

Teach patient/family:
• To take with food or milk; avoid alcohol
• To protect susp from freezing and shake well before taking
• That drug may cause drowsiness; instruct client to seek aid in walking and other activities; advise client not to drive or operate machinery while on medication
• That diabetics should monitor blood glucose level
• That drug may turn urine rust-yellow to brown

◆ = Nursing alert   🖉 = Herb-drug interaction   🚫 = Do not crush

nitroglycerin (R)

(nye-troe-gli'ser-in)

Deponit, Minitran, Nitrek, Nitro-Bid, Nitro-Bid IV, Nitro-Bid Plateau Caps, Nitrocine, Nitrocine Timecaps, Nitrodisc, Nitro-Dur, Nitrogard, nitroglycerin, nitroglycerin transdermal, Nitroglyn, Nitrol, Nitrolingual, Nitrong, Nitrostat, Transderm-Nitro, Tridil

Func. class.: Coronary vasodilator, antianginal

Chem. class.: Nitrate

Action: Decreases preload, afterload, which is responsible for decreasing left ventricular end-diastolic pressure, systemic vascular resistance; dilates coronary arteries, improves blood flow

Uses: Chronic stable angina pectoris, prophylaxis of angina pain, CHF associated with acute MI, controlled hypotension in surgical procedures

Dosage and routes:

• *Adult:* **SL** dissolve tab under tongue when pain begins; may repeat q5min until relief occurs; take no more than 3 tabs/15 min; use 1 tab prophylactically 5-10 min before activities; **SUS CAP** q6-12h on empty stomach; **TOP** 1-2 in q8h, increase to 4 in q4h as needed; **IV** 5 µg/min, then increase by 5 µg/min q3-5min; if no response after 20 µg/min, increase by 10-20 µg/min until desired response; **TRANS** apply a pad qd to a site free of hair; remove patch hs to provide 10-12h nitrate-free interval to avoid tolerance

• *Child:* **IV** initial: 0.25-0.5 µg/kg/min, titrate to patient response, usual dose 1-3 µg/kg/min

Available forms: Buccal tabs 1, 2, 3 mg; aero 0.4 mg/metered spray; sus rel caps 2.5, 6.5, 9, 13 mg; tabs, sus rel 2.6, 6.5, 9 mg; inj 0.5, 5, mg/ml; SL tabs 0.15, 0.3, 0.4, 0.6 mg; trans oint 2%; trans syst 0.1, 0.2, 0.3, 0.4, 0.6 mg/24 hr; inj sol 25 mg/250 ml, 50 mg/250 ml, 50 mg/500 ml, 100 mg/500 ml, 200 mg/500 ml; patch 22.4, 44.8, 67.2 mg

Side effects/adverse reactions:

CV: Postural hypotension, tachycardia, ***collapse,*** syncope

GI: Nausea, vomiting

INTEG: Pallor, sweating, rash

CNS: Headache, flushing, dizziness

Contraindications: Hypersensitivity to this drug or nitrites, severe anemia, increased intracranial pressure, cerebral hemorrhage

Precautions: Postural hypotension, pregnancy (C), lactation

Pharmacokinetics:

SUS REL: Onset 20-45 min, duration 3-8 hr

SL: Onset 1-3 min, duration 30 min

TRANS: Onset ½-1 hr, duration 12-24 hr

IV: Onset 1-2 min, duration 3-5 min

TRANSMUC: Onset 3 min, duration 3-5 hr

AEROSOL: Onset 2 min, duration 30-60 min

TOP OINT: Onset 30-60 min, duration 2-12 hr

Metabolized by liver, excreted in urine, half-life 1-4 min

Interactions:

• Increased effects: β-blockers, diuretics, antihypertensives, anticoagulants, alcohol

• Decreased heparin: IV nitroglycerin

NURSING CONSIDERATIONS

Assess:

• Orthostatic B/P, pulse

• Pain: duration, time started, activity being performed, character

• Tolerance if taken over long period

• Headache, light-headedness, decreased B/P; may indicate a need for decreased dosage

Administer:
• With 8 oz H_2O on empty stomach (oral tablet) 1 hr before or 2 hr after meals
• Trans tab should be placed between cheek and gum line
• Topical ointment should be measured on papers supplied
• Apply a new TD patch qd and remove after 12-14 hr to prevent tolerance

IV
• Diluted in amount specified D_5 or NS for infusion; use glass infusion bottles, nonpolyvinyl chloride infusion tubing; titrate to patient response; do not use filters

Additive compatibilities: Alteplase, aminophylline, dobutamine, dopamine, enalaprilat, furosemide, lidocaine, verapamil

Syringe compatibilities: Heparin

Y-site compatibilities: Amiodarone, amrinone, atracurium, cefmetazole, diltiazem, dobutamine, dopamine, epinephrine, esmolol, famotidine, fentanyl, fluconazole, furosemide, haloperidol, heparin, hydromorphone, insulin (regular), labetalol, lidocaine, lorazepam, midazolam, milrinone, morphine, nicardipine, norepinephrine, pancuronium, propofol, ranitidine, sodium nitroprusside, streptokinase, tacrolimus, theophylline, thiopental, vecuronium, warfarin

Evaluate:
• Therapeutic response: decrease, prevention of anginal pain

Teach patient/family:
• To place buccal tab between lip and gum above incisors or between cheek and gum
🚫 That sus rel must be swallowed whole, not chewed
• That SL should be dissolved under tongue, not swallowed
• That aerosol should be sprayed under tongue, not inhaled
• To use inhaler only when lying down
• Not to inhale spray
• To keep tabs in original container
• If 3 SL tabs in 15 min do not relieve pain, to seek immediate medical attention
• To avoid alcohol
• That drug may cause headache; tolerance usually develops; use nonnarcotic analgesic
• That drug may be taken before stressful activity: exercise, sexual activity
• That SL may sting when drug comes in contact with mucous membranes
• To avoid hazardous activities if dizziness occurs
• To comply with complete medical regimen
• To make position changes slowly to prevent fainting

---

nitroprusside (℞)

(nye-troe-pruss′ide)
Nitropress, sodium nitroprusside

Func. class.: Antihypertensive
Chem. class.: Peripheral vasodilator

Action: Directly relaxes arteriolar, venous smooth muscle, resulting in reduction in cardiac preload, afterload

Uses: Hypertensive crisis, to decrease bleeding by creating hypotension during surgery, acute CHF, cardiogenic shock

Dosage and routes:
• *Adult:* IV INF dissolve 50 mg in 2-3 ml of D_5W, then dilute in 250-

---

◆ = Nursing alert   ✐ = Herb-drug interaction   🚫 = Do not crush

1000 ml of D$_5$W; run at 0.5-8 µg/kg/min
• *Child:* **IV** 0.3-0.5 µg/kg/min, titrate to response
Available forms: Inj 50 mg
Side effects/adverse reactions:
GI: Nausea, vomiting, abdominal pain
CNS: Dizziness, headache, agitation, twitching, decreased reflexes, **LOC,** restlessness
EENT: Tinnitus, blurred vision
GU: Impotence
INTEG: Pain, irritation at injection site, sweating
CV: Palpitation, severe hypotension, dyspnea
MISC: Cyanide, thiocyanate toxicity
Contraindications: Hypersensitivity, hypertension (compensatory)
Precautions: Pregnancy (C), lactation, children, fluid, electrolyte imbalances, hepatic disease, renal disease, hypothyroidism, elderly
Pharmacokinetics:
IV: Onset 1-2 min, duration 1-10 min, half-life 4 days in patients with abnormal renal function; metabolized in liver, excreted in urine
Interactions:
• Severe hypotension: ganglionic blockers, volatile liquid anesthetics, halothane, enflurane, circulatory depressants
NURSING CONSIDERATIONS
Assess:
• Electrolytes: K, Na, Cl, CO$_2$, CBC, serum glucose, serum methemoglobin if pulmonary O$_2$ levels are decreased
• Renal function studies: catecholamines, BUN, creatinine
• Hepatic function studies: AST (SGOT), ALT (SGPT), alk phosphatase
• B/P by direct means if possible; check ECG continuously; pulse; jugular vein distention; PCWP

• Weight qd, I&O
• Thiocyanate, lactate, cyanide levels if on long-term treatment
• Nausea, vomiting, diarrhea
• Edema in feet, legs daily; skin turgor, dryness of mucous membranes for hydration status
• Rales, dyspnea, orthopnea q30min
• For decrease in bicarbonate, Pco$_2$ blood pH, acidosis
Administer:
IV
• Depending on B/P reading q15min
• IV after diluting 50 mg/2-3 ml of D$_5$W, further dilute in 250 ml of D$_5$W; use an infusion pump only; wrap bottle with aluminum foil to protect from light; observe for color change in the infusion; discard if highly discolored (blue, green, dark red); titrate to patient response
Syringe compatibilities: Heparin
Y-site compatibilities: Amrinone, atracurium, diltiazem, dobutamine, dopamine, enalaprilat, famotidine, lidocaine, nitroglycerin, pancuronium, tacrolimus, theophylline, vecuronium
Evaluate:
• Therapeutic response: decreased B/P, absence of bleeding
Teach patient/family:
• To report headache, dizziness, loss of hearing, blurred vision, dyspnea, faintness
Treatment of overdose: Administer amyl nitrite inhalation until 3% sodium nitrate solution can be prepared for IV administration, then inject sodium thiosulfate IV, correct drop in B/P with vasopressor

nizatidine

(ni-za'ti-deen)

Axid

Func. class.: H$_2$-receptor antagonist

Chem. class.: Substituted thiazole

Action: Blocks H$_2$-receptors, thereby reducing gastric acid output

Uses: Benign gastric and duodenal ulceration, prevention of duodenal ulcer recurrence, symptomatic relief of gastroesophageal reflux

Dosage and routes:

Renal dose

• CrCl 20-50 ml/min give 150 mg/day; CrCl <20 ml/min give 150 mg qod

Gastric and duodenal ulcer

• *Adult:* **PO** 300 mg at night or 150 mg bid for 4-8 wk; maintenance 150 mg at night for up to 1 yr

Gastroesophageal reflux

• *Adult:* **PO** 150-300 mg bid for up to 12 wk

Available forms: Caps 150 mg, 300 mg

Side effects/adverse reactions:

CNS: Headache, somnolence, confusion, abnormal dreams, dizziness

ENDO: Gynecomastia

HEMA: **Thrombocytopenia**

INTEG: Pruritus, sweating, urticaria, exfoliative dermatitis

MS: Myalgia

RESP: **Bronchospasm, laryngeal edema**

METAB: Hyperuricemia

GI: Elevated liver enzymes, hepatitis, jaundice, nausea

CV: Cardiac dysrhythmias, ***cardiac arrest***

Contraindications: Hypersensitivity

Precautions: Renal or hepatic impairment (reduce dose in renal impairment), pregnancy (C), lactation

Pharmacokinetics: Partially metabolized by liver, excreted by kidneys, plasma half-life 1½ hr, 70% absorbed orally, small amount (0.1% of plasma concentration) enters breast milk, 35% bound to plasma proteins

NURSING CONSIDERATIONS

Assess:

• Gastric pH (>5 should be maintained)

• Fluid balance, I&O

Administer:

PO

• With meals for prolonged drug effect; antacids 1 hr before or 1 hr after drug

Evaluate:

• Mental status, confusion, dizziness, depression, anxiety, weakness, tremors, psychosis, diarrhea, jaundice, report immediately

• For GI symptoms: nausea, vomiting, diarrhea, cramps

Teach patient/family:

• That gynecomastia, impotence may occur, are reversible

• To avoid driving or other hazardous activities until patient is stabilized on this medication; dizziness may occur

• To avoid black pepper, caffeine, alcohol, harsh spices, extremes in temp of food

• To avoid OTC preparations: aspirin, cough, cold preparations

Treatment of overdose: Symptomatic and supportive therapy is recommended; activated charcoal, emesis or lavage may reduce absorption

norepinephrine (℞)

(nor-ep-i-nef′rin)
Levophed
Func. class.: Adrenergic
Chem. class.: Catecholamine

Action: Causes increased contractility and heart rate by acting on β-receptors in heart; also acts on α-receptors, causing vasoconstriction in blood vessels; B/P is elevated, coronary blood flow improves, cardiac output increases

Uses: Acute hypotension, shock

Dosage and routes:
• *Adult:* IV INF 8-12 μg/min titrated to B/P
• *Child:* IV INF 0.05-0.1 μg/kg/min titrated to B/P

Available forms: Inj 1 mg/ml

Side effects/adverse reactions:
CNS: Headache, anxiety, dizziness, insomnia, restlessness, tremor
CV: Palpitations, tachycardia, hypertension, ectopic beats, angina
GI: Nausea, vomiting
INTEG. Necrosis, tissue sloughing with extravasation, ***gangrene***
RESP: Dyspnea
GU: Decreased urine output

Contraindications: Hypersensitivity, ventricular fibrillation, tachydysrhythmias, pheochromocytoma

Precautions: Lactation, arterial embolism, peripheral vascular disease, hypertension, hyperthyroidism, elderly, heart disease, pregnancy (C)

Pharmacokinetics:
IV: Onset 1-2 min; metabolized in liver; excreted in urine (inactive metabolites); crosses placenta

Interactions:
• Severe hypertension: guanethidine
• Do not use within 2 wk of MAOIs, or hypertensive crisis may result

• Dysrhythmias: general anesthetics, bretylium
• Decreased action of norepinephrine: α-blockers
• Increased B/P: oxytocics
• Increased pressor effect: tricyclic antidepressant, MAOIs
• Incompatible with alkaline solutions: Na, HCO_3

NURSING CONSIDERATIONS
Assess:
• I&O ratio; notify prescriber if output <30 ml/hr
• ECG during administration continuously; if B/P increases, drug is decreased
• B/P and pulse q2-3min after parenteral route
• CVP or PWP during infusion if possible
• For paresthesias and coldness of extremities; peripheral blood flow may decrease
• Injection site: tissue sloughing; administer phentolamine mixed with 0.9% NaCl
• Sulfite sensitivity, which may be life-threatening

Administer:
• Plasma expanders for hypovolemia
• IV after diluting with 500-1000 ml D_5W or D_5/0.9% NaCl; average dilution is 4 ml/1000 ml diluent; give as infusion 2-3 ml/min; titrate to response
• Using 2-bottle setup so drug may be discontinued while IV is still running; use infusion pump

Additive compatibilities: Amikacin, calcium chloride, calcium gluconate, cimetidine, corticotropin, dimenhydrinate, dobutamine, heparin, hydrocortisone, magnesium sulfate, meropenem, methylprednisolone, multivitamins, netilmicin, potassium chloride, succinylcholine, verapamil, vit B/C

N

Syringe compatibilities: Heparin

Y-site compatibilities: Amiodarone, amrinone, diltiazem, dobutamine, dopamine, epinephrine, esmolol, famotidine, fentanyl, furosemide, haloperidol, heparin, hydrocortisone, hydromorphone, labetalol, lorazepam, meropenem, midazolam, milrinone, morphine, nicardipine, nitroglycerin, potassium chloride, propofol, ranitidine, vecuronium, vit B/C

Perform/provide:
• Storage of reconstituted sol if refrigerated no longer than 24 hr
• Do not use discolored sol

Evaluate:
• Therapeutic response: increased B/P with stabilization

Teach patient/family:
• The reason for drug administration and to report dyspnea, dizziness, chest pain

Treatment of overdose: Administer fluids, electrolyte replacement

---

norethindrone (Ŗ)
(nor-eth-in′drone)
Micronor, Norlutin, Nor-QD
Func. class.: Progestogen
Chem. class.: Progesterone derivative

Action: Inhibits secretion of pituitary gonadotropins, which prevents follicular maturation, ovulation; stimulates growth of mammary tissue; antineoplastic action against endometrial cancer

Uses: Uterine bleeding (abnormal), amenorrhea, endometriosis

Dosage and routes:
• *Adult:* **PO** 5-20 mg qd days 5-25 of menstrual cycle

Endometriosis
• *Adult:* **PO** 10 mg qd × 2 wk, then increased by 5 mg qd × 2 wk, up to 30 mg qd

Available forms: Tabs 5 mg

Side effects/adverse reactions:

CNS: Dizziness, headache, migraines, depression, fatigue

CV: Hypotension, ***thrombophlebitis,*** edema, ***thromboembolism, stroke, pulmonary embolism, MI***

GI: Nausea, vomiting, anorexia, cramps, increased weight, ***cholestatic jaundice***

EENT: Diplopia

GU: Amenorrhea, cervical erosion, breakthrough bleeding, dysmenorrhea, vaginal candidiasis, breast changes, (gynecomastia, testicular atrophy, impotence), endometriosis, ***spontaneous abortion***

INTEG: Rash, urticaria, acne, hirsutism, alopecia, oily skin, seborrhea, purpura, melasma

META: Hyperglycemia

Contraindications: Breast cancer, hypersensitivity, thromboembolic disorders, reproductive cancer, genital bleeding (abnormal, undiagnosed), pregnancy (X)

Precautions: Lactation, hypertension, asthma, blood dyscrasias, gallbladder disease, CHF, diabetes mellitus, bone disease, depression, migraine headache, convulsive disorders, hepatic disease, renal disease, family history of breast or reproductive tract cancer

Pharmacokinetics:
PO: Duration 24 hr, excreted in urine, feces, metabolized in liver

Lab test interferences:
Increase: Alk phosphatase, nitrogen (urine), pregnanediol, amino acids, factors VII, VIII, IX, X
Decrease: GTT, HDL

NURSING CONSIDERATIONS
Assess:
• Weight qd: notify prescriber of weekly weight gain >5 lb
• B/P at beginning of treatment and periodically

⬥ = Nursing alert   ▉ = Herb-drug interaction   ⊘ = Do not crush

- I&O ratio; be alert for decreasing urinary output, increasing edema
- Liver function studies: ALT (SGPT), AST (SGOT), bilirubin, periodically during long-term therapy
- Edema, hypertension, cardiac symptoms, jaundice
- Mental status: affect, mood, behavioral changes, depression
- Hypercalcemia

Administer:
- Titrated dose; use lowest effective dose
- Oil solution inj deep in large muscle mass (IM), rotate sites
- In one dose in AM
- With food or milk to decrease GI symptoms
- After warming to dissolve crystals

Perform/provide:
- Storage in dark area

Evaluate:
- Therapeutic response: decreased abnormal uterine bleeding, absence of amenorrhea

Teach patient/family:
- About cushingoid symptoms
- To report breast lumps, vaginal bleeding, edema, jaundice, dark urine, clay-colored stools, dyspnea, headache, blurred vision, abdominal pain, numbness or stiffness in legs, chest pain; male to report impotence or gynecomastia
- To report suspected pregnancy

---

norfloxacin (℞)

(nor-flox'-a-sin)
Chibroxin, Noroxin
Func. class.: Urinary antiinfective
Chem. class.: Fluoroquinolone

Action: Interferes with conversion of intermediate DNA fragments into high-molecular-weight DNA in bacteria, inhibits DNA gyrase

Uses: Adult urinary tract infections (including complicated) caused by *E. coli, E. cloacae, P. mirabilis, K. pneumoniae,* group D strep, indole-positive *Proteus, C. freundii, S. aureus;* uncomplicated gonorrhea, ocular infection

Dosage and routes:
Renal dose
- CrCl <30 ml/min 400 mg **PO** qid
Uncomplicated infections
- *Adult:* **PO** 400 mg bid × 3-10 days 1 hr before or 2 hr after meals
Complicated infections
- *Adult:* **PO** 400 mg bid × 10-21 days; 400 mg qd × 7-10 days in impaired renal function
Uncomplicated gonorrhea
- *Adult:* **PO** 800 mg as a single dose
Ocular infection
- *Adult and child:* **OPHTH** 1 gtt qid, may increase to 1 gtt q2h for severe infections
Prostatitis
- *Adult:* **PO** 400 mg bid × 4 wk
Available forms: Tabs 400 mg; ophth sol 3 mg/ml

Side effects/adverse reactions:
CNS: Headache, dizziness, fatigue, somnolence, depression, insomnia
GI: Nausea, constipation, increased ALT (SGPT), AST (SGOT), flatulence, heartburn, vomiting, diarrhea, dry mouth
INTEG: Rash
EENT: Visual disturbances

Contraindications: Hypersensitivity to quinolones

Precautions: Pregnancy (C), lactation, children, renal disease, seizure disorders

Pharmacokinetics: Peak 1 hr, half-life 3-4 hr; steady state 2 days; excreted in urine as active drug, metabolites

Interactions:
- Decreased effect of norfloxacin:

N

antacids, calcium, antineoplastics, nitrofurantoin
- Decreased effect: phenytoin
- Increased toxicity: digoxin, warfarin, caffeine, theophylline, cyclosporine
- Increased norfloxacin levels: cimetidine, probenecid

Lab test interferences:
Increase: AST (SGOT), ALT (SGPT), BUN, creatinine, alk phosphatase

NURSING CONSIDERATIONS
Assess:
- Kidney, liver function studies: BUN, creatinine, AST (SGOT), ALT (SGPT)
- I&O ratio; urine pH, <5.5 is ideal
- CNS symptoms: insomnia, vertigo, headache, agitation, confusion
- Allergic reactions: fever, flushing, rash, urticaria, pruritus

Administer:
PO
- After clean-catch urine for C&S
- Two daily doses if urine output is high or if patient has diabetes

Evaluate:
- Therapeutic response: decreased pain, frequency, urgency, C&S, absence of infection

Teach patient/family:
- That fluid intake must be 3 L/day to avoid crystallization in kidneys
- That if dizziness occurs, to walk, perform activities with assistance
- To complete full course of drug therapy
- To contact prescriber if adverse reaction occurs
- To take 1 hr before or 2 hr after meals; not to take antacids with or within 2 hr of this drug; to sip water or use hard candy for dry mouth

---

norgestrel (℞)
(nor-jess'trel)
Ovrette, Ovral*
Func. class.: Progestogen
Chem. class.: Progesterone derivative

Action: Inhibits secretion of pituitary gonadotropins, which prevents follicular maturation, ovulation, stimulates growth of mammary tissue, antineoplastic action against endometrial cancer

Uses: Female contraception

Dosage and routes:
- *Adult:* PO 1 tab qd
Available forms: Tabs 0.35, 0.075 mg

Side effects/adverse reactions:
CNS: Dizziness, headache, migraines, depression, fatigue
CV: Hypotension, *thrombophlebitis,* edema, *thromboembolism, stroke, pulmonary embolism, myocardial infarction*
GI: Nausea, vomiting, anorexia, cramps, increased weight, *cholestatic jaundice*
EENT: Diplopia
GU: Amenorrhea, cervical erosion, breakthrough bleeding, dysmenorrhea, vaginal candidiasis, breast changes, *gynecomastia, testicular atrophy, impotence,* endometriosis, *spontaneous abortion*
INTEG: Rash, urticaria, acne, hirsutism, alopecia, oily skin, seborrhea, purpura, melasma
META: Hyperglycemia

Contraindications: Breast cancer, hypersensitivity, thromboembolic disorders, reproductive cancer, genital bleeding (abnormal, undiagnosed), cerebral hemorrhage, pregnancy (X)

Precautions: Lactation, hypertension, asthma, blood dyscrasias, gall-bladder disease, CHF, diabetes mellitus, bone disease, depression, migraine headache, convulsive disorders, hepatic disease, renal disease, family history of breast or reproductive tract cancer

Pharmacokinetics:

PO: Duration 24 hr; excreted in urine, feces; metabolized in liver

Lab test interferences:

Increase: Alk phosphatase, nitrogen (urine), pregnanediol, amino acids, factors VII, VIII, IX, X

Decrease: GTT, HDL

NURSING CONSIDERATIONS

Assess:

• Weight qd; notify prescriber of weekly weight gain >5 lb

• B/P at beginning of treatment and periodically

• I&O ratio; be alert for decreasing urinary output, increasing edema

• Liver function studies: ALT (SGPT), AST (SGOT), bilirubin, periodically during long-term therapy

• Edema, hypertension, cardiac symptoms, jaundice

• Mental status: affect, mood, behavioral changes, depression

• Hypercalcemia

Administer:

• Titrated dose; use lowest effective dose

• In one dose in AM

• With food or milk to decrease GI symptoms

• After warming to dissolve crystals

Perform/provide:

• Storage in dark area

Evaluate:

• Therapeutic response: absence of pregnancy

Teach patient/family:

• About cushingoid symptoms

• To report breast lumps, vaginal-bleeding, edema, jaundice, dark urine, clay-colored stools, dyspnea, headache, blurred vision, abdominal pain, numbness or stiffness in legs, chest pain

• To report suspected pregnancy

• To monitor blood sugar if diabetic

nortriptyline (R)

(nor-trip'ti-leen)

Aventyl, Pamelor

Func. class.: Antidepressant—tricyclic

Chem. class.: Dibenzocyclo-heptene—secondary amine

Action: Blocks reuptake of norepinephrine, serotonin into nerve endings, increasing action of norepinephrine, serotonin in nerve cells

Uses: Major depression

Investigational uses: Chronic pain management

Dosage and routes:

• *Adult:* PO 25 mg tid or qid, may increase to 150 mg/day; may give daily dose hs

• *Geriatric:* PO 10-25 mg q hs, increase by 10-25 mg at weekly intervals to desired dose; usual maintenance 75 mg

Available forms: Caps 10, 25, 50, 75 mg; sol 10 mg/5 ml

Side effects/adverse reactions:

*HEMA: **Agranulocytosis, thrombocytopenia, eosinophilia, leukopenia***

CNS: Dizziness, drowsiness, confusion, headache, anxiety, tremors, stimulation, weakness, insomnia, nightmares, EPS (elderly), increased psychiatric symptoms

GI: Constipation, dry mouth, nausea, vomiting, ***paralytic ileus,*** increased appetite, cramps, epigastric

N

distress, jaundice, *hepatitis,* stomatitis

*GU: Retention, **acute renal failure***
INTEG: Rash, urticaria, sweating, pruritus, photosensitivity
*CV: Orthostatic hypotension, ECG changes, tachycardia, **hypertension,*** palpitations
EENT: Blurred vision, tinnitus, mydriasis
Contraindications: Hypersensitivity to tricyclic antidepressants, recovery phase of MI, convulsive disorders, prostatic hypertrophy
Precautions: Suicidal patients, severe depression, increased intraocular pressure, narrow-angle glaucoma, urinary retention, cardiac disease, hepatic disease, hyperthyroidism, electroshock therapy, elective surgery, pregnancy (C), lactation
Pharmacokinetics:
PO: Steady state 4-19 days; metabolized by liver; excreted by kidneys; crosses placenta; excreted in breast milk; half-life 18-28 hr
Interactions:
• Decreased effects of guanethidine, clonidine, indirect-acting sympathomimetics (ephedrine)
• Increased effects of direct-acting sympathomimetics (epinephrine), alcohol, barbiturates, benzodiazepines, CNS depressants
• Hyperpyretic crisis, convulsions, hypertensive episode: MAOI
🌿 Increased anticholinergic effect: belladonna leaf/root, henbane leaf
🌿 Increased antidepressant action: scopolia root
Lab test interferences:
Increase: Serum bilirubin, blood glucose, alk phosphatase
False increase: Urinary catecholamines
Decrease: VMA, 5-HIAA

NURSING CONSIDERATIONS
Assess:
• B/P (lying, standing), pulse q4h; if systolic B/P drops 20 mm Hg, hold drug, notify prescriber; take vital signs q4h in patients with cardiovascular disease
• Blood studies: CBC, leukocytes, differential, cardiac enzymes if patient is receiving long-term therapy
• Hepatic studies: AST (SGOT), ALT (SGPT), bilirubin
• Weight qwk; appetite may increase with drug
• ECG for flattening of T wave, bundle branch block, AV block, dysrhythmias in cardiac patients
• EPS primarily in elderly: rigidity, dystonia, akathisia
• Mental status changes: mood, sensorium, affect, suicidal tendencies, increase in psychiatric symptoms, depression, panic
• Urinary retention, constipation; constipation is more likely to occur in children
◆ Withdrawal symptoms: headache, nausea, vomiting, muscle pain, weakness; do not usually occur unless drug was discontinued abruptly
• Alcohol intake; if alcohol is consumed, hold dose until AM
Administer:
• Increased fluids, bulk in diet if constipation occurs
• With food, milk for GI symptoms
• Dosage hs for oversedation during day; may take entire dose hs; elderly may not tolerate once/day dosing
• Gum, hard candy, frequent sips of water for dry mouth
• Concentrate with fruit juice, water, or milk to disguise taste
Perform/provide:
• Storage in tight, light-resistant container at room temp
• Assistance with ambulation dur-

◆ = Nursing alert   🌿 = Herb-drug interaction   🚫 = Do not crush

ing beginning therapy, since drowsiness/dizziness occurs
• Safety measures including side rails, primarily for elderly
• Checking to see if PO medication swallowed

Evaluate:
• Therapeutic response: decreased depression

Teach patient/family:
• That therapeutic effects may take 2-3 wk
• To use caution in driving, other activities requiring alertness because of drowsiness, dizziness, blurred vision
• To avoid alcohol ingestion, other CNS depressants
• Not to discontinue medication quickly after long-term use; may cause nausea, headache, malaise
• To wear sunscreen or large hat, since photosensitivity occurs

Treatment of overdose: ECG monitoring; induce emesis; lavage, activated charcoal; administer anticonvulsant

---

nystatin (℞)

(nye-stat′in)
Mycostatin, Mycostatin Pastilles, Nadostine*, nystatin
Func. class.: Antifungal
Chem. class.: Amphoteric polyene

Action: Interferes with fungal DNA replication; binds sterols in fungal cell membrane, which increases permeability, leaking of cell nutrients
Uses: *Candida* species causing oral, vaginal, intestinal infections

Dosage and routes:
Oral infection
• *Adult:* **SUSP** 400,000-600,000 U qid, swish and swallow
• *Child and infant >3 mo:* **SUSP** 250,000-500,000 U qid

• *Newborn and premature infant:* **SUSP** 100,000 U qid
GI infection
• *Adult:* **PO** 500,000-1,000,000 U tid

Available forms: Tabs 500,000 U; powder 50 million, 150 million, 500 million, 1 billion, 2 billion, 5 billion U; susp 100,000 U per ml

Side effects/adverse reactions:
INTEG: Rash, urticaria (rare)
GI: Nausea, vomiting, anorexia, diarrhea, cramps

Contraindications: Hypersensitivity
Precautions: Pregnancy (C)
Pharmacokinetics:
PO: Little absorption, excreted in feces

NURSING CONSIDERATIONS
Assess:
• For allergic reaction: rash, urticaria; drug may have to be discontinued
• For predisposing factors: antibiotic therapy, pregnancy, diabetes mellitus, sexual partner infection (vaginal infections)

Administer:
• Oral susp dose by placing ½ in each cheek, then swallow
• Topical dose after cleansing area; mouth may be swabbed

Perform/provide:
• Storage in refrigerator for oral susp; tabs in tight, light-resistant containers at room temp

Evaluate:
• Therapeutic response: culture negative for *Candida*

Teach patient/family:
• That long-term therapy may be needed to clear infection; to complete entire course of medication
• Proper hygiene: changing socks if feet are infected; using no commercial mouthwashes for mouth infection

---

- Shake susp before measuring each dose
- To avoid getting preparation on hands
- To wear light-day pad for vaginal preparations
- To avoid tight shoes, bandages when using on feet
- To avoid sexual contact during treatment to minimize reinfection
- To notify prescriber of irritation; drug may have to be discontinued
- That relief from itching may occur after 24-72 hr

---

ofloxacin (Rx)
(o-flox′a-sin)
Floxin, Floxin IV, Occuflox
Func. class.: Antiinfective
Chem. class.: Fluoroquinolone

Action: Interferes with conversion of intermediate DNA fragments into high-molecular-weight DNA in bacteria, inhibits DNA gyrase

Uses: Treatment of lower respiratory tract infections (pneumonia, bronchitis), genitourinary infections (prostatitis, UTIs) caused by *E. coli, K. pneumoniae, C. trachomatis, N. gonorrhoeae;* skin and skin structure infections; conjunctivitis (ophth)

Dosage and routes:
Renal dose
- CrCl 10-50 ml/min give q24h; CrCl <10 ml/min give ½ of dose q24h

Lower respiratory tract infections/skin and skin structure infections
- *Adult:* **PO, IV** 400 mg q12h × 10 days

Cervicitis, urethritis
- *Adult:* **PO, IV** 300 mg q12h × 7 days

Prostatitis
- *Adult:* **PO, IV** 300 mg q12h × 6 wk

Acute, uncomplicated gonorrhea
- *Adult:* **PO, IV** 400 mg as a single dose

Conjunctivitis
- *Adult and child:* **OPHTH** 1-2 gtt q2-4h × 2 days, then qid × 5 days

Urinary tract infection
- *Adult:* **PO, IV** 200-400 mg q12h × 3-10 days

Available forms: Tabs 200, 300, 400 mg; 4 mg/ml (IV); ophth sol 0.3%

Side effects/adverse reactions:
CNS: Dizziness, headache, fatigue, somnolence, depression, insomnia, lethargy, malaise
GI: Diarrhea, nausea, vomiting, anorexia, flatulence, heartburn, dry mouth, increased AST (SGOT), ALT (SGPT), abdominal pain, constipation
INTEG: Rash, pruritus
EENT: Visual disturbances

Contraindications: Hypersensitivity to quinolones

Precautions: Pregnancy (C), lactation, children, elderly, renal disease, seizure disorders, excessive sunlight

Pharmacokinetics:
PO: Peak 1-2 hr, half-life 9 hr, steady state 2 days; excreted in urine as active drug, metabolites; 90%-95% bioavailability

Interactions:
- Decreased effects of ofloxacin: antacids, nitrofurantoin, sucralfate, iron salts, zinc salts, calcium
- Increased ofloxacin levels: probenecid, cimetidine
- Increased effects of warfarin, cyclosporine, caffeine, theophylline, procainamide

NURSING CONSIDERATIONS
Assess:
- Kidney, liver function studies: BUN, creatinine, AST (SGOT), ALT (SGPT)
- I&O ratio; urine pH <5.5 is ideal

• CNS symptoms: insomnia, vertigo, headache, agitation, confusion
• Allergic reactions: rash, flushing, urticaria, pruritus

Administer:

PO

• 2 hr before or 2 hr after antacids, calcium, iron, zinc products
• After clean-catch urine for C&S

IV

• Over 1 hr or more

Additive compatibilities: Amoxicillin, ceftazidime, clindamycin, gentamicin, piperacillin, tobramycin, vancomycin

Syringe compatibilities: Cefotaxime

Y-site compatibilities: Ampicillin, granisetron, propofol, thiotepa

Perform/provide:

• Limited intake of alkaline foods, drugs: milk, dairy products, peanuts, vegetables, alkaline antacids, sodium bicarbonate
• Storage for 2 wk refrigerated or 6 mo frozen after reconstitution

Evaluate:

• Therapeutic response: negative C&S; absence of redness, swelling (ophth)

Teach patient/family:

• That fluid intake must be 3 L/day to avoid crystallization in kidneys
• That if dizziness or lightheadedness occurs, ambulate, perform activities with assistance
• To complete full course of therapy
• To notify prescriber of adverse reactions or tendon pain
• To avoid iron- or mineral-containing supplements within 2 hr before or after dose

olanzapine
(oh-lanz′a-peen)
Zyprexa
Func. class.: Antipsychotic, neuroleptic
Chem. class.: Thienbenzodiazepine

Action: Unknown; may mediate antipsychotic activity by both dopamine and serotonin type 2 (5HT2) antagonist; also, may antagonize muscarinic receptors, histaminic (H_1)- and α-adrenergic receptors

Uses: Psychotic disorders

Dosage and routes:

• *Adult:* **PO** 5-10 mg initially qd, may increase dosage by 5 mg at 1 wk or more intervals
• *Elderly:* **PO** 5 mg, may increase cautiously at 1 wk intervals

Available forms: Tab 5, 7.5, 10 mg

Side effects/adverse reactions:

CV: Orthostatic hypotension, tachycardia, chest pain
EENT: Blurred vision
GI: Dry mouth, nausea, vomiting, anorexia, constipation, abdominal pain, weight gain
GU: Urinary retention, urinary frequency, enuresis, impotence, amenorrhea, gynecomastia, breast engorgement, premenstrual syndrome
INTEG: Rash
RESP: Dyspnea, rhinitis, cough, pharyngitis
CNS: EPS: pseudoparkinsonism, akathisia, dystonia, tardive dyskinesia, seizures, headache, ***neuroleptic malignant syndrome (rare)***, fever, insomnia, somnolence, agitation, nervousness, hostility, dizziness, hypertonia, tremor, euphoria
MS: Joint pain, twitching

Contraindications: Hypersensitivity

Precautions: Pregnancy (C), lactation, hypertension, hepatic disease, cardiac disease, elderly

Pharmacokinetics: Well absorbed, peak 6 hr, metabolized by liver, excreted in urine, 93% bound to plasma proteins

Interactions:

• Oversedation: other CNS depressants, alcohol, barbiturate anesthetics, antihistamines, sedatives/hypnotics, antidepressants

• Decreased levels of olanzapine: carbamazepine

• Increased hypotension: antihypertensives

• Decreased antiparkinson activity: levodopa, bromocriptine

• Increased anticholinergic effects: anticholinergics

Lab test interferences:

Increase: Liver function test, prolactin, CPK

NURSING CONSIDERATIONS
Assess:

• Mental status: orientation, mood, behavior, presence of hallucinations and type before initial administration and monthly

• Swallowing of PO medication: check for hoarding or giving of medication to other patients

• I&O ratio; palpate bladder if low urinary output occurs, especially in elderly

• Bilirubin, CBC, liver function studies monthly

• Urinalysis recommended before, during prolonged therapy

• Affect, orientation, LOC, reflexes, gait, coordination, sleep pattern disturbances

• B/P sitting, standing, lying: take pulse and respirations q4h during initial treatment; establish baseline before starting treatment; report drops of 30 mm Hg; obtain baseline ECG

• Dizziness, faintness, palpitations, tachycardia on rising

◆ For neuroleptic malignant syndrome: hyperpyrexia, muscle rigidity, increased CPK, altered mental status, for acute dystonia (check chewing, swallowing, eyes, pill rolling)

• EPS, including akathisia (inability to sit still, no pattern to movements), tardive dyskinesia (bizarre movements of the jaw, mouth, tongue, extremities), pseudoparkinsonism (rigidity, tremors, pill rolling, shuffling gait)

• Skin turgor daily

• Constipation, urinary retention daily; increase bulk, H_2O in diet

Administer:

• Antiparkinsonian agent for EPS

• Decreased dose in elderly

• PO with full glass of water, milk; or with food to decrease GI upset

Perform/provide:

• Decreased stimuli by dimming light, avoiding loud noises

• Supervised ambulation until stabilized on medication; do not involve in strenuous exercise program because fainting is possible; patient should not stand still for long periods

• Increased fluids to prevent constipation

• Sips of water, candy, gum for dry mouth

• Storage in tight, light-resistant container

Evaluate:

• Therapeutic response: decrease in emotional excitement, hallucinations, delusion, paranoia, reorganization of patterns of thought, speech

Teach patient/family:

• To use good oral hygiene; frequent rinsing of mouth, sugarless gum for dry mouth

• To avoid hazardous activities until drug response is determined

• That orthostatic hypotension occurs often and to rise from sitting or lying position gradually

• To avoid hot tubs, hot showers, tub baths, since hypotension may occur

• To avoid abrupt withdrawal of this drug, or EPS may result; drug should be withdrawn slowly

• To avoid OTC preparations (cough, hay fever, cold) unless approved by prescriber, since serious drug interactions may occur; avoid use with alcohol, CNS depressants; increased drowsiness may occur

• That in hot weather, heat stroke may occur; take extra precautions to stay cool

Treatment of overdose: Lavage if orally ingested; provide airway; do not induce vomiting or use epinephrine

---

olsalazine (℞)

(ohl-sal'ah-zeen)
Dipentum
Func. class.: Antiinflammatory
Chem. class.: Salicylate derivative

Action: Bioconverted to 5-aminosalicylic acid, which decreases inflammation

Uses: Maintenance of remission of ulcerative colitis in patients intolerant to sulfasalazine

Dosage and routes:
• *Adult:* PO 1 g/day in 2 divided doses

Available forms: Tabs 250 mg

Side effects/adverse reactions:
EENT: Dry mouth, dry eyes, watery eyes, blurred vision
SYST: Anaphylaxis
GI: Nausea, vomiting, abdominal pain, stomatitis, hepatitis, pancreatitis, diarrhea, bloating

CNS: Headache, insomnia, hallucinations, depression, vertigo, fatigue, drug fever, chills, dizziness, drowsiness, tremors
HEMA: Leukopenia, neutropenia, thrombocytopenia, agranulocytosis, anemia
INTEG: Rash, dermatitis, urticaria, *Stevens-Johnson syndrome,* erythema, photosensitivity, alopecia
GU: Frequency, dysuria, hematuria, impotence
CV: Allergic myocarditis, 2nd degree heart block, hypertension, peripheral edema, chest pain, palpitations
RESP: Bronchospasm, shortness of breath

Contraindications: Hypersensitivity to salicylates

Precautions: Pregnancy (C), child <14 yr, lactation; impaired hepatic, renal function, severe allergy, bronchial asthma

Pharmacokinetics:
PO: Partially absorbed, peak 1½ hr, half-life 5-10 hr, excreted in urine as 5-aminosalicylic acid and metabolites, crosses placenta

Lab test interferences:
False positive: Urinary glucose test

NURSING CONSIDERATIONS
Assess:
• I&O ratio: note color, character, pH of urine in treatment for UTIs; output should be 800 ml less than intake; if urine is highly acidic, alkalization may be needed

• Kidney function studies: BUN, creatinine, urinalysis (long-term therapy)

• Blood dyscrasias: skin rash, fever, sore throat, bruising, bleeding, fatigue, joint pain

• Allergic reaction: rash, dermatitis, urticaria, pruritus, dyspnea, bronchospasm

---

Administer:

- With food in evenly divided doses
- Medication after C&S; repeat C&S after full course of medication
- With resuscitative equipment available; severe allergic reactions may occur
- Total daily dose evenly spaced to minimize GI intolerance

Perform/provide:

- Storage in tight, light-resistant container at room temp

Evaluate:

- Therapeutic response: absence of fever, mucus in stools

---

omeprazole (℞)

(oh-mep′ray-zole)

Losec*, Prilosec

Func. class.: Antisecretory compound

Chem. class.: Benzimidazole

Action: Suppresses gastric secretion by inhibiting hydrogen/potassium ATPase enzyme system in gastric parietal cell; characterized as gastric acid pump inhibitor, since it blocks final step of acid production

Uses: Gastroesophageal reflux disease (GERD), severe erosive esophagitis, poorly responsive systemic GERD, pathologic hypersecretory conditions (Zollinger-Ellison syndrome, systemic mastocytosis, multiple endocrine adenomas); treatment of active duodenal ulcers with or without antiinfectives for *H. pylori*

Dosage and routes:

Active duodenal ulcers

- *Adult:* **PO** 20 mg qd × 4-8 wk

Severe erosive esophagitis/poorly responsive GERD

- *Adult:* **PO** 20 mg qd × 4-8 wk

Pathologic hypersecretory conditions

- *Adult:* **PO** 60 mg/day; may increase to 120 mg tid; daily doses >80 mg should be divided

Available forms: Caps, delayed rel 10, 20 mg

Side effects/adverse reactions:

CNS: Headache, dizziness, asthenia

GI: Diarrhea, abdominal pain, vomiting, nausea, constipation, flatulence, acid regurgitation, abdominal swelling, anorexia, irritable colon, esophageal candidiasis, dry mouth

RESP: Upper respiratory infections, cough, epistaxis

INTEG: Rash, dry skin, urticaria, pruritus, alopecia

META: Hypoglycemia, increased hepatic enzymes, weight gain

EENT: Tinnitus, taste perversion

CV: Chest pain, angina, tachycardia, bradycardia, palpitations, peripheral edema

GU: UTI, frequency, increased creatinine, *proteinuria, hematuria,* testicular pain, glycosuria

HEMA: Pancytopenia, thrombocytopenia, neutropenia, leukocytosis, anemia

MISC: Back pain, fever, fatigue, malaise

Contraindications: Hypersensitivity

Precautions: Pregnancy (C), lactation, children

Pharmacokinetics: Peak ½-3½ hr, half-life ½-1 hr, protein binding 95%, eliminated in urine as metabolites and in feces; in elderly elimination rate decreased, bioavailability increased

Interactions:

- Increased serum levels of omeprazole: diazepam, phenytoin
- Possible increased bleeding: warfarin

◆ = Nursing alert   ▌= Herb-drug interaction   ◯ = Do not crush

NURSING CONSIDERATIONS
Assess:
- GI system: bowel sounds q8h, abdomen for pain, swelling, anorexia
- Hepatic enzymes: AST (SGOT), ALT (SGPT), alk phosphatase during treatment

Administer:

🚫 Before eating; swallow capsule whole; do not break, crush, or chew

Evaluate:
- Therapeutic response: absence of epigastric pain, swelling, fullness

Teach patient/family:
- To report severe diarrhea; drug may have to be discontinued
- That diabetic patient should know hypoglycemia may occur
- To avoid hazardous activities; dizziness may occur
- To avoid alcohol, salicylates, ibuprofen; may cause GI irritation

---

ondansetron (℞)

(on-dan-seh'tron)
Zofran
Func. class.: Antiemetic
Chem. class.: 5-HT3 receptor antagonist

Action: Prevents nausea, vomiting by blocking serotonin peripherally, centrally, and in the small intestine

Uses: Prevention of nausea, vomiting associated with cancer chemotherapy, radiotherapy, and prevention of postoperative nausea, vomiting

Dosage and routes:
Hepatic dose
- Max dose 8 mg qd

Prevention of nausea/vomiting of cancer chemotherapy
- *Adult and child 4-18 yr:* IV 0.15 mg/kg infused over 15 min, 30 min before start of cancer chemotherapy; 0.15 mg/kg given 4 hr and 8 hr after first dose or 32 mg as a single dose;

dilute in 50 ml of D$_5$W or 0.9% NaCl before giving

Prevention of nausea/vomiting of radiotherapy
- *Adult:* PO 8 mg tid

Prevention of postoperative nausea/vomiting
- *Adult:* IV 4 mg undiluted over >30 sec

Available forms: Inj 2 mg/ml, 32 mg/50 ml (premixed), tabs 4, 8 mg

Side effects/adverse reactions:

GI: Diarrhea, constipation, abdominal pain

CNS: Headache, dizziness, drowsiness, fatigue, extrapyramidal syndrome

*MISC: Rash, **bronchospasm** (rare), MS pain, wound problems, shivering, fever, hypoxia, urinary retention*

Contraindications: Hypersensitivity

Precautions: Pregnancy (B), lactation, children, elderly

Pharmacokinetics:
IV: Mean elimination half-life 3.5-4.7 hr, plasma protein binding 70%-76%; extensively metabolized in the liver

NURSING CONSIDERATIONS
Assess:
- For absence of nausea, vomiting during chemotherapy
- Hypersensitivity reaction: rash, bronchospasm

Administer:
IV
- After diluting a single dose in 50 ml NS or D$_5$W, 0.45% or NS and given over 15 min

Additive compatibilities: Cisplatin, cyclophosphamide, cytarabine, dacarbazine, dexamethasone, doxorubicin, etoposide, fluconazole, hydromorphone, meperidine, methotrexate, morphine

Solution compatibilities: May also be diluted with D$_5$W, lactated

---

Ringer's, D_5/0.9% NaCl, D_5/0.45% NaCl

Y-site compatibilities: Aldesleukin, amifostine, amikacin, aztreonam, bleomycin, carboplatin, carmustine, cefazolin, cefmetazole, cefotaxime, cefoxitin, ceftazidime, ceftizoxime, cefuroxime, chlorpromazine, cimetidine, cisplatin, cladribine, clindamycin, cyclophosphamide, cytarabine, dacarbazine, dactinomycin, daunorubicin, dexamethasone, diphenhydramine, dopamine, doxorubicin, doxycycline, droperidol, etoposide, famotidine, filgrastim, floxuridine, fluconazole, fludarabine, gallium, gentamicin, haloperidol, heparin, hydrocortisone, hydromorphone, hydroxyzine, ifosfamide, imipenem/cilastatin, magnesium sulfate, mannitol, mechlorethamine, melphalan, meperidine, mesna, methotrexate, metoclopramide, miconazole, mitomycin, mitoxantrone, morphine, paclitaxel, pentostatin, piperacillin/tazobactam, potassium chloride, prochlorperazine, promethazine, ranitidine, sodium acetate, streptozocin, teniposide, thiotepa, ticarcillin, ticarcillin/clavulanate, vancomycin, vinblastine, vincristine, vinorelbine, zidovudine

Perform/provide:

• Storage at room temp 48 hr after dilution

Evaluate:

• Therapeutic response: absence of nausea, vomiting during cancer chemotherapy

Teach patient/family:

• To report diarrhea, constipation, rash, or changes in respirations

opium tincture/camphorated opium tincture

(oh'pee-um)

Opium Tincture Deodorized, Pantopan, Paregoric, Paregorique*

Func. class.: Antidiarrheal
Chem. class.: Opium, opium and morphine

Controlled Substance Schedule III/II (depending on amount of opium)

Action: Antiperistaltic activity

Uses: Diarrhea (cause undetermined); withdrawal symptoms in infants born to addicted mothers

Dosage and routes:

• *Adult:* **PO** 0.3-1 ml qid, not to exceed 6 ml/day (tincture) or 5-10 ml qd-qid (camphorated)

• *Child:* **PO** 0.25-0.5 ml/kg qd-qid (camphorated)

Withdrawal

• *Neonate:* **PO** 1:25 dilution, 3-6 gtt q3-6h (tincture), dosage adjustment to control symptoms

Available forms: Liq 2 mg morphine equivalent per 5 ml

Side effects/adverse reactions:

CNS: Dizziness, drowsiness, fainting, flushing, physical dependency, *CNS depression*

GI: Nausea, vomiting, constipation, abdominal pain

Contraindications: Hypersensitivity, severe ulcerative colitis, pseudomembranous colitis

Precautions: Liver disease, addiction proneness, prostatic hypertrophy (severe), pregnancy (B)

Pharmacokinetics:

PO: Duration 4 hr, half-life 2-3 hr; metabolized in liver; excreted in urine

Interactions:
- Increased action of both drugs: other CNS depressants
- Increased CNS toxicity: cimetidine

NURSING CONSIDERATIONS
Assess:
- Electrolytes (K, Na, Cl) if on long-term therapy
- Skin turgor q8h if dehydration is suspected
- Bowel pattern before; for rebound constipation
- Response after 48 hr; if no response, drug should be discontinued
- Dehydration in children
- Abdominal distention; toxic megacolon may occur in ulcerative colitis

Administer:
- Undiluted with water
- For 48 hr only

Evaluate:
- Therapeutic response: decreased diarrhea

Teach patient/family:
- To avoid OTC products (cough, cold, hay fever preparations) unless directed by prescriber
- Not to exceed recommended dose
- That drug may be habit forming
- To avoid hazardous activities; drowsiness may occur

---

oral contraceptives (℞)

Func. class.: Hormone
Chem. class.: Estrogen, progestin combinations

Action: Prevents ovulation by suppressing FSH, LH; *monophasic:* estrogen/progestin (fixed dose) used during a 21-day cycle; ovulation is inhibited by suppression of FSH and LH; thickness of cervical mucus and endometrial lining prevents preg-

nancy; *biphasic:* ovulation is inhibited by suppression of FSH and LH; alteration of cervical mucus, endometrial lining prevents pregnancy; *triphasic:* ovulation is inhibited by suppression of FSH and LH; change of cervical mucus, endometrial lining prevents pregnancy; variable doses of estrogen/progestin combinations may be similar to natural hormonal fluctuations; *progestin-only pill and implant:* change of cervical mucus and endometrial lining prevents pregnancy; ovulation may be suppressed

Uses: To prevent pregnancy, endometriosis, hypermenorrhea

Dosage and routes:
- *Adult:* **PO** 1 qd starting on day 5 of menstrual cycle; day 1 is 1st day of period

20/21 tablet packs
- *Adult:* **PO** 1 qd starting on day 7 of menstrual cycle; day 1 is 1st day of period, then on 20 or 21 days, off 7 days

28 tablet packs
- *Adult:* **PO** 1 qd continuously

Biphasic
- *Adult:* 1 qd × 10 days, then next color 1 qd × 11 days

Triphasic
- *Adult:* 1 qd; check package insert

Endometriosis
- *Adult:* **PO** 1 qd × 20 days from day 5 to 24 of cycle

Available forms: Check specific brand

Side effects/adverse reactions:
GI: Nausea, vomiting, cramps, diarrhea, bloating, constipation, change in appetite, ***cholestatic jaundice***

INTEG: Chloasma, melasma, acne, rash, urticaria, erythema, pruritus, hirsutism, alopecia, photosensitivity

CV: Increased B/P, thromboembolic conditions, fluid retention, edema

---

ENDO: Decreased glucose tolerance, increased TBG, PBI, T_4, T_3

GU: Breakthrough bleeding, amenorrhea, spotting, dysmenorrhea, galactorrhea, endocervical hyperplasia, vaginitis, cystitis-like syndrome, breast change

CNS: Depression, fatigue, dizziness, nervousness, anxiety, headache

EENT: Optic neuritis, retinal thrombosis, cataracts

HEMA: Increased fibrinogen, clotting factor

Contraindications: Pregnancy (X), lactation, reproductive cancer, thrombophlebitis, MI, hepatic tumors, hepatic disease, CAD, women 40 and over, CVA

Precautions: Depression, hypertension, renal disease, seizure disorders, lupus erythematosus, rheumatic disease, migraine headache, amenorrhea, irregular menses, breast cancer (fibrocystic), gallbladder disease, diabetes mellitus, heavy smoking, acute mononucleosis, sickle cell disease

Pharmacokinetics: Excreted in breast milk

Interactions:
• Decreased effectiveness of oral contraceptives: anticonvulsants, rifampin, analgesics, antibiotics, antihistamines, chenodiol, griseofulvin
• Decreased action of oral anticoagulants
• Increased clotting: aminocaproic acid

Lab test interferences:
Increase: Pro-time; clotting factors VII, VIII, IX, X; TBG, PBI, T_4, platelet aggregability, BSP, triglycerides, bilirubin, AST (SGOT), ALT (SGPT)

Decrease: T_3, antithrombin III, folate, metyrapone test, GTT, 17-OHCS

NURSING CONSIDERATIONS
Assess:
• Glucose, thyroid function, liver function tests
• Reproductive changes: change in breasts, tumors, positive Pap smear; drug should be discontinued

Administer:
• PO with food for GI symptoms; give at same time each day
• Subdermal implant of 6 caps effective for 5 yr; then should be removed
• IM inj deep in large muscle mass after shaking suspension; ensure patient not pregnant if injections are 2 wk or more apart

Evaluate:
• Therapeutic response: absence of pregnancy, endometriosis, hypermenorrhea

Teach patient/family:
• About detection of clots using Homan's sign
• To use sunscreen or avoid sunlight; photosensitivity can occur
• To take at same time each day to ensure equal drug level
• To report GI symptoms that occur after 4 mo
• To use another birth control method during 1st week of oral contraceptive use
• To take another tablet as soon as possible if one is missed
• That after drug is discontinued, pregnancy may not occur for several months
• To report abdominal pain, change in vision, shortness of breath, change in menstrual flow, spotting, breakthrough bleeding, breast lumps, swelling, headache, severe leg pain
• That continuing medical care is needed: Pap smear and gynecologic examinations q6mo
• To notify health care providers and dentists of oral contraceptive use

---

orphenadrine (℞)

(or-fen'a-dreen)

Banflex, Flexoject, Flexon, Marflex, Myolin, Neocyten, Norflex, O-Flex, Orphenadrine Citrate, Orphenate

Func. class.: Skeletal muscle relaxant, central-acting; anticholinergic

Chem. class.: Tertiary amine

Action: Acts centrally on skeletal muscle to relax, inhibit muscle spasm

Uses: Pain in musculoskeletal disorders

Dosage and routes:
• *Adult:* **PO** 100 mg bid; **IM/IV** 60 mg q12h

Available forms: Tabs 100 mg; tabs, sus rel 100 mg; inj 30 mg/ml

Side effects/adverse reactions:

*HEMA: **Aplastic anemia***

CNS: Dizziness, weakness, fatigue, drowsiness, headache, disorientation, insomnia, stimulation, hallucination, agitation

EENT: Nasal congestion, blurred vision, increased intraocular pressure, mydriasis

CV: Orthostatic hypotension, tachycardia

GI: Nausea, vomiting, constipation, dry mouth

GU: Urinary frequency, hesitancy, retention

INTEG: Rash, pruritus, urticaria

Contraindications: Hypersensitivity, narrow-angle glaucoma, GI obstruction, myasthenia gravis, stenosing peptic ulcer, bladder neck obstruction, cardiospasm

Precautions: Pregnancy (C), children, cardiac disease, tachycardia, elderly

Pharmacokinetics:

PO: Peak 2 hr, duration 4-6 hr, half-life 14 hr; metabolized in liver, excreted in urine (unchanged)

Interactions:
• Increased CNS effects: propoxyphene, other anticholinergics, oral contraceptives
• Incompatibility unknown

NURSING CONSIDERATIONS

Assess:
• Monitor VS q10-15min during administration
• Blood studies: CBC, WBC, differential; blood dyscrasias may occur (rare)
• I&O ratio; check for urinary retention, frequency, hesitancy
• Dosage: even slight overdose can cause toxicity
• Allergic reactions: rash, fever, respiratory distress
• Blood dyscrasias: fever, bleeding, fatigue (rare)
• CNS symptoms: dizziness, drowsiness, psychiatric symptoms; more common in elderly

Administer:
• With meals for GI symptoms

IV
• IV undiluted, or diluted in 5-10 ml sterile H_2O for inj; give 60 mg or less over 5 min
• May cause paradoxic initial bradycardia; usually disappears in 2 min

Perform/provide:
• Assistance with ambulation if dizziness/drowsiness occurs

Evaluate:
• Therapeutic response: decreased rigidity, spasms

Teach patient/family:
• Not to discontinue medication quickly; insomnia, nausea, headache will occur
• Not to take with alcohol, other CNS depressants
• To avoid altering activities while taking this drug
• To avoid hazardous activities if drowsiness/dizziness occurs

- To avoid using OTC medication: cough preparations, antihistamines, unless directed by prescriber
- To use gum, frequent sips of water for dry mouth

oxacillin (R)

(ox-a-sill'in)

Bactocill, oxacillin sodium, Prostaphilin

Func. class.: Broad-spectrum antiinfective

Chem. class.: Penicillinaseresistant penicillin

Action: Interferes with cell wall replication of susceptible organisms; osmotically unstable cell wall swells, bursts from osmotic pressure

Uses: Effective for gram-positive cocci *(S. aureus, S. pneumoniae),* infections caused by penicillinase-producing *Staphylococcus*

Dosage and routes:
- *Adult:* **PO** 2-6 g/day in divided doses q4-6h; **IM/IV** 2-12 g/day in divided doses q4-6h
- *Child:* **PO** 50-100 mg/kg/day in divided doses q6h; **IM/IV** 50-100 mg/kg/day in divided doses q4-6h

Available forms: Caps 250, 500 mg; powder for oral susp 250 mg/5 ml; powder for inj 250, 500 mg, 1, 2, 4, 10 g; inf 1, 2 g

Side effects/adverse reactions:

HEMA: Anemia, increased bleeding time, **bone marrow depression, granulocytopenia**

GI: Nausea, vomiting, diarrhea, increased AST (SGOT), ALT (SGPT), abdominal pain, glossitis, colitis

GU: **Oliguria, proteinuria, hematuria,** *vaginitis, moniliasis,* **glomerulonephritis**

CNS: Lethargy, hallucinations, anxiety, depression, twitching, **coma, convulsions**

Contraindications: Hypersensitivity to penicillins

Precautions: Pregnancy (B), hypersensitivity to cephalosporins, neonates

Pharmacokinetics:

PO/IM: Peak 30-60 min, duration 4-6 hr

IV: Peak 5 min, duration 4-6 hr, half-life 30-60 min

Metabolized in the liver; excreted in urine, bile, breast milk; crosses placenta

Interactions:
- Decreased antimicrobial effectiveness of oxacillin: tetracyclines
- Decreased effect of oral contraceptives
- Increased oxacillin concentrations: aspirin, probenecid, disulfiram

Lab test interferences:

False positive: Urine glucose, urine protein

NURSING CONSIDERATIONS

Assess:
- I&O ratio; report hematuria, oliguria, since penicillin in high doses is nephrotoxic

◆ Any patient with compromised renal system, since drug is excreted slowly in poor renal system function; toxicity may occur rapidly
- Liver studies: AST (SGOT), ALT (SGPT)
- Blood studies: WBC, RBC, Hct/Hgb, bleeding time
- Renal studies: urinalysis, protein
- C&S before therapy; drug may be given as soon as culture is taken
- Bowel pattern before and during treatment
- Skin eruptions after administration of penicillin to 1 wk after discontinuing drug
- Respiratory status: rate, character, wheezing, tightness in chest
- Allergies before initiation of treatment, and reaction of each medication; highlight allergies on chart

◆ = Nursing alert   *Ɱ* = Herb-drug interaction   Ⓞ = Do not crush

Administer:
• Drug after C&S completed
• PO with full glass of water 1 hr before or 2 hr after meals
• IM inj deep in gluteal muscle

IV
• After diluting 500 mg or less/5 ml sterile H_2O or NaCl for inj; may dilute further in D_5W, NS, LR and give 1 g over 10 min; may be given as infusion over 6 hr

Additive compatibilities: Cephapirin, chloramphenicol, dopamine, potassium chloride, sodium bicarbonate

Y-site compatibilities: Acyclovir, cyclophosphamide, diltiazem, famotidine, fluconazole, foscarnet, heparin, hydrocortisone, hydromorphone, labetalol, magnesium sulfate, meperidine, methotrexate, morphine, perphenazine, potassium chloride, tacrolimus, vit B/C, zidovudine

Perform/provide:
• Adrenalin, suction, tracheostomy set, endotracheal intubation equipment
• Scratch test to assess allergy, after securing order from prescriber; usually done when penicillin is only drug of choice
• Storage in air-tight container; refrigerate reconstituted sol up to 2 wk

Evaluate:
• Therapeutic response: absence of fever, draining wounds

Teach patient/family:
• All aspects of drug therapy, including need to complete course of medication to ensure organism death (10-14 days); culture may be taken after completed course
• To report sore throat, fever, fatigue (may indicate superinfection); persistent diarrhea
• To wear or carry Medic Alert ID if allergic to penicillins

• To take on empty stomach with a full glass of water

Treatment of anaphylaxis: Withdraw drug, maintain airway, administer epinephrine, aminophylline, O_2, IV corticosteroids

---

oxamniquine (℞)
(ox-am′ni-kwin)
Vansil
Func. class.: Anthelmintic
Chem. class.: Tetrahydroquinone derivative

Action: Causes paralysis, contraction, leading to dislodgement of suckers; they are carried to liver, where phagocytosis takes place

Uses: Schistosomiasis

Dosage and routes:
• *Adult and child >30 kg:* **PO** 12-15 mg/kg as single dose
• *Child <30 kg:* **PO** 20 mg/kg in 2 divided doses q2-8h

Available forms: Caps 250 mg

Side effects/adverse reactions:
INTEG: Rash, pruritus, urticaria
CNS: *Dizziness, headache, drowsiness,* insomnia, **convulsions,** hallucinations, personality changes, stimulation
EENT: Bad taste, oral irritation
GI: Nausea, vomiting, anorexia, abdominal pain
HEMA: Increased sedimentation rate, reticulocyte count, increase or decrease in leukocytes

Contraindications: Hypersensitivity

Precautions: Pregnancy (C), lactation, seizure disorders

Pharmacokinetics:
PO: Peak 1-1½ hr, half-life 1-2½ hr; excreted in urine (unchanged/metabolites)

Lab test interferences:
Interference: Urinalysis

NURSING CONSIDERATIONS
Assess:
• Stools during entire treatment, 1, 3 mo after treatment; specimens must be sent to lab while still warm
• For allergic reaction: rash, itching, urticaria
• For infection in other family members, since infection from person to person is common

Administer:
• PO after meals to avoid GI symptoms

Perform/provide:
• Storage in tight container, cool environment

Evaluate:
• Therapeutic response: expulsion of worms, 3 negative stool cultures after completion of treatment

Teach patient/family:
• Proper hygiene after stool, including hand-washing technique; tell patient not to put fingers in mouth
• That infected person should sleep alone; not to shake bed linen; change bed linen daily; wash in hot water
• To clean toilet qd with disinfectant (green soap)
• The need for compliance with dosage schedule, duration of treatment
• That urine may turn orange or red
• To avoid hazardous activities since drowsiness occurs
• That seizures may recur in patient who is controlled on medication

---

oxandrolone (R)

(ox-an'droe-lone)
Oxandrin, oxandrolone
Func. class.: Androgenic anabolic steroid
Chem. class.: Halogenated testosterone derivative

Action: Increases weight by building body tissue, increases potassium, phosphorus, chloride, nitrogen levels, increases bone development

Uses: Tissue building after steroid therapy, osteoporosis, prolonged immobility

Dosage and routes:
• *Adult:* **PO** 2.5 mg bid-qid, not to exceed 20 mg qd × 2-3 wk
• *Child:* **PO** 0.25 mg/kg/day × 2-4 wk, not to exceed 3 mo

Available forms: Tabs 2.5 mg

Side effects/adverse reactions:
INTEG: Rash, acneiform lesions, oily hair, skin, flushing, sweating, acne vulgaris, alopecia, hirsutism
CNS: Dizziness, headache, fatigue, tremors, paresthesias, flushing, sweating, anxiety, lability, insomnia
MS: Cramps, spasms
CV: Increased B/P
GU: **Hematuria,** amenorrhea, vaginitis, decreased libido, decreased breast size, clitoral hypertrophy, testicular atrophy
GI: Nausea, vomiting, constipation, weight gain, *cholestatic jaundice*
EENT: Carpal tunnel syndrome, conjunctival edema, nasal congestion
ENDO: Abnormal GT

Contraindications: Severe renal, severe cardiac, severe hepatic disease, hypersensitivity, pregnancy (X), lactation, genital bleeding (abnormal)

Precautions: Diabetes mellitus, CV disease, MI

Pharmacokinetics:
PO: Metabolized in liver, excreted in urine, breast milk, crosses placenta

Interactions:
• Increased effects of oral antidiabetics, oxyphenbutazone
• Increased PT: anticoagulants
• Edema: ACTH, adrenal steroids
• Decreased effects of insulin

 = Nursing alert   = Herb-drug interaction   = Do not crush

Lab test interferences:

Increase: Serum cholesterol, blood glucose, urine glucose

Decrease: Serum Ca, serum K, T_4, T_3, thyroid ^{131}I uptake test, urine 17-OHCS, 17-KS, PBI, BSP

NURSING CONSIDERATIONS

Assess:

• Weight qd; notify prescriber if weekly weight gain is >5 lb

• B/P q4h

• I&O ratio; be alert for decreasing urinary output, increasing edema

• Growth rate in children, since growth rate may be uneven (linear/bone growth) in long-term use

• Electrolytes: K, Na, Cl, Ca; cholesterol

• Liver function studies: ALT (SGPT), AST (SGOT), bilirubin

• Edema, hypertension, cardiac symptoms, jaundice

• Mental status: affect, mood, behavioral changes, aggression

• Signs of masculinization in female: increased libido, deepening of voice, decreased breast tissue, enlarged clitoris, menstrual irregularities; male: gynecomastia, impotence, testicular atrophy

• Hypercalcemia: lethargy, polyuria, polydipsia, nausea, vomiting, constipation; drug may have to be decreased

• Hypoglycemia in diabetics, since oral anticoagulant action is decreased

Administer:

• Titrated dose, use lowest effective dose

Perform/provide:

• Diet with increased calories and protein; decrease Na for edema

Evaluate:

• Therapeutic response: occurs in 4-6 wk in osteoporosis

Teach patient/family:

• That drug must be combined with complete health plan: diet, rest, exercise

• To notify prescriber if therapeutic response decreases

• Not to discontinue abruptly

• About change in sex characteristics

• That women should report menstrual irregularities

• That 1-3 mo course is necessary for response in breast cancer

• The proper procedure for use of buccal tablets (requires 30-60 min to dissolve, change absorption site with each dose; do not eat, drink, chew, or smoke while tablet is in place)

---

oxaprozin (℞)

(ox-a-proe′zin)

Daypro

Func. class.: Nonsteroidal antiinflammatory

Chem. class.: Propionic acid derivative

Action: May inhibit prostaglandin synthesis by decreasing enzyme needed for biosynthesis, analgesic, antiinflammatory

Uses: Acute and long-term management of osteoarthritis, rheumatoid arthritis

Dosage and routes:

• *Adult:* **PO** 1200 mg qd; maximum dose 1800 mg/day or 26 mg/kg, whichever is lower

Available forms: Caplets 600 mg

Side effects/adverse reactions:

*MISC: **Anaphylaxis, angioneurotic edema***

GI: Nausea, anorexia, vomiting, diarrhea, jaundice, ***cholestatic hepatitis,*** constipation, flatulence, cramps, dry mouth, peptic ulcer, ***GI bleeding***

CNS: Dizziness, headache, drowsiness, fatigue, tremors, confusion, insomnia, anxiety, depression

---

CV: Tachycardia, peripheral edema, palpitations, dysrhythmias
INTEG: Purpura, rash, pruritus, sweating
*GU: **Nephrotoxicity: dysuria, hematuria, oliguria, azotemia***
*HEMA: **Increased bleeding time***
EENT: Tinnitus, hearing loss, blurred vision

Contraindications: Hypersensitivity, asthma, patients in whom aspirin and iodides have induced symptoms of allergic reactions or asthma

Precautions: Pregnancy (B) 1st and 2nd trimester, lactation, children, bleeding disorders, GI disorders, cardiac disorders, hypersensitivity to other antiinflammatory agents, severe renal and hepatic disease, elderly, CHF

Pharmacokinetics:
PO: Onset 1 wk, peak unknown, duration unknown, half-life 40-50 hr; metabolized in liver; excreted in urine (metabolites), breast milk; 99% plasma protein binding

Interactions:
• Oxaprozin may decrease effects of loop diuretics and β-blockers
• May increase the action or toxicity of warfarin, phenytoin, lithium, methotrexate
• May increase effects of oxaprozin: phenobarbital, probenecid

NURSING CONSIDERATIONS
Assess:
• Pain: frequency, intensity, characteristics; relief of pain after med
• Asthma, aspirin hypersensitivity, oronasal polyps; increased hypersensitivity reactions
• Renal, liver, blood studies: BUN, creatinine, AST (SGOT), ALT (SGPT), Hgb, before treatment, periodically thereafter
• Audiometric, ophthalmic exam before, during, after treatment
• For eye, ear problems: blurred vision, tinnitus; may indicate toxicity

Administer:
• With food to decrease GI symptoms
Perform/provide:
• Storage at room temp
Evaluate:
• Therapeutic response: decreased pain, stiffness in joints, decreased swelling in joints, ability to move more easily
Teach patient/family:
• To report blurred vision, ringing, roaring in ears; may indicate toxicity
• To avoid driving, other hazardous activities if dizziness/drowsiness occurs
• To report change in urine pattern, increased weight, edema, increased pain in joints, fever, blood in urine; indicates nephrotoxicity
• That therapeutic effects may take up to 1 mo
• To take with a full glass of water to enhance absorption

---

oxazepam (℞)
(ox-ay′ze-pam)
Apo-Oxazepam*, Novoxapam*, oxazepam, Ox-Pam*, Serax, Zapex*
Func. class.: Sedative/hypnotic; antianxiety
Chem. class.: Benzodiazepine

Controlled Substance Schedule IV
Action: Potentiates the actions of GABA, especially in limbic system and reticular formation
Uses: Anxiety, alcohol withdrawal
Dosage and routes:
Anxiety
• *Adult:* **PO** 10-30 mg tid-qid
Alcohol withdrawal
• *Adult:* **PO** 15-30 mg tid-qid
Available forms: Caps 10, 15, 30 mg; tabs 10, 15, 30 mg

Side effects/adverse reactions:

CNS: Dizziness, drowsiness, confusion, headache, anxiety, tremors, fatigue, depression, insomnia, hallucinations, paradoxical excitement, transient amnesia
GI: Nausea, vomiting, anorexia
INTEG: Rash, dermatitis, itching
*CV: Orthostatic hypotension, **ECG changes, tachycardia,*** hypotension
EENT: Blurred vision, tinnitus, mydriasis

Contraindications: Hypersensitivity to benzodiazepines, narrow-angle glaucoma, psychosis, pregnancy (D), lactation, child <12 yr

Precautions: Elderly, debilitated, hepatic disease, renal disease

Pharmacokinetics:

PO: Peak 2-4 hr, metabolized by liver, excreted by kidneys, half-life 5-15 hr

Interactions:

• Decreased effects of oxazepam: oral contraceptives, valproic acid
• Increased effects of oxazepam: CNS depressants, alcohol, disulfiram, oral contraceptives

Lab test interferences:

Increase: AST (SGOT), ALT (SGPT), serum bilirubin
Decrease: RAIU
False increase: 17-OHCS

NURSING CONSIDERATIONS

Assess:

• B/P (lying, standing), pulse; if systolic B/P drops 20 mm Hg, hold drug, notify prescriber
• Blood studies: CBC during long-term therapy; blood dyscrasias have occurred rarely
• Hepatic studies: AST (SGOT), ALT (SGPT), bilirubin, creatinine, LDH, alk phosphatase
• Mental status: mood, sensorium, affect, sleeping pattern, drowsiness, dizziness
◆ Physical dependency, withdrawal symptoms: headache, nausea, vomiting, muscle pain, weakness, tremors, convulsions (long-term use)
• Suicidal tendencies

Administer:

PO
• With food, milk for GI symptoms
• Sugarless gum, hard candy, frequent sips of water for dry mouth

Perform/provide:

• Assistance with ambulation during beginning therapy; drowsiness/dizziness occurs
• Safety measures, including side rails
• Check to see if PO medication has been swallowed

Evaluate:

• Therapeutic response: decreased anxiety, restlessness, insomnia

Teach patient/family:

• That drug may be taken with food
• That medication is not to be used for everyday stress or used longer than 4 mo unless directed by prescriber; not to take more than prescribed dose; may be habit forming
• To avoid OTC preparations (cough, cold, hay fever) unless approved by prescriber
• To avoid driving, activities that require alertness, since drowsiness may occur
• To avoid alcohol ingestion, other psychotropic medications unless directed by prescriber
• Not to discontinue medication abruptly after long-term use
• To rise slowly, or fainting may occur, especially elderly
• That drowsiness may worsen at beginning of treatment

Treatment of overdose: Lavage, VS, supportive care, flumazenil

---

oxidized cellulose (℞)
Oxycel, Surgicel
Func. class.: Hemostatic
Chem. class.: Cellulose product

Action: Absorbs blood, acts as an artificial clot, swells as it contacts with blood, conforms readily to surface

Uses: Hemostasis in surgery, oral surgery, exodontia

Dosage and routes:
• *Adult and child:* **TOP** apply using sterile technique as needed, remove after bleeding stops, if possible, or leave in place if needed

Available forms: TOP knitted fabric as strips, pads, pledgets

Side effects/adverse reactions:
EENT: Sneezing, burning in epistaxis
INTEG: Burning, stinging, encapsulation of fluid, foreign bodies
CNS: Headache in epistaxis

Contraindications: Hypersensitivity, large artery hemorrhage, oozing surfaces, implantation in bone deficit, placement around optic nerve, and chiasm

NURSING CONSIDERATIONS
Assess:
• Allergy: fever, rash, itching, burning, stinging

Administer:
TOP
• Dry; use only amount needed to control bleeding
• Loosely; remove excess before closure in surgery; irrigate first, then remove using sterile technique
• Using sterile technique; cannot be resterilized

Evaluate:
• Therapeutic response: decreased bleeding in surgery

oxtriphylline (℞)
(ox-trye'fi-lin)
Apo-Oxtriphylline*, Choledyl*, Choledyl SA, Novotriphyl*, oxtriphylline
Func. class.: Bronchodilator, spasmolytic
Chem. class.: Choline salt of theophylline

Action: Relaxes smooth muscle of respiratory system by blocking phosphodiesterase, which increases cyclic AMP; 64% theophylline

Uses: Acute bronchial asthma, reversible bronchospasm in chronic bronchitis and COPD

Dosage and routes:
• *Adult and child >12 yr:* **PO** 200 mg qid or sus action q12h
• *Child 2-12 yr:* **PO** 4 mg/kg q6h; may be increased to desired response, therapeutic level

Available forms: Elix 100 mg/5 ml; syr 50 mg/5 ml; tabs 100, 200, 400, 600 mg; sus action tabs 400, 600 mg

Side effects/adverse reactions:
CNS: Anxiety, restlessness, insomnia, dizziness, **convulsions,** headache, light-headedness
CV: Palpitations, sinus tachycardia, hypotension
GI: Nausea, vomiting, anorexia, diarrhea, bitter taste, dyspepsia
RESP: Increased rate
INTEG: Flushing, urticaria, alopecia

Contraindications: Hypersensitivity to xanthines, tachydysrhythmias

Precautions: Elderly, CHF, cor pulmonale, hepatic disease, active peptic ulcer disease, diabetes mellitus, hyperthyroidism, hypertension, children, pregnancy (C), glaucoma, prostatic hypertrophy

Pharmacokinetics:
ELIXIR: Peak 1 hr
PO-SA: Peak 4-7 hr, duration 8-12 hr

◆ = Nursing alert   ⫸ = Herb-drug interaction   ⊘ = Do not crush

Metabolized in liver; excreted in urine, breast milk; crosses placenta
Interactions:

• Increased action of oxtriphylline: cimetidine, erythromycin, troleandomycin, oral contraceptive, propranolol

• May increase effects of anticoagulants, coffee (caffeine items)

• Cardiotoxicity: β-blockers

• Decreased effect of lithium

• Decreased theophylline level: rifampin, phenytoin

🖋 Increased action of both: ephedra
NURSING CONSIDERATIONS
Assess:

• Therapeutic blood levels; toxicity may occur with small increase above therapeutic level

• Therapeutic theophylline levels: 11-20 μg/ml

• Smoking: reduces effects of theophyllines, requiring larger doses

• Respiratory rate, rhythm, depth; auscultate lung fields bilaterally; notify prescriber of abnormalities

• Allergic reactions: rash, urticaria, drug should be discontinued
Administer:

• PO after meals to decrease GI symptoms; absorption may be affected

• After meals, hs
Perform/provide:

• Storage in closed container away from heat; protect elixir from light
Evaluate:

• Therapeutic response: absence of dyspnea, wheezing
Teach patient/family:

🚫 Not to break, crush, or chew tab

• To check OTC medications, prescription medications for ephedrine, which will increase stimulation

• To avoid hazardous activities; dizziness may occur

• If GI upset occurs, to take drug

with 8 oz water; avoid food; absorption may be decreased

• To notify prescriber of toxicity: nausea, vomiting, anxiety, convulsions, insomnia, rapid pulse

• To notify prescriber of change in smoking habit; may need to change dose; encourage not to smoke

---

oxybutynin (℞)

(ox-i-byoo'ti-nin)
Ditropan, oxybutynin chloride
Func. class.: Spasmolytic
Chem. class.: Synthetic tertiary amine

Action: Relaxes smooth muscles in urinary tract by inhibiting acetylcholine at postganglionic sites
Uses: Antispasmodic for neurogenic bladder
Dosage and routes:

• *Adult:* PO 5 mg bid-tid, not to exceed 5 mg qid

• *Geriatric:* PO 2.5-5 mg tid, increase by 2.5 mg q several days

• *Child >5 yr:* PO 5 mg bid, not to exceed 5 mg tid

• *Child 1-5 yr:* PO 0.2 mg/kg/dose 2-4 ×/day
Available forms: Syrup 5 mg/5 ml; tabs 5 mg
Side effects/adverse reactions:
*CNS: Anxiety, restlessness, dizziness, **convulsions**, headache, drowsiness, confusion*
CV: Palpitations, sinus tachycardia, hypotension
GI: Nausea, vomiting, anorexia, abdominal pain, constipation
GU: Dysuria, retention, hesitancy
EENT: Blurred vision, increased intraocular tension, dry mouth, throat
Contraindications: Hypersensitivity, GI obstruction, GI hemorrhage, GU obstruction, glaucoma, severe

colitis, myasthenia gravis, unstable CV status in acute hemorrhage

Precautions: Pregnancy (B), lactation, suspected glaucoma, children <12 yr, elderly

Pharmacokinetics: Onset ½-1 hr, peak 3-4 hr, duration 6-10 hr; metabolized by liver, excreted in urine

Interactions:

• Increased levels of atenolol, digoxin, nitrofurantoin, oxybutynin
• Decreased levels of acetaminophen, haloperidol, levodopa
• Increased or decreased levels of phenothiazines

NURSING CONSIDERATIONS

Assess:

• Urinary patterns: distention, nocturia, frequency, urgency, incontinence
• Allergic reactions: rash, urticaria; if these occur, drug should be discontinued
• CNS effects: confusion, anxiety; anticholinergic effects in the elderly

Evaluate:

• Urinary status: dysuria, frequency, nocturia, incontinence

Teach patient/family:

• To avoid hazardous activities; dizziness may occur
• To avoid OTC medications with alcohol, other CNS depressants
• To prevent photophobia by wearing sunglasses

oxycodone (Ṟ)

(ox-i-koe′done)

Oxycocet*, Oxycodan*, OxyIR, Oxycodone/Aspirin Endodan*, Percocet, Percodan, Percodan-Demi, Roxicet, Roxicodone, Roxilox, Roxiprin Oxycodone/Acetaminophen Endocet*, Supeudol*, Tylox

Func. class.: Narcotic analgesic

Chem. class.: Opiate, semisynthetic derivative

Controlled Substance Schedule II

Action: Inhibits ascending pain pathways in CNS, increases pain threshold, alters pain perception

Uses: Moderate to severe pain

Dosage and routes:

• *Adult:* **PO** 5 mg q4-6h or 10 mg tid or qid prn
• *Child:* **PO** 0.05-0.15 mg/kg/dose up to 5 mg/dose q4-6h

Available forms: Oxycodone supp 10, 20 mg; tabs 5 mg; caps, immediate rel 5 mg; oral sol conc 20 mg/ml; oxycodone with acetaminophen tabs 5 mg/325 mg; cap 5 mg/500 mg; oral sol 5 mg/325 mg/5 ml; oxycodone with aspirin 2.44 mg/325 mg, 4.88/325 mg

Side effects/adverse reactions:

CNS: Drowsiness, dizziness, confusion, headache, sedation, euphoria

GI: Nausea, vomiting, anorexia, constipation, cramps

GU: Increased urinary output, dysuria, urinary retention

INTEG: Rash, urticaria, bruising, flushing, diaphoresis, pruritus

EENT: Tinnitus, blurred vision, miosis, diplopia

CV: Palpitations, bradycardia, change in B/P

RESP: Respiratory depression

Contraindications: Hypersensitivity, addiction (narcotic)

Precautions: Addictive personality, pregnancy (B), lactation, increased intracranial pressure, MI (acute), severe heart disease, respiratory depression, hepatic disease, renal disease, child <18 yr

Pharmacokinetics:
PO: Onset 15-30 min, peak 1 hr, duration 4-6 hr; detoxified by liver, excreted in urine, crosses placenta, excreted in breast milk

Interactions:
• Increased effects with other CNS depressants: alcohol, narcotics, sedative/hypnotics, antipsychotics, skeletal muscle relaxants

Lab test interferences:
Increase: Amylase

NURSING CONSIDERATIONS
Assess:
• I&O ratio; check for decreasing output; may indicate urinary retention
• CNS changes: dizziness, drowsiness, hallucinations, euphoria, LOC, pupil reaction
• Allergic reactions: rash, urticaria
• Respiratory dysfunction: respiratory depression, character, rate, rhythm; notify prescriber if respirations are <10/min
• Need for pain medication by pain, sedation scoring; physical dependence

Administer:
• With antiemetic if nausea, vomiting occur
• When pain is beginning to return; determine dosage interval by response

Perform/provide:
• Storage in light-resistant area at room temp
• Assistance with ambulation
• Safety measures: side rails, nightlight, call bell within easy reach

Evaluate:
• Therapeutic response: decrease in pain

Teach patient/family:
• To report any symptoms of CNS changes, allergic reactions
• That physical dependency may result from extended use
• That withdrawal symptoms may occur: nausea, vomiting, cramps, fever, faintness, anorexia

Treatment of overdose: Naloxone (Narcan) 0.2-0.8 mg IV, O_2, IV fluids, vasopressors

---

oxymetholone (℞)

(ox-i-meth'oh-lone)
Anadrol-50, Anapolon 50*

Func. class.: Androgenic anabolic steroid

Chem. class.: Halogenated testosterone derivative

Action: Increases weight by building body tissue, increases potassium, phosphorus, chloride, and nitrogen levels, increases bone development

Uses: Tissue building after steroid therapy, osteoporosis, aplastic anemia, anemias caused by deficient RBC production

Dosage and routes:
Aplastic anemia
• *Adult and child:* **PO** 1-5 mg/kg/day, titrated to patient response, not to exceed 3 mo

Osteoporosis/tissue building (possible indication)
• *Adult:* **PO** 5-15 mg/day, not to exceed 30 mg/day or 3 mo
• *Child >6 yr:* **PO** up to 10 mg/day, not to exceed 1 mo
• *Child <6 yr:* **PO** 1.25 mg qd-qid, not to exceed 1 mo

Available forms: Tabs 50 mg

Side effects/adverse reactions:
INTEG: Rash, acneiform lesions, oily hair, skin, flushing, sweating, acne vulgaris, alopecia, hirsutism

---

CNS: Dizziness, headache, fatigue, tremors, paresthesias, flushing, sweating, anxiety, lability, insomnia

MS: Cramps, spasms

CV: Increased B/P

*GU: **Hematuria,*** amenorrhea, vaginitis, decreased libido, decreased breast size, clitoral hypertrophy, testicular atrophy

GI: Nausea, vomiting, constipation, weight gain, ***cholestatic jaundice***

EENT: Carpal tunnel syndrome, conjunctival edema, nasal congestion

ENDO: Abnormal GTT

Contraindications: Severe renal, severe cardiac, severe hepatic disease, hypersensitivity, pregnancy (X), lactation, genital bleeding (abnormal)

Precautions: Diabetes mellitus, CV disease, MI

Pharmacokinetics:

PO: Metabolized in liver, excreted in urine, crosses placenta, excreted in breast milk

Interactions:
• Increased effects of oral antidiabetics, oxyphenbutazone
• Increased PT: anticoagulants
• Edema: ACTH, adrenal steroids
• Decreased effects of insulin

Lab test interferences:

Increase: Serum cholesterol, blood glucose, urine glucose

Decrease: Serum Ca, serum K, T_4, T_3, thyroid ^{131}I uptake test, urine 17-OHCS, 17-KS, PBI, BSP

NURSING CONSIDERATIONS

Assess:
• Weight qd, notify prescriber of weekly weight gain >5 lb
• B/P q4h
• I&O ratio; be alert for decreasing urinary output, increasing edema
• Growth rate in children, since growth rate may be uneven (linear/bone growth) with extended use

• Electrolytes: K, Na, Cl, Ca; cholesterol
• Liver function studies: ALT (SGPT), AST (SGOT), bilirubin
• Edema, hypertension, cardiac symptoms, jaundice
• Mental status: affect, mood, behavioral changes, aggression
• Signs of masculinization in female: increased libido, deepening of voice, breast tissue, enlarged clitoris, menstrual irregularities; male: gynecomastia, impotence, testicular atrophy
• Hypercalcemia: lethargy, polyuria, polydipsia, nausea, vomiting, constipation; drug may have to be decreased
• Hypoglycemia in diabetics; oral antidiabetic action is increased

Administer:
• Titrated dose; use lowest effective dose

Perform/provide:
• Diet with increased calories, protein; decreased Na for edema

Evaluate:
• Therapeutic response: occurs in 4-6 wk in osteoporosis

Teach patient/family:
• That drug must be combined with complete health plan: diet, rest, exercise
• To notify prescriber if therapeutic response decreases
• Not to discontinue abruptly
• About changes in sex characteristics
• That women should report menstrual irregularities
• That 1-3 mo course is necessary for response in breast cancer
• The correct procedure for use of buccal tablets (requires 30-60 min to dissolve; change absorption site with each dose; do not eat, drink, chew, or smoke while tablet is in place)

oxymorphone (℞)

(ox-i-mor'fone)

Numorphan

Func. class.: Narcotic analgesic

Chem. class.: Opiate, semisynthetic phenanthrene derivative

Controlled Substance Schedule II

Action: Inhibits ascending pain pathways in CNS, increases pain threshold, alters pain perception

Uses: Moderate to severe pain

Dosage and routes:

• *Adult:* **IM/SC** 1-1.5 mg q4-6h prn; **IV** 0.5 mg q4-6h prn; **RECT** 2.5-5 mg q4-6h prn

Labor analgesia

• *Adult:* **IM:** 0.5-1 mg

Available forms: Inj 1, 1.5 mg/ml; supp 5 mg

Side effects/adverse reactions:

CNS: Drowsiness, dizziness, confusion, headache, sedation, euphoria (elderly)

GI: Nausea, vomiting, anorexia, constipation, cramps

GU: Increased urinary output, dysuria, urinary retention

INTEG: Rash, urticaria, bruising, flushing, diaphoresis, pruritus

EENT: Tinnitus, blurred vision, miosis, diplopia

CV: Palpitations, bradycardia, change in B/P

*RESP: **Respiratory depression***

Contraindications: Hypersensitivity, addiction (narcotic)

Precautions: Addictive personality, pregnancy (B), lactation, increased intracranial pressure, MI (acute), severe heart disease, respiratory depression, hepatic disease, renal disease, child <18 yr

Pharmacokinetics:

SC/IM: Onset 10-15 min, peak 1½ hr, duration, 3-6 hr

IV: Onset 5-10 min, peak 15-30 min, duration 3-6 hr

RECT: Onset 15-30 min, duration 3-6 hr

Metabolized by liver, excreted in urine, crosses placenta

Interactions:

• Increased effects with other CNS depressants: alcohol, narcotics, sedative/hypnotics, antipsychotics, skeletal muscle relaxants

Lab test interferences:

Increase: Amylase

NURSING CONSIDERATIONS

Assess:

• I&O ratio for decreasing output; may indicate urinary retention

• CNS changes: dizziness, drowsiness, hallucinations, euphoria, LOC, pupil reaction

• Allergic reactions: rash, urticaria

• Respiratory dysfunction: respiratory depression, character, rate, rhythm; notify prescriber if respirations are <10/min

• Need for pain medication, physical dependence

Administer:

• With antiemetic for nausea, vomiting

• When pain is beginning to return; determine interval by response

IV

• After diluting with 5 ml sterile H₂O or NS for inj; give over 2-5 min through Y-tube or 3-way stopcock

Syringe compatibilities: Glycopyrrolate, hydroxyzine, ranitidine

Perform/provide:

• Storage in light-resistant area at room temp

• Assistance with ambulation

• Safety measures: side rails, nightlight, call bell within easy reach

Evaluate:

• Therapeutic response: decrease in pain

Teach patient/family:
• To report any symptoms of CNS changes, allergic reactions
• That physical dependency may result from extended use
• That withdrawal symptoms may occur: nausea, vomiting, cramps, fever, faintness, anorexia
Treatment of overdose: Naloxone (Narcan) 0.2-0.8 mg IV, O_2, IV fluids, vasopressors

---

oxyphenbutazone (℞)

(ox-i-fen-byoo'ta-zone)
Oxybutazone*, oxyphenbutazone*
Func. class.: Nonsteroidal antiinflammatory
Chem. class.: Pyrazolone derivative

Action: Inhibits prostaglandin synthesis by decreasing an enzyme needed for biosynthesis; analgesic, antiinflammatory, antipyretic
Uses: Mild to moderate pain, osteoarthritis, rheumatoid arthritis
Dosage and routes:
Pain
• *Adult:* **PO** 100-200 mg tid-qid
Acute arthritis
• *Adult:* **PO** 400 mg, then 100 mg q4h × 4 days or until desired response
Available forms: Tabs 100 mg
Side effects/adverse reactions:
GI: Nausea, anorexia, vomiting, diarrhea, jaundice, *cholestatic hepatitis,* constipation, flatulence, cramps, dry mouth, peptic ulcer
CNS: Dizziness, drowsiness, fatigue, tremors, confusion, insomnia, anxiety, depression
CV: Tachycardia, peripheral edema, palpitations, dysrhythmias, hypertension, cardiac decompensation
INTEG: Purpura, rash, pruritus, sweating

*GU: **Nephrotoxicity: dysuria, hematuria, oliguria, azotemia***
*HEMA: **Blood dyscrasias,** bone marrow suppression
EENT: Tinnitus, hearing loss, blurred vision
Contraindications: Hypersensitivity, asthma, severe renal disease, severe hepatic disease, pregnancy (D), children <14 yr, ulcer disease
Precautions: Lactation, children, bleeding disorders, GI disorders, cardiac disorders, hypersensitivity to other antiinflammatory agents
Pharmacokinetics:
PO: Peak 2 hr, half-life 3-3½ hr, metabolized in liver, excreted in urine (metabolites), breast milk
Interactions:
• Increased action of warfarin, phenytoin, sulfonamides

NURSING CONSIDERATIONS
Assess:
• Renal, liver, blood studies: BUN, creatinine, AST (SGOT), ALT (SGPT), Hgb before treatment, periodically thereafter
• Audiometric, ophthalmic exam before, during, after treatment
• For eye, ear problems: blurred vision, tinnitus (may indicate toxicity)
Administer:
• With food to decrease GI symptoms; best to take on empty stomach to facilitate absorption
Perform/provide:
• Storage at room temp
Evaluate:
• Therapeutic response: decreased pain, stiffness, swelling in joints, ability to move more easily
Teach patient/family:
• To report blurred vision, ringing, roaring in ears (may indicate toxicity)
• To avoid driving, other hazardous activities if dizzy or drowsy
• To report change in urine pattern,

---

weight increase, edema, pain increase in joints, fever, blood in urine (indicates nephrotoxicity)
• That therapeutic effects may take up to 1 mo

---

oxytetracycline (℞)

(ox-i-tet-ra-sye'kleen)
Oxytetracycline HCl, Terramycin, Terramycin IM, Uri-Tet
Func. class.: Broad-spectrum antiinfective
Chem. class.: Tetracycline

Action: Inhibits protein synthesis, phosphorylation in microorganisms by binding to 30S ribosomal subunits, reversibly binding to 50S ribosomal subunits; bacteriostatic artificial clot

Uses: Syphilis, chlamydia trachomatis, gonorrhea, lymphogranuloma venereum, uncommon gram-positive/negative organisms, rickettsial infections

Dosage and routes:
• *Adult:* **PO** 250-500 mg q6h; **IM** 100 mg q8h or 150 mg q12h
• *Child >8 yr:* **PO** 25-50 mg/kg day in divided doses q6h; **IM** 15-25 mg/kg/day in divided doses q8-12h

Gonorrhea
• *Adult:* **PO** 1.5 g, then 500 mg qid for a total of 9 g

Chlamydia trachomatis
• *Adult:* **PO** 500 mg qid × 7 days

Syphilis
• *Adult:* **PO** 2-3 g in divided doses × 10-15 days up to 30-40 g total
• Dosage adjustment necessary in renal impairment

Available forms: Caps 250 mg; inj 50, 125 mg/ml

Side effects/adverse reactions:
CNS: Fever
HEMA: Eosinophilia, neutropenia, ***thrombocytopenia, leukocytosis, hemolytic anemia***
EENT: Dysphagia, glossitis, decreased calcification of deciduous teeth, oral candidiasis
GI: Nausea, abdominal pain, *vomiting, diarrhea,* anorexia, enterocolitis, ***hepatotoxicity,*** flatulence, abdominal cramps, epigastric burning, stomatitis
CV: Pericarditis
GU: Increased BUN
*INTEG: Rash, urticaria, photosensitivity, increased pigmentation, **exfoliative dermatitis,*** pruritus, angioedema, pain at injection site

Contraindications: Hypersensitivity to tetracyclines, children <8 yr, pregnancy (D)

Precautions: Renal disease, hepatic disease, lactation

Pharmacokinetics:
PO: Peak 2-4 hr, half-life 6-12 hr; excreted in urine, bile, feces in active form; crosses placenta; 20%-40% protein bound

Interactions:
• Decreased effect of oxytetracycline: antacids, NaHCO₃, dairy products, alkali products, iron, kaolin/pectin, cimetidine, barbiturates, carbamazepine, phenytoin
• Increased effect: warfarin
• Decreased effect: penicillins, oral contraceptives
• Nephrotoxicity: methoxyflurane
⬤ Increased action of oxytetracycline: bromelain

Lab test interferences:
False negative: Urine glucose with Clinistix or Tes-Tape
False increase: Urinary catecholamines

NURSING CONSIDERATIONS
Assess:
• I&O ratio
• Blood studies: PT, CBC, AST

(SGOT), ALT (SGPT), BUN, creatinine
• Signs of anemia: Hct, Hgb, fatigue
• Allergic reactions: rash, itching, pruritus, angioedema
• Nausea, vomiting, diarrhea; administer antiemetic, antacids as ordered
• Overgrowth of infection: fever, malaise, redness, pain, swelling, drainage, perineal itching, diarrhea, changes in cough or sputum

Administer:

PO
🚫 With a full glass of water; do not break, crush, or chew caps

IM
• IM inj, deep only
• After C&S obtained
• 2 hr before or after laxative or ferrous products, 3 hr after antacid

Perform/provide:
• Storage in tight, light-resistant container at room temp

Evaluate:
• Therapeutic response: decreased temp, absence of lesions, negative C&S

Teach patient/family:
• To avoid sunlight; sunscreen does not seem to decrease photosensitivity
• If diabetic, use blood glucose testing
• That all prescribed medication must be taken to prevent superinfection
• To avoid milk products, to take with a full glass of water

---

oxytocin, synthetic injection (℞)

(ox-i-toe′sin)
Pitocin, Syntocinon
Func. class.: Oxytocic
Chem. class.: Hormone

Action: Acts directly on myofibrils, producing uterine contraction; stimulates milk ejection by the breast

Uses: Stimulation, induction of labor; missed or incomplete abortion; postpartum bleeding

Dosage and routes:
Postpartum hemorrhage
• *Adult:* IV 10 U infused at 20-40 µU/min
• *Adult:* IM 10 U after delivery of placenta
Fetal stress test
• *Adult:* IV 0.5 µU/min, increase q20min until 3 contractions within 10 min
Stimulation of labor
• *Adult:* IV 0.5-2 µU/min, increase by 1-2 µU q15-60min until contractions occur; then decrease dose
Incomplete abortion
• *Adult:* IV INF 10 U/500 ml D_5W or 0.9% NaCl at 20-40 µU/min
Available forms: Inj 10 µU/ml

Side effects/adverse reactions:
CNS: Hypertension, *convulsions, tetanic contractions*
CV: Hypotension, dysrhythmias, increased pulse, bradycardia, tachycardia, PVC
FETUS: Dysrhythmias, jaundice, hypoxia, *intracranial hemorrhage*
GI: Anorexia, nausea, vomiting, constipation
GU: Abruptio placentae, decreased uterine blood flow
HEMA: Increased hyperbilirubinemia
INTEG: Rash
RESP: Asphyxia

 = Nursing alert   = Herb-drug interaction   = Do not crush

Contraindications: Hypersensitivity, serum toxemia, cephalopelvic disproportion, fetal distress, hypertonic uterus

Precautions: Cervical/uterine surgery, uterine sepsis, primipara >35 yr, 1st, 2nd stage of labor

Pharmacokinetics:

IM: Onset 3-7 min, duration 1 hr, half-life 12-17 min

IV: Onset 1 min, duration 30 min, half-life 12-17 min

Interactions:

• Hypertension: vasopressors

🖊 Hypertension: ephedra

NURSING CONSIDERATIONS

Assess:

• I&O ratio

• Respiration

• B/P, pulse; watch for changes that may indicate hemorrhage

• Respiratory rate, rhythm, depth; notify prescriber of abnormalities

• Length, intensity, duration of contraction; notify prescriber of contractions lasting over 1 min or absence of contractions; turn patient on her side

• FHTs, fetal distress; watch for acceleration, deceleration; notify prescriber if problems occur; fetal presentation, pelvic dimensions; turn patient on left side if FHT change in rate

⬥ For signs and symptoms of water intoxication; confusion, anuria, drowsiness, headache

Administer:

Labor induction

• After diluting 10 U/L of 0.9% NS or D_5 NS run at 1-2 µU/min at 15-30 min intervals to begin normal labor; dilute 10-40 µU/min, titrate to control postpartum bleeding; dilute 10 U/500 ml sol; run 10 U-20 µU/ml; administer by only 1 route at a time; use inf pump; rotate inf to provide mixing; do not shake

Control of postpartum bleeding

• Dilute 10-40 U/1 L of sol, run at 10-20 µU/min; adjust rate as needed

• With crash cart available on unit (Mg^+SO_4 at bedside)

Additive compatibilities: Chloramphenicol, metaraminol, netilmicin, sodium bicarbonate, thiopental, verapamil

Y-site compatibilities: Heparin, hydrocortisone, insulin (regular), meperidine, morphine, potassium chloride, vit B/C, warfarin

Evaluate:

• Therapeutic response: stimulation of labor, control of postpartum bleeding

Teach patient/family:

• To report increased blood loss, abdominal cramps, fever, foul-smelling lochia

• That contractions will be similar to menstrual cramps, gradually increasing in intensity

---

oxytocin, synthetic nasal (℞)

(ox-i-toe′sin)

Func. class.: Oxytocic hormone

Action: Acts directly on myofibrils, producing uterine contraction; stimulates milk ejection by the breast

Uses: Postpartum breast engorgement, initial milk letdown

Dosage and routes:

• *Adult:* **NAS SPRAY** 1 spray into one or both nostrils q2-3min before breastfeeding; **NAS DROPS** 3 gtt into one or both nostrils q2-3min before breastfeeding

Available forms: Nas spray 40 U/ml; nas drops

Side effects/adverse reactions:

• None

Pharmacokinetics: Onset 5-10 min, half-life 1 min

Side effects: *italics* = common; ***bold italics*** = life-threatening

Interactions:
• Hypertension: vasopressors
🖋 Hypertension: ephedra

NURSING CONSIDERATIONS
Assess:
• I&O ratio
• Environment conducive to letdown reflex

Evaluate:
• Therapeutic response: stimulation of milk ejection

Teach patient/family:
• To blow nose before administering; not to touch dropper to inside of nares
• To rinse dropper with warm water after each use
• Not to overuse

---

paclitaxel (℞)
(pa-kli-tax′el)
Taxol
Func. class.: Misc. antineoplastic
Chem. class.: Natural diterpene

Action: Inhibits reorganization of microtubule network needed for interphase and mitotic cellular functions; also causes abnormal bundles of microtubules during cell cycle and multiple esters of microtubules during mitosis

Uses: Metastatic carcinoma of the ovary, breast; AIDS-related Kaposi's sarcoma (2nd-line)

Investigational uses: Advanced head, neck, small-cell lung cancer; non-Hodgkin's lymphoma, adenocarcinoma of the upper GI tract, hormone-refractory prostate cancer

Dosage and routes:
Ovarian carcinoma
• *Adult:* IV INF 135 mg/m^2 given over 24 hr q3wk or 175 mg/m^2 over 3 hr q3wk

Breast carcinoma
• *Adult:* IV INF 175 mg/m^2 over 3 hr q3wk

AIDS-related Kaposi's sarcoma
• *Adult:* IV INF 135 mg/m^2 over 3 hr q3wk or 100 mg/m^2 over 3 hr q2wk

Available forms: Inj 30 mg/5 ml vial

Side effects/adverse reactions:
*HEMA: **Neutropenia, leukopenia, thrombocytopenia, anemia,** bleeding, infections*
*SYST: **Hypersensitivity reactions, anaphylaxis***
CV: Bradycardia, *hypotension,* abnormal ECG
NEURO: Peripheral neuropathy
MS: Arthralgia, myalgia
GI: Nausea, vomiting, diarrhea, mucositis, increased bilirubin, alk phosphatase, AST (SGOT)
INTEG: Alopecia

Contraindications: Hypersensitivity to paclitaxel or other drugs with polyoxyethylated castor oil, neutropenia of <1500/mm^3, pregnancy (D)

Precautions: Children, lactation; hepatic, cardiovascular disease; CNS disorder

Pharmacokinetics: 89%-98% of drug is serum protein bound, metabolized in liver, excreted in bile and urine; terminal half-life 5.3-17.4 hr

Interactions:
• Increased myelosuppression: cisplatin
• Decreased metabolism of paclitaxel: ketoconazole, verapamil, diazepam, cyclosporine, teniposide, etoposide, quinidine, dexamethasone, vincristine, testosterone
• Increased doxorubicin levels: doxorubicin

NURSING CONSIDERATIONS
Assess:
• CBC, differential, platelet count qwk; withhold drug if WBC is <4000

◆ = Nursing alert   🖋 = Herb-drug interaction   🚫 = Do not crush

or platelet count is 100,000, neutrophil is <1500/mm³; notify prescriber

• Monitor temp q4h (may indicate beginning infection)

• Liver function tests before, during therapy (bilirubin, AST [SGOT], alk phosphatase) prn or qmo

• VS during 1st hr of infusion, check IV site for signs of infiltration

• Hypersensitive reactions including hypotension, dyspnea, angioedema, generalized urticaria; discontinue infusion immediately

• Bleeding: hematuria, guaiac, bruising or petechiae, mucosa or orifices q8h; obtain prescription for viscous lidocaine (Xylocaine)

• Food preferences; list likes, dislikes

• Effects of alopecia on body image; discuss feelings about body changes

Administer:

• Antiemetic 30-60 min before giving drug and prn

• Antibiotics for prophylaxis of infection

IV

• After diluting in 0.9% NaCl, D₅, D₅ and 0.9% NaCl, D₅LR to a concentration of 0.3-1.2 mg/ml

• Using an in-line filter <0.22 μm

• After premedicating with dexamethasone 20 mg PO 12 hr and 6 hr before paclitaxel, diphenhydramine 50 mg IV ½-1 hr before paclitaxel and cimetidine 300 mg or ranitidine 50 mg IV ½-1 hr before paclitaxel

• Using only glass bottles, polypropylene, polyolefin bags and administration sets; do not use PVC infusion bags or sets

• Using gloves and cytotoxic handling precautions

Y-site compatibilities: Acyclovir, amikacin, aminophylline, ampicillin/sulbactam, bleomycin, butorphanol, calcium chloride, carboplatin, cefepime, cefotetan, ceftazidime, ceftriaxone, cimetidine, cisplatin, cladribine, cyclophosphamide, cytarabine, dacarbazine, dexamethasone, diphenhydramine, doxorubicin, droperidol, etoposide, famotidine, floxuridine, fluconazole, fluorouracil, furosemide, ganciclovir, gentamicin, granisetron, haloperidol, heparin, hydrocortisone, hydromorphone, ifosfamide, lorazepam, magnesium sulfate, mannitol, meperidine, mesna, methotrexate, metoclopramide, morphine, nalbuphine, ondansetron, pentostatin, potassium chloride, prochlorperazine, propofol, ranitidine, sodium bicarbonate, thiotepa, vancomycin, vinblastine, vincristine, zidovudine

Perform/provide:

• Confirmation that dexamethasone was given 12 hr and 6 hr before infusion begins

• Storage of prepared sol up to 27 hr in refrigeration

Evaluate:

• Therapeutic response: decreased tumor size, spread of malignancy

Teach patient/family:

• To report signs of infection: fever, sore throat, flu symptoms

• To report signs of anemia: fatigue, headache, faintness, shortness of breath, irritability

• To report bleeding; avoid use of razors, commercial mouthwash

• To avoid use of aspirin, ibuprofen

• To report any complaints or side effects to nurse or prescriber

• That hair may be lost during treatment; a wig or hairpiece may make patient feel better; new hair may be different in color, texture

• About side effects and what to do about them

• That pain in muscles and joints 2-5 days after infusion is common

pamidronate (R)

(pam-i-drone'ate)
Aredia
Func. class.: Bone-resorption inhibitor
Chem. class.: Bisphosphonate

Action: Absorbs calcium phosphate crystals in bone and may directly block dissolution of hydroxyappetite crystals of bone; inhibits bone resorption, apparently without inhibiting bone formation and mineralization

Uses: Moderate to severe hypercalcemia associated with malignancy with or without bone metastases, osteolytic lesions in breast cancer patients

Dosage and routes:
• *Adult:* **IV INF** 60-90 mg in moderate hypercalcemia, 90 mg in severe hypercalcemia over 24 hr
Available forms: Inj 30, 60, 90 mg

Side effects/adverse reactions:
INTEG: Redness, swelling, induration, pain on palpation at site of catheter insertion
META: Anemia, hypokalemia, hypomagnesemia, hypophosphatemia
GI: Abdominal pain, anorexia, constipation, nausea, vomiting
MS: Bone pain
CV: Hypertension
GU: UTI, fluid overload

Contraindications: Hypersensitivity to bisphosphonates
Precautions: Children, nursing mothers, pregnancy (C), renal dysfunction
Pharmacokinetics: Rapidly cleared from circulation and taken up mainly by bones, eliminated primarily by kidneys
Interactions:
• Do not mix with Ca-containing infusion sol such as Ringer's sol

NURSING CONSIDERATIONS
Assess:
• Renal studies and Ca, P, Mg, K
• For hypercalcemia: paresthesia, twitching, laryngospasm, Chvostek's, Trousseau's signs
Administer:
• After reconstituting by adding 10 ml of sterile water for inj to each vial, then adding to 1000 ml of sterile 0.45%, 0.9% NaCl, D_5W, run over 24 hr
Perform/provide:
• Storage of infusion sol up to 24 hr at room temp
• Reconstituted sol with sterile water may be stored under refrigeration for up to 24 hr
Evaluate:
• Therapeutic response: decreased Ca levels

pancreatin (R)

(pan'kree-a-tin)
Elzyme 303 Enseals
Func. class.: Digestant
Chem. class.: Pancreatic enzyme concentrate—bovine\porcine

Action: Pancreatic enzyme needed for breakdown of substances released from the pancreas
Uses: Exocrine pancreatic secretion insufficiency, cystic fibrosis (digestive aid)
Dosage and routes:
• *Adult:* **PO** 8000-24,000 USP U with meals
Available forms: Tabs 650, 2000, 12,000 U
Side effects/adverse reactions:
GI: Anorexia, nausea, vomiting, diarrhea, glossitis, anal soreness
GU: Hyperuricuria, hyperuricemia
INTEG: Rash, hypersensitivity
EENT: Buccal soreness

 = Nursing alert   = Herb-drug interaction   = Do not crush

Contraindications: Hypersensitivity to pork, chronic pancreatic disease

Precautions: Pregnancy (C), lactation

Interactions:

• Decreased absorption: cimetidine, antacids, oral iron

NURSING CONSIDERATIONS
Assess:

• I&O ratio; watch for increasing urinary output

• Fecal fat, nitrogen, pro-time, Ca during treatment

• For polyuria, polydipsia, polyphagia (may indicate diabetes mellitus)

• For allergy to pork

Administer:

PO

• After antacid or H₂-blockers; decreased pH inactivates drug

🚫 Whole; do not break, crush, or chew (enteric coated)

• Low-fat diet for GI symptoms

Perform/provide:

• Storage in tight container at room temp

Evaluate:

• Therapeutic response: relief of GI symptoms

---

pancrelipase (℞)

(pan-kre-li′pase)

Cotazym, Cotazym Capsules, Cotazym-S Capsules, Creon Capsules, Festal II Tablets, Ilozyme, Ku-Zyme HP Capsules, Pancrease Capsules, Pancrease MT 4, Pancrease MT 10, Pancrease MT 16, Ultrase MT 12, Ultrase MT 20, Ultrase MT 24, Viokase Powder, Viokase Tablets, Zymase

Func. class.: Digestant

Chem. class.: Pancreatic enzyme—bovine/porcine

Action: Pancreatic enzyme needed for breakdown of substances released from the pancreas

Uses: Exocrine pancreatic secretion insufficiency, cystic fibrosis (digestive aid), steatorrhea, pancreatic enzyme deficiency

Dosage and routes:

• *Adult and child:* **PO** 1-3 caps/tabs ac or with meals, or 1 cap/tab with snack or 1-2 powder pkt ac

Available forms: Tabs 8000, 11,000, 30,000 U; caps 8000, 30,000 U; enteric coated caps 4000, 5000, 20,000, 25,000 U; powder 16,800 U

Side effects/adverse reactions:

GI: Anorexia, nausea, vomiting, diarrhea

GU: Hyperuricuria, hyperuricemia

Contraindications: Allergy to pork, chronic pancreatic disease

Precautions: Pregnancy (C)

Interactions:

• Decreased absorption: cimetidine, antacids, oral iron

NURSING CONSIDERATIONS
Assess:

• For appropriate height, weight development; may be delayed

• I&O ratio; watch for increasing urinary output

P

• Fecal fat, nitrogen, pro-time during treatment
• For polyuria, polydipsia, polyphagia (may indicate diabetes mellitus)

Administer:
• After antacid or cimetidine; decreased pH inactivates drug
• Powder mixed in prepared fruit juice for infants, children
 Whole; do not break, crush, or chew (enteric coated)
• Low-fat diet for GI symptoms
• Powder mixed with pureed fruit; take tabs with or before food

Perform/provide:
• Storage in tight container at room temp

Evaluate:
• Therapeutic response: improved digestion of carbohydrates, protein, fat; absence of steatorrhea

Teach patient/family:
• Not to inhale powder; may be very irritating to mucous membranes; some powder may irritate skin
• To take with 8 oz water or more, not to allow to sit in mouth, have patient sit up during administration
• To notify prescriber of allergic reactions, abdominal pain, cramping, or blood in the urine

---

pancuronium (℞)
(pan-kyoo-roe′nee-um)
pancuronium Bromide, Pavulon
Func. class.: Neuromuscular blocker (nondepolarizing)
Chem. class.: Synthetic curariform

Action: Inhibits transmission of nerve impulses by binding with cholinergic receptor sites, antagonizing action of acetylcholine
Uses: Facilitation of endotracheal intubation, skeletal muscle relaxation during mechanical ventilation, surgery, or general anesthesia

Dosage and routes:
• *Adult:* IV 0.04-0.1 mg/kg, then 0.01 mg/kg q½-1h
• *Child >10 yr:* IV 0.04-0.1 mg/kg, then ⅕ initial dose q½-1h
Available forms: Inj 1, 2 mg/ml

Side effects/adverse reactions:
CV: Bradycardia; tachycardia; increased, decreased B/P; ventricular extrasystoles
RESP: ***Prolonged apnea, bronchospasm, cyanosis, respiratory depression***
EENT: Increased secretions
MS: Weakness to prolonged skeletal muscle relaxation
INTEG: Rash, flushing, pruritus, urticaria, sweating, salivation

Contraindications: Hypersensitivity to bromide ion
Precautions: Pregnancy (C), renal disease, cardiac disease, lactation, children <2 yr, electrolyte imbalances, dehydration, neuromuscular disease, respiratory disease

Pharmacokinetics:
IV: Onset 30-45 sec, peak 3-5 min; metabolized (small amounts), excreted in urine (unchanged), crosses placenta

Interactions:
• Increased neuromuscular blockade: aminoglycosides, clindamycin, lincomycin, quinidine, local anesthetics, polymyxin antibiotics, lithium, narcotic analgesics, thiazides, enflurane, isoflurane
• Dysrhythmias: theophylline

Lab test interferences:
Decrease: Cholinesterase

NURSING CONSIDERATIONS
Assess:
• For electrolyte imbalances (K, Mg); may lead to increased action of this drug

---

 ⬥ = Nursing alert   🦠 = Herb-drug interaction   🚫 = Do not crush

• Vital signs (B/P, pulse, respirations, airway) until fully recovered; rate, depth, pattern of respirations, strength of hand grip
• I&O ratio; check for urinary retention, frequency, hesitancy
• Recovery: decreased paralysis of face, diaphragm, leg, arm, rest of body; allow to recover fully before neuro assessment
• Allergic reactions: rash, fever, respiratory distress, pruritus, drug should be discontinued

Administer:
IV, direct
• With diazepam or morphine when used for therapeutic paralysis; this drug provides no sedation
• Using nerve stimulator by anesthesiologist to determine neuromuscular blockade
• Atropine to counteract muscarinic effects
• After succinylcholine effects subside
• Anticholinesterase to reverse neuromuscular blockade
• IV undiluted, give over 1-2 min (only by qualified persons)

Additive compatibilities: Verapamil
Syringe compatibilities: Heparin
Y-site compatibilities: Aminophylline, cefazolin, cefuroxime, cimetidine, dobutamine, dopamine, epinephrine, esmolol, fentanyl, fluconazole, gentamicin, heparin, hydrocortisone, isoproterenol, lorazepam, midazolam, morphine, nitroglycerin, nitroprusside, ranitidine, sulfamethoxazole/trimethoprim, vancomycin

Perform/provide:
• Storage in refrigerator; do not store in plastic; use only fresh sol
• Reassurance if communication is difficult during recovery from neuromuscular blockade

• Frequent (q2h) instillation of artificial tears and covering eyes to prevent drying of cornea
Evaluate:
• Therapeutic response: paralysis of jaw, eyelid, head, neck, rest of body
Treatment of overdose: Edrophonium or neostigmine, atropine, monitor VS; may require mechanical ventilation

---

paroxetine (℞)

(par-ox'e-teen)
Paxil
Func. class.: Antidepressant, serotonin reuptake inhibitor
Chem. class.: Phenylpiperidine derivative

Action: Inhibits CNS neuron uptake of serotonin but not of norepinephrine or dopamine
Uses: Major depressive disorder, obsessive-compulsive disorder, panic disorder
Investigational uses: Diabetic neuropathy, headaches, premature ejaculation

Dosage and routes:
• *Geriatric:* **PO** 10 mg qd, increase by 10 mg to desired dose, max 40 mg/day
• *Adult:* **PO** 20 mg qd in AM; after 4 wk if no clinical improvement is noted, dose may be increased by 10 mg/day qwk to desired response, not to exceed 50 mg/day
Obsessive-compulsive disorder
• *Adult:* **PO** 40 mg/day in AM, start with 20 mg/day, increase 10 mg/day increments, max 60 mg/day
Panic disorder
• *Adult:* **PO** 40 mg/day, start with 10 mg/day and increase in 10 mg/day increments, max 60 mg/day
Available forms: Tabs 10, 20, 30, 40 mg

P

Side effects/adverse reactions:

CNS: Headache, nervousness, insomnia, drowsiness, anxiety, tremor, dizziness, fatigue, sedation, abnormal dreams, agitation, apathy, euphoria, hallucinations, delusions, psychosis

GI: Nausea, diarrhea, dry mouth, anorexia, dyspepsia, constipation, cramps, vomiting, taste changes, flatulence, decreased appetite

INTEG: Sweating, rash

RESP: Infection, pharyngitis, nasal congestion, sinus headache, sinusitis, cough, dyspnea

CV: Vasodilation, postural hypotension, palpitations

MS: Pain, arthritis, myalgia, myopathy, myosthenia

GU: Dysmenorrhea, decreased libido, urinary frequency, UTI, amenorrhea, cystitis, impotence, abnormal ejaculation

EENT: Visual changes

SYST: Asthenia, fever

Contraindications: Hypersensitivity, patients taking MAOIs

Precautions: Pregnancy (B), lactation, children, elderly, seizure history, patients with history of mania, renal and hepatic disease

Pharmacokinetics:

PO: Peak 5.2 hr; metabolized in liver, unchanged drugs and metabolites excreted in feces and urine; half-life 21 hr; protein binding 95%

Interactions:

• Increased bleeding: warfarin
• Do not use with MAOIs
• Cimetidine increases paroxetine plasma levels
• Increased agitation: L-tryptophan
• Phenobarbital and phenytoin decrease paroxetine levels
• Increased side effects: highly protein-bound drugs
• Paroxetine may decrease digoxin levels
• Increased theophylline levels: theophylline

Lab test interferences:

Increase: Serum bilirubin, blood glucose, alk phosphatase

Decrease: VMA, 5-HIAA

False increase: Urinary catecholamines

NURSING CONSIDERATIONS

Assess:

• Mental status: mood, sensorium, affect, suicidal tendencies, increase in psychiatric symptoms, depression, panic
• B/P (lying/standing), pulse q4h; if systolic B/P drops 20 mm Hg, hold drug, notify prescriber; take vital signs q4h in patients with cardiovascular disease
• Blood studies: CBC, leukocytes, differential, cardiac enzymes if patient is receiving long-term therapy
• Hepatic studies: AST (SGOT), ALT (SGPT), bilirubin, creatinine
• Weight qwk; appetite may decrease with drug
• ECG for flattening of T wave, bundle branch, AV block, dysrhythmias in cardiac patients
• EPS primarily in elderly: rigidity, dystonia, akathisia
• Urinary retention, constipation
• Withdrawal symptoms: headache, nausea, vomiting, muscle pain, weakness; not usual unless drug discontinued abruptly
• Alcohol intake; if alcohol is consumed, hold dose until morning

Administer:

• Increased fluids, bulk in diet for constipation, urinary retention
• With food, milk for GI symptoms
• Crushed if patient is unable to swallow medication whole
• Dosage hs for oversedation during day; may take entire dose hs; elderly may not tolerate once/day dosing

---

◆ = Nursing alert   ∥ = Herb-drug interaction   ⊗ = Do not crush

• Gum, hard candy, frequent sips of water for dry mouth

Perform/provide:

• Storage at room temp; do not freeze

• Assistance with ambulation during therapy, since drowsiness, dizziness occur

• Safety measures including side rails, primarily in elderly

• Checking to see if PO medication swallowed

Evaluate:

• Therapeutic response: decreased depression

Teach patient/family:

• That therapeutic effect may take 1-4 wk

• To use caution in driving, other activities requiring alertness because of drowsiness, dizziness, blurred vision

• Not to discontinue medication quickly after long-term use; may cause nausea, headache, malaise

• To avoid alcohol ingestion, other CNS depressants

Treatment of overdose: Airway, for seizures give diazepam, symptomatic treatment

---

pegaspargase (R)

(peg-as'per-gase)

Elspar, Oncaspar

Func. class.: Antineoplastic

Chem. class.: E. coli enzyme

Action: Indirectly inhibits protein synthesis in tumor cells; without amino acid, DNA, RNA synthesis is halted; asparagine, protein synthesis is halted; G$_1$ phase; cell-cycle specific; a nonvesicant; a modified version of L-asparginase

Uses: Acute lymphocytic leukemia in combination with other antineoplastics

Dosage and routes:

In combination

• *Adult and child with BSA ≥0.6 m^2:*
IV/IM 2500 IU/m^2 q14 days, run **IV** over 2 hr in 100 ml of NaCl or D$_5$ through a running **IV**; **IM** should be no more than 2 ml in one inj site

• *Child with BSA <0.6 m^2:* **IV/IM** 82.5 IU/kg q14 days

Sole induction

• *Adult·* **IV** 2500 IU/m^2 q14 days

Available forms: Inj 750 IU/ml in a phosphate buffered saline sol

Side effects/adverse reactions:

SYST: **Anaphylaxis, hypersensitivity**

HEMA: **Thrombocytopenia, leukopenia, myelosuppression, anemia, decreased clotting factors, pancytopenia**

GI: Nausea, vomiting, anorexia, cramps, stomatitis, **hepatotoxicity, pancreatitis,** *diarrhea*

GU: Urinary retention, **renal failure,** glycosuria, polyuria, azotemia, uric acid neuropathy

INTEG: Rash, urticaria, chills, fever

ENDO: Hyperglycemia

RESP: **Fibrosis, pulmonary infiltrate, severe bronchospasm**

CV: Chest pain, **hypertension**

CNS: Neuritis, dizziness, headache, **coma,** depression, fatigue, confusion, hallucinations, seizures

Contraindications: Hypersensitivity, infant, pregnancy (D), lactation, pancreatitis

Precautions: Renal disease, hepatic disease, pregnancy (C), CNS disease

Pharmacokinetics: Unknown

Interactions:

• Decreased action of methotrexate

• Do not use with radiation

• Coagulation factor imbalances: heparin, warfarin, aspirin, NSAIDs

• Considered incompatible with other drugs in syringe or sol

NURSING CONSIDERATIONS
Assess:
◆ For signs and symptoms of pancreatitis (nausea, vomiting, severe abdominal pain), anaphylaxis (bronchospasm, dyspnea), cyanosis

• CBC, differential, platelet count qwk; withhold drug if WBC count is <4000 or platelet count is <75,000; notify prescriber of results

• Pulmonary function tests, chest x-ray studies before and during therapy; chest x-ray film should be obtained q2wk during treatment, watch for severe bronchospasm, fibrosis, pulmonary infiltrate

• Renal function studies: BUN, serum uric acid, ammonia, urine CrCl, electrolytes before and during therapy

• I&O ratio; report fall in urine output of 30 ml/hr, may indicate renal failure

• Temp q4h (may indicate beginning infection)

• Liver function tests before and during therapy (bilirubin, AST [SGOT], ALT [SGPT], LDH) as needed or monthly, hepatotoxicity can occur

• RBC, Hct, Hgb; may be decreased

• Serum, urine glucose levels, glycosuria can occur

• Bleeding: hematuria, stool guaiac, bruising or petechiae, mucosa or orifices q8h

• Dyspnea, rales, nonproductive cough, chest pain, tachypnea, fatigue, increased pulse, pallor, lethargy, swelling around eyes or lips; anaphylaxis may occur

• B/P, since hypertension can occur

• Food preferences; list likes, dislikes

• Yellow skin, sclera; dark urine, clay-colored stools, itchy skin, abdominal pain, fever, diarrhea

• Local irritation, pain, burning, discoloration at injection site

• Symptoms of severe allergic reaction: rash, pruritus, urticaria, purpuric skin lesions, itching, flushing, dyspnea

• Frequency of stools, characteristics; cramping, acidosis; signs of dehydration: rapid respirations, poor skin turgor, decreased urine output, dry skin, restlessness, weakness

Administer:
• Transfusion for severe anemia

• Antispasmodic if GI symptoms occur

• Allopurinol or sodium bicarbonate to reduce uric acid levels, alkalinization of urine

IV infusion
• Using 21, 23, 25G needle; administer by slow IV infusion via Y-tube or 3-way stopcock of flowing D_5W or NS infusion over 2 hr after diluting

Perform/provide:
• Deep-breathing exercises with patient tid-qid; place in semi-Fowler's position

• Increase fluid intake to 2-3 L/day to prevent urate deposits, calculi formation

• Diet low in purines: no organ meats (kidney, liver), dried beans, peas to maintain alkaline urine

• Rinsing of mouth tid-qid with water, club soda

• Brushing of teeth bid-tid with soft brush or cotton-tipped applicator for stomatitis; use unwaxed dental floss

• Warm compresses at injection site for inflammation

• Nutritious diet with iron, vitamin supplements

• HOB raised to facilitate breathing

Evaluate:
• Therapeutic response: decreased exacerbations in acute lymphocytic leukemia

◆ = Nursing alert   🖋 = Herb-drug interaction   🚫 = Do not crush

Teach patient/family:
• To report any complaints or side effects to nurse or prescriber
• To report any changes in breathing or coughing
Treatment of anaphylaxis: Administer epinephrine, diphenhydramine, IV corticosteroids

---

pemoline (℞)

(pem'oh-leen)

Cylert, Cylert Chewable

Func. class.: Cerebral stimulant

Chem. class.: Oxazolidinone derivative

Controlled Substance Schedule IV

Action: Exact mechanism unknown; may act through dopaminergic mechanisms; produces CNS stimulation and a paradoxic effect in ADHD

Uses: Attention deficit hyperactivity disorder

Investigational uses: Schizophrenia, fatigue, depression

Dosage and routes:
• *Child >6 yr:* **PO** 37.5 mg in AM, increasing by 18.75 mg/wk, not to exceed 112.5 mg/day
Available forms: Tabs 18.75, 37.5, 75 mg; chewable tabs 37.5 mg

Side effects/adverse reactions:

MISC: Rashes, growth suppression in children

CNS: Hyperactivity, insomnia, restlessness, dizziness, depression, headache, stimulation, irritability, aggressiveness, hallucinations, *seizures, Gilles de la Tourette's syndrome,* drowsiness, dyskinetic movements

GI: Nausea, anorexia, diarrhea, abdominal pain, increased liver enzymes, *hepatitis,* jaundice, weight loss

CV: Tachycardia

Contraindications: Hypersensitivity, hepatic insufficiency

Precautions: Renal disease, pregnancy (B), lactation, drug abuse, child <6 yr, psychosis, tics, seizure disorder

Pharmacokinetics:

PO: Peak 2-4 hr, duration 8 hr, metabolized (50%) by liver, excreted (40%) by kidneys, half-life 10-30 hr

NURSING CONSIDERATIONS

Assess:
• Hepatic function studies: ALT (SGPT), AST (SGOT), bilirubin; renal, creatinine
• Child for growth retardation
• Mental status: mood, sensorium, affect, stimulation, insomnia, aggressiveness

Administer:

PO
• At least 6 hr before hs

Evaluate:
• Therapeutic response: decreased hyperactivity

Teach patient/family:
• To decrease caffeine consumption (coffee, tea, cola, chocolate); may increase irritability, stimulation
• To avoid OTC preparations unless approved by prescriber
• To withdraw over several wk
• To avoid alcohol ingestion
• To avoid hazardous activities until patient is stabilized
• That therapeutic effect may take 2-4 wk

P

PENICILLINS

penicillin G benzathine (℞)

(pen-i-sill'in)

Bicillin C-R, Bicillin C-R 900/300, Bicillin L-A, Megacillin*, Permapen

penicillin G potassium (℞)

Acrocillin, Burcillin-G, Deltapen, Megacillin*, Novopen G*, Pentids, Pfizerpen

penicillin G procaine (℞)

Crysticillin A.S., Duracillin A.S., Pfizerpen-AS, Wycillin

penicillin G sodium (℞)

Crystapen*, Pfizerpen*

penicillin V potassium (℞)

Apo-Pen-VK*, Betapen-VK, Deltapen-VK, Ledercillin-VK, Novopen-VK*, Penapar-VK, Pen-Vee K*, PVFK*, Robicillin-VK, Uticillin-VK, V-Cillin K, Veetids

Func. class.: Broad-spectrum antiinfective

Chem. class.: Natural penicillin

Action: Interferes with cell wall replication of susceptible organisms; osmotically unstable cell wall swells, bursts from osmotic pressure, results in cell death

Uses: Respiratory infections, scarlet fever, erysipelas, otitis media, pneumonia, skin and soft tissue infections, gonorrhea; effective for gram-positive cocci (*Staphylococcus, S. pyogenes, S. viridans, S. faecalis, S. bovis, S. pneumoniae*), gram-negative cocci (*N. gonorrhoeae*), gram-positive bacilli (*Actinomyces, B. anthracis, C. perfringens, C. tetani, Corynebacterium diphtheriae, L. monocytogenes*), gram-negative bacilli (*E. coli, P. mirabilis, Salmonella, Shigella, Enterobacter, S. moniliformis*), spirochetes (*T. pallidum*)

Dosage and routes:

Penicillin G benzathine

Early syphilis

• *Adult:* **IM** 2.4 million U in single dose

Congenital syphilis

• *Child <2 yr:* **IM** 50,000 U/kg in single dose

Prophylaxis of rheumatic fever, glomerulonephritis

• *Adult and child >60 lb:* **IM** 1.2 million U in single dose qmo or 600,000 U q2wk

• *Child <60 lb:* **IM** 600,000 U in single dose

Upper respiratory infections (group A streptococcal)

• *Adult:* **IM** 1.2 million U in single dose

• *Child >27 kg:* **IM** 900,000 U in single dose

• *Child <27 kg:* **IM** 300,000-600,000 g in single dose

Available forms: Inj 300,000, 600,000 U/ml; tabs 200,000 U

Penicillin G potassium

• Dosage reduction indicated in renal impairment (CrCl <50 ml/min)

Pneumococcal/streptococcal infections (mild to moderate)

• *Adult:* **IM/IV** 2-24 million U in divided doses q4h

• *Child <12 yr:* **IV** 100,000-400,000 U/kg/day in 4-6 divided doses

Available forms: Inj 1, 2, 3 million U/50 ml

Penicillin G procaine

Renal dose

• CrCl 10-30 ml/min give q8-12h; CrCl <10 ml/min give q12-18h

Moderate to severe infections

• *Adult and child:* **IM** 600,000-1.2

million U in 1 or 2 doses/day for 10 days to 2 wk
• *Newborn:* 50,000 U/kg **IM** once daily
Gonorrhea
• *Adult and child >12 yr:* **IM** 4.8 million U in two injections given 30 min after probenecid 1 g
Available forms: Inj 300,000, 500,000, 600,000 U/ml; 600,000 U/1.2 ml, 1,200,000 U/dose; 2,400,000 U/dose
Penicillin G sodium
• Dosage reduction indicated in renal impairment (CrCl <50 ml/min)
Moderate to severe infections
• *Adult:* **IM/IV** 2 million-24 million U/day in divided doses q4h
• *Child:* **IM/IV** 50,000-400,000 U/kg/day in divided doses q4-12h
Dental surgery prophylaxis for endocarditis
• *Adult:* **IM/IV** 2 million U ½-1 hr before procedure, then 1 million U 6 hr after procedure
Available forms: Inj 1 million, 5 million, 20 million U
Penicillin V potassium
• Dosage reduction indicated in renal impairment (CrCl <50 ml/min)
Pneumococcal/staphylococcal infections
• *Adult:* **PO** 250-500 mg q6h
• *Child <12 yr:* **PO** 25-50 mg/kg/day in divided doses q6-8h
Streptococcal infections
• *Adult:* **PO** 125-250 mg q6-8h × 10 days
Prevention of recurrence of rheumatic fever/chorea
• *Adult:* **PO** 125-250 mg bid continuously
• *Child <5 yr:* **PO** 125 mg bid
• *Child >5 yr:* **PO** 250 mg bid
Vincent's gingivitis/pharyngitis
• *Adult:* **PO** 500 mg q6h
Available forms: Tabs 125, 250, 500 mg; film-coated tabs 250, 500

mg; powder for oral susp 125, 250 mg/5 ml
Side effects/adverse reactions:
HEMA: Anemia; increased bleeding time; **bone marrow depression, granulocytopenia**
GI: Nausea, vomiting, diarrhea, increased AST (SGOT), ALT (SGPT), abdominal pain, glossitis, colitis
GU: Oliguria, proteinuria, hematuria, vaginitis, moniliasis, glomerulonephritis
CNS: Lethargy, hallucinations, anxiety, depression, twitching, *coma, convulsions*
META: Hyperkalemia, hypokalemia, alkalosis, hypernatremia
MISC: Local pain, tenderness and fever with IM injection
Contraindications: Hypersensitivity to penicillins; neonates
Precautions: Hypersensitivity to cephalosporins, pregnancy (B), lactation, severe renal disease
Pharmacokinetics:
Penicillin G benzathine
IM: Very slow absorption, duration 21-28 days, half-life 30-60 min; excreted in urine, feces, breast milk; crosses placenta
Penicillin G potassium
IV: Peak immediate
IM: Peak ¼-½ hr
PO: Peak 1 hr, duration 6 hr
Excreted in urine unchanged, excreted in breast milk, crosses placenta, half-life 30-60 min
Penicillin G procaine
IM: Peak 1-4 hr, duration 15 hr, excreted in urine
Penicillin G sodium
IM: Peak 1-3 hr, duration 6 hr; excreted in urine
Penicillin V potassium
PO: Peak 30-60 min, duration 6-8 hr, half-life 30 min, excreted in urine, breast milk

Interactions:
- Decreased antimicrobial effect of penicillin: tetracyclines
- Increased penicillin concentrations: aspirin, probenecid
- Decreased effect of oral contraceptives
- Increased effect of heparin

Lab test interferences:

False positive: Urine glucose, urine protein

NURSING CONSIDERATIONS
Assess:
- I&O ratio; report hematuria, oliguria, since penicillin in high doses is nephrotoxic
- ⬥ Any patient with compromised renal system, since drug is excreted slowly in poor renal system function; toxicity may occur rapidly
- Liver studies: AST (SGOT), ALT (SGPT)
- Blood studies: WBC, RBC, H&H, bleeding time
- Renal studies: urinalysis, protein, blood
- C&S before therapy; drug may be given as soon as culture is taken
- Bowel pattern before and during treatment
- Skin eruptions after administration of penicillin to 1 wk after discontinuing drug
- Respiratory status: rate, character, wheezing, tightness in chest
- Allergies before initiation of treatment, reaction of each medication; highlight allergies on chart; because of prolonged action, allergic reaction may be prolonged and severe

Administer:
Penicillin G benzathine
- Drug after C&S completed
- After shaking well, deep IM inj in large muscle mass; avoid intravascular inj, aspirate

Penicillin G potassium
- Drug after C&S

Additive compatibilities: Ascorbic acid, calcium chloride, calcium gluconate, cephapirin, chloramphenicol, cimetidine, clindamycin, colistimethate, corticotropin, dimenhydrinate, diphenhydramine, ephedrine, erythromycin, furosemide, hydrocortisone, kanamycin, lidocaine, magnesium sulfate, methicillin, methylprednisolone, metronidazole, polymyxin B, prednisolone, potassium chloride, procaine, prochlorperazine, ranitidine, verapamil

Syringe compatibilities: Heparin

Y-site compatibilities: Acyclovir, amiodarone, cyclophosphamide, diltiazem, enalaprilat, esmolol, fluconazole, foscarnet, heparin, hydromorphone, labetalol, magnesium sulfate, meperidine, morphine, perphenazine, potassium chloride, tacrolimus, theophylline, verapamil, vit B/C

Penicillin G procaine
- Drug after C&S
- Deep IM inj avoid intravascular inj, aspirate

Penicillin G sodium
- IV after diluting with sterile H_2O; shake; follow manufacturer's instructions for dilution; may be added to 0.9% NaCl; give by continuous inf, usually over 12 hr
- Drug after C&S

Additive compatibilities: Calcium chloride, calcium gluconate, chloramphenicol, clindamycin, colistimethate, diphenhydramine, erythromycin, furosemide, gentamicin, hydrocortisone, kanamycin, methicillin, polymyxin B, prednisolone, procaine, ranitidine, verapamil, vit B/C

Syringe compatibilities: Aminoglycosides, chloramphenicol, cimetidine, colistimethate, gentamicin, heparin, kanamycin, lincomycin, polymyxin B, streptomycin

Penicillin V potassium
- Orally on empty stomach for best absorption
- Drug after C&S

Perform/provide:
- Adrenaline, suction, tracheostomy set, endotracheal intubation equipment
- Adequate fluid intake (2L) during diarrhea episodes
- Scratch test to assess allergy after securing order from prescriber; usually done when penicillin is only drug of choice
- Storage in dry, tight container; oral susp refrigerated 2 wk, 1 wk at room temp

Evaluate:
- Therapeutic response: absence of fever, draining wounds
- Allergies before initiation of treatment, reaction of each medication; highlight allergies on chart; hypersensitivity reaction may be delayed

Teach patient/family:
- To report sore throat, fever, fatigue; may indicate superinfection
- To wear or carry Medic Alert ID if allergic to penicillins
- To report diarrhea, prevent dehydration
- To shake susp well before each dose; store in refrigerator for up to 2 wk

Treatment of anaphylaxis: Withdraw drug; maintain airway; administer epinephrine, aminophylline, O_2, IV corticosteroids

---

pentamidine (℞)

(pen-tam′i-deen)
Nebupent, Pentam 300, Pentacarinat*, Pneumopent
Func. class.: Antiprotozoal
Chem. class.: Aromatic diamide derivative

Action: Interferes with DNA/RNA synthesis in protozoa

Uses: Treatment/prevention of *P. carinii* infections

Dosage and routes:
- *Adult and child:* **IV/IM** 4 mg/kg/day × 2 wk; **NEB** 600 mg/6ml **NS** via specific nebulizer given q4wk for prevention

Available forms: Inj, aerosol 300 mg/vial

Side effects/adverse reactions:
CV: Hypotension, ventricular tachycardia, ECG abnormalities
HEMA: Anemia, *leukopenia, thrombocytopenia*
INTEG: Sterile abscess, pain at injection site, pruritus, urticaria, *rash*
GU: Acute renal failure, increased serum creatinine, renal toxicity
GI: Nausea, vomiting, anorexia; increased AST (SGOT), ALT (SGPT); *acute pancreatitis,* metallic taste
CNS: Disorientation, hallucinations, *dizziness,* confusion
RESP: Cough, shortness of breath, *bronchospasm* (with aerosol)
MISC: Fatigue, chills, night sweats
META: Hyperkalemia, hypocalcemia, hypoglycemia

Precautions: Blood dyscrasias, hepatic disease, renal disease, diabetes mellitus, cardiac disease, hypocalcemia, pregnancy (C), hypertension, hypotension, lactation, children

Pharmacokinetics: Excreted unchanged in urine (66%)

Interactions:
- Nephrotoxicity: aminoglycosides,

P

amphotericin B, colistin, cisplatin, methoxyflurane, polymyxin B, vancomycin

NURSING CONSIDERATIONS

Assess:
- Blood studies, blood glucose, CBC, platelets
- I&O ratio; report hematuria, oliguria
- ECG for cardiac dysrhythmias
- Patient should be lying down when receiving drug; severe hypotension may develop; monitor B/P during administration and until B/P stable

◆ Any patient with compromised renal system; drug is excreted slowly in poor renal system function; toxicity may occur rapidly

- Liver studies: AST (SGOT), ALT (SGPT)
- Renal studies: urinalysis, BUN, creatinine; nephrotoxicity may occur
- Signs of infection, anemia
- Bowel pattern before, during treatment
- Sterile abscess, pain at injection site
- Respiratory status: rate, character, wheezing, dyspnea
- Dizziness, confusion, hallucination
- Allergies before treatment, reaction of each medication; place allergies on chart in bright red letters; notify all people giving drugs

Administer:
- Inhalation through nebulizer; mix contents in 6 ml of sterile H_2O; do not use low pressure (<20 psi); flow rate should be 5-7 L/min (40-50 psi) air or O_2 source over 30-45 min until chamber is empty
- IM diluted in 3 ml sterile H_2O; give deep IM; painful by this route

IV
- By intermittent inf over 60 min
- Do not mix with NS

Y-site compatibilities: Diltiazem, zidovudine

Perform/provide:
- Storage in refrigerator protected from light

Evaluate:
- Therapeutic response: decreased temp, ability to breathe

Teach patient/family:
- To report sore throat, fever, fatigue; may indicate superinfection
- To maintain adequate fluid intake

pentazocine (℞)

(pen-taz'oh-seen)
Talwin, Talwin NX

Func. class.: Narcotic analgesic, antagonist

Chem. class.: Synthetic benzomorphan

Controlled Substance Schedule IV
Action: Inhibits ascending pain pathways in CNS, increases pain threshold, alters pain perception
Uses: Moderate to severe pain
Dosage and routes:
Renal dose
- CrCl 10-50 ml/min give q24-36h; CrCl <10 ml/min give q48h
- *Adult:* **PO** 50-100 mg q3-4h prn, not to exceed 600 mg/day; **IV/IM/SC** 30 mg q3-4h prn, not to exceed 360 mg/day
Available forms: Inj 30 mg/ml; tabs 50 mg
Side effects/adverse reactions:
CNS: Drowsiness, dizziness, confusion, headache, sedation, euphoria, hallucinations, dreaming
GI: Nausea, vomiting, anorexia, constipation, *cramps*
GU: Increased urinary output, dysuria, retention
INTEG: Rash, urticaria, bruising, flushing, diaphoresis, pruritus, severe irritation at injection sites

---

◆ = Nursing alert　　🌿 = Herb-drug interaction　　🚫 = Do not crush

pentazocine 773

EENT: Tinnitus, blurred vision, miosis, diplopia
CV: Palpitations, bradycardia, change in B/P, tachycardia, increased B/P (high doses)
RESP: Respiratory depression
Contraindications: Hypersensitivity, addiction (narcotic)
Precautions: Addictive personality, pregnancy (C), lactation, increased intracranial pressure, MI (acute), severe heart disease, respiratory depression, hepatic disease, renal disease, seizure disorder, child <18 yr, head trauma
Pharmacokinetics:
SC/IM: Onset 15-30 min, peak 1-2 hr, duration 2-4 hr
IV: Onset 2-3 min, duration 4-6 hr
Metabolized by liver, excreted by kidneys, crosses placenta, half-life 2-3 hr, extensive first-pass metabolism with less than 20% entering circulation
Interactions:
• Increased effects: CNS depressants; alcohol, sedative/hypnotics, antipsychotics, skeletal muscle relaxants
• Decreased effects: narcotics
Lab test interferences:
Increase: Amylase
NURSING CONSIDERATIONS
Assess:
• I&O ratio; check for decreasing output; may indicate urinary retention
• For withdrawal symptoms in narcotic-dependent patients
• Pulmonary embolism, abscesses, ulcerations, vascular occlusion, WBC
• CNS changes: dizziness, drowsiness, hallucinations, euphoria, LOC, pupil reaction
• Allergic reactions: rash, urticaria
• Respiratory dysfunction: respiratory depression, character, rate, rhythm; notify prescriber if respirations are <10/min
• Need for pain medication, physical dependence
Administer:
• With antiemetic if nausea, vomiting occur
• When pain is beginning to return; determine dosage interval by patient response
IV
• Undiluted or diluted 5 mg/ml of sterile H_2O for inj; give 5 mg or less over 1 min
Syringe compatibilities: Atropine, benzquinamide, butorphanol, chlorpromazine, cimetidine, dimenhydrinate, diphenhydramine, droperidol, fentanyl, hydromorphone, hydroxyzine, meperidine, metoclopramide, morphine, perphenazine, prochlorperazine, promazine, promethazine, ranitidine, scopolamine
Y-site compatibilities: Heparin, hydrocortisone, potassium chloride, vit B/C
Perform/provide:
• Storage in light-resistant area at room temp
• Assistance with ambulation
• Safety measures: side rails, nightlight, call bell within easy reach
Evaluate:
• Therapeutic response: decrease in pain
Teach patient/family:
• To report any symptoms of CNS changes, allergic reactions
• That physical dependency may result from extended use
• That withdrawal symptoms may occur: nausea, vomiting, cramps, fever, faintness, anorexia
Treatment of overdose: Naloxone (Narcan) 0.2-0.8 mg IV, O_2, IV fluids, vasopressors

P

---
* = Canada only   Side effects: *italics* = common; ***bold italics*** = life-threatening

pentobarbital (℞)

(pen-toe-bar′bi-tal)
Nembutal, Nembutal Sodium, Nembutal Sodium Solution, Nova-Rectal*, pentobarbital sodium, Pentogen*

Func. class.: Sedative/hypnotic barbiturate

Chem. class.: Barbitone, short acting

Controlled Substance Schedule II (USA), Schedule G (Canada)

Action: Depresses activity in brain cells, primarily in reticular activating system in brain stem; selectively depresses neurons in posterior hypothalamus, limbic structures

Uses: Insomnia, sedation, preoperative medication, increased intracranial pressure, dental anesthetic

Dosage and routes:
• *Adult:* **PO** 100-200 mg hs; **IM** 150-200 mg hs; **IV** 100 mg initially, then up to 500 mg; **RECT** 120-200 mg hs
• *Child:* **IM** 2-6 mg, not to exceed 100 mg; **PO** 2-6 mg/kg/day in divided doses; **PO** preoperatively 2-6 mg/kg, max 100 mg/dose; **IV** 100 mg (hypnotic/anticonvulsant)
• *Child 2 mo-1 yr:* **RECT** 30 mg
• *Child 1-4 yr:* **RECT** 30-60 mg
• *Child 5-12 yr:* **RECT** 60 mg
• *Child 12-14 yr:* **RECT** 60-120 mg
Available forms: Caps 50, 100 mg; elix 18.2 mg/5 ml; powder, rect supp 30, 60, 120, 200 mg; inj 50 mg/ml

Side effects/adverse reactions:

CNS: Lethargy, drowsiness, hangover, dizziness, paradoxical stimulation in elderly and children, lightheadedness, dependence, *CNS depression,* mental depression, slurred speech
GI: Nausea, vomiting, diarrhea, constipation

INTEG: Rash, urticaria, pain, abscesses at injection site, angioedema, thrombophlebitis, *Stevens-Johnson syndrome*
CV: Hypotension, bradycardia
RESP: Respiratory depression, apnea, laryngospasm, bronchospasm
HEMA: Agranulocytosis, thrombocytopenia, megaloblastic anemia (long-term treatment)

Contraindications: Hypersensitivity to barbiturates, pregnancy (D), respiratory depression, addiction to barbiturates; severe liver, renal impairment; porphyria, uncontrolled pain

Precautions: Anemia, lactation, hepatic disease, renal disease, hypertension, elderly, acute/chronic pain

Pharmacokinetics:
PO: Onset 15-30 min, duration 4-6 hr
RECT: Onset slow, duration 4-6 hr
Metabolized by liver, excreted by kidneys (metabolites); half-life 15-48 hr

Interactions:
• Increased CNS depression: alcohol, MAOIs, sedatives, narcotics
• Decreased effect of oral anticoagulants, corticosteroids, griseofulvin, quinidine
• Increased half-life of doxycycline

Lab test interferences:
False increase: Sulfobromophthalein

NURSING CONSIDERATIONS
Assess:
• VS q30min after parenteral route for 2 hr
• Blood studies: Hct, Hgb, RBCs, serum folate, vit D (long-term therapy); pro-time in patients receiving anticoagulants
• Hepatic studies: AST (SGOT), ALT (SGPT), bilirubin; if increased, drug is usually discontinued
• Mental status: mood, sensorium, affect, memory (long, short)

◆ = Nursing alert   🖊 = Herb-drug interaction   ⊘ = Do not crush

• Physical dependency: more frequent requests for medication, shakes, anxiety

⬧ Barbiturate toxicity: hypotension; pupillary constriction; cold, clammy skin; cyanosis of lips; insomnia; nausea; vomiting; hallucinations; delirium; weakness; coma; mild symptoms may occur in 8-12 hr without drug

• Respiratory dysfunction: respiratory depression, character, rate, rhythm; hold drug if respirations are <10/min or if pupils are dilated

• Blood dyscrasias: fever, sore throat, bruising, rash, jaundice, epistaxis

Administer:

• After removal of cigarettes to prevent fires

• IM inj deep in large muscle mass to prevent tissue sloughing and abscesses; do not inject more than 5 ml in one site

• After trying conservative measures for insomnia

• ½-1 hr before hs for sleeplessness

• On empty stomach for best absorption

• For <14 days, since not effective after that; tolerance develops

• Crushed or whole

• Alone; do not mix with other drugs or inject if there is precipitate

IV

• After mixing with sterile H_2O for injection, inject within 30 min of preparation

• IV undiluted or dilute in sterile H_2O, LR, NaCl, give 50 mg or less/min; titrate to patient response; use only clear sol; avoid extravasation

• IV only with resuscitative equipment available; administer at <100 mg/min (only by qualified personnel)

Additive compatibilities: Amikacin, aminophylline, calcium chloride, cephapirin, chloramphenicol, dimenhydrinate, erythromycin lactobionate, lidocaine, thiopental, verapamil

Syringe compatibilities: Aminophylline, ephedrine, hydromorphone, neostigmine, scopolamine, sodium bicarbonate, thiopental

Y-site compatibilities: Acyclovir, insulin (regular), propofol

Perform/provide:

• Assistance with ambulation after receiving dose

• Safety measures: night-light, call bell within easy reach

• Checking to see if PO medication has been swallowed

• Storage of suppositories in refrigerator; do not use aqueous solutions that contain precipitate

Evaluate:

• Therapeutic response: ability to sleep at night, less early morning awakening if taking drug for insomnia, or decrease in number, severity of seizures if taking drug for seizure disorder

Teach patient/family:

• That hangover is common

• That drug is indicated only for short-term treatment of insomnia; probably ineffective after 2 wk

• That physical dependency may result from extended use (45-90 days depending on dose)

• To avoid driving, other activities requiring alertness

• To avoid alcohol ingestion, CNS depressants; serious CNS depression may result

• Not to discontinue medication quickly after long-term use; drug should be tapered over 1-2 wk

• To tell all prescribers that a barbiturate is being taken

• That withdrawal insomnia may occur after short-term use; not to start using drug again; insomnia will improve in 1-3 nights

P

• That effects may take 2 nights for benefits to be noticed

• Alternative measures to improve sleep (reading, exercise several hr before hs, warm bath, warm milk, TV, self-hypnosis, deep breathing)

Treatment of overdose: Lavage, activated charcoal, warming blanket, vital signs, hemodialysis, I&O ratio

---

pentosan polysulfate sodium

(pen'toh-san' pol-ee-sul'fate)
Elmiron
Func. class.: Urinary analgesic

Action: Low-molecular-weight heparinlike compound; mechanism of action for interstitial cystitis is unknown; may act as a buffer on bladder wall mucosal membrane

Uses: UTI used with a urinary antiinfective

Dosage and routes:
• *Adult:* **PO** 100 mg tid
Available forms: Caps 100 mg
Side effects/adverse reactions:
HEMA: **Thrombocytopenia, leukopenia, increased PT, PTT**
CNS: Headache, depression
GI: Nausea, vomiting, diarrhea, anorexia
INTEG: Rash, alopecia
Contraindications: Hypersensitivity
Precautions: Pregnancy (B), renal disease, lactation, children <16 yr, bleeding disorders
Pharmacokinetics: Metabolized by liver, excreted by kidneys, half-life 4.8 hr

NURSING CONSIDERATIONS
Assess:
• Urinary status: burning pain, itching, urgency, frequency, hematuria; before and after completion of treatment

• Allergic reactions: rash, drug may have to be discontinued

Administer:
🚫 To patient whole, do not break, crush, or chew caps, give with water 1 hr ac or 2 hr pc

Evaluate:
• Therapeutic response: decrease in pain of cystitis

Teach patient/family:
• Not to exceed recommended dosage
• To discontinue after pain is relieved but continue to take concurrent prescribed antibiotic until finished

---

pentostatin (℞)

(pen-toh-stat'in)
Nipent
Func. class.: Antineoplastic, enzyme inhibitor
Chem. class.: *Streptomyces antibioticus* derivative

Action: Inhibits the enzyme adenosine deaminase (ADA), which is able to block DNA synthesis and some RNA synthesis

Uses: α-interferon-refractory hairy cell leukemia, chronic lymphocytic leukemia

Dosage and routes:
• *Adult:* **IV** 4 mg/m^2 every other wk; may be given **IV BOL,** or diluted in a larger volume and given over 20-30 min

Available forms: Inj 10 mg/vial

Side effects/adverse reactions:
CNS: Headache, anxiety, confusion, depression, dizziness, insomnia, nervousness, paresthesia
RESP: Cough, upper respiratory infection, bronchitis, dyspnea, epistaxis, pneumonia, pharyngitis, rhinitis, sinusitis
SYST: Fever, infection, fatigue, pain,

---

allergic reaction, chills, ***death, sepsis,*** chest pain, flu syndrome
HEMA: ***Leukopenia, anemia, thrombocytopenia, ecchymosis, lymphadenopathy,*** petechiae
GI: Nausea, vomiting, anorexia, diarrhea, constipation, flatulence, stomatitis, elevated liver function tests
INTEG: Rash, eczema, dry skin, pruritus, sweating, herpes simplex/zoster
GU: ***Hematuria,*** dysuria, increased BUN/creatinine
Contraindications: Hypersensitivity to this drug or mannitol
Precautions: Renal disease, pregnancy (C), lactation, children, bone marrow depression
Pharmacokinetics:
IV: Elimination half-life 5.7 hr, low protein binding, 90% excreted in urine unchanged or as metabolites
Interactions:
• Fatal pulmonary toxicity: fludarabine
• Increased adverse reactions: vidarabine
Lab test interferences:
Increase: Uric acid

NURSING CONSIDERATIONS
Assess:
• CBC, differential, platelet count qwk; withhold drug if WBC is <4000/mm^3 or platelet count is <75,000/mm^3; notify prescriber
• Renal function studies, BUN, serum uric acid, urine CrCl, electrolytes before, during therapy
• I&O ratio; report fall in urine output to <30 ml/hr
• Monitor temp q4h; fever may indicate beginning infection
• Liver function tests before, during therapy: bilirubin, AST (SGOT), ALT (SGPT), alk phosphatase, prn or qmo
• Bleeding: hematuria, guaiac stools, bruising, petechiae, mucosa or orifices q8h

• Effects of alopecia on body image; discuss feelings about body changes
• Inflammation of mucosa, breaks in skin
• Yellow skin and sclera, dark urine, clay-colored stools, itchy skin, abdominal pain, fever, diarrhea
• Buccal cavity q8h for dryness, sores, ulceration, white patches, oral pain, bleeding, dysphagia
• Local irritation, pain, burning at injection site
• Symptoms of severe allergic reaction: rash, pruritus, urticaria, purpuric skin lesions, itching, flushing
• GI symptoms: frequency of stools, cramping
• Acidosis, signs of dehydration; rapid respiration, poor skin turgor, decreased urine output, dry skin, restlessness, weakness
Administer:
• Antiemetic 30-60 min before giving drug to prevent vomiting
• Antibiotics as ordered for prophylaxis of infection
IV
• After diluting, use with 5 ml sterile H$_2$O for injection and mix thoroughly (2 mg/ml); may be given by bolus or diluted in 25-50 ml 5% dextrose, or 0.9% NaCl (0.33 or 0.18 mg/ml)
Solution compatibilities: D$_5$W, 0.9% NaCl, LR
Y-site compatibilities: Fludarabine, melphalan, ondansetron, paclitaxel, sargramostim
Perform/provide:
• Hydrocortisone, sodium thiosulfate to infiltration area, and ice compress after stopping infusion
• Strict hand-washing technique, gloves, protective covering
• Liquid diet: carbonated beverages; gelatin may be added if patient is not nauseated or vomiting

P

---

* = Canada only   Side effects: *italics* = common; ***bold italics*** = life-threatening

• Rinsing of mouth tid-qid with water, club soda; brushing of teeth bid-qid with soft brush or cotton-tipped applicators for stomatitis; use unwaxed dental floss

• Storage in refrigerator; reconstituted or diluted sol may be stored at room temp up to 8 hr

Evaluate:

• Therapeutic response: decrease in tumor size, spread of malignancy

Teach patient/family:

• To report any complaints, side effects to nurse or prescriber

• That hair may be lost during treatment and wig or hairpiece may make patient feel better; tell patient that new hair may be different in color, texture

• To avoid foods with citric acid, hot or rough texture

• To report any bleeding, white spots, ulcerations in mouth to prescriber; tell patient to examine mouth qd

• To avoid crowds and sources of infection when granulocyte count is low

---

pentoxifylline (℞)

(pen-tox′ih-fill-in)
Trental

Func. class.: Hemorrheologic agent

Chem. class.: Dimethylxanthine derivative

Action: Decreases blood viscosity, stimulates prostacyclin formation, increases blood flow by increasing flexibility of RBCs; decreases RBC hyperaggregation; reduces platelet aggregation, decreases fibrinogen concentration

Uses: Intermittent claudication related to chronic occlusive vascular disease

Investigational uses: Cerebrovascular insufficiency, diabetic neuropathies, TIAs, leg ulcers, strokes

Dosage and routes:

• *Adult:* **PO** 400 mg tid with meals

Available forms: Tabs, controlled release 400 mg

Side effects/adverse reactions:

MISC: Epistaxis, flulike symptoms, laryngitis, nasal congestion, ***leukopenia,*** malaise, weight changes

EENT: Blurred vision, earache, increased salivation, sore throat, conjunctivitis

CNS: Headache, anxiety, *tremors,* confusion, *dizziness*

GI: Dyspepsia, nausea, vomiting, anorexia, bloating, belching, constipation, cholecystitis, dry mouth, thirst, bad taste

INTEG: Rash, pruritus, urticaria, brittle fingernails

CV: Angina, dysrhythmias, palpitation, hypotension, chest pain, dyspnea, edema

Contraindications: Hypersensitivity to this drug or xanthines, retinal/cerebral hemorrhage

Precautions: Pregnancy (C), angina pectoris, cardiac disease, lactation, children, impaired renal function, recent surgery, peptic ulceration

Pharmacokinetics:

PO: Peak 1 hr, half-life ½-1 hr, degradation in liver, excreted in urine

Interactions:

• Increased bleeding: warfarin

• Increased theophylline level: theophylline

NURSING CONSIDERATIONS

Assess:

• B/P, respirations of patient also taking antihypertensives

Administer:

• With meals to prevent GI upset

🚫 Do not break, crush, or chew cont rel tabs

 = Nursing alert   = Herb-drug interaction   🚫 = Do not crush

Evaluate:

• Therapeutic response: decreased pain, cramping, increased ambulation

Teach patient/family:

• That therapeutic response may take 2-4 wk

• That decreased fats, increased cholesterol, increased exercise, decreased smoking are necessary to correct condition

• To observe feet for arterial insufficiency

• To use cotton socks, well-fitted shoes; not to go barefoot

• To watch for bleeding, bruises, petechiae, epistaxis

---

perphenazine (℞)

(per-fen'a-zeen)

Apo-Perphenazine*, perphenazine, Phenazine, PMS Perphenazine*, Trilafon

Func. class.: Antipsychotic, neuroleptic

Chem. class.: Phenothiazine piperidine

Action: Depresses cerebral cortex, hypothalamus, limbic system, which control activity, aggression; blocks neurotransmission produced by dopamine at synapse; exhibits strong α-adrenergic, anticholinergic blocking action; as antiemetic inhibits medullary chemoreceptor trigger zone; mechanism for antipsychotic effects is unclear

Uses: Psychotic disorders, schizophrenia, nausea, vomiting

Dosage and routes:

• *Geriatric:* **PO** 2-4 mg qd-bid, increase by 2-4 mg/wk to desired dose

Nausea/vomiting

• *Adult and child >12 yr:* **IM** 5-10 mg prn, max 15 mg in ambulatory patients, 30 mg in hospitalized patients; **PO** 8-16 mg/day in divided

doses, up to 24 mg; **IV** not to exceed 5 mg, give diluted or slow **IV** drip

Psychiatric use in hospitalized patients

• *Adult:* **PO** 8-16 mg bid-qid, gradually increased to desired dose, not to exceed 64 mg/day; **IM** 5 mg q6h, not to exceed 30 mg/day

• *Child >12 yr:* **PO** 6-12 mg in divided doses

Nonhospitalized patients

• *Adult:* **PO** 4-8 mg tid or 8-32 mg repeat-action bid; **IM** 5 mg q6h

Available forms: Tabs 2, 4, 8, 16 mg; oral sol 16 mg/5ml; inj 5 mg/ml

Side effects/adverse reactions:

RESP: **Laryngospasm,** dyspnea, *respiratory depression*

CNS: EPS: pseudoparkinsonism, akathisia, dystonia, tardive dyskinesia, **seizures,** *headache*

HEMA: Anemia, **leukopenia, leukocytosis, agranulocytosis**

INTEG: Rash, photosensitivity, dermatitis

EENT: Blurred vision, glaucoma

GI: Dry mouth, nausea, vomiting, anorexia, constipation, diarrhea, jaundice, weight gain

GU: Urinary retention, urinary frequency, enuresis, impotence, amenorrhea, gynecomastia

CV: Orthostatic hypotension (elderly), **cardiac arrest,** ECG changes, **tachycardia**

Contraindications: Hypersensitivity, blood dyscrasias, coma, child <12 yr, brain damage, bone marrow depression

Precautions: Pregnancy (C), lactation, seizure disorders, hypertension, hepatic disease, cardiac disease, elderly

Pharmacokinetics:

PO: Onset erratic, peak 2-4 hr

IM: Onset 10 min, peak 1-2 hr; duration 6 hr, occasionally 12-24 hr

Metabolized by liver; excreted in urine, breast milk; crosses placenta

P

Interactions:

• Oversedation: other CNS depressants, alcohol, barbiturate anesthetics

• Toxicity: epinephrine

• Decreased absorption: aluminum hydroxide or magnesium hydroxide antacids

• Decreased effects of lithium, levodopa

• Increased effects of both drugs: β-adrenergic blockers, alcohol

• Increased anticholinergic effects: anticholinergics

🍂 Increased anticholinergic effect: henbane leaf

Lab test interferences:

Increase: Liver function tests, cardiac enzymes, cholesterol, blood glucose, prolactin, bilirubin, PBI, cholinesterase, ^{131}I

Decrease: Hormones (blood, urine)

False positive: Pregnancy tests, PKU

False negative: Urinary steroids, 17-OHCS

NURSING CONSIDERATIONS

Assess:

• Mental status before initial administration

• Swallowing of PO medication; check for hoarding or giving of medication to other patients

• I&O ratio; palpate bladder if urinary output is low

• Bilirubin, CBC, liver function studies qmo

• Urinalysis is recommended before and during prolonged therapy

• Affect, orientation, LOC, reflexes, gait, coordination, sleep pattern disturbances

• B/P standing and lying; also include pulse, respirations q4h during initial treatment; establish baseline before starting treatment; report drops of 30 mm Hg

• Dizziness, faintness, palpitations, tachycardia on rising

• EPS including akathisia (inability to sit still, no pattern to movements), tardive dyskinesia (bizarre movements of jaw, mouth, tongue, extremities), pseudoparkinsonism (rigidity, tremors, pill rolling, shuffling gait)

• Skin turgor daily

◆ For neuroleptic malignant syndrome: hyperthermia, altered mental status, increased CPK, muscle rigidity

• Constipation, urinary retention daily; increase bulk, water in diet

Administer:

• Antiparkinsonian agent on order from prescriber for EPS

• Concentrate mixed in water, orange, pineapple, apricot, prune, tomato, grapefruit juice; do not mix with caffeine beverages (coffee, cola), tannics (tea), or pectinates (apple juice), since incompatibility may result; use 60 ml diluent for each 5 ml of concentrate

🚫 Repeat-action tablets whole; do not break, crush, or chew

• IM inj into large muscle mass

IV

• After diluting each 5 mg/9 ml of NaCl, shake, give 0.5 mg or less (1 ml = 0.5 mg) over 1 min; may be further diluted and infused

Additive compatibilities: Ascorbic acid, ethacrynate, netilmicin

Syringe compatibilities: Atropine, benztropine, butorphanol, chlorpromazine, cimetidine, dimenhydrinate, diphenhydramine, droperidol, fentanyl, hydroxyzine, meperidine, methotrimeprazine, metoclopramide, morphine, pentazocine, prochlorperazine, promethazine, ranitidine, scopolamine

Y-site compatibilities: Acyclovir, amikacin, ampicillin, azlocillin, cefamandole, cefazolin, cefotaxime, cefoxitin, cefuroxime, cephalothin, cephapirin, chloramphenicol, clindamycin, doxycycline, erythromycin, famotidine, gentamicin, kanamycin, metronidazole, mezlocillin, minocycline, moxalactam, nafcillin, oxacillin, penicillin G potassium, piperacillin, tacrolimus, ticarcillin, ticarcillin/clavulanate, tobramycin, trimethoprim/sulfamethoxazole, vancomycin

Perform/provide:

• Decreased sensory input by dimming lights, avoiding loud noises
• Supervised ambulation until stabilized on medication; do not involve in strenuous exercise program because fainting is possible; patient should not stand still for long periods
• Increased fluids to prevent constipation
• Sips of water, candy, gum for dry mouth
• Storage in tight, light-resistant container

Evaluate:

• Therapeutic response: decrease in emotional excitement, hallucinations, delusions, paranoia, reorganization of patterns of thought, speech

Teach patient/family:

• That orthostatic hypotension occurs frequently and to rise from sitting or lying position gradually; to avoid hazardous activities until stabilized on medication
• To remain lying down after IM inj for at least 30 min
• To avoid hot tubs, hot showers, tub baths, since hypotension may occur
• To avoid abrupt withdrawal of this drug, or EPS may result; drug should be withdrawn slowly
• To avoid OTC preparations (cough, hay fever, cold) unless approved by prescriber, since serious drug interactions may occur; avoid use with alcohol or CNS depressants; increased drowsiness may occur
• To use a sunscreen
• About compliance with drug regimen
• About necessity for meticulous oral hygiene, since oral candidiasis may occur
• To report sore throat, malaise, fever, bleeding, mouth sores; if these occur, CBC should be drawn and drug discontinued
• In hot weather, that heat stroke may occur; to take extra precautions to stay cool

Treatment of overdose: Lavage if orally ingested; provide an airway; *do not induce vomiting*

---

phenazopyridine
(℞, OTC)

(fen-az-oh-peer′i-deen)
Azo-Standard, Baridium, Phenazo*, phenazopyridine HCl, Prodium, Pyridiate, Pyridate No. 2, Pyridium, Urogesic

Func. class.: Nonnarcotic analgesic

Chem. class.: Azodye

Action: Exerts analgesic, anesthetic action on the urinary tract mucosa

Uses: Urinary tract irritation, infection used with a urinary antiinfective

Dosage and routes:
Renal dose
• Do not use in CrCl <50 ml/min
• *Adult:* **PO** 100-200 mg tid × 2 days or less when used with antibacterial for UTI
• *Child 6-12 yr:* **PO** 12 mg/kg/24 hr in divided doses × 2 days

Available forms: Tabs 95, 100, 200 mg

Side effects/adverse reactions:
HEMA: ***Thrombocytopenia, agranu-***

locytosis, leukopenia, neutropenia,
hemolytic anemia, methemoglobin-
emia
CNS: Headache
GI: Nausea, vomiting, diarrhea,
heartburn, anorexia, **hepatic toxic-**
ity
INTEG: Rash, skin pigmentation, pru-
ritus
GU: **Renal toxicity,** *orange-red urine*
Contraindications: Hypersensitiv-
ity, renal insufficiency
Precautions: Pregnancy (B), lacta-
tion, children <12 yr
Pharmacokinetics:
Metabolized by liver, excreted by
kidneys, crosses placenta, duration
6-8 hr
Lab test interferences:
Interference: Urinalysis
NURSING CONSIDERATIONS
Assess:
• Urinary status: burning, pain, itch-
ing, urgency, frequency, hematuria,
before/after treatment completed
• Liver function studies: AST
(SGOT), ALT (SGPT), bilirubin if
patient is on long-term therapy
◆ Hepatotoxicity: dark urine, clay-
colored stools, yellow skin and
sclera, itching, abdominal pain, fe-
ver, diarrhea if patient is on long-
term therapy
• Allergic reactions: rash, urticaria;
drug may have to be discontinued
Administer:
PO
• To patient crushed or whole; chew-
able tablets may be chewed
• With food or milk to decrease gas-
tric symptoms
Evaluate:
• Therapeutic response: decrease in
pain
Teach patient/family:
• To report any symptoms of hepa-
totoxicity
• Not to exceed recommended dosage and to take with meals

• To discontinue after pain is relieved but continue to take concurrent prescribed antibiotic until finished
• That urine may turn red-orange;
may stain clothing or contact lenses
Treatment of overdose: Methylene blue 1-2 mg/kg IV or 100-200
mg vit C PO

---

phenelzine (R̶x̶)
(fen'el-zeen)
Nardil
Func. class.: Antidepressant,
MAOI
Chem. class.: Hydrazine

Action: Increases concentrations of
endogenous epinephrine, norepinephrine, serotonin, dopamine in
storage sites in CNS by inhibition of
MAO; increased concentration reduces depression
Uses: Depression, when uncontrolled by other means
Investigational uses: Bulimia, cocaine addiction, migraines, seasonal
affective disorder, panic disorder
Dosage and routes:
• *Adult:* **PO** 45 mg/day in divided
doses; may increase to 60 mg/day;
dose should be reduced to 15 mg/
day, not to exceed 90 mg/day
• *Geriatric:* **PO** 7.5 mg qd, increase
by 7.5-15 mg q3-4 days
Available forms: Tabs 15 mg
Side effects/adverse reactions:
HEMA: **Anemia**
CNS: Dizziness, drowsiness, confusion, headache, anxiety, tremors,
stimulation, weakness, hyperreflexia, mania, insomnia, fatigue,
weight gain
GI: Constipation, dry mouth, nausea, vomiting, *anorexia,* diarrhea,
weight gain
GU: Change in libido, frequency

◆ = Nursing alert   ▰ = Herb-drug interaction   ⊘ = Do not crush

INTEG: Rash, flushing, increased perspiration

CV: Orthostatic hypotension, hypertension, dysrhythmias, **hypertensive crisis**

EENT: Blurred vision

ENDO: **SIADH-like syndrome**

Contraindications: Hypersensitivity to MAOIs, hypertension, CHF, severe hepatic disease, pheochromocytoma, severe renal disease, severe cardiac disease

Precautions: Suicidal patients, convulsive disorders, severe depression, schizophrenia, hyperactivity, diabetes mellitus, pregnancy (C)

Pharmacokinetics: Metabolized by liver, excreted by kidneys

Interactions:

• Increased hypotension: thiazide diuretics

• Confusion, shivering, hyperreflexia: L-tryptophan

• Toxicity: sumatriptan, sulfonamide

• Decreased serotonin, norepinephrine: rauwolfia alkaloids

• Increased pressor effects: guanethidine, clonidine, indirect-acting or mixed sympathomimetics (ephedrine)

• Increased effects of direct-acting sympathomimetics (epinephrine): alcohol, barbiturates, benzodiazepines, CNS depressants, levodopa

• Hyperpyretic crisis, convulsions, hypertensive episode: tricyclic antidepressants, SSRIs, meperidine

• Increased hypoglycemic effect: antidiabetics

Drug/food

• Avoid tyramine foods

🌶 Increased sympathomimetic action: ephedra

🌶 Hypertension: Brewer's yeast

NURSING CONSIDERATIONS

Assess:

• B/P (lying, standing), pulse; if systolic B/P drops 20 mm Hg, hold drug, notify prescriber

• Blood studies: CBC, leukocytes, cardiac enzymes (long-term therapy)

• Hepatic studies: ALT (SGPT), AST (SGOT), bilirubin; hepatotoxicity may occur

⬦ Toxicity: increased headache, palpitation; discontinue drug immediately; prodromal signs of hypertensive crisis

• Mental status changes: mood, sensorium, affect, memory (long, short); increase in psychiatric symptoms

• Urinary retention, constipation, edema; take weight qwk

• Withdrawal symptoms: headache, nausea, vomiting, muscle pain, weakness

Administer:

PO

• Increased fluids, bulk in diet for constipation

• With food, milk for GI symptoms

• Crushed if patient cannot swallow medication whole

• Dosage hs for oversedation during day

• Gum, hard candy, or frequent sips of water for dry mouth

• Phentolamine for severe hypertension

Perform/provide:

• Storage in tight container in cool environment

• Ambulation assistance at start of therapy, since drowsiness/dizziness occurs, especially elderly

• Safety measures including side rails

• Checking to see if PO medication swallowed

Evaluate:

• Therapeutic response: decreased depression

Teach patient/family:

• That therapeutic effects may take 1-4 wk

• To avoid driving, other activities requiring alertness

• To avoid alcohol ingestion, CNS

depressants, OTC medications: cold, weight loss, hay fever, cough syrup
• Not to discontinue medication quickly after long-term use
• To avoid high-tyramine foods: cheese (aged), sour cream, beer, wine, pickled products, liver, raisins, bananas, figs, avocados, meat tenderizers, chocolate, yogurt; increased caffeine
• To report headache, palpitation, neck stiffness, dizziness, constriction in chest, throat

Treatment of overdose: Lavage, activated charcoal, monitor electrolytes, vital signs, diazepam IV, NaHCO$_3$

---

phenobarbital (R)

(fee-noe-bar'bi-tal)
Barbita, Luminal, Phenobarbital, Phenobarbital Sodium, Solfoton
Func. class.: Anticonvulsant
Chem. class.: Barbiturate

Controlled Substance Schedule IV
Action: Decreases impulse transmission; increases seizure threshold at cerebral cortex level
Uses: All forms of epilepsy, status epilepticus, febrile seizures in children, sedation, insomnia
Investigational uses: Hyperbilirubinemia, chronic cholestasis
Dosage and routes:
Seizures
• *Adult:* **PO** 100-200 mg/day in divided doses tid or total dose hs
• *Child:* **PO** 4-6 mg/kg/day in divided doses q12h; may be given as single dose
Status epilepticus
• *Adult:* **IV INF** 10 mg/kg; run no faster than 50/mg/min; may give up to 20 mg/kg
• *Child:* **IV INF** 5-10 mg/kg; may

repeat q10-15min up to 20 mg/kg; run no faster than 50 mg/min
Insomnia
• *Adult:* **PO/IM** 100-320 mg
• *Child:* **PO/IM** 3-6 mg/kg
Sedation
• *Adult:* **PO** 30-120 mg/day in 2-3 divided doses
• *Child:* **PO** 6 mg/kg/day in 3 divided doses
Preoperative sedation
• *Adult:* **IM** 100-200 mg 1-1½ hr before surgery
• *Child:* **PO** 6 mg/kg/day in 3 divided doses
Hyperbilirubinemia
• *Neonate:* **PO** 7 mg/kg/day on days 1-5 after birth; **IM** 5 mg/kg/day on day 1, then **PO** on days 2-7 after birth
Chronic cholestasis
• *Adult:* **PO** 90-180 mg/day in 2-3 divided doses
• *Child <12 yr:* **PO** 3-12 mg/kg/day in 2-3 divided doses
Available forms: Caps 16 mg; elix 15, 20 mg/5 ml; tabs 8, 15, 16, 30, 32, 60, 65, 100 mg; inj 30, 60, 65, 130 mg/ml
Side effects/adverse reactions:
CNS: Paradoxic excitement (elderly), drowsiness, lethargy, hangover headache, flushing, hallucinations, ***coma***
GI: Nausea, vomiting, diarrhea, constipation
INTEG: Rash, urticaria, ***Stevens-Johnson syndrome, angioedema,*** local pain, swelling, necrosis, ***thrombophlebitis***
Contraindications: Hypersensitivity to barbiturates, porphyria, hepatic disease, respiratory disease, nephritis, hyperthyroidism, diabetes mellitus, elderly, lactation, pregnancy (D)
Precautions: Anemia
Pharmacokinetics:
IV: Onset 5 min, peak 30 min, duration 4-6 hr

 = Nursing alert　　　✦ = Herb-drug interaction　　　⊘ = Do not crush

IM/SC: Onset 10-30 min, duration 4-6 hr

PO: Onset 20-60 min, peak 8-12 hr, duration 6-10 hr

Metabolized by liver; crosses placenta; excreted in urine, breast milk; half-life 53-118 hr

Interactions:

• Increased effects: CNS depression, alcohol, chloramphenicol, valproic acid, disulfiram, nondepolarizing skeletal muscle relaxants, sulfonamides

• Decreased effects: theophylline, oral anticoagulants, corticosteroids, metronidazole, doxycycline, quinidine

• Increased orthostatic hypotension: furosemide

NURSING CONSIDERATIONS

Assess:

• Mental status: mood, sensorium, affect, memory (long, short)

• Respiratory depression

• Blood dyscrasias: fever, sore throat, bruising, rash, jaundice

• Convulsion activity: type, duration, precipitating factors

• Blood studies, liver function tests during long-term treatment

• Therapeutic blood level periodically: 15-40 µg/ml

• Respiratory status: rate, rhythm, depth

Administer:

• Give IM inj deep in large muscle mass to prevent tissue sloughing; use < 5 ml in each site

IV

• Slow IV after dilution with at least 10 ml sterile H_2O for inj regardless of dose; give 65 mg or less/min; titrate to patient response

Additive compatibilities: Amikacin, aminophylline, calcium chloride, calcium gluconate, cephapirin, colistimethate, dimenhydrinate, meropenem, polymyxin B, sodium bicarbonate, thiopental, verapamil

Solution compatibilities: D_5W, $D_{10}W$, 0.45% NaCl, 0.9% NaCl, Ringer's, dextrose/saline combinations, dextrose/Ringer's, dextrose/LR combinations, sodium lactate

Syringe compatibilities: Heparin

Y-site compatibilities: Enalaprilat, meropenem, propofol, sufentanil

Perform/provide:

• Supervision of ambulation for dizziness, drowsiness

Evaluate:

• Therapeutic response: decreased seizures, increased sedation

Teach patient/family:

• To use exactly as ordered

• To avoid other CNS depressants, including alcohol

• To avoid hazardous activities until stabilized on drug; drowsiness may occur

• Never to withdraw drug abruptly; withdrawal symptoms may occur

• That therapeutic effects (PO) may not be seen for 2-3 wk

Treatment of overdose: Calcium gluconate IV

P

---

phentolamine (R)

(fen-tole'a-meen)

Regitine, Roytine*

Func. class.: Antihypertensive

Chem. class.: α-adrenergic blocker

Action: α-adrenergic blocker, binds to α-adrenergic receptors, dilating peripheral blood vessels, lowering peripheral resistances, lowering blood pressure

Uses: Hypertension, pheochromocytoma, prevention, treatment of dermal necrosis following extravasation of norepinephrine or dopamine, impotence

---

Dosage and routes:

Treatment of hypertensive episodes in pheochromocytoma

• *Adult:* **IV/IM,** 5 mg, repeat if necessary

• *Child:* **IV/IM,** 1 mg, repeat if necessary

Prevention, treatment of necrosis

• *Adult and child:* 5-10 mg/10 ml **NS** injected into area of norepinephrine extravasation within 12 hr

• *Neonate:* 2.5-5 mg

Impotence (adjunct)

• *Adult:* Intracavernosal 0.5-1 mg with 30 mg papaverine given 1, 2, or 3 treatments/wk

Available forms: Inj 5 mg/ml; tabs 25, 50 mg (only injectable form available in US)

Side effects/adverse reactions:

GI: Dry mouth, nausea, vomiting, diarrhea, abdominal pain

CV: Hypotension, tachycardia, angina, dysrhythmias, **MI**

CNS: Dizziness, flushing, weakness

EENT: Nasal congestion

Contraindications: Hypersensitivity, MI, coronary insufficiency, angina

Precautions: Pregnancy (C), lactation

Pharmacokinetics:

IV: Peak 2 min, duration 10-15 min

IM: Peak 15-20 min, duration 3-4 hr Metabolized in liver, excreted in urine

Interactions:

• Increased effects of epinephrine, antihypertensives

NURSING CONSIDERATIONS

Assess:

• Electrolytes: K, Na, Cl, CO_2

• Weight qd, I&O

• B/P lying, standing before starting treatment, q4h after

• Nausea, vomiting, diarrhea, edema in feet, legs daily; skin turgor, dryness of mucous membranes for hydration status, postural hypotension, cardiac system: pulse, ECG

Administer:

• Gum, frequent rinsing of mouth, or hard candy for dry mouth

• With vasopressor available

• After discontinuing all medication for 24 hr

IV

• After diluting 5 mg/1 ml sterile H_2O for inj; may be further diluted with 5-10 ml sterile H_2O for inj; give 5 mg or less/min

• 10 mg/L may be added to norepinephrine in IV sol for prevention of dermal necrosis

Additive compatibilities: Dobutamine, verapamil

Syringe compatibilities: Papaverine

Y-site compatibilities: Amiodarone

Evaluate:

• Therapeutic response: decreased B/P

Teach patient/family:

• That bed rest is required during treatment, 1 hr after

Treatment of overdose: Administer norepinephrine; discontinue drug

---

phenylbutyrate (℞)

(fen-ill-byoo′te-rate)

Buphenyl

Func. class.: Nitrogen excretion product

Action: Provides an alternate method for waste nitrogen excretion; similar to urea

Uses: Cycle disorders; urea cycle disorders with CPS, OTC, AAS

Dosage and routes:

• *Adult and child:* **PO** 450-600 mg/kg/day <20 kg or 9.9-13 g/m²/day in larger persons. May use powder via mouth, NG tube, gastrostomy tube mixed with solid or liquid food

---

 = Nursing alert   = Herb-drug interaction   ⊘ = Do not crush

Available forms: Tabs 500 mg; powder 3.2 g (3 g phenylbutyrate) per tsp, 9.1 g (8.6 g phenylbutyrate) per tsp

Side effects/adverse reactions:
GU: Amenorrhea, menstrual changes
GI: Decreased appetite, taste aversion, abdominal pain, nausea, vomiting, constipation, rectal bleeding, peptic ulcer
MISC.: Body odor
CV: Dysrhythmias
HEMA: Aplastic anemia
CNS: Depression, *neurotoxicity,* headache

Contraindications: Hypersensitivity, acute hyperammonemia

Precautions: CHF, severe renal insufficiency, hepatic disease, pregnancy (C), lactation, children, preexisting neurologic impairment

Pharmacokinetics: Absorption within 1 hr, excreted via kidneys within 24 hr

Interactions:
• Increased plasma ammonia levels: corticosteroids, haloperidol, valproate
• Renal excretion may be affected: probenecid

NURSING CONSIDERATIONS
Assess:
• And maintain levels of ammonia, arginine, branched-chain amino acids and serum proteins: glutamine levels should be <1000 cmol/L; monitor drug levels of: phenylbutyrate, phenylacetate, phenylactylglutamine
• For neurotoxicity and aplastic anemia; drug should be discontinued

Evaluate:
• Therapeutic response: decreased ammonia levels

---

phenylephrine (℞)
(fen-ill-ef´rin)
Neo-Synephrine
Func. class.: Adrenergic, direct-acting
Chem. class.: Substituted phenylethylamine

Action: Powerful and selective (α_1) receptor agonist causing contraction of blood vessels

Uses: Hypotension, paroxysmal supraventricular tachycardia, shock, maintain B/P during spinal anesthesia

Dosage and routes:
Hypotension
• *Adult:* **SC/IM** 2-5 mg, may repeat q10-15 min if needed; **IV** 0.1-0.5 mg, may repeat q10-15 min if needed
• *Child:* **IM/SC** 0.1 mg/kg/dose q1-2h prn

PVCs
• *Adult:* **IV BOL** 0.5 mg given rapidly, not to exceed prior dose by >0.1 mg; total dose >1 mg

Shock
• *Adult:* **IV INF** 100-180 µg/min (if 20 gtt/ml inf device), then maint of 40-60 µg/min (if 20 gtt/ml inf device)
• *Child:* **IV BOL** 5-20 µg/kg/dose q10-15; **IV INF** 0.1-0.5 µg/kg/min

Available forms: Inj 1% (10 mg/ml)

Side effects/adverse reactions:
CNS: Headache, anxiety, tremor, insomnia, dizziness
CV: Palpitations, tachycardia, hypertension, ectopic beats, angina, reflex bradycardia
GI: Nausea, vomiting
INTEG: Necrosis, tissue sloughing with extravasation, *gangrene*

Contraindications: Hypersensitivity, ventricular fibrillation, tachydysrhythmias, pheochromocytoma, narrow-angle glaucoma

Precautions: Pregnancy (C), lactation, arterial embolism, peripheral vascular disease, elderly, hyperthyroidism, bradycardia, myocardial disease, severe arteriosclerosis

Pharmacokinetics:

IV: Duration 20-30 min

IM/SC: Duration 45-60 min

Interactions:

• Do not use within 2 wk of MAOIs, or hypertensive crisis may result

• Dysrhythmias: general anesthetics, bretylium

• Decreased action of phenylephrine: α-blockers

• Increase in B/P: oxytocics

• Increased pressor effect: tricyclic antidepressant, MAOIs, guanethidine

NURSING CONSIDERATIONS

Assess:

• I&O ratio; notify prescriber if output <30 ml/hr

• ECG during administration continuously; if B/P increases, drug is decreased

• B/P and pulse q5min after parenteral route

• CVP or PWP during inf if possible

• For paresthesias and coldness of extremities; peripheral blood flow may decrease

Administer:

IV

• Plasma expanders for hypovolemia

• IV after diluting 1 mg/9 ml sterile H_2O for inj; give dose over ½-1 min; may be diluted 10 mg/500 ml of D_5W or NS; titrate to response (normal B/P); check for extravasation, check site for infiltration, use infusion pump

Additive compatibilities: Chloramphenicol, dobutamine, lidocaine, potassium chloride, sodium bicarbonate

Y-site compatibilities: Amiodarone, amrinone, famotidine, haloperidol, zidovudine

Perform/provide:

• Storage of reconstituted sol if refrigerated for no longer than 24 hr

• Discard discolored sol

Evaluate:

• Therapeutic response: increased B/P with stabilization

Teach patient/family:

• The reason for administration

• To report pain at infusion site immediately

Treatment of overdose: Administer an α-blocker

---

phenytoin (℞)

(fen'i-toh-in)

Dilantin, Dilantin Capsules, DiPhen, Diphenylhydantoin, Diphenylan, Phenytoin oral suspension

Func. class.: Anticonvulsant; antidysrhythmic (IB)

Chem. class.: Hydantoin

Action: Inhibits spread of seizure activity in motor cortex by altering ion transport; increases AV conduction

Uses: Generalized tonic-clonic seizures; status epilepticus; nonepileptic seizures associated with Reye's syndrome or after head trauma; migraines, trigeminal neuralgia, Bell's palsy, ventricular dysrhythmias uncontrolled by antidysrhythmics

Dosage and routes:

Renal dose

• Do not use loading dose CrCl <10 ml/min or hepatic failure

Seizures

• *Adult:* IV loading dose 900 mg-1.5 g run not faster than 50 mg/min; if patient has received phenytoin, 100-300 mg run not faster than 50

 = Nursing alert   = Herb-drug interaction   **🚫** = Do not crush

mg/min; **PO** loading dose 900 mg-1.5 g divided tid, then 300 mg/day (extended) or divided tid (extended/prompt)
• *Child:* **IV** loading dose 15 mg/kg run not faster than 50 mg/min; if patient has received phenytoin, 5-7 mg/kg run not faster than 50 mg/min; may repeat in 30 min; **PO** loading dose of 15 mg/kg divided q8-12h, then 5-7 mg/kg in divided doses q12h

Status epilepticus
• *Adult:* **IV** 15-20 mg/kg, max 25-50 mg/min, may give 100 mg q6-8h thereafter
• *Child:* **IV** 15-20 mg/kg given 1-3 mg/kg/min

Neuritic pain
• *Adult:* **PO** 200-400 mg/day

Ventricular dysrhythmias
• *Adult:* **PO** loading dose 1 g divided over 24 hr, then 500 mg/day × 2 days; **IV** 250 mg over 5 min until dysrhythmias subside or until 1 g is given, or 100 mg q15min until dysrhythmias subside or until 1 g given
• *Child:* **PO** 3-8 mg/kg or 250 mg/m²/day as single dose or 2 divided doses; **IV** 3-8 mg/kg over several min, or 250 mg/m²/day as single dose or 2 divided doses

Available forms: Susp 30, 125 mg/5 ml; tabs, chewable 50 mg; inj 50 mg/ml; caps ext rel 30, 100 mg; caps prompt 30*, 100 mg

Side effects/adverse reactions:
CNS: Drowsiness, dizziness, insomnia, paresthesias, depression, suicidal tendencies, aggression, headache, confusion, slurred speech
CV: Hypotension, *ventricular fibrillation*
EENT: Nystagmus, diplopia, blurred vision
GI: Nausea, vomiting, constipation, anorexia, weight loss, *hepatitis*, jaundice, gingival hyperplasia

GU: **Nephritis,** urine discoloration
HEMA: **Agranulocytosis, leukopenia, aplastic anemia, thrombocytopenia, megaloblastic anemia**
INTEG: Rash, *lupus erythematosus, Stevens-Johnson syndrome,* hirsutism
SYST: Hypocalcemia

Contraindications: Hypersensitivity, psychiatric condition, pregnancy (D), bradycardia, SA and AV block, Stokes-Adams syndrome, hepatic failure

Precautions: Allergies, hepatic disease, renal disease, elderly, petit mal seizures

Pharmacokinetics:
PO-ER: Onset 2-24 hr, peak 4-12 hr, duration 12-36 hr
IV: Onset 1-2 hr, duration 12-24 hr
PO: Onset 2-24 hr, peak 1½-2½ hr, duration 6-12 hr
Metabolized by liver, excreted by kidneys; highly protein-bound, half-life 22 hr

Interactions:
• Decreased effects of phenytoin: alcohol (chronic use), antihistamines, antacids, antineoplastics, CNS depressants, rifampin, folic acid
• Increased effect of phenytoin: low plasma albumin levels

🖉 Increased potassium loss, increased antidysrhythmic action: aloe, buckthorn bark/berry, cascara sagrada bark, senna pod/leaf

Lab test interferences:
Decrease: Dexamethasone, metyrapone test serum, PBI, urinary steroids
Increase: Glucose, alk phosphatase, BSP

NURSING CONSIDERATIONS
Assess:
• Drug level: toxic level 30-50 µg/ml, ther level: 7.5-20 µg/ml, wait ≥1 wk to draw levels

• Blood studies: CBC, platelets q2wk until stabilized, then qmo × 12, then q3mo; discontinue drug if neutrophils <1600/mm³; renal function: albumin conc

• Mental status: mood, sensorium, affect, memory (long, short)

• Respiratory depression; rate, depth, character

• Blood dyscrasias: fever, sore throat, bruising, rash, jaundice

Administer:

• Shake susp well before each dose

• G tube/NG tube: dilute susp prior to administration, flush tube with 20 ml H₂O after dose

IV

• After diluting with diluent provided (2.2 ml/100 mg, 5.2 ml/250 mg) (1 ml/50 mg); shake; place vial in warm water to dissolve powder; give through Y-tube or 3-way stopcock; inject slowly <50 mg/min; clear IV tubing first with NS sol; use in-line filter; discard 4 hr after preparation; inject into large veins to prevent purple glove syndrome

Additive compatibilities: Bleomycin, sodium bicarbonate, verapamil

Y-site compatibilities: Esmolol, famotidine, fluconazole, foscarnet, tacrolimus

Evaluate:

• Therapeutic response; decrease in severity of seizures, ventricular dysrhythmias

Teach patient/family:

• To take PO doses divided with or after meals to decrease adverse effects

• That if diabetic, urine glucose should be monitored

• That urine may turn pink

• Not to discontinue drug abruptly; seizures may occur

• Proper brushing of teeth using a soft toothbrush, flossing to prevent gingival hyperplasia; need to see dentist frequently

• To avoid hazardous activities until stabilized on drug

• To carry Medic Alert ID stating drug use

• That heavy use of alcohol may diminish effect of drug; to avoid OTC medications

• Not to change brands or forms once stabilized on therapy; brands may vary

---

phytonadione (vit K₁) (℞)

(fye-toe-na-dye′one)
AquaMEPHYTON, Konakion, Mephyton
Func. class.: Vit K₁, fat-soluble vitamin

Action: Needed for adequate blood clotting (factors II, VII, IX, X)

Uses: Vit K malabsorption, hypoprothrombinemia, prevention of hypoprothrombinemia caused by oral anticoagulants, prevention of hemorrhagic disease of the newborn

Dosage and routes:

Hypoprothrombinemia caused by vit K malabsorption

• *Adult:* **PO/IM** 2-25 mg, may repeat or increase to 50 mg

• *Child:* **PO/IM** 5-10 mg

• *Infant:* **PO/IM** 2 mg

Prevention of hemorrhagic disease of the newborn

• *Neonate:* **SC/IM** 0.5-1 mg after birth, repeat in 6-8 hr if required

Hypoprothrombinemia caused by oral anticoagulants

• *Adult and child:* **PO/SC/IM** 2.5-10 mg, may repeat 12-48 hr after **PO** dose or 6-8 hr after **SC/IM** dose, based on PT

Available forms: Tabs 5 mg; inj 2 mg, 10 mg/ml aqueous colloidal (IM, IV); inj aqueous dispersion 2, 10 mg/ml, (IM)

Side effects/adverse reactions:
CNS: Headache, ***brain damage*** (large doses)
GI: Nausea, decreased liver function tests
HEMA: ***Hemolytic anemia, hemoglobinuria, hyperbilirubinemia***
INTEG: Rash, urticaria

Contraindications: Hypersensitivity, severe hepatic disease, last few wk of pregnancy

Precautions: Pregnancy (C), neonates

Pharmacokinetics:
PO/Inj: Metabolized, crosses placenta

Interactions:
• Decreased action of phytonadione: cholestyramine, mineral oil
• Decreased action of oral anticoagulants

NURSING CONSIDERATIONS
Assess:
• Pro-time during treatment (2-sec deviation from control time, bleeding time, and clotting time); monitor for bleeding, pulse, and B/P
• Nutritional status: liver (beef), spinach, tomatoes, coffee, asparagus, broccoli, cabbage, lettuce, greens

Administer:
IV
• After diluting with D₅NS 10 ml or more; give 1 mg/min or more
• IV only when other routes not possible (deaths have occurred)

Additive compatibilities: Amikacin, calcium gluceptate, cephapirin, chloramphenicol, cimetidine, netilmicin, sodium bicarbonate

Syringe compatibilities: Doxapram

Y-site compatibilities: Ampicillin, epinephrine, famotidine, heparin, hydrocortisone, potassium chloride, tolazoline, vit B/C

Perform/provide:
• Storage in tight, light-resistant container

Evaluate:
• Therapeutic response: decreased bleeding tendencies, decreased protime, decreased clotting time

Teach patient/family:
• Not to take other supplements unless directed by prescriber
• The necessary foods for diet
• To avoid IM injections, use soft toothbrush, don't floss, use electric razor until coagulation defect corrected
• To report symptoms of bleeding
• Not to use OTC medications unless approved by prescriber
• The importance of frequent lab tests to monitor coagulation factors

---

pindolol (℞)
(pin'doe-lole)
Visken
Func. class.: Antihypertensive
Chem. class.: Nonselective β-blocker

Action: Competitively blocks stimulation of β-adrenergic receptor within vascular smooth muscle; (decreases rate of SA node discharge, increases recovery time), slows conduction of AV node, decreases heart rate, which decreases O₂ consumption in myocardium; also decreases renin-aldosterone-angiotensin system, at high doses inhibits β-2 receptors in bronchial system

Uses: Mild to moderate hypertension

Investigational uses: Mitral valve prolapse, hypertrophic cardiomyopathy, angina pectoris, ventricular dysrhythmias, anxiety

Dosage and routes:
• *Adult:* **PO** 5 mg bid, usual dose 15 mg/day (5 mg tid), may increase by 10 mg/day q3-4wk to a max of 60 mg/day

• *Geriatric:* **PO** 5 mg qd, increase by 5 mg q3-4wk

Available forms: Tabs 5, 10 mg

Side effects/adverse reactions:

CV: Hypotension, bradycardia, *CHF,* edema, chest pain, palpitation, claudication, tachycardia, *AV block*

CNS: Insomnia, dizziness, hallucinations, anxiety, fatigue

GI: Nausea, vomiting, *ischemic colitis,* diarrhea, *abdominal pain, mesenteric arterial thrombosis*

INTEG: Rash, alopecia, pruritus, fever

HEMA: Agranulocytosis, thrombocytopenia, purpura

EENT: Visual changes, sore throat, *double vision;* dry, burning eyes

GU: Impotence, urinary frequency

RESP: **Bronchospasm,** *dyspnea,* cough, rales

MISC: Joint pain, muscle pain

Contraindications: Hypersensitivity to β-blockers, cardiogenic shock; 2nd, 3rd degree heart block; sinus bradycardia, CHF, cardiac failure, bronchial asthma

Precautions: Major surgery, pregnancy (B), lactation, diabetes mellitus, renal disease, thyroid disease, COPD, well-compensated heart failure, CAD, nonallergic bronchospasm

Pharmacokinetics:

PO: Peak 2-4 wk; half-life 3-4 hr, excreted 30%-45% unchanged; 60%-65% metabolized by liver; excreted in breast milk

Interactions:

• Increased hypotension, bradycardia: reserpine, hydralazine, methyldopa, prazosin, anticholinergics

• Decreased antihypertensive effects: indomethacin, sympathomimetics, thyroid

• Increased hypoglycemic effect: insulin

• Decreased bronchodilation: theophyllines, β₂-agonists

• Decreased hypoglycemic effect: sulfonylureas

Lab test interferences:

Increase: Liver function tests, renal function tests

NURSING CONSIDERATIONS
Assess:

• I&O, weight qd

• B/P during initial treatment, periodically thereafter; pulse q4h, note rate, rhythm, quality

• Apical, radial pulse before administration; notify prescriber of any significant changes

• Baselines in renal, liver function tests before therapy begins

• Edema in feet, legs qd

• Skin turgor, dryness of mucous membranes for hydration status

Administer:

• PO ac, hs; tablet may be crushed or swallowed whole

• Reduced dosage in renal dysfunction

Perform/provide:

• Storage in dry area at room temp; do not freeze

Evaluate:

• Therapeutic response: decreased B/P after 1-2 wk

Teach patient/family:

• To take with or immediately after meals

• Not to discontinue drug abruptly; taper over 2 wk; may cause precipitate angina

• Not to use OTC products containing α-adrenergic stimulants (nasal decongestants, OTC cold preparations) unless directed by prescriber

• To report bradycardia, dizziness, confusion, depression, fever, sore throat, shortness of breath to prescriber

• To take pulse at home; to notify prescriber if pulse <50 BPM

• To avoid alcohol, smoking, Na

◆ = Nursing alert   ∅ = Herb-drug interaction   ⊘ = Do not crush

• To comply with weight control, dietary adjustments, modified exercise program

• To carry Medic Alert ID to identify drug, allergies

• To avoid hazardous activities if dizziness is present

• To report symptoms of CHF: difficult breathing, especially on exertion or when lying down, night cough, swelling of extremities

• To take medication at bedtime to prevent orthostatic hypotension

• To wear support hose to minimize effects of orthostatic hypotension

Treatment of overdose: Lavage, IV atropine for bradycardia, IV theophylline for bronchospasm, digitalis, O_2, diuretic for cardiac failure, hemodialysis, hypotension; give vasopressor (norepinephrine)

---

pipecuronium (℞)

(pip-e-kyoor-oh′nee-um)
Arduran
Func. class.: Neuromuscular blocker (nondepolarizing)
Chem. class.: Synthetic curariform

Action: Inhibits transmission of nerve impulses by binding with cholinergic receptor sites, antagonizing action of acetylcholine

Uses: Facilitation of endotracheal intubation; skeletal muscle relaxation during mechanical ventilation, surgery, or general anesthesia

Dosage and routes:

• *Adult:* **IV** dosage is individualized, in patients with normal renal function who are not obese, initial dose is 70-85 μg/kg; maintenance dose ranges from 10-15 μg/kg

• *Child 1-14 yr:* **IV** 57 μg/kg

• *Child 3 mo-1 yr:* **IV** 40 μg/kg

Available forms: Inj 10 mg vials

Side effects/adverse reactions:

CV: Bradycardia, tachycardia, increased or decreased B/P, ventricular extrasystole, *myocardial ischemia, cardiovascular accident, thrombosis, atrial fibrillation*

RESP: Prolonged apnea, bronchospasm, cyanosis, respiratory depression

GU: Anuria

EENT: Increased secretions

CNS: Hypesthesia, CNS depression

MS: Weakness to prolonged skeletal muscle relaxation

INTEG: Rash, urticaria

META: Hypoglycemia, hyperkalemia, increased creatinine

Contraindications: Hypersensitivity to bromide ion

Precautions: Pregnancy (C), renal disease, cardiac disease, lactation, children <3 mo, fluid and electrolyte imbalances, neuromuscular diseases, respiratory disease, obesity

Pharmacokinetics:

IV: Onset 30-45 sec, peak 3-5 min; metabolized (small amounts), excreted in urine (unchanged), crosses placenta

Interactions:

• Increased neuromuscular blockade: aminoglycosides, quinidine, local anesthetics, polymyxin antibiotics, enflurane, isoflurane, tetracyclines, halothane, magnesium, colistin

NURSING CONSIDERATIONS

Assess:

• For electrolyte imbalances (K, Mg); may lead to increased action of this drug

• Vital signs (B/P, pulse, respirations, airway) until fully recovered; rate, depth, pattern of respirations; strength of hand grip

• I&O ratio; check for urinary retention, frequency, hesitancy

---

Side effects: *italics* = common; ***bold italics*** = life-threatening

• Recovery: decreased paralysis of face, diaphragm, leg, arm, rest of body
• Allergic reactions: rash, fever, respiratory distress, pruritus; drug should be discontinued

Administer:
• Using nerve stimulator by anesthesiologist to determine neuromuscular blockade
• Atropine to counteract muscarinic effects
• After succinylcholine effects subside
• Anticholinesterase to reverse neuromuscular blockade

IV
• By slow IV over 1-2 min (only by qualified persons, usually an anesthesiologist)
• Only fresh sol

Perform/provide:
• Storage in refrigerator; do not store in plastic container or syringe
• Reassurance if communication is difficult during recovery from neuromuscular blockade
• Use of reconstituted sol within 24 hr or discard
• Frequent (q2h) instillation of artificial tears and covering eyes to prevent drying of cornea

Evaluate:
• Therapeutic response: paralysis of jaw, eyelid, head, neck, rest of body

Treatment of overdose: Neostigmine, atropine; monitor VS; may require mechanical ventilation

---

piperacillin (℞)
(pip′er-ah-sill′in)
Pipracil
Func. class.: Broad-spectrum antiinfective
Chem. class.: Extended-spectrum penicillin

Action: Interferes with cell wall replication of susceptible organisms; osmotically unstable cell wall swells and bursts from osmotic pressure

Uses: Respiratory, skin, urinary tract, bone infections; gonorrhea; pneumonia; effective for gram-positive cocci *(S. aureus, S. pyogenes, S. viridans, S. faecalis, S. bovis, S. pneumoniae),* gram-negative cocci *(N. gonorrhoeae, N. meningitidis),* gram-positive bacilli *(C. perfringens, C. tetani),* gram-negative bacilli *(Bacteroides, F. nucleatum, E. coli, Klebsiella, P. mirabilis, M. morganii, P. vulgaris, P. rettgeri, Enterobacter, Citrobacter, P. aeruginosa, Serratia, Acinetobacter, Peptococcus, Peptostreptococcus, Eubacterium)*

Dosage and routes:
Renal dose
• CrCl 20-40 ml/min give q8h; CrCl <20 ml/min give q12h
Systemic infections
• *Adult and child >12 yr:* **IM/IV** 2-4 g q4-6h (2 g/site **IM**)
• *Child<12 yr:* **IM/IV** 200-300 mg/kg/day in divided doses q4-6h
Prophylaxis of surgical infections
• *Adult:* **IV** 2 g ½-1 hr before procedure; may be repeated during surgery or after surgery
Available forms: Inj 2, 3, 4, 40 g; inf 2, 3, 4 g

Side effects/adverse reactions:
HEMA: Anemia, increased bleeding time, **bone marrow depression,** thrombocytopenia

---

 = Nursing alert   / = Herb-drug interaction   🚫 = Do not crush

GI: Nausea, vomiting, diarrhea; increased AST (SGOT), ALT (SGPT); abdominal pain, glossitis, colitis

GU: Oliguria, proteinuria, hematuria, vaginitis, moniliasis, glomerulonephritis

CNS: Lethargy, hallucinations, anxiety, depression, twitching, *coma, convulsions*

META: Hypokalemia, hypernatremia

Contraindications: Hypersensitivity to penicillins

Precautions: Pregnancy (B), lactation, hypersensitivity to cephalosporins; CHF, renal disease

Pharmacokinetics:
IM: Peak 30-50 min
IV: Peak 20-30 min
Half-life 0.7-1.33 hr; excreted in urine, bile, breast milk; crosses placenta

Interactions:
• Increased effect of neuromuscular blockers, heparin
• Decreased antimicrobial effect of piperacillin: tetracyclines (with high concentrations of piperacillin), aminoglycosides
• Increased piperacillin concentrations: aspirin, probenecid

Lab test interferences:
False positive: Urine glucose, urine protein, Coombs' test

NURSING CONSIDERATIONS
Assess:
• I&O ratio; report hematuria, oliguria, since penicillin in high doses is nephrotoxic

◆ Any patient with compromised renal system, since drug is excreted slowly in poor renal system function; toxicity may occur rapidly
• Liver studies: AST (SGOT), ALT (SGPT)
• Blood studies: WBC, RBC, Hgb, Hct, bleeding time

• Renal studies: urinalysis, protein, blood, BUN, creatinine
• C&S before drug therapy; drug may be taken as soon as culture is taken
• Bowel pattern before and during treatment
• Skin eruptions after administration of penicillin to 1 wk after discontinuing drug
• Respiratory status: rate, character, wheezing, tightness in chest
• Allergies before initiation of treatment, reaction of each medication; highlight allergies on chart

Administer:
• Drug after C&S completed
IV
• After diluting 1 g or less/5 ml or more sterile H_2O or 0.9% NaCl; shake; give dose over 3-5 min; may further dilute to 50-100 ml with D_5W, 0.9% NS, and give over ½ hr; discontinue primary IV

Additive compatibilities: Ciprofloxacin, clindamycin, flucloxacillin, fluconazole, hydrocortisone, ofloxacin, potassium chloride, verapamil

Syringe compatibilities: Heparin
Y-site compatibilities: Acyclovir, allopurinol, amifostine, aztreonam, ciprofloxacin, cyclophosphamide, diltiazem, enalaprilat, esmolol, famotidine, fludarabine, foscarnet, gallium, granisetron, heparin, hydromorphone, IL-2, labetalol, lorazepam, magnesium sulfate, melphalan, meperidine, midazolam, morphine, perphenazine, propofol, ranitidine, tacrolimus, teniposide, theophylline, thiotepa, verapamil, zidovudine

Perform/provide:
• Adrenaline, suction, tracheostomy set, endotracheal intubation equipment on unit
• Adequate intake of fluids (2 L) during diarrhea episodes

P

• Scratch test to assess allergy after securing order from prescriber; usually done when penicillin is only drug of choice

• Storage of reconstituted sol 24 hr at room temp or 7 days refrigerated

Evaluate:

• Therapeutic response: absence of fever, purulent drainage, redness, inflammation

Teach patient/family:

• That culture may be taken after completed course of medication

• To report sore throat, fever, fatigue; may indicate superinfection

• To wear or carry Medic Alert ID if allergic to penicillins

• To notify nurse of diarrhea

Treatment of anaphylaxis: Withdraw drug, maintain airway, administer epinephrine, aminophylline, O₂, IV corticosteroids

---

piperacillin and tazobactam (℞)

(pip′er-ah-sill′in & ta-zoe-bak′tam)

Zosyn

Func. class.: Antiinfective, broad-spectrum

Chem. class.: Extended-spectrum penicillin, β-lactamase inhibitor

---

Action: Interferes with cell wall replication of susceptible organisms; osmotically unstable cell wall swells and bursts from osmotic pressure

Uses: Moderate to severe infections: piperacillin-resistant, β-lactamase-producing strains causing infections in respiratory, skin, urinary tract, bone, gonorrhea, pneumonia; effective for resistant *S. aureus*, resistant *E. coli, B. fragilis, B. ovatus, H. influenzae, B. thetaiotaomicron, B. vulgatus*

Dosage and routes:
Renal dose

• CrCl 20-40 ml/min give 2.25 g q6h; CrCl <20 ml/min give 2.25 g q8h

• *Adult:* **IV INF** 6-12 g/day given 2.25 g q8h to 3.375 g q6h over 30 min × 7-10 days

Nosocomial pneumonia:

• *Adult:* 3.375g q4h with an aminoglycoside; continue aminoglycoside only if *P. aeruginosa* is isolated

Available forms: Powder for inj 2 g piperacillin/0.25 g tazobactam, 3 g piperacillin/0.375 g tazobactam, 4 g piperacillin/0.5 g tazobactam

Side effects/adverse reactions:

CNS: Lethargy, hallucinations, anxiety, depression, twitching, *coma, convulsions,* insomnia, headache, fever, dizziness

GI: Nausea, vomiting, diarrhea; increased AST (SGOT), ALT (SGPT); abdominal pain, glossitis, colitis, constipation

GU: Oliguria, proteinuria, hematuria, vaginitis, moniliasis, glomerulonephritis

HEMA: Anemia, increased bleeding time, *bone marrow depression*

META: Hypokalemia, hypernatremia

CV: Hypertension

INTEG: Rash, pruritus

Contraindications: Hypersensitivity to penicillins, neonates

Precautions: Pregnancy (B), lactation, hypersensitivity to cephalosporins, CHF

Pharmacokinetics:

IV: Peak completion of IV, duration 6 hr

Half-life 0.7-1.2 hr; excreted in urine, bile, breast milk; crosses placenta; 33% bound to plasma proteins

Interactions:

• Increased effect of neuromuscular blockers, heparin

• Decreased antimicrobial effect of

◆ = Nursing alert   ⬛ = Herb-drug interaction   ⊗ = Do not crush piperacillin: tetracyclines, aminoglycosides IV

• Increased piperacillin concentrations: aspirin, probenecid

Lab test interferences:

False positive: Urine glucose, urine protein, Coombs' test

Decrease: Hct, Hgb, electrolytes

Increase: Platelet count, eosinophilia, neutropenia, leukopenia, serum creatinine, PTT, AST (SGOT), ALT (SGPT), alk phosphatase, bilirubin, BUN, electrolytes

NURSING CONSIDERATIONS

Assess:

• I&O ratio; report hematuria, oliguria, since penicillin in high doses is nephrotoxic

◆ Any patient with compromised renal system, since drug is excreted slowly in poor renal system function; toxicity may occur rapidly

• Liver studies: AST (SGOT), ALT (SGPT)

• Blood studies: WBC, RBC, Hct, Hgb, bleeding time

• Renal studies: urinalysis, protein, blood, BUN, creatinine

• C&S before drug therapy; drug may be given as soon as culture is taken

• Bowel pattern before and during treatment

• Skin eruptions after administration of penicillin to 1 wk after discontinuing drug

• Respiratory status: rate, character, wheezing, tightness in chest

• Allergies before initiation of treatment, reaction of each medication; highlight allergies on chart

Administer:

• Drug after C&S is complete

IV

• After diluting 5 ml 0.9% NaCl for injection or sterile H_2O for injection, dextran 6% in NS, dextrose 5%, KCl 40 mEq, bacteriostatic saline/parabens, bacteriostatic saline/

benzyl alcohol, bacteriostatic H_2O/benzyl alcohol per 1 g piperacillin; shake well; further dilute in at least 50 ml compatible IV sol and run as int inf over at least 30 min

Y-site compatibilities: Aminophylline, aztreonam, bleomycin, bumetanide, buprenorphine, butorphanol, calcium gluconate, carboplatin, carmustine, cefepime, cimetidine, clindamycin, cyclophosphamide, cytarabine, dexamethasone, diphenhydramine, dopamine, enalaprilat, etoposide, floxuridine, fluconazole, fludarabine, fluorouracil, furosemide, gallium, granisetron, heparin, hydrocortisone, hydromorphone, ifosfamide, leucovorin, lorazepam, magnesium sulfate, mannitol, meperidine, mesna, methotrexate, methylprednisolone, metoclopramide, metronidazole, morphine, ondansetron, plicamycin, potassium chloride, ranitidine, sargramostim, sodium bicarbonate, thiotepa, trimethoprim/sulfamethoxazole, vinblastine, vincristine, zidovudine

Perform/provide:

• Adrenaline, suction, tracheostomy set, endotracheal intubation equipment on unit

• Adequate intake of fluids (2 L) during diarrhea episodes

• Scratch test to assess allergy on order from prescriber; usually when penicillin is only drug of choice

• Discard after 24 hr if stored at room temp or after 48 hr if refrigerated; use single-dose vials immediately after reconstitution; stable in ambulatory IV pump for 12 hr

Evaluate:

• Therapeutic response: absence of fever, purulent drainage, redness, inflammation; culture shows decreased organisms

Teach patient/family:

• That culture may be taken after completed course of medication

• To report sore throat, fever, fatigue; may indicate superinfection
• To wear or carry Medic Alert ID if allergic to penicillins
• To notify nurse of diarrhea

Treatment of overdose: Withdraw drug, maintain airway, administer epinephrine, aminophylline, O_2, IV corticosteroids for anaphylaxis

---

pirbuterol (Ŗ)

(peer-byoo'ter-ole)
Maxair
Func. class.: Bronchodilator
Chem. class.: β-adrenergic agonist

Action: Causes bronchodilation with little effect on heart rate by action on β-receptors, causing increased cAMP and relaxation of smooth muscle

Uses: Reversible bronchospasm (prevention, treatment) including asthma; may be given with theophylline or steroids

Dosage and routes:
• *Adult and child >12 yr:* **AEROSOL** 1-2 **INH** (0.4 mg) q4-6h; do not exceed 12 **INH**/day

Available forms: Aerosol delivery 0.2 mg pirbuterol/actuation

Side effects/adverse reactions:
CNS: Tremors, anxiety, insomnia, headache, dizziness, stimulation, restlessness, hallucinations, drowsiness, irritability
EENT: Dry nose and mouth, irritation of nose, throat
CV: Palpitations, tachycardia, hypertension, angina, hypotension, dysrhythmias
GI: Gastritis, nausea, vomiting, anorexia
MS: Muscle cramps
RESP: **Bronchospasm,** dyspnea, coughing

Contraindications: Hypersensitivity to sympathomimetics, tachycardia

Precautions: Lactation, pregnancy (C), cardiac disorders, hyperthyroidism, diabetes mellitus, prostatic hypertrophy

Pharmacokinetics:
INH: Onset 3 min, peak ½-1 hr, duration 5 hr

Interactions:
• Increased action of other aerosol bronchodilators
• Increased action of pirbuterol: tricyclic antidepressants, antihistamines, sodium levothyroxine
• Decreased action of pirbuterol: β-blockers
• Increased dysrhythmias: halogenated hydrocarbon anesthetics
🍵 Increased action of both: ephedra

NURSING CONSIDERATIONS

Assess:
• Respiratory function: vital capacity, forced expiratory volume, ABGs, B/P

Administer:
• After shaking; exhale, place mouthpiece in mouth, inhale slowly, hold breath, remove, exhale slowly
• Gum, sips of water for dry mouth

Perform/provide:
• Storage in light-resistant container; do not expose to temps over 86° F (30° C)

Evaluate:
• Therapeutic response: absence of dyspnea, wheezing over 1 hr

Teach patient/family:
• Not to use OTC medications; extra stimulation may occur
• Use of inhaler; review package insert with patient
• To avoid getting aerosol in eyes
• To wash inhaler in warm water and dry qd, rinse mouth after use; if used with inhalers containing glucocorticosteroids, wait 5 min before using steroid inhaler

---

◆ = Nursing alert   🍵 = Herb-drug interaction   🚫 = Do not crush

- About all aspects of drug; avoid smoking, smoke-filled rooms, persons with respiratory infections
- To keep fluid intake >2 L/day to liquefy thick secretions

Treatment of overdose: Administer a β-adrenergic blocker

---

piroxicam (R)

(peer-ox'i-kam)
Apo-Piroxicam*, Feldene*, novopirocam*

Func. class.: Nonsteroidal antiinflammatory
Chem. class.: Oxicam derivative

Action: Inhibits prostaglandin synthesis by decreasing an enzyme needed for biosynthesis; has analgesic, antiinflammatory, antipyretic properties

Uses: Mild to moderate pain, osteoarthritis, rheumatoid arthritis

Dosage and routes:
- *Adult:* PO 20 mg qd or 10 mg bid

Available forms: Caps 10, 20 mg

Side effects/adverse reactions:
GI: Nausea, anorexia, vomiting, diarrhea, jaundice, ***cholestatic hepatitis,*** constipation, flatulence, cramps, dry mouth, peptic ulcer, ***bleeding, ulceration, perforation***
CNS: Dizziness, drowsiness, fatigue, tremors, confusion, insomnia, anxiety, depression, *headache*
CV: Tachycardia, peripheral edema, palpitations, dysrhythmias
INTEG: Purpura, rash, pruritus, sweating, photosensitivity
*GU: **Nephrotoxicity: dysuria, hematuria, oliguria, azotemia***
*HEMA: **Blood dyscrasias***
EENT: Tinnitus, hearing loss, blurred vision

Contraindications: Hypersensitivity, asthma, severe renal disease, severe hepatic disease, ulcer disease, cardiac disease

Precautions: Pregnancy (C), lactation, children, bleeding disorders, GI disorders, cardiac disorders, hypersensitivity to other antiinflammatory agents, CHF

Pharmacokinetics:
PO: Peak 2 hr, half-life 50 hr; metabolized in liver; excreted in urine (metabolites), breast milk; 99% protein binding

Interactions:
- Increased action of warfarin, phenytoin, sulfonamides

NURSING CONSIDERATIONS
Assess:
- Renal, liver, blood studies: BUN, creatinine, AST (SGOT), ALT (SGPT), Hgb, before treatment, periodically thereafter
- Audiometric, ophthalmic exam before, during, after treatment
- For eye, ear problems: blurred vision, tinnitus (may indicate toxicity)

Administer:
- With food to decrease GI symptoms; best to take on empty stomach to facilitate absorption; take drug same time qd

Perform/provide:
- Storage at room temp

Evaluate:
- Therapeutic response: decreased pain, stiffness, swelling in joints; ability to move more easily

Teach patient/family:
- 🚫 Not to break, crush, or chew caps
- To report blurred vision or ringing, roaring in ears (may indicate toxicity)
- To avoid driving, other hazardous activities if dizzy or drowsy
- That patient should drink at least 6-8 glasses of water/day
- To report change in urine pattern, weight increase, edema, pain in-

---

crease in joints, fever, blood in urine (indicates nephrotoxicity)
• That therapeutic effects may take up to 1 mo
• To avoid ASA, other OTC meds, alcohol; advise patient to use sunscreen

plasma protein fraction (℞)

Plasmanate, Plasma Plex, Plasmatein, PPF Protenate
Func. class.: Blood derivative
Chem. class.: Human plasma in NaCl

Action: Exerts similar oncotic pressure as human plasma, expands blood volume

Uses: Hypovolemic shock, hypoproteinemia, ARDS, preoperative cardiopulmonary bypass, acute liver failure, nephrotic syndrome

Dosage and routes:

Hypovolemia
• *Adult:* IV INF 250-500 ml (12.5-25 g protein), not to exceed 10 ml/min
• *Child:* IV INF 22-33 ml/kg at 5-10 ml/min

Hypoproteinemia
• *Adult:* IV INF 1000-1500 ml qd, not to exceed 8 ml/min

Available forms: Inj 50 mg/ml

Side effects/adverse reactions:

GI: Nausea, vomiting, increased salivation
INTEG: Rash, urticaria, cyanosis
CNS: Fever, chills, headache, paresthesias, flushing
RESP: Altered respirations, dyspnea, **pulmonary edema**
CV: **Fluid overload,** hypotension, erratic pulse

Contraindications: Hypersensitivity, CHF, severe anemia, renal insufficiency

Precautions: Decreased salt intake, decreased cardiac reserve, lack of albumin deficiency, hepatic disease, renal disease, pregnancy (C)

Pharmacokinetics: Metabolized as a protein/energy source

Lab test interferences:

False increase: Alk phosphatase

NURSING CONSIDERATIONS

Assess:
• Blood studies: Hct, Hgb, electrolytes, serum protein; if serum protein declines, dyspnea, hypoxemia can result
• B/P (decreased), pulse (erratic), respiration during infusion
• I&O ratio; urinary output may decrease
• CVP, pulmonary wedge pressure (increases if overload occurs)
• Allergy: fever, rash, itching, chills, flushing, urticaria, nausea, vomiting, or hypotension requires discontinuation of infusion; use new lot if therapy reinstituted

➡ Increased CVP reading: distended neck veins indicate circulatory overload; SOB, anxiety, insomnia, expiratory rales, frothy blood-tinged cough, cyanosis indicate pulmonary overload

Administer:

IV
• No dilution required; use infusion pump, use large-gauge needle (≥20G), discard unused portion, infuse slowly
• Within 4 hr of opening

Additive compatibilities: Carbohydrate and electrolyte sol, whole blood, packed red blood cells, chloramphenicol, tetracycline

Perform/provide:
• Adequate hydration before administration
• Storage—check type of albumin, date; may have to refrigerate

---

Evaluate:
• Therapeutic response: increased B/P, decreased edema, increased serum albumin

---

plicamycin (℞)

(ply-ka-my′sin)
mithramycin, Mithracin
Func. class.: Antineoplastic, antibiotic; hypocalcemic
Chem. class.: Crystalline aglycone

Action: Inhibits DNA, RNA, protein synthesis; derived from *Streptomyces plicatus;* replication is decreased by binding to DNA; demonstrates calcium-lowering effect not related to its tumoricidal activity; also acts on osteoclasts and blocks action of parathyroid hormone; a vesicant

Uses: Testicular cancer, hypercalcemia, hypercalciuria, symptomatic treatment of advanced neoplasms

Dosage and routes:
Testicular tumors
• *Adult:* IV 25-30 µg/kg/day × 8-10 days, not to exceed 30 µg/kg/day
Hypercalcemia/hypercalciuria
• *Adult:* IV 25 µg/kg/day × 3-4 days, repeat at intervals of 1 wk
Available forms: Inj 2.5 mg/vial powder

Side effects/adverse reactions:
META: Decreased serum Ca, P, K
*HEMA: **Hemorrhage, thrombocytopenia,** decreased pro-time, WBC count*
GI: Nausea, vomiting, anorexia, diarrhea, stomatitis, increased liver enzymes
GU: Increased BUN, creatinine; ***proteinuria***
INTEG: Rash, cellulitis, ***extravasation,*** facial flushing
CNS: Drowsiness, weakness, lethargy, headache, flushing, fever, depression

Contraindications: Hypersensitivity, thrombocytopenia, bone marrow depression, bleeding disorders, pregnancy (X), lactation

Precautions: Renal disease, hepatic disease, electrolyte imbalances

Pharmacokinetics: Crosses blood-brain barrier, excreted in urine; little known about pharmacokinetics

Interactions:
• Increased toxicity: other antineoplastics or radiation

NURSING CONSIDERATIONS
Assess:
• CBC, differential, platelet count qwk; withhold drug if WBC is <4000/mm^3 or platelet count is <50,000/mm^3; notify prescriber
• Renal function studies: BUN, serum uric acid, urine CrCl, electrolytes before, during therapy
• I&O ratio; report urine output <30 ml/hr
• Monitor temp q4h; fever may indicate beginning infection
• Liver function tests before, during therapy: bilirubin, AST (SGOT), ALT (SGPT), alk phosphatase prn or qmo
• Alkalosis if severe vomiting is present
◆ Toxicity: facial flushing, epistaxis, increased pro-time, thrombocytopenia; drug should be discontinued
• Bleeding: hematuria, guaiac stools, bruising or petechiae, mucosa or orifices q8h
• Food preferences; list likes, dislikes
• Inflammation of mucosa, breaks in skin
• Yellow skin, sclera; dark urine, clay-colored stools, itchy skin, abdominal pain, fever, diarrhea
• Buccal cavity q8h for dryness, sores, ulceration, white patches, oral pain, bleeding, dysphagia

---

• Local irritation, pain, burning at injection site
• Frequency of stools, characteristics, cramping
• Acidosis, signs of dehydration: rapid respirations, poor skin turgor, decreased urine output, dry skin, restlessness, weakness

Administer:
• Antiemetic 30-60 min before giving drug and 4-10 hr after treatment to prevent vomiting
• Transfusion for anemia
• Antispasmodic for diarrhea, phenothiazine for nausea and vomiting

IV
• Direct over 30 min
• IV dilute 2.5 mg/4.9 ml of sterile H_2O; (500 µg/ml) dilute single dose in 1000 ml of D_5W run over 4-6 hr
• EDTA for extravasation, apply ice compress
• Slow IV infusion using 20G, 21G needle

Y-site compatibilities: Allopurinol, amifostine, aztreonam, filgrastim, granisetron, melphalan, piperacillin/tazobactam, teniposide, thiotepa, vinorelbine

Perform/provide:
• Liquid diet: carbonated beverages; gelatin may be added if patient is not nauseated or vomiting
• Rinsing of mouth tid-qid with water; brushing of teeth with baking soda bid-tid with soft brush or cotton-tipped applicator for stomatitis; unwaxed dental floss
• Usage immediately after mixing

Evaluate:
• Therapeutic response: decreased tumor size, spread of malignancy

Teach patient/family:
• To report any complaints or side effects to nurse or prescriber
• To avoid foods with citric acid, hot or rough texture
• To report to prescriber any bleeding, white spots, ulcerations in the mouth; tell patient to examine mouth qd
• To avoid driving, activities requiring alertness; drowsiness may occur
• To report leg cramps, tingling of fingertips, weakness; may indicate hypocalcemia
• To avoid crowds, persons with infections when granulocyte count is low

---

podophyllum resin (R_X)
(poe-doe-fil'um rez'in)
Pod-Ben-25,   Podocon-25, Podofilm*, Podofin
Func. class.: Keratolytic
Chem. class.: Podophyllum derivative

Action: Arrests mitosis by binding to tubulin, protein subunit of spindle microtubules; also interferes with movements of chromosomes

Uses: Venereal warts, keratoses, multiple superficial epitheliomatoses

Dosage and routes:
Warts
• *Adult:* **TOP** cover wart, cover with wax paper, bandage for 1-4 hr, wash, may repeat qwk if needed

Keratoses/epitheliomatoses
• *Adult:* **TOP** apply qd with applicator, let dry, remove tissue, may reapply if needed

Available forms: Sol 11.5%, 25%

Side effects/adverse reactions:
HEMA: **Thrombocytopenia, leukopenia**
INTEG: Irritation of unaffected areas
CNS: Peripheral neuropathy
MISC: Paresthesia, nausea, vomiting, diarrhea, abdominal pain, confusion, dizziness, ***stupor, convulsions, coma, death***

Contraindications: Hypersensi-

---

tivity, pregnancy (X), bleeding, lactation, poor blood circulation, diabetes

Interactions:

• Necrosis of skin: when used with other keratolytic

NURSING CONSIDERATIONS
Assess:

• Platelets, WBC if systemic absorption occurs

• Allergic reactions: irritation, redness, itching, stinging, burning; drug should be discontinued

• Blood dyscrasias if systemic absorption is suspected: decrease platelets

⬧ CNS toxicity: peripheral neuropathy; drug should be discontinued

Administer:

• Only to affected area; cover normal skin with petrolatum for protection; do not apply to broken or inflamed skin; applied only by prescriber; not dispensed to patient

• Only to small areas or for short periods, or absorption (systemic) may occur

Evaluate:

• Therapeutic response: decrease in size, number of lesions

Teach patient/family:

• That discomfort will begin after 24 hr, subside in 2-4 days

• To use soap and water to clean area and remove drug

---

poliovirus vaccine, live, oral, trivalent (℞)
Orimune, OPV
Func. class.: Vaccine

Action: Produces specific antibodies for poliomyelitis
Uses: Prevention of polio
Dosage and routes:
• *Adult and child >2 yr:* **PO** 0.5 ml,

given q8wk × 2 doses, then 0.5 ml ½-1 yr after dose 2
• *Infant:* **PO** 0.5 ml at 2, 4, 18 mo; booster at 4-6 yr; may also be given: **IPV** at 2, 4 mo, then **OPV** at 12-18 mo, booster at 4-6 yr
Available forms: Oral vaccine; IPV
Side effects/adverse reactions:
*SYST: **Paralysis***
Contraindications: Hypersensitivity, active infection, allergy to neomycin/streptomycin, immunosuppression, vomiting, or diarrhea
Precautions: Pregnancy
Interactions:
• Do not use TB skin test or other live virus vaccines within 6 wk of vaccine
• Do not use within 3 mo of transfusion of whole blood, plasma, or use with immune serum globulin
NURSING CONSIDERATIONS
Assess:
• For anaphylaxis: inability to breathe, bronchospasm
Administer:
• Only **PO**
• Do not administer within 1 mo of other live virus vaccines
Perform/provide:
• Storage at 7° F (−13° C)
• Written record of immunization
Evaluate:
• For history of allergies, skin conditions (eczema, psoriasis, dermatitis), reactions to vaccinations

---

polymyxin B (℞)
(pol-ee-mix'in)
Aerosporin, polymyxin B Sulfate
Func. class.: Antiinfective-misc.
Chem. class.: Polymyxin

Action: Interferes with phospholipids, penetrates cell wall; immediately changes bacterial membrane, causing leakage of essential metabolites

Uses: Serious *P. aeruginosa, E. aerogenes, K. pneumoniae, E. coli, H. influenzae* infections or when other antibiotics cannot be used; septicemia, meningitis, UTIs

Dosage and routes:

• *Adult and child:* **IV INF** 15,000-25,000 U/kg/day in divided doses q12h

P. aeruginosa/H. influenzae

• *Adult and child >2 yr:* **INTRATHECAL** 50,000 U/day × 3-4 days, then 50,000 U/qod × 2 wk after CSF negative, glucose normal

• *Child <2 yr:* **INTRATHECAL** 20,000 U/day × 3-4 days, then 25,000 U/qod × 2 wk after CSF negative

Available forms: Inj 500,000 U

Side effects/adverse reactions:

INTEG: Urticaria, pain at inj site, phlebitis, flushing

CNS: Dizziness, confusion, weakness, drowsiness, paresthesia, slurred speech, ***coma, seizures,*** headache, stiff neck, irritability

RESP: ***Paralysis***

GU: ***Proteinuria, hematuria, azotemia, leukocyturia***

SYST: ***Anaphylaxis,*** superinfection

Contraindications: Hypersensitivity, severe renal disease

Precautions: Pregnancy (B)

Pharmacokinetics:

IM: Peak 2 hr, half-life 4½-6 hr, excreted in urine unchanged (60%)

IV: Data not available

Interactions:

• Increased skeletal muscle relaxation: anesthetics, neuromuscular blockers (tubocurarine decamethonium, succinylcholine, gallamine)

• Increased nephrotoxicity, neurotoxicity: aminoglycosides

NURSING CONSIDERATIONS

Assess:

• I&O ratio; report hematuria, oliguria

◆ Any patient with compromised renal system; drug is excreted slowly in poor renal system function; toxicity may occur rapidly; monitor BUN, creatinine

• Renal studies: urinalysis, protein, blood

• C&S before drug therapy; drug may be given as soon as culture is taken; C&S may be done after completion of therapy

• Skin eruptions, itching; drug should be discontinued

• Respiratory status: rate, character, dyspnea, symptoms of neuromuscular blockade, tightness in chest; discontinue drug

• Allergies before initiation of treatment, reaction of each medication; place allergies on chart in bright red letters; notify all people giving drugs

• For flushing of face, dizziness, disorientation, weakness, paresthesia, blurred vision, slurred speech, restlessness, irritability; indicate neurotoxicity

• For headache, fever, stiff neck; after intrathecal administration, indicate meningeal irritation

Administer:

• Intrathecal after reconstituting with 10 ml NS to yield 50,000 U/ml

IV

• After diluting 500,000 U/5 ml sterile H_2O or NS for inj (100,000 U/ml), then dilute each dose with 300-500 ml D_5W as cont inf over 60-90 min

Additive compatibilities: Amikacin, ascorbic acid, colistimethate, diphenhydramine, erythromycin, hydrocortisone, kanamycin, methicillin, penicillin G potassium or sodium, phenobarbital, ranitidine, vit B/C

Syringe compatibilities: Methicillin, penicillin G sodium
Y-site compatibilities: Esmolol
Perform/provide:

• Storage in dark area at room temp
• Do not use procaine HCl in intrathecal injection
• Adrenaline, suction, tracheostomy set, endotracheal intubation equipment on unit
Evaluate:

• Therapeutic response: absence of fever, purulent drainage, C&S negative
Teach patient/family:

• To report sore throat, fever, fatigue; may indicate superinfection
• To report dizziness, ringing in ears, loss of hearing, or muscle weakness
Treatment of overdose: Withdraw drug, maintain airway, administer epinephrine, aminophylline, O_2, IV corticosteroids

---

porfimer (℞)

(pour'fih-mur)

Photofiln

Func. class.: Antineoplastic-miscellaneous

Action: Used in photodynamic treatment of tumors (PDT); antitumor and cytotoxic actions are light and O_2 dependent; used with 630 nm laser light

Uses: Esophageal cancer (completely obstructing)
Dosage and routes:

• *Adult:* IV 2 mg/kg, then illumination with laser light 40-50 hr after inj; a second laser light application may be given 96-120 hr after inj; may repeat q30 days × 3
Available forms: Cake/powder for inj 75 mg
Side effects/adverse reactions:

CV: Hypotension, hypertension,

atrial fibrillation, **cardiac failure,** *tachycardia*
GI: Abdominal pain, constipation, diarrhea, dyspepsia, dysphagia, eructation, esophageal edema/ bleeding, hematemesis, melena, nausea, vomiting, anorexia
CNS: Anxiety, confusion, insomnia
RESP: **Pleural effusion,** pneumonia, dyspnea, respiratory insufficiency, **tracheoesophageal fistula**
MISC: Dehydration, weight decrease, anemia, photosensitivity reaction, UTI, moniliasis
Contraindications: Porphyria, porphyrin allergy (porfimer); tracheoesophageal, bronchoesophageal fistula; major blood vessels with eroding tumors (PDT)
Precautions: Elderly, pregnancy (C), lactation, children
Pharmacokinetics: Half-life 250 hr, 90% protein bound
Interactions:

• Increased photosensitivity: tetracyclines, sulfonamides, phenothiazines, sulfonylureas, thiazides, griseofulvin
NURSING CONSIDERATIONS
Assess:

• Ocular sensitivity: sensitivity to sun, bright lights, car headlights, patients should wear dark sunglasses with an average light transmittance of <4%
• Chest pain: may be so severe as to necessitate opiate analgesics
• For extravasation at inj site: take care to protect from light
Administer:

• As a single slow IV inj over 3-5 min at 2 mg/kg; reconstitute each vial with 31.8 ml D_5 or 0.9% NaCl (2.5 mg/ml), shake well; do not mix with other drugs or sol; protect from light and use immediately
• Laser light is initiated 630 nm wave length laser light

Side effects: *italics* = common; ***bold italics*** = life-threatening

Perform/provide:

• Wiping of spills with damp cloth, avoid skin/eye contact, use rubber gloves, eye protection, dispose of material in polyethylene bag according to policy

• To report chest pain, eye sensitivity

• To wear sunglasses with average white light transmittance of <4%

---

potassium bicarbonate/ potassium acetate/ potassium chloride/ potassium gluconate/ potassium phosphate (OTC, ℞)

Cena-K, Effer-K, Gen-K, K+10, K+ Care, Kaochlor, Kaochlor S-F, Kaon-Cl, Kaon-Cl-10, Kao-Nor, Kato, Kay Ciel, Kaylixir, K-Dur 10, K-Dur 20, K-G Elixir, K-Lease, Klor, Klor-Con, Klor-Con 8, Klor-Con 10, Klor-Con/25, Klortrix, Klorvess, K-Lyte, K-Lyte/Cl, K-Lyte DS, K-Norm, K-Tab, Micro-K, Micro KLS, My-K Elixir, Potachlor, Potage, Potasalan, potassium chloride, potassium gluconate, Rum-K, Slow-K, Ten-K, Tri-K, Twin-K, Urocit-K

Func. class.: Electrolyte
Chem. class.: Potassium

Action: Needed for adequate transmission of nerve impulses and cardiac contraction, renal function, intracellular ion maintenance
Uses: Prevention and treatment of hypokalemia
Dosage and routes:
Potassium bicarbonate
• *Adult:* **PO** dissolve 25-50 mEq in water qd-qid

Potassium acetate—hypokalemia
• *Adult and child:* **PO** 40-100 mEq/ day in divided doses 2-4 days
Hypokalemia (prevention)
• *Adult and child:* **PO** 20 mEq/day in 2-4 divided doses
Potassium chloride
• *Adult:* **PO** 40-100 mEq in divided doses tid-qid; **IV** 20 mEq/hr when diluted as 40 mEq/1000 ml, not to exceed 150 mEq/day
• *Child:* **PO** 2-4 mEq/kg/day
Potassium gluconate
• *Adult:* **PO** 40-100 mEq in divided doses tid-qid
Potassium phosphate
• *Adult:* **IV** 1 mEq/hr in sol of 60 mEq/L, not to exceed 150 mEq/day; **PO** 40-100 mEq/day in divided doses
• *Child:* **IV** max rate of inf 1 mEq/ kg/hr
Available forms: Tabs for sol 6.5, 25 mEq; caps, ext rel 8, 10 mEq; powder for sol 3.3, 5, 6.7, 10, 13.3 mEq/5 ml; tabs 2, 4, 5, 13.4 mEq; tabs, ext rel 6.7, 8, 10 mEq; elix 6.7 mEq/5 ml; oral sol 2.375 mEq/5 ml; inj for prep of IV 1.5, 2, 2.4, 3, 3.2, 4.4, 4.7 mEq/ml
Side effects/adverse reactions:
CNS: Confusion
CV: Bradycardia, *cardiac depression, dysrhythmias, arrest, peaking T waves, lowered R and depressed RST, prolonged P-R interval, widened QRS complex*
GI: Nausea, vomiting, cramps, pain, *diarrhea,* ulceration of small bowel
GU: Oliguria
INTEG: Cold extremities, rash
Contraindications: Renal disease (severe), severe hemolytic disease, Addison's disease, hyperkalemia, acute dehydration, extensive tissue breakdown
Precautions: Cardiac disease, K-sparing diuretic therapy, systemic acidosis, pregnancy (A)

◆ = Nursing alert   🌿 = Herb-drug interaction   🚫 = Do not crush

Pharmacokinetics:

PO: Excreted by kidneys and in feces; onset of action ≈30 min

IV: Immediate onset of action

Interactions:

• Hyperkalemia: potassium phosphate IV and products containing Ca or Mg; K-sparing, diuretic, or other K products

NURSING CONSIDERATIONS

Assess:

• ECG for peaking T waves, lowered R, depressed RST, prolonged P-R interval, widening QRS complex, hyperkalemia; drug should be reduced or discontinued

• K level during treatment (3.5-5 mg/dl is normal level)

• I&O ratio; watch for decreased urinary output; notify prescriber immediately

• Cardiac status: rate, rhythm, CVP, PWP, PAWP, if being monitored directly

Administer:

PO

• With meal or pc; dissolve effervescent tabs, powder in 8 oz cold water or juice; do not give IM, SC

IV

• Through large-bore needle to decrease vein inflammation; check for extravasation

• In large vein, avoiding scalp vein in child (IV)

• IV after diluting in large volume of IV sol and give as an inf, slowly by IV inf to prevent toxicity; never give IV bolus or IM

Potassium acetate

Additive compatibilities: Metoclopramide

Y-site compatibilities: Ciprofloxacin

Potassium chloride

Additive compatibilities: Aminophylline, amiodarone, atracurium, bretylium, calcium gluconate, cefepime, cephalothin, cephapirin, chloramphenicol, cimetidine, ciprofloxacin, clindamycin, cloxacillin, corticotropin, cytarabine, dimenhydrinate, dopamine, enalaprilat, erythromycin, floxacillin, fluconazole, furosemide, heparin, hydrocortisone, isoproterenol, lidocaine, metaraminol, methicillin, methyldopate, metoclopramide, mitoxantrone, nafcillin, netilmicin, norepinephrine, oxacillin, penicillin G potassium, phenylephrine, piperacillin, ranitidine, sodium bicarbonate, thiopental, vancomycin, verapamil, vit B/C

Y-site compatibilities: Acyclovir, aldesleukin, allopurinol, amifostine, aminophylline, amiodarone, ampicillin, amrinone, atropine, aztreonam, betamethasone, calcium gluconate, cefmetazole, cephalothin, cephapirin, chlordiazepoxide, chlorpromazine, ciprofloxacin, cladribine, cyanocobalamin, dexamethasone, digoxin, diltiazem, diphenhydramine, dobutamine, dopamine, droperidol, edrophonium, enalaprilat, epinephrine, esmolol, estrogens, ethacrynate, famotidine, fentanyl, filgrastim, fludarabine, fluorouracil, furosemide, gallium, granisetron, heparin, hydralazine, idarubicin, indomethacin, insulin (regular), isoproterenol, kanamycin, labetalol, lidocaine, lorazepam, magnesium sulfate, melphalan, meperidine, methicillin, methoxamine, methylergonovine, midazolam, minocycline, morphine, neostigmine, norepinephrine, ondansetron, oxacillin, oxytocin, paclitaxel, penicillin G potassium, pentazocine, phytonadione, piperacillin/tazobactam, prednisolone, procainamide, prochlorperazine, propofol, propranolol, pyridostigmine, sargramostim, scopolamine, sodium bicarbonate, succinylcholine, tacrolimus, teniposide, theophylline, thiotepa, trimethaphan, trimethobenzamide, vinorelbine, zidovudine

Perform/provide:

• Storage at room temp

Evaluate:

• Therapeutic response: absence of fatigue, muscle weakness; decreased thirst and urinary output; cardiac changes

Teach patient/family:

• To add potassium-rich foods to diet: bananas, orange juice, avocados; whole grains, broccoli, carrots, prunes, cocoa after this medication is discontinued

• To avoid OTC products: antacids, salt substitutes, analgesics, vitamin preparations, unless specifically directed by prescriber

• To report hyperkalemia symptoms (lethargy, confusion, diarrhea, nausea, vomiting, fainting, decreased output) or continued hypokalemia symptoms (fatigue, weakness, polyuria, polydipsia, cardiac changes)

• To take capsules with full glass of liquid

• To dissolve powder or tablet completely in at least 120 ml water or juice

🚫 Not to chew time-rel or ext-rel preparations

• Importance of regular follow-up visits

---

potassium iodide (℞)

Pima, potassium iodide solution, SSKI, Thyro-Block

Func. class.: Thyroid hormone antagonist

Chem. class.: Iodine product

Action: Inhibits secretion of thyroid hormone, fosters colloid accumulation in thyroid follicles, decreases vascularity of gland

Uses: Preparation for thyroidectomy, thyrotoxic crisis, neonatal thyrotoxicosis, radiation protectant, thyroid storm

Dosage and routes:

Thyrotoxic crisis

• *Adult and child:* PO 1 ml in water tid after meals (strong iodine sol)

Preparation for thyroidectomy

• *Adult and child:* PO 0.1-0.3 ml tid (strong iodine sol) or 5 gtt in water tid pc × 2-3 wk before surgery (potassium iodide sol)

Available forms: Sol 5%, 10%, 21 mg/gtt; tabs 130, 300 mg; inj 10%, 20%; oral syr 325 mg/5 ml; tabs 130 mg*

Side effects/adverse reactions:

ENDO: Hypothyroidism, hyperthyroid adenoma

INTEG: Rash, urticaria, *angineurotic edema,* acne, mucosal hemorrhage, fever

CNS: Headache, confusion, paresthesias

GI: Nausea, diarrhea, vomiting, small-bowel lesions, upper gastric pain

MS: Myalgia, arthralgia, weakness

EENT: Metallic taste, stomatitis, salivation, periorbital edema, sore teeth and gums, cold symptoms

Contraindications: Hypersensitivity to iodine, pulmonary edema, pulmonary TB, pregnancy (D)

Precautions: Lactation, children

Pharmacokinetics:

PO: Onset 24-48 hr, peak 10-15 days after continuous therapy, uptake by thyroid gland or excreted in urine; crosses placenta

Interactions:

• Hypothyroidism: lithium, other antithyroid agents

Lab test interferences:

Interference: Urinary 17-OHCS

NURSING CONSIDERATIONS

Assess:

• Pulse, B/P, temp

• I&O ratio; check for edema: puffy

 = Nursing alert   = Herb-drug interaction 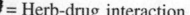 = Do not crush

hands, feet, periorbit; indicate hypothyroidism
• Weight qd; same clothing, scale, time of day
• T_3, T_4, which is increased; serum TSH, which is decreased; free thyroxine index, which is increased if dosage is too low; discontinue drug 3-4 wk before RAIU

◆ Overdose: peripheral edema, heat intolerance, diaphoresis, palpitations, dysrhythmias, severe tachycardia, fever, delirium, CNS irritability
• Hypersensitivity: rash; enlarged cervical lymph nodes may indicate drug should be discontinued
• Hypoprothrombinemia: bleeding, petechiae, ecchymosis
• Clinical response: after 3 wk should include increased weight, pulse; decreased T_4

Administer:
• Strong iodine solution after diluting with water or juice to improve taste
• Through straw to prevent tooth discoloration
• With meals to decrease GI upset
• At same time each day to maintain drug level
• Lowest dose that relieves symptoms, discontinue before RAIU

Perform/provide:
• Fluids to 3-4 L/day, unless contraindicated

Evaluate:
• Therapeutic response: weight gain, decreased pulse, T_4, size of thyroid gland

Teach patient/family:
• To abstain from breastfeeding after delivery
• To keep graph of weight, pulse, mood
• To avoid OTC products that contain iodine
• That seafood, other iodine products may be restricted

• Not to discontinue this medication abruptly; thyroid crisis may occur; stress response
• That response may take several mo if thyroid is large
• To discontinue drug, notify prescriber of fever, rash, metallic taste, swelling of throat; burning of mouth, throat; sore gums, teeth; severe GI distress, enlargement of thyroid, cold symptoms

---

povidone iodine (OTC)

(poe'vi-done)
Acu-Dyne, Betadine, Biodine Topical 1%, Efo-Dine, Iodex Regular, Mallisol, Operand Povidone-Iodine, Pharmadine, Polydine, Proviodine*
Func. class.: Disinfectant
Chem. class.: Iodophor

Action: Destroys a wide variety of microorganisms by local irritation, germicidal action
Uses: Cleansing wounds, disinfection, preoperative skin preparation
Dosage and routes:
• *Adult and child:* Use **SOL** as needed, topical only
Available forms: Top sol 1.5%, 3%
Side effects/adverse reactions:
*GU: **Renal damage***
*META: **Metabolic acidosis***
INTEG: Irritation
Contraindications: Hypersensitivity to iodine, pregnancy (vaginal antiseptic) (D)
Precautions: Extensive burns
Interactions:
• Do not use with alcohol or hydrogen peroxide
NURSING CONSIDERATIONS
Assess:
• For allergies to seafood; drug should not be used

Perform/provide:
• Storage in tight, light-resistant container
• Bandaging of areas if needed
Evaluate:
• Area of the body involved: irritation, rash, breaks, dryness, scales
Teach patient/family:
• To discontinue use if rash, irritation, or redness occurs

---

pramipexole (℞)

(pra-mi-pex′ol)
Mirapex
Func. class.: Antiparkinson agent
Chem. class.: Dopamine-receptor agonist, non-ergot

Action: Selective agonist for D_2 receptors (presynaptic/postsynaptic sites); binding at D_3 receptor contributes to antiparkinson effects
Uses: Parkinsonism
Dosage and routes:
Maintenance treatment
• *Adult:* **PO** 1.5-4.5 mg qd in 3 divided doses
Initial treatment
• *Adult:* **PO** from a starting dose of 0.375 mg/day given in 3 divided doses; increase gradually at 5-7 day intervals until total daily dose of 4.5 mg is reached
Available forms: Tabs 0.125, 0.25, 1.0, 1.5 mg
Side effects/adverse reactions:
HEMA: Hemolytic anemia, leukopenia, agranulocytosis
CNS: Agitation, insomnia, psychosis, hallucination, depression, dizziness
GI: Nausea, anorexia, constipation
CV: Orthostatic hypotension
GU: Impotence
EENT: Blurred vision

Contraindications: Hypersensitivity
Precautions: Renal disease, cardiac disease, MI with dysrhythmias, affective disorders, psychosis
Pharmacokinetics: Minimally metabolized
Interactions:
• Increased pramipexole levels: levodopa, cimetidine, ranitidine, diltiazem, triamterene, verapamil, quinidine
• Decreased pramipexole levels: dopamine antagonists
⬆ Decreased effect of pramipexole: chaste tree fruit
NURSING CONSIDERATIONS
Assess:
• Renal function studies
• Involuntary movements in parkinsonism: akinesia, tremors, staggering gait, muscle rigidity, drooling
• B/P, respiration during initial treatment; hypo/hypertension should be reported
• Mental status: affect, mood, behavioral changes, depression; complete suicide assessment
Administer:
• Drug until NPO before surgery
• Adjust dosage to patient response
• With meals
Perform/provide:
• Assistance with ambulation during beginning therapy
• Testing for diabetes mellitus, acromegaly if on long-term therapy
Evaluate:
• Therapeutic response: decrease in akathisia, increased mood
Teach patient/family:
• That therapeutic effects may take several wk to a few mo
• To change positions slowly to prevent orthostatic hypotension
• To use drug exactly as prescribed: if drug is discontinued abruptly, parkinsonian crisis may occur

---

pravastatin (℞)

(pra′va-sta-tin)
Pravachol
Func. class.: Antilipidemic

Action: Inhibits HMG-CoA reductase enzyme, which reduces cholesterol synthesis

Uses: As an adjunct in primary hypercholesterolemia (types IIa, IIb), to reduce the risk of recurrent MI, atherosclerosis

Dosage and routes:
• *Adult:* **PO** 10-20 mg qd at hs (range 10-40 mg qd)
• *Elderly/renal hepatic disease:* **PO** 10 mg/day

Available forms: Tabs 10, 20, 40 mg

Side effects/adverse reactions:
INTEG: Rash, pruritus
GI: Nausea, constipation, diarrhea, dyspepsia, flatus, abdominal pain, heartburn, *liver dysfunction,* pancreatitis, *hepatitis*
EENT: Lens opacities, common cold, rhinitis, cough
MS: Muscle cramps, myalgia, *myositis, rhabdomyolysis*
CNS: Headache, dizziness, psychic disturbances

Contraindications: Hypersensitivity, pregnancy (X), lactation, active liver disease

Precautions: Past liver disease, alcoholism, severe acute infections, trauma, hypotension, uncontrolled seizure disorders, severe metabolic disorders, electrolyte imbalances

Pharmacokinetics: Peak 1-1½ hr; metabolized by the liver, highly protein bound; excreted in urine, feces, breast milk; crosses placenta

Interactions:
• Increased risk for myopathy: erythromycin, niacin, cyclosporine, gemfibrozil, clofibrate, clarithromycin, itraconazole, protease inhibitors
• Increased effects of warfarin
• Decreased bioavailability of pravastatin: bile acid sequestrants

Lab test interferences:
Increase: CPK, liver function tests

NURSING CONSIDERATIONS
Assess:
• Whether patient is pregnant
• Fasting lipid profile: LDL, HDL, TG, Chol
• Liver function studies: baseline, q6wk during the first 3 mo, q8wk for remainder of yr, then q6mo; AST, ALT, liver function tests may increase
• Renal studies in patients with compromised renal system: BUN, I&O ratio, creatinine

Administer:
• Without regard to meals, hs

Perform/provide:
• Storage in cool environment in tight container protected from light

Evaluate:
• Therapeutic response: decrease in cholesterol to desired level after 8 wk

Teach patient/family:
• That blood work will be necessary during treatment
• To report blurred vision, severe GI symptoms, dizziness, headache, muscle pain, fever
• That regimen will continue: low-cholesterol diet, exercise program

praziquantel (℞)

(pray-zi-kwon′tel)
Biltricide
Func. class.: Anthelmintic
Chem. class.: Pyrazinoisoquinoline derivative

Action: Causes contraction, paralysis, leading to dislodgement of suckers; they are carried to liver, where phagocytosis takes place

Uses: Schistosomiasis, liver flukes, lung flukes, intestinal flukes, tapeworms

Dosage and routes:
• *Adult and child >4 yr:* **PO** 20 mg/kg q4-6h × 1 day
Available forms: Tabs 600 mg

Side effects/adverse reactions:
INTEG: Rash, pruritus, urticaria, internal hypertension
CNS: Dizziness, headache, drowsiness, malaise, increased seizure activity, fever, sweating
GI: Nausea, vomiting, anorexia, diarrhea, abdominal pain, increased liver enzymes

Contraindications: Hypersensitivity, lactation

Precautions: Child <4 yr, seizure disorders, pregnancy (B)

Pharmacokinetics:
PO: Peak 1-3 hr, half-life 48-90 min; metabolized by liver (metabolites); excreted in urine, breast milk; enters CSF

NURSING CONSIDERATIONS
Assess:
• Liver function tests: AST (SGOT), ALT (SGPT); watch for increase
• Stools during entire treatment, 1, 3 mo after treatment; specimens must be sent to lab while still warm
• For allergic reaction: rash, urticaria, pruritus
• For diarrhea during expulsion of worms
⬥ For CSF reaction: headache, high fever; drug should be discontinued, prescriber notified

Administer:
• Corticosteroids as ordered to reduce CNS effects (cerebral cysticercosis)
• Laxatives before treatment to cleanse bowel
• PO with liquids during meals to avoid GI symptoms

🚫 Whole; do not break, crush, or chew

Perform/provide:
• Storage in tight container in cool environment

Evaluate:
• Therapeutic response: expulsion of worms, 3 negative stool cultures after completion of treatment

Teach patient/family:
• To avoid driving, hazardous activities on day of treatment and day after treatment
• Proper hygiene after BM, including hand-washing technique; tell patient not to put fingers in mouth
• That tablets taste very bitter; keeping in mouth too long may cause gagging/vomiting
• The need for compliance with dosage schedule, duration of treatment
• To refrain from breastfeeding on day of treatment, 72 hr after

Treatment of overdose: Fast-acting laxative

---

prazosin (℞)
(pray'zoe-sin)
Minipress, Prazosin
Func. class.: Antihypertensive
Chem. class.: α₁-adrenergic blocker

Action: Peripheral blood vessels dilate, peripheral resistance drops; reduction in blood pressure results from α-adrenergic receptors being blocked

Uses: Hypertension, refractory CHF, Raynaud's vasospasm

Investigational uses: Benign prostatic hypertrophy to decrease urine outflow obstruction

Dosage and routes:
• *Adult:* **PO** 1 mg bid or tid, increasing to 20 mg qd in divided doses if required; usual range 6-15

⬥ = Nursing alert   🌿 = Herb-drug interaction   🚫 = Do not crush

mg/day, not to exceed 1 mg initially; max 20-40 mg/day
• *Child:* **PO** 5 µg/kg/dose, titrate up to 25 µg/kg/dose if needed, usual dosing interval q6h
Available forms: Caps 1, 2, 5 mg
Side effects/adverse reactions:
CV: Palpitations, orthostatic hypotension, tachycardia, edema, rebound hypertension
CNS: Dizziness, headache, drowsiness, anxiety, depression, vertigo, weakness, fatigue
GI: Nausea, vomiting, diarrhea, constipation, abdominal pain
GU: Urinary frequency, incontinence, impotence, priapism, H_2O, sodium retention
EENT: Blurred vision, epistaxis, tinnitus, dry mouth, red sclera
Contraindications: Hypersensitivity
Precautions: Pregnancy (C), children
Pharmacokinetics:
PO: Onset 2 hr, peak 1-3 hr, duration 6-12 hr, half-life 2-3 hr, metabolized in liver, excreted via bile, feces (>90%), in urine (<10%)
Interactions:
• Increased hypotensive effects: β-blockers, nitroglycerin
• Decreased effect: indomethacin
Lab test interferences:
Increase: Urinary norepinephrine, VMA
NURSING CONSIDERATIONS
Assess:
• B/P (sitting, standing) during initial treatment, periodically thereafter
• Pulse, jugular venous distention q4h
• BUN, uric acid if on long-term therapy
• Weight qd, I&O
• Edema in feet, legs qd

• Skin turgor, dryness of mucous membranes for hydration status
• Rales, dyspnea, orthopnea q30min
Perform/provide:
• Storage in tight container in cool environment
Evaluate:
• Therapeutic response: decreased B/P
Teach patient/family:
• That fainting occasionally occurs after 1st dose; do not drive or operate machinery for 4 hr after 1st dose, or take 1st dose at bedtime
Treatment of overdose: Administer volume expanders or vasopressors, discontinue drug, place in supine position

prednisolone/ prednisolone acetate/ prednisolone phosphate/ prednisolone tebutate (℞)
(pred-niss'oh-lone)
Articulose-50, Delta-Cortef, Hydeltrasol, Hydeltra-T.B.A., Key-Pred 25, Key-Pred 50, Key-Pred SP, Pediapred, Predaject-50, Predalone 50, Predalone-T.B.A., Predcor-25, Predcor-50, Prednisolone, Prednisolone Acetate, Prednisol TBA, Prelone
Func. class.: Corticosteroid
Chem. class.: Glucocorticoid, immediate acting

Action: Decreases inflammation by suppression of migration of polymorphonuclear leukocytes, fibroblasts; reversal to increase capillary permeability and lysosomal stabilization
Uses: Severe inflammation, immunosuppression, neoplasms

Dosage and routes:
- *Adult:* **PO** 2.5-15 mg bid-qid; **IM** 2-30 mg (acetate, phosphate) q12h; **IV** 2-30 mg (phosphate) q12h; 2-30 mg in joint or soft tissue (phosphate), 4-40 mg in joint of lesion (tebutate), 0.25-1 ml qwk in joints (acetate-phosphate)

Asthma/antiinflammatory
- *Child:* **PO** 1-2 mg/kg/day; **IV** 2-4 mg/kg/day

Available forms: Tabs 5 mg; inj 25, 50, 100 mg/ml acetate; inj 20 mg/ml tebutate; inj 20 mg/ml phosphate; inj 80 mg/ml acetate/phosphate

Side effects/adverse reactions:
INTEG: Acne, poor wound healing, ecchymosis, petechiae
CNS: **Depression,** flushing, sweating, headache, mood changes
CV: Hypertension, **circulatory collapse, thrombophlebitis, embolism,** tachycardia
HEMA: **Thrombocytopenia**
MS: Fractures, osteoporosis, weakness
GI: Diarrhea, nausea, abdominal distention, **GI hemorrhage,** increased appetite, *pancreatitis*
EENT: Fungal infections, increased intraocular pressure, blurred vision
Contraindications: Psychosis, hypersensitivity, idiopathic thrombocytopenia, acute glomerulonephritis, amebiasis, fungal infections, nonasthmatic bronchial disease, child <2 yr
Precautions: Pregnancy (C), diabetes mellitus, glaucoma, osteoporosis, seizure disorders, ulcerative colitis, CHF, myasthenia gravis
Pharmacokinetics:
PO: Peak 1-2 hr, duration 2 days
IM: Peak 3-45 hr
Interactions:
- Decreased action of prednisolone: cholestyramine, colestipol, barbiturates, rifampin, ephedrine, phenytoin, theophylline
- Decreased effects of anticoagulants, anticonvulsants, antidiabetics, ambenonium, neostigmine, isoniazid, toxoids, vaccines, anticholinesterases, salicylates, somatrem
- Increased side effects: alcohol, salicylates, indomethacin, amphotericin B, digitalis, cyclosporine, diuretics
- Increased action of prednisolone: salicylates, estrogens, indomethacin, oral contraceptives, ketoconazole, macrolide antibiotics

/ Potassium deficiency: aloe, buckthorn bark/berry, cascara sagrada bark, senna pod/leaf

Lab test interferences:
Increase: Cholesterol, Na, blood glucose, uric acid, Ca, urine glucose
Decrease: Ca, K, T_4, T_3, thyroid ^{131}I uptake test, urine 17-OHCS, 17-KS, PBI
False negative: Skin allergy tests

NURSING CONSIDERATIONS
Assess:
- K, blood sugar, urine glucose while on long-term therapy; hypokalemia and hyperglycemia
- Weight qd; notify prescriber if weekly gain >5 lb
- B/P q4h, pulse; notify prescriber if chest pain occurs
- I&O ratio; be alert for decreasing urinary output, increasing edema
- Plasma cortisol levels (long-term therapy) (normal level: 138-635 nmol/L SI units when drawn at 8 AM)
- Infection: increased temp, WBC, even after withdrawal of medication; drug masks infection
- K depletion: paresthesias, fatigue, nausea, vomiting, depression, polyuria, dysrhythmias, weakness
- Edema, hypertension, cardiac symptoms
- Mental status: affect, mood, behavioral changes, aggression

Administer:

• After shaking suspension (parenteral)

• Titrated dose; use lowest effective dose

• IM inj deep in large muscle mass; rotate sites; avoid deltoid; use 21G needle

• In one dose in AM to prevent adrenal suppression; avoid SC administration; may damage tissue

• With food or milk to decrease GI symptoms

IV

• Undiluted or added to NaCl or D_5 and given by IV inf; give 10 mg or less/1 min; decrease rate if burning occurs

Additive compatibilities: Ascorbic acid, cephalothin, cytarabine, erythromycin, fluorouracil, heparin, methicillin, penicillin G potassium, penicillin G sodium, vit B/C

Y-site compatibilities: Ciprofloxacin, heparin/hydrocortisone, potassium chloride, vit B/C

Perform/provide:

• Assistance with ambulation to patient with bone tissue disease to prevent fractures

Evaluate:

• Therapeutic response: ease of respirations, decreased inflammation

Teach patient/family:

• That ID as steroid user should be carried

• To notify prescriber if therapeutic response decreases; dosage adjustment may be needed

• Not to discontinue abruptly; adrenal crisis can result

• To avoid OTC products: salicylates, alcohol in cough products, cold preparations unless directed by prescriber

• About cushingoid symptoms

• The symptoms of adrenal insufficiency: nausea, anorexia, fatigue, dizziness, dyspnea, weakness, joint pain

---

prednisone (R)

(pred'ni-sone)
Apo-Prednisone*, Deltasone*, Liquid Pred, Meticorten, Orasone, Panasol-S, Prednicen-M, Prednisone, Sterapred, Winpred

Func. class.: Corticosteroid
Chem. class.: Intermediate-acting glucocorticoid

Action: Decreases inflammation by suppression of migration of polymorphonuclear leukocytes, fibroblasts, reversal to increase capillary permeability, and lysosomal stabilization

Uses: Severe inflammation, immunosuppression, neoplasms, multiple sclerosis, collagen disorders, dermatologic disorders

Dosage and routes:

• *Adult:* PO 1.5-2.5 mg bid-qid, then qd or qod; maintenance up to 250 mg/day

• *Child:* PO 0.05-2 mg/kg/day divided 1-4 ×/day

Nephrosis

• *Child 18 mo-4 yr:* 7.5-10 mg qid initially

• *Child 4-10 yr:* 15 mg qid initially

• *Child >10 yr:* 20 mg qid initially

Multiple sclerosis

• *Adult:* PO 200 mg/day × 1 wk, then 80 mg qod × 1 mo

Available forms: Tabs 1, 2.5, 5, 10, 20, 25, 50 mg; oral sol 5 mg/5 ml; syr 5 mg/5 ml

Side effects/adverse reactions:

CNS: Depression, flushing, sweating, headache, mood changes

CV: Hypertension, *circulatory collapse, thrombophlebitis, embolism,* tachycardia

---

816 prednisone

EENT: Fungal infections, increased intraocular pressure, blurred vision
GI: Diarrhea, nausea, abdominal distention, **GI hemorrhage,** increased appetite, pancreatitis
HEMA: **Thrombocytopenia**
INTEG: Acne, poor wound healing, ecchymosis, petechiae
MS: Fractures, osteoporosis, weakness

Contraindications: Psychosis, hypersensitivity, idiopathic thrombocytopenia, acute glomerulonephritis, amebiasis, fungal infections, nonasthmatic bronchial disease, child <2 yr, AIDS, TB

Precautions: Pregnancy (C), diabetes mellitus, glaucoma, osteoporosis, seizure disorders, ulcerative colitis, CHF, myasthenia gravis, renal disease, esophagitis, peptic ulcer

Pharmacokinetics:
PO: Well absorbed PO, peak 1-2 hr, duration 1-1½ days, half-life 3½-4 hr
Crosses placenta, enters breast milk, metabolized by liver after conversion

Interactions:
• Decreased action of prednisone: cholestyramine, colestipol, barbiturates, rifampin, ephedrine, phenytoin, theophylline
• Decreased effects of anticoagulants, anticonvulsants, antidiabetics, ambenonium, neostigmine, isoniazid, toxoids, vaccines, anticholinesterases, salicylates, somatrem
• Increased side effects: alcohol, salicylates, indomethacin, amphotericin B, digitalis, cyclosporine, diuretics
• Increased action of prednisone: salicylates, estrogens, indomethacin, oral contraceptives, ketoconazole, macrolide antibiotics
 Potassium deficiency: aloe, buckthorn bark/berry, rhubarb root, senna leaf/fruits

Lab test interferences:
Increase: Cholesterol, Na, blood glucose, uric acid, Ca, urine glucose
Decrease: Ca, K, T_4, T_3, thyroid ^{131}I uptake test, urine 17-OHCS, 17-KS, PBI
False negative: Skin allergy tests

NURSING CONSIDERATIONS
Assess:
• Adrenal insufficiency: nausea, vomiting, anorexia, confusion, hypotension
• K, blood sugar, urine glucose while on long-term therapy; hypokalemia and hyperglycemia
• Weight qd; notify prescriber of weekly gain >5 lb
• B/P q4h, pulse; notify prescriber of chest pain; monitor for rales, crackles, dyspnea if edema is present
• I&O ratio; be alert for decreasing urinary output, increasing edema
• Plasma cortisol (long-term therapy) (normal: 138-635 nmol/L SI units drawn at 8 AM)
• Infection: increased temp, WBC, even after withdrawal of medication; drug masks infection
• K depletion: paresthesias, fatigue, nausea, vomiting, depression, polyuria, dysrhythmias, weakness
• Edema, hypertension, cardiac symptoms
• Mental status: affect, mood, behavioral changes, aggression

Administer:
• Titrated dose; use lowest effective dose
• With food or milk to decrease GI symptoms

Perform/provide:
• Assistance with ambulation to patient with bone tissue disease to prevent fractures

Evaluate:
• Therapeutic response: ease of respirations, decreased inflammation

Teach patient/family:
• That ID as steroid user should be

---

carried; information on drug being taken and condition

• To notify prescriber if therapeutic response decreases; dosage adjustment may be needed

• To avoid vaccinations

• Not to discontinue abruptly, or adrenal crisis can result

• To avoid OTC products: salicylates, alcohol in cough products, cold preparations unless directed by prescriber

• About cushingoid symptoms: moon face, weight gain

• That drug causes immunosuppression; to report any symptoms of infection (fever, sore throat, cough)

• The symptoms of adrenal insufficiency: nausea, anorexia, fatigue, dizziness, dyspnea, weakness, joint pain

---

primaquine (Ṛ)
(prim'a-kween)

Func. class.: Antimalarial
Chem. class.: Synthetic 8-aminoquinolone

Action: Unknown; thought to destroy exoerythrocytic forms by gametocidal action

Uses: Malaria caused by *P. vivax,* in combination with clindamycin for *Pneumocystis carinii* pneumonia

Dosage and routes:

• *Adult:* PO 15 mg (base) qd × 2 wk; 26.3-mg tab is 15-mg base

• *Child:* PO 0.3 mg/kg qd × 2 wk

Available forms: Tabs 26.3 mg

Side effects/adverse reactions:

INTEG: Pruritus, skin eruptions

CNS: Headache

EENT: Blurred vision, difficulty focusing

GI: Nausea, vomiting, anorexia, cramps

CV: Hypertension

*HEMA: **Agranulocytosis, granulocytopenia, leukopenia, hemolytic anemia, leukocytosis,** mild anemia, **methemoglobinemia***

Contraindications: Hypersensitivity, anemia, lupus erythematosus, methemoglobinemia, porphyria, rheumatoid arthritis, methemoglobin reductase deficiency, G6PD deficiency

Precautions: Pregnancy (C)

Pharmacokinetics:

PO: Metabolized by liver (metabolites), half-life 3.7-9.6 hr

Interactions:

• Toxicity: quinacrine

NURSING CONSIDERATIONS
Assess:

• Ophthalmic test if long-term treatment or drug dosage >150 mg/day

• Liver studies qwk: AST, ALT, bilirubin, if on long-term therapy

• Blood studies: CBC; blood dyscrasias occur

• Allergic reactions: pruritus, rash, urticaria

• Blood dyscrasias: malaise, fever, bruising, bleeding (rare)

• For renal status: dark urine, hematuria, decreased output

➡ For hemolytic reaction: chills, fever, chest pain, cyanosis; drug should be discontinued immediately

Administer:

PO

• Before or after meals at same time each day to maintain drug level

Evaluate:

• Therapeutic response: decreased symptoms of malaria

Teach patient/family:

• To report visual problems, fever, fatigue, dark urine, bruising, bleeding; may indicate blood dyscrasias

• To complete full course of therapy

primidone (℞)
(pri'mi-done)
Apo-Primidone*, Myidone*, Mysoline, primidone, Sertan*
Func. class.: Anticonvulsant
Chem. class.: Barbiturate derivative

Action: Raises seizure threshold by conversion of drug to phenobarbital, decreases neuron firing

Uses: Generalized tonic-clonic (grand mal), complex-partial psychomotor seizures

Dosage and routes:
• *Adult and child >8 yr:* **PO** 250 mg/day; may increase by 250 mg/wk, not to exceed 2 g/day in divided doses qid
• *Child <8 yr:* **PO** 125 mg/day; may increase by 125 mg/wk, not to exceed 1 g/day in divided doses qid
Available forms: Tabs 50, 250 mg; susp 250 mg/5 ml; chew tabs 125 mg*

Side effects/adverse reactions:
*HEMA: **Thrombocytopenia, leukopenia, neutropenia, eosinophilia, megaloblastic anemia,** decreased serum folate level, lymphadenopathy*
CNS: Stimulation, drowsiness, dizziness, confusion, sedation, headache, flushing, hallucinations, coma, psychosis, ataxia, vertigo
GI: Nausea, vomiting, anorexia, hepatitis
INTEG: Rash, edema, alopecia, lupuslike syndrome
EENT: Diplopia, nystagmus, edema of eyelids
GU: Impotence

Contraindications: Hypersensitivity, porphyria, pregnancy (D)

Precautions: COPD, hepatic disease, renal disease, hyperactive children

Pharmacokinetics:
PO: Peak 4 hr; excreted by kidneys, in breast milk; half-life 3-24 hr

Interactions:
• Primidone levels are decreased by acetazolamide, succinimides, carbamazepine
• Primidone levels are increased by: isoniazid, nicotinamide, hydantoins
• Increased blood levels: alcohol, heparin, CNS depressants, isoniazid, phenytoin, phenobarbital

NURSING CONSIDERATIONS
Assess:
• For seizures, folic acid deficiency
• Drug level: therapeutic level 5-12 µg/ml; CBC should be done q6mo
• Mental status: mood, sensorium, affect, memory (long, short)
• Respiratory depression, wheezing
• Blood dyscrasias: fever, sore throat, bruising, rash, jaundice

Administer:
PO
• After shaking liquid susp well
• With food for GI upset
• Tablets crushed and mixed with food or fluid for swallowing difficulties

Evaluate:
• Therapeutic response: decreased seizures

Teach patient/family:
• Not to withdraw drug quickly; withdrawal symptoms may occur
• To avoid hazardous activities until stabilized on drug
• To carry Medic Alert ID with condition and medication
• To recognize the signs of blood dyscrasias; when to notify prescriber
• To avoid alcohol, CNS depressants

◆ = Nursing alert　　　🖋 = Herb-drug interaction　　　🛇 = Do not crush

probenecid (℞)

(proe-ben′e-sid)

Benemid, Benuryl*, probenecid

Func. class.: Uricosuric

Chem. class.: Sulfonamide derivative

Action: Inhibits tubular reabsorption of urates, with increased excretion of uric acids

Uses: Gonorrhea, hyperuricemia in gout, gouty arthritis, adjunct to cephalosporin or penicillin treatment

Dosage and routes:

Renal dose

• Avoid use if CrCl <30 ml/min

Gonorrhea

• *Adult:* **PO** 1 g with 3.5 g ampicillin or 1 g ½ hr before 4.8 million U of aqueous penicillin G procaine injected into 2 sites **IM**

Gout/gouty arthritis

• *Adult:* **PO** 250 mg bid for 1 wk, then 500 mg bid, not to exceed 2 g/day; maintenance: 500 mg/day × 6 mo

Adjunct in penicillin/cephalosporin treatment

• *Adult and child >50 kg:* **PO** 500 mg qid

• *Child <50 kg:* **PO** 25 mg/kg, then 40 mg/kg in divided doses qid

Available forms: Tabs 0.5 g

Side effects/adverse reactions:

CNS: Drowsiness, headache

CV: Bradycardia

GU: Glycosuria, thirst, frequency, **nephrotic syndrome**

GI: Gastric irritation, nausea, vomiting, anorexia, **hepatic necrosis**

INTEG: Rash, dermatitis, pruritus, fever

META: Acidosis, hypokalemia, hyperchloremia, hyperglycemia

RESP: **Apnea,** irregular respirations

Contraindications: Hypersensitivity, severe hepatic disease, severe renal disease, CrCl <50 mg/min, history of uric acid calculus

Precautions: Pregnancy (B), child <2 yr

Pharmacokinetics:

PO: Peak 2-4 hr, duration 8 hr, half-life 5-8 hr; metabolized by liver; excreted in urine

Interactions:

• Increased effect of acyclovir, barbiturates, allopurinol, benzodiazepines, dyphylline, zidovudine

• Increased toxicity: sulfa drugs, dapsone, clofibrate, indomethacin, rifampin, naproxen, methotrexate, pantothenic acid

• Decreased action of probenecid: salicylates

Lab test interferences:

False positive: Urine glucose with copper sulfate test (Clinitest)

Increase: BSP/urinary PSP, theophylline levels

NURSING CONSIDERATIONS

Assess:

• Uric acid levels (3-7 mg/dl); mobility, joint pain, swelling

• Respiratory rate, rhythm, depth; notify prescriber of abnormalities

• Electrolytes, CO_2 before, during treatment

• Urine pH, output, glucose during beginning treatment

◆ For CNS symptoms; confusion, twitching, hyperreflexia, stimulation, headache; may indicate overdose

Administer:

• After meals or with milk if GI symptoms occur

• Increase fluid intake to 2-3 L/day to prevent urinary calculi

Evaluate:

• Therapeutic response: absence of pain, stiffness in joints

Teach patient/family:

• To avoid OTC preparations (aspirin) unless directed by prescriber

procainamide (R)

(proe-kane-ah'mide)
procainamide, Procanbid, Procan SR, Promine, Pronestyl, Pronestyl-SR, Rhythmin
Func. class.: Antidysrhythmic (Class IA)
Chem. class.: Procaine HCl amide analog

Action: Depresses excitability of cardiac muscle to electrical stimulation and slows conduction in atrium, bundle of His, and ventricle

Uses: PVCs, atrial fibrillation, PAT, ventricular tachycardia, atrial dysrhythmias, ventricular tachycardia

Dosage and routes:

Renal dose
• CrCl 10-50 ml/min give q6-12h; CrCl <10 ml/min give q8-24h

Atrial fibrillation/PAT
• *Adult:* **PO** 1-1.25 g, may give another 750 mg if needed; if no response, 500 mg-1g q2h until desired response; maintenance 50 mg/kg in divided doses q6h

Ventricular tachycardia
• *Adult:* **PO** 1g; maintenance 50 mg/kg/day given in 3 hr intervals; **SUS REL TABS** 500 mg-1.25 g q6h

Other dysrhythmias
• *Adult:* **IV BOL** 100 mg q5min, given 25-50 mg/min, not to exceed 500 mg; or 17 mg/kg total then **IV INF** 2-6 mg/min

Available forms: Caps 250, 375, 500 mg; tabs 250, 375, 500 mg; tabs sus rel 250, 500, 750, 1000 mg; inj 100, 500 mg/ml

Side effects/adverse reactions:

CNS: Headache, dizziness, confusion, psychosis, restlessness, irritability, weakness
GI: Nausea, vomiting, anorexia, diarrhea, hepatomegaly

*CV: Hypotension, **heart block, cardiovascular collapse, arrest***
HEMA: SLE syndrome, **agranulocytosis, thrombocytopenia, neutropenia, hemolytic anemia**
INTEG: Rash, urticaria, edema, swelling (rare), pruritus

Contraindications: Hypersensitivity, myasthenia gravis, severe heart block

Precautions: Pregnancy (C), lactation, children, renal disease, liver disease, CHF, respiratory depression

Pharmacokinetics:

PO: Peak 1-2 hr, duration 3 hr (8 hr extended)
IM: Peak 10-60 min, duration 3 hr; half-life 3 hr
Metabolized in liver to active metabolites, excreted unchanged by kidneys (60%)

Interactions:
• Increased effects of neuromuscular blockers, anticholinergics, antihypertensives
• Increased procainamide effects: cimetidine
• Decreased effects of procainamide: barbiturates
• Increased toxicity: other antidysrhythmics
 Increased anticholinergic effect: henbane leaf

NURSING CONSIDERATIONS

Assess:
• ECG continuously if using IV to determine increased PR or QRS segments; discontinue immediately; watch for increased ventricular ectopic beats, maximum need to rebolus
• Blood levels, 3-10 μg/ml or NAPA levels
• CBC q2wk × 3 mo
• B/P continuously for fluctuations
• I&O ratio; electrolytes (K, Na, Cl)
• Malignant hyperthermia: tachy-

pnea, tachycardia, changes in B/P, fever
• Cardiac rate, rhythm, character
• Respiratory status: rate, rhythm, character, lung fields; bilateral rales may occur in CHF patient; watch for respiratory depression
• CNS effects: dizziness, confusion, psychosis, paresthesias, convulsions; drug should be discontinued
• Increased respiration, increased pulse; drug should be discontinued

Administer:
IM
• IM injection in deltoid; aspirate to avoid intravascular administration
IV
• After diluting 100 mg/ml of D_5W or sterile H_2O for inj; give 20 mg or less/1 min; may dilute 1 g/250-500 ml D_5W, run at 2-6 mg/min
• Check IV site q8h for infiltration or extravasation

Additive compatibilities: Amiodarone, atracurium, dobutamine, flumazenil, lidocaine, netilmicin, verapamil

Solution compatibilities: D_5W, D_5/0.9% NaCl, 0.45% NaCl, 0.9% NaCl, water for inj

Y-site compatibilities: Amiodarone, famotidine, heparin, hydrocortisone, potassium chloride, ranitidine, vit B/C

Evaluate:
• Therapeutic response: decreased dysrhythmias

Teach patient/family:
• That wax matrix may appear in stools
• Not to discontinue without healthcare provider's advice

---

procaine (℞)
(proe'kane)
Novocain, Unicaine
Func. class.: Local anesthetic
Chem. class.: Ester

Action: Competes with calcium for sites in nerve membrane that control sodium transport across cell membrane; decreases rise of depolarization phase of action potential

Uses: Spinal anesthesia, epidural, peripheral nerve block, perineum, lower extremities, infiltration

Dosage and routes:
Vary by route of anesthesia
Available forms: Inj 1%, 2%, 10%

Side effects/adverse reactions:
CNS: Anxiety, restlessness, *convulsions, loss of consciousness,* drowsiness, disorientation, tremors, shivering
CV: ***Myocardial depression, cardiac arrest, dysrhythmias,*** bradycardia, hypotension, hypertension, fetal bradycardia
GI: Nausea, vomiting
EENT: Blurred vision, tinnitus, pupil constriction
INTEG: Rash, urticaria, allergic reactions, edema, burning, skin discoloration at injection site, tissue necrosis
RESP: ***Status asthmaticus, respiratory arrest, anaphylaxis***

Contraindications: Hypersensitivity, child <12 yr, elderly, severe liver disease

Precautions: Elderly, severe drug allergies, pregnancy (C)

Pharmacokinetics: Onset 2-5 min, duration 1 hr; metabolized by liver, excreted in urine (metabolites)

Interactions:
• Dysrhythmias: epinephrine, halothane, enflurane

P

- Hypertension: MAOIs, tricyclic antidepressants, phenothiazines
- Decreased action of procaine: chloroprocaine

NURSING CONSIDERATIONS
Assess:

- B/P, pulse, respiration during treatment
- Fetal heart tones if drug is used during labor
- Allergic reactions: rash, urticaria, itching
- Cardiac status: ECG for dysrhythmias, pulse, B/P during anesthesia

Administer:

- Only drugs that are not cloudy, do not contain precipitate
- Only with crash cart, resuscitative equipment nearby
- Only drugs without preservatives for epidural or caudal anesthesia

Additive compatibilities: Ascorbic acid, cephalothin, hydrocortisone, methicillin, penicillin G potassium, penicillin G sodium, vit B/C

Syringe compatibilities: Ampicillin, cloxacillin, glycopyrrolate, hydroxyzine, methicillin

Perform/provide:

- Use of new sol; discard unused portions

Evaluate:

- Therapeutic response: anesthesia necessary for procedure

Treatment of overdose: Airway, O$_2$, vasopressor, IV fluids, anticonvulsants for seizures

---

procarbazine (R)
(proe-kar′ba-zeen)
Matulane, Natulan*
Func. class.: Antineoplastic, alkylating agent
Chem. class.: Hydrazine derivative

Action: Inhibits DNA, RNA, protein synthesis; has multiple sites of action; a nonvesicant

Uses: Lymphoma, Hodgkin's disease, cancers resistant to other therapy

Investigational uses: Brain, lung malignancies, other lymphomas, multiple myeloma, malignant melanoma, polycythemia vera

- *Adult:* **PO** 2-4 mg/kg/day for first wk; maintain dosage of 4-6 mg/kg/day until platelets and WBC fall; after recovery, 1-2 mg/kg/day
- *Child:* **PO** 50 mg/m^2/day for 7 days, then 100 mg/m^2 until desired response, leukopenia, or thrombocytopenia occurs; 50 mg/day is maintenance after bone marrow recovery

Available forms: Caps 50 mg
Side effects/adverse reactions:
HEMA: ***Thrombocytopenia, anemia, leukopenia, myelosuppression, bleeding tendencies,*** purpura, petechiae, epistaxis
GI: Nausea, vomiting, anorexia, diarrhea, constipation, dry mouth, stomatitis
EENT: Retinal hemorrhage, nystagmus, photophobia, diplopia
INTEG: Rash, pruritus, dermatitis, alopecia, herpes, hyperpigmentation
CNS: Headache, dizziness, insomnia, hallucinations, confusion, coma, pain, chills, fever, sweating, paresthesias
RESP: Cough, pneumonitis

◆ = Nursing alert   ∥ = Herb-drug interaction   ⊘ = Do not crush

MS: Arthralgias, myalgias

GU: Azoospermia, cessation of menses

Contraindications: Hypersensitivity, pregnancy (D), thrombocytopenia, bone marrow depression

Precautions: Renal disease, hepatic disease, radiation therapy

Pharmacokinetics: Half-life 1 hr; concentrates in liver, kidney, skin; metabolized in liver, excreted in urine

Interactions:
• Increased CNS depression: barbiturates, antihistamines, narcotics, hypotensive agents, phenothiazines
• Disulfiram-like reaction: ethyl alcohol, MAOIs, tricyclic antidepressants, tyramine foods, sympathomimetic drugs
• Hypertension: guanethidine, levodopa, methyldopa, reserpine
• Increased hypoglycemia: insulin, oral hypoglycemics

NURSING CONSIDERATIONS

Assess:
• CBC, differential, platelet count qwk; withhold drug if WBC is <4000/mm³ or platelet count is <100,000/mm³; notify prescriber
• Renal function studies: BUN, serum uric acid, urine CrCl, electrolytes before, during therapy
• I&O ratio, report fall in urine output to <30 ml/hr
• Monitor temp q4h; fever may indicate beginning infection
• Liver function tests before, during therapy: bilirubin, AST, ALT, alk phosphatase prn or q1no
• CNS changes: confusion, paresthesias, neuropathies, drug should be discontinued
◆ Toxicity: facial flushing, epistaxis, increased pro-time, thrombocytopenia; drug should be discontinued
• Bleeding: hematuria, guaiac stools, bruising or petechiae, mucosa or orifices q8h

• Food preferences; list likes, dislikes
• Effects of alopecia on body image; discuss feelings about body changes
• Inflammation of mucosa, breaks in skin
• Yellow skin, sclera; dark urine, clay-colored stools, itchy skin, abdominal pain, fever, diarrhea
• Buccal cavity q8h for dryness, sores or ulceration, white patches, oral pain, bleeding, dysphagia
• Alkalosis if vomiting is severe
• GI symptoms: frequency of stools, cramping
• Acidosis, signs of dehydration: rapid respirations, poor skin turgor, decreased urine output, dry skin, restlessness, weakness

Administer:
• In divided doses and at hs to minimize nausea and vomiting
• Nonphenothiazine antiemetic 30-60 min before giving drug and 4-10 hr after treatment to prevent vomiting
• Transfusion for anemia
• Antispasmodic for GI symptoms

Perform/provide:
• Liquid diet: carbonated beverages; gelatin may be added if patient is not nauseated or vomiting
• Storage in tight, light-resistant container in cool environment

Evaluate:
• Therapeutic response: decreased tumor size, spread of malignancy

Teach patient/family:
• To report any complaints, side effects to nurse or prescriber; cough, shortness of breath, fever, chills, sore throat, bleeding, bruising, vomiting blood; black, tarry stools
• That hair may be lost during treatment and wig or hairpiece may make patient feel better; tell patient that new hair may be different in color, texture

• To avoid foods with citric acid, hot or rough texture
• To report any bleeding, white spots, ulcerations in mouth to prescriber; tell patient to examine mouth qd
• To avoid driving, activities requiring alertness; dizziness may occur
• That contraceptive measures are recommended during therapy
• To avoid ingestion of alcohol, tyramine-containing foods; cold, hay fever, weight-reducing products may cause serious drug interactions
• To avoid crowds, persons with infections if granulocytes are low

---

prochlorperazine (R)

(proe-klor-pair'a-zeen)
Chlorpazine, Compa-Z, Compazine, Contranzine, Provacin*, Stemetil*, Ultrazine
Func. class.: Antiemetic, antipsychotic
Chem. class.: Phenothiazine, piperazine derivative

Action: Acts centrally by blocking chemoreceptor trigger zone, which in turn acts on vomiting center
Uses: Nausea, vomiting
Dosage and routes:
Postoperative nausea/vomiting
• *Adult:* **IM** 5-10 mg 1-2 hr before anesthesia; may repeat in 30 min; **IV** 5-10 mg 15-30 min before anesthesia; **IV INF** 20 mg/L D_5W or **NS** 15-30 min before anesthesia, not to exceed 40 mg/day
Severe nausea/vomiting
• *Adult:* **PO** 5-10 mg tid-qid; **SUS REL** 15 mg qd in AM or 10 mg q12h; **RECT** 25 mg/bid; **IM** 5-10 mg; may repeat q4h, not to exceed 40 mg/day
• *Child 18-39 kg:* **PO** 2.5 mg tid or 5 mg bid, not to exceed 15 mg/day; **IM** 0.132 mg/kg

• *Child 14-17 kg:* **PO/RECT** 2.5 mg bid-tid, not to exceed 10 mg/day; **IM** 0.132 mg/kg
• *Child 9-13 kg:* **PO/RECT** 2.5 mg qd-bid, not to exceed 7.5 mg/day; **IM** 0.132 mg/kg
Available forms: Syr 5 mg/ml; inj 5 mg/ml; tabs 5, 10, 25 mg; caps, sus rel 10, 15, 30 mg; supp 2.5, 5, 25 mg
Side effects/adverse reactions:
CNS: **Neuroleptic malignant syndrome,** *extrapyramidal reactions, tardive dyskinesia, euphoria, **depression,** EPS,* restlessness, tremor, dizziness
GI: Nausea, vomiting, anorexia, dry mouth, diarrhea, constipation, weight loss, metallic taste, cramps
CV: **Circulatory failure, tachycardia**
RESP: **Respiratory depression**
Contraindications: Hypersensitivity to phenothiazines, coma, seizure, encephalopathy, bone marrow depression
Precautions: Children <2 yr, pregnancy (C), elderly, lactation
Pharmacokinetics:
PO: Onset 30-40 min, duration 3-4 hr
SUS REL: Onset 30-40 min, duration 10-12 hr
RECT: Onset 60 min, duration 3-4 hr
IM: Onset 10-20 min, duration 12 hr
Metabolized by liver; excreted in urine, breast milk; crosses placenta
Interactions:
• Decreased effect of prochlorperazine: barbiturates, antacids
• Increased anticholinergic action: anticholinergics, antiparkinson drugs, antidepressants
🍃 Increased anticholinergic effect: henbane leaf
Lab test interferences:
Increase: Liver function tests, cardiac enzymes, cholesterol, blood glucose, prolactin, bilirubin, PBI, ^{131}I,

---

◆ = Nursing alert   🍃 = Herb-drug interaction   🚫 = Do not crush

alk phosphatase, leukocytes, granulocytes, platelets
Decrease: Hormones (blood and urine)
False positive: Pregnancy tests, PKU, urine bilirubin
False negative: Urinary steroids, 17-OHCS, pregnancy tests

NURSING CONSIDERATIONS
Assess:

• EPS: abnormal movement, tardive dyskinesia, akathisia
• VS, B/P; check patients with cardiac disease more often
• Respiratory status before, during, after administration of emetic; check rate, rhythm, character; respiratory depression can occur rapidly with elderly or debilitated patients

Administer:

• IM injection in large muscle mass; aspirate to avoid IV administration

IV

• Keep patient recumbent for ½ hr
• IV after diluting 5 mg/9 ml of NaCl for inj (0.5 mg/ml); give 5 mg or less/min; may dilute 10-20 mg/L NaCl and give as infusion; can cause contact dermatitis

Additive compatibilities: Amikacin, ascorbic acid, dexamethasone, dimenhydrinate, erythromycin, ethacrynate, lidocaine, nafcillin, sodium bicarbonate, vit B/C

Syringe compatibilities: Atropine, butorphanol, chlorpromazine, cimetidine, diamorphine, diphenhydramine, droperidol, fentanyl, glycopyrrolate, hydroxyzine, meperidine, metoclopramide, nalbuphine, pentazocine, perphenazine, promazine, promethazine, ranitidine, scopolamine, sufentanil

Y-site compatibilities: Amsacrine, calcium gluconate, cisplatin, cladribine, cyclophosphamide, cytarabine, doxorubicin, fluconazole, granisetron, heparin, hydrocortisone, melphalan, methotrexate, ondansetron, paclitaxel, potassium chloride, propofol, sargramostim, sufentanil, teniposide, thiotepa, vinorelbine, vit B/C

Evaluate:

• Therapeutic response: absence of nausea, vomiting

Teach patient/family:

• To avoid hazardous activities, activities requiring alertness; dizziness may occur
• To avoid alcohol
• Not to double or skip doses
• That urine may be pink to reddish brown
• To report dark urine, clay-colored stools, bleeding, bruising, rash, blurred vision

---

procyclidine (R)

(proc-sye'kli-deen)
Kemadrin, Procyclid*
Func. class.: Cholinergic blocker
Chem. class.: Tertiary amine

Action: Centrally acting anticholinergic

Uses: Parkinson symptoms, extrapyramidal disorders

Dosage and routes:

• *Adult:* **PO** 2.5 mg tid pc, titrated to patient response

Available forms: Tabs 5 mg

Side effects/adverse reactions:

MS: Weakness, cramping
INTEG: Rash, urticaria, dermatoses
MISC: Fever, flushing, decreased sweating, hyperthermia, *heat stroke*, numbness of fingers
CNS: Confusion, anxiety, restlessness, irritability, delusions, hallucinations, headache, sedation, depression, incoherence, dizziness, lightheadedness, memory loss
EENT: Blurred vision, photophobia, dilated pupils, difficulty swallow-

826   progesterone

ing, mydriasis, increased intraocular tension, angle-closure glaucoma
CV: Palpitations, tachycardia, postural hypotension, bradycardia
GI: Dryness of mouth, constipation, nausea, vomiting, abdominal distress, *paralytic ileus, epigastric distress*
GU: Hesitancy, retention, dysuria
Contraindications: Hypersensitivity, narrow-angle glaucoma, myasthenia gravis, GI/GU obstruction, child <3 yr, megacolon, stenosing peptic ulcer, prostatic hypertrophy
Precautions: Pregnancy (C), elderly, lactation, tachycardia, children, kidney, liver disease, drug abuse, hypotension, hypertension, psychiatric patients, prostatic hypertrophy
Pharmacokinetics:
PO: Onset 30-45 min, duration 4-6 hr
Interactions:
• Decreased action of haloperidol, levodopa
• Increased anticholinergic effect: antihistamines, MAOIs, phenothiazines, amantadine

NURSING CONSIDERATIONS
Assess:
• Response if patient receiving anticholinergic agents
• I&O ratio; retention commonly causes decreased urinary output
• Heart rate, rhythm, B/P
• Parkinsonism: shuffling gait, muscle rigidity, involuntary movements (elderly)
• Urinary hesitancy, retention; palpate bladder if retention occurs (elderly)
• Constipation, especially elderly; increase fluids, bulk, exercise; if this occurs, palpate abdomen
• For tolerance over long-term therapy; dose may have to be increased or changed

• Mental status: affect, mood, CNS depression, worsening of mental symptoms during early therapy (elderly)
Administer:
• With or after meals for GI upset; may give with fluids other than water
• At hs to avoid daytime drowsiness in patient with parkinsonism
Perform/provide:
• Storage at room temp in tight container
• Hard candy, frequent drinks, sugarless gum to relieve dry mouth
Evaluate:
• Therapeutic response: decreased involuntary movements
Teach patient/family:
• Not to discontinue this drug abruptly; to taper off over 1 wk
• To avoid driving, other hazardous activities; drowsiness may occur
• To avoid OTC medication: cough, cold preparations with alcohol, antihistamines unless directed by prescriber
• To avoid alcohol

---

progesterone (℞)
(proe-jess'ter-one)
Crinone, Progestacert, progesterone, Progesterone in Oil
Func. class.: Progestogen
Chem. class.: Progesterone derivative

Action: Inhibits secretion of pituitary gonadotropins, which prevents follicular maturation, ovulation; stimulates growth of mammary tissue; antineoplastic action against endometrial cancer
Uses: Contraception, amenorrhea, premenstrual syndrome, abnormal uterine bleeding

---

 = Nursing alert   = Herb-drug interaction   = Do not crush

Dosage and routes:
Infertility
• *Adult:* **VAG** 90 mg g d
Amenorrhea/uterine bleeding
• *Adult:* **IM** 5-10 mg qd × 6-8 doses
Contraception
• *Adult:* **INSERT** 1 in uterine cavity, active for 1 yr
PMS
• *Adult:* **RECT SUPP/VAG SUPP** 200-400 mg
Available forms: Inj 50 mg/ml; powder micronized, vag gel 8%, intrauterine system
Side effects/adverse reactions:
CNS: Dizziness, headache, migraines, depression, fatigue
CV: Hypotension, ***thrombophlebitis,*** edema, ***thromboembolism, stroke, pulmonary embolism, MI***
GI: Nausea, vomiting, anorexia, cramps, increased weight, ***cholestatic jaundice***
EENT: Diplopia
GU: Amenorrhea, cervical erosion, breakthrough bleeding, dysmenorrhea, vaginal candidiasis, breast changes, *gynecomastia, testicular atrophy, impotence,* endometriosis, ***spontaneous abortion***
INTEG: Rash, urticaria, acne, hirsutism, alopecia, oily skin, seborrhea, purpura, melasma
META: Hyperglycemia
Contraindications: Breast cancer, hypersensitivity, thromboembolic disorders, reproductive cancer, genital bleeding (abnormal, undiagnosed), cerebral hemorrhage, pregnancy (X)
Precautions: Lactation, hypertension, asthma, blood dyscrasias, gallbladder disease, CHF, diabetes mellitus, bone disease, depression, migraine headache, convulsive disorders, hepatic disease, renal disease, family history of breast or reproductive tract cancer

Pharmacokinetics:
IM, Rect, Vag: Duration 24 hr
Excreted in urine, feces; metabolized in liver
Lab test interferences:
Increase: Alk phosphatase, nitrogen (urine), pregnanediol, amino acids, factors VII, VIII, IX, X
Decrease: GTT, HDL

NURSING CONSIDERATIONS
Assess:
• Weight qd; notify prescriber of weekly weight gain >5 lb
• B/P at beginning of treatment and periodically
• I&O ratio; be alert for decreasing urinary output, increasing edema
• Liver function studies: ALT (SGPT), AST (SGOT), bilirubin periodically during long-term therapy
• Edema, hypertension, cardiac symptoms, jaundice
• Mental status: affect, mood, behavioral changes, depression
• Hypercalcemia
Administer:
• Titrated dose, use lowest effective dose
• Oil solution deep in large muscle mass IM; rotate sites
• After warming to dissolve crystals
• In one dose in AM
• With food or milk to decrease GI symptoms
Perform/provide:
• Storage in dark area
Evaluate:
• Therapeutic response: decreased abnormal uterine bleeding, absence of amenorrhea
Teach patient/family:
• To report breast lumps, vaginal bleeding, edema, jaundice, dark urine, clay-colored stools, dyspnea, headache, blurred vision, abdominal pain, numbness or stiffness in legs, chest pain

P

- To report suspected pregnancy
- To monitor blood sugar if diabetic

---

promazine (℞)

(proe′ma-zeen)
Promanyl, promazine, Prozine, Sparine

Func. class.: Antipsychotic, neuroleptic

Chem. class.: Phenothiazine, aliphatic

Action: Depresses cerebral cortex, hypothalamus, limbic system, which control activity, aggression; blocks neurotransmission produced by dopamine at synapse; exhibits a strong α-adrenergic, anticholinergic blocking action; as antiemetic, inhibits medullary chemoreceptor trigger zone; mechanism for antipsychotic effects is unclear

Uses: Psychotic disorders, schizophrenia, nausea, vomiting, alcohol withdrawal

Dosage and routes:

Psychosis
- *Adult:* **PO** 10-200 mg q4-6h, max dose 1 g/day; **IM** 50-150 mg, followed in 30 min with additional dose up to a total dose of 300 mg
- *Geriatric:* **PO** 25 mg qd-bid, increase by 25 mg q4-7 days
- *Child >12 yr:* **PO** 10-25 mg q4-6h

Nausea/vomiting
- *Adult:* **PO** 25-50 mg q4-6h; **IM** 50 mg; **IV** not recommended, but may use in concentrations of <25 mg/ml

Available forms: Tabs 25, 50, 100 mg; inj 25, 50 mg/ml

Side effects/adverse reactions:

RESP: **Laryngospasm,** dyspnea, *respiratory depression*

*CNS: EPS: pseudoparkinsonism, akathisia, dystonia, tardive dyski-nesia, drowsiness, headache, **seizures***

HEMA: Anemia, **leukopenia, leukocytosis, agranulocytosis**

INTEG: Rash, photosensitivity, dermatitis

EENT: Blurred vision, glaucoma, dry eyes

GI: Dry mouth, nausea, vomiting, anorexia, constipation, diarrhea, jaundice, weight gain

GU: Urinary retention, urinary frequency, enuresis, impotence, amenorrhea, gynecomastia

*CV: Orthostatic hypotension, **cardiac arrest,** ECG changes, **tachycardia***

Contraindications: Hypersensitivity, blood dyscrasias, coma, child <12 yr, brain damage, bone marrow depression, glaucoma

Precautions: Pregnancy (C), lactation, seizure disorders, hypertension, hepatic or cardiac disease

Pharmacokinetics:

PO: Onset erratic, peak 2-4 hr

IM: Onset 15 min, peak 1 hr, duration 4-6 hr; metabolized by liver; excreted in urine, breast milk; crosses placenta

Interactions:
- Oversedation: other CNS depressants, alcohol, barbiturate anesthetics
- Toxicity: epinephrine
- Decreased absorption: aluminum hydroxide, magnesium hydroxide antacids
- Decreased effects of lithium, levodopa
- Increased effects of both drugs: β-adrenergic blockers, alcohol
- Increased anticholinergic effects: anticholinergics

🌿 Increased anticholinergic effect: henbane leaf

Lab test interferences:

Increase: Liver function tests, car-

◆ = Nursing alert   🌿 = Herb-drug interaction   ⊘ = Do not crush

diac enzymes, cholesterol, blood glucose, prolactin, bilirubin, PBI, cholinesterase, ^{131}I

Decrease: Hormones (blood and urine)

False positive: Pregnancy tests, PKU

False negative: Urinary steroids, 17-OHCS, pregnancy tests

NURSING CONSIDERATIONS
Assess:
• Mental status before initial administration
• Swallowing of PO medication; check for hoarding or giving of medication to other patients
• I&O ratio; palpate bladder if urinary output is low
• Bilirubin, CBC, liver function studies qmo
• Urinalysis is recommended before and during prolonged therapy
• Affect, orientation, LOC, reflexes, gait, coordination, sleep pattern disturbances
• B/P standing and lying; also include pulse, respirations, q4h during initial treatment; establish baseline before starting treatment; report drops of 30 mm Hg
• Dizziness, faintness, palpitations, tachycardia on rising
• EPS including akathisia (inability to sit still, no pattern to movements), tardive dyskinesia (bizarre movements of jaw, mouth, tongue, extremities), pseudoparkinsonism (rigidity, tremors, pill rolling, shuffling gait)
◆ For neuroleptic malignant syndrome: muscle rigidity, altered mental status, hyperthermia, increased CPK
• Skin turgor qd
• Constipation, urinary retention qd; increase bulk, water in diet

Administer:
• Reduced dose in elderly
• Antiparkinsonian agent on order from prescriber for EPS

• Syrup mixed in citrus- or chocolate-flavored drinks
• IM inj into large muscle mass

IV
• IV undiluted; give at 25 mg/min or less over 1 min; may dilute 25-60 mg/9 ml NaCl for inj

Additive compatibilities: Chloramphenicol, erythromycin, ethacrynate, heparin, lidocaine, metaraminol, methyldopate

Syringe compatibilities: Atropine, chlorpromazine, cimetidine, diphenhydramine, droperidol, fentanyl, glycopyrrolate, hydroxyzine, meperidine, metoclopramide, midazolam, morphine, pentazocine, prochlorperazine, promethazine, scopolamine

Perform/provide:
• Decreased sensory input by dimming lights, avoiding loud noises
• Supervised ambulation until stabilized on medication; do not involve in strenuous exercise program because fainting is possible; patient should not stand still for long periods
• Increased fluids to prevent constipation
• Sips of water, candy, gum for dry mouth
• Storage in air-tight, light-resistant container; avoid contact with hands

Evaluate:
• Therapeutic response: decrease in emotional excitement, hallucinations, delusions, paranoia; reorganization of patterns of thought, speech

Teach patient/family:
• That orthostatic hypotension occurs frequently and to rise from sitting or lying position gradually, to avoid hazardous activities until stabilized on medication
• To remain lying down for at least 30 min after IM injection

P

• To avoid hot tubs, hot showers, tub baths; hypotension may occur
• To avoid abrupt withdrawal of this drug, or EPS may result; drug should be withdrawn slowly
• To avoid OTC preparations (cough, hay fever, cold) unless approved by prescriber, since serious drug interactions may occur; avoid use with alcohol, CNS depressants; increased drowsiness may occur
• To use a sunscreen
• About compliance with drug regimen
• About EPS and necessity for meticulous oral hygiene, since oral candidiasis may occur
• To report sore throat, malaise, fever, bleeding, mouth sores; CBC should be drawn and drug discontinued
• That in hot weather, heat stroke may occur; take extra precautions to stay cool

Treatment of overdose: Lavage if orally ingested; provide an airway; do not induce vomiting

---

promethazine (℞)

(proe-meth′a-zeen)
Anergan 50, Phenergan, Phenergan Fortis, Phenergan Plain, promethazine HCl
Func. class.: Antihistamine, H_1-receptor antagonist
Chem. class.: Phenothiazine derivative

Action: Acts on blood vessels, GI, respiratory system by competing with histamine for H_1-receptor site; decreases allergic response by blocking histamine

Uses: Motion sickness, rhinitis, allergy symptoms, sedation, nausea, preoperative and postoperative sedation

Dosage and routes:
Nausea
• *Adult:* **PO/IM/IV** 10-25 mg; may repeat 12.5-25 mg q4-6h
• *Child >2 yr:* **PO/IM** 0.25-0.5 mg/kg q4-6h
Motion sickness
• *Adult:* **PO** 25 mg bid, give ½-1 hr before departure
• *Child >2 yr:* **PO/IM/RECT** 12.5-25 mg bid, give ½-1 hr before departure
Allergy/rhinitis
• *Adult:* **PO** 12.5 mg qid, or 25 mg hs
• *Child >2 yr:* **PO** 6.25-12.5 mg tid or 25 mg hs
Sedation
• *Adult:* **PO/IM** 25-50 mg hs
• *Child >2 yr:* **PO/IM/RECT** 12.5-25 mg hs
Sedation (preoperative/postoperative)
• *Adult:* **PO/IM/IV** 25-50 mg
• *Child >2 yr:* **PO/IM/IV** 12.5-25 mg

Available forms: Tabs 12.5, 25, 50 mg; supp 12.5, 25, 50 mg; inj 25, 50 mg/ml, syrup 6.25 mg/5 ml

Side effects/adverse reactions:
CNS: Dizziness, drowsiness, poor coordination, fatigue, anxiety, euphoria, confusion, paresthesia, neuritis, EPS
CV: Hypotension, palpitations, tachycardia
RESP: Increased thick secretions, wheezing, chest tightness, ***apnea in neonates, infants, young children***
*HEMA: **Thrombocytopenia, agranulocytosis, hemolytic anemia***
GI: Constipation, dry mouth, nausea, vomiting, anorexia, diarrhea
INTEG: Rash, urticaria, photosensitivity

 = Nursing alert   = Herb-drug interaction   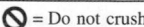 = Do not crush

GU: *Retention,* dysuria, frequency
EENT: Blurred vision, dilated pupils, tinnitus, nasal stuffiness; dry nose, throat, mouth; photosensitivity

Contraindications: Hypersensitivity to H_1-receptor antagonist, acute asthma attack, lower respiratory tract disease

Precautions: Increased intraocular pressure, renal disease, cardiac disease, hypertension, bronchial asthma, seizure disorder, stenosed peptic ulcers, hyperthyroidism, prostatic hypertrophy, bladder neck obstruction, pregnancy (C)

Pharmacokinetics:
PO: Onset 20 min, duration 4-6 hr; metabolized in liver; excreted by kidneys, GI tract (inactive metabolites)

Interactions:
• Increased CNS depression: barbiturates, narcotics, hypnotics, tricyclic antidepressants, alcohol
• Decreased effect of oral anticoagulants, heparin
• Increased effect of promethazine: MAOIs
🍴 Increased anticholinergic effect: henbane leaf

Lab test interferences:
False negative: Skin allergy test
False positive: Urine pregnancy test

NURSING CONSIDERATIONS
Assess:
• I&O ratio; be alert for urinary retention, frequency, dysuria; drug should be discontinued
• CBC during long-term therapy; blood dyscrasias
• Respiratory status: rate, rhythm, increase in bronchial secretions, wheezing, chest tightness
• Cardiac status: palpitations, increased pulse, hypotension

Administer:
• With meals for GI symptoms; absorption may slightly decrease
• IM inj deep in large muscle; rotate site
• When used for motion sickness, 30 min before travel
IV
• After diluting each 25-50 mg/9 ml of NaCl for inj; give 25 mg or less/2 min

Additive compatibilities: Amikacin, ascorbic acid, chloroquine, hydromorphone, netilmicin, vit B/C

Syringe compatibilities: Atropine, butorphanol, chlorpromazine, cimetidine, diphenhydramine, droperidol, fentanyl, glycopyrrolate, hydromorphone, hydroxyzine, meperidine, metoclopramide, midazolam, pentazocine, perphenazine, prochlorperazine, promazine, ranitidine, scopolamine

Y-site compatibilities: Amifostine, amsacrine, aztreonam, ciprofloxacin, cisplatin, cladribine, cyclophosphamide, cytarabine, doxorubicin, filgrastim, fluconazole, fludarabine, granisetron, melphalan, ondansetron, sargramostim, teniposide, thiotepa, vinorelbine

Perform/provide:
• Hard candy, gum, frequent rinsing of mouth for dryness
• Storage in tight, light-resistant container

Evaluate:
• Therapeutic response: absence of running, congested nose, rashes, absence of motion sickness, nausea; sedation

Teach patient/family:
• That drug may cause photosensitivity; to avoid prolonged sunlight
• To notify prescriber of confusion, sedation, hypotension
• To avoid driving, other hazardous activity if drowsy

• To avoid concurrent use of alcohol, other CNS depressants
Treatment of overdose: Administer ipecac syrup or lavage, diazepam, vasopressors, barbiturates (short-acting)

---

propafenone (℞)

(pro-pah-fen'ohn)
Rythmol
Func. class.: Antidysrhythmic, (Class Ic)

Action: Slows conduction velocity; reduces membrane responsiveness; inhibits automaticity; increases ratio of effective refractory period to action potential duration; β-blocking activity

Uses: Life-threatening dysrhythmias, sustained ventricular tachycardia

Dosage and routes:
• *Adult:* **PO** 300-900 mg/day in divided doses, 150 mg q8h; allow a 3-4 day interval before increasing dose

Available forms: Tabs 150, 300 mg

Side effects/adverse reactions:
INTEG: Rash
CV: Dysrhythmias, bradycardia, prodysrhythmia, palpitations, AV block, intraventricular conduction delay, AV dissociation, *CHF, sudden death, atrial flutter*
HEMA: *Leukopenia, agranulocytosis, granulocytopenia, thrombocytopenia,* anemia
CNS: Headache, dizziness, abnormal dreams, syncope, confusion, *seizures*
GI: Nausea, vomiting, constipation, dyspepsia, cholestasis, *hepatitis,* abnormal liver function studies, dry mouth
RESP: Dyspnea
EENT: Blurred vision, altered taste, tinnitus

Contraindications: 2nd- or 3rd-degree AV block, right bundle branch block, cardiogenic shock, hypersensitivity, bradycardia, uncontrolled CHF, sick-sinus syndrome, marked hypotension, bronchospastic disorders

Precautions: CHF, hypokalemia, hyperkalemia, recent MI, nonallergic bronchospasm, pregnancy (C), lactation, children, hepatic or renal disease

Pharmacokinetics: Peak 3-5 hr, half-life 2-10 hr; metabolized in liver; excreted in urine (metabolite)

Interactions:
• Increased effect of propafenone: cimetidine, quinidine
• Increased anticoagulation: warfarin
• Increased digoxin level: digoxin
• Increased β-blocker effect: propranolol, metoprolol
• Increased cyclosporine levels: cyclosporine
• Decreased propafenone effect: rifampin
🌿 Decreased potassium, increased antidysrhythmic action: aloe, buckthorn bark/berry, cascara sagrada bark, senna pod/leaf

Lab test interferences:
Increase: CPK

NURSING CONSIDERATIONS
Assess:
• GI status: bowel pattern, number of stools
• Cardiac status: rate, rhythm, quality
• Chest x-ray film, pulmonary function test during treatment
• I&O ratio; check for decreasing output
• B/P for fluctuations
• Lung fields; bilateral rales may occur in CHF patient
• Increased respiration, increased pulse; drug should be discontinued

---

◆ = Nursing alert   🌿 = Herb-drug interaction   🚫 = Do not crush

◆ Toxicity: fine tremors, dizziness
• Cardiac function: respiratory rate, rhythm, character continuously
Evaluate:
• Therapeutic response: absence of dysrhythmias
Treatment of overdose: O_2, artificial ventilation, ECG; administer dopamine for circulatory depression, diazepam or thiopental for convulsions

---

propantheline (℞)

(proe-pan'the-leen)
Norpanth, Pro-Banthine, Propanthel*, propantheline bromide
Func. class.: GI anticholinergic
Chem. class.: Synthetic quaternary ammonium compound

Action: Inhibits muscarinic actions of acetylcholine at postganglionic parasympathetic neuroeffector sites
Uses: Treatment of peptic ulcer disease, irritable bowel syndrome, duodenography, urinary incontinence
Investigational uses: Antispasmodic uses
Dosage and routes:
• *Adult:* **PO** 15 mg tid ac, 30 mg hs
• *Elderly:* **PO** 7.5 mg tid ac
Available forms: Tabs 7.5, 15 mg
Side effects/adverse reactions:
CNS: Confusion, stimulation in elderly, headache, insomnia, dizziness, drowsiness, anxiety, weakness, hallucinations
*GI: Dry mouth, constipation, **paralytic ileus,** heartburn, nausea, vomiting, dysphagia, absence of taste
GU: Hesitancy, retention, impotence
CV: Palpitations, tachycardia, orthostatic hypotension (elderly)
EENT: Blurred vision, photophobia, mydriasis, cycloplegia, increased ocular tension

INTEG: Urticaria, rash, pruritus, anhidrosis, fever, allergic reactions
Contraindications: Hypersensitivity to anticholinergics, narrow-angle glaucoma, GI obstruction, myasthenia gravis, paralytic ileus, GI atony, toxic megacolon
Precautions: Hyperthyroidism, coronary artery disease, dysrhythmias, CHF, ulcerative colitis, hypertension, hiatal hernia, hepatic disease, renal disease, pregnancy (C), urinary retention, prostatic hypertrophy, elderly
Pharmacokinetics:
PO: Onset 30-45 min, duration 6 hr; metabolized by liver, GI system; excreted in urine, bile
Interactions:
• Increased anticholinergic effect: amantadine, tricyclic antidepressants, MAOIs, H_1-antihistamines
• Decreased effect of phenothiazines, levodopa, ketoconazole
NURSING CONSIDERATIONS
Assess:
• VS, cardiac status: checking for dysrhythmias, increased rate, palpitations
• I&O ratio; check for urinary retention or hesitancy
• GI complaints: pain, bleeding (frank or occult), nausea, vomiting, anorexia
Administer:
• ½-1 hr ac for better absorption
• Decreased dose to elderly patients; metabolism may be slowed
• Gum, hard candy, frequent rinsing for dry mouth
Perform/provide:
• Storage in tight container protected from light
• Increased fluids, bulk, exercise to decrease constipation
Evaluate:
• Therapeutic response: absence of epigastric pain, bleeding, nausea, vomiting

---

Teach patient/family:
• To avoid driving, other hazardous activities until stabilized on medication; may cause blurred vision; to use caution when standing due to orthostatic hypotension
• To avoid alcohol, other CNS depressants; will enhance sedating properties of this drug
• To drink plenty of fluids
• To report dysphagia

---

propofol (℞)
(pro'poh-fole)
Diprivan, Disoprofol
Func. class.: General anesthetic

Action: Produces dose-dependent CNS depression; action is unknown
Uses: Induction or maintenance of anesthesia as part of balanced anesthetic technique; sedation in mechanically ventilated patients
Dosage and routes:
Induction
• *Adult:* **IV** 2-2.5 mg/kg, approximately 40 mg q10sec until induction onset
• *Child ≥3 yr:* **IV** 2.5-3.5 mg/kg over 20-30 sec
• *Elderly:* **IV** 1-1.5 mg/kg, approximately 20 mg q10sec until induction onset
Maintenance
• *Adult:* **IV** 0.1-0.2 mg/kg/min (6-12 mg/kg/hr)
• *Child ≥3 yr:* **IV** 0.125-0.3 mg/kg/min (7.5-18 mg/kg/hr)
• *Elderly:* **IV** 0.05-0.1 mg/kg/min (3-6 mg/kg/hr)
Critical care sedatives
• *Adult:* **IV** 5 μg/kg over 5 min; may give 5-10 μg/kg/min over 5-10 min until desired response
Available forms: Inj 10 mg/ml in 20 ml ampule, 50-cc and 100-cc vials

Side effects/adverse reactions:
CNS: Movement, headache, jerking, fever, dizziness, shivering, tremor, confusion, somnolence, paresthesia, agitation, abnormal dreams, euphoria, fatigue
GI: Nausea, vomiting, abdominal cramping, dry mouth, swallowing, hypersalivation
MS: Myalgia
GU: Urine retention, green urine
EENT: Blurred vision, tinnitus, eye pain, strange taste
CV: Bradycardia, hypotension, hypertension, PVC, PAC, tachycardia, abnormal ECG, ST segment depression, *asystole*
RESP: Apnea, cough, *hiccups,* dyspnea, hypoventilation, sneezing, wheezing, tachypnea, hypoxia
INTEG: Flushing, phlebitis, hives, burning/stinging at injection site
Contraindications: Hypersensitivity, hyperlipidemia
Precautions: Elderly, respiratory depression, severe respiratory disorders, cardiac dysrhythmias, pregnancy (B), labor and delivery, lactation, children
Pharmacokinetics: Onset 40 sec, rapid distribution, half-life 1-8 min, terminal elimination half-life 5-10 hr; 70% excreted in urine; metabolized in liver by conjugation to inactive metabolites
Interactions:
• Increased CNS depression: alcohol, narcotics, sedative/hypnotics, antipsychotics, skeletal muscle relaxants, inhalational anesthetics
• Do not administer with other drugs
NURSING CONSIDERATIONS
Assess:
• Injection site: phlebitis, burning, stinging
• ECG for changes: PVC, PAC, ST segment changes

◆ = Nursing alert　　🖋 = Herb-drug interaction　　🚫 = Do not crush

- CNS changes: movement, jerking, tremors, dizziness, LOC, pupil reaction
- Allergic reactions: hives
- Respiratory dysfunction: respiratory depression, character, rate, rhythm; notify prescriber if respirations are <10/min

Administer:

IV

- After diluting with D_5W mixed in lipid base; use only glass containers when mixing, not stable in plastic
- By IV only
- Alone; do not mix with other agents before using
- Only with resuscitative equipment available
- Only by qualified persons trained in anesthesia

Syringe compatibilities: Thiopental

Y-site compatibilities: Acyclovir, alfentanil, amikacin, aminophylline, ampicillin, amrinone, aztreonam, bumetanide, buprenorphine, butorphanol, calcium gluconate, carboplatin, cefazolin, cefonicid, cefoperazone, cefotaxime, cefotetan, cefoxitin, ceftazidime, ceftizoxime, ceftriaxone, cefuroxime, chlorpromazine, cimetidine, ciprofloxacin, cisplatin, clindamycin, cyclophosphamide, cyclosporine, cytarabine, dexamethasone, digoxin, diphenhydramine, dobutamine, dopamine, doxorubicin, doxycycline, droperidol, enalaprilat, ephedrine, epinephrine, esmolol, famotidine, fentanyl, fluconazole, fluorouracil, furosemide, ganciclovir, glycopyrrolate, granisetron, haloperidol, heparin, hydrocortisone, hydromorphone, hydroxyzine, ifosfamide, imipenem-cilastatin, insulin, isoproterenol, ketamine, labetalol, levorphanol, lidocaine, lorazepam, magnesium sulfate, mannitol, meperidine, metoclopramide, mezlocillin, miconazole, morphine, nafcillin, nalbuphine, naloxone, nitroglycerin, norepinephrine, ofloxacin, paclitaxel, pentobarbital, phenobarbital, piperacillin, potassium chloride, prochlorperazine, propranolol, ranitidine, scopolamine, sodium bicarbonate, sodium nitroprusside, succinylcholine, sufentanil, ticarcillin, ticarcillin/clavulanate, vancomycin, vecuronium, verapamil

Perform/provide:

- Storage in light-resistant area at room temp
- Safety measures: side rails, nightlight, call bell within easy reach

Evaluate:

- Therapeutic response: induction of anesthesia

Treatment of overdose: Discontinue drug; administer vasopressor agents or anticholinergics, artificial ventilation

---

propoxyphene (℞)

(proe-pox′i-feen)

Benophene, Cotanal, Darvocet-N, Darvon, Darvon-N, Darvon-N Compound*, Darvon Compound-65, Dolane AP, Dolene, Doraphen, Doraphen Compound, Doxapap-N, Doxaphene, D-Rex, E-Lor, Genagesic, Margesic A C, Novapropoxyn*, Novopropoxy Compound*, Pancet Propacet, Profene, Pro-Pox, Pro-Pox Plus, Pro-Pox with APAP, Propoxycon, propoxyphene/acetaminophen, propoxyphene/aspirin/caffeine, propoxyphene HCl; Propoxyphene with APAP, Wygesic

Func. class.: Narcotic analgesic
Chem. class.: Synthetic opiate

Controlled Substance Schedule IV
Action: Depresses pain impulse

Side effects: *italics* = common; ***bold italics*** = life-threatening

transmission at the spinal cord level by interacting with opioid receptors

Uses: Mild to moderate pain

Dosage and routes:
• *Adult:* **PO** 65 mg q4h prn (HCl)
• *Adult:* **PO** 100 mg q4h prn (napsylate)

Available forms: Propoxyphene HCl Caps 65 mg, tabs 65 mg*; propoxyphene napsylate tabs 50, 100 mg; caps 100 mg*; oral susp 50 mg/5 ml propoxyphene HCl; acetaminophen tabs 65 mg/650 mg; propoxyphene napsylate/acetaminophen tabs 50 mg/325 mg, 100 mg/ 650 mg; propoxyphene/aspirin/caffeine cap 65 mg/389 mg/32.4 mg

Side effects/adverse reactions:
CNS: Drowsiness, dizziness, confusion, headache, sedation, euphoria, **convulsions, hyperthermia** (elderly)
GI: Nausea, vomiting, anorexia, constipation, cramps
GU: Urinary retention, dysuria
INTEG: Rash, urticaria, bruising, flushing, diaphoresis, pruritus
EENT: Tinnitus, blurred vision, miosis, diplopia
CV: Palpitations, bradycardia, change in B/P, *dysrhythmias*
RESP: Respiratory depression

Contraindications: Hypersensitivity to ASA products (some preparations), addiction (narcotic)

Precautions: Addictive personality, pregnancy (C), lactation, increased intracranial pressure, MI (acute), severe heart disease, respiratory depression, hepatic disease, renal disease, child <18 yr, elderly

Pharmacokinetics:
PO: Onset ½-1 hr, peak 2-2½ hr, duration 4-6 hr
Metabolized by liver, excreted by kidneys (as metabolites), crosses placenta, excreted in breast milk, half-life 6-12 hr (metabolites)

Interactions:
• Increased effects with other CNS depressants: alcohol, narcotics, sedative/hypnotics, antipsychotics, skeletal muscle relaxants

Lab test interferences:
Increase: Amylase

NURSING CONSIDERATIONS
Assess:
• I&O ratio; check for decreasing output; may indicate retention
• CNS changes: dizziness, drowsiness, hallucinations, euphoria, loss of consciousness, pupil reaction
• Allergic reactions: rash, urticaria
• Respiratory dysfunction: respiratory depression, character, rate, rhythm; notify prescriber if respirations are <10/min
• Need for pain medication; physical dependence

Administer:
• With antiemetic for nausea, vomiting
• When pain is beginning to return; determine dosage interval by response

Perform/provide:
• Storage in light-resistant area at room temp
• Assistance with ambulation
• Safety measures: side rails, nightlight, call bell within easy reach

Evaluate:
• Therapeutic response: decrease in pain

Teach patient/family:
• To report any symptoms of CNS changes, allergic reactions
• That physical dependency may result when used for extended periods; not to exceed dose
• That withdrawal symptoms may occur: nausea, vomiting, cramps, fever, faintness, anorexia

Treatment of overdose: Naloxone (Narcan) 0.2-0.8 mg IV, O$_2$, IV fluids, vasopressors

---

➡ = Nursing alert   🖋 = Herb-drug interaction   🚫 = Do not crush

propranolol (℞)

(proe-pran'oh-lole)

Apo-Propranolol*, Detensol*, Inderal, Inderal LA, Inderal 10, Inderal 20, Inderal 40, Inderal 60, Inderal 80, propranolol HCl, Propranolol Intensol, Novo-Pranol*

Func. class.: Antihypertensive, antianginal

Chem. class.: β-Adrenergic blocker

Action: Nonselective β-blocker with negative inotropic, chronotropic, dromotropic properties

Uses: Chronic stable angina pectoris, hypertension, supraventricular dysrhythmias, migraine, prophylaxis, MI, pheochromocytoma, essential tremor, tetralogy of Fallot, cyanotic spells

Investigational uses. Mitral valve prolapse, anxiety, dysrhythmias associated with thyrotoxicosis

Dosage and routes:

Dysrhythmias
• *Adult:* **PO** 10-30 mg tid-qid; **IV BOL** 0.5-3 mg give 1 mg/min; may repeat in 2 min, may repeat q4h thereafter
• *Child:* **PO** 0.5-1 mg/kg/day divided q6-8h; **IV** 0.01-0.1 mg/kg

Hypertension
• *Adult:* **PO** 40 mg bid or 80 mg qd **(EXT REL)** initially; usual dose 120-240 mg/day bid-tid or 120-160 mg qd **(EXT REL)**
• *Child:* **PO** 0.5-1 mg/kg/day divided q6-12h

Angina
• *Adult:* **PO** 80-320 mg in divided doses bid-qid or 80 mg qd **(EXT REL)**; usual dose 160 mg qd **(EXT REL)**

MI prophylaxis
• *Adult:* **PO** 180-240 mg/day tid-qid starting 5 day to 2 wk after MI

Pheochromocytoma
• *Adult:* **PO** 60 mg/day × 3 days preoperatively in divided doses or 30 mg/day in divided doses (inoperable tumor)

Migraine
• *Adult:* **PO** 80 mg/day (EXT REL) or in divided doses; may increase to 160-240 mg/day in divided doses
• *Child:* **PO** 0.6-1.5 mg/kg/day divided q8h **PO**

Essential tremor
• *Adult:* **PO** 40 mg bid; usual dose 120 mg/day

Tetralogy of Fallot
• *Child:* **PO** 1-2 mg/kg/dose q6h

Available forms: Caps, ext rel 60, 80, 120, 160 mg; tabs 10, 20, 40, 60, 80, 90 mg; inj 1 mg/ml; oral sol 4 mg/ml, 8 mg/ml; conc oral sol 80 mg/ml

Side effects/adverse reactions:

RESP: Dyspnea, respiratory dysfunction, *bronchospasm*
CV: Bradycardia, hypotension, ***CHF***, palpitations, AV block, peripheral vascular insufficiency, vasodilation
HEMA: ***Agranulocytosis, thrombocytopenia***
GI: Nausea, vomiting, diarrhea, colitis, constipation, cramps, dry mouth, hepatomegaly, gastric pain, acute pancreatitis
GU: Impotence, decreased libido, UTIs
MS: Joint pain, arthralgia, muscle cramps, pain
MISC: Facial swelling, weight change, Raynaud's phenomenon
INTEG: Rash, pruritus, fever
CNS: Depression, hallucinations, dizziness, fatigue, lethargy, paresthesias, bizarre dreams, disorientation
EENT: Sore throat, *laryngospasm*, blurred vision, dry eyes

META: Hyperglycemia, hypoglycemia

Contraindications: Hypersensitivity to this drug, cardiac failure, cardiogenic shock, 2nd- or 3rd-degree heart block, bronchospastic disease, sinus bradycardia, CHF

Precautions: Diabetes mellitus, pregnancy (C), renal disease, lactation, hyperthyroidism, COPD, hepatic disease, children, myasthenia gravis, peripheral vascular disease, hypotension, CHF

Pharmacokinetics:

PO: Onset 30 min, peak 1-1½ hr, duration 6-12 hr

PO-ER: Peak 6 hr, duration 24 hr

IV: Onset 2 min, peak 15 min, duration 3-6 hr; immediate rel half-life 3-5 hr; ext rel half-life 8-11 hr; metabolized by liver; crosses placenta, blood-brain barrier; excreted in breast milk

Interactions:

• AV block: digitalis, calcium channel blockers

• Increased negative inotropic effects: verapamil, disopyramide

• Increased effects of reserpine, digitalis, neuromuscular blocking agents

• Decreased β-blocking effects: norepinephrine, isoproterenol, barbiturates, rifampin, dopamine, dobutamine, smoking

• Increased β-blocking effect: cimetidine

• Increased hypotension: quinidine, haloperidol, hydralazine

Lab test interferences:

Increase: Serum K, serum uric acid, ALT (SGPT)/AST (SGOT), alk phosphatase, LDH

Decrease: Blood glucose

NURSING CONSIDERATIONS

Assess:

• B/P, pulse, respirations during beginning therapy; notify prescriber if pulse <50 BPM

• Weight qd; report gain of 5 lb

• I&O ratio, CrCl if kidney damage is diagnosed

• ECG if using as antidysrhythmic

• Hepatic enzymes: AST (SGOT), ALT (SGPT), bilirubin

• Angina pain: duration, time started, activity being performed, character

• Tolerance (long-term use)

• Headache, light-headedness, decreased B/P; may indicate a need for decreased dosage

Administer:

• With 8 oz water on empty stomach

• Do not give with aluminum-containing antacid; may decrease GI absorption

IV

• IV undiluted or diluted 10 ml D_5W for inj; give 1 mg or less/min; may be diluted in 50 ml NaCl and run 1 mg over 10-15 min

Additive compatibilities: Dobutamine, verapamil

Solution compatibilities: 0.9% NaCl, 0.45 NaCl, Ringer's, D_5W, D_5/0.9% NaCl, D_5/0.45% NaCl

Syringe compatibilities: Amrinone, benzquinamide, milrinone

Y-site compatibilities: Alteplase, amrinone, heparin, hydrocortisone, meperidine, milrinone, morphine, potassium chloride, propofol, tacrolimus, vit B/C

Perform/provide:

• Protection from light (injection)

Evaluate:

• Therapeutic response: decreased B/P, dysrhythmias

Teach patient/family:

• Not to discontinue abruptly, to take drug at same time each day; to decrease dosage over 2 wk to prevent cardiac damage

• To avoid OTC drugs unless approved by prescriber

◆ = Nursing alert   ∥ = Herb-drug interaction   ⊘ = Do not crush

- To avoid hazardous activities if dizzy
- The importance of compliance with complete medical regimen
- To make position changes slowly to prevent fainting

---

propylthiouracil (℞)

(proe-pill-thye-oh yoor'a-sill)
propylthiouracil, Propyl-Thyra-cil*, PTU
Func. class.: Thyroid hormone antagonist (antithyroid)
Chem. class.: Thioamide

Action: Blocks synthesis peripherally of T_3, T_4 (triiodothyronine, thyroxine), inhibits organification of iodine

Uses: Preparation for thyroidectomy, thyrotoxic crisis, hyperthyroidism, thyroid storm

Dosage and routes:
Thyrotoxic crisis
- *Adult and child:* PO same as hyperthyroidism with iodine and propranolol

Preparation for thyroidectomy
- *Adult:* 600-1200 mg/day
- *Child:* 10 mg/kg/day in divided doses

Hyperthyroidism
- *Adult:* PO 100 mg tid increasing to 300 mg q8h if condition is severe; continue to euthyroid state, then 100 mg qd-tid
- *Child >10 yr:* PO 100 mg tid; continue to euthyroid state, then 25 mg tid to 100 mg bid
- *Child 6-10 yr:* PO 50-150 mg in divided doses q8h
- *Neonate:* PO 10 mg/kg/day in divided doses

Available forms: Tabs 50 mg

Side effects/adverse reactions:
INTEG: Rash, urticaria, pruritus, alopecia, hyperpigmentation, lupus-like syndrome
GU: Nephritis
CNS: Drowsiness, headache, vertigo, fever, paresthesias, neuritis
HEMA: Agranulocytosis, leukopenia, thrombocytopenia, hypothrombinemia, lymphadenopathy, bleeding, vasculitis, periarteritis
GI: Nausea, diarrhea, vomiting, jaundice, hepatitis, loss of taste
MS: Myalgia, arthralgia, nocturnal muscle cramps, osteoporosis

Contraindications: Hypersensitivity, pregnancy (D), lactation

Precautions: Infection, bone marrow depression, hepatic disease

Pharmacokinetics:
PO: Onset up to 3 wk, peak 6-10 wk, duration 1 wk to 1 mo, half-life 1-2 hr; excreted in urine, bile, breast milk; crosses placenta; concentration in thyroid gland

Interactions:
- Increased anticoagulant effect: heparin, oral anticoagulants
- Bone marrow depression: radiation, antineoplastics
- Additive effects: potassium/sodium iodide, lithium
- Agranulocytosis: phenothiazines

Lab test interferences:
Increase: Pro-time, AST (SGOT), ALT (SGPT), alk phosphatase

NURSING CONSIDERATIONS
Assess:
- Pulse, B/P, temp
- I&O ratio; check for edema: puffy hands, feet, periorbits; indicates hypothyroidism
- Weight qd; same clothing, scale, time of day
- T_3, T_4, which are increased; serum TSH, which is decreased; free thyroxine index, which is increased if dosage is too low; discontinue drug 3-4 wk before RAIU
- Blood work: CBC for blood dys-

P

crasias: leukopenia, thrombocytopenia, agranulocytosis; LFTs

◆Overdose: peripheral edema, heat intolerance, diaphoresis, palpitations, dysrhythmias, severe tachycardia, increased temp, delirium, CNS irritability

• Hypersensitivity: rash, enlarged cervical lymph nodes; drug may have to be discontinued

• Hypoprothrombinemia: bleeding, petechiae, ecchymosis

• Clinical response: after 3 wk should include increased weight, pulse; decreased T_4

• Bone marrow depression: sore throat, fever, fatigue

Administer:

• With meals to decrease GI upset

• At same time each day to maintain drug level

• Lowest dose that relieves symptoms

Perform/provide:

• Storage in light-resistant container

• Fluids to 3-4 L/day, unless contraindicated

Evaluate:

• Therapeutic response: weight gain, decreased pulse, decreased T_4, decreased B/P

Teach patient/family:

• To abstain from breastfeeding after delivery

• To take pulse qd

• To report redness, swelling, sore throat, mouth lesions, which indicate blood dyscrasias

• To keep graph of weight, pulse, mood

• To avoid OTC products that contain iodine

• That seafood, other iodine products may be restricted

• Not to discontinue this medication abruptly; thyroid crisis may occur; stress response

• That response may take several months if thyroid is large

• The symptoms/signs of overdose: periorbital edema, cold intolerance, mental depression

• The symptoms of inadequate dose: tachycardia, diarrhea, fever, irritability

• To take medication as prescribed; not to skip or double dose; missed doses should be taken when remembered up to 1 hr before next dose

• To carry Medic Alert ID listing condition, medication

---

protamine (℞)

(proe′ta-meen)

Func. class.: Heparin antagonist

Chem. class.: Low-molecular-weight protein

Action: Binds heparin, making it ineffective

Uses: Heparin overdose

Dosage and routes:

• *Adult and child:* IV 1 mg of protamine/90-115 U heparin given; administer slowly 1-3 min; give undiluted to 1%, not to exceed 50 mg/10 min

Available forms: Inj 10 mg/ml

Side effects/adverse reactions:

CV: Hypotension, bradycardia, *circulatory collapse*

GI: Nausea, vomiting, anorexia

INTEG: Rash, dermatitis, urticaria

CNS: Lassitude

HEMA: Bleeding, *anaphylaxis*

RESP: Dyspnea, *pulmonary edema, severe respiratory distress*

Contraindications: Hypersensitivity

Precautions: Pregnancy (C), lactation, children, allergy to fish

Pharmacokinetics:

IV: Onset 5 min, duration 2 hr

◆ = Nursing alert   ∅ = Herb-drug interaction   ⊘ = Do not crush

NURSING CONSIDERATIONS
Assess:
- Blood studies (Hct, platelets, occult blood in stools) q3mo
- Coagulation tests (APTT, ACT) 15 min after dose, then in several hours
- VS, B/P, pulse after 30 min; plus 3 hr after dose
- Skin rash, urticaria, dermatitis
- Allergy to fish; use with caution

Administer:
IV
- After diluting 50 mg/5 ml sterile bacteriostatic H_2O for inj; shake, give 20 mg or less over 1-3 min; may further dilute with equal volume of NaCl or D_5W and run over 2-3 hr; titrate to APTT, ACT; use infusion pump

Additive compatibilities: Cimetidine, ranitidine, verapamil

Perform/provide:
- Storage at 36°-46° F (2°-8° C)

Evaluate:
- Therapeutic response: reversal of heparin overdose

---

protriptyline (R)
(proc-trip'tih-leen)
Triptil*, Vivactil
Func. class.: Tricyclic antidepressant
Chem. class.: Dibenzocycloheptene—secondary amine

Action: Blocks reuptake of norepinephrine, serotonin into nerve endings, increasing action of norepinephrine, serotonin in nerve cells

Uses: Depression

Dosage and routes:
- *Adult:* PO 15-40 mg/day in divided doses; may increase to 60 mg/day
- *Geriatric:* PO 5-10 mg/day, increase q3-7 days by 5-10 mg

Available forms: Tabs 5, 10 mg

Side effects/adverse reactions:
*HEMA: **Agranulocytosis, thrombocytopenia, eosinophilia, leukopenia***
CNS: Dizziness, drowsiness, confusion, headache, anxiety, tremors, stimulation, weakness, insomnia, nightmares, EPS (elderly), increased psychiatric symptoms, paresthesia, seizures
GI: Diarrhea, dry mouth, nausea, vomiting, ***paralytic ileus,*** increased appetite, cramps, epigastric distress, jaundice, ***hepatitis,*** stomatitis, constipation
*GU: Retention, **acute renal failure***
INTEG: Rash, urticaria, sweating, pruritus, photosensitivity
*CV: Orthostatic hypotension, ECG changes, tachycardia, **hypertension,** palpitations
EENT: Blurred vision, tinnitus, mydriasis

Contraindications: Hypersensitivity to tricyclic antidepressants, recovery phase of MI, convulsive disorders, prostatic hypertrophy

Precautions: Suicidal patients, severe depression, increased intraocular pressure, narrow-angle glaucoma, urinary retention, cardiac disease, hepatic disease, hyperthyroidism, electroshock therapy, elective surgery, pregnancy (C), elderly

Pharmacokinetics:
PO: Onset 15-30 min, peak 24-30 hr, duration 4-6 hr; therapeutic effect 2-3 wk; metabolized by liver, excreted by kidneys, crosses placenta, half-life 54-98 hr

Interactions:
- Decreased effects of guanethidine, clonidine, indirect-acting sympathomimetics (ephedrine)
- Increased effects of direct-acting sympathomimetics (epinephrine), alcohol, barbiturates, benzodiazepines, CNS depressants

• Hyperpyretic crisis, convulsions, hypertensive episode: MAOI (pargyline [Eutonyl])

🍃 Increased anticholinergic effect: belladonna leaf/root, henbane leaf

🍃 Increased antidepressant action: scopolia root

Lab test interferences:

Increase: Serum bilirubin, blood glucose, alk phosphatase

False increase: Urinary catecholamines

Decrease: VMA, 5-HIAA

NURSING CONSIDERATIONS
Assess:

• B/P (lying, standing), pulse q4h; if systolic B/P drops 20 mm Hg, hold drug, notify prescriber; take vital signs q4h in patients with cardiovascular disease

• Blood studies: CBC, leukocytes, differential, cardiac enzymes (long-term therapy)

• Hepatic studies: AST (SGOT), ALT (SGPT), bilirubin

• Weight qwk; appetite may increase with drug

• ECG for flattening of T wave, bundle branch block, AV block, dysrhythmias in cardiac patients

• EPS primarily in elderly: rigidity, dystonia, akathisia

• Mental status changes: mood, sensorium, affect, suicidal tendencies, increase in psychiatric symptoms: depression, panic

• Urinary retention, constipation; constipation most likely in children/elderly

• Withdrawal symptoms: headache, nausea, vomiting, muscle pain, weakness; not usual unless discontinued abruptly

• Alcohol consumption; hold dose until morning

Administer:

PO

• Increased fluids, bulk in diet if constipation occurs

• With food, milk for GI symptoms

• Dosage hs if oversedation occurs during day; may take entire dose hs; elderly may not tolerate once/day dosing

• Gum, hard candy, or frequent sips of water for dry mouth

Perform/provide:

• Storage in tight, light-resistant container at room temp

• Assistance with ambulation during beginning therapy for drowsiness/dizziness

• Safety measures including side rails, primarily in elderly

• Checking to see if PO medication swallowed

Evaluate:

• Therapeutic response: decreased depression

Teach patient/family:

• That therapeutic effects may take 2-3 wk

• To use caution in driving, other activities requiring alertness because of drowsiness, dizziness, blurred vision

• To avoid alcohol ingestion, other CNS depressants

• Not to discontinue medication quickly after long-term use; may cause nausea, headache, malaise

• To wear sunscreen or large hat

Treatment of overdose: ECG monitoring; induce emesis; lavage, activated charcoal; administer anticonvulsant

pseudoephedrine
(OTC, ℞)

(soo-doe-e-fed′rin)

Allerid, Children's Sudafed, Decofed Syrup, DeFed-60, Dorcol Children's Decongestant, Drixoral Non-Drowsy Formula, Eltor*, Efidac/24, Genaphed, Halofed, Myfedrine, Novafed, Pedia Care Infant's Decongestant, pseudoephedrine HCl, Pseudogest Decongestant, Pseudo Syrup, Sinustat, Sudafed, Sudafed 12 hour, Sudrin

Func. class.: Adrenergic
Chem. class.: Substituted phenylethylamine

Action: Primary activity through α-effects on respiratory mucosal membranes reducing congestion hyperemia, edema; minimal bronchodilation secondary to β-effects

Uses: Nasal decongestant, adjunct in otitis media; with antihistamines

Dosage and routes:
• *Adult:* PO 60 mg q6h; EXT REL 60-120 mg q12h or q24h
• *Geriatric:* PO 30-60 mg q6h prn
• *Child 6-12 yr:* PO 30 mg q6h, not to exceed 120 mg/day
• *Child 2-6 yr:* PO 15 mg q6h, not to exceed 60 mg/day

Available forms: Caps, ext rel 120, 240 mg; oral sol 15 mg, 30 mg/5 ml; drops 7.5 mg/0.8 ml; tabs 30, 60 mg; caps 60 mg; tabs, ext rel 120 mg

Side effects/adverse reactions:
CNS: Tremors, anxiety, insomnia, headache, dizziness, hallucinations, *seizures* (elderly)
EENT: Dry nose, irritation of nose and throat
CV: Palpitations, tachycardia, hypertension, chest pain, *dysrhythmias*

GI: Anorexia, nausea, vomiting, dry mouth
GU: Dysuria

Contraindications: Hypersensitivity to sympathomimetics, narrow-angle glaucoma

Precautions: Pregnancy (C), cardiac disorders, hyperthyroidism, diabetes mellitus, prostatic hypertrophy, lactation, hypertension

Pharmacokinetics:
PO: Onset 15-30 min, duration 4-6 hr, 8-12 hr (ext rel); metabolized in liver, excreted in feces and breast milk

Interactions:
• Do not use with MAOIs or tricyclic antidepressants; hypertensive crisis may occur
• Decreased effect of this drug: methyldopa, urinary acidifiers, rauwolfia alkaloids
• Increased effect of this drug: urinary alkalizers

NURSING CONSIDERATIONS
Assess:
• For nasal congestion; auscultate lung sounds; check for tenacious bronchial secretions
• B/P, pulse throughout treatment
• For CNS side effects in the elderly: excitation, seizures, hallucinations

Perform/provide:
• Storage at room temp

Evaluate:
• Therapeutic response: decreased nasal congestion

Teach patient/family:
• The reason for drug administration
• Not to use continuously, or more than recommended dose; rebound congestion may occur
• To check with prescriber before using other drugs, as drug interactions may occur

• To avoid taking near hs; stimulation can occur
• Not to use if stimulation, restlessness, or tremors occur
• That use in children may cause excessive agitation

---

psyllium (OTC, ℞)

(sill'ee-um)

Cillium, Effer-Syllium, Fiberall, Fiberall Natural Flavor and Orange Flavor, Hydrocil Instant Powder, Karacil*, Konsyl-D, Metamucil, Metamucil Instant Mix Lemon Lime, Metamucil Instant Mix Orange, Metamucil Orange Flavor, Metamucil Sugar Free, Metamucil Sugar Free Orange Flavor, Modane Bulk, Natural Vegetable Reguloid, Perdiem, Pro-Lax, Prodiem Plain*, Reguloid Natural, Reguloid Orange, Reguloid Sugar Free Orange, Reguloid Sugar Free Regular, Serutan, Siblin, Syllact, V-Lax

Func. class.: Bulk laxative
Chem. class.: Psyllium colloid

Action: Bulk-forming laxative
Uses: Chronic constipation, ulcerative colitis, irritable bowel syndrome

Dosage and routes:
• *Adult:* **PO** 1-2 tsp in 8 oz H_2O bid or tid, then 8 oz H_2O or 1 premeasured packet in 8 oz H_2O bid or tid, then 8 oz H_2O
• *Child >6 yr:* **PO** 1 tsp in 4 oz H_2O hs

Available forms: Chew pieces 1.7 g/piece; powder 309, 390, 430, 450, 486, 500, 600, 630, 654, 672, 791, 919, 950 mg/g, 1 g/g; granules 2.5 g/dose

Side effects/adverse reactions:
GI: Nausea, vomiting, anorexia, diarrhea, cramps

Contraindications: Hypersensitivity, intestinal obstruction, abdominal pain, nausea/vomiting, fecal impaction
Precautions: Pregnancy (C)
Pharmacokinetics: Excreted in feces, not absorbed in GI tract

NURSING CONSIDERATIONS
Assess:
• Blood, urine electrolytes if used often
• I&O ratio to identify fluid loss
• Cause of constipation; fluids, bulk, exercise missing
• Cramping, rectal bleeding, nausea, vomiting; drug should be discontinued
Administer:
PO
• Alone for better absorption
• In morning or evening (oral dose)
• After mixing with H_2O immediately before use
• With 8 oz H_2O or juice followed by another 8 oz of fluid
Evaluate:
• Therapeutic response: decrease in constipation or decreased diarrhea in colitis
Teach patient/family:
• To maintain adequate fluid consumption
• That normal bowel movements do not always occur daily
• Not to use in presence of abdominal pain, nausea, vomiting
• To notify prescriber if constipation unrelieved or if symptoms of electrolyte imbalance occur: muscle cramps, pain, weakness, dizziness, excessive thirst

---

◆ = Nursing alert   ∥ = Herb-drug interaction   ⊘ = Do not crush

pyrantel (℞)

(pie-ran'tel)

Antiminth, Combantrin*, Pin-X, Reese's Pinworm

Func. class.: Anthelmintic

Chem. class.: Pyrimidine derivative

Action: Causes paralysis in worm by neuroblockade via stimulation of ganglionic receptors; worms expelled by normal peristalsis

Uses: Pinworms, roundworms, hookworms

Dosage and routes:

• *Adult and child >2 yr:* **PO** 11 mg/kg as single dose, not to exceed 1 g; repeat in 2 wk for pinworms; 11 mg/kg as a single dose × 3 days

Available forms: Oral susp 250 mg/5 ml

Side effects/adverse reactions:

INTEG: Rash

CNS: Dizziness, headache, drowsiness, insomnia, fever, weakness

GI: Nausea, vomiting, anorexia, diarrhea, distention, abdominal cramps

Contraindications: Hypersensitivity

Precautions: Seizure disorders, hepatic disease, dehydration, anemia, child <2 yr, pregnancy (C)

Pharmacokinetics:

PO: Peak 1-3 hr; metabolized in liver; excreted in feces, urine (unchanged/metabolites)

Interactions:

• Antagonizes effect of pyrantel: piperazine

NURSING CONSIDERATIONS

Assess:

• Stools during entire treatment; specimens must be sent to lab while still warm

• For allergic reaction: rash

• For diarrhea during expulsion of worms

Administer:

PO

• After meals to avoid GI symptoms

• After shaking suspension

Perform/provide:

• Storage in tight, light-resistant container in cool environment

Evaluate:

• Therapeutic response: expulsion of worms, 3 negative stool cultures after completion of treatment

Teach patient/family:

• Proper hygiene after BM, including hand-washing technique; tell patient not to put fingers in mouth

• That infected person should sleep alone; not to shake bed linen; to change bed linen qd, wash in hot water

• To clean toilet qd with disinfectant (green soap solution)

• The need for compliance with dosage schedule, duration of treatment

• To drink fruit juice to help expel worms

• To wear shoes, wash all fruits, vegetables well before eating

pyrazinamide (℞)

(peer-a-zin'a-mide)

PMS Pyrazinamide*, pyrazinamide, Tebrazid™

Func. class.: Antitubercular agent

Chem. class.: Pyrazinoic acid amine, nicoturimide analog

Action: Bactericidal interference with lipid, nucleic acid biosynthesis

Uses: Tuberculosis, as an adjunct when other drugs are not feasible

Dosage and routes:

• *Adult:* **PO** 20-35 mg/kg/day qd or in divided dose not to exceed 3 g/day

• *Child:* **PO** 15-30 mg/kg/day qd or divided bid, max 1.5 g/day

P

Available forms: Tabs 500 mg
Side effects/adverse reactions:
INTEG: Photosensitivity, urticaria
CNS: Headache
GI: **Hepatotoxicity,** abnormal liver function tests, peptic ulcer
GU: Urinary difficulty, increased uric acid, nausea, vomiting, anorexia
HEMA: **Hemolytic anemia**
Contraindications: Hypersensitivity, severe hepatic damage
Precautions: Pregnancy (C), child <13 yr
Pharmacokinetics:
PO: Peak 2 hr, half-life 9-10 hr; metabolized in liver, excreted in urine (metabolites/unchanged drug)
Lab test interferences:
Increase: PBI
Decrease: 17-KS

NURSING CONSIDERATIONS
Assess:
• Signs of anemia: Hct, Hgb, fatigue
• Temp; if >101° F (38° C), drug should be reduced
• Liver studies qwk: ALT (SGPT), AST (SGOT), bilirubin
• Renal status before, qmo: BUN, creatinine, output, sp gr, urinalysis, uric acid
• Hepatic status: decreased appetite, jaundice, dark urine, fatigue
Administer:
PO
• With meals for GI symptoms
• After C&S is completed; qmo to detect resistance
Evaluate:
• Therapeutic response: decreased symptoms of TB, culture negative
Teach patient/family:
• That compliance with dosage schedule, length is necessary
• To avoid alcohol
• To report fever, loss of appetite, malaise, nausea, vomiting, darkened urine, pale stools

pyrethrins (℞)
(pie′rih-thrins)
A-200 Pyrinate, Barc, Pyrinyl, RID, TISIT, Triple X
Func. class.: Pediculocide
Chem. class.: Pyrethrin/piperonyl butoxide/petroleum distillate

Action: Causes paralysis, death of organism by acting as a contact poison
Uses: Head, body, pubic lice; nits; scabies
Dosage and routes:
• *Adult and child:* Apply undiluted to infested area; allow application to remain no longer than 10 min, wash thoroughly with warm water, soap, or shampoo; remove dead lice, eggs with fine-toothed comb; do not exceed 2 consecutive applications within 24 hr; may repeat in 7-10 days
• *Adult and child:* CREAM/LOTION wash area with soap, water; remove visible crusts, apply to skin surfaces, remove with soap, water in 8-12 hr; may reapply in 1 wk if needed; SHAMPOO using 30 ml, work into lather, rub for 5 min, rinse, dry with towel
Available forms: Gel, liq, shampoo, cream, lotion
Side effects/adverse reactions:
INTEG: Irritation, pruritus, urticaria, eczema
Contraindications: Hypersensitivity, inflammation of skin, abrasions, or breaks in skin
Precautions: Child/infant, ragweed sensitivity, pregnancy (C)
NURSING CONSIDERATIONS
Administer:
• To body areas, scalp only; do not apply to face, lips, mouth, eyes, any

◆ = Nursing alert   ✇ = Herb-drug interaction   ⊘ = Do not crush

mucous membrane, anus, or meatus; apply from neck down for body lice
• Topical corticosteroids as ordered to decrease contact dermatitis
• Lotions of menthol or phenol to control itching
• Topical antibiotics for infection
Perform/provide:
• Storage in tight container
• Isolation until areas on skin, scalp have cleared and treatment is complete
• Removal of nits by using a fine-toothed comb rinsed in vinegar after treatment
Evaluate:
• Therapeutic response: decreased nits, crusts
Teach patient/family:
• To discontinue use, notify prescriber of irritation or infection
• To flush with water in case of contact with eyes
• To wash all inhabitants' clothing, bed linen using insecticide; preventive treatment may be required of all persons living in same house, using lotion or shampoo to decrease spread of infection
• That itching may continue 4-6 wk
• That drug must be reapplied if accidentally washed off, or treatment will be ineffective
• To use externally only
• To treat sexual partners simultaneously

---

pyridostigmine (℞)

(peer-id-oh-stig′meen)
Mestinon, Mestinon SR*, Mestinon Timespan, Regonol
Func. class.: Cholinergic; anticholinesterase
Chem. class.: Tertiary amine carbamate

Action: Inhibits destruction of acetylcholine, which increases concentration at sites where acetylcholine is released; this facilitates transmission of impulses across myoneural junction

Uses: Nondepolarizing muscle relaxant antagonist, myasthenia gravis

Dosage and routes:

Myasthenia gravis
• *Adult:* **PO** 60-180 mg bid-qid, not to exceed 1.5 g/day; **IM/IV** 2 mg or ¹/₃₀ of **PO** dose; **SUS REL** 180-540 mg qd or bid at intervals of at least 6 hr
• *Child:* 7 mg/kg/day in 5-6 divided doses

Nondepolarizing neuromuscular blocker antagonist
• *Adult:* 0.6-1.2 mg **IV** atropine, then 10-30 mg
• *Child:* 0.1-0.25 mg/kg/dose

Available forms: Tabs 60 mg; tabs, sus rel 180 mg; syr 60 mg/5 ml; inj 5 mg/ml

Side effects/adverse reactions:
INTEG: Rash, urticaria, flushing
CNS: Dizziness, headache, sweating, weakness, *convulsions,* incoordination, paralysis, drowsiness, LOC
GI: Nausea, diarrhea, vomiting, cramps, increased salivary and gastric secretions, peristalsis
CV: Tachycardia, dysrhythmias, bradycardia, AV block, hypotension, ECG changes, *cardiac arrest,* syncope

P

GU: Frequency, incontinence, urgency

*RESP: **Respiratory depression, bronchospasm, constriction, laryngospasm, respiratory arrest***

EENT: Miosis, blurred vision, lacrimation, visual changes

Contraindications: Bradycardia; hypotension; obstruction of intestine, renal system; bromide sensitivity

Precautions: Seizure disorders, bronchial asthma, coronary occlusion, hyperthyroidism, dysrhythmias, peptic ulcer, megacolon, poor GI motility, pregnancy (C)

Pharmacokinetics:

PO: Onset 20-30 min, duration 3-6 hr

IM/IV/SC: Onset 2-15 min, duration 2½-4 hr; metabolized in liver, excreted in urine

Interactions:

• Decreased action: gallamine, metocurine, pancuronium, tubocurarine, atropine

• Increased action: decamethonium, succinylcholine

• Decreased action of pyridostigmine: aminoglycosides, anesthetics, procainamide, quinidine, mecamylamine, polymyxin, magnesium, corticosteroids, antidysrhythmics

NURSING CONSIDERATIONS

Assess:

• VS, respiration q8h

• I&O ratio; check for urinary retention or incontinence

• Bradycardia, hypotension, bronchospasm, headache, dizziness, convulsions, respiratory depression; drug should be discontinued if toxicity occurs

Administer:

• Only with atropine sulfate available for cholinergic crisis

• Only after all other cholinergics have been discontinued

• Increased doses for tolerance

• Larger doses after exercise or fatigue

• On empty stomach for better absorption

IV

• Undiluted, give through Y-tube or 3-way stopcock, give 0.5 mg or less/min

Syringe compatibilities: Glycopyrrolate

Y-site compatibilities: Heparin, hydrocortisone, potassium chloride, vit B/C

Perform/provide:

• Storage at room temp

Evaluate:

• Therapeutic response: increased muscle strength, hand grasp, improved gait, absence of labored breathing (if severe)

Teach patient/family:

🚫 Not to break, crush, or chew sus rel prep

• That drug is not a cure, only relieves symptoms

• To wear Medic Alert ID specifying myasthenia gravis, drugs taken

Treatment of overdose: Discontinue drug, atropine 1-4 mg IV

---

pyridoxine (vit B₆) (℞)

(peer-i-dox′een)

Beesix, Hexa-Betalin, Nestrex, Pyridoxine HCl, Rodex TD, Vitamin B₆

Func. class.: Vit B₆, water soluble

Action: Needed for fat, protein, carbohydrate metabolism; enhances glycogen release from liver and muscle tissue; needed as coenzyme for metabolic transformations of a variety of amino acids

Uses: Vit B₆ deficiency of inborn errors of metabolism, seizures, iso-

---

◆ = Nursing alert　　🖋 = Herb-drug interaction　　🚫 = Do not crush

niazid therapy, oral contraceptives, alcoholic polyneuritis

Dosage and routes:

Vit B₆ deficiency
- *Adult:* **PO/IM/IV** 2.5-10 mg until corrected, then 2-5 mg qd
- *Child:* **PO/IM/IV** 100 mg until desired response

Inborn errors of metabolism
- *Adult:* **IM/IV/PO** 600 mg or less qd, then 50 mg qd for life
- *Child:* **IM/PO/IV** 100 mg, then 2-10 mg **IM** or 10-100 mg **PO** qd

Deficiency caused by isoniazid
- *Adult:* **PO** 100 mg qd × 3 wk, then 50 mg qd
- *Child:* **PO** 5-25 mg/day × 3 wk, then 1.5-2.5 mg/day

Prevention of deficiency caused by isoniazid
- *Adult:* **PO** 10-50 mg qd
- *Child:* **PO** 0.5-1.5 mg qd
- *Infant:* **PO** 0.1-0.5 mg qd

Available forms: Tabs 10, 25, 50, 100, 200, 250, 500 mg; tabs, time rel 500 mg; inj 100 mg/ml; oral caps 500 mg

Side effects/adverse reactions:
CNS: Paresthesia, flushing, warmth, lethargy (rare with normal renal function)
INTEG: Pain at injection site

Contraindications: Hypersensitivity

Precautions: Pregnancy (A), lactation, child, Parkinson's disease

Pharmacokinetics:
PO/Inj: Half-life 2-3 wk, metabolized in liver, excreted in urine

Interactions:
- Decreased effects of levodopa
- Decreased effects of pyridoxine: oral contraceptives, isoniazid, cycloserine, hydralazine, penicillamine

NURSING CONSIDERATIONS
Assess:
- Pyridoxine levels throughout treatment

- Nutritional status: yeast, liver, legumes, bananas, green vegetables, whole grains

Administer:
- IM, rotate sites; burning or stinging at site may occur
- Z-track to minimize pain

IV
- Undiluted or added to most IV sol; give 50 mg or less/1 min if undiluted

Syringe compatibilities: Doxapram

Perform/provide:
- Storage in tight, light resistant container

Evaluate:
- Therapeutic response: absence of nausea, vomiting, anorexia, skin lesions, glossitis, stomatitis, edema, convulsions, restlessness, paresthesia

Teach patient/family:
- To avoid vitamin supplements unless directed by prescriber
- To keep out of children's reach
- To increase meat, bananas, potatoes, lima beans, whole grain cereals
- To discuss birth control status with prescriber

---

pyrimethamine (R)
(peer-i-meth'a-meen)
Daraprim, Fansidar (with sulfadoxine)
Func. class.: Antimalarial
Chem. class.: Folic acid antagonist

Action: Inhibits folic acid metabolism in parasite, prevents transmission by stopping growth of fertilized gametes

Uses: Malaria prophylaxis, *P. vivax*

Investigational uses: *Pneumocystis carinii* pneumonia as an adjunct

Dosage and routes:
Prophylaxis of malaria
- *Adult:* **PO** 1 tab qwk or 2 tabs q2wk (Fansidar)
- *Child 9-14 yr:* **PO** ¾ tab qwk or 1½ tabs q2wk (Fansidar)
- *Child >10 yr:* **PO** 25 mg qwk
- *Child 4-10 yr:* **PO** 12.5 mg qwk
- *Child 4-8 yr:* **PO** ½ tab qwk or 1 tab q2wk (Fansidar)
- *Child <4 yr:* **PO** ¼ tab qwk or ½ tab q2wk (Fansidar)
- *Child <4 yr:* **PO** 6.25 mg qwk

Acute attacks of malaria
- *Adult:* **PO** 2-3 tabs as a single dose (Fansidar) alone or with quinine or primaquine
- *Child 9-14 yr:* 2 tabs
- *Child 4-8 yr:* 1 tab
- *Child <4 yr:* ½ tab

Toxoplasmosis
- *Adult:* **PO** 100 mg, then 25 mg qd × 4-5 wk, with 1 g sulfadoxine q6h
- *Child:* **PO** 1 mg/kg, then 0.25 mg/kg qd × 4-5 wk, with sulfadoxine 100 mg/kg/day in divided doses q6h

Toxoplasmosis in AIDS patients
- *Adult:* **PO** 100-200 mg/day × 1-2 days, then 50-100 mg/day × 3-6 wk, then 25-50 mg/day for life (given with clindamycin or sulfadiazine)

Available forms: Tabs 25 mg; combo tabs 500 mg sulfadoxine/25 mg pyrimethamine

Side effects/adverse reactions:
RESP: **Respiratory failure**
INTEG: Skin eruptions, photosensitivity
CNS: Stimulation, irritability, **convulsions,** tremors, ataxia, fatigue
GI: Nausea, vomiting, cramps, anorexia, diarrhea, atrophic glossitis, gastritis
HEMA: **Thrombocytopenia, leukopenia, pancytopenia, megaloblastic anemia,** decreased folic acid, **agranulocytosis**
Contraindications: Hypersensitivity, chloroquine-resistant malaria, megaloblastic anemia caused by folate deficiency

Precautions: Blood dyscrasias, seizure disorder, pregnancy (C), lactation, G6PD disease, renal, hepatic disease

Pharmacokinetics:
PO: Peak 2 hr, half-life 111 hr; metabolized in liver, highly protein bound, excreted in urine (metabolites)

Interactions:
- Synergistic action: paraaminobenzoic acid or folic acid
- Increased bone marrow suppression: antibiotics

NURSING CONSIDERATIONS
Assess:
- Folic acid level; megaloblastic anemia occurs
- Blood studies, CBC, platelets, since blood dyscrasias occur; twice weekly if dosage is increased
- ⬥ For toxicity: vomiting, anorexia, seizure, blood dyscrasia, glossitis; drug should be discontinued immediately

Administer:
- Leucovorin IM 3-9 mg/day × 3 days if folic acid deficiency occurs
- Before or after meals at same time each day to maintain drug level, to decrease GI symptoms

Perform/provide:
- Storage in tight, light-resistant container

Evaluate:
- Therapeutic response: decreased symptoms of malaria

Teach patient/family:
- To report visual problems, fever, fatigue, bruising, bleeding; may indicate blood dyscrasias

Treatment of overdose: Gastric lavage, short-acting barbiturate, leucovorin, respiratory support if needed

---

⬥ = Nursing alert　　🌿 = Herb-drug interaction　　🚫 = Do not crush

quazepam (℞)

(kway'ze-pam)

Doral

Func. class.: Sedative-hypnotic

Chem. class.: Benzodiazepine derivative

Controlled Substance Schedule IV

Action: Produces CNS depression at the limbic, thalamic, hypothalamic levels of CNS; may be mediated by neurotransmitter γ-aminobutyric acid (GABA); results are sedation, hypnosis, skeletal muscle relaxation, anticonvulsant activity, anxiolytic action

Uses: Insomnia

Dosage and routes:

• *Adult:* **PO** 15 mg hs, then 7.5-15 mg hs

• *Elderly:* **PO** 15 mg hs × 2 days, then 7.5 mg hs

Available forms: Tabs 7.5, 15 mg

Side effects/adverse reactions:

HEMA: **Leukopenia, granulocytopenia** (rare)

CNS: Lethargy, drowsiness, daytime sedation, dizziness, confusion, lightheadedness, headache, anxiety, irritability, weakness, tremor, depression

GI: Nausea, vomiting, diarrhea, heartburn, abdominal pain, constipation, anorexia, taste alteration

CV: Chest pain, pulse changes, palpitations, tachycardia

MISC: Joint pain, congestion, dermatitis, sweating

Contraindications: Hypersensitivity to benzodiazepines, pregnancy (X), lactation

Precautions: Hepatic or renal disease, suicidal individuals, drug abuse, elderly, psychosis, child <18 yr, depression, pulmonary insufficiency

Pharmacokinetics:

PO: Onset 15-45 min, duration 7-8 hr; metabolized by liver, excreted by kidneys (inactive/active metabolites), crosses placenta, excreted in breast milk

Interactions:

• Increased effects of quazepam: cimetidine, disulfiram

• Decreased effects: smoking, rifampin, theophylline with increased levels of phenytoin and digoxin

• Increased CNS depression: alcohol, CNS depressants

• Decreased effect of quazepam: antacids

⚕ Increased CNS depression: kava kava

Lab test interferences:

Increase: AST (SGOT), ALT (SGPT), serum bilirubin

Decrease: RAI uptake

NURSING CONSIDERATIONS

Assess:

• Blood studies: Hct, Hgb, RBCs (if on long-term therapy)

• Hepatic studies: AST (SGOT), ALT (SGPT), bilirubin

• Mental status: mood, sensorium, affect, memory (long, short)

• Blood dyscrasias: fever, sore throat, bruising, rash, jaundice, epistaxis (rare)

• Type of sleep problem: falling asleep, staying asleep

Administer:

• After removal of cigarettes to prevent fires

• After trying conservative measures for insomnia

• ½-1 hr before hs for sleeplessness

• On empty stomach for fast onset, but may be taken with food if GI symptoms occur

Perform/provide:

• Assistance with ambulation after receiving dose

- Safety measures: night-light, call bell within easy reach
- Checking to see if PO medication has been swallowed
- Storage in tight container in cool environment

Evaluate:

- Therapeutic response: ability to sleep at night, decreased amount of early morning awakening

Teach patient/family:

- To avoid driving or other activities requiring alertness until drug is stabilized
- To avoid alcohol ingestion, CNS depressants; serious CNS depression may result
- That effects may take 2 nights for benefits to be noticed
- Alternative measures to improve sleep: reading, exercise several hr before hs, warm bath, warm milk, TV, self-hypnosis, deep breathing
- That hangover is common in elderly but less common than with barbiturates

Treatment of overdose: Lavage, activated charcoal; monitor electrolytes, vital signs

---

quetiapine (Ŗ)

(kwe-tie'a-peen)

Seroquel

Func. class.: Antipsychotic/neuroleptic

Action: Functions as an antagonist at multiple neurotransmitter receptors in the brain including $5HT_{1A}$, $5HT_2$, dopamine D_1, D_2, H_1, and adrenergic $alpha_1$, $alpha_2$ receptors

Uses: Psychotic disorders

Dosage and routes:

- *Adult:* **PO** 25 mg bid, with incremental increases of 25 mg bid-tid on days 2 and 3 to a dose of 300-400 mg qd given bid-tid

Available forms: Tabs 25, 100, 200 mg

Side effects/adverse reactions:

CNS: EPS, pseudoparkinsonism, akathisia, dystonia, tardive dyskinesia; drowsiness, insomnia, agitation, anxiety, *headache, seizures,* **neuroleptic malignant syndrome,** *dizziness*

CV: Orthostatic hypotension, **tachycardia**

GI: Nausea, anorexia, constipation, abdominal pain, dry mouth

RESP: Rhinitis

INTEG: Rash

MISC: Asthenia, back pain, fever, ear pain

Contraindications: Hypersensitivity

Precautions: Children, pregnancy (C), hepatic disease, elderly, breast cancer, lactation, long-term use, seizures, dementia

Pharmacokinetics:

PO: Extensively metabolized by liver half-life ≥6 hr; peak 1½ hr

Interactions:

- Decreased clearance of quetiapine: cimetidine
- Increased clearance of quetiapine: phenytoin, thioridazine, barbiturates, glucocorticoids
- Decreased clearance of lorazepam: lorazepam
- Decreased clearance of levodopa: levodopa
- Decreased effects of dopamine agonists: dopamine agonists

NURSING CONSIDERATIONS

Assess:

- Mental status before initial administration
- Swallowing of PO medication: check for hoarding or giving of medication to other patients
- I&O ratio; palpate bladder if urinary output is low
- Bilirubin, CBC, liver function studies qmo

• Urinalysis before, during prolonged therapy

• Affect, orientation, LOC, reflexes, gait, coordination, sleep pattern disturbances

• B/P standing and lying; also pulse, respirations; take these q4h during initial treatment; establish baseline before starting treatment; report drops of 30 mm Hg; watch for ECG changes

• Dizziness, faintness, palpitations, tachycardia on rising

• EPS, including akathisia (inability to sit still, no pattern to movements), tardive dyskinesia (bizarre movements of the jaw, mouth, tongue, extremities), pseudoparkinsonism (rigidity, tremors, pill rolling, shuffling gait)

◆ For neuroleptic malignant syndrome: hyperthermia, increased CPK, altered mental status, muscle rigidity

• Skin turgor qd

• Constipation, urinary retention qd; if these occur, increase bulk and water in the diet

Administer:

• Reduced dose in elderly

• Antiparkinsonian agent on order from prescriber, to be used for EPS

Perform/provide:

• Decreased stimulus by dimming lights, avoiding loud noises

• Supervised ambulation until patient is stabilized on medication; do not involve in strenuous exercise program because fainting is possible; patient should not stand still for a long time

• Increased fluids to prevent constipation

• Sips of water, candy, gum for dry mouth

• Storage in tight, light-resistant container

Evaluate:

• Therapeutic response: decrease in

emotional excitement, hallucinations, delusions, paranoia,; reorganization of patterns of thought, speech

---

quinapril (R)

(kwin′a-pril)
Accupril
Func. class.: Antihypertensive
Chem. class.: Angiotensin-converting enzyme (ACE) inhibitor

Action: Selectively suppresses renin-angiotensin-aldosterone system; inhibits ACE, prevents conversion of angiotensin I to angiotensin II; results in dilation of arterial, venous vessels

Uses: Hypertension, alone or in combination with thiazide diuretics; systolic CHF

Dosage and routes:
Renal dose

• CrCl 30-60 ml/min 5 mg/day initially; CrCl <30 ml/min 2.5 mg/day initially

Hypertension

• *Adult:* PO 10 mg qd initially, then 20-80 mg/day divided bid or qd

• *Geriatric:* PO 2.5-5 mg qd, increase by 2.5-5 mg at weekly intervals to desired dose

Congestive heart failure

• *Adult:* PO 2.5 mg initially, then 5-40 mg/day maintenance qd or in 2 divided doses

Available forms: Tabs 5, 10, 20, 40 mg

Side effects/adverse reactions:

CV: Hypotension, postural hypotension, syncope, palpitations, angina pectoris, MI, tachycardia, vasodilation

GU: Increased BUN, creatinine, decreased libido, impotence, urinary tract infection

---

HEMA: **Thrombocytopenia, agranulocytosis**
INTEG: **Angioedema,** rash, sweating, photosensitivity, pruritus
RESP: Cough, bronchitis
META: Hyperkalemia
GI: Nausea, constipation, vomiting, gastritis, GI hemorrhage, dry mouth
CNS: Headache, dizziness, fatigue, somnolence, depression, malaise, nervousness, vertigo
MISC: Back pain, amblyopia, pharyngitis
MS: Arthralgia, arthritis, myalgia
Contraindications: Hypersensitivity to ACE inhibitors, pregnancy (D), children
Precautions: Impaired renal, liver function, dialysis patients, hypovolemia, blood dyscrasias, COPD, asthma, elderly, lactation
Pharmacokinetics:
PO: Peak ½-1 hr, serum protein binding 97%, half-life 2 hr, metabolized by liver (metabolites), metabolites excreted in urine
Interactions:
• Increased hypotension: diuretics, other antihypertensives, ganglionic blockers, adrenergic blockers, phenothiazines
• Use caution with vasodilators, hydralazine, prazosin, potassium-sparing diuretics, sympathomimetics, K supplements
• Decreased absorption of tetracycline
• Reduced hypotensive effect of quinapril: indomethacin
• Increased toxicity: lithium, digoxin
Lab test interferences:
False positive: Urine acetone

NURSING CONSIDERATIONS
Assess:
• Blood studies: neutrophils, decreased platelets
• B/P, orthostatic hypotension, syncope

• Renal studies: protein, BUN, creatinine; watch for increased levels; may indicate nephrotic syndrome
• Baselines in renal, liver function tests before therapy begins
• K levels; hyperkalemia is rare
• Edema in feet, legs qd
• Allergic reactions: rash, fever, pruritus, urticaria; drug should be discontinued if antihistamines fail to help
• Renal symptoms: polyuria, oliguria, frequency, dysuria
Administer:
• IV infusion of 0.9% NaCl (as ordered) to expand fluid volume if severe hypotension occurs
Perform/provide:
• Supine or Trendelenburg position for severe hypotension
Evaluate:
• Therapeutic response: decrease in B/P
Teach patient/family:
• To take 1 hr before meals; not to take antacids within 1-2 hr of quinapril
• Not to discontinue drug abruptly
• Not to use OTC products (cough, cold, allergy); not to use salt substitutes containing potassium unless directed by prescriber
• To comply with dosage schedule, even if feeling better
• To rise slowly to sitting or standing position to minimize orthostatic hypotension
• To notify prescriber of mouth sores, sore throat, fever, swelling of hands or feet, irregular heartbeat, chest pain, persistent dry cough
• To report excessive perspiration, dehydration, vomiting, diarrhea; may lead to fall in B/P
• That drug may cause dizziness, fainting, light-headedness; may occur during first few days of therapy

---

• That drug may cause skin rash or impaired taste perception
• How to take B/P, and normal readings for age group
Treatment of overdose: 0.9% NaCl IV inf

---

quinestrol (Ŗ)
(kwin-ess'trole)
Estrovis
Func. class.: Estrogen
Chem. class.: Nonsteroidal synthetic estrogen

Action: Needed for adequate functioning of female reproductive system; affects release of pituitary gonadotropins, inhibits ovulation, promotes adequate calcium use in bone structures

Uses: Menopause, atrophic vaginitis, kraurosis vulvae, female castration, female hypogonadism, primary ovarian failure

Dosage and routes:
• *Adult:* PO 100 μg qd × 1 wk, then 100 μg qwk starting 2 wk after beginning treatment; may increase to 200 μg/wk
Available forms: Tabs 100 μg

Side effects/adverse reactions:
CNS: Dizziness, headache, migraine, depression
CV: Hypotension, thrombophlebitis, edema, *thromboembolism, stroke, pulmonary embolism, MI*
GI: *Nausea,* vomiting, diarrhea, anorexia, *pancreatitis,* cramps, constipation, increased appetite, increased weight, *cholestatic jaundice*
EENT: Contact lens intolerance, increased myopia, astigmatism
GU: Amenorrhea, cervical erosion, breakthrough bleeding, dysmenorrhea, vaginal candidiasis, breast changes, *gynecomastia, testicular atrophy, impotence*
INTEG: Rash, urticaria, acne, hirsutism, alopecia, oily skin, seborrhea, purpura, melasma
META: Folic acid deficiency, hypercalcemia, hyperglycemia

Contraindications: Breast cancer, thromboembolic disorders, reproductive cancer, genital bleeding (abnormal, undiagnosed), pregnancy (X), lactation

Precautions: Hypertension, asthma, blood dyscrasias, gallbladder disease, CHF, diabetes mellitus, bone disease, depression, migraine headache, convulsive disorders, hepatic disease, renal disease, family history of cancer of breast or reproductive tract

Pharmacokinetics:
PO: Degraded in liver; excreted in urine, breast milk; crosses placenta

Interactions:
• Decreased action of anticoagulants, oral hypoglycemics
• Toxicity: tricyclic antidepressants
• Decreased action of quinestrol: anticonvulsants, barbiturates, phenylbutazone, rifampin
• Increased action of corticosteroids

NURSING CONSIDERATIONS

Assess:
• Urine glucose in patient with diabetes; urine glucose may rise
• Weight qd; notify prescriber of weekly gain >5 lb; if increase, diuretic may be ordered
• B/P q4h; watch for increase caused by H_2O, Na retention
• I&O ratio; be alert for decreasing urinary output, increasing edema
• Liver function studies, including AST, ALT, bilirubin, alk phosphatase
• Edema, hypertension, cardiac symptoms, jaundice, calcemia
• Mental status: affect or mood, behavioral changes, aggression

---

Administer:
• Titrated dose; use lowest effective dose
• With food or milk to decrease GI symptoms

Evaluate:
• Therapeutic response: reversal of menopause or decrease in tumor size in prostatic cancer

Teach patient/family:
• To weigh qwk, report gain >5 lb
• To report breast lumps, vaginal bleeding, edema, jaundice, dark urine, clay-colored stools, dyspnea, headache, blurred vision, abdominal pain, numbness or stiffness in legs, chest pain; male to report impotence or gynecomastia

---

quinidine (℞)

(kwin'i-deen)
Apo-Quinidine*, Cardioquin; Cin-Quin*, Novoquinidin*, Quinaglute, Quinalan, Quinidex Extentabs, quinidine gluconate; quinidine sulfate, Quinora

Func. class.: Antidysrhythmic (Class Ia)

Chem. class.: Quinine dextro-isomer

Action: Prolongs duration of action potential and effective refractory period, thus decreasing myocardial excitability; anticholinergic properties

Uses: PVCs, atrial fibrillation, PAT, ventricular tachycardia, atrial dysrhythmias

Investigational uses: Malaria/IV quinidine gluconate

Dosage and routes:

Quinidine sulfate

Atrial fibrillation/flutter
• *Adult:* PO 200 mg q2-3h × 5-8 doses; may increase qd until sinus rhythm is restored; max 4 g/day given only after digitalization

Paroxysmal supraventricular tachycardia
• *Adult:* PO 400-600 mg q2-3h, then 200-300 mg q6-8h or 300-600 mg q8-12h (SUS REL)

Premature atrial/ventricular contraction
• *Adult:* PO 200-300 mg q6-8h or 300-600 mg (SUS REL) q8-12h; max 4 g/day
• *Child:* PO 6 mg/kg or 180 mg/m² 5×/day

Quinidine gluconate
• *Adult:* PO 324-660 mg q6-12h (SUS REL); **IM** 600 mg, then 400 mg q2h; **IV** give 16 mg/min

Quinidine polygalacturonate
• *Adult:* **PO** 275-825 mg q3-4h × 4 doses, then increase by 137.5-275 mg; repeat up to 4× until dysrhythmias decreased
• *Child:* PO 8.25 mg/kg (247.5 mg/ m²) 5×/day

Available forms: Gluconate tabs sus rel 324, 330 mg; inj gluconate 80 mg/ml; sulfate tabs 200, 300 mg; tabs sus rel 300 mg; polygalacturonate tabs 275 mg

Side effects/adverse reactions:
CNS: Headache, dizziness, involuntary movement, confusion, psychosis, restlessness, irritability, syncope, excitement

EENT: Cinchonism: tinnitus, blurred vision, hearing loss, mydriasis, disturbed color vision

GI: Nausea, vomiting, anorexia, *diarrhea,* **hepatotoxicity**

CV: Hypotension, bradycardia, PVCs, **heart block, cardiovascular collapse, arrest,** torsades de pointes

HEMA: **Thrombocytopenia,** hemolytic anemia, agranulocytosis, hypoprothrombinemia

RESP: Dyspnea, **respiratory depression**

 = Nursing alert   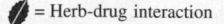 = Herb-drug interaction   🚫 = Do not crush

INTEG: Rash, urticaria, angioedema, swelling, photosensitivity

Contraindications: Hypersensitivity, blood dyscrasias, severe heart block, myasthenia gravis

Precautions: Pregnancy (C), lactation, children, renal disease, K imbalance, liver disease, CHF, respiratory depression

Pharmacokinetics:

PO: Peak 0.5-6 hr, duration 6-8 hr; half-life 6-7 hr, metabolized in liver, excreted unchanged by kidneys

Interactions:

• Increased effects of neuromuscular blockers, digoxin, warfarin

• Increased effects of quinidine: cimetidine, propranolol, thiazides, sodium bicarbonate, carbonic anhydrase inhibitors, antacids, hydroxide suspensions, amiodarone

• May decrease effects of quinidine: barbiturates, phenytoin, rifampin, nifedipine

• Additive vagolytic effect: anticholinergic blockers

• Additive cardiac depression: other antidysrhythmics, phenothiazines, reserpine

🌿 Potassium deficiency, increased antidysrhythmic action: aloe, buckthorn bark/berry, cascara sagrada bark, senna pod/leaf

Lab test interferences:

Increase: CPK

NURSING CONSIDERATIONS

Assess:

• ECG continuously to determine increased PR or QRS segments, QT interval; discontinue or reduce dose

• Blood levels (therapeutic level 2-6 μg/ml)

• B/P continuously for fluctuations

• Cinchonism: tinnitus, headache, nausea, dizziness, fever, vertigo, tremor; may lead to hearing loss

• Cardiac status: rate, rhythm, character, continuously

• Respiratory status: rate, rhythm, lung fields for rales; increased respiration, increased pulse; drug should be discontinued

• CNS effects: dizziness, confusion, psychosis, paresthesias, convulsions; drug should be discontinued

Administer:

• IM inj in deltoid; aspirate to avoid intravascular administration

• AV node blocker (digoxin, verapamil) before starting quinidine to avoid increased ventricular rate

IV

• After diluting 800 mg/40 ml or more D_5; give 16 mg or less over 1 min as inf; use inf pump

Additive compatibilities: Bretylium, cimetidine, milrinone, ranitidine, verapamil

Y-site compatibilities: Diazepam, milrinone

Evaluate:

• Therapeutic response: decreased dysrhythmias

Treatment of overdose: O_2, artificial ventilation, ECG, administer dopamine for circulatory depression, diazepam or thiopental for convulsions

---

quinine (otc, ℞)

(kwye′nine)

Formula Q, Legatrin, M-Kya, Novoquine*, Quinamm, Quinine Sulfate, Quiphile, Q-Vel

Func. class.: Antimalarial

Chem. class.: Cinchona tree alkaloid

Action: Inhibits parasite replications, transcription of DNA to RNA by forming complexes with DNA of parasite

Uses: *Plasmodium falciparum* malaria, nocturnal leg cramps

Dosage and routes:

• *Adult:* PO 650 mg q8h × 10 days,

given with pyrimethamine 25 mg q12h × 3 days, with sulfadiazine 500 mg qid × 5 days
• *Child:* **PO** 25 mg/kg/day divided q8h for 3-7 days
Leg cramps
• *Adult:* **PO** 250-300 mg hs
Available forms: Caps 130, 195, 200, 300, 325 mg; tabs 260, 325 mg
Side effects/adverse reactions:
RESP: Dyspnea
INTEG: Pruritus, pigmentary changes, skin eruptions, lichen planuslike eruptions, flushing, facial edema, sweating
*HEMA: **Thrombocytopenia, purpura, hypothrombinemia, hemolysis***
CNS: Headache, stimulation, fatigue, irritability, *convulsions,* bad dreams, dizziness, fever, confusion, anxiety
EENT: Blurred vision, corneal changes, retinal changes, difficulty focusing, tinnitus, vertigo, deafness, photophobia, diplopia, night blindness
GU: Renal tubular damage, *anuria*
GI: Nausea, vomiting, anorexia, diarrhea, epigastric pain
CV: Angina, dysrhythmias, tachycardia, hypotension, *acute circulatory failure*
ENDO: Hypoglycemia
Contraindications: Hypersensitivity, G6PD deficiency, retinal field changes, pregnancy (X)
Precautions: Blood dyscrasias, severe GI disease, neurologic disease, severe hepatic disease, psoriasis, cardiac dysrhythmias, tinnitus
Pharmacokinetics:
PO: Peak 1-3 hr, metabolized in liver, excreted in urine, half-life 4-5 hr
Interactions:
• Toxicity: $NaHCO_3$, acetazolamide
• Decreased absorption: magnesium or aluminum salts

• Increased levels of digoxin, digitoxin, neuromuscular blockers, other anticoagulants
Lab test interferences:
Increase: 17-KS
Interference: 17-OHCS
NURSING CONSIDERATIONS
Assess:
• B/P, pulse, watch for hypotension, tachycardia
• Liver studies qwk: ALT (SGPT), AST (SGOT), bilirubin
• Blood studies, CBC, since blood dyscrasias occur
• For cinchonism: nausea, blurred vision, tinnitus, headache, difficulty focusing
Administer:
• Before or after meals at same time each day to maintain level
Perform/provide:
• Storage in tight, light-resistant container
Evaluate:
• Therapeutic response: decreased symptoms of malaria
Teach patient/family:
• To avoid OTC preparations: cold preparations, tonic water

---

rabies immune globulin, human (℞)
Hyperab, Imogam
Func. class.: Immune serum
Chem. class.: IgG

Action: Provides passive immunity; given with HDCV; may be used regardless of time of bite, treatment
Uses: Exposure to rabies
Dosage and routes:
• *Adult and child:* **IM** 20 IU/kg given at same time as 1st rabies vaccine; infiltrate wound with ½ dose, then administer rest **IM,** 1 ml dose of vaccine on each of days 3, 7, 14, 28 after 1st dose

---

◆ = Nursing alert   ∥ = Herb-drug interaction   ⃠ = Do not crush

Available forms: Inj 125 IU/ml
Side effects/adverse reactions:
INTEG: Pain at injection site, rash, pruritus
MS: Arthralgia
SYST: Lymphadenopathy, **anaphylaxis,** fever
CNS: Headache, fatigue, malaise
GI: Abdominal pain
Contraindications: Hypersensitivity to equine products and thimerosal
Interactions:
• Decreased action of rabies immune globulin: corticosteroids, immunosuppressants
NURSING CONSIDERATIONS
Administer:
• Test dose: dilute drug either with 1:100 or 1:1000 0.9% NaCl for inj, inj 0.1 ml 0.9% NaCl in other arm intradermally, check for wheal [dG]10 mm after 10 min; if present, drug should not be used
• Only with epinephrine 1:1000, resuscitative equipment available
• As soon as possible after exposure
Perform/provide:
• Storage at 36°-46°F (2°-8°C)
Evaluate:
• Allergic reactions: dyspnea, rash, pruritus, eruptions
Teach patient/family:
• That pain, swelling, itching may occur at injection site
• To take acetaminophen to alleviate headache, fever, and pain

---

radioactive iodine (sodium iodide)
¹³¹I (℞)

Func. class.: Antithyroid
Chem. class.: Radiopharmaceutical

Action: Converted to protein-bound iodine by thyroid gland for use when needed

Uses:
High dose: Thyroid cancer, hyperthyroidism
Low dose: Visualization to determine thyroid cancer, diagnostic aid in thyroid function studies
Dosage and routes:
Thyroid cancer
• Adult: **PO** 50-150 mCi, may repeat depending on clinical status
Hyperthyroidism
• Adult: **PO** 4-10 mCi, depending on serum thyroxine level
Available forms: Caps 1-50, 0.8-100 mCi; oral sol 7.05 mCi/ml, 3.5-150 mCi/vial
Side effects/adverse reactions:
ENDO: Hypothyroidism, **hyperthyroid adenoma,** transient thyroiditis
INTEG: Alopecia
HEMA: **Eosinophilia, lymphedema, leukemia, bone marrow depression, leukopenia,** anemia
GI: Nausea, diarrhea, vomiting
EENT: Sore throat, cough
Contraindications: Recent MI, lactation, large nodular goiter, pregnancy (X), age <30 yr, vomiting/diarrhea, acute hyperthyroidism, use of thyroid drugs, lactation
Pharmacokinetics:
PO: Onset 3-6 days; excreted in urine, sweat, feces, breast milk; crosses placenta; excreted in 56 days
Interactions:
• Hypothyroidism: lithium
• Decreased uptake if recent intake of stable iodine, thyroid, antithyroid drugs
NURSING CONSIDERATIONS
Assess:
• Weight qd in same clothing, scale, time of day
• Blood work, including CBC for blood dyscrasias (leukopenia, thrombocytopenia, agranulocytosis)
• Overdose: peripheral edema, heat intolerance, diaphoresis, palpitations, dysrhythmias, severe tachy-

R

cardia, increased temp, delirium, CNS irritability
- Hypersensitivity: rash, enlarged cervical lymph nodes; drug may have to be discontinued
- Hypoprothrombinemia: bleeding, petechiae, ecchymosis
- Clinical response: after 3 wk should include increased weight, pulse; decreased T_4
- Bone marrow depression: sore throat, fever, fatigue

Administer:
- Only after discontinuing all other antithyroid agents × 5-7 days
- After NPO overnight, food delays action
- During or within 10 days after menstruation

Perform/provide:
- Limited contact with patient ½ hr/day for each person
- Adequate rest after treatment
- Fluids to 3-4 L/day for 48 hr to remove agent from body

Evaluate:
- Therapeutic response: weight gain, decreased pulse, decreased T_4, B/P

Teach patient/family:
- To empty bladder often during treatment; avoids irradiation of gonads
- To report redness, swelling, sore throat, mouth lesions; indicate blood dyscrasias
- To avoid extended contact with children, spouse for 1 wk
- That bathroom may be used by entire family
- Not to take antithyroid agents but propranolol, which decreases hyperthyroid symptoms, until total effect of taking ^{131}I has occurred (about 6 wk)
- To avoid coughing, expectorating for 24 hr (saliva and vomitus are highly radioactive for 6-8 hr)

ramipril (℞)

(ra-mi'pril)

Altace

Func. class.: Antihypertensive

Chem. class.: Angiotensin-converting enzyme inhibitor (ACE)

Action: Selectively suppresses renin-angiotensin-aldosterone system; inhibits ACE, prevents conversion of angiotensin I to angiotensin II; results in dilation of arterial, venous vessels

Uses: Hypertension, alone or in combination with thiazide diuretics; CHF (post MI)

Dosage and routes:
- *Adult:* **PO** 2.5 mg qd initially, then 2.5-20 mg/day divided bid or qd; *renal impairment:* 1.25 mg qd with CrCl <40 ml/min/1.73 m², increase as needed to max or 5 mg/day

CHF
- *Adult:* **PO** 1.25-2.5 mg bid; may increase to 5 mg bid

Available forms: Caps 1.25, 2.5, 5, 10 mg

Side effects/adverse reactions:

CV: Hypotension, chest pain, palpitations, angina, syncope, dysrhythmia

GU: Proteinuria, increased BUN, creatinine, impotence

HEMA: Decreased Hct, Hgb, *eosinophilia, leukopenia*

INTEG: Angioedema, rash, sweating, photosensitivity, pruritus

RESP: Cough, dyspnea

META: Hyperkalemia

GI: Nausea, constipation, vomiting, dyspepsia, dysphagia, anorexia, diarrhea, abdominal pain

CNS: Headache, dizziness, anxiety, insomnia, paresthesia, fatigue, depression, malaise, vertigo, *convulsions,* hearing loss

MS: Arthralgia, arthritis, myalgia

 = Nursing alert   = Herb-drug interaction   ⊘ = Do not crush

Contraindications: Hypersensitivity to ACE inhibitors, pregnancy (D), lactation, children

Precautions: Impaired renal, liver function; dialysis patients, hypovolemia, blood dyscrasias, CHF, COPD, asthma, elderly, renal artery stenosis

Pharmacokinetics:

PO: Peak ½-1 hr, serum protein binding 97%, half-life 1-2 hr, metabolized by liver (metabolites excreted in urine, feces)

Interactions:

• Increased hypotension: diuretics, other antihypertensives, ganglionic blockers, adrenergic blockers
• Increased toxicity: vasodilators, hydralazine, prazosin, K-sparing diuretics, sympathomimetics, K supplements
• Decreased absorption: antacids
• Decreased antihypertensive effect: indomethacin
• Increased serum levels of digoxin, lithium
• Increased hypersensitivity: allopurinol

Lab test interferences:

False positive: Urine acetone

NURSING CONSIDERATIONS

Assess:

• Blood studies: neutrophils, decreased platelets
• B/P, orthostatic hypotension, syncope
• Renal studies: protein, BUN, creatinine; increased levels may indicate nephrotic syndrome
• Baselines in renal, liver function tests before therapy begins
• K levels, although hyperkalemia rarely occurs
• Dipstick of urine for protein qd in first morning specimen; if protein is increased, a 24-hr urinary protein should be collected
• Edema in feet, legs qd

• Allergic reactions: rash, fever, pruritus, urticaria; drug should be discontinued if antihistamines fail to help
• Renal symptoms: polyuria, oliguria, frequency, dysuria

Administer:

• IV inf 0.9% NaCl (as ordered) to expand fluid volume if severe hypotension occurs
• Caps can be opened and added to food

Perform/provide:

• Storage in tight container at 48° F (30° C) or less
• Supine or Trendelenburg position for severe hypotension

Evaluate:

• Therapeutic response: decrease in B/P

Teach patient/family:

• Not to discontinue drug abruptly
• Not to use OTC products (cough, cold, allergy) unless directed by prescriber; not to use salt substitutes containing potassium without consulting prescriber
• To comply with dosage schedule, even if feeling better
• To rise slowly to sitting or standing position to minimize orthostatic hypotension
• To notify prescriber of mouth sores, sore throat, fever, swelling of hands or feet, irregular heartbeat, chest pain
• To report excessive perspiration, dehydration, vomiting, diarrhea; may lead to fall in B/P
• That drug may cause dizziness, fainting, light-headedness; may occur during first few days of therapy
• That drug may cause skin rash or impaired perspiration
• How to take B/P, and normal readings for age group

Treatment of overdose: 0.9% NaCl IV inf, hemodialysis

R

ranitidine (R, OTC)

(ra-nit'i-deen)
Apo-Ranitidine*, Tritec, Zantac, Zantac C*, Zantac EFFERdose
Func. class.: H$_2$-histamine receptor antagonist

Action: Inhibits histamine at H$_2$-receptor site in parietal cells, which inhibits gastric acid secretion

Uses: Duodenal ulcer, Zollinger-Ellison syndrome, gastric ulcers, hypersecretory conditions, gastroesophageal reflux disease, stress ulcers, erosive esophagitis (maintenance), active duodenal ulcers with *Helicobacter pylori* in combination with clarithromycin

Investigational uses: Prevention of aspiration pneumonitis, stress ulcers, upper GI bleeding

Dosage and routes:
Renal dose
• CrCl <50 ml/min give **PO** q24h give **IM/IV** q8-24h
Duodenal ulcer
• *Adult:* **PO** 150 mg bid, maintenance 150 hs
Zollinger-Ellison syndrome
• *Adult:* **PO** 150 mg bid, may increase if needed
Gastric ulcer
• *Adult:* **PO** 150 mg bid × 6 wk, then 150 mg hs
GERD
• *Adult:* **PO** 150 mg bid
Erosive esophagitis
• *Adult:* **PO** 150 mg qid
• *Adult:* **PO** 150 mg bid, 300 mg hs; **IM** 50 mg q6-8h; **IV BOL** 50 mg diluted to 20 ml over 5 min q6-8h; **IV INT INF** 50 mg/100 ml D$_5$ over 15-20 min q6-8h
• *Child:* **PO** 4-5 mg/kg/day divided q8-12h, max 6 mg/kg/day or 300 mg; **IV** 2-4 mg/kg/day divided q6-8h

Available forms: Tabs 150, 300 mg; tabs, effervescent 150 mg; inj 0.5, 25 mg/ml; caps 150, 300 mg; syr 15 mg/ml; granules, effervescent 150 mg

Side effects/adverse reactions:
CNS: Headache, sleeplessness, dizziness, confusion, agitation, depression, hallucination (elderly)
GI: Constipation, abdominal pain, diarrhea, nausea, vomiting, *hepatotoxicity*
GU: Impotence, gynecomastia
CV: Tachycardia, bradycardia, PVCs
EENT: Blurred vision, increased ocular pressure
INTEG: Urticaria, rash, fever

Contraindications: Hypersensitivity

Precautions: Pregnancy (B), lactation, child <12 yr, hepatic disease, renal disease

Pharmacokinetics:
PO: Peak 2-3 hr, duration 8-12 hr; metabolized by liver; excreted in urine, breast milk; half-life 2-3 hr

Interactions:
• Increased absorption, toxicity: anticoagulants, sulfonylureas, procainamide
• Decreased absorption of ranitidine: antacids, diazepam, anticholinergics, metoclopramide

Lab test interferences:
Increase: AST (SGOT), ALT (SGPT), alk phosphatase, creatinine, LDH, bilirubin
False positive: Urine protein

NURSING CONSIDERATIONS
Assess:
• Gastric pH (>5 should be maintained)
• I&O ratio, BUN, creatinine
• Mental status: confusion, dizziness, depression, anxiety, weakness,

 = Nursing alert   = Herb-drug interaction   = Do not crush

tremors, psychosis, diarrhea, abdominal discomfort, jaundice; report immediately
• GI complaints: nausea, vomiting, diarrhea, cramps

Administer:
• With meals for prolonged effect
• Antacids 1 hr before or 1 hr after ranitidine

IV
• IV after diluting 50 mg/20 ml NS, D_5W, $D_{10}W$, LR, $NaCO_3$ 5% and give 50 mg or less/5 min or more; may dilute 50 mg/50-100 ml of 0.9% NaCl, D_5W, $D_{10}W$, LR, $NaCO_3$ 5% and give over 15-20 min

Additive compatibilities: Acetazolamide, amikacin, aminophylline, chloramphenicol, chlorothiazide, ciprofloxacin, colistimethate, dexamethasone, digoxin, dobutamine, dopamine, doxycycline, epinephrine, erythromycin, floxacillin, fluconazole/ondansetron, flumazenil, furosemide, gentamicin, heparin, insulin (regular), isoproterenol, lidocaine, lincomycin, meropenem, methylprednisolone, moxalactam, penicillin G potassium, penicillin G sodium, polymyxin B, potassium chloride, protamine, quinidine, sodium nitroprusside, ticarcillin, tobramycin, vancomycin

Syringe compatibilities: Atropine, cyclizine, dexamethasone, dimenhydrinate, diphenhydramine, dobutamine, dopamine, fentanyl, glycopyrrolate, hydromorphone, isoproterenol, meperidine, metoclopramide, morphine, nalbuphine, oxymorphone, pentazocine, perphenazine, prochlorperazine, promethazine, scopolamine

Y-site compatibilities: Acyclovir, aldesleukin, allopurinol, amifostine, aminophylline, amsacrine, atracurium, aztreonam, bretylium, cefepime, cefmetazole, ceftazidime, ciprofloxacin, cisplatin, cladribine, cyclophosphamide, cytarabine, diltiazem, dobutamine, dopamine, doxorubicin, enalaprilat, epinephrine, esmolol, fentanyl, filgrastim, fluconazole, fludarabine, foscarnet, furosemide, gallium, granisetron, heparin, hydromorphone, idarubicin, labetalol, lorazepam, melphalan, meperidine, methotrexate, midazolam, milrinone, morphine, nicardipine, nitroglycerin, norepinephrine, ondansetron, paclitaxel, pancuronium, piperacillin, piperacillin/tazobactam, procainamide, propofol, sargramostim, tacrolimus, teniposide, theophylline, thiopental, thiotepa, vecuronium, vinorelbine, warfarin, zidovudine

Perform/provide:
• Storage at room temp

Evaluate:
• Therapeutic response: decreased abdominal pain

Teach patient/family:
• That gynecomastia, impotence may occur but are reversible
• To avoid driving, other hazardous activities until stabilized on this medication
• To avoid black pepper, caffeine, alcohol, harsh spices, extremes in temp of food
• That drug must be continued for prescribed time to be effective

R

---

remifentanil (R̶)

(rem-ih-fin′ta-nill)

Ultiva

Func. class.: Narcotic agonist analgesic

Chem. class.: Mu-opioid agonist

Action: Inhibits ascending pain pathways in limbic system, thalamus, midbrain, hypothalamus

Uses: In combination with other drugs in general anesthesia, as a primary anesthetic in general surgery

Dosage and routes:

• *Adult:* Induction **IV** 0.5-1 µg/kg/min with a hypnotic or volative agent

Available forms: Powder for inj-lyophilized

Side effects/adverse reactions:

CNS: Drowsiness, *dizziness,* confusion, *headache,* sedation, euphoria, delirium, agitation, anxiety

GI: Nausea, vomiting, anorexia, constipation, cramps, dry mouth

GU: Urinary retention, dysuria

INTEG: Rash, urticaria, bruising, flushing, diaphoresis, pruritus

EENT: Tinnitus, blurred vision, miosis, diplopia

CV: Palpitations, *bradycardia,* change in B/P, facial flushing, syncope, *asystole*

RESP: Respiratory depression, apnea

MS: Rigidity

Contraindications: Child <12 yr, hypersensitivity

Precautions: Pregnancy (C), lactation, increased intracranial pressure, acute MI, severe heart disease, renal disease, hepatic disease, asthma, respiratory conditions, convulsive disorders, elderly

Pharmacokinetics: Unknown

Interactions:

• Respiratory depression, hypotension, profound sedation: alcohol, sedatives, hypnotics, or other CNS depressants; antihistamines, phenothiazines

 Increased CNS depression: kava kava

NURSING CONSIDERATIONS

Assess:

• I&O ratio, check for decreasing output; may indicate urinary retention, especially in elderly

• CNS changes; dizziness, drowsiness, hallucinations, euphoria, LOC, pupil reaction

• Allergic reactions: rash, urticaria

• Respiratory dysfunction: respiratory depression, character, rate, rhythm; notify prescriber if respirations are <12/min; CV status; bradycardia, syncope

• Use pain scoring to determine pain perception

Administer:

• Direct IV over 1½-3 min; use tuberculin syringe

Perform/provide:

• Storage in light-resistant area at room temp

Evaluate:

• Therapeutic response: maintenance of anesthesia

Teach patient/family:

• To call for assistance when ambulating or smoking; drowsiness, dizziness may occur

• Advise patient to make position changes slowly to prevent orthostatic hypotension

---

reserpine (℞)

(re-ser′peen)

Novoreserpine*, Reserfia*, reserpine, Serpasil

Func. class.: Antihypertensive

Chem. class.: Antiadrenergic agent, peripheral action

Action: Inhibits norepinephrine release, depleting norepinephrine stores in adrenergic nerve endings

Uses: Hypertension

Dosage and routes:

• *Adult:* **PO** 0.25-0.5 mg qd × 1-2 wk, then 0.1-0.25 mg qd maintenance

• *Geriatric:* **PO** 0.05 mg qd, increase by 0.05 weekly to desired dose

Available forms: Tabs 0.1, 0.25 mg

◆ = Nursing alert   = Herb-drug interaction   ◯ = Do not crush

Side effects/adverse reactions:
CV: Bradycardia, chest pain, dysrhythmias, prolonged bleeding time, *thrombocytopenia,* purpura
CNS: Drowsiness, fatigue, lethargy, dizziness, depression, anxiety, headache, increased dreaming, nightmares, convulsions, parkinsonism, EPS (high doses)
GI: Nausea, vomiting, cramps, peptic ulcer, dry mouth, increased appetite, anorexia
INTEG: Rash, purpura, alopecia, flushing, warm feeling, pruritus, ecchymosis
EENT: Lacrimation, miosis, blurred vision, ptosis, dry mouth, epistaxis
GU: Impotence, dysuria, nocturia, Na and H_2O retention, edema, breast engorgement, galactorrhea, gynecomastia
RESP: Bronchospasm, dyspnea, cough, rales
Contraindications: Hypersensitivity, depression, suicidal patients, active peptic ulcer disease, ulcerative colitis, pregnancy (D), Parkinson's disease
Precautions: Lactation, seizure disorders, renal disease
Pharmacokinetics:
PO: Peak 4 hr, duration 2-6 wk; half-life 50-100 hr; metabolized by liver; excreted in urine, feces, breast milk; crosses placenta; blood-brain barrier
Interactions:
• Increased hypotension: diuretics, hypotension, β-blockers, methotrimeprazine
• Dysrhythmias: cardiac glycosides
• Increased cardiac depression: quinidine, procainamide
• Excitation, hypertension: MAOIs, avoid use
• Increased CNS depression: barbiturates, alcohol, narcotics

• Increased pressor effects: epinephrine, isoproterenol, norepinephrine
• Decreased pressor effects: ephedrine, amphetamine
Lab test interferences:
Increase: VMA excretion, 5-HIAA excretion
Interferences: 17-OHCS, 17-KS
NURSING CONSIDERATIONS
Assess:
• Renal function studies in renal impairment (BUN, creatinine)
• Bleeding time; check for ecchymosis, thrombocytopenia, purpura
• I&O in renal disease patient
• Cardiac status: B/P, pulse; watch for hypotension, bradycardia
• Edema in feet, legs qd; take weight qd
• Skin turgor, dryness of mucous membranes for hydration status
• Symptoms of CHF: edema, dyspnea, wet rales
Evaluate:
• Therapeutic response: decreased hypertension
Teach patient/family:
• To avoid driving, hazardous activities if drowsiness occurs
• Not to discontinue drug abruptly
• Not to use OTC products (cough, cold preparations) unless directed by prescriber
• To report bradycardia, dizziness, confusion, depression, fever, sore throat
• That impotence, gynecomastia may occur but are reversible
• To rise slowly to sitting or standing position to minimize orthostatic hypotension
• That therapeutic effect may take 2-4 wk
Treatment of overdose: Lavage, IV atropine for bradycardia, supportive therapy

R

respiratory syncytial virus immune globulin (RSV-IGIV) (℞)

RespiGam

Func. class.: Immune serums
Chem. class.: Immunoglobulin G (IgG)

Action: High titer of neutralizing antibody against RSV (respiratory syncytial virus)

Uses: Prevention of serious lower respiratory tract infection caused by RSV in children <2 yr with bronchopulmonary dysplasia, or premature birth

Dosage and routes:
• *Child:* <2 yr **IV INF** 1.5 ml/kg/hr × 15 min, then 3 ml/kg/hr 15-30 min; then 6 ml/kg/hr from 30 min to end of **INF**

Available forms: Inj 2500 mg RSV immunoglobulin

Side effects/adverse reactions:
RESP: **Respiratory distress, hypoxia,** tachypnea, rales, wheezing
CNS: Fever
CV: Hypertension, tachycardia, fluid overload
GI: Diarrhea, gastroenteritis, vomiting
MISC.: Rash, overdose effect, inflammation at inj site

Contraindications: Hypersensitivity to this drug or other human immunoglobulin preparations, IgA deficiency

Precautions: Pregnancy (C), fluid overload

Pharmacokinetics: Unknown

Interactions:
• Interference with immune response in: MMR, DPT, *H. influenzae b*

NURSING CONSIDERATIONS

Assess:
• VS for increases in heart rate, respiratory rate, retractions, rales; a loop diuretic may be needed for fluid overload
• For aseptic meningitis syndrome (AMS): severe headache, drowsiness, photophobia, fever, painful eye movements, nausea, vomiting, muscle rigidity, discontinue RSV-IGIV if these occur

Administer:

IV inf
• Do not admix; begin inf within 6 hr and complete within 12 hr after the single-use vial is entered

Perform/provide:
• Refrigerated storage, do not freeze, do not shake vial, discard after use
• The reason for IV inf and expected results

Rh₀(D) immune globulin, human (℞)

Gamulin Rh, Hydro Rho-D, HypoRho-D, MICRhoGAM, Mini-Dose, Mini-Gamulin RH, Rhesonatre Rho-Gam

Func. class.: Immunizing agent
Chem. class.: IgG

Action: Suppresses immune response of nonsensitized Rh₀ (D or Dᵘ)-negative patients who are exposed to Rh₀ (D or Dᵘ)-positive blood

Uses: Prevention of isoimmunization in Rh-negative women given Rh-positive blood after abortions, miscarriages, amniocentesis

Dosage and routes:
Prior delivery
• *Adult:* **IM** 1 vial (standard dose) at 26-28 wk, 1 vial (standard dose) 72 hr after delivery
Pregnancy termination <13 wk
• *Adult:* **IM** 1 vial (microdose) within 72 hr

Following delivery
• *Adult:* **IM** 1 vial if fetal-packed RBCs <15 ml, or 2 vials if fetal-packed RBCs >15 ml; given within 72 hr of delivery or miscarriage
Transfusion error
• *Adult:* **IM** give within 72 hr
Available forms: Inj single-dose vial (50 µg/vial-microdose; 300 µg/vial-standard)
Side effects/adverse reactions:
INTEG: Irritation at inj site, fever
CNS: Lethargy
MS: Myalgia
Contraindications: Previous immunization with this drug, Rh_o (O)-positive/D^u-positive patient
NURSING CONSIDERATIONS
Assess:
• Allergies, reactions to immunizations; previous immunization with this drug
Administer:
IM
• After sending newborn's cord blood to lab after delivery for crossmatch, type; infant must be Rh-positive, with Rh-negative mother
• IM inj in deltoid; aspirate
• Only equal lot numbers of drug, cross-match
• Only MICRhoGAM for abortions or miscarriages <12 wk unless fetus or father is Rh ; unless patient is Rh_o (D)-positive, D^u-positive, Rh antibodies are present
Perform/provide:
• Storage in refrigerator
Evaluate:
• Rh_o (D) sensitivity in transfusion error, prevention of erythroblastosis fetalis
Teach patient/family:
• How drug works; that drug must be given after subsequent deliveries if subsequent babies are Rh positive

riboflavin (vit B₂)
(OTC)
(rye'boh-flay-vin)
Func. class.: Vit B₂, water soluble

Action: Needed for respiratory reactions by catalyzing proteins and for normal vision
Uses: Vit B₂ deficiency or polyneuritis; cheilosis adjunct with thiamine
Dosage and routes:
• *Adult and child >12 yr:* **PO** 5-50 mg qd in divided doses
• *Child <12 yr:* **PO** 2-10 mg qd, then 0.6 mg/1000 calories ingested
Available forms: Tabs 10, 25, 50, 100 mg
Side effects/adverse reactions:
GU: Yellow discoloration of urine (large doses)
Contraindications: Child <12 yr
Precautions: Pregnancy (A)
Pharmacokinetics:
PO: Half-life 65-85 min, 60% protein bound, unused amounts excreted in urine (unchanged)
Interactions:
• Decreased action of tetracyclines
Lab test interferences:
• May cause false elevations of urinary catecholamines
NURSING CONSIDERATIONS
Assess:
• Nutritional status: liver, eggs, dairy products, yeast, whole grain, green vegetables
Administer:
• With food for better absorption
Perform/provide:
• Storage in air-tight, light-resistant container
Evaluate:
• Therapeutic response: absence of headache, GI problems, cheilosis,

R

skin lesions, depression, burning, itchy eyes, anemia

Teach patient/family:
- That urine may turn bright yellow
- About addition of needed foods that are rich in riboflavin
- To avoid alcohol

---

rifabutin (℞)
(riff′a-byoo-ten)
Mycobutin

Func. class.: Antimycobacterial agent

Chem. class.: Rifamycin S derivative

Action: Inhibits DNA-dependent RNA polymerase in susceptible strains of *E. coli* and *B. subtilis;* mechanism of action against *M. avium* unknown

Uses: Prevention of *M. avium* complex in patients with advanced HIV infection

Dosage and routes:
- *Adult:* 300 mg qd (may take as 150 mg bid)

Available forms: Caps 150 mg

Side effects/adverse reactions:

INTEG: Rash

MS: Asthenia, arthralgia, myalgia

MISC: Flulike syndrome, shortness of breath, chest pressure

GI: Nausea, vomiting, anorexia, diarrhea, heartburn, hepatitis

GU: Hematuria, *discolored urine*

CNS: Headache, fatigue, anxiety, confusion, insomnia

HEMA: **Hemolytic anemia, eosinophilia, thrombocytopenia, leukopenia**

Contraindications: Hypersensitivity, active TB, WBC <1000 or platelet count <50,000

Precautions: Pregnancy (B), lactation, hepatic disease, blood dyscrasias, children

Pharmacokinetics:
PO: Peak 2-3 hr, duration >24 hr, half-life 3 hr; metabolized in liver (active/inactive metabolites), excreted in urine primarily as metabolites

Interactions:
- Decreased action: barbiturates, clofibrate, corticosteroids, dapsone, anticoagulants, sulfonylureas, estrogens, digitoxin and digoxin, oral contraceptives, theophylline, β-blockers, verapamil, cyclosporine, zidovudine, ketoconazole
- Rifabutin does not appear to alter the acetylation of isoniazid

Lab test interferences:
Interference: Folate level, vit B_{12}, BSP, gallbladder studies

NURSING CONSIDERATIONS
Assess:
- CBC for neutropenia, thrombocytopenia, eosinophilia
- For acute TB: chest x-ray, sputum culture, blood culture, biopsy of lymph nodes, PPD; drug should not be given for acute TB
- Signs of anemia: Hct, Hgb, fatigue
- Liver studies qwk: ALT (SGPT), AST (SGOT), bilirubin
- Renal status before, qmo: BUN, creatinine, output, specific gravity, urinalysis
- Hepatic studies: decreased appetite, jaundice, dark urine, fatigue

Administer:
- With food if GI upset occurs; better to take on empty stomach 1 hr ac or 2 hr pc, fat foods slow absorption
- Antiemetic if vomiting occurs
- After C&S is completed; qmo to detect resistance

Evaluate:
- Therapeutic response: not used for active TB because of risk of development of resistance to rifampin; culture negative

---

 = Nursing alert   ⫸ = Herb-drug interaction   🚫 = Do not crush

Teach patient/family:

• That patients using oral contraceptives should consider using nonhormonal methods of birth control, since rifabutin may decrease their efficacy

• That compliance with dosage schedule, duration is necessary

• That scheduled appointments must be kept; relapse may occur

• That urine, feces, saliva, sputum, sweat, tears may be colored redorange; soft contact lenses may be permanently stained

• To report flulike symptoms: excessive fatigue, anorexia, vomiting, sore throat; unusual bleeding, yellowish discoloration of skin, eyes

---

rifampin (℞)

(rif´am-pin)
Rifadin, Rifampicin, Rimactane, Rofact*
Func. class.: Antitubercular
Chem. class.: Rifamycin B derivative

Action: Inhibits DNA-dependent polymerase, decreases tubercle bacilli replication

Uses: Pulmonary tuberculosis, meningococcal carriers (prevention)

Dosage and routes:

Tuberculosis

• *Adult:* **PO/IV** 600 mg/day as single dose 1 hr ac or 2 hr pc or 10 mg/kg/day

• *Child >5 yr:* **PO/IV** 10-20 mg/kg/day as single dose 1 hr ac or 2 hr pc, not to exceed 600 mg/day, with other antituberculars

Meningococcal carriers

• *Adult:* **PO/IV** 600 mg bid × 2 days

• *Child >5 yr:* **PO/IV** 10 mg/kg bid × 2 days, not to exceed 600 mg/dose

• *Infant 3 mo-1 yr:* 5 mg/kg **PO** bid for 2 days

Available forms: Caps 150, 300 mg; inj 600 mg/vial

Side effects/adverse reactions:

INTEG: Rash, pruritus, urticaria

EENT: Visual disturbances

MS: Atoxia, weakness

MISC: Flulike syndrome, menstrual disturbances, edema, shortness of breath

GI: Nausea, vomiting, anorexia, diarrhea, **pseudomembranous colitis,** *heartburn,* sore mouth and tongue, **pancreatitis**

GU: **Hematuria, acute renal failure, hemoglobinuria**

CNS: Headache, fatigue, anxiety, drowsiness, confusion

HEMA: **Hemolytic anemia, eosinophilia, thrombocytopenia, leukopenia**

Contraindications: Hypersensitivity

Precautions: Pregnancy (C), lactation, hepatic disease, blood dyscrasias

Pharmacokinetics:

PO: Peak 2-3 hr, duration >24 hr, half-life 3 hr; metabolized in liver (active/inactive metabolites), excreted in urine as free drug (30% crosses placenta), excreted in breast milk

Interactions:

• Decreased action: barbiturates, clofibrate, corticosteroids, dapsone, anticoagulants, antidiabetics, hormones, digoxin, PAS, alcohol, oral contraceptives, verapamil, diltiazem, nifedipine, cyclosporine, haloperidol, theophylline, chloramphenicol, acetaminophen, benzodiazepines, phenytoin, sulfonamides, beta-blockers, doxycycline, fluoroquinolones, zidovudine

• Hepatotoxicity: isoniazid

• Incompatible with sodium lactate

Lab test interferences:

Interference: Folate level, vit B_{12}, BSP, gallbladder studies

R

NURSING CONSIDERATIONS
Assess:

- For infection: sputum culture, lung sounds
- Signs of anemia: Hct, Hgb, fatigue
- Liver studies qwk: ALT (SGPT), AST (SGOT), bilirubin
- Renal status before, qmo: BUN, creatinine, output, specific gravity, urinalysis
- Hepatic status: decreased appetite, jaundice, dark urine, fatigue

Administer:

- After C&S is completed; qmo to detect resistance

PO

- On empty stomach, 1 hr ac or 2 hr pc
- Antiemetic if vomiting occurs

IV

- After diluting each 600 mg/10 ml of sterile water for inj (60 mg/ml), agitate, withdraw dose and dilute in 100 ml or 500 ml of D_5W or 0.9% NaCl given as an inf over 3 hr, or if diluted in 100 ml, give over ½ hr

Evaluate:

- Therapeutic response: decreased symptoms of TB, culture negative

Teach patient/family:

- That compliance with dosage schedule, duration is necessary
- That scheduled appointments must be kept; relapse may occur
- To avoid alcohol
- That urine, feces, saliva, sputum, sweat, tears may be colored red-orange; soft contact lenses may be permanently stained
- To report flulike symptoms: excessive fatigue, anorexia, vomiting, sore throat; unusual bleeding, yellowish discoloration of skin, eyes

---

riluzole (℞)

(rill'you-zole)
Rilutek
Func. class.: ALS agent
Chem. class.: Benzathiazole

Action: Unknown; may act by inhibiting glutamate, interfering with binding of amino acid receptors, and inactivating of voltage-dependent sodium channels

Uses: Amyotropic lateral sclerosis (ALS)

Dosage and routes:

- *Adult:* **PO** 50 mg q12h, take 1 hr ac or 2 hr pc

Available forms: Tabs 50 mg

Side effects/adverse reactions:

GI: Nausea, vomiting, dyspepsia, anorexia, diarrhea, flatulence, stomatitis, dry mouth

*HEMA: **Neutropenia***

CNS: Hypertonia, depression, dizziness, insomnia, somnolence, vertigo

INTEG: Pruritus, eczema, alopecia, ***exfoliative dermatitis***

RESP: Decreased lung function, rhinitis, increased cough

CV: Hypertension, tachycardia, phlebitis, palpitation, postural hypertension

GU: UTI, dysuria

Contraindications: Hypersensitivity

Precautions: Neutropenia, renal disease, hepatic disease, elderly, pregnancy (C), lactation, children

Pharmacokinetics: Well absorbed, extensively metabolized by the liver, excretion in urine/feces

Interactions:

- Decreased elimination of riluzole: caffeine, theophylline, amitriptyline, quinolones
- Increased elimination of riluzole:

◆ = Nursing alert   ✏ = Herb-drug interaction   🚫 = Do not crush

cigarette smoking, rifampin, omeprazole, charcoal-broiled food

NURSING CONSIDERATIONS
Assess:
• LFTs: SGPT, SGOT, bilirubin,
GGT, baseline and qmo × 3 mo,
then q3mo; monitor liver chemis-
tries
• For neutropenia <500/mm³

Administer:
• 1 hr ac or 2 hr pc; a high fat meal
decreases absorption

Teach patient/family:
• To report febrile illness, which may
indicate neutropenia
• The reason for drug and expected
results

---

rimantadine (℞)

(ri-man'tah dcen)
Flumadine
Func. class.: Synthetic antiviral
Chem. class.: Tricyclic amine

Action: Prevents uncoating of
nucleic acid in viral cell, preventing
penetration of virus to host; causes
release of dopamine from neurons
Uses: Prophylaxis or treatment of
influenza type A

Dosage and routes:
Influenza type A
Prophylaxis
• *Adult:* PO 100 mg bid; in renal,
hepatic disease, lower dose to 100
mg/day
• *Child <10 yr:* PO 5 mg/kg/day,
not to exceed 150 mg
Treatment
• *Adult:* PO 100 mg bid; in renal or
hepatic disease, lower dose to 100
mg/day; start treatment at onset of
symptoms, continue for at least 1 wk
• *Geriatric:* PO 100 mg/day
Available forms: Tabs 100 mg; syr
50 mg/5 ml

Side effects/adverse reactions:
CNS: Headache, dizziness, fatigue,
depression, hallucinations, tremors,
convulsions, insomnia, *poor concentration,* asthenia, gait abnormalities, *anxiety, confusion*
CV: Pallor, palpitations, *hypotension, edema*
EENT: Tinnitus, taste abnormality,
eye pain
GI: Nausea, vomiting, constipation,
dry mouth, anorexia, abdominal
pain, diarrhea, dyspepsia
INTEG: Rash
Contraindications: Hypersensitivity
Precautions: Epilepsy, hepatic disease, renal disease, pregnancy (C),
lactation, child <1 yr
Pharmacokinetics:
PO: Peak 6 hr, elimination half-life
25½ hr, plasma protein binding
(40%)
Interactions:
• Decreased peak concentration of
rimantadine: acetaminophen, aspirin
• Increased rimantadine concentration: cimetidine

NURSING CONSIDERATIONS
Assess:
• I&O ratio; report frequency, hesitancy in renal disease
• Bowel pattern before, during treatment
• CNS effect in elderly or patients
with severe hepatic/renal disease
• Skin eruptions, photosensitivity after administration of drug
• Respiratory status: rate, character,
wheezing, tightness in chest
• Allergies before initiation of treatment, reaction of each medication;
list allergies on chart in bright red
letters
• Signs of infection

Administer:
• Within 48 hr of exposure to influenza; continue for 10 days after
contact

R

• At least 4 hr before hs to prevent insomnia

• After meals for better absorption, to decrease GI symptoms

• In divided doses to prevent CNS disturbances: headache, dizziness, fatigue, drowsiness

Perform/provide:

• Storage in tight, dry container

Evaluate:

• Therapeutic response: absence of fever, malaise, cough, dyspnea in infection

Teach patient/family:

• About aspects of drug therapy: need to report dyspnea, dizziness, poor concentration, behavioral changes

• To avoid hazardous activities if dizziness occurs

Treatment of overdose: Withdraw drug, maintain airway, administer epinephrine, aminophylline, O₂, IV corticosteroids, physostigmine

---

risperidone (℞)

(ris-pehr'ih-dohn)
Risperdal
Func. class.: Antipsychotic/ neuroleptic
Chem. class.: Benzisoxazole derivative

Action: Unknown; may be mediated through both dopamine type 2 (D_2) and serotonin type 2 ($5-HT_2$) antagonism

Uses: Psychotic disorders

Dosage and routes:

• *Adult:* **PO** 1 mg bid, with incremental increases of 1 mg bid on days 2 and 3 to a dose of 3 mg bid by day 3; then do not increase dose for at least 1 wk

• *Geriatric:* **PO** 0.5 mg qd-bid, increase by 1 mg qwk

Available forms: Tabs 1, 2, 3, 4 mg; oral sol 1 mg/ml

Side effects/adverse reactions:

CNS: EPS, pseudoparkinsonism, akathisia, dystonia, tardive dyskinesia; drowsiness, insomnia, agitation, anxiety, headache, seizures, **neuroleptic malignant syndrome**

CV: Orthostatic hypotension, **tachycardia**

EENT: Blurred vision

GI: Nausea, vomiting, anorexia, constipation, jaundice, weight gain

RESP: Rhinitis

Contraindications: Hypersensitivity, lactation, seizure disorders

Precautions: Children, renal disease, pregnancy (C), hepatic disease, elderly, breast cancer

Pharmacokinetics:

PO: Extensively metabolized by liver to a major active metabolite, plasma protein binding 90%

Interactions:

• Increased sedation: other CNS depressants, alcohol

• Increased EPS: other antipsychotics, lithium

• Increased excretion of risperidone: carbamazepine

🖊 Increased CNS depression: kava kava

Lab test interferences: Not known

NURSING CONSIDERATIONS

Assess:

• Mental status before initial administration

• Swallowing of PO medication; check for hoarding or giving of medication to other patients

• I&O ratio; palpate bladder if urinary output is low

• Bilirubin, CBC, liver function studies qmo

• Urinalysis before, during prolonged therapy

• Affect, orientation, LOC, reflexes, gait, coordination, sleep pattern disturbances

---

- B/P standing and lying; also pulse, respirations; take these q4h during initial treatment; establish baseline before starting treatment; report drops of 30 mm Hg; watch for ECG changes
- Dizziness, faintness, palpitations, tachycardia on rising
- EPS, including akathisia (inability to sit still, no pattern to movements), tardive dyskinesia (bizarre movements of the jaw, mouth, tongue, extremities), pseudoparkinsonism (rigidity, tremors, pill rolling, shuffling gait)

◆ For neuroleptic malignant syndrome: hyperthermia, increased CPK, altered mental status, muscle rigidity
- Skin turgor qd
- Constipation, urinary retention qd; if these occur, increase bulk and water in diet

Administer:
- Reduced dose in elderly
- Antiparkinsonian agent on order from prescriber, to be used for EPS

Perform/provide:
- Decreased stimulus by dimming lights, avoiding loud noises
- Supervised ambulation until patient is stabilized on medication; do not involve in strenuous exercise program because fainting is possible; patient should not stand still for a long time
- Increased fluids to prevent constipation
- Sips of water, candy, gum for dry mouth
- Storage in tight, light-resistant container

Evaluate:
- Therapeutic response: decrease in emotional excitement, hallucinations, delusions, paranoia; reorganization of patterns of thought, speech

Teach patient/family:
- That orthostatic hypotension may occur and to rise from sitting or lying position gradually
- To avoid hot tubs, hot showers, tub baths; hypotension may occur
- To avoid abrupt withdrawal of this drug; EPS may result; drug should be withdrawn slowly
- To avoid OTC preparations (cough, hay fever, cold) unless approved by prescriber, since serious drug interactions may occur; avoid use with alcohol, CNS depressants; increased drowsiness may occur
- To avoid hazardous activities if drowsy or dizzy
- Compliance with drug regimen
- To report impaired vision, tremors, muscle twitching
- In hot weather, that heat stroke may occur; take extra precautions to stay cool

Treatment of overdose: Lavage if orally ingested; provide airway; *do not induce vomiting*

ritodrine (℞)

(rih'toh-dreen)
ritodrine, Yutopar
Func. class.: Tocolytic, uterine relaxant
Chem. class.: β₂-adrenergic agonist

Action: Reduces frequency, intensity of uterine contractions by stimulation of the β₂-receptors in uterine smooth muscle
Uses: Management of preterm labor
Dosage and routes:
Adult: **IV INF** 150 mg/500 ml (0.3 mg/ml) given 0.1 mg/min, increased gradually by 0.05 mg/min q10min until desired response

Available forms: Inj 10 mg/ml, 15 mg/ml

Side effects/adverse reactions:

MISC: Erythema, rash, dyspnea, hyperventilation, glycosuria, *lactic acidosis*

META: Hyperglycemia, hypokalemia

CNS: Headache, restlessness, anxiety, nervousness, sweating, chills, drowsiness, tremor

GI: Nausea, vomiting, anorexia, malaise, bloating, constipation, diarrhea

CV: Altered maternal, fetal heart rate, B/P, dysrhythmias, palpitations, chest pain, maternal pulmonary edema

Contraindications: Hypersensitivity, eclampsia, hypertension, dysrhythmias, thyrotoxicosis, before 20th wk of pregnancy, antepartum hemorrhage, intrauterine fetal death, maternal cardiac disease, pulmonary hypertension, uncontrolled diabetes, pheochromocytoma, bronchial asthma

Precautions: Migraine, sulfite sensitivity, pregnancy-induced hypertension, diabetes

Pharmacokinetics:

IV: Immediate, distribution half-life 6 min, 2nd phase 1½-2½ hr, elimination phase >10 hr; metabolized in liver; 90% excreted in urine; crosses placenta

Interactions:

• Pulmonary edema: corticosteroids
• Increased CV effects of ritodrine: magnesium sulfate, diazoxide, meperidine, potent general anesthetics
• Increased effects of sympathomimetic amines
• Systemic hypertension: atropine
• Decreased action of ritodrine: β-blockers
• Considered incompatible with any drug in sol or syringe

Lab test interferences:

Increase: Blood glucose, free fatty acids, insulin, GTT

Decrease: K

NURSING CONSIDERATIONS
Assess:

• Maternal, fetal heart tones during infusion
• Intensity, length of uterine contractions
• Fluid intake to prevent fluid overload; discontinue if this occurs
• Blood glucose in diabetics

Administer:

• Only clear sol
• After dilution: 150 mg/500 ml D₅W or NS, give at 0.3 mg/ml
• Using infusion pump

Perform/provide:

• Positioning of patient in left lateral recumbent position to decrease hypotension, increase renal blood flow

Evaluate:

• Therapeutic response: decreased intensity, length of contraction, absence of preterm labor, decreased B/P

Teach patient/family:

• To remain in bed during infusion

---

ritonavir (℞)

(ri-toe′na-veer)
Norvir
Func. class.: Antiviral
Chem. class.: Petidomimetic inhibitor

Action: Inhibits human immunodeficiency virus (HIV) protease and prevents maturation of the infectious virus

Uses: HIV in combination with zidovudine, ddc or alone

Dosage and routes:

• *Adult:* PO 600 mg bid. If nausea occurs begin dose at ½ and gradually increase

---

◆ = Nursing alert   ⫻ = Herb-drug interaction   ⊘ = Do not crush

• *Child:* **PO** 250 mg/m^2 bid, titrate upward to 400 mg/m^2 bid

Available forms: Caps 100 mg; oral sol 80 mg/ml

Side effects/adverse reactions:

GI: Diarrhea, buccal mucosa ulceration, abdominal pain, *nausea,* taste perversion, dry mouth, dizziness, insomnia, headache, vomiting

CNS: Paresthesia, *headache,* vomiting

INTEG: Rash

MS: Pain

MISC.: Asthenia

Contraindications: Hypersensitivity

Precautions: Liver disease, pregnancy (B), lactation, children

Pharmacokinetics: Well absorbed; 98% protein binding, hepatic metabolism

Interactions:

• Increased ritonavir levels: fluconazole

• Decreased ritonavir levels: rifamycins, nevirapine

• Increased level of both drugs: clarithromycin, ddI

• Toxicity: amiodarone, astemizole, benzodiazepines, bepridil, bupropion, cisapride, clozapine, desipramine, flecainide, meperidine, piroxicam, propafenone, propoxyphene, quinidine, saquinavir, terfenadine, zolpidem

• Decreased theophylline, sulfamethoxazole, zidovudine, ethinyl estradiol levels when used with ritonavir

Lab test interferences:

Increase: ALT, GGT, PT, triglycerides

Decrease: HCT, RBC

NURSING CONSIDERATIONS

Assess:

• Signs of infection, anemia

• Liver studies: ALT, AST

• C&S before drug therapy; drug may be taken as soon as culture is taken; repeat C&S after treatment; determine the presence of other sexually transmitted diseases

• Bowel pattern before, during treatment; if severe abdominal pain with bleeding occurs, drug should be discontinued; monitor hydration

• Skin eruptions; rash

• Allergies before treatment, reaction to each medication; place allergies on chart

Teach patient/family:

• To take as prescribed; if dose is missed, take as soon as remembered up to 1 hr before next dose; do not double dose

• That drug must be taken in equal intervals around the clock to maintain blood levels for duration of therapy

• To take with food; mix liquid formulation with chocolate milk or liquid nutritional supplement

---

rocuronium (℞)

(rō kyur oh′nium)

Zemuron

Func. class.: Neuromuscular blocker (nondepolarizing)

Chem. class.: Biquaternary ammonium ester

Action: Inhibits transmission of nerve impulses by binding with cholinergic receptor sites, antagonizing action of acetylcholine

Uses: Facilitation of endotracheal intubation, skeletal muscle relaxation during mechanical ventilation, surgery, or general anesthesia

Dosage and routes:

Intubation

• *Adult and child:* **IV** 0.6 mg/kg

Available forms: Inj 10 mg/ml

Side effects/adverse reactions:

CV: Bradycardia, tachycardia, change in B/P

RESP: ***Prolonged apnea, broncho-spasm, cyanosis, respiratory depression***

GI: Nausea, vomiting

INTEG: Rash, flushing, pruritus, urticaria

Contraindications: Hypersensitivity

Precautions: Pregnancy (C), cardiac disease, lactation, child <2 yr, electrolyte imbalances, dehydration, neuromuscular disease, respiratory disease

Pharmacokinetics: Half-life 71-203 min, duration ½ hr

Interactions:

• Blocked action of rocuronium: phenylephrine

• Increased effect of rocuronium: anesthetics

NURSING CONSIDERATIONS
Assess:

• For electrolyte imbalances (K, Mg), before drug is used; electrolyte imbalances may lead to increased action of this drug

• Vital signs (B/P, pulse, respirations, airway) until fully recovered; rate, depth, pattern of respirations, strength of hand grip; patient should be intubated before use

• Recovery: decreased paralysis of face, diaphragm, leg, arm, rest of body; residual weakness and respiratory problems may occur during recovery

• Allergic reactions: rash, fever, respiratory distress, pruritus; drug should be discontinued

Administer:

• Using peripheral nerve stimulator by anesthesiologist to determine neuromuscular blockade; deep tendon reflexes should be monitored during extended use

• Undiluted direct IV over 2 min (only by qualified person, usually anesthesiologist); do not administer IM

• Maintenance q20-45min after 1st dose; titrate to response

Perform/provide:

• Storage in light-resistant area

• Reassurance if communication is difficult during recovery from neuromuscular blockade

Evaluate:

• Therapeutic response: paralysis of jaw, eyelid, head, neck, rest of body as evaluated by peripheral nerve stimulator

Teach patient/family:

• About all procedures or treatments; patient will remain conscious if anesthesia is not given also

Treatment of overdose: Edrophonium or neostigmine, atropine, monitor VS; may require mechanical ventilation

---

ropinirole (℞)

(roh-pin'ih-role)
Requip

Func. class.: Antiparkinson agent

Chem. class.: Dopamine-receptor agonist, non-ergot

Action: Selective agonist for D_2 receptors (presynaptic/postsynaptic sites); binding at D_3 receptor contributes to antiparkinson effects

Uses: Parkinsonism

Dosage and routes:

• *Adult:* **PO** 0.25 mg tid, titrate weekly to a max of 24 mg/day

Available forms: Tabs 0.25, 0.5, 1, 2, 5 mg

Side effects/adverse reactions:

HEMA: ***Hemolytic anemia, leukopenia, agranulocytosis***

CNS: Agitation, insomnia, psychosis, hallucination, dystonia, depression, dizziness

GI: Nausea, vomiting, anorexia, dry mouth, constipation, dyspepsia, flatulence

---

◆ = Nursing alert   🖋 = Herb-drug interaction   ⊘ = Do not crush

INTEG: Rash, sweating
CV: Orthostatic hypotension, tachycardia, hypertension, hypotension, syncope, palpitations
EENT: Blurred vision
GU: Impotence, urinary frequency
RESP: Pharyngitis, rhinitis, sinusitis, bronchitis, dyspnea
Contraindications: Hypersensitivity
Precautions: Renal disease, cardiac disease, dysrhythmias, affective disorder, psychosis
Pharmacokinetics:
PO: Half-life 6 hr
Interactions:
• Increased ropinirole effect: cimetidine, ciprofloxacin, diltiazem, enoxacin, erythromycin, fluvoxamine, mexiletine, norfloxacin, tacrine
🍂 Decreased ropinirole action: chaste tree fruit
NURSING CONSIDERATIONS
Assess:
• Involuntary movements in parkinsonism: akinesia, tremors, staggering gait, muscle rigidity, drooling
• B/P, respiration during initial treatment; hypo/hypertension should be reported
• Mental status: affect, mood, behavioral changes, depression; complete suicide assessment
Administer:
• Drug until NPO before surgery
• Adjust dosage to patient response
• With meals
Perform/provide:
• Assistance with ambulation during beginning therapy
• Testing for diabetes mellitus, acromegaly if on long-term therapy
Evaluate:
• Therapeutic response: decrease in akathisia, increased mood
Teach patient/family:
• That therapeutic effects may take several wk to a few mo

• To change positions slowly to prevent orthostatic hypotension
• To use drug exactly as prescribed; if drug is discontinued abruptly, parkinsonian crisis may occur

---

ropivacaine (℞)
(roe-pi′va-kane)
Naropin
Func. class.: Local anesthetic
Chem. class.: Amide

Action: Competes with calcium for sites in nerve membrane that control sodium transport across cell membrane; decreases rise of depolarization phase of action potential
Uses: Peripheral nerve block, caudal anesthesia, central neural block, vaginal block
Dosage and routes:
• Varies with route of anesthesia
Available forms: Inj 2, 5, 7.5 mg/ml
Side effects/adverse reactions:
CNS: Anxiety, restlessness, *convulsions, loss of consciousness,* drowsiness, disorientation, tremors, shivering
CV: Myocardial depression, cardiac arrest, dysrhythmias, bradycardia, hypotension, hypertension, *fetal bradycardia*
GI: Nausea, vomiting
EENT: Blurred vision, tinnitus, pupil constriction
INTEG: Rash, urticaria, allergic reactions, edema, burning, skin discoloration at injection site, tissue necrosis
RESP: Status asthmaticus, respiratory arrest, anaphylaxis
Contraindications: Hypersensitivity, child <12 yr, elderly, severe liver disease
Precautions: Severe drug allergies, pregnancy (B)
Pharmacokinetics: Onset 2-8 min,

R

duration 3-6 hr; metabolized by liver, excreted in urine (metabolites)
Interactions:
• Dysrhythmias: epinephrine, halothane, enflurane
• Hypertension: MAOIs, tricyclic antidepressants, phenothiazines
• Decreased action of ropivacaine chloroprocaine
NURSING CONSIDERATIONS
Assess:
• B/P, pulse, respiration during treatment
• Fetal heart tones during labor
• Allergic reactions: rash, urticaria, itching
• Cardiac status: ECG for dysrhythmias, pulse, B/P during anesthesia
Administer:
• Only with crash cart, resuscitative equipment nearby
• Only drugs without preservatives for epidural or caudal anesthesia
Perform/provide:
• Use of new sol; discard unused portions
Evaluate:
• Therapeutic response: anesthesia necessary for procedure
Treatment of overdose: Airway, O_2, vasopressor, IV fluids, anticonvulsants for seizures

---

salicylic acid (OTC, ℞)
(sal-i-sil'ik)
Calicylic Creme, Clear Away, Clear Away Plantar, Compound W, Duofilm, Freezone, Gordofilm, Hydrisalic, Keralyt, Lactisol, Lactisol Forte, Mediplast, Mosco, Occlusal, Occlusal HP, Off-Ezy Wart Remover, Panscol, Paplex Ultra, Pediapatch, Sal-Acid, Salacid 25%, Salacid 60%, Salactic Film, Salicylic Acid Creme 60%, Sal Plant, Trans-Ver-Sal, Trans-Plantar, Vergogel Duoplant for Feet, Verukan HP Paplex, Viranol, Viranol Gel Ultra, Wart-Off, Wart Remover
Func. class.: Keratolytic

Action: Corrects abnormal keratinization and causes peeling of skin
Uses: Dandruff, seborrheic dermatitis, psoriasis, multiple superficial epitheliomatoses; wart removal, corns, calluses
Dosage and routes:
• *Adult:* **TOP** apply as needed, cover at night
Available forms: Powder, cream 2%, 2.5%, 10%; gel 6%, 17%; oint 3%, 25%, 60%; plaster 40%; pledgets 0.5%; shampoo 2%, 4%; sol 13.6%, 17%; stick 2%; susp 2%, liquid 12%, 16.7%, 17%, 20%, 26%
Side effects/adverse reactions:
INTEG: Irritation, drying
*CNS: **Salicylism:** hearing loss, tinnitus, dizziness, confusion, headache, hyperventilation*
Contraindications: Hypersensitivity, diabetes, impaired circulation, use on moles, genital or facial warts
Precautions: Pregnancy (C), diabetes

◆ = Nursing alert   ∥ = Herb-drug interaction   ⊘ = Do not crush

NURSING CONSIDERATIONS
Assess:
• Platelets, WBC if systemic absorption occurs
• Salicylism: tinnitus, hearing loss, dizziness, confusion, headache, hyperventilation
• Allergic reactions: irritation, redness

Administer:
• Only to intact skin; do not use on inflamed, denuded skin
• After wetting skin; wash thoroughly each AM after treatment
• With occlusive dressing to increase absorption; apply more often to areas where occlusion is impossible

Evaluate:
• Therapeutic response: decrease in dandruff, size of lesions

Teach patient/family:
• To avoid contact with eyes, mucous membranes
• To apply lotion if drying occurs
• To avoid applying to large areas; salicylate toxicity may occur

---

salmeterol (℞)
(sal-met′er-ole)
Serevent
Func. class.: β₂-adrenergic agonist

Action: Causes bronchodilation by action on β₂ (pulmonary) receptors by increasing levels of cAMP, which relaxes smooth muscle; with very little effect on heart rate, maintains improvement in FEV from 3 to 12 hr; prevents nocturnal asthma symptoms

Uses: Prevention of exercise-induced asthma, bronchospasm

Dosage and routes:
• *Adult:* INH 2 puffs bid (AM and PM)

Available forms: Aerosol

Side effects/adverse reactions:
CNS: Tremors, anxiety, insomnia, headache, dizziness, stimulation, restlessness, hallucinations, flushing, irritability
CV: Palpitations, tachycardia, hypertension, angina, hypotension, dysrhythmias
EENT: Dry nose, irritation of nose and throat
GI: Heartburn, nausea, vomiting
MS: Muscle cramps
RESP: **Bronchospasm**

Contraindications: Hypersensitivity to sympathomimetics, tachydysrhythmias, severe cardiac disease

Precautions: Lactation, pregnancy (C), cardiac disorders, hyperthyroidism, diabetes mellitus, hypertension, prostatic hypertrophy, narrow-angle glaucoma, seizures

Pharmacokinetics:
INH: Onset 5-15 min, peak 4 hr, duration 12 hr, metabolized in liver, excreted in urine, breast milk; crosses placenta; blood-brain barrier

Interactions:
• Increased action of aerosol bronchodilators
• Increased action of salmeterol: tricyclic antidepressants, MAOIs
• May inhibit action of salmeterol: other β-blockers

NURSING CONSIDERATIONS
Assess:
• Respiratory function: vital capacity, forced expiratory volume, ABGs, lung sounds, heart rate and rhythm

Administer:
• After shaking; exhale, place mouthpiece in mouth, inhale slowly, hold breath, remove, exhale slowly
• Gum, sips of water for dry mouth
• Using spacing device for pediatric/geriatric patients

Perform/provide:
• Storage in light-resistant container;

S

do not expose to temps over 86° F (30° C)

Evaluate:

• Therapeutic response: absence of dyspnea, wheezing

Teach patient/family:

• Not to use OTC medications; extra stimulation may occur

• Use of inhaler; review package insert with patient

• To avoid getting aerosol in eyes

• To wash inhaler in warm water qd and dry

• To avoid smoking, smoke-filled rooms, persons with respiratory infections

Treatment of overdose: β_2-adrenergic blocker

---

salsalate (℞)

(sal'sah-late)

Amigesic, Argesic-SA, Arthra-G, Disalcid, Mono-Gesic, Salflex, salsalate, Salsitab

Func. class.: Nonnarcotic analgesic, nonsteroidal antiinflammatory

Chem. class.: Salicylate

Action: Blocks formation of peripheral prostaglandins, which cause pain and inflammation; antipyretic action results from inhibition of hypothalamic heat-regulating center; does not inhibit platelet aggregation

Uses: Mild to moderate pain or fever, including arthritis, juvenile rheumatoid arthritis

Dosage and routes:

• *Adult:* **PO** 3 g/day in divided doses

Available forms: Caps 500 mg; tabs 500, 750 mg

Side effects/adverse reactions:

*HEMA: **Thrombocytopenia, agranulocytosis, leukopenia, neutropenia, hemolytic anemia,*** increased protime

CNS: Stimulation, drowsiness, dizziness, confusion, ***convulsions,*** headache, flushing, hallucinations, ***coma***

GI: Nausea, vomiting, GI bleeding, diarrhea, heartburn, anorexia, ***hepatotoxicity***

INTEG: Rash, urticaria, bruising

EENT: Tinnitus, hearing loss

CV: Rapid pulse, ***pulmonary edema***

RESP: Wheezing, hyperpnea

ENDO: Hypoglycemia, hyponatremia, hypokalemia, alteration in acid-base balance

Contraindications: Hypersensitivity to salicylates, NSAIDs, GI bleeding, bleeding disorders, children <3 yr, vit K deficiency

Precautions: Anemia, hepatic disease, renal disease, Hodgkin's disease, pregnancy (C), lactation, elderly

Pharmacokinetics: Metabolized by liver; excreted by kidneys; half-life 1 hr; highly protein bound; crosses blood-brain barrier and placenta slowly

Interactions:

• Decreased effects of salsalate: antacids, steroids, urinary alkalizers

• Increased blood loss: alcohol, heparin, ibuprofen, warfarin

• Increased effects of anticoagulants, insulin, methotrexate, probenecid, penicillins, phenytoin

• Decreased effects of spironolactone, sulfinpyrazone, sulfonamides, loop diuretics

• Toxic effects: PABA

• Decreased blood sugar levels: salicylates

Drug/food

• Foods cause acidic urine, may increase salsalate levels

Lab test interferences:

Increase: Coagulation studies, liver function studies, serum uric acid, amylase, CO_2, urinary protein

---

 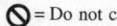

Decrease: Serum K, PBI, cholesterol, blood glucose

Interference: Urine catecholamines, pregnancy test

NURSING CONSIDERATIONS
Assess:
• Pain: frequency, intensity, characteristics; relief of pain after medication
• For asthma, aspirin hypersensitivity, nasal polyps; may develop hypersensitivity to this product
• Liver function studies: AST, ALT, bilirubin (long-term therapy)
• Renal function studies: BUN, urine creatinine (long-term therapy)
• Blood studies: CBC, Hct, Hgb, pro-time (long-term therapy)
• I&O ratio; decreasing output may indicate renal failure (long-term therapy)
• Hepatotoxicity, dark urine, clay-colored stools; yellow skin, sclera; itching, abdominal pain, fever, diarrhea (long-term therapy)
• Allergic reactions: rash, urticaria; drug may have to be discontinued
• Ototoxicity: tinnitus, ringing, roaring in ears; audiometric testing is needed before, after long-term therapy
• Visual changes: blurring, halos, corneal and retinal damage
• Edema in feet, ankles, legs
• Drug history; many interactions
Administer:
• To patient crushed or whole; chewable tablets may be chewed
• With food or milk to decrease gastric symptoms; give 30 min before or 2 hr after meals
• With full glass of water
Evaluate:
• Therapeutic response: decreased pain, fever
Teach patient/family:
• To report any symptoms of hepatotoxicity, renal toxicity, visual changes, ototoxicity, allergic reactions (long-term therapy)
• Not to exceed recommended dosage; acute poisoning may result
• To read label on other OTC drugs; many contain aspirin
• That therapeutic response takes 2 wk (arthritis)
• To avoid alcohol ingestion; GI bleeding may occur
• To watch for signs of bleeding: dark stools

Treatment of overdose: Lavage, activated charcoal, monitor electrolytes, VS

---

saquinavir (℞)
(sa-quen'ah-veer)
Invirase, Fortovase
Func. class.: Antiviral
Chem. class.: Synthetic peptide-like substrate analog

Action: Inhibits human immunodeficiency virus (HIV) protease, which prevents maturation of the infectious virus

Uses: HIV in combination with AZT, zalcitabine, ddc

Dosage and routes:
• *Adult:* **PO** 600 mg (hard cap) or 1200 mg (soft cap) tid within 2 hr after a full meal; given with either zalcitabine 0.75 mg tid or zidovudine 200 mg tid

Available forms: Caps 200 mg (soft); 200 mg (hard)

Side effects/adverse reactions:
GI: Diarrhea, buccal mucosa ulceration, *abdominal pain, nausea*
CNS: Paresthesia, headache
INTEG: Rash
MS: Pain
MISC.: Asthenia, hyperglycemia
Contraindications: Hypersensitivity

Precautions: Liver disease, pregnancy (B), lactation, children

Pharmacokinetics: Absorption increased with food, protein binding 98%, extensive first-pass metabolism

• Toxicity: astemizole, terfenadine, cisapride, ergots, midazolam, triazolam, dapsone, quinidine, calcium channel blockers, clindamycin

Interactions:

• Increased saquinavir levels: ketoconazole

• Decreased saquinavir levels: rifamycins

Drug/food

• Increased bioavailability after high-fat meal

Lab test interferences:
CPK, glucose (low)

NURSING CONSIDERATIONS
Assess:

• Signs of infection, anemia

• Liver function studies: ALT, AST

• C&S before drug therapy; drug may be taken as soon as culture is taken; repeat C&S after treatment; determine the presence of other sexually transmitted diseases

• Bowel pattern before, during treatment; if severe abdominal pain with bleeding occurs, drug should be discontinued; monitor hydration

• Skin eruptions, rash, urticaria, itching

• Allergies before treatment, reaction of each medication; place allergies on chart

Teach patient/family:

• To take as prescribed within 2 hr of a full meal; if dose is missed, take as soon as remembered up to 1 hr before next dose; do not double dose

• That drug must be taken in equal intervals around the clock to maintain blood levels for duration of therapy

---

sargramostim (℞)

(sar-gram′oh-stim)

Leukine, Prokine, rhu GM-CSF, recombinant human

Func. class.: Biologic modifier: cytokine

Action: Stimulates proliferation and differentiation of hematopoietic progenitor cells (granulocytes, macrophages)

Uses: Acceleration of myeloid recovery in patients with non-Hodgkin's lymphoma, acute lymphoblastic leukemia, autologous bone marrow transplantation in Hodgkin's disease; bone marrow transplantation failure or engraftment delay

Dosage and routes:
Myeloid reconstitution after autologous bone marrow transplantation

• *Adult:* IV 250 µg/m²/day × 3 wk; give over 2 hr, 2-4 hr after autologous bone marrow infusion, not less than 24 hr after last dose of antineoplastics and 12 hr after last dose of radiotherapy, bone marrow transplantation failure, or engraftment delay

Acceleration of myeloid recovery

• *Adult:* IV 250 µg/m²/day × 14 days; give over 2 hr; may repeat in 7 days, may repeat 500 µg/m²/day × 14 days after another 7 days if no improvement

Available forms: Powder for inj lyophilized 250, 500 µg

Side effects/adverse reactions:

CNS: Fever, malaise, CNS disorder, weakness, chills

GI: Nausea, vomiting, diarrhea, anorexia, ***GI hemorrhage,*** stomatitis, ***liver damage***

HEMA: ***Blood dyscrasias, hemorrhage***

 = Nursing alert   = Herb-drug interaction   ⊘ = Do not crush

INTEG: Alopecia, rash, peripheral edema

GU: Urinary tract disorder, abnormal kidney function

RESP: Dyspnea

CV: Supraventricular tachycardia, peripheral edema, *pericardial effusion*

Contraindications: Hypersensitivity to GM-CSF, yeast products; excessive leukemic myeloid blast in bone marrow, peripheral blood

Precautions: Pregnancy (C), lactation, child; renal, hepatic, lung disease; cardiac disease; pleural, pericardial effusions

Pharmacokinetics: Half-life 2 hr, detected within 5 min after administration, peak 2 hr

Interactions:

• Do not use this drug concomitantly with antineoplastics

• Increased myeloproliferation: lithium, corticosteroids

NURSING CONSIDERATIONS

Assess:

• Blood studies: CBC, differential count before treatment and twice weekly; leukocytosis may occur (WBC >50,000 cells/mm^3, ANC >20,000 cells/mm^3)

• Renal and hepatic studies before treatment: BUN, creatinine, urinalysis; AST (SGOT), ALT (SGPT), alk phosphatase; twice weekly monitoring is needed in renal, hepatic disease

• For hypersensitivity, rashes, local inj site reactions; usually transient

• For increased fluid retention in cardiac disease

Administer:

IV

• After reconstituting with 1 ml sterile water for inj without preservative; do not reenter vial; discard unused portion; direct reconstitution sol at side of vial; rotate contents; do not shake

• Dilute in 0.9% NaCl inj to prepare IV inf; if final concentration is <10 μg/ml, add human albumin to make a final concentration of 0.1% to NaCl before adding sargramostim to prevent adsorption; for a final concentration of 0.1% albumin, add 1 mg human albumin/1 ml 0.9% NaCl inj run over 2 hr; give within 6 hr after reconstitution

Y-site compatibilities: Amikacin, aminophylline, aztreonam, bleomycin, butorphanol, calcium gluconate, carboplatin, carmustine, cefazolin, cefepime, cefotaxime, cefotetan, ceftizoxime, ceftriaxone, cefuroxime, cimetidine, cisplatin, clindamycin, cyclophosphamide, cyclosporine, cytarabine, dacarbazine, dactinomycin, dexamethasone, diphenhydramine, dopamine, doxorubicin, doxycycline, droperidol, etoposide, famotidine, fentanyl, floxuridine, fluconazole, fluorouracil, furosemide, gentamicin, granisetron, heparin, idarubicin, ifosfamide, immune globulin, magnesium sulfate, mannitol, mechlorethamine, meperidine, mesna, methotrexate, metoclopramide, metronidazole, mezlocillin, miconazole, minocycline, mitoxantrone, netilmicin, pentostatin, piperacillin/tazobactam, potassium chloride, prochlorperazine, promethazine, ranitidine, teniposide, ticarcillin, ticarcillin/clavulanate, trimethoprim/sulfamethoxazole, vinblastine, vincristine, zidovudine

Perform/provide:

• Storage in refrigerator; do not freeze

Evaluate:

• Therapeutic response: WBC and differential recovery

---

scopolamine (℞)

(skoe-pol′a-meen)

Func. class.: Cholinergic blocker
Chem. class.: Belladonna alkaloid

Action: Inhibits acetylcholine at receptor sites in autonomic nervous system, which controls secretions, free acids in stomach; blocks central muscarinic receptors, which decreases involuntary movements

Uses: Reduction of secretions before surgery, calm delirium, motion sickness, parkinsonian symptoms

Dosage and routes:

Parkinsonian symptoms

• *Adult:* **IM/SC/IV** 0.3-0.6 mg tid-qid using dilution provided
• *Child:* **SC** 0.006 mg/kg tid-qid or 0.2 mg/m^2

Preoperatively

• *Adult:* **SC** 0.4-0.6 mg

Available forms: Inj 0.3, 0.4, 0.86, 1 mg/ml

Side effects/adverse reactions:

CNS: Confusion, anxiety, restlessness, irritability, delusions, hallucinations, headache, sedation, depression, incoherence, dizziness, excitement, delirium, flushing, weakness
INTEG: Urticaria
MISC: Suppression of lactation, nasal congestion, decreased sweating
EENT: Blurred vision, photophobia, dilated pupils, difficulty swallowing, mydriasis, cycloplegia
CV: Palpitations, tachycardia, postural hypotension, paradoxic bradycardia
GI: Dryness of mouth, constipation, nausea, vomiting, abdominal distress, *paralytic ileus*
GU: Hesitancy, retention

Contraindications: Hypersensitivity, narrow-angle glaucoma, myasthenia gravis, GI/GU obstruction, hypersensitivity to belladonna, barbiturates

Precautions: Pregnancy (C), elderly, lactation, prostatic hypertrophy, CHF, hypertension, dysrhythmia, children, gastric ulcer

Pharmacokinetics:

SC/IM: Peak 30-45 min, duration 7 hr
IV: Peak 10-15 min, duration 4 hr
Excreted in urine, bile, feces (unchanged)

Interactions:

• Increased anticholinergic effect: alcohol, narcotics, antihistamines, phenothiazines, tricyclics

NURSING CONSIDERATIONS

Assess:

• I&O ratio; retention commonly causes decreased urinary output
• Parkinsonism, EPS: shuffling gait, muscle rigidity, involuntary movements
• Urinary hesitancy, retention; palpate bladder if retention occurs
• Constipation; increase fluids, bulk, exercise if this occurs
• For tolerance over long-term therapy; dose may have to be increased or changed
• Mental status: affect, mood, CNS depression, worsening of mental symptoms during early therapy

Administer:

• Parenteral dose with patient recumbent to prevent postural hypotension
• Parenteral dose slowly; keep in bed for at least 1 hr after dose
• With or after meals for GI upset; may give with fluids other than H_2O
• At hs to avoid daytime drowsiness in patient with parkinsonism
• With analgesic to avoid behavioral changes when given as a preop

Additive compatibilities: Floxacil-

 = Nursing alert   = Herb-drug interaction   = Do not crush

lin, furosemide, meperidine, succinylcholine

Syringe compatibilities: Atropine, benzquinamide, butorphanol, chlorpromazine, cimetidine, diamorphine, dimenhydrinate, diphenhydramine, droperidol, fentanyl, glycopyrrolate, hydromorphone, hydroxyzine, meperidine, metoclopramide, midazolam, morphine, nalbuphine, pentazocine, pentobarbital, perphenazine, prochlorperazine, promazine, promethazine, ranitidine, sufentanil, thiopental

Y-site compatibilities: Heparin, hydrocortisone, potassium chloride, propofol, sufentanil, vit B/C

Perform/provide:
• Storage at room temp in light-resistant container
• Hard candy, frequent drinks, sugarless gum to relieve dry mouth

Evaluate:
• Therapeutic response: decreased secretions

Teach patient/family:
• Not to discontinue this drug abruptly; to taper off over 1 wk
• To avoid driving, other hazardous activities; drowsiness may occur
• To avoid OTC medication: cough, cold preparations with alcohol, antihistamines unless directed by prescriber

---

scopolamine (℞) (transdermal)

(skoe-pol′-a-meen)

Transderm-Scop

Func. class.: Antiemetic, anticholinergic

Chem. class.: Belladonna alkaloid

Action: Competitive antagonism of acetylcholine at receptor site in eye, smooth muscle, cardiac muscle, glandular cells; inhibition of vestibular input to the CNS, resulting in inhibition of vomiting reflex

Uses: Prevention of motion sickness

Dosage and routes:
• *Adult:* PATCH 1 placed behind ear 4-5 hr before travel, reapply q3 day, alternate ears
Not recommended for children

Available forms: Patch, 0.5 mg delivered in 72 hr

Side effects/adverse reactions:
INTEG: Rash, erythema
GU: Difficult urination
CNS: Dizziness, drowsiness, confusion, disorientation, memory disturbances, hallucinations
EENT: Blurred vision, altered depth perception, *dilated pupils,* photophobia, *dry mouth;* dry, itchy, red eyes; acute narrow-angle glaucoma

Contraindications: Hypersensitivity, glaucoma

Precautions: Children, elderly, pregnancy (C); pyloric, urinary, bladder neck, intestinal obstruction; liver, kidney disease

Pharmacokinetics:
Patch: Onset 4-5 hr, duration 72 hr

Interactions:
• Increased anticholinergic effects: antihistamines, antidepressants

NURSING CONSIDERATIONS
Teach patient/family:
• To avoid hazardous activities, activities requiring alertness; dizziness may occur
• To wash, dry hands before and after applying to surface behind ear
• To change patch q72h
• To apply at least 4 hr before traveling
• If blurred vision, severe dizziness, drowsiness occurs, to discontinue use, use another type of antiemetic

- To read label of all OTC medications; if any scopolamine is found in product, avoid use
- To keep out of children's reach

---

secobarbital (℞)

(see-koe-bar'bi-tal)
Secobarbital Sodium, Secogen Sodium*, Seconal Sodium, Seconal Sodium Pulvules, Seral*, Secretin-Ferring

Func. class.: Sedative/hypnotic-barbiturate

Chem. class.: Barbitone (short acting)

Controlled Substance Schedule II (USA), Schedule G (Canada)

Action: Depresses activity in brain cells primarily in reticular activating system in brain stem; selectively depresses neurons in posterior hypothalamus, limbic structures; decreases seizure activity by inhibition of epileptic activity in CNS

Uses: Insomnia, sedation, preoperative medication, status epilepticus, acute tetanus convulsions

Dosage and routes:

Insomnia
- *Adult:* **PO/IM** 100-200 mg hs
- *Child:* **IM** 3-5 mg/kg, not to exceed 100 mg, not to inject >5 ml in one site; **RECT** 4-5 mg/kg

Sedation/preoperatively
- *Adult:* **PO** 200-300 mg 1-2 hr preoperatively
- *Child:* **PO** 50-100 mg 1-2 hr preoperatively; **RECT** 4-5 mg/kg 1-2 hr preoperatively

Status epilepticus
- *Adult and child:* **IM/IV** 250-350 mg

Acute psychotic agitation
- *Adult and child:* **IM/IV** 5.5 mg/kg q3-4h

Available forms: Caps 50, 100 mg;

tabs 100 mg; inj 50 mg/ml; powder, rect supp 200 mg

Side effects/adverse reactions:

CNS: Lethargy, drowsiness, hangover, dizziness, paradoxical stimulation in elderly and children, lightheadedness, dependency, CNS depression, mental depression, slurred speech

GI: Nausea, vomiting, diarrhea, constipation

INTEG: Rash, urticaria, pain, abscesses at injection site, angioedema, thrombophlebitis, ***Stevens-Johnson syndrome***

CV: Hypotension, bradycardia

RESP: Depression, ***apnea, laryngospasm, bronchospasm***

HEMA: ***Agranulocytosis, thrombocytopenia, megaloblastic anemia*** (long-term treatment)

Contraindications: Hypersensitivity to barbiturates, pregnancy (D), respiratory depression, addiction to barbiturates, severe liver impairment, porphyria, uncontrolled severe pain

Precautions: Anemia, lactation, hepatic disease, renal disease, hypertension, elderly, acute/chronic pain

Pharmacokinetics:

IM: Onset 10-15 min, duration 4-6 hr

RECT: Onset slow, duration 3-6 hr; metabolized by liver, excreted by kidneys (metabolites); half-life 15-40 hr

Interactions:
- Do not mix with other drugs in sol or syringe
- Increased CNS depression: alcohol, MAOIs, sedatives, narcotics
- Decreased effect of oral anticoagulants, corticosteroids, griseofulvin, quinidine
- Decreased half-life of doxycycline
- ⚗ Increased CNS depression: kava kava

⬧ = Nursing alert   ⚗ = Herb-drug interaction   ⊘ = Do not crush

Lab test interferences:
False increase: Sulfobromophthalein

NURSING CONSIDERATIONS
Assess:
• VS q30min after parenteral route for 2 hr
• Blood studies: Hct, Hgb, RBCs, serum folate, vit D (if on long-term therapy); pro-time in patients receiving anticoagulants
• Hepatic studies: AST, ALT, bilirubin; if increased, drug is usually discontinued
• Unresolved pain; drug may cause severe stimulation if pain is present
• Mental status: mood, sensorium, affect, memory (long, short)
• Physical dependency: frequent requests for medication, shakes, anxiety
◆ Barbiturate toxicity: hypotension; pulmonary constriction; cold, clammy skin; cyanosis of lips; insomnia; nausea; vomiting; hallucinations; delirium; weakness; mild symptoms may occur in 8-12 hr without drug
• Respiratory dysfunction: depression, character, rate, rhythm; hold drug if respirations <10/min or if pupils dilated
• Blood dyscrasias: fever, sore throat, bruising, rash, jaundice, epistaxis
• Perianal irritation if rectal forms used

Administer:
• After removal of cigarettes to prevent fires
• IM inj deep in large muscle mass to prevent tissue sloughing and abscesses
• After conservative measures for insomnia have been tried
• ½-1 hr before hs for sleeplessness
• On empty stomach for best absorption

• For <14 days, since drug is not effective after that; tolerance develops
• Crushed or whole
• Alone; do not mix with other drugs or inject if there is precipitate
• After cleansing enema is given rectally preoperatively in children
IV
• After diluting with sterile H_2O for inj; rotate; give 50 mg or less over 1 min; titrate to response
• Within 30 min of mixing with sterile water for inj; reconstitute after rotating ampule; do not shake; do not use cloudy sol; may be given directly or indirectly
• IV only with resuscitative equipment available; administer at <100 mg/min (only by qualified personnel)
Additive compatibilities: Amikacin, aminophylline
Perform/provide:
• Assistance with ambulation after receiving dose
• Safety measures: side rails, nightlight, call bell within easy reach
• Checking to see if PO medication has been swallowed
• Storage of suppositories in refrigerator; do not use aqueous sol containing precipitate
Evaluate:
• Therapeutic response: ability to sleep at night, decreased early morning awakening if taking drug for insomnia, or decrease in number, severity of seizures if taking drug for seizure disorder
Teach patient/family:
• That morning hangover is common
• That drug is indicated only for short-term treatment of insomnia, probably ineffective after 2 wk
• That physical dependency may result when used for extended periods (45-90 days depending on dose)

S

• To avoid driving, other activities requiring alertness

• To avoid alcohol ingestion, CNS depressants; serious CNS depression may result

• Not to discontinue medication quickly after long-term use; drug should be tapered over 1-2 wk

• To tell all prescribers that barbiturate is being taken

• That withdrawal insomnia may occur after short-term use; not to start using drug again; insomnia will improve in 1-3 nights; may experience increased dreaming

• That effects may take 2 nights for benefits to be noticed

• Alternative measures to improve sleep (reading, exercise several hr before hs, warm bath, warm milk, TV, self-hypnosis, deep breathing)

Treatment of overdose: Lavage, activated charcoal, warming blanket, vital signs, hemodialysis, I&O ratio

---

selegiline (℞)

(se-le'ji-leen)

Carbex, Eldepryl, SD-Deprenyl

Func. class.: Antiparkinson agent

Chem. class.: Levorotatory acetylenic derivative of phenethylamine

---

Action: Increased dopaminergic activity by inhibition of MAO type B activity; not fully understood

Uses: Adjunct management of Parkinson's disease in patients being treated with levodopa/carbidopa who had poor response to therapy

Investigational uses: Alzheimer's disease

Dosage and routes:

• *Adult:* **PO** 10 mg/day in divided doses 5 mg at breakfast and lunch; after 2-3 days begin to reduce dose of levodopa/carbidopa 10%-30%

Available forms: Tabs 5 mg, caps 5 mg

Side effects/adverse reactions:

CNS: Increased tremors, chorea, restlessness, blepharospasm, increased bradykinesia, grimacing, tardive dyskinesia, dystonic symptoms, involuntary movements, increased apraxia, hallucinations, dizziness, mood changes, nightmares, delusions, lethargy, apathy, overstimulation, sleep disturbances, headache, migraine, numbness, muscle cramps, confusion, anxiety, tiredness, vertigo, personality change, back/leg pain

CV: Orthostatic hypotension, hypertension, dysrhythmia, palpitations, angina pectoris, hypotension, *tachycardia,* edema, *sinus bradycardia,* syncope

GI: Nausea, vomiting, constipation, weight loss, anorexia, diarrhea, heartburn, rectal bleeding, poor appetite, dysphagia

GU: Slow urination, nocturia, prostatic hypertrophy, hesitation, retention, frequency, sexual dysfunction

INTEG: Increased sweating, alopecia, hematoma, rash, photosensitivity, facial hair

RESP: Asthma, shortness of breath

EENT: Diplopia, dry mouth, blurred vision, tinnitus

Contraindications: Hypersensitivity

Precautions: Pregnancy (C), lactation, children

Pharmacokinetics: Rapidly absorbed, peak ½-2 hr; rapidly metabolized (active metabolites: N-desmethyldeprenyl, amphetamine, methamphetamine), metabolites excreted in urine

---

◆ = Nursing alert   ⫽ = Herb-drug interaction   🛇 = Do not crush

Interactions:
• **Fatal interaction:** Opioids (especially meperidine); do not administer together
• Increased side effects of: levodopa/carbidopa
• Serotonin syndrome (confusion, seizures, fever, hypertension, agitation): fluoxetine, paroxitine, sertraline, fluvoxamine (discontinue 5 wk prior to selegiline)
• **Drug/food interaction:** Tyramine foods may increase hypertensive reactions
🖋 May decrease selegiline action: chaste tree fruit

Lab test interferences:
False positive: Urine ketones, urine glucose
False negative: Urine glucose (glucose oxidase)
False increase: Uric acid, urine protein
Decrease: VMA

NURSING CONSIDERATIONS
Assess:
• Decreased parkinsonian symptoms: rigidity, unsteady gait, weakness, tremors
• B/P, respiration throughout treatment
• Mental status: affect, mood behavioral changes, depression; perform suicide assessment
Administer:
• Drug until NPO before surgery
• Adjusting dosage to response
• With meals; limit protein taken with drug
• At doses <10 mg/day because of risks associated with nonselective inhibition of MAO
Perform/provide:
• Assistance with ambulation during beginning therapy
Evaluate:
• Therapeutic response: decrease in akathisia, improved mood

Teach patient/family:
• To change positions slowly to prevent orthostatic hypotension
• To report side effects: twitching, eye spasms; indicate overdose
• To use drug exactly as prescribed; if discontinued abruptly, parkinsonian crisis may occur
• To avoid foods high in tyramine: cheese, pickled products, wine, beer, large amounts of caffeine
• Not to exceed recommended dose of 10 mg; might precipitate hypertensive crisis; report severe headache, other unusual symptoms
Treatment of overdose: IV fluids for hypertension, IV dilute pressure agent for B/P titration

senna (OTC)
(sen'na)
Black Draught, Dr. Caldwell Senna Laxative, Fletcher's Castoria, Gentlax, Senexon, Senna-Gen, Senokot, Senokot xtra, Senolax
Func. class.: Laxative-stimulant
Chem. class.: Anthraquinone

Action: Stimulates peristalsis by action on Auerbach's plexus; softens feces by increasing water, electrolytes in large intestine
Uses: Acute constipation; bowel preparation for surgery or examination
Dosage and routes:
• *Adult:* **PO** 1-8 tabs (Senokot)/day or ½ to 4 tsp of granules (1 tsp-4 ml) added to water or juice; **RECT SUPP** 1-2 hs; **SYR** 1-4 tsp hs, 7.5-15 ml; (Black Draught) ¾ oz dissolved in 2.5 oz liquid given between 2-4 PM the day before procedure (X-Prep)
• *Child >27 kg:* ½ adult dose; do not use Black Draught for children

• *Child 1 mo-1 yr:* **SYR** 1.25-2.5 ml (Senokot) hs

Available forms: Supp 625 mg, 30 mg sennosides; powder 662 mg/g, 6, 15 mg sennosides/3g; tabs 8.6 mg sennosides, 180 mg; oral sol 3 mg sennosides/ml

Side effects/adverse reactions:

GI: Nausea, vomiting, anorexia, cramps, diarrhea, flatulence
META: Hypocalcemia, enteropathy, alkalosis, hypokalemia, *tetany*
GU: Pink, red or brown, black urine
Contraindications: Hypersensitivity, GI bleeding, obstruction, CHF, lactation, abdominal pain, nausea/ vomiting, appendicitis, acute surgical abdomen
Precautions: Pregnancy (C)
Pharmacokinetics:
PO: Onset 6-24 hr; metabolized by liver, excreted in feces
Interactions:
• Do not use with disulfiram (Antabuse)

NURSING CONSIDERATIONS
Assess:
• Stool: color, consistency, amount
• Blood, urine electrolytes if drug is used often
• I&O ratio to identify fluid loss
• Cause of constipation: fluids, bulk, exercise missing
• Cramping, rectal bleeding, nausea, vomiting; drug should be discontinued
Administer:
• In morning or evening (oral dose) with full glass of water
• Dissolve granules in water or juice before administration
• On empty stomach for more rapid results
• Shake oral sol before giving
Evaluate:
• Therapeutic response: decrease in constipation

Teach patient/family:
• That urine, feces may turn yellow-brown to red
• Not to use laxatives for long-term therapy; bowel tone will be lost
• That normal bowel movements do not always occur daily
• Not to use in presence of abdominal pain, nausea, vomiting
• To notify prescriber if constipation unrelieved or of symptoms of electrolyte imbalance: muscle cramps, pain, weakness, dizziness, excessive thirst

---

sertraline (Ŗ)

(ser′tra-leen)
Zoloft
Func. class.: Antidepressant
Chem. class.: SSRI

Action: Inhibits serotonin reuptake in CNS; increases action of serotonin; does not affect dopamine, norepinephrine
Uses: Major depression, obsessive-compulsive disorder (OCD)
Dosage and routes:
• *Adult:* **PO** 50 mg qd; may increase to max of 200 mg/day; do not change dose at intervals of <1 wk; administer qd in AM or PM
• *Geriatric:* **PO** 25 mg qd, increase by 25 mg q3 days to desired dose
Available forms: Tabs 25, 50, 100 mg
Side effects/adverse reactions:
CNS: Insomnia, agitation, somnolence, dizziness, headache, tremor, fatigue, paresthesia, twitching, confusion, ataxia, gait abnormality (elderly)
GU: Male sexual dysfunction, micturition disorder
GI: Diarrhea, nausea, constipation, anorexia, dry mouth, dyspepsia, *vomiting, flatulence*

◆ = Nursing alert   ⫽ = Herb-drug interaction   ⊘ = Do not crush

CV: Palpitations, chest pain
EENT: Vision abnormalities
INTEG: Increased sweating, rash, hot flashes
ENDO: SIADH (elderly)

Contraindications: Hypersensitivity to this drug or SSRIs

Precautions: Pregnancy (B), lactation, elderly, hepatic, renal disease, epilepsy

Pharmacokinetics:
PO: Peak 4.5-8.4 hr; steady state 1 wk; plasma protein binding 99%, elimination half-life 26-104 hr, extensively metabolized, metabolite excreted in urine, bile

Interactions:
• Increased effects of: antidepressants (tricyclics), diazepam, tolbutamide, warfarin, benzodiazepines
• Fatal reactions: MAOIs
• Increased sertraline levels: cimetidine
• Altered lithium levels: lithium

💋 Potentiation of SSRI: St. John's wort; do not use together

Lab test interferences:
Increase: AST (SGOT), ALT (SGPT)

NURSING CONSIDERATIONS
Assess:
• Mental status: mood, sensorium, affect, suicidal tendencies, increase in psychiatric symptoms, depression, panic
• B/P (lying/standing), pulse q4h; if systolic B/P drops 20 mm Hg, hold drug, notify prescriber; take vital signs q4h in patients with cardiovascular disease
• Weight qwk; appetite may decrease with drug
• Urinary retention, constipation, especially in elderly
• Alcohol consumption; hold dose until morning

Administer:
• Increased fluids, bulk in diet for constipation, urinary retention
• With food, milk for GI symptoms
• Crushed if patient is unable to swallow medication whole
• Gum, hard candy, frequent sips of water for dry mouth

Perform/provide:
• Storage at room temp; do not freeze
• Assistance with ambulation during therapy, since drowsiness, dizziness occur
• Safety measures, including side rails, primarily for elderly
• Checking to see that PO medication is swallowed

Evaluate:
• Therapeutic response: significant improvement in depression, OCS

Teach patient/family:
• That therapeutic effect may take 1 wk
• To use caution in driving, other activities requiring alertness; drowsiness, dizziness, blurred vision may occur
• Not to discontinue medication quickly after long-term use; may cause nausea, headache, malaise
• To avoid alcohol, other CNS depressants
• To notify prescriber if pregnant or plan to become pregnant or breastfeed

---

sildenafil (℞)
(sil-den'a-fill)
Viagra
Func. class: Erectile agent
Chem. class: Selective inhibitor of cGMP-PDE5

Action: Enhances the effect of nitric oxide (NO) by inhibiting phosphodiesterase type 5 (PDE5), which is necessary for degrading cGMP in the corpus cavernosum

Uses: Treatment of erectile dysfunction

Dosage and routes:
• *Adult:* **PO** 50 mg 1 hr before sexual activity; may be increased to 100 mg or decreased to 25 mg; max once/day

Available forms: Tabs 25, 50, 100 mg

Side effects/adverse reactions:
CNS: Headache, flushing, dizziness
MISC.: Dyspepsia, nasal congestion, UTI, abnormal vision, diarrhea, rash

Contraindication: Hypersensitivity

Precautions: Anatomical penile deformities, sickle cell anemia, leukemia, multiple myeloma, pregnancy (B)

Pharmacokinetics: Rapidly absorbed; bioavailability 40%; metabolized by liver (active metabolites); terminal half-life 4 hr, peak ½-1½ hr; reduced absorption with high fat meal; excreted feces, urine

Interactions:
• Increased sildenafil levels: cimetidine, erythromycin, ketoconazole, itraconazole
• Decreased sildenafil levels: rifampin

NURSING CONSIDERATIONS
Assess:
• Use of organic nitrates that should not be used with this drug

Administer:
PO
• Approximately 1 hr before sexual activity, do not use more than once a day

Teach patient/family:
• That drug does not protect against sexually transmitted diseases, including HIV
• That drug absorption is reduced with a high fat meal

---

silver nitrate (℞)
Func. class.: Keratolytic

Action: Antiinfective, astringent, caustic

Uses: Cauterization of lesions, warts, burns (low concentrations)

Dosage and routes:
• *Adult and child:* **TOP** apply to area to be treated

Available forms: Sticks, sol 10%, 25%, 50%

Side effects/adverse reactions:
INTEG: Skin discoloration

Contraindications: Hypersensitivity

Interactions:
• Not to be used with alkalies, phosphates, thimerosal, benzalkonium chloride, halogenated acids

NURSING CONSIDERATIONS
Administer:
• After moistening stick with water
• To burns using a wet dressing (low concentrations 0.125%)

Perform/provide:
• Storage in cool area

Evaluate:
• Therapeutic response: absence of lesions, healing of burned areas

Teach patient/family:
• To avoid contact with clothing, unaffected areas; discoloration may occur

---

silver protein, mild (℞, OTC)
Argyrol S.S. 10%, Argyrol S.S. 20%

Func. class.: Disinfectant
Chem. class.: Silver colloidal compound

Action: Destroys gram-positive, gram-negative organisms
Uses: Eye, nose, throat, swelling, infection

 = Nursing alert   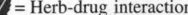 = Herb-drug interaction   ⊗ = Do not crush

Dosage and routes:
• *Adult and child:* **TOP** sol use as needed
Available forms: Top sol 5%, 10%, 25%; eyedrops 20%
Side effects/adverse reactions:
INTEG: Irritation, discolored tissue
Contraindications: Hypersensitivity
Precautions: Pregnancy (C)
NURSING CONSIDERATIONS
Administer:
• To area to be treated only; do not apply to healthy skin
Perform/provide:
• Storage in tight container
Evaluate:
• Area of body involved: irritation, rash, breaks, dryness, scales

---

simethicone (OTC, ℞)
(si-meth'i-kone)
Extra Strength Gas-X, Flatulex Gas Relief, Gas-X, Majur Con, Mylanta Gas, Myllcon, Mylicon 80, Ovol*, Phazyme, Phazyme 95, Phazyme 125
Func. class.: Antiflatulent

Action: Disperses, prevents gas pockets in GI system; does not decrease gas production
Uses: Flatulence
Dosage and routes:
• *Adult and child >12 yr:* **PO** 40-100 mg pc, hs
• *Infants:* **PO** 20 mg qid
Available forms: Chew tabs 40, 80 mg; tabs 50, 60, 95, 125 mg; drops 40 mg/0.6 ml; caps 125 mg
Side effects/adverse reactions:
GI: Belching, rectal flatus
Contraindications: Hypersensitivity
Precautions: Pregnancy (C)
NURSING CONSIDERATIONS
Assess:
• Reason for excess gas production,

decreased bowel sounds, recent surgery, other GI conditions
Administer:
• After meals, hs; shake susp well before giving; chew tabs should be chewed
Evaluate:
• Therapeutic response: absence of flatulence
Teach patient/family:
• That tablets must be chewed
• To shake suspension well before pouring

---

simvastatin (℞)
(sim-va-sta'tin)
Zocor
Func. class.: Antilipidemic
Chem. class.: HMG-CoA reductase inhibitor

Action: Inhibits HMG-CoA reductase enzyme, which reduces cholesterol synthesis
Uses: As an adjunct in primary hypercholesterolemia (types IIa, IIb), coronary artery disease
Dosage and routes:
• *Adult:* **PO** 5-10 mg qd in PM initially; usual range 5-40 mg/day qd in PM, not to exceed 40 mg/day; dosage adjustments may be made in 4-wk intervals or more
• *Elderly/renal disease:* **PO** 5 mg/day
Available forms: Tabs 5, 10, 20, 40 mg
Side effects/adverse reactions:
INTEG: Rash, pruritus, alopecia
GI: Nausea, constipation, diarrhea, dyspepsia, flatus, abdominal pain, heartburn, *liver dysfunction,* pancreatitis
EENT: Lens opacities
MS: Muscle cramps, myalgia, ***myositis, rhabdomyolysis***
CNS: Headache, tremor, vertigo, peripheral neuropathy

S

Contraindications: Hypersensitivity, pregnancy (X), lactation, active liver disease

Precautions: Past liver disease, alcoholism, severe acute infections, trauma, hypotension, uncontrolled seizure disorders, severe metabolic disorders, electrolyte imbalances

Pharmacokinetics: Peak 1-2½ hr, metabolized in liver (active metabolites), highly protein bound, excreted primarily in bile, feces

Interactions:
- Increased effects of warfarin
- Increased myalgia, myositis: cyclosporine, gemfibrozil, niacin, erythromycin
- Increased serum level of digoxin

Lab test interferences:
Increase: CPK, liver function tests

NURSING CONSIDERATIONS

Assess:
- 12 hr fasting lipid profile: LDL, ADL, TG, Chol at 6-8 wk, and q6mo
- Liver function studies q1-2mo during the first 1½ yr of treatment; AST (SGOT), ALT (SGPT), liver function tests may increase
- Renal studies in patients with compromised renal system: BUN, I&O ratio, creatinine
- Eyes with slit lamp before, 1 mo after treatment begins, annually; lens opacities may occur

Administer:
- Total daily dose in evening

Perform/provide:
- Storage in cool environment in tight container protected from light

Evaluate:
- Therapeutic response: decrease in cholesterol to desired level after 8 wk

Teach patient/family:
- That blood work and eye exam will be necessary during treatment
- To report blurred vision, severe GI symptoms, dizziness, headache
- That previously prescribed regimen will continue: low-cholesterol diet, exercise program

---

sodium bicarbonate (OTC)

Arm & Hammer Pure Baking Soda, Bellans, Citrocarbonate, Soda Mint

Func. class.: Alkalinizer
Chem. class.: NaHCO$_3$

Action: Orally neutralizes gastric acid, which forms water, NaCl, CO$_2$; increases plasma bicarbonate, which buffers H$^+$-ion concentration; reverses acidosis IV

Uses: Acidosis (metabolic), cardiac arrest, alkalinization (systemic/urinary) antacid

Dosage and routes:

Acidosis, metabolic
- *Adult and child:* **IV INF** 2-5 mEq/kg over 4-8 hr depending on CO$_2$, pH

Cardiac arrest
- *Adult and child:* **IV BOL** 1 mEq/kg, then 0.5 mEq/kg q10 min, then doses based on ABGs
- *Infant:* **IV INF** not to exceed 8 mEq/kg/day based on ABGs (4.2% sol)

Alkalinization of urine
- *Adult:* **PO** 325 mg-2 g qid or 48 mEq (4g), then 12-24 mEq q4h
- *Child:* **PO** 12-120 mg/kg/day (1-10 mEq/kg)

Antacid
- *Adult:* **PO** 300 mg-2 g chewed, taken with H$_2$O qd-qid

Available forms: Tabs 300, 325, 600, 650 mg; inj 4%, 4.2%, 5%, 7.5%, 8.4%

Side effects/adverse reactions:
CNS: Irritability, headache, confusion, stimulation, tremors, *twitch-*

 = Nursing alert   ✏ = Herb-drug interaction   ⊘ = Do not crush

*ing, hyperreflexia, **tetany,** weakness, **convulsions** of alkalosis

CV: Irregular pulse, **cardiac arrest,** water retention, edema, weight gain

GI: Flatulence, *belching, distention, **paralytic ileus,*** acid rebound

META: Alkalosis

GU: Calculi

RESP: Shallow, slow respirations; cyanosis, ***apnea***

Contraindications: Hypertension, peptic ulcer, renal disease, hypocalcemia

Precautions: CHF, cirrhosis, toxemia, renal disease, pregnancy (C)

Pharmacokinetics:

PO: Onset 2 min, duration 10 min

IV: Onset 15 min, duration 1-2 hr, excreted in urine

Interactions:

• Increased effects: amphetamines, mecamylamine, quinine, quinidine, pseudoephedrine, flecainide, anorexiants

• Decreased effects: lithium, chlorpropamide, barbiturates, salicylates, benzodiazepines

• Increased Na and decreased K: corticosteroids

⚫ Decreased action of sodium bicarbonate: oak bark

Lab test interferences:

Increase: Urinary urobilinogen

False positive: Urinary protein, blood lactate

NURSING CONSIDERATIONS

Assess:

• Respiratory and pulse rate, rhythm, depth, lung sounds; notify prescriber of abnormalities

• Fluid balance (I&O, weight qd, edema); notify prescriber of fluid overload

• Electrolytes, blood pH, PO_2, HCO_3, during treatment; ABGs frequently during emergencies

• Urine pH, urinary output, during beginning treatment

• Extravasation with IV administration (tissue sloughing, ulceration, and necrosis)

• Weight qd with initial therapy

• Alkalosis: irritability, confusion, twitching, hyperreflexia stimulation, slow respirations, cyanosis, irregular pulse

• Milk-alkali syndrome: confusion, headache, nausea, vomiting, anorexia, urinary stones, hypercalcemia

• For GI perforation secondary to CO_2 in GI tract; may lead to perforation if ulcer is severe enough

Administer:

IV

• In prepared sol or diluted in an equal amount of compatible sol given 2-5 mEq/kg over 4-8 hr, not to exceed 50 mEq/hr; slower rate in children

Additive compatibilities: Amikacin, aminophylline, amobarbital, amphotericin B, atropine, bretylium, calcium chloride, calcium gluceptate, cefoxitin, ceftazidime, cephalothin, cephapirin, chloramphenicol, chlorothiazide, cimetidine, clindamycin, cytarabine, droperidol/fentanyl, ergonovine, erythromycin, esmolol, floxacillin, furosemide, heparin, hyaluronidase, hydrocortisone, kanamycin, lidocaine, mannitol, metaraminol, methotrexate, methyldopate, multivitamins, nafcillin, nalmefene, netilmicin, nizatidine, ofloxacin, oxacillin, oxytocin, phenobarbital, phenylephrine, phenytoin, phytonadione, potassium chloride, prochlorperazine, thiopental, verapamil

Syringe compatibilities: Milrinone, pentobarbital

Y-site compatibilities: Acyclovir, amifostine, asparaginase, aztreonam, cefepime, cefmetazole, ceftriaxone, cladribine, cyclophosphamide, cytarabine, daunorubicin, dexamethasone, dexchlorpheniramine, doxorubicin, etoposide, famotidine, filgrastim, fludarabine, gallium, granisetron, heparin, ifosfamide, indomethacin sodium trihydrate, insulin, melphalan, mesna, methylprednisolone, morphine, paclitaxel, piperacillin/tazobactam, potassium chloride, propofol, tacrolimus, teniposide, thiotepa, tolazoline, vancomycin, vit B/C

Evaluate:

• Therapeutic response: ABGs, electrolytes, blood pH, HCO_3 WNL

Teach patient/family:

• To chew antacid tablets and drink 8 oz water

• Not to take antacid with milk, or milk-alkali syndrome may result

• Not to use antacid for more than 2 wk

• To notify prescriber if indigestion is accompanied by chest pain, dyspnea, diarrhea, dark, tarry stools

• About sodium-restricted diet; to avoid use of baking soda for indigestion

---

sodium biphosphate/ sodium phosphate
(OTC)

Fleet Enema, Phospho-Soda
Func. class.: Laxative, saline

Action: Increases water absorption in the small intestine by osmotic action, laxative effect occurs by increased peristalsis and water retention

Uses: Constipation, bowel or rectal preparation for surgery, exam

Dosage and routes:

• *Adult:* **PO** 20-30 ml (Phospho-Soda)

• *Child:* **PO** 5-15 ml (Phospho-Soda)

• *Adult and child >12 yr:* **RECT** 1 enema (118 ml)

• *Child 2-12 yr:* **RECT** ½ enema (59 ml)

Available forms: Enema 7 g phosphate/19 g biphosphate/118 ml; oral sol 18 g phosphate/48 g biphosphate/100 ml

Side effects/adverse reactions:

GI: Nausea, cramps, diarrhea

META: Electrolyte, fluid imbalances

Contraindications: Hypersensitivity, rectal fissures, abdominal pain, nausea/vomiting, appendicitis, acute surgical abdomen, ulcerated hemorrhoids, Na-restricted diets (Sal-Hepatica, Phospho-Soda)

Precautions: Pregnancy (C)

Pharmacokinetics: Excreted in feces

NURSING CONSIDERATIONS

Assess:

• Stools: color, amount, consistency

• Bowel pattern, bowel sounds, flatulence, distention, fever, dietary patterns, exercise

• Blood, urine electrolytes if drug is used often by patient

• Cramping, rectal bleeding, nausea, vomiting; if these symptoms occur, drug should be discontinued

Administer:

• Alone for better absorption; do not take within 1 hr of other drugs

Evaluate:

• Therapeutic response: decrease in constipation

Teach patient/family:

• Not to use laxatives for long-term therapy; bowel tone will be lost

• That normal bowel movements do not always occur daily

• Not to use in presence of abdominal pain, nausea, vomiting

• To notify prescriber if constipa-

---

tion unrelieved or if symptoms of electrolyte imbalance occur: muscle cramps, pain, weakness, dizziness, excessive thirst
• To maintain fluid consumption

• To report double vision, rapid change in vision, appearance of floating spots, acute redness of eyes

---

sodium chloride, hypertonic (otc, ℞)
Adsorbonac Ophthalmic Solution, AK-NaCl, Dey-Pak Sodium Chloride 3% and 10%, Muro-128 Ophthalmic, Muroptic-S
Func. class.: Miscellaneous ophthalmic agent
Chem. class.: Hyperosmolar ophthalmic

Action: Reduces corneal edema by osmosis of water through semipermeable corneal epithelium
Uses: Reduces corneal edema
Dosage and routes:
• *Adult:* **INSTILL** 1-2 gtt q3-4h or ointment hs
Available forms: Sol 2%, 5%; oint 5%
Side effects/adverse reactions:
EENT: Stinging
Contraindications: Hypersensitivity
NURSING CONSIDERATIONS
Administer:
• By instillation; medication should not be shared with others
Perform/provide:
• Storage in tight container at room temperature
Evaluate:
• Therapeutic response: decreased corneal edema
Teach patient/family:
• The correct method of instillation, including pressure on lacrimal sac for 1 min, and not to touch dropper to eye
• That blurred vision is common with ointment

---

sodium hyaluronate (hylan G-F20) (℞)
(so dee-um hy-al yur'o-nate)
Hyalgan, Synvisc
Func. class.: Joint agent

Action: Improves elasticity and viscosity of synovial fluid
Uses: Osteoarthritis of the knee
Dosages and routes:
• *Adult:* Intra-articular **INJ:** 2 ml injected qwk into affected knee, for a total treatment cycle of 3-5 inj/treatment cycle
Side effects/adverse reactions:
Local: Pain at inj site, pruritus
SYST: Headache
Contraindications: Hypersensitivity to hyaluronan, infections in area to be injected
Precautions: Pregnancy, lactation, children
NURSING CONSIDERATIONS
Assess:
• Site for bruising, swelling, pain

---

sodium polystyrene sulfonate (℞)
(po-lee-stye'reen)
Kayexalate, SPS Suspension
Func. class.: Potassium-removing resin
Chem. class.: Cation exchange resin

Action: Removes potassium by exchanging sodium for potassium in body primarily in large intestine
Uses: Hyperkalemia in conjunction with other measures
Dosage and routes:
• *Adult:* **PO** 15 g qd-qid; **RECT**

---

enema 30-50 g/100 ml of sorbitol warmed to body temp q6h
• *Child:* **PO/RECT** 1 mEq of K exchanged/g of resin, approximate dose 1g/kg q6h

Available forms: Susp 15 g polystyrene sulfonate, 21.5 ml sorbitol, 15 g (65 mEq) Na/60 ml; powder 15 g/4 level tsp

Side effects/adverse reactions:
GI: Constipation, anorexia, nausea, vomiting, diarrhea (sorbitol), fecal impaction, gastric irritation
META: Hypocalcemia, hypokalemia, hypomagnesemia, Na retention

Precautions: Pregnancy (C), renal failure, CHF, severe edema, severe hypertension

Interactions:
• Decreased effect of sodium polystyrene: antacids, laxatives

NURSING CONSIDERATIONS
Assess:
• Bowel function qd
• Hypotension: confusion, irritability, muscular pain, weakness
• Serum K, Ca, Mg, Na, acid-base balance

Administer:
• Oral dose as susp mixed with H_2O or syr (20-100 ml)
• Mild laxative as ordered to prevent constipation, fecal impaction
• Sorbitol as ordered to prevent constipation
• Retention enema after mixing with warm water; introduce by gravity, continue stirring, flush with 100 ml of fluid, clamp, and leave in place

Perform/provide:
• Retention of enema for at least ½-1 hr
• Irrigation of colon after enema with 1-2 qt nonsodium sol, drain
• Storage of freshly prepared sol 24 hr at room temp

Evaluate:
• Therapeutic response: K level WNL

---

sodium thiosalicylate (℞)
Rexolate, Tusal

Func. class.: Nonnarcotic analgesic
Chem. class.: Salicylate

Action: Blocks pain impulses in CNS that occur in response to inhibition of prostaglandin synthesis; antipyretic action results from inhibition of hypothalamic heat-regulating center

Uses: Mild to moderate pain (rheumatic fever, acute gout)

Dosage and routes:
Pain
• *Adult:* **IM** 50-100 mg qd or qod
Rheumatic fever
• *Adult:* **IM** 100-150 mg q4-6h × 3 days, then 100 mg bid
Arthritis
• *Adult:* **IM** 100 mg/day
Available forms: Inj 50 mg/ml

Side effects/adverse reactions:
HEMA: **Thrombocytopenia, agranulocytosis, leukopenia, neutropenia, hemolytic anemia,** increased protime
CNS: Stimulation, drowsiness, dizziness, confusion, **convulsions,** headache, flushing, hallucinations, coma
GI: Nausea, vomiting, GI bleeding, diarrhea, heartburn, anorexia, **hepatitis**
INTEG: Rash, urticaria, bruising
EENT: Tinnitus, hearing loss
CV: Rapid pulse, **pulmonary edema**
RESP: Wheezing, hyperpnea
ENDO: Hypoglycemia, hyponatremia, hypokalemia

Contraindications: Hypersensitivity to salicylates, GI bleeding, bleeding disorders, children <3 yr, vit K deficiency, peptic ulcer

---

Precautions: Anemia, hepatic disease, renal disease, Hodgkin's disease, pregnancy (C), lactation

Pharmacokinetics:
PO: Onset 15-30 min, peak 1-2 hr, duration 4-6 hr
Metabolized by liver, excreted by kidneys, crosses placenta, excreted in breast milk, half-life 1-3½ hr

Interactions:
• Decreased effects of sodium thiosalicylate: antacids, steroids, urinary alkalizers
• Increased blood loss: alcohol, heparin
• Increased effects of anticoagulants, insulin, methotrexate
• Decreased effects of probenecid, spironolactone, sulfinpyrazone, sulfonamides
• Toxic effects: PABA
🖋 Increased CNS depression: kava kava

Lab test interferences:
Increase: Coagulation studies, liver function studies, serum uric acid, amylase, CO_2, urinary protein
Decrease: Serum K, PBI, cholesterol, blood glucose
Interference: Urine catecholamines, pregnancy test

NURSING CONSIDERATIONS
Assess:
• Liver function studies: ALT, AST, bilirubin (long-term therapy)
• Renal function studies: BUN, urine creatinine (long-term therapy)
• Blood studies: CBC, Hct, Hgb, pro-time (long-term therapy)
• I&O ratio; decreasing output may indicate renal failure (long-term therapy)
• Hepatotoxicity: dark urine, clay-colored stools, yellow skin, sclera, itching, abdominal pain, fever, diarrhea (long-term therapy)
• Allergic reactions: rash, urticaria; drug may have to be discontinued

• Renal dysfunction: decreased urine output
• Ototoxicity: tinnitus, ringing, roaring in ears; audiometric testing is needed before, after long-term therapy
• Visual changes: blurring, halos, corneal, retinal damage
• Edema in feet, ankles, legs
• Prior drug history; many drug interactions

Evaluate:
• Therapeutic response: less pain

Teach patient/family:
• To report any symptoms of hepatotoxicity, renal toxicity, visual changes, ototoxicity, allergic reactions (long-term therapy)
• Not to exceed recommended dosage; acute poisoning may result
• To read label on other OTC drugs; many contain aspirin
• That therapeutic response takes 2 wk (arthritis)
• To avoid alcohol ingestion; GI bleeding may occur

Treatment of overdose: Lavage, activated charcoal, monitor electrolytes, VS

---

somatotropin (℞)

(soe-ma-toe-troe'pin)
Genotropin, Humatrope, Norditropin, Nutropin, Nutropin AQ, Serostim
Func. class.: Pituitary hormone
Chem. class.: Growth hormone

Action: Stimulates growth; somatotropin similar to natural growth hormone; both preparations developed by recombinant DNA

Uses: Pituitary growth hormone deficiency (hypopituitary dwarfism), children with human growth hormone deficiency, AIDS wasting syn-

---

drome, cachexia, adults with somatotropin deficiency syndrome (SDS)

Dosage and routes:

Genotropin

SC 0.16-0.24 mg/kg/wk divided into 6 or 7 inj, give in abd, thigh, buttocks

Humatrope

SC/IM 0.18 mg/kg divided into equal doses either on 3 alternate days or 6 ×/wk, max wk dose is 0.3 mg/kg

Nutropin/Nutropin AQ (Growth hormone deficiency)

SC 0.3 mg/kg/wk

Serostim

SC at hs >55 kg, 6 mg; 45-55 kg, 5 mg; 35-45 kg, 4 mg

Norditropin

SC 0.024-0.034 mg/kg 6-7 ×/wk

Available forms: Powder for inj (lyophilized) 1.5 mg (4 IU/ml), 4 mg (12 IU/vial), 5 mg (13 IU/vial), 5 mg (15 IU/vial), 5 mg (15 IU/vial) rDNA origin, 5.8 mg (15 IU/ml), 6 mg (18 IU/ml), 8 mg (24 IU/vial), 10 mg (26 IU/vial); inj 10 mg (30 IU/vial)

Side effects/adverse reactions:

GU: Hypercalciuria

INTEG: Rash, urticaria, pain; inflammation at injection site

CNS: Headache, growth of intracranial tumor

ENDO: Hyperglycemia, ketosis, hypothyroidism

SYST: Antibodies to growth hormone

MS: Tissue swelling, joint and muscle pain

Contraindications: Hypersensitivity to benzyl alcohol, closed epiphyses, intracranial lesions

Precautions: Diabetes mellitus, hypothyroidism, pregnancy (C)

Pharmacokinetics: Half-life 15-60 min, duration 7 days; metabolized in liver

Interactions:

• Decreased growth: glucocorticosteroids

• Epiphyseal closure: androgens, thyroid hormones

NURSING CONSIDERATIONS

Assess:

• Growth hormone antibodies if patient fails to respond to therapy

• Thyroid function tests: T_3, T_4, T_7, TSH to identify hypothyroidism

• Allergic reaction: rash, itching, fever, nausea, wheezing

• Hypercalciuria: urinary stones; groin, flank pain; nausea, vomiting, frequency, hematuria, chills

• Growth rate of child at intervals during treatment

Administer:

IM

• Rotate injection site

• Norditropin: after reconstituting 4 or 8 mg/2 ml diluent

• Humatrope: 5 mg/1.5-5 ml diluent, do not shake

• Nutropin/Nutropin AQ: reconstitute 5 mg/1-5 ml or 10 mg/1-10 ml bacteriostatic water for inj (benzyl alcohol preserved)

Perform/provide:

• Storage in refrigerator for <1 mo, if reconstituted <1 wk; do not use discolored or cloudy sol

Evaluate:

• Therapeutic response: growth in children

Teach patient/family:

• That treatment may continue for years; regular assessments are required

◆ = Nursing alert   🖊 = Herb-drug interaction   🚫 = Do not crush

sotalol (R)

(sot'ah-lahl)
Betapace, Sotacar*
Func. class.: Antidysrhythmic
group II, III
Chem. class.: Nonselective
β-blocker

Action: Blockade of β₁- and β₂-receptors leads to antidysrhythmic effect, prolongs action potential in myocardial fibers without affecting conduction, prolongs QT interval, no effect on QRS duration

Uses: Life-threatening ventricular dysrhythmias

Dosage and routes:

Renal dose

• CrCl 30-60 ml/min give q24h; CrCl 10-29 ml/min give q36-48h; CrCl <10 ml/min individualize dose

• *Adult:* PO initial 80 mg bid, may increase to 240-320 mg/day

Available forms: Tabs 80, 160, 240 mg

Side effects/adverse reactions:

CV: Orthostatic hypotension, bradycardia, CHF, chest pain, ventricular dysrhythmias, AV block, peripheral vascular insufficiency, palpitations, prodysrhythmia, torsades de pointes

CNS: Dizziness, mental changes, drowsiness, fatigue, headache, catatonia, depression, anxiety, nightmares, paresthesia, lethargy, insomnia, decreased concentration

GI: Nausea, vomiting, diarrhea, dry mouth, flatulence, constipation, anorexia

INTEG: Rash, alopecia, urticaria, pruritus, fever

HEMA: Agranulocytosis, thrombocytopenic purpura (rare), thrombocytopenia, leukopenia

EENT: Tinnitus, visual changes, sore throat, double vision; dry, burning eyes

GU: Impotence, dysuria, ejaculatory failure, urinary retention

RESP: Bronchospasm, dyspnea, wheezing, nasal stuffiness, pharyngitis

MS: Joint pain, arthralgia, muscle cramps, pain

MISC.: Facial swelling, decreased exercise tolerance, weight change, Raynaud's disease

Contraindications: Hypersensitivity to β-blockers, cardiogenic shock, heart block (2nd or 3rd degree), sinus bradycardia, CHF, bronchial asthma, congenital or acquired long QT syndrome

Precautions: Major surgery, pregnancy (B), lactation, diabetes mellitus, renal disease, thyroid disease, COPD, well-compensated heart failure, CAD, nonallergic bronchospasm, electrolyte disturbances, bradycardia, cardiac dysrhythmias, peripheral vascular disease

Pharmacokinetics:

PO: Onset 1-2 hr, peak 2-4 hr, duration 8-12 hr, half-life 12 hr; metabolized by liver (metabolites inactive), excreted unchanged in urine, crosses placenta, excreted in breast milk

Interactions:

• Increased hypotension: diuretics, other antihypertensives, nitroglycerin, prazosin

• Decreased β-blocker effects: sympathomimetics, nonsteroidal antiinflammatory agents, salicylates

• Increased hypoglycemia effect: insulin

• Increased effects of lidocaine

• Decreased bronchodilating effects of theophylline

• Decreased hypoglycemic effects of sulfonylureas

🖉 Potassium deficiency, increased antidysrhythmic effect: aloe, buckthorn bark/berry, cascara sagrada bark, senna pod/leaf

S

Lab test interferences:
- *False increase:* Urinary catecholamines
- *Interference:* Glucose, insulin tolerance tests

NURSING CONSIDERATIONS
Assess:
- I&O, weight qd
- B/P, pulse q4h; note rate, rhythm, quality
- Apical/radial pulse before administration: notify prescriber of any significant changes
- Baselines in renal, liver function tests before therapy begins
- Edema in feet, legs qd
- Skin turgor, dryness of mucous membranes for hydration status

Administer:
- PO: ac, hs; tablet may be crushed or swallowed whole
- Reduced dosage in renal dysfunction

Perform/provide:
- Storage in dry area at room temp; do not freeze

Evaluate:
- Therapeutic response: absence of life-threatening dysrhythmias

Teach patient/family:
- Not to discontinue drug abruptly; taper over 2 wk or may precipitate angina
- Not to use OTC products containing α-adrenergic stimulants (nasal decongestants, OTC cold preparations) unless directed by prescriber
- To report bradycardia, dizziness, confusion, depression, fever
- To take pulse at home; advise when to notify prescriber
- To avoid alcohol, smoking, sodium intake
- To carry Medic Alert ID to identify drug being taken, allergies
- To avoid hazardous activities if dizziness is present
- To report symptoms of CHF including: difficulty in breathing, especially on exertion or when lying down; night cough, swelling of extremities
- To take medication to minimize orthostatic hypotension
- To wear support hose to minimize effects of orthostatic hypotension

Treatment of overdose: Lavage, IV atropine for bradycardia, IV theophylline for bronchospasm, digitalis, O_2, diuretic for cardiac failure; hemodialysis is useful for removal; administer vasopressor (norepinephrine) for hypotension, isoproterenol for heart block

---

sparfloxacin
(spar-floks′a-sin)
Zagam
Func. class.: Antiinfective
Chem. class.: Fluoroquinolone

Action: Interferes with conversion of intermediate DNA fragments into high-molecular-weight DNA in bacteria; DNA-gyrase inhibitor

Uses: Community-acquired pneumonia; chronic bronchitis caused by *C. pneumoniae, H. influenzae, H. parainfluenzae, M. catarrhalis*

Dosage and routes:
Renal dose
- CrCl <50 ml/min day 1:400 mg then 200 mg qod day 2-10
- *Adult:* **PO** 400 mg loading dose, then 200 mg q24h × 10 days

Available forms: Tabs 200 mg

Side effects/adverse reactions:
*HEMA: **Leukopenia,*** eosinophilia, anemia

CNS: Headache, dizziness, insomnia

GI: Nausea, flatulence, *vomiting,* diarrhea, *abdominal pain, **pseudomembranous colitis***

CV: QT interval prolongation, vasodilation

◆ = Nursing alert   🖊 = Herb-drug interaction   ⊘ = Do not crush

INTEG: Rash, pruritus, photosensitivity

Contraindications: Hypersensitivity to quinolones, photosensitivity

Precautions: Pregnancy (C), lactation, children, renal disease, seizure disorders

Pharmacokinetics: Slow, erratic absorption, widely distributed; metabolized by liver, excreted in urine, feces; half-life 20 hr

Interactions:

• Decreased absorption of sparfloxacin: zinc, antacids, calcium

• Decreased effect: phenytoin

• Increased toxicity: caffeine, theophylline, cyclosporine, warfarin

• Increased sparfloxacin levels: cimetidine, probenecid

Lab test interferences:

Increase: AST (SGOT), ALT (SGPT)

NURSING CONSIDERATIONS

Assess:

• For previous sensitivity reaction

• For signs and symptoms of infection: characteristics of sputum, WBC > 10,000/mm^3, fever; obtain baseline information before and during treatment

• C&S before beginning drug therapy to identify if correct treatment has been initiated

• For allergic reactions: rash, urticaria, pruritus, chills, fever, joint pain; may occur a few days after therapy begins; epinephrine and resuscitation equipment should be available for anaphylactic reaction

• Blood studies: AST (SGOT), ALT (SGPT), alk phosphatase if patient is on long-term therapy

• Bowel pattern qd; if severe diarrhea occurs, drug should be discontinued

• For overgrowth of infection: perineal itching, fever, malaise, redness, pain, swelling, drainage, rash, diarrhea, change in cough, sputum

Administer:

• As directed only

• 4 hr before or 2 hr after antacids, zinc, calcium

Evaluate:

• Therapeutic response: absence of signs/symptoms of infection (WBC <10,000/mm^3, temp WNL)

Teach patient/family:

• To contact prescriber if vaginal itching, loose, foul-smelling stools, furry tongue occur; may indicate superinfection; report itching, rash, pruritus, urticaria

• To take all medication prescribed for the length of time ordered; drug must be taken as directed to maintain blood levels; do not give medication to others

• To notify prescriber of diarrhea with blood or pus

• To drink plenty of liquids

• To take 4 hr before or 2 hr after antacids, dairy products, zinc products

• To avoid direct sunlight

---

spectinomycin (℞)

(spek-ti-noe-mye'sin)

Trobicin

Func. class.: Antiinfective

Chem. class.: Aminocyclitol

Action: Inhibits bacterial synthesis by binding to 30S subunit on ribosomes

Uses: Gonorrhea

Dosage and routes:

• *Adult:* IM 2-4 g as single dose

Available forms: Inj 2, 4 g

Side effects/adverse reactions:

CNS: Dizziness, chills, fever, insomnia, headache, anxiety

HEMA: Anemia

GI: Nausea, vomiting, increased BUN

GU: Decreased urine output

INTEG: Pain at injection site, urticaria, rash, pruritus, fever

Contraindications: Hypersensitivity, syphilis

Precautions: Pregnancy (B), infants, children

Pharmacokinetics:

IM: Peak 1-2 hr, duration >8 hr, half-life 1-3 hr, excreted in urine (active form)

NURSING CONSIDERATIONS

Assess:

• Gonorrhea culture after treatment
• I&O ratio; report decreased output
• Liver studies: AST (SGOT), ALT (SGPT), serum alk phosphatase following multiple doses
• Blood studies: Hct, Hgb, BUN if multiple doses given
• Serologic test for gonorrhea 3 mo after treatment
• Allergies before treatment, reaction of each medication

Administer:

IM

• After shaking vial
• IM inj deep into large muscle mass (gluteus muscle only)
• With 20G needle; no more than 5 ml per site

Perform/provide:

• Storage at room temp; discard reconstituted sol after 24 hr
• Treatment of partner; report infection

Evaluate:

• Therapeutic response: negative gonorrhea culture after treatment

---

spironolactone (℞)

(speer'on-oh-lak'tone)

Aldactone

Func. class.: Potassium-sparing diuretic

Chem. class.: Aldosterone antagonist

Action: Competes with aldosterone at receptor sites in distal tubule, resulting in excretion of sodium chloride, water, retention of potassium, phosphate

Uses: Edema of CHF, hypertension, diuretic-induced hypokalemia, primary hyperaldosteronism (diagnosis, short-term treatment, long-term treatment), edema of nephrotic syndrome, cirrhosis of the liver with ascites

Edema/hypertension

• *Adult:* **PO** 25-200 mg/qd in single or divided doses

Edema

• *Child:* **PO** 3.3 mg/kg/day in single or divided doses

Hypertension

• *Child:* **PO** 1-2 mg/kg bid

Hypokalemia

• *Adult:* **PO** 25-100 mg/day; if **PO**, K supplements must not be used

Primary hyperaldosteronism diagnosis

• *Adult:* **PO** 400 mg/day × 4 days or 4 wk depending on test, then 100-400 mg/day maintenance

Available forms: Tabs 25, 50, 100 mg

Side effects/adverse reactions:

CNS: Headache, confusion, drowsiness, lethargy, ataxia

GI: Diarrhea, cramps, ***bleeding,*** gastritis, *vomiting,* anorexia, nausea

INTEG: Rash, pruritus, urticaria

ENDO: Impotence, gynecomastia, irregular menses, amenorrhea, post-

---

◆ = Nursing alert   ✦ = Herb-drug interaction   ⊘ = Do not crush menopausal bleeding, hirsutism, deepening voice

HEMA: **Agranulocytosis**
ELECT: Hyperchloremic metabolic acidosis, **hyperkalemia,** hyponatremia

Contraindications: Hypersensitivity, anuria, severe renal disease, hyperkalemia, pregnancy (D)

Precautions: Dehydration, hepatic disease, lactation, renal impairment

Pharmacokinetics:
PO: Onset 24-48 hr, peak 48-72 hr; metabolized in liver, excreted in urine, crosses placenta

Interactions:
• Decreased effect of anticoagulants
• Increased action of antihypertensives, digitalis, lithium
• Increased hyperkalemia: K-sparing diuretics, K products, ACE inhibitors, salt substitutes
• Decreased effect of spironolactone, ASA

Lab test interferences:
Interference: 17-OHCS, 17-KS, radioimmunoassay, digoxin assay

NURSING CONSIDERATIONS
Assess:
• Electrolytes: Na, Cl, K, BUN, serum creatinine, ABGs, CBC
• Weight, I&O qd to determine fluid loss; effect of drug may be decreased if used qd, ECG periodically (long-term therapy)
• Signs of metabolic acidosis: drowsiness, restlessness
• Rashes, temperature qd
• Confusion, especially in elderly; take safety precautions if needed
• Hydration: skin turgor, thirst, dry mucous membranes

Administer:
• In AM to avoid interference with sleep
• With food; if nausea occurs, absorption may be decreased slightly

Evaluate:
• Therapeutic response: improvement in edema of feet, legs, sacral area qd if medication is being used in CHF

Teach patient/family:
• To avoid foods with high K⁺ content: oranges, bananas, salt substitutes, dried apricots, dates
• That drowsiness, ataxia, mental confusion may occur; observe caution in driving
• To notify prescriber of cramps, diarrhea, lethargy, thirst, headache, skin rash, menstrual abnormalities, deepening voice, breast enlargement

Treatment of overdose: Lavage if taken orally; monitor electrolytes, administer IV fluids, monitor hydration, renal, CV status

---

stanozolol (℞)
(stan-oh′zoe′lole)
Winstrol
Func. class.: Androgenic anabolic steroid
Chem. class.: Halogenated testosterone derivative

Action: Increases weight by building body tissue; increases potassium, phosphorus, chloride, and nitrogen levels; increases bone development

Uses: Prevention of hereditary angioedema, aplastic anemia to increase hemoglobin

Dosage and routes:
Aplastic anemia (possibly effective)
• *Adult:* **PO** 2 mg tid
• *Child 6-12 yr:* **PO** up to 2 mg tid
• *Child <6 yr:* **PO** 1 mg bid
Angioedema
• *Adult:* **PO** 2 mg tid, then decrease q1-3mo, down to 2 mg qd or q2d

Available forms: Tabs 2 mg

Side effects/adverse reactions:

INTEG: Rash, acneiform lesions; oily hair, skin; flushing, sweating, acne vulgaris, alopecia, hirsutism

CNS: Dizziness, headache, fatigue, tremors, paresthesias, flushing, sweating, anxiety, lability, insomnia, carpal tunnel syndrome

MS: Cramps, spasms

CV: Increased B/P

GU: **Hematuria,** amenorrhea, vaginitis, decreased libido, decreased breast size, clitoral hypertrophy, testicular atrophy

GI: Nausea, vomiting, constipation, weight gain, *cholestatic jaundice*

EENT: Conjunctival edema, nasal congestion

ENDO: Abnormal GTT

Contraindications: Severe renal, severe cardiac, and severe hepatic disease; hypersensitivity, pregnancy (X), lactation, genital bleeding (abnormal)

Precautions: Diabetes mellitus, CV disease, MI

Pharmacokinetics:

PO: Metabolized in liver, excreted in urine, crosses placenta, excreted in breast milk

Interactions:

• Increased effects of oral antidiabetics, oxyphenbutazone

• Increased PT: anticoagulants

• Edema: ACTH, adrenal steroids

• Decreased effects of insulin

Lab test interferences:

Increase: Serum cholesterol, blood glucose, urine glucose

Decrease: Serum Ca, serum K, T_4, T_3, thyroid ^{131}I uptake test, urine 17-OHCS

NURSING CONSIDERATIONS

Assess:

• Weight qd, notify prescriber if weekly weight gain is >5 lb

• B/P q4h

• I&O ratio; be alert for decreasing urinary output, increasing edema

• Growth rate in children; growth rate may be uneven (linear/bone growth) (extended use)

• Electrolytes: K, Na, Cl, Ca; cholesterol

• Liver function studies: ALT (SGPT), AST (SGOT), bilirubin

• Edema, hypertension, cardiac symptoms, jaundice

• Mental status: affect, mood, behavioral changes, aggression

• Signs of masculinization in female: increased libido, deepening of voice, decreased breast tissue, enlarged clitoris, menstrual irregularities; male: gynecomastia, impotence, testicular atrophy

• Hypercalcemia: lethargy, polyuria, polydipsia, nausea, vomiting, constipation; dosage may have to be decreased

• Hypoglycemia in diabetics, since oral antidiabetic action is increased

Administer:

• Titrated dose; use lowest effective dose

Perform/provide:

• Diet with increased calories and protein; decrease Na for edema

• Supportive drug of anemia

Evaluate:

• Therapeutic response: 4-6 wk in osteoporosis

Teach patient/family:

• That drug must be combined with complete health plan: diet, rest, exercise

• To notify prescriber if therapeutic response decreases

• Not to discontinue abruptly

• About change in sex characteristics

• Women to report menstrual irregularities

• That 1-3-mo course is necessary for response in breast cancer

• The correct procedure for use of

 = Nursing alert   = Herb-drug interaction   ⊘ = Do not crush

buccal tablets (requires 30-60 min to dissolve; change absorption site with each dose; do not eat, drink, chew, or smoke while tablet is in place)

---

stavudine (℞)

(sta′vyoo-deen)
Zerit
Func. class.: Antiviral
Chem. class.: Thymidine nucleoside

Action: Prevents replication of HIV by the inhibition of the enzyme reverse transcriptase, causes DNA chain termination

Uses: Treatment of advanced HIV infection not responsive to other antivirals

Dosage and routes:
Renal dose
• *Wt >60 kg:* CrCl 26-50 ml/min 20 mg q12h; CrCl 10-25 ml/min 20 mg q24h
• *Wt <60 kg:* CrCl 26-50 ml/min 15 mg q12h; CrCl 10-25 ml/min 15 mg q24h
• *Adult >60 kg:* **PO** 40 mg q12h
• *Adult <60 kg:* 30 mg q12h
• *Child:* 2 mg/kg/day divided q12h
Available forms: Caps 15, 20, 30, 40 mg; PO powder for sol 1 mg/ml
Side effects/adverse reactions:
HEMA: **Bone marrow suppression**
CNS: Peripheral neuropathy, insomnia, anxiety, neuropathy, depression, dizziness, confusion, headache, chills/fever, malaise
GI: **Hepatotoxicity,** diarrhea, nausea, vomiting, anorexia, dyspepsia, constipation, stomatitis
MS: Myalgia, arthralgia
CV: Chest pain, vasodilation, hypertension
RESP: Dyspnea, pneumonia, asthma

INTEG: Rash, sweating, pruritus, benign neoplasms
EENT: Conjunctivitis, abnormal vision
Contraindications: Hypersensitivity to this drug or zidovudine, didanosine, zalcitabine; severe peripheral neuropathy
Precautions: Advanced HIV infection, pregnancy (C), lactation, bone marrow suppression; renal, liver disease, peripheral neuropathy, hypersensitivity to zidovudine, didanosine, zalcitabine
Interactions:
• Increased myelosuppression: other myelosuppressants
Pharmacokinetics: Excreted in urine, breast milk; peak 1 hr; half-life: elimination: 1-1.6 hr, intracellular: 3-3.5 hr
NURSING CONSIDERATIONS
Assess:
• Liver studies: AST (SGOT), ALT (SGPT)
• Blood studies: WBC, differential, RBC, Hct, Hgb, platelets
• Renal studies: urinalysis, protein, blood
• C&S before drug therapy; drug may be given as soon as culture is taken
• Bowel pattern before, during treatment
• Weakness, tremors, confusion, dizziness; drug may have to be decreased or discontinued
Administer:
• With or without meals; absorption does not appear to be lowered when taken with food
Teach patient/family:
• The signs of peripheral neuropathy: burning, weakness, pain, prickling feeling in the extremities
• That drug should not be given with antineoplastics
• That drug is not a cure for AIDS, but will control symptoms

• To call prescriber if sore throat, swollen lymph nodes, malaise, fever occur; other drugs may be needed to prevent other infections
• That even with this drug, patient may pass AIDS virus to others
• That follow-up visits are necessary; serious toxicity may occur; blood counts must be done q2wk
• To take q12h around clock
• That serious drug interactions may occur if OTC products are ingested; see prescriber before taking aspirin, acetaminophen, indomethacin
• That drug may cause fainting or dizziness

Evaluate:
• Therapeutic response: decreased symptoms of HIV

---

streptokinase (℞)

(strep-toe-kye'nase)
Kabikinase, Streptase
Func. class.: Thrombolytic enzyme
Chem. class.: β-hemolytic streptococcus filtrate (purified)

Action: Activates conversion of plasminogen to plasmin (fibrinolysin): plasmin breaks down clots (fibrin), fibrinogen, factors V, VII; occlusion of venous access lines
Uses: Deep-vein thrombosis, pulmonary embolism, arterial thrombosis, arterial embolism, arteriovenous cannula occlusion, lysis of coronary artery thrombi after MI, acute evolving transmural MI
Dosage and routes:
Lysis of coronary artery thrombi
• *Adult:* **IC** 20,000 IU, then 2000 IU/min over 1 hr as **IV INF**
Arteriovenous cannula occlusion
• *Adult:* **IV INF** 250,000 IU/2 ml sol into occluded limb of cannula run over ½ hr; clamp for 2 hr; as-

pirate contents; flush with NaCl sol and reconnect
***Thrombosis/embolism/DVT/
pulmonary embolism***
• *Adult:* **IV INF** 250,000 IU over ½ hr, then 100,000 IU/hr for 72 hr for deep-vein thrombosis; 100,000 IU/hr over 24-72 hr for pulmonary embolism; 100,000 IU/hr × 24-72 hr for arterial thrombosis or embolism
Acute evolving transmural MI
• *Adult:* **IV INF** 1,500,000 IU diluted to a volume of 45 ml; give within 1 hr; intracoronary **INF** 20,000 IU by **BOL,** then 2,000 IU/min × 1 hr, total dose 140,000 IU
Available forms: Powder for inj, lyophilized, 250,000, 750,000, 1,500,000 IU/vial
Side effects/adverse reactions:
CV: Dysrhythmias, hypotension, noncardiogenic pulmonary edema, *pulmonary embolism*
CNS: Headache, fever
EENT: Periorbital edema
GI: Nausea
HEMA: Decreased Hct, *bleeding*
INTEG: Rash, urticaria, phlebitis at IV inf site, itching, flushing
MS: Low back pain
RESP: Altered respirations, SOB, *bronchospasm*
SYST: **GI, GU, intracranial, retroperitoneal bleeding, surface bleeding, anaphylaxis**
Contraindications: Hypersensitivity, active bleeding, intraspinal surgery, CNS neoplasms, ulcerative colitis, enteritis, severe hypertension, severe renal disease, hepatic disease, hypocoagulation, COPD, subacute bacterial endocarditis, rheumatic valvular disease, cerebral embolism/thrombosis/hemorrhage, intraarterial diagnostic procedure or surgery (10 days), recent major surgery
Precautions: Arterial emboli from left side of heart, pregnancy (C)

Pharmacokinetics:

IV: Onset immediate, duration <12 hr; half-life <20 min; excreted in bile, urine

Interactions:

• Bleeding potential: aspirin, indomethacin, phenylbutazone, anticoagulants

Lab test interferences:

Increase: PT, aPTT, TT

Decrease: Plasminogen, fibrinogen

NURSING CONSIDERATIONS

Assess:

• Allergy: fever, rash, itching, chills; mild reaction may be treated with antihistamines

➡ For bleeding during 1st hr of treatment; hematuria, hematemesis, bleeding from mucous membranes, epistaxis, ecchymosis; may require tranfusion (rare); continue to assess for bleeding for 24 hr

• Blood studies (Hct, platelets, PTT, PT, TT, aPTT) before starting therapy; PT or aPTT must be less than 2× control before starting therapy; PTT or PT q3-4h during treatment

• For hypersensitive reactions: fever, rash, dyspnea; drug should be discontinued; for streptokinase reactions previously

• VS, B/P, pulse, respirations, neuro signs, temp at least q4h; temp >104° F (40° C) indicates internal bleeding; cardiac rhythm following intracoronary administration; systolic pressure increase >25 mm Hg should be reported to prescriber

➡ For neurologic changes that may indicate intracranial bleeding

➡ Retroperitoneal bleeding: back pain, leg weakness, diminished pulses

• For Guillain-Barré syndrome that may occur after treatment with this drug

• For respiratory depression

Administer:

IV

• As soon as thrombi identified; not useful for thrombi over 1 wk old

• Cryoprecipitate or fresh frozen plasma if bleeding occurs

• Loading dose at beginning of therapy; may require increased loading doses

• Heparin after fibrinogen level >100 mg/dl; heparin infusion to increase PTT to 1.5-2 × baseline for 3-7 days; IV heparin with loading dose is recommended after discontinuing streptokinase to prevent redevelopment of thrombi

• After reconstituting with 5 ml NS or D_5W; do not shake; further dilute to total volume of 45 ml; may be diluted to 500 ml in 45 ml increments; may dilute vial in 15 ml NS, further dilute 750,000 IU/50 ml NS or D_5W; further dilute 1,500,000 IU dose/100 ml or more

• About 10% patients have high streptococcal antibody titers requiring increased loading doses

• IV therapy using 0.8 µm filter

Y-site compatibilities: Dobutamine, dopamine, heparin, lidocaine, nitroglycerin

Perform/provide:

• Storage of reconstituted sol in refrigerator; discard after 24 hr

• Bed rest during entire course of treatment

• Avoidance of venous or arterial puncture, inj, rectal temp; any invasive treatment

• Treatment of fever with acetaminophen or aspirin

• Pressure for 30 sec to minor bleeding sites; inform prescriber if this does not attain hemostasis; apply pressure dressing

Evaluate:

• Therapeutic response: resolution of thrombosis, embolism

---

* = Canada only Side effects: *italics* = common; ***bold italics*** = life-threatening

streptomycin (℞)

(strep-toe-mye'sin)

Func. class.: Antiinfective/antitubercular

Chem. class.: Aminoglycoside

Action: Interferes with protein synthesis in bacterial cell by binding to ribosomal subunit, causing inaccurate peptide sequence to form in protein chain, causing bacterial death

Uses: Sensitive strains of *M. tuberculosis,* nontuberculous infections caused by sensitive strains of *Y. pestis, Brucella, H. influenzae, K. pneumoniae, E. coli, E. aerogenes, S. viridans, F. tularensis, Proteus*

Dosage and routes:

Tuberculosis

• *Adult:* IM 1 g qd × 2-3 mo, then 1 g 2-3 ×/week with other antitubercular drugs

• *Child:* IM 20-40 mg/kg/day in divided doses with other antitubercular drugs; max 15 mg/kg/day

Streptococcal endocarditis

• *Adult:* IM 1 g q12h × 1 wk with penicillin, then 500 mg bid × 1 wk

Enterococcal endocarditis

• *Adult:* IM 1 g q12h × 2 wk, then 500 mg q12h × 4 wk with penicillin, max 15 mg/kg/day

Available forms: Inj 1 g, 400 mg/ml

Side effects/adverse reactions:

GU: Oliguria, hematuria, renal damage, azotemia, renal failure, nephrotoxicity

CNS: Confusion, depression, numbness, tremors, *convulsions,* muscle twitching, *neurotoxicity*

EENT: Ototoxicity, deafness, visual disturbances

HEMA: Agranulocytosis, thrombocytopenia, leukopenia, eosinophilia, anemia

GI: Nausea, vomiting, anorexia, increased ALT (SGPT), AST (SGOT), bilirubin; hepatomegaly, *hepatic necrosis,* splenomegaly

CV: Hypotension, myocarditis, palpitations

INTEG: Rash, burning, urticaria, dermatitis, alopecia

Contraindications: Severe renal disease, hypersensitivity

Precautions: Neonates, mild renal disease, pregnancy (B), myasthenia gravis, lactation, hearing deficit, elderly, Parkinson's disease

Pharmacokinetics:

IM: Onset rapid, peak 1-2 hr; plasma half-life 2-2½ hr; not metabolized, excreted unchanged in urine, crosses placental barrier, poor penetration into CSF, small amounts enter breast milk

Interactions:

• Increased ototoxicity, neurotoxicity, nephrotoxicity: other aminoglycosides, amphotericin B, polymyxin, vancomycin, ethacrynic acid, furosemide, mannitol, methoxyflurane, cisplatin, cephalosporins, bacitracin

• Increased effects: nondepolarizing muscle relaxants, succinylcholine, warfarin

NURSING CONSIDERATIONS

Assess:

• Weight before treatment; calculation of dosage is usually based on ideal body weight, but may be calculated on actual body weight

• I&O ratio, urinalysis qd for proteinuria, cells, casts; report sudden change in urine output

• Serum peak 20-30 min after IM injection, trough level drawn 8 hr; acceptable levels—peak 5-25 μg/ml, trough should not be >5 μg/ml

• Urine pH if drug is used for UTI; urine should be kept alkaline

• Renal impairment by collecting urine for CrCl testing, BUN, serum

---

 = Nursing alert   = Herb-drug interaction   ⊘ = Do not crush

creatinine; lower dosage should be given in renal impairment (CrCl <80 ml/min), monitor electrolytes: K, Na, Cl, Mg
• Deafness by audiometric testing, ringing, roaring in ears, vertigo; assess hearing before, during, after treatment
• Dehydration: high specific gravity, decrease in skin turgor, dry mucous membranes, dark urine
• Overgrowth of infection: fever, malaise, redness, pain, swelling, perineal itching, diarrhea, stomatitis, change in cough, sputum
• C&S before starting treatment to identify infecting organism
• Vestibular dysfunction: nausea, vomiting, dizziness, headache; drug should be discontinued if severe
• Inj sites for redness, swelling, abscesses; use warm compresses at site

Administer:
• IM inj in large muscle mass; rotate inj sites
• Drug in evenly spaced doses to maintain blood level

Additive compatibilities: Bleomycin

Syringe compatibilities: Penicillin G sodium

Y-site compatibilities: Esmolol

Perform/provide:
• Adequate fluids of 2-3 L/day unless contraindicated to prevent irritation of tubules
• Supervised ambulation, other safety measures with vestibular dysfunction

Evaluate:
• Therapeutic effect: absence of fever, draining wounds, negative C&S after treatment

Teach patient/family:
• To report headache, dizziness, symptoms of overgrowth of infection, renal impairment

• To report loss of hearing, ringing, roaring in ears, fullness in head
Treatment of overdose: Hemodialysis; monitor serum levels of drug

---

succimer (Ŗ)
(sux'i-mer)
Chemet
Func. class.: Heavy metal antagonist
Chem. class.: Chelating agent

Action: Binds with ions of lead to form a water-soluble complex excreted by kidneys

Uses: Lead poisoning in children with lead levels above 45 µg/dl; may be beneficial in mercury, arsenic poisoning

Dosage and routes:
• *Child:* **PO** 10 mg/kg or 350 mg/m^2 q8h × 5 days, then 10 mg/kg or 350 mg/m^2 q12h × 2 wk; another course may be required depending on lead levels; allow 2 wk between courses
Available forms: Caps 100 mg

Side effects/adverse reactions:
SYST: Back, stomach, head, rib, flank pain; abdominal cramps, chills, fever, flulike symptoms, head cold, headache
HEMA: **Increased platelets, intermittent eosinophilia**
GU: **Proteinuria,** decreased urination, voiding difficulties
INTEG: Rash, urticaria, pruritus
META: Increased AST (SGOT), ALT (SGPT), alk phosphatase, cholesterol
GI: Nausea, vomiting, diarrhea, metallic taste, anorexia
CNS: Drowsiness, dizziness, paresthesia, sensorimotor neuropathy
EENT: Otitis media, watery eyes, film in eyes, plugged ears
RESP: Sore throat, rhinorrhea, nasal congestion, cough

Contraindications: Hypersensitivity

Precautions: Pregnancy (C), lactation, children <1 yr

Pharmacokinetics:

PO: Peak 1-2 hr, 49% excreted (39% in feces, 9% urine, 1% as CO_2 from lungs)

Interactions:

• Not recommended concurrently with other chelating agents

NURSING CONSIDERATIONS

Assess:

• Hepatic, renal studies: ALT (SGPT), AST (SGOT), alk phosphatase, BUN, creatinine, serum lead level

• I&O

• For lead sources in home, school

• Allergic reactions: rash, pruritus, urticaria; drug should be discontinued if antihistamines fail to help

Administer:

PO

• To children who cannot swallow capsule by separating the capsule and sprinkling content on food or in a spoon followed by a drink

Perform/provide:

• Adequate fluids; check hydration status qd

Evaluate:

• Therapeutic response: decrease in serum lead level

Teach patient/family:

• That therapeutic effect may take 1-3 mo

• To report urticaria, rash

---

succinylcholine (R)

(suk-sin-ill-koe'leen)

Anectine, Anectine Flo-Pack, Quelicin, succinylcholine chloride, Sucostrin, Suxamethonium

Func. class.: Neuromuscular blocker (depolarizing-ultra short)

Action: Inhibits transmission of nerve impulses by binding with cholinergic receptor sites, antagonizing action of acetylcholine; causes release of histamine

Uses: Facilitation of endotracheal intubation, skeletal muscle relaxation during orthopedic manipulations

Dosage and routes:

• *Adult:* **IV** 25-75 mg, then 2.5 mg/min as needed; **IM** 2.5 mg/kg, not to exceed 150 mg

• *Child:* **IV/IM** 1-2 mg/kg, not to exceed 150 mg **IM**

Available forms: Inj 20, 50, 100 mg/ml; powder for inj 100, 500 mg/vial, 1 g/vial

Side effects/adverse reactions:

CV: Bradycardia, tachycardia; increased, decreased B/P; *sinus arrest, dysrhythmias*

RESP: Prolonged apnea, bronchospasm, cyanosis, respiratory depression

EENT: Increased secretions, increased intraocular pressure

MS: Weakness, muscle pain, fasciculations, prolonged relaxation

HEMA: Myoglobulinemia

INTEG: Rash, flushing, pruritus, urticaria

Contraindications: Hypersensitivity, malignant hyperthermia, decreased plasma pseudocholinesterase, penetrating eye injuries, acute narrow-angle glaucoma

Precautions: Pregnancy (C), car-

◆ = Nursing alert   ∥ = Herb-drug interaction   ⊘ = Do not crush

diac disease, severe burns, fractures—fasciculations may increase damage—lactation, children <2 yr, electrolyte imbalances, dehydration, neuromuscular disease, respiratory disease, collagen diseases, glaucoma, eye surgery, elderly or debilitated patients

Pharmacokinetics:

IV: Onset 1 min, peak 2-3 min, duration 6-10 min

IM: Onset 2-3 min

Hydrolyzed in urine (active/inactive metabolites)

Interactions:

• Increased neuromuscular blockade: aminoglycosides, clindamycin, lincomycin, quinidine, local anesthetics, polymyxin antibiotics, lithium, narcotic analgesics, thiazides, enflurane, isoflurane, Mg salts, oxytocin

• Dysrhythmias: theophylline

NURSING CONSIDERATIONS

Assess:

• For electrolyte imbalances (K, Mg); may lead to increased action of this drug

• Vital signs (B/P, pulse, respirations, airway) until fully recovered; rate, depth, pattern of respirations, strength of hand grip

• I&O ratio; check for urinary retention, frequency, hesitancy

• Recovery: decreased paralysis of face, diaphragm, leg, arm, rest of body

• Allergic reactions: rash, fever, respiratory distress, pruritus; drug should be discontinued

Administer:

• Deep IM inj, preferably high in deltoid muscle

IV

• Using nerve stimulator by anesthesiologist to determine neuromuscular blockade

• Anticholinesterase to reverse neuromuscular blockade

• IV inf; dilute 1-2 mg/ml in D_5, isotonic saline sol, give 0.5-10 mg/min, titrate to response; may be given directly over 1 min

Additive compatibilities: Amikacin, cephapirin, isoproterenol, meperidine, methyldopa, morphine, norepinephrine, scopolamine

Syringe compatibilities: Heparin

Y-site compatibilities: Etomidate, heparin, potassium chloride, propofol, vit B/C

Perform/provide:

• Storage in refrigerator, powder at room temp; close tightly

• Reassurance if communication is difficult during recovery from neuromuscular blockade; postoperative stiffness is normal, soon subsides

Evaluate:

• Therapeutic response: paralysis of jaw, eyelid, head, neck, rest of body

Treatment of overdose: Edrophonium or neostigmine, atropine, monitor VS; may require mechanical ventilation

---

sucralfate (℞)

(soo-kral'fate)

Carafate, Sulcrate*

Func. class.: Protectant

Chem. class.: Aluminum hydroxide, sulfated sucrose

Action: Forms a complex that adheres to ulcer site, adsorbs pepsin

Uses: Duodenal ulcer, oral mucositis, stomatitis after radiation of head and neck

Investigational uses: Gastric ulcers, gastroesophageal reflux

Dosage and routes:

• *Adult:* PO 1 g qid 1 hr ac, hs

• *Child:* PO 40-80 mg/kg/day

Available forms: Tabs 1 g; oral susp
500 mg/5 ml
Side effects/adverse reactions:
CNS: Drowsiness, dizziness
GI: Dry mouth, constipation, nau-
sea, gastric pain, vomiting
INTEG: Urticaria, rash, pruritus
Contraindications: Hypersensitiv-
ity
Precautions: Pregnancy (B), lacta-
tion, children, renal failure
Pharmacokinetics:
PO: Duration up to 5 hr
Interactions:
• Decreased action of tetracyclines,
phenytoin, fat-soluble vitamins, ci-
metidine, digoxin, ketoconazole,
ranitidine, theophylline
• Decreased absorption of fluoro-
quinolones
• Decreased absorption of sucral-
fate: antacids
NURSING CONSIDERATIONS
Assess:
• Gastric pH (>5 should be main-
tained)
Administer:
PO
• On an empty stomach, 1 hr before
meals and hs
Perform/provide:
• Storage at room temp
Evaluate:
• Therapeutic response: absence of
pain, GI complaints
Teach patient/family:
• To avoid black pepper, caffeine,
alcohol, harsh spices, extremes in
temp of food
• To take on empty stomach
• To take full course of therapy
• To avoid antacids within ½ hr of
drug

---

sufentanil (℞)
(soo-fen′ta-nil)
Sufenta
Func. class.: Narcotic analgesic
Chem. class.: Opiate, synthetic

Controlled Substance Schedule II
Action: Inhibits ascending pain
pathways in CNS, increases
pain threshold, alters pain percep-
tion
Uses: Primary anesthetic, adjunct
to general anesthetic
Dosage and routes:
Primary anesthetic
• *Adult:* **IV** 8-30 µg/kg given with
100% O_2, a muscle relaxant
Adjunct
• *Adult:* **IV** 1-8 µg/kg given with
nitrous oxide/O_2
Available forms: Inj 50 µg/ml
Side effects/adverse reactions:
*CNS: Drowsiness, dizziness, confu-
sion, headache, sedation, euphoria*
*GI: Nausea, vomiting, anorexia, con-
stipation, cramps*
GU: Increased urinary output, dys-
uria, urinary retention
INTEG: Rash, urticaria, bruising,
flushing, diaphoresis, pruritus
EENT: Tinnitus, blurred vision, mio-
sis, diplopia
CV: Palpitations, bradycardia, change
in B/P
RESP: Respiratory depression
Contraindications: Hypersensitiv-
ity, addiction (narcotic)
Precautions: Addictive personality, pregnancy (C), lactation, increased intracranial pressure, MI
(acute), severe heart disease, respiratory depression, hepatic disease,
renal disease, child <18 yr
Pharmacokinetics: Onset 1½-3 hr,
half-life 2½ hr
Interactions:
• Increased effects with other CNS

---

depressants: alcohol, narcotics, sedative/hypnotics, antipsychotics, skeletal muscle relaxants, antihistamines

🚫 Increased CNS depression: kava kava

Lab test interferences:

Increase: Amylase

NURSING CONSIDERATIONS

Assess:

• I&O ratio; decreasing output may indicate urinary retention

• CNS changes: dizziness, drowsiness, hallucinations, euphoria, LOC, pupil reaction

• Allergic reactions: rash, urticaria

• Respiratory dysfunction: respiratory depression, character, rate, rhythm; notify prescriber if respirations are <10/min

• Need for pain medication, physical dependence

Administer:

• With antiemetic if nausea, vomiting occur

IV

• Undiluted over 1-2 min or give as inf

Perform/provide:

• Storage in light-resistant area at room temp

• Safety measures: side rails, night light, call bell within easy reach

Evaluate:

• Therapeutic response: maintenance of anesthesia

Teach patient/family:

• To report any symptoms of CNS changes, allergic reactions

Treatment of overdose: Naloxone (Narcan) 0.2-0.8 mg IV, O$_2$, IV fluids, vasopressors

---

sulfadiazine (R)

(sul-fa-dye′a-zeen)

Sulfadiazine

Func. class.: Antiinfective

Chem. class.: Sulfonamide, intermediate acting

Action: Interferes with bacterial biosynthesis of proteins by competitive antagonism of PABA

Uses: UTIs, rheumatic fever prophylaxis, with pyrimethamine for *Toxoplasma gondii* encephalitis, chancroid, inclusion conjunctivitis, malaria, meningitis, *H. influenzae,* meningococeal meningitis, nocardiosis, acute otitis media, trachoma

Dosage and routes:

UTIs

• *Adult:* **PO** 2-4 g, then 1-2 g q6h × 10 days

• *Child:* **PO** 75 mg/kg or 2 g/m^2, then 150 mg/kg/day or 4 g/m^2 in 4-6 divided doses, max 6 g/day

Rheumatic fever prophylaxis

• *Child >30 kg:* **PO** 1 g qd

• *Child <30 kg:* **PO** 500 mg qd

Available forms: Tabs 500 mg

Side effects/adverse reactions:

SYST: Anaphylaxis

GI: Nausea, vomiting, abdominal pain, stomatitis, *hepatitis, glossitis,* pancreatitis, diarrhea, *enterocolitis,* anorexia

CNS: Headache, insomnia, hallucinations, depression, vertigo, fatigue, anxiety, convulsions, drug fever, chills, drowsiness

HEMA: Leukopenia, thrombocytopenia, agranulocytosis, hemolytic anemia, aplastic anemia

INTEG: Rash, dermatitis, urticaria, *Stevens-Johnson syndrome,* erythema, photosensitivity, alopecia

GU: Renal failure, toxic nephrosis, increased BUN, creatinine, crystalluria, hematuria, proteinuria

S

CV: Allergic myocarditis

Contraindications: Hypersensitivity to sulfonamides, sulfonylureas, thiazide and loop diuretics, salicylates, sunscreens with PABA, lactation, infants < 2 mo (except congenital toxoplasmosis), pregnancy at term, porphyria

Precautions: Pregnancy (B), impaired hepatic function, severe allergy, bronchial asthma, renal dysfunction

Pharmacokinetics:

PO: Rapidly absorbed, onset ½ hr; peak 3-6 hr, 30%-50% bound to plasma proteins, half-life 8-10 hr; excreted in urine, breast milk; crosses placenta, metabolized in liver

Interactions:

• Increased hypoglycemic response: sulfonylurea agents

• Increased anticoagulant effects: warfarin

• Decreased renal excretion of: methotrexate

• Decreased hepatic clearance of: phenytoin

• Increased effects of: barbiturates, tolbutamide, uricosurics

• Increased drug-free concentrations: indomethacin, probenecid, salicylates

• Increased thrombocytopenia: thiazide diuretics

• Increased nephrotoxicity; cyclosporine

Lab test interferences:

False positive: Urinary glucose test (Benedict's method)

NURSING CONSIDERATIONS

Assess:

• I&O ratio; note color, character, pH of urine if drug administered for UTIs; output should be 800 ml less than intake; if urine is highly acidic, alkalization may be needed

• Kidney function studies: BUN, creatinine, urinalysis (long-term therapy)

• Blood dyscrasias: skin rash, fever, sore throat, bruising, bleeding, fatigue, joint pain, monitor CBC before and periodically

• Allergic reaction: rash, dermatitis, urticaria, pruritus, dyspnea, bronchospasm

Administer:

• On an empty stomach

• With full glass of H_2O to maintain adequate hydration; increase fluids to 2 L/day to decrease crystallization in kidneys

• Medication after C&S; repeat C&S after full course of medication

Perform/provide:

• Storage in tight, light-resistant container at room temp

Evaluate:

• Therapeutic response: absence of pain, fever, C&S negative

Teach patient/family:

• To take each oral dose with full glass of water to prevent crystalluria

• To complete full course of treatment to prevent superinfection

• To avoid sunlight or use sunscreen to prevent burns

• To avoid OTC medication (aspirin, vit C) unless directed by prescriber

• To notify prescriber of skin rash, sore throat, fever, mouth sores, unusual bruising, bleeding

---

sulfamethizole (℞)

(sul-fa-meth'i-zole)

Thiosulfil Forte

Func. class.: Antiinfective

Chem. class.: Sulfonamide, short acting

Action: Interferes with bacterial biosynthesis of proteins by competitive antagonism of PABA

Uses: UTIs

 = Nursing alert   = Herb-drug interaction   = Do not crush

Dosage and routes:
- *Adult:* **PO** 0.5-1 g tid-qid
- *Child >2 mo:* **PO** 30-45 mg/kg/day in divided doses q6h

Available forms: Tabs 500 mg

Side effects/adverse reactions:

*SYST: **Anaphylaxis***

GI: Nausea, vomiting, abdominal pain, stomatitis, ***hepatitis***, glossitis, pancreatitis, diarrhea, ***enterocolitis***

CNS: Headache, confusion, insomnia, hallucinations, depression, vertigo, fatigue, anxiety, ***convulsions***, drug fever, chills

*HEMA: **Leukopenia, neutropenia, thrombocytopenia, agranulocytosis, hemolytic anemia***

INTEG: Rash, dermatitis, urticaria, ***Stevens-Johnson syndrome***, erythema, photosensitivity

*GU: **Renal failure, toxic nephrosis,*** increased BUN, creatinine, crystalluria

*CV: **Allergic myocarditis***

Contraindications: Hypersensitivity to sulfonamides, sulfonylureas, thiazide/loop diuretics, salicylates, sunscreens with PABA, lactation, infants < 2 mo (except congenital toxoplasmosis), pregnancy at term

Precautions: Pregnancy (B), lactation, impaired hepatic function, severe allergy, bronchial asthma

Pharmacokinetics:

PO: Rapidly absorbed, peak 2 hr, 90% bound to plasma proteins; excreted in urine, breast milk; crosses placenta

Interactions:
- Increased effects of: barbiturates, tolbutamide, uricosurics
- Increased drug-free concentrations: indomethacin, probenecid, salicylates
- Increased thrombocytopenia: thiazide diuretics
- Increased nephrotoxicity: cyclosporine
- Increased hypoglycemic response: sulfonylurea agents
- Increased anticoagulant effects: warfarin
- Decreased renal excretion of methotrexate
- Decreased hepatic clearance of phenytoin

Lab test interferences:

False positive: Urinary glucose test (Benedict's method)

NURSING CONSIDERATIONS

Assess:
- I&O ratio; note color, character, pH of urine if drug administered for UTIs; output should be 800 ml less than intake; if urine is highly acidic, alkalization may be needed
- Kidney function studies: BUN, creatinine, urinalysis if on long-term therapy
- Blood dyscrasias: skin rash, fever, sore throat, bruising, bleeding, fatigue, joint pain, monitor CBC before and periodically
- Allergic reaction: rash, dermatitis, urticaria, pruritus, dyspnea, bronchospasm

Administer:
- With full glass of H_2O to maintain adequate hydration; increase fluids to 2 L/day to decrease crystallization in kidneys
- Medication after C&S; repeat C&S after full course of medication

Perform/provide:
- Storage in tight, light-resistant container at room temp

Evaluate:
- Therapeutic response: absence of pain, fever, C&S negative

Teach patient/family:
- To take each oral dose with full glass of H_2O to prevent crystalluria
- To complete full course of treatment to prevent superinfection
- To avoid sunlight or use sunscreen to prevent burns
- To avoid OTC medication (aspi-

rin, vit C) unless directed by prescriber
• To notify prescriber of skin rash, sore throat, fever, mouth sores, unusual bruising, bleeding

---

sulfamethoxazole (℞)

(sul-fa-meth-ox′a-zole)
Apo-Sulfamethoxazole*, Gantanol
Func. class.: Antiinfective
Chem. class.: Sulfonamide, intermediate acting

Action: Interferes with bacterial biosynthesis of proteins by competitive antagonism of PABA

Uses: UTIs, chancroid, inclusion conjunctivitis, malaria, meningococcal meningitis, nocardiosis, acute otitis media, toxoplasmosis, trachoma

Dosage and routes:
Renal dose
• CrCl <50 ml/min give 50% of dose
• *Adult:* **PO** 2 g, then 1 g bid or tid for 7-10 days
• *Child >2 mo:* **PO** 50-60 mg/kg × 1 dose then 25-30 mg/kg bid, not to exceed 75 mg/kg/day

Lymphogranuloma venereum
• *Adult:* **PO** 1 g bid × 14 days

Available forms: Tabs 500 mg; oral susp 500 mg/5 ml

Side effects/adverse reactions:
*SYST: **Anaphylaxis***
GI: Nausea, vomiting, abdominal pain, stomatitis, ***hepatitis,*** glossitis, pancreatitis, diarrhea, ***enterocolitis,*** anorexia
CNS: Headache, insomnia, hallucinations, depression, vertigo, fatigue, anxiety, convulsions, drug fever, chills, drowsiness
*HEMA: **Leukopenia, thrombocytopenia, agranulocytosis, hemolytic anemia, aplastic anemia***

INTEG: Rash, dermatitis, urticaria, ***Stevens-Johnson syndrome,*** erythema, photosensitivity, alopecia
*GU: **Renal failure, toxic nephrosis,*** increased BUN, creatinine, crystalluria, hematuria, proteinuria
*CV: **Allergic myocarditis***

Contraindications: Hypersensitivity to sulfonamides, sulfonylureas, thiazide and loop diuretics, salicylates, sunscreens with PABA, lactation, infants < 2 mo (except congenital toxoplasmosis), pregnancy at term, porphyria

Precautions: Pregnancy (B), lactation, impaired hepatic/renal function, severe allergy, bronchial asthma

Pharmacokinetics:
PO: Poorly absorbed, peak 3-4 hr, 50%-70% bound to plasma proteins, half-life 7-12 hr; excreted in urine (unchanged 90%), breast milk; crosses placenta

Interactions:
• Increased effects of: barbiturates, uricosurics
• Increased drug-free concentrations: indomethacin, probenecid, salicylates
• Increased thrombocytopenia: thiazide diuretics
• Increased nephrotoxicity: cyclosporine
• Increased hypoglycemic response: sulfonylurea agents
• Increased anticoagulant effects: warfarin
• Decreased renal excretion of methotrexate
• Decreased hepatic clearance of phenytoin

Lab test interferences:
False positive: Urinary glucose test (Benedict's method)

NURSING CONSIDERATIONS
Assess:
• I&O ratio; note color, character, pH of urine if drug administered for

---

UTIs; output should be 800 ml less than intake; if urine is highly acidic, alkalization may be needed
• Kidney function studies: BUN, creatinine, urinalysis (long-term therapy)
• Blood dyscrasias: skin rash, fever, sore throat, bruising, bleeding, fatigue, joint pain, monitor CBC before and periodically
• Allergic reaction: rash, dermatitis, urticaria, pruritus, dyspnea, bronchospasm

Administer:

PO
• On empty stomach
• With full glass of H_2O to maintain adequate hydration; increase fluids to 2 L/day to decrease crystallization in kidneys
• Medication after C&S; repeat C&S after full course of medication

Perform/provide:
• Storage in tight, light-resistant container at room temp

Evaluate:
• Therapeutic response: absence of pain, fever, C&S negative

Teach patient/family:
• To take each oral dose with full glass of H_2O to prevent crystalluria
• To complete full course of treatment to prevent superinfection
• To avoid sunlight or use sunscreen to prevent burns
• To avoid OTC medication (aspirin, vit C) unless directed by prescriber
• To notify prescriber of skin rash, sore throat, fever, mouth sores, unusual bruising, bleeding

sulfasalazine (℞)

(sul-fa-sal'a-zeen)
Azulfidine, Azulfidine EN-Tabs, PMS-Sulfasalazine*, S.A.S.*, Salazopyrin*, sulfasalazine
Func. class.: Antiinflammatory
Chem. class.: Sulfonamide

Action: Prodrug to deliver sulfapyridine and 5-aminosalicylic acid to colon; antiinflammatory in connective tissue also

Uses: Ulcerative colitis; rheumatoid arthritis in patients who inadequately respond to or are intolerant of analgesics/NSAIDs

Investigational uses: Ankylosing spondylitis, collagenous colitis, Crohn's disease, psoriasis

Dosage and routes:

Renal dose
• CrCl 10-30 ml/min give bid; CrCl <10 ml/min give qd
• *Adult.* **PO** 3-4 g/day in divided doses; maintenance 1.5-2 g/day in divided doses q6h
• *Child >2 yr:* **PO** 40-60 mg/kg/day in 4-6 divided doses, then 20-30 mg/kg/day in 4 doses, max 2 g/day

Rheumatoid arthritis
• *Adult:* **PO** 2g/day in evenly divided doses, initiate treatment with a lower dose of enteric-coated tab

Available forms: Tabs 500 mg; oral susp 250 mg/5ml; enteric-coated tabs, 500 mg

Side effects/adverse reactions:

*SYST: **Anaphylaxis***

GI: Nausea, vomiting, abdominal pain, stomatitis, ***hepatitis,*** glossitis, pancreatitis, diarrhea

CNS: Headache, confusion, insomnia, hallucinations, depression, vertigo, fatigue, anxiety, ***convulsions,*** drug fever, chills

*HEMA: **Leukopenia, neutropenia,***

S

thrombocytopenia, agranulocytosis, hemolytic anemia
INTEG: Rash, dermatitis, urticaria, *Stevens-Johnson syndrome,* erythema, photosensitivity
GU: Renal failure, toxic nephrosis, increased BUN, creatinine, crystalluria
CV: Allergic myocarditis
Contraindications: Hypersensitivity to sulfonamides or salicylates, pregnancy at term, child <2 yr, intestinal, urinary obstruction
Precautions: Pregnancy (C), lactation, impaired hepatic function, severe allergy, bronchial asthma, impaired renal function
Pharmacokinetics:
PO: Partially absorbed, peak 1½-6 hr, duration 6-12 hr, half-life 6 hr, excreted in urine as sulfasalazine (15%), sulfapyridine (60%), 5-aminosalicylic acid and metabolites (20%-33%), in breast milk; crosses placenta
Interactions:
• Decreased absorption of digoxin
• Increased hypoglycemic response: oral hypoglycemics
• Increased anticoagulant effects: oral anticoagulants
• Decreased renal excretion of methotrexate
• Decreased hepatic clearance of phenytoin
• Drug/food: decreased iron/folic acid absorption
Lab test interferences:
False positive: Urinary glucose test
NURSING CONSIDERATIONS
Assess:
• Kidney function studies: BUN, creatinine, urinalysis (long-term therapy)
• Blood dyscrasias: skin rash, fever, sore throat, bruising, bleeding, fatigue, joint pain; monitor CBC before and q3mo

• Allergic reaction: rash, dermatitis, urticaria, pruritus, dyspnea, bronchospasm
Administer:
• With full glass of H_2O to maintain adequate hydration; increase fluids to 2 L/day to decrease crystallization in kidneys
• Total daily dose in evenly spaced doses and after meals to help minimize GI intolerance
Perform/provide:
• Storage in tight, light-resistant container at room temp
Evaluate:
• Therapeutic response: absence of fever, mucus in stools, pain in joints
Teach patient/family:
• To take each oral dose with full glass of H_2O to prevent crystalluria
• That contact lens, urine/skin may be yellow-orange
• To complete full course of treatment to prevent superinfection
• To avoid sunlight or use sunscreen to prevent burns
• To notify prescriber of skin rash, sore throat, fever, mouth sores, unusual bruising, bleeding

---

sulfinpyrazone (℞)
(sul-fin-peer′a-zone)
Anturane, Sulfinpyrazone
Func. class.: Uricosuric
Chem. class.: Pyrazolone

Action: Inhibits tubular reabsorption of urates, with increased excretion of uric acid; inhibits prostaglandin synthesis, which decreases platelet aggregation
Uses: Inhibition of platelet aggregation, gout
Dosage and routes:
Inhibition of platelet aggregation
• *Adult:* **PO** 200 mg qid

 = Nursing alert   = Herb-drug interaction   = Do not crush

Gout/gouty arthritis
• *Adult:* **PO** 100-200 mg bid × 1 wk, then 200-400 mg bid, not to exceed 800 mg/day
Available forms: Tabs 100 mg; caps 200 mg
Side effects/adverse reactions:
CNS: Dizziness, ***convulsions, coma***
EENT: Tinnitus
GU: Renal calculi, hypoglycemia
*GI: Gastric irritation, nausea, vomiting, anorexia, **hepatic necrosis,** GI bleeding*
INTEG: Rash, dermatitis, pruritus, fever, photosensitivity
*HEMA: **Agranulocytosis** (rare)*
*RESP: **Apnea,** irregular respirations*
Contraindications: Hypersensitivity to pyrazolone derivatives, blood dyscrasias, CrCl <50 ml/min, active peptic ulcer, GI inflammation
Precautions: Pregnancy (C)
Pharmacokinetics:
PO: Peak 1-2 hr, duration 4-6 hr, half-life 4 hr; metabolized by liver, excreted in urine
Interactions:
• Increased toxicity: acetaminophen
• Increased effects of: warfarin, tolbutamide
• Decreased effects of: verapamil, theophylline
• Decreased effects of sulfinpyrazone: salicylates, niacin
Lab test interferences:
Increase: PSP, aminohippuric acid
False positive: Clinitest
NURSING CONSIDERATIONS
Assess:
• Uric acid levels (3-7 mg/dl); joint mobility, pain, swelling
• Respiratory rate, rhythm, depth; notify prescriber of abnormalities
• Renal function
• Bleeding tendencies, RBC, Hct
• I&O
• Electrolytes, CO_2 before, during treatment

• Urine pH, output, glucose during beginning treatment
Administer:
• With glass of milk
• With food for GI symptoms
• Increased fluids to prevent calculi; alkalinization of urine may be required
Evaluate:
• Therapeutic response: absence of pain, stiffness in joints
Teach patient/family:
• To avoid aspirin, alcohol, high-purine diet

---

sulfisoxazole (℞)
(sul-fi-sox′a-zole)
Gantrisin, Novosoxazole*, sulfisoxazole
Func. class.: Antiinfective
Chem. class.: Sulfonamide, short acting

Action: Interferes with bacterial biosynthesis of proteins by competitive antagonism of PABA
Uses: Urinary tract, systemic infections; chancroid; trachoma; toxoplasmosis; acute otitis media, malaria, *H. influenzae* meningitis, meningococcal meningitis, nocardiosis, eye infections
Dosage and routes:
Renal dose
• CrCl 10-50 ml/min give q8-12h; CrCl <10 ml/min give q12-24h
• *Adult:* **PO** 2-4 g loading dose, then 1-2 g qid × 7-10 days
• *Child >2 mo:* **PO** 75 mg/kg or 2 g/m^2 loading dose, then 120-150 mg/kg/day or 4 g/m^2/day in divided doses q6h, not to exceed 6 g/day
Available forms: Tabs 500 mg
Side effects/adverse reactions:
*SYST: **Anaphylaxis***
*GI: Nausea, vomiting, abdominal pain, stomatitis, **hepatitis,** glossitis,*

pancreatitis, diarrhea, *enterocolitis,* anorexia

CNS: Headache, insomnia, hallucinations, depression, vertigo, fatigue, anxiety, *convulsions,* drug fever, chills, drowsiness

HEMA: Leukopenia, thrombocytopenia, agranulocytosis, hemolytic anemia, aplastic anemia

INTEG: Rash, dermatitis, urticaria, *Stevens-Johnson syndrome,* erythema, photosensitivity, alopecia

GU: Renal failure, toxic nephrosis, increased BUN, creatinine, crystalluria, hematuria, proteinuria

CV: Allergic myocarditis

Contraindications: Hypersensitivity to sulfonamides and sulfonylureas, thiazide and loop diuretics, salicylates; sunscreen with PABA, lactation, infants < 2 mo (except congenital toxoplasmosis), pregnancy at term, porphyria

Precautions: Pregnancy (B), lactation, impaired hepatic/renal function, severe allergy, bronchial asthma

Pharmacokinetics:

PO: Rapidly absorbed, peak 2-4 hr, 85% protein bound; half-life 4-7 hr, excreted in urine, crosses placenta

Interactions:

• Increased effects of: barbiturates, tolbutamide, uricosurics

• Increased drug-free concentrations: indomethacin, probenecid, salicylates

• Increased thrombocytopenia: thiazides

• Increased nephrotoxicity: cyclosporine

• Increased hypoglycemic response: sulfonylurea agents

• Increased anticoagulant effect: warfarin

• Decreased renal excretion of methotrexate

• Decreased hepatic clearance of phenytoin

Lab test interferences:

False positive: Urinary glucose test

NURSING CONSIDERATIONS

Assess:

• I&O ratio; note color, character, pH of urine if drug administered for UTIs; output should be 800 ml less than intake; if urine is highly acidic, alkalization may be needed

• Kidney function studies: BUN, creatinine, urinalysis (long-term therapy)

• Blood dyscrasias: skin rash, fever, sore throat, bruising, bleeding, fatigue, joint pain, monitor CBC before and periodically

• Allergic reaction: rash, dermatitis, urticaria, pruritus, dyspnea, bronchospasm

Administer:

• On an empty stomach

• With full glass of H_2O to maintain adequate hydration; increase fluids to 2 L/day to decrease crystallization in kidneys

• Medication after C&S; repeat C&S after full course of medication

Perform/provide:

• Storage in tight, light-resistant container at room temp

Evaluate:

• Therapeutic response: absence of pain, fever, C&S negative

Teach patient/family:

• To take each oral dose with full glass of H_2O to prevent crystalluria

• To complete full course of treatment to prevent superinfection

• To avoid sunlight or use sunscreen to prevent burns; avoid hazardous activities if dizziness occurs

• To avoid OTC medication (aspirin, vit C) unless directed by prescriber

• To notify prescriber of skin rash, sore throat, fever, mouth sores, unusual bruising, bleeding

---

 = Nursing alert   = Herb-drug interaction $\bigcirc$ = Do not crush

sulindac (℞)

(sul-in'dak)
Apo-Sulin*, Clinoril, NovoSundac*, sulindac

Func. class.: Nonsteroidal antiinflammatory

Chem. class.: Indeneacetic acid derivative

Action: Inhibits prostaglandin synthesis by decreasing an enzyme needed for biosynthesis; analgesic, antiinflammatory, antipyretic

Uses: Mild to moderate pain, osteoarthritis; rheumatoid, gouty arthritis; ankylosing spondylitis

Dosage and routes:

Arthritis
• *Adult:* **PO** 150 mg bid, may increase to 200 mg bid

Bursitis/acute arthritis
• *Adult:* **PO** 200 mg bid × 1-2 wk, then reduce dose

Available forms: Tabs 150, 200 mg

Side effects/adverse reactions:

GI: Nausea, anorexia, vomiting, diarrhea, jaundice, *cholestatic hepatitis,* constipation, flatulence, cramps, dry mouth, peptic ulcer, *bleeding, ulceration, perforation*

CNS: Dizziness, drowsiness, fatigue, tremors, confusion, insomnia, anxicty, depression, headache

CV: Tachycardia, peripheral edema, palpitations, dysrhythmias

INTEG: Purpura, rash, pruritus, sweating, photosensitivity

GU: Nephrotoxicity: dysuria, hematuria, oliguria, azotemia

HEMA: Blood dyscrasias with prolonged use

EENT: Tinnitus, hearing loss, blurred vision

Contraindications: Hypersensitivity, asthma, severe renal disease, severe hepatic disease, active ulcers

Precautions: Pregnancy (C), lactation, child, bleeding disorders, GI disorders, cardiac disorders, hypersensitivity to other antiinflammatory agents, renal disease

Pharmacokinetics:

PO: Peak 2 hr, half-life 3-3½ hr; metabolized in liver; excreted in urine (metabolites), breast milk; 93% protein binding

Interactions:
• Increased action of warfarin, phenytoin, sulfonamides, salicylates

NURSING CONSIDERATIONS

Assess:
• Pain: frequency, intensity, characteristics, relief after med
• Asthma, aspirin hypersensitivity, nasal polyps; increased hypersensitivity
• Renal, liver, blood studies: BUN, creatinine, AST, ALT, Hgb, before treatment, periodically thereafter
• Have B/P checked qmo; drug causes Na retention
• Audiometric, ophthalmic exam before, during, after treatment
• For eye, ear problems: blurred vision, tinnitus may indicate toxicity

Administer:
• With food to decrease GI symptoms; best to take on empty stomach to facilitate absorption; tablet may be crushed

Perform/provide:
• Storage at room temp

Evaluate:
• Therapeutic response: decreased pain, stiffness, swelling in joints, ability to move more easily

Teach patient/family:
• To report blurred vision or ringing, roaring in ears (may indicate toxicity)
• To avoid driving, other hazardous activities if dizzy or drowsy
• To report change in urine pattern, weight increase, edema, pain in-

crease in joints, fever, blood in urine (indicates nephrotoxicity)
• That therapeutic effects may take up to 1 mo
• To avoid alcohol and aspirin
• To take with full glass of water
• To use sunscreen

---

sumatriptan (℞)

(soo-ma-trip′tan)
Imitrex
Func. class.: Migraine agent
Chem. class.: 5-HT$_1$-like receptor agonist

Action: Binds selectively to the vascular 5-HT$_1$ receptor subtype, exerts antimigraine effect; causes vasoconstriction in cranial arteries

Uses: Acute treatment of migraine with or without aura and cluster headache

Dosage and routes:
• *Adult:* **SC** 6 mg or less; may repeat in 1 hr; not to exceed 12 mg/24 hr; **PO** 25 mg with fluids, max 100 mg; **NASAL** one dose of 5, 10, or 20 mg in one nostril, may repeat in 2 hr, max 40 mg/24hr or >5 mo

Available forms: Inj 6 mg (12 mg/ml); tabs 25, 50 mg, nasal spray 5 mg/100 mcl-U dose spray device, 20 mg/100 mcl-U

Side effects/adverse reactions:

NEURO: Tingling, hot sensation, burning, feeling of pressure, tightness, numbness, dizziness, sedation, headache, anxiety, fatigue, cold sensation
CV: Flushing
RESP: Chest tightness, pressure
EENT: Throat, mouth, nasal discomfort; vision changes
GI: Abdominal discomfort
MS: Weakness, neck stiffness, myalgia

INTEG: Injection site reaction, sweating

Contraindications: Angina pectoris, history of MI, documented silent ischemia, Prinzmetal's angina, ischemic heart disease, IV use, concurrent ergotamine-containing preparations, uncontrolled hypertension, hypersensitivity, basilar or hemiplegic migraine

Precautions: Postmenopausal women, men >40 yr, risk factors for CAD, hypercholesterolemia, obesity, diabetes, impaired hepatic or renal function, pregnancy (C), lactation, children, elderly

Pharmacokinetics: Onset of pain relief 10 min-2 hr, peak 10-20 min, 10%-20% plasma protein binding, metabolized in the liver (metabolite), excreted in urine, feces

Interactions:
• Extended vasospastic effects: ergot, ergot derivatives

NURSING CONSIDERATIONS
Assess:
• B/P; signs/symptoms of coronary vasospasms
• Tingling, hot sensation, burning, feeling of pressure, numbness, flushing, injection site reaction
• For stress level, activity, recreation, coping mechanisms
• Neurologic status: LOC, blurring vision, nausea, vomiting, tingling in extremities preceding headache
• Ingestion of tyramine foods (pickled products, beer, wine, aged cheese), food additives, preservatives, colorings, artificial sweeteners, chocolate, caffeine, which may precipitate these types of headaches

Administer:
• SC only just below the skin; avoid IM or IV administration
🚫 PO, swallow whole

Perform/provide:
• Quiet, calm environment with de-

🔸 = Nursing alert   ⚗ = Herb-drug interaction   🚫 = Do not crush creased stimulation for noise, bright light, excessive talking

Evaluate:

• Therapeutic response: decrease in frequency, severity of migraine

Teach patient/family:

• The use of self-dosing system; not to exceed 12 mg/24 hr

• To report any side effects to prescriber

• To use contraception while taking drug

• To use nasal spray: one spray in one nostril, may repeat if headache returns, do not repeat if pain continues after 1st dose

---

tacrine (tetrahydroaminoacridine, THA) (℞)

(tack'rin)
Cognex
Func. class.: Reversible cholinesterase

Action: Elevates acetylcholine concentrations (cerebral cortex) by slowing degradation of acetylcholine released in cholinergic neurons; does not alter underlying dementia

Uses: Treatment of mild to moderate dementia in Alzheimer's disease

Dosage and routes:

• *Adult:* **PO** 10 mg qid × 6 wk, then 20 mg qid × 6 wk, increase at 6-wk intervals if patient tolerating drug well and if transaminase is WNL

Available forms: Caps 10, 20, 30, 40 mg

Side effects/adverse reactions:

CNS: Dizziness, confusion, insomnia, tremor, *ataxia, somnolence, anxiety, agitation, depression, hallucinations, hostility, abnormal thinking,* chills, fever

CV: Hypotension or hypertension

GI: Nausea, vomiting, anorexia, abdominal pain, constipation, dyspepsia, flatulence

GU: Frequency, UTI, incontinence

INTEG: Rash, flushing

RESP: Rhinitis, URI, cough, pharyngitis

Contraindications: Hypersensitivity to this drug or acridine derivatives, patients treated with this drug who developed jaundice with a total bilirubin of >3 mg/dl

Precautions: Sick sinus syndrome, history of ulcers, GI bleeding, hepatic disease, bladder obstruction, asthma, pregnancy (C), lactation, children

Pharmacokinetics: Rapidly absorbed PO, 55% bound to plasma proteins, metabolized to metabolites, elimination half-life 2-4 hr

Interactions:

• Decreased activity of anticholinergics

• Increased elimination half-life of theophylline

• Synergistic effect: succinylcholine, cholinesterase inhibitors, cholinergic agonists

NURSING CONSIDERATIONS

Assess:

• B/P: hypotension, hypertension

• Mental status: affect, mood, behavioral changes, depression; complete suicide assessment; hallucinations, confusion

• GI status: nausea, vomiting, anorexia, constipation, abdominal pain; add bulk, increase fluids for constipation

• GU status: urinary frequency, incontinence

• Serum ALT qo wk × 16 wk, then qo mo × 2 mo, then q3mo

• Weekly ALT × 6 wks if dose is increased

Administer:

• Between meals; may be given with meals for GI symptoms

T

- Dosage adjusted to response no more than q6wk

Perform/provide:

- Assistance with ambulation during beginning therapy; dizziness, ataxia may occur

Evaluate:

- Therapeutic response: decrease in confusion, improved mood

Teach patient/family:

- To report side effects: twitching, eye spasms; indicate overdose
- To use drug exactly as prescribed: at regular intervals, preferably between meals; may be taken with meals for GI upset; drug is not a cure
- To notify prescriber of nausea, vomiting, diarrhea (dose increase or beginning treatment), or rash; very dark or very light stools, jaundice (delayed onset)
- Not to increase or abruptly decrease dose; serious consequences may result

Treatment of overdose: Withdraw drug, administer tertiary anticholinergics, provide supportive care

---

tacrolimus (℞)

(tak-roe-li'mus)
Prograf
Func. class.: Immunosuppressant
Chem. class.: Macrolide

Action: Produces immunosuppression by inhibiting T-lymphocytes

Uses: Organ transplants to prevent rejection

Dosage and routes:

- *Adult and child:* **IV** 0.15 mg/kg/day × 3 days then **PO** 0.15 mg/kg bid; adjust dose in renal impairment

Available forms: Inj 5 mg/ml; caps 1, 5 mg

Side effects/adverse reactions:

HEMA: **Anemia, leukocytosis, thrombocytopenia, purpura**

GI: Nausea, vomiting, diarrhea, constipation

CV: Hypertension

CNS: Tremors, headache, insomnia, paresthesia, chills, fever

GU: UTIs, **albuminuria, hematuria, proteinuria, renal failure**

META: Hirsutism, hyperglycemia, hyperkalemia, hyperuricemia, hypokalemia, hypomagnesemia

RESP: **Pleural effusion, atelectasis,** dyspnea

INTEG: Rash, flushing, itching, alopecia

EENT: Blurred vision, photophobia

Contraindications: Hypersensitivity to this drug or to some kinds of castor oil

Precautions: Severe renal, hepatic disease; pregnancy (C), diabetes mellitus, hyperkalemia, hyperuricemia, lymphomas, lactation, children <12, hypertension

Pharmacokinetics: Extensively metabolized, half-life 10 hr, 75% protein binding

Interactions:

- Increased toxicity: aminoglycosides, cisplatin, cyclosporine
- Increased blood levels: antifungals, calcium channel blockers, cimetidine, danazol, erythromycin
- Decreased blood levels: carbamazepine, phenobarbital, phenytoin, rifamycin
- Decreased effect of: vaccines

NURSING CONSIDERATIONS

Assess:

- Blood studies: Hgb, WBC, platelets during treatment qmo; if leukocytes <3000/mm^3 or platelets <100,000/mm^3, drug should be discontinued or reduced; decreased hemoglobin level may indicate bone marrow suppression
- Liver function studies: alk phos-

◆ = Nursing alert   🥄 = Herb-drug interaction   Ⓝ = Do not crush phatase, AST (SGOT), ALT (SGPT), amylase, bilirubin, and for hepatotoxicity: dark urine, jaundice, itching, light-colored stools; drug should be discontinued

Administer:
• All medications PO if possible, avoiding IM injections; bleeding may occur
• With meals to reduce GI upset; nausea is common
• For several days before transplant surgery; patients should be placed in protective isolation

IV
• After diluting in 0.9% NaCl or D_5W to 0.004 to 0.02 mg/ml as a continuous infusion

Additive compatibilities: Cimetidine

Y-site compatibilities: Acyclovir, aminophylline, amphotericin B, ampicillin, ampicillin/sulbactam, benztropine, calcium gluconate, cefazolin, cefotetan, ceftazidime, ceftriaxone, cefuroxime, chloramphenicol, cimetidine, ciprofloxacin, clindamycin, dexamethasone, digoxin, diphenhydramine, dobutamine, dopamine, doxycycline, erythromycin, esmolol, fluconazole, furosemide, ganciclovir, gentamicin, haloperidol, heparin, hydrocortisone, imipenem/cilastatin, insulin (regular), isoproterenol, leucovorin, lorazepam, methylprednisolone, metoclopramide, metronidazole, mezlocillin, multivitamins, nitroglycerin, oxacillin, penicillin G potassium, perphenazine, phenytoin, piperacillin, potassium chloride, propranolol, ranitidine, sodium bicarbonate, sodium nitroprusside, trimethoprim-sulfamethoxazole, vancomycin

Evaluate:
• Therapeutic response: absence of graft rejection; immunosuppression in autoimmune disorders

Teach patient/family:
• To report fever, rash, severe diarrhea, chills, sore throat, fatigue; serious infections may occur; clay-colored stools, cramping (hepatotoxicity)
• To avoid crowds, persons with known infections to reduce risk of infection

---

talbutal (℞)
(tal'byoo-tal)
Lotusate
Func. class.: Sedative/hypnotic barbiturate (intermediate acting)
Chem. class.: Barbitone

Controlled Substance Schedule II (USA), Schedule G (Canada)
Action: Depresses activity in brain cells, primarily in reticular activating system in brain stem; selectively depresses neurons in posterior hypothalamus, limbic structures
Uses: Insomnia, short-term only
Dosage and routes:
• *Adult:* PO 120 mg hs
Available forms: Tabs 120 mg
Side effects/adverse reactions:
CNS: Lethargy, drowsiness, hangover, dizziness, paradoxical stimulation in elderly and children, lightheadedness, dependency, CNS depression, mental depression, slurred speech
GI: Nausea, vomiting, diarrhea, constipation
INTEG: Rash, urticaria, pain, abscesses at injection site, angioedema, thrombophlebitis, ***Stevens-Johnson syndrome***
CV: Hypotension, bradycardia
RESP: Depression, apnea, ***laryngospasm, bronchospasm***
*HEMA: **Agranulocytosis, thrombocytopenia, megaloblastic anemia*** (long-term treatment)

Contraindications: Hypersensitivity to barbiturates, respiratory depression, addiction to barbiturates, severe liver impairment, porphyria, pregnancy (D), uncontrolled severe pain

Precautions: Anemia, lactation, hepatic disease, renal disease, hypertension, elderly, acute/chronic pain

Pharmacokinetics: Onset 30-45 min, duration 4-6 hr; metabolized by liver, excreted by kidneys (metabolites)

Interactions:

• Increased CNS depression: alcohol, MAOIs, sedatives, narcotics

• Decreased effect of oral anticoagulants, corticosteroids, griseofulvin, quinidine

• Decreased half-life of doxycycline

🖊 Increased CNS depression: kava kava

Lab test interferences:

False increase: Sulfobromophthalein

NURSING CONSIDERATIONS

Assess:

• Blood studies: Hct, Hgb, RBCs, if blood dyscrasias are suspected

• Hepatic studies: AST, ALT, bilirubin, if hepatic damage has occurred

• Mental status: mood, sensorium, affect, memory (long, short)

• Physical dependency: frequent requests for medication, shakes, anxiety

◆ Barbiturate toxicity: hypotension; pupillary constriction; cold, clammy skin; cyanosis of lips; insomnia; nausea; vomiting; hallucinations; delirium; weakness; mild symptoms may occur in 8-12 hr without drug

• Respiratory dysfunction: respiratory depression, character, rate, rhythm; hold drug if respirations are <10/min or if pupils are dilated (rare)

• Blood dyscrasias: fever, sore throat, bruising, rash, jaundice, epistaxis (rare)

Administer:

• After removal of cigarettes to prevent fires

• After trying conservative measures for insomnia

• ½-1 hr before hs for sleeplessness

• On empty stomach for best absorption

• For <14 days; drug not effective after that; tolerance develops

• Crushed or whole

Perform/provide:

• Assistance with ambulation after receiving dose

• Safety measures: side rails, nightlight, call bell within easy reach

• Checking to see if PO medication has been swallowed

• Storage in tight container in cool environment

Evaluate:

• Therapeutic response: ability to sleep at night, decreased amount of early morning awakening

Teach patient/family:

• That AM hangover is common

• That drug is indicated only for short-term treatment of insomnia, is probably ineffective after 2 wk

• That physical dependency may result when used for extended periods (45-90 days depending on dose)

• To avoid driving, other activities requiring alertness; sleep occurs within 45-60 min, lasts 6-8 hr

• To avoid alcohol ingestion, CNS depressants; serious CNS depression may result

• To tell all prescribers that barbiturate is being taken

• That withdrawal insomnia may occur after short-term use; not to start using drug again; insomnia will improve in 1-3 nights; may experience increased dreaming

---

◆ = Nursing alert   🖊 = Herb-drug interaction   🚫 = Do not crush

• That effects may take 2 nights for benefits to be noticed

• Alternative measures to improve sleep (reading, exercise several hours before hs, warm bath, warm milk, TV, self-hypnosis, deep breathing)

Treatment of overdose: Lavage, activated charcoal, warming blanket, vital signs, hemodialysis, I&O ratio

---

tamoxifen (℞)

(ta-mox'i-fen)

Nolvadex Nolvadex D*, Novo-Tamoxifen*, Tamofen*, Tamone*

Func. class.: Antineoplastic

Chem. class.: Antiestrogen hormone

Action: Inhibits cell division by binding to cytoplasmic estrogen receptors; resembles normal cell complex but inhibits DNA synthesis and estrogen response of target tissue

Uses: Advanced breast carcinoma not responsive to other therapy in estrogen-receptor-positive patients (usually postmenopausal)

Investigational uses: Prevention of breast cancer

Dosage and routes:

• *Adult:* **PO** 10-20 mg bid

Available forms: Tabs 10, 20 mg

Side effects/adverse reactions:

*HEMA: **Thrombocytopenia, leukopenia,** DVT, PE*

GI: Nausea, vomiting, altered taste (anorexia)

GU: Vaginal bleeding, pruritus vulvae

INTEG: Rash, alopecia

CV: Chest pain

CNS: Hot flashes, headache, lightheadedness, depression

META: Hypercalcemia

EENT: Ocular lesions, retinopathy, corneal opacity, blurred vision (high doses)

Contraindications: Hypersensitivity, pregnancy (D)

Precautions: Leukopenia, thrombocytopenia, lactation, cataracts

Pharmacokinetics:

PO: Peak 4-7 hr, half-life 7 days (1 wk terminal), excreted primarily in feces

Lab test interferences:

Increase: Serum Ca

NURSING CONSIDERATIONS

Assess:

• CBC, differential, platelet count qwk; withhold drug if WBC is <3500 or platelet count is <100,000; notify prescriber

• Bleeding: hematuria, guaiac, bruising, petechiae, mucosa or orifices q8h

• Food preferences; list likes, dislikes

• Effects of alopecia on body image; discuss feelings about body changes

◆ Symptoms indicating severe allergic reactions: rash, pruritus, urticaria, purpuric skin lesions, itching, flushing

Administer:

• Antacid before oral agent; give drug after evening meal, before bedtime

• Antiemetic 30-60 min before giving drug to prevent vomiting

Perform/provide:

• Liquid diet, if needed, including cola, Jell-O; dry toast or crackers may be added if patient is not nauseated or vomiting

• Increase fluid intake to 2-3 L/day to prevent dehydration

• Nutritious diet with iron, vitamin supplements as ordered

• Storage in light-resistant container at room temp

Evaluate:
• Therapeutic response: decreased tumor size, spread of malignancy

Teach patient/family:
• To report any complaints, side effects to prescriber
• That vaginal bleeding, pruritus, hot flashes are reversible after discontinuing treatment
• To report immediately decreased visual acuity, which may be irreversible; stress need for routine eye exams; care providers should be told about tamoxifen therapy
• To report vaginal bleeding immediately
• That tumor flare—increase in size of tumor, increased bone pain—may occur and will subside rapidly; may take analgesics for pain
• That premenopausal women must use mechanical birth control because ovulation may be induced
• That hair may be lost during treatment; a wig or hairpiece may make patient feel better; new hair may be different in color, texture

---

tamsulosin (℞)

(tam-sue-lo'sen)
Flomax
Func. class.: Selective α₁-adrenergic blocker
Chem. class.: Sulfamoylphenethylamine derivative

Action: Binds preferentially to α_{1A} adrenoceptor subtype located mainly in the prostate

Uses: Symptoms of benign prostatic hyperplasia

Dosage and routes:
• *Adult:* **PO** 0.4 mg qd, increasing up to 0.8 mg qd if required
Available forms: Tabs 0.4 mg

Side effects/adverse reactions:
CV: Chest pain

CNS: Dizziness, headache, asthenia
GI: Nausea, diarrhea
GU: Decreased libido, abnormal ejaculation
EENT: Amblyopia
MS: Back pain
RESP: Rhinitis, pharyngitis, cough

Contraindications: Hypersensitivity

Precautions: Pregnancy (C), children, lactation, hepatic disease, coronary artery disease, severe renal disease

Pharmacokinetics:
PO: Onset 2 hr, peak 2-6 hr, duration 6-12 hr; half-life 9-15 hr; metabolized in liver; excreted via urine; extensively protein bound (98%)

Interactions:
• Not to be taken with: prazosin, terazosin, doxazosin

NURSING CONSIDERATIONS
Assess:
• CBC with diff and liver function studies; B/P and heart rate
• BUN, uric acid, urodynamic studies (urinary flow rates, residual volume)

Administer:
PO
🚫 Whole; do not chew or crush tablets; may be given with food

Perform/provide:
• Storage in tight container in cool environment

Evaluate:
• Therapeutic response: decreased symptoms of benign prostatic hyperplasia

Teach patient/family:
• Not to drive or operate machinery for 4 hr after first dose or after dosage increase

---

temazepam (R)

(te-maz′e-pam)
Razepam, Restoril, temazepam
Func. class.: Sedative-hypnotic
Chem. class.: Benzodiazepine

Controlled Substance Schedule IV (USA), Schedule F (Canada)
Action: Produces CNS depression at limbic, thalamic, hypothalamic levels of the CNS; may be mediated by neurotransmitter γ-aminobutyric acid (GABA); results are sedation, hypnosis, skeletal muscle relaxation, anticonvulsant activity, anxiolytic action
Uses: Insomnia
Dosage and routes:
• *Adult:* **PO** 15-30 mg hs
Available forms: Caps 7.5, 15, 30 mg
Side effects/adverse reactions:
*HEMA: **Leukopenia, granulocytopenia** (rare)*
CNS: Lethargy, drowsiness, daytime sedation, dizziness, confusion, lightheadedness, headache, anxiety, irritability
GI: Nausea, vomiting, diarrhea, heartburn, abdominal pain, constipation, anorexia
CV: Chest pain, pulse changes
Contraindications: Hypersensitivity to benzodiazepines, pregnancy (X), lactation, intermittent porphyria
Precautions: Anemia, hepatic disease, renal disease, suicidal individuals, drug abuse, elderly, psychosis, child <15 yr, acute narrow-angle glaucoma, seizure disorders
Pharmacokinetics:
PO: Onset 30-45 min, duration 6-8 hr, half-life 10-20 hr; metabolized by liver, excreted by kidneys, crosses placenta, excreted in breast milk

Interactions:
• Increased effects of cimetidine, disulfiram, oral contraceptives
• Increased action of both drugs: alcohol, CNS depressants
• Decreased effect of antacids, theophylline, smoking, rifampin
⚠ Increased CNS depression: kava kava
Lab test interferences:
Increase: ALT (SGPT), AST (SGOT), serum bilirubin
Decrease: RAI uptake
False increase: Urinary 17-OHCS
NURSING CONSIDERATIONS
Assess:
• Blood studies: Hct, Hgb, RBCs (long-term therapy)
• Hepatic studies: AST (SGPT), ALT (SGOT), bilirubin (long-term therapy)
• Mental status: mood, sensorium, affect, memory (long, short)
• Blood dyscrasias: fever, sore throat, bruising, rash, jaundice, epistaxis (rare)
• Type of sleep problem: falling asleep, staying asleep
Administer:
• After removal of cigarettes to prevent fires
• After trying conservative measures for insomnia
• ½-1 hr before hs for sleeplessness
• On empty stomach for fast onset, but may be taken with food if GI symptoms occur
Perform/provide:
• Assistance with ambulation after receiving dose
• Safety measures: night-light, call bell within easy reach
• Checking to see if PO medication has been swallowed
• Storage in tight container in cool environment
Evaluate:
• Therapeutic response: ability to

sleep at night, decreased early morning awakening if taking drug for insomnia

Teach patient/family:
• To avoid driving, other activities requiring alertness until stabilized
• To avoid alcohol ingestion, CNS depressants; serious CNS depression may result
• That effects may take 2 nights for benefits to be noticed
• Alternative measures to improve sleep: reading, exercise several hours before hs, warm bath, warm milk, TV, self-hypnosis, deep breathing
• That hangover, memory impairment are common in elderly but less common than with barbiturates

Treatment of overdose: Lavage, activated charcoal; monitor electrolytes, VS

---

terazosin (R)

(ter-ay′zoe-sin)
Hytrin
Func. class.: Antihypertensive
Chem. class.: Peripherally acting adrenergic blocker

Action: Decreases total vascular resistance, which is responsible for a decrease in B/P; this occurs by blockade of α_1-adrenoreceptors

Uses: Hypertension, as a single agent or in combination with diuretics or β-blockers, BPH

Dosage and routes:
• *Adult:* **PO** 1 mg hs, may increase dose slowly to desired response; not to exceed 20 mg/day
Available forms: Tabs 1, 2, 5, 10 mg

Side effects/adverse reactions:
CV: Palpitations, orthostatic hypotension, tachycardia, edema, rebound hypertension

CNS: Dizziness, headache, drowsiness, anxiety, depression, vertigo, weakness, fatigue
GI: Nausea, vomiting, diarrhea, constipation, abdominal pain
GU: Urinary frequency, incontinence, impotence, priapism
EENT: Blurred vision, epistaxis, tinnitus, dry mouth, red sclera, nasal congestion, sinusitis
RESP: Dyspnea

Contraindications: Hypersensitivity

Precautions: Pregnancy (C), children, lactation

Pharmacokinetics: Peak 1 hr, half-life 9-12 hr, highly bound to plasma proteins; metabolized in liver, excreted in urine, feces

Interactions:
• Increased hypotensive effects: β-blockers, nitroglycerin, verapamil, nifedipine

NURSING CONSIDERATIONS

Assess:
• Urinary symptoms associated with BPH
• Orthostatic B/P, pulse, jugular venous distention q4h
• BUN, uric acid if on long-term therapy
• Weight qd, I&O
• Skin turgor, dryness of mucous membranes for hydration status
• Rales, dyspnea, orthopnea q30min

Perform/provide:
• Cool storage in tight container

Evaluate:
• Therapeutic response: decreased B/P, edema in feet, legs, decreased symptoms of BPH

Teach patient/family:
• That fainting occasionally occurs after first dose; not to drive or operate machinery for 4 hr after first dose or after an increase in dose; or take first dose hs

---

◆ = Nursing alert   🌿 = Herb-drug interaction   🚫 = Do not crush

• To rise slowly from sitting/lying position

---

terbinafine (℞)

(ter-bin'a-feen)
Lamisil
Func. class.: Topical antifungal
Chem. class.: Synthetic allyl amine derivative

Action: Interferes with cell membrane permeability in fungi such as *T. rubrum, T. mentagrophytes, T. tonsurans, E. floccosum, M. canis, M. audouinii, M. gypseum, Candida,* broad-spectrum antifungal

Uses: (TOP) Tinea cruris, tinea corporis, tinca pedis; (oral) onychomycosis of the toenail or fingernail due to dermatophytes

Investigational uses: Cutaneous candidiasis, tinea versicolor

Dosage and routes:
Topical
• Massage into affected area, surrounding area qd or bid, continue for 7-14 days, not to exceed 4 wk
Oral
• *Fingernail:* 250 mg/day × 6 wk
• *Toenail:* 250 mg/day × 12 wk
Available forms: Cream 1%, tabs 250 mg

Side effects/adverse reactions:
Topical
INTEG: Burning, stinging, dryness, itching, local irritation
Oral
HEME: **Neutropenia**
GI: Diarrhea, dyspepsia, abdominal pain, nausea
INTEG: Rash, pruritus, urticaria, **Stevens-Johnson syndrome**
MISC: Headache, liver enzyme changes, taste, visual disturbance
Contraindications: Hypersensitivity

Precautions: Pregnancy (B), lactation, children, liver/renal disease

Interactions:
• Decreased terbinafine clearance: cimetidine, terfenadine
• Increased terbinafine clearance: rifampin
• Increased clearance of: cyclosporine

NURSING CONSIDERATIONS
Assess:
• For continuing infection: increased size, number of lesions
Administer:
• To affected area, surrounding area; do not cover with occlusive dressings
Perform/provide:
• Storage below 30° C (86° F)
Evaluate:
• Therapeutic response: decrease in size, number of lesions
Teach patient/family:
• To wear cotton clothing
• To use clean towel, dry well
• To avoid contact with mucous membranes
• Not to cover areas unless directed by prescriber
• To report excessive itching, burning
• How to apply; massage cream into affected area and surrounding skin in AM, PM; effects observed within 1 wk, continue 1-2 wk after symptoms decrease

---

terbutaline (℞)

(ter-byoo'te-leen)
Brethaire, Brethine, Bricanyl
Func. class.: Selective β_2-agonist; bronchodilator
Chem. class.: Catecholamine

Action: Relaxes bronchial smooth muscle by direct action on β_2-adrenergic receptors through accu-

---

Side effects: *italics* = common; ***bold italics*** = life-threatening

mulation of cAMP at β-adrenergic receptor sites; bronchodilation, diuresis, CNS, cardiac stimulation occur; relaxes uterine smooth muscle

Uses: Bronchospasm, hyperkalemia

Investigational uses: Premature labor

Dosage and routes:

Bronchospasm

• *Adult and child >12 yr:* **INH** 2 puffs q1min, then q4-6h; **PO** 2.5-5 mg q8h; **SC** 0.25 mg q8h

Premature labor

• *Adult:* **IV INF** 10 µg/min, increased by 5 µg q10min, not to exceed 25 µg/min; **SC** 0.25 mg q1h; **PO** 5 mg q4h × 48 hr, then 5 mg q6h as maintenance

Available forms: Tabs 2.5, 5 mg; aerosol 0.2 mg/actuation; inj 1 mg/ml

Side effects/adverse reactions:

CNS: Tremors, anxiety, insomnia, headache, dizziness, stimulation

CV: Palpitations, tachycardia, hypertension, dysrhythmias, *cardiac arrest*

GI: Nausea, vomiting

Contraindications: Hypersensitivity to sympathomimetics, narrow-angle glaucoma, tachydysrhythmias

Precautions: Pregnancy (B), cardiac disorders, hyperthyroidism, diabetes mellitus, prostatic hypertension, lactation, elderly, hypertension, glaucoma

Pharmacokinetics:

PO: Onset ½ hr, peak 1-2 hr, duration 4-8 hr

SC: Onset 6-15 min, peak ½-1 hr, duration 1½-4 hr

INH: Onset 5-30 min, peak 1-2 hr, duration 3-6 hr

Interactions:

• Increased effects of both drugs: other sympathomimetics

• Decreased action: β-blockers

• Hypertensive crisis: MAOIs

• Incompatible with bleomycin

NURSING CONSIDERATIONS

Assess:

• Respiratory function: vital capacity, forced expiratory volume, ABGs, B/P, pulse, respiratory pattern, lung sounds, sputum before and after treatment

• Tolerance over long-term therapy; dose may have to be changed; monitor for rebound bronchospasm

Administer:

• With food; may be crushed

• 2 hr before hs to avoid sleeplessness

IV

• IV after diluting each 5 mg/1 L D₅W for inf

• IV, run 5 µg/min; may increase 5 µg q10min, titrate to response; after ½-1 hr taper dose by 5 µg; switch to PO as soon as possible

Additive compatibilities: Aminophylline

Syringe compatibilities: Doxapram

Y-site compatibilities: Insulin (regular)

Perform/provide:

• Storage at room temp; do not use discolored sol

Evaluate:

• Therapeutic response: absence of dyspnea, wheezing

Teach patient/family:

• Not to use OTC medications; extra stimulation may occur

• The use of inhaler; review package insert with patient

• To avoid getting aerosol in eyes; burning, stinging will occur

• To wash inhaler in warm water and dry qd, rinse mouth after use

• All aspects of drug; avoid smoking, smoke-filled rooms, persons with respiratory infections

• To increase fluids >2 L/day; allow 15 min between inhalation of this drug and inhaler containing steroid

• To take on time; if missed, do not make up after 1 hr; wait until next dose

Treatment of overdose: Administer an α-blocker, then norepinephrine for severe hypotension

---

testolactone (℞)

(tess-toe-lak′tone)
Teslac
Func. class.: Antineoplastic
Chem. class.: Androgen hormone

Action: Acts on adrenal cortex to suppress activity; reduces estrone synthesis

Uses: Advanced breast carcinoma in postmenopausal women; prostatic cancer

Dosage and routes:
• *Adult:* **PO** 250 mg qid
Available forms: Tabs 50 mg

Side effects/adverse reactions:
GI: Nausea, vomiting, anorexia, glossitis
GU: Urinary retention, ***renal failure***
INTEG: Rash, nail changes, facial hair growth
CV: Orthostatic hypertension, edema
CNS: Paresthesias, dizziness
EENT: Deepening voice
META: Hypercalcemia

Contraindications: Hypersensitivity, premenopausal women, carcinoma of male breast

Precautions: Renal disease, hypercalcemia, cardiac disease, pregnancy (C)

Pharmacokinetics: None known

Interactions:
• Enhanced effects of oral anticoagulants

Lab test interferences:
Increase: Urinary 17-OHCS
Decrease: Estradiol

NURSING CONSIDERATIONS
Assess:
• CA$^+$ levels
• B/P q4h; tell patient to rise slowly from sitting or lying down
• Food preferences; list likes, dislikes
• Edema in feet; joint, stomach pain; shaking
◆ Symptoms indicating severe allergic reaction: rash, pruritus, urticaria, purpuric skin lesions, itching, flushing
• Anorexia, nausea, vomiting, constipation, weakness, loss of muscle tone (indicating hypercalcemia)

Administer:
PO
• For 1 mo or longer for desired response

Evaluate:
• Therapeutic response: decreased tumor size, spread of malignancy

Teach patient/family:
• To recognize and report signs of hepatotoxicity, hypercalcemia, virilization (in females), bleeding if on anticoagulants

T

testosterone (Ŗ)

Andro-Cyp 100, Andro-Cyp 200, Andro L.A. 200, Androderm, Andronate 100, Andronate 200, Delatest, Delatestryl, depAndro 100, depAndro 200, Depotest 100, Depotest 200, Depo-Testosterone, Duratest-100, Duratest-200, Durathate-200, Everone 100, Everone 200, Testex, Testone LA 100, Testone LA 200, testosterone cypionate, testosterone enanthate, testosterone propionate, Testred Cypionate, Testrin PA, Testoderm Transdermal

Func. class.: Androgenic anabolic steroid

Chem. class.: Halogenated testosterone derivative

Action: Increases weight by building body tissue, increases potassium, phosphorus, chloride, nitrogen levels, bone development

Uses: Female breast cancer, eunuchoidism, male climacteric, oligospermia, impotence, osteoporosis, weight loss in AIDS patients, vulvar dystrophies

Dosage and routes:
Replacement
• *Adult:* **IM** 25-50 mg 2-3 ×/wk (base or propionate) or 50-400 mg q2-4wk (enanthate or cypionate)
• *Adult:* **trans testoderm** 4-6 mg applied q24h; **Androderm**-5 mg applied q24h
Breast cancer
• *Adult:* **IM** 50-100 mg 3 ×/wk (propionate) or 200-400 mg q2-4wk (cypionate or enanthate)
Delayed male puberty
• *Child >12 yr:* **IM** up to 100 mg/mo for up to 6 mo
Available forms: Propionate inj 25, 50, 100 mg/ml, transdermal patches: Testoderm 4 mg/day (30 patches), 6 mg/day (30 patches), Androderm 2.5 mg/day (60 patches), 5 mg/day (60 patches); enanthate inj 100, 200 mg/ml; cypionate inj 50, 100, 200 mg/ml; 4, 6 mg/day

Side effects/adverse reactions:
INTEG: Rash, acneiform lesions, oily hair and skin, flushing, sweating, acne vulgaris, alopecia, hirsutism
CNS: Dizziness, headache, fatigue, tremors, paresthesias, flushing, sweating, anxiety, lability, insomnia, carpal tunnel syndrome
MS: Cramps, spasms
CV: Increased B/P
GU: Hematuria, amenorrhea, vaginitis, decreased libido, decreased breast size, clitoral hypertrophy, testicular atrophy
GI: Nausea, vomiting, constipation, weight gain, *cholestatic jaundice*
EENT: Conjunctival edema, nasal congestion
ENDO: Abnormal GTT

Contraindications: Severe renal, severe cardiac, severe hepatic disease, hypersensitivity, pregnancy (X), lactation, genital bleeding (rare)

Precautions: Diabetes mellitus, CV disease, MI

Pharmacokinetics:
PO: Metabolized in liver, excreted in urine, breast milk; crosses placenta

Interactions:
• Increased effects of oral antidiabetics, oxyphenbutazone
• Increased PT: anticoagulants
• Edema: ACTH, adrenal steroids
• Decreased effects of insulin

Lab test interferences:
Increase: Serum cholesterol, blood glucose, urine glucose
Decrease: Serum Ca, serum K, T_4, T_3, thyroid ^{131}I uptake test, urine 17-OHCS, 17-KS, PBI

NURSING CONSIDERATIONS
Assess:
- Weight qd; notify prescriber if weekly weight gain is >5 lb
- B/P q4h
- I&O ratio; be alert for decreasing urinary output, increasing edema
- Growth rate in children; growth rate may be uneven (linear/bone growth) with extended use
- Electrolytes: K, Na, Cl, Ca; cholesterol
- Liver function studies: ALT (SGPT), AST (SGOT), bilirubin
- Edema, hypertension, cardiac symptoms, jaundice
- Mental status: affect, mood, behavioral changes, aggression
- Signs of masculinization in female: increased libido, deepening of voice, decreased breast tissue, enlarged clitoris, menstrual irregularities; male: gynecomastia, impotence, testicular atrophy
- Hypercalcemia: lethargy, polyuria, polydipsia, nausea, vomiting, constipation, drug may have to be decreased
- Hypoglycemia in diabetics; oral antidiabetic action is increased

Administer:
- Titrated dose; use lowest effective dose
- IM inj deep into upper outer quadrant of gluteal muscle
- Transdermal patches: Testoderm to skin of scrotum; Androderm to skin of back, upper arms, thighs, abdomen; area must be dry-shaved; may be reapplied after bathing, swimming

Perform/provide:
- Diet with increased calories, protein; decrease Na if edema occurs

Evaluate:
- Therapeutic response: 4-6 wk in osteoporosis

Teach patient/family:
- That drug must be combined with complete health plan: diet, rest, exercise
- To notify prescriber if therapeutic response decreases; if edema occurs
- Not to discontinue abruptly
- About changes in sex characteristics
- That women should report menstrual irregularities, voice changes, acne, facial hair growth
- That 1-3-mo course is necessary for response in breast cancer
- The procedure for use of buccal tablets (requires 30-60 min to dissolve, change absorption site with each dose; not to eat, drink, chew, or smoke while tablet is in place)
- The proper application of patches

---

tetanus toxoid, adsorbed/tetanus toxoid (R)
Func. class.: Toxoid

Action: Produces specific antibodies to tetanus

Uses: Tetanus toxoid: used for prophylactic treatment of wounds

Dosage and routes:
- *Adult and child:* **IM** 0.5 ml q4-6 wk × 2 doses, then 0.5 ml 1 yr after dose 2 (adsorbed); **SC/IM** 0.5 ml q4-8wk × 3 doses, then 0.5 ml ½-1 yr after dose 3, booster dose 0.5 ml q10yr

Available forms: Inj adsorbed IM 5, 10 LfU/0.5 ml; inj IM, SC 4, 5 LfU/0.5 ml

Side effects/adverse reactions:
GI: Nausea, vomiting, anorexia
INTEG: Skin abscess, urticaria, itching, swelling, erythema, induration at injection site
CV: Tachycardia, hypotension
SYST: Lymphadenitis, **anaphylaxis**
CNS: Crying, fretfulness, fever, drowsiness

Contraindications: Hypersensitivity, active infection, poliomyelitis outbreak, immunosuppression

Precautions: Pregnancy (C), elderly

NURSING CONSIDERATIONS
Assess:
• For skin reactions: swelling, rash, urticaria
• For history of allergies, skin conditions (eczema, psoriasis, dermatitis), reactions to vaccinations
• For anaphylaxis: inability to breathe, bronchospasm

Administer:
• At least 4 wk apart × 3 doses for children >6 wk old
• Only with epinephrine 1:1000 on unit to treat laryngospasm

Perform/provide:
• Written record of immunization

Teach patient/family:
• That doses are given at least 4 wk apart × 3 doses; booster needed at 10-yr intervals

---

tetracaine (℞)
(tet′ra-kane)
Pontocaine
Func. class.: Local anesthetic
Chem. class.: Ester

Action: Competes with calcium for sites in nerve membrane that control sodium transport across cell membrane; decreases rise of depolarization phase of action potential

Uses: Spinal anesthesia, epidural and peripheral nerve block, perineum, lower extremities

Dosage and routes:
Varies with route of anesthesia
Available forms: Inj 0.2%, 0.3%, 1%; powder

Side effects/adverse reactions:
CNS: Anxiety, restlessness, *convulsions, LOC,* drowsiness, disorientation, tremors, shivering
CV: Myocardial depression, car-

diac arrest, dysrhythmias, bradycardia, hypotension, hypertension, fetal bradycardia
GI: Nausea, vomiting
EENT: Blurred vision, tinnitus, pupil constriction
INTEG: Rash, urticaria, allergic reactions, edema, burning, skin discoloration at injection site, tissue necrosis
RESP: Status asthmaticus, respiratory arrest, anaphylaxis

Contraindications: Hypersensitivity, severe liver disease, heart block
Precautions: Elderly, severe drug allergies, pregnancy (C), lactation, children
Pharmacokinetics: Onset 15 min, duration 3 hr; metabolized by liver, excreted in urine (metabolites)
Interactions:
• Dysrhythmias: epinephrine, halothane, enflurane
• Hypertension: MAOIs, tricyclic antidepressants, phenothiazines
• Decreased action of tetracaine: chloroprocaine
• Decreased action of sulfonamides

NURSING CONSIDERATIONS
Assess:
• B/P, pulse, respiration during treatment
• Fetal heart tones during labor
• Allergic reactions: rash, urticaria, itching
• Cardiac status: ECG for dysrhythmias, pulse, B/P, during anesthesia

Administer:
• Only if not cloudy, does not contain precipitate
• Only with crash cart, resuscitative equipment nearby
• Only without preservatives for epidural or caudal anesthesia

Perform/provide:
• Use of new sol, discard unused portions, store in refrigerator

---

Evaluate:
• Therapeutic response: anesthesia necessary for procedure

Treatment of overdose: Airway, O_2, vasopressor, IV fluids, anticonvulsants for seizures

---

tetracycline (℞)

(tet-ra-sye′kleen)

Achromycin, Achromycin V, Alatel, Apo-Tetra*, Nor-Tet, Novotetra*, Nu-Tetra*, Panmycin, Robitet, Sumycin 250, Sumycin 500, Sumycin Syrup, Teline, Teline 500, Tetracap, tetracycline HCl, tetracycline HCl Syrup, Tetracyn, Tetralan 250, Tetralan 500, Tetralan Syrup, Tetralean*, Tetram

Func. class.: Broad-spectrum antiinfective

Chem. class.: Tetracycline

Action: Inhibits protein synthesis and phosphorylation in microorganisms; bacteriostatic

Uses: Syphilis, *Chlamydia trachomatis,* gonorrhea, lymphogranuloma venereum; uncommon gram-positive, gram-negative organisms; rickettsial infections

Dosage and routes:
• *Adult:* PO 250-500 mg q6h
• *Child >8 yr:* PO 25-50 mg/kg/day in divided doses q6h
Gonorrhea
• *Adult:* PO 1.5 g, then 500 mg qid for a total of 9 g over 7 days
Chlamydia trachomatis
• *Adult:* PO 500 mg qid × 7 days
Syphilis
• *Adult:* PO 2-3 g in divided doses × 10-15 days; if syphilis duration > 1 yr, must treat 30 days
Brucellosis
• *Adult:* PO 500 mg qid × 3 wk with

1 g streptomycin **IM** 2 × /day × 1 wk, and 1 × /day the second wk
Urethral syndrome in women
• *Adult:* PO 500 mg qid × 7 days
Acne
• *Adult:* 1 g/day in divided doses; maintenance 125-500 mg/day

Available forms: Oral susp 125 mg/5 ml; caps 100, 200, 500 mg; tabs 100, 250, 500 mg

Side effects/adverse reactions:
CNS: Fever, headache, paresthesia
HEMA: Eosinophilia, neutropenia, thrombocytopenia, leukocytosis, hemolytic anemia
EENT: Dysphagia, glossitis, decreased calcification, discoloration of deciduous teeth, oral candidiasis, oral ulcers
GI: Nausea, abdominal pain, *vomiting, diarrhea,* anorexia, enterocolitis, *hepatotoxicity,* flatulence, abdominal cramps, epigastric burning, stomatitis
CV: Pericarditis
GU: Increased BUN
INTEG: Rash, urticaria, photosensitivity, increased pigmentation, exfoliative dermatitis, pruritus, *angioedema*

Contraindications: Hypersensitivity to tetracyclines, children <8 yr, pregnancy (D), lactation

Precautions: Renal disease, hepatic disease

Pharmacokinetics:
PO: Peak 2-3 hr, duration 6 hr, half-life 6-10 hr; excreted in urine, breast milk; crosses placenta; 20%-60% protein bound

Interactions:
• Decreased effect of tetracycline: antacids, $NaHCO_3$, dairy products, alkali products, iron, kaolin/pectin, cimetidine
• Increased effect: warfarin, digoxin
• Decreased effect of penicillins, oral contraceptives
• Nephrotoxicity: methoxyflurane

Lab test interferences:

False negative: Urine glucose with Clinistix or Tes-Tape

False increase: Urinary catecholamines

NURSING CONSIDERATIONS

Assess:

• Signs of anemia: Hct, Hgb, fatigue

• I&O ratio

• Blood studies: PT, CBC, AST (SGOT), ALT (SGPT), BUN, creatinine

• Allergic reactions: rash, itching, pruritus, angioedema

• Nausea, vomiting, diarrhea; administer antiemetic, antacids as ordered

• Overgrowth of infection: fever, malaise, redness, pain, swelling, drainage, perineal itching, diarrhea, changes in cough or sputum

Administer:

• After C&S obtained

• 2 hr before or after iron products; 3 hr after antacid or kaolin/pectin products

Perform/provide:

• Storage in tight, light-resistant container at room temp

Evaluate:

• Therapeutic response: decreased temp, absence of lesions, negative C&S

Teach patient/family:

• To avoid sun exposure; sunscreen does not seem to decrease photosensitivity

• That diabetic should avoid use of Clinistix, Diastix, or Tes-Tape for urine glucose testing

• That all prescribed medication must be taken to prevent superinfection

• To avoid milk products, antacids, or separate by 2 hr; take with a full glass of water

---

theophylline (R)

(thee-off'i-lin)

Accurbron, Aerolate III, Aerolate Jr., Aerolate Slo-Phyllin, Aerolate Sr., Aquaphyllin, Asmalix, Bronkodyl, Constant-T, Elixomin, Elixophyllin, Elixophyllin SR, Lanophyllin, Quibron-T Dividose, Quibron-T/SR Dividose, Respbid, Slo-bid Gyrocaps, Slo-Phyllin Gyrocaps, Sustaire, Theolair-SR, Theo-24, Theobid Duracaps, Theobid Jr. Duracaps, Theochron, Theoclear-80, Theoclear L.A., Theo-Dur, Theo-Dur Sprinkle, Theolair, Theolair-SR, Theophylline, Theophylline and 5% Dextrose, Theophylline Extended Release, Theophylline Oral, Theophylline S.R., Theo-Sav, Theospan-SR, Theostat 80, Theovent, Theox, T-Phyl, Uniphyl

Func. class.: Spasmolytic

Chem. class.: Xanthine, ethylenediamide

Action: Relaxes smooth muscle of respiratory system by blocking phosphodiesterase, which increases cAMP

Uses: Bronchial asthma, bronchospasm of COPD, chronic bronchitis

Dosage and routes:

Bronchospasm, bronchial asthma

• *Adult:* PO 100-200 mg q6h; dosage must be individualized; **RECT** 250-500 mg q8-12h

• *Child:* PO 50-100 mg q6h, not to exceed 12 mg/kg/24 hr

COPD, chronic bronchitis

• *Adult:* PO 330-660 mg q6-8h pc (sodium glycinate)

• *Child 1-9 yr:* PO 5 mg/kg loading dose, then 4 mg/kg q6h

• *Child 9-16 yr:* PO 5 mg/kg loading dose, then 3 mg/kg q6h

 = Nursing alert   = Herb-drug interaction   = Do not crush

Apnea of prematurity
- *Neonate:* 2-10 mg/kg/day divided q8-12h (usual loading dose is 4 mg/kg **PO**)

Available forms: Caps 50, 100, 200, 250 mg; tabs 100, 125, 200, 225, 250, 300 mg; tabs, time-release 100, 200, 250, 300, 400, 500 mg; caps, time-release 50, 65, 100, 125, 130, 200, 250, 260, 300, 400, 500 mg; elix 80, 11.25 mg/15 ml; sol 80 mg/15 ml; liq 80, 150, 160 mg/15 ml; susp 300 mg/15 ml

Side effects/adverse reactions:

CNS: Anxiety, restlessness, insomnia, dizziness, convulsions, headache, light-headedness, muscle twitching, tremors

CV: Palpitations, sinus tachycardia, hypotension, other dysrhythmias, fluid retention with tachycardia

ENDO: Hyperglycemia

GI: Nausea, vomiting, anorexia, diarrhea, bitter taste, dyspepsia, gastric distress

RESP: Increased rate

INTEG: Flushing, urticaria

Contraindications: Hypersensitivity to xanthines, tachydysrhythmias

Precautions: Elderly, CHF, cor pulmonale, hepatic disease, active peptic ulcer disease, diabetes mellitus, hyperthyroidism, hypertension, children, pregnancy (C)

Pharmacokinetics:

PO: Peak 2 hr

SOL: Peak 1 hr

Metabolized in liver, excreted in urine and breast milk, crosses placenta

Interactions:
- Decreased theophylline level: phenytoin, phenobarbital, carbamazepine, rifampin, smoking
- Increased action of theophylline: cimetidine, propranolol, erythromycin, troleandomycin, ciprofloxacin, oral contraceptives

- May increase effects of anticoagulants
- Cardiotoxicity: β-blockers
- Decreased effect of lithium

NURSING CONSIDERATIONS

Assess:

◆ Theophylline blood levels (therapeutic level is 5-15 µg/ml); toxicity may occur with small increase above 20 µg/ml
- Monitor I&O; diuresis occurs; elderly or child may be dehydrated
- Signs of toxicity: irritability, insomnia, restlessness, tremors, nausea, vomiting
- Respiratory rate, rhythm, depth; auscultate lung fields bilaterally; notify prescriber of abnormalities
- Allergic reactions: rash, urticaria; drug should be discontinued

Administer:
- PO after meals for GI symptoms; absorption may be affected

IV

Additive compatibilities: Cefepime, chlorpromazine, fluconazole, furosemide, hydrocortisone, lidocaine, methylprednisolone, verapamil

Y-site compatibilities: Acyclovir, ampicillin, ampicillin/sulbactam, aztreonam, cefazolin, cefotetan, ceftazidime, ceftriaxone, cimetidine, clindamycin, dexamethasone, diltiazem, dobutamine, dopamine, doxycycline, erythromycin, famotidine, fluconazole, gentamicin, haloperidol, heparin, hydrocortisone, lidocaine, methyldopa, methylprednisolone, metronidazole, midazolam, nafcillin, nitroglycerin, penicillin G potassium, piperacillin, potassium chloride, ranitidine, sodium nitroprusside, ticarcillin, ticarcillin/clavulanate, tobramycin, vancomycin

Evaluate:
- Therapeutic response: ability to breathe more easily

Teach patient/family:
• To check OTC medications, current prescription medications for ephedrine, which will increase stimulation; to avoid alcohol, caffeine
• To avoid hazardous activities; dizziness may occur
• That if GI upset occurs, to take drug with 8 oz H_2O; avoid food; absorption may be decreased
🚫 Not to break, crush, chew, or dissolve slow-release products
• That contents of bead-filled capsule may be sprinkled over food for children's use
• To notify prescriber of toxicity: nausea, vomiting, anxiety, insomnia, convulsions
• To notify prescriber of change in smoking habit; dosage may have to be changed

---

thiabendazole (℞)

(thye-a-ben´da-zole)
Mintezol
Func. class.: Antihelmintic
Chem. class.: Benzimidazole derivative

Action: Inhibits anaerobic metabolism, disrupts microtubules
Uses: Pinworm, roundworm, threadworm, whipworm, trichinosis, hookworm, cutaneous larva migrans (creeping eruption)
Dosage and routes:
• *Adult and child:* **PO** 25 mg/kg in 2 doses qd × 2-5 days, not to exceed 3 g/day
Available forms: Tabs, chew 500 mg; oral susp 500 mg/5 ml
Side effects/adverse reactions:
SYST: Anaphylaxis
GU: Hematuria, nephrotoxicity, enuresis, abnormal smell of urine

INTEG: Rash, pruritus, erythema, *Stevens-Johnson syndrome*
CNS: Dizziness, headache, drowsiness, fever, flushing, ***convulsions,*** behavioral changes
EENT: Tinnitus, blurred vision, xanthopsia
GI: Nausea, vomiting, anorexia, diarrhea, jaundice, liver damage, epigastric distress
CV: Hypotension, bradycardia
Contraindications: Hypersensitivity
Precautions: Severe malnutrition, hepatic disease, renal disease, anemia, severe dehydration, child <14 kg, pregnancy (C)
Pharmacokinetics:
PO: Peak 1-2 hr, metabolized completely by liver, excreted in feces and urine

NURSING CONSIDERATIONS
Assess:
• Stools periodically during entire treatment
Administer:
• Susp after shaking
• PO after meals to avoid GI symptoms
Perform/provide:
• Storage in tight container
Evaluate:
• Therapeutic response: stools negative for helminths
Teach patient/family:
• Proper hygiene after BM, including hand-washing technique; tell patient not to put fingers in mouth
• That infected person should sleep alone; not to shake bed linen; to change bed linen qd
• To clean toilet qd with disinfectant (green soap solution)
• The need for compliance with dosage schedule, duration of treatment
• To drink fruit juice to remove mucus that intestinal tapeworms burrow in; aids in expulsion of worms

---

◆ = Nursing alert   🌿 = Herb-drug interaction   🚫 = Do not crush

• To avoid hazardous activities if drowsiness occurs
Treatment of overdose: Induce emesis or gastric lavage

---

thiamine (vit B₁)
(PO-OTC, IM-℞)
Betaxin⁺, Betalin S, Biamine, Revitonus, Thiamilate, thiamine HCl
Func. class.: Vit B₁
Chem. class.: Water soluble

Action: Needed for pyruvate metabolism, carbohydrate metabolism
Uses: Vit B₁ deficiency or polyneuritis, cheilosis adjunct with thiamine beriberi, Wernicke-Korsakoff syndrome, pellagra, metabolic disorders
Dosage and routes:
Beriberi
• *Adult:* **IM** 10-500 mg tid × 2 wk, then 5-10 mg qd × 1 mo
• *Child.* **IM** 10-50 mg qd × 4-6 wk
Anemia/alcoholism/pregnancy/pellagra
• *Adult:* **PO** 100 mg qd
• *Child:* **PO** 10-50 mg qd in divided doses
Beriberi with cardiac failure
• *Adult and child:* **IV** 100-500 mg
Wernicke-Korsakoff syndrome
• *Adult:* **IV** 500 mg or less, then 100 mg bid
Available forms: Tabs 50, 100, 250, 500 mg; inj 100 mg/ml; enteric coated tabs 20 mg
Side effects/adverse reactions:
CNS: Weakness, restlessness
GI: Hemorrhage, *nausea, diarrhea*
CV: Collapse, pulmonary edema, hypotension
INTEG: Angioneurotic edema, cyanosis, sweating, warmth
SYST: Anaphylaxis
EENT: Tightness of throat

Contraindications: Hypersensitivity
Precautions: Pregnancy (A)
Pharmacokinetics:
PO/INJ: Unused amounts excreted in urine (unchanged)
NURSING CONSIDERATIONS
Assess:
• Thiamine levels throughout treatment
• Nutritional status: yeast, beef, liver, whole or enriched grains, legumes
Administer:
• By IM injection; rotate sites if pain and inflammation occur; do not mix with alkaline sols; Z-track to minimize pain
IV
• Undiluted over 5 min or diluted with IV sol and given as an inf at 100 mg or less/5 min or more
Syringe compatibilities: Doxapram
Y-site compatibilities: Famotidine
Perform/provide:
• Storage in tight, light-resistant container
• Application of cold to help decrease pain
Evaluate:
• Therapeutic response: absence of nausea, vomiting, anorexia, insomnia, tachycardia, paresthesias, depression, muscle weakness
Teach patient/family:
• The necessary foods to be included in diet: yeast, beef, liver, legumes, whole grain

---

thiethylperazine (℞)
(thye eth-il-per′a-zeen)
Norzine, Torecan
Func. class.: Antiemetic
Chem. class.: Phenothiazine, piperazine derivative

Action: Acts centrally by blocking chemoreceptor trigger zone, which in turn acts on vomiting center

---

Uses: Nausea, vomiting
Dosage and routes:
• *Adult:* **PO/IM/RECT** 10 mg/qd-tid
Available forms: Tabs 10 mg; supp 10 mg; inj 5 mg/ml
Side effects/adverse reactions:
GU: Urinary retention, dark urine
CNS: Euphoria, depression, restlessness, tremor, EPS, *convulsions,* drowsiness
GI: Nausea, vomiting, anorexia, dry mouth, diarrhea, constipation, weight loss, metallic taste, cramps
CV: Circulatory failure, tachycardia, postural hypotension, ECG changes
RESP: Respiratory depression
Contraindications: Hypersensitivity to phenothiazines, coma, seizure, encephalopathy, bone marrow depression
Precautions: Children <2 yr, pregnancy (C), elderly, lactation
Pharmacokinetics:
PO: Onset 45-60 min
RECT: Onset 45-60 min, metabolized by liver, crosses placenta, excreted in urine, breast milk
Interactions:
• Decreased effect of thiethylperazine: barbiturates, antacids
• Increased anticholinergic action: anticholinergics, antiparkinson drugs, antidepressants
NURSING CONSIDERATIONS
Assess:
• VS, B/P; check patients with cardiac disease more often
• Respiratory status before, during, after administration of emetic; check rate, rhythm, character; respiratory depression can occur rapidly with elderly or debilitated patients
Administer:
• IM inj in large muscle mass; aspirate to avoid IV administration;

patient should remain recumbent 1 hr after inj
Syringe compatibilities: Butorphanol, hydromorphone, midazolam, ranitidine
Y-site compatibilities: Aldesleukin
Evaluate:
• Therapeutic response: absence of nausea, vomiting
Teach patient/family:
• To avoid hazardous activities, activities requiring alertness; dizziness may occur

---

thioguanine (6-TG) (℞)

(thye-oh-gwah′neen)
thioguanine, Lanvis*
Func. class.: Antineoplastic-antimetabolite
Chem. class.: Purine analog

Action: Interferes with synthesis, utilization of purine nucleotides; S phase of cell cycle specific
Uses: Acute leukemias, chronic granulocytic leukemia, lymphomas, multiple myeloma, solid tumors
Dosage and routes:
• *Adult and child:* **PO** 2 mg/kg/day, then increase slowly to 3 mg/kg/day after 4 wk
Available forms: Tabs 40 mg
Side effects/adverse reactions:
HEMA: Thrombocytopenia, leukopenia, myelosuppression, anemia
GI: Nausea, vomiting, anorexia, diarrhea, stomatitis, *hepatotoxicity,* gastritis, jaundice
GU: Renal failure, hyperuricemia, oliguria
INTEG: Rash, dermatitis, dry skin
Contraindications: Prior drug resistance, leukopenia (<2500/mm³), thrombocytopenia (<100,000/mm³), anemia, pregnancy (D)

Precautions: Liver disease

Pharmacokinetics: Oral form absorbed only 30%, metabolized in liver, only small amounts excreted in urine (unchanged)

Interactions:

• Increased toxicity: radiation, other antineoplastics

Lab test interferences:

Increase: Uric acid (blood, urine)

NURSING CONSIDERATIONS

Assess:

• CBC, differential, platelet count qwk; withhold drug if WBC is <3500/mm^3 or platelet count is <100,000/mm^3; notify prescriber; drug should be discontinued

• Renal function studies: BUN, serum uric acid, urine CrCl, electrolytes before, during therapy

• I&O ratio; report fall in urine output to <30 ml/hr

• Monitor temp q4h; fever may indicate beginning infection

• Liver function tests before, during therapy: bilirubin, alk phosphatase, AST (SGOT), ALT (SGPT)

• Bleeding time, coagulation time during treatment

• Bleeding: hematuria, guaiac, bruising, petechiae, mucosa or orifices q8h

• Food preferences; list likes, dislikes

• Hepatotoxicity: yellow skin, sclera; dark urine, clay colored stools, pruritus, abdominal pain, fever, diarrhea

• Buccal cavity q8h for dryness, sores, ulceration, white patches, oral pain, bleeding, dysphagia

◆ Symptoms indicating severe allergic reaction: rash, urticaria, itching, flushing

Administer:

• Antacid before oral agent; give drug after evening meal before bedtime

• Antiemetic 30-60 min before giving drug to prevent vomiting

• Allopurinol or sodium bicarbonate to maintain uric acid levels, alkalinization of urine

• Antibiotics for prophylaxis of infection

• Topical or systemic analgesics for pain

• Transfusion for anemia

Perform/provide:

• Strict medical asepsis, protective isolation if WBC levels are low

• Liquid diet: carbonated beverage, Jell-O; dry toast, crackers may be added when patient is not nauseated or vomiting

• Increase fluid intake to 2-3 L/day to prevent urate deposits, calculi formation, unless contraindicated

• Diet low in purines: no organ meats (kidney, liver), dried beans, peas to maintain alkaline urine

• Rinsing of mouth tid-qid with water, club soda, brushing of teeth bid-tid with soft brush or cotton-tipped applicators for stomatitis; use unwaxed dental floss

• Nutritious diet with iron, vitamin supplements as ordered

• Storage in tightly closed container in cool environment

Evaluate:

• Therapeutic response: decreased tumor size, spread of malignancy

Teach patient/family:

• Why protective isolation precautions are needed

• To report any complaints, side effects to prescriber: black tarry stools, chills, fever, sore throat, bleeding, bruising, cough, shortness of breath, dark, bloody urine

• To avoid foods with citric acid, hot or rough texture if stomatitis is present

• To report stomatitis: any bleeding,

white spots, ulcerations in mouth; to examine mouth qd, report symptoms

• That contraceptive measures are recommended during therapy

• To drink 10-12 (8 oz) glasses of fluid/day

---

thiopental (℞)

(thye-oh-pen'tal)
Pentothal, thiopental sodium
Func. class.: General anesthetic
Chem. class.: Barbiturate

Controlled Substance Schedule III

Action: Acts in reticular-activating system to produce anesthesia, raises seizure threshold

Uses: Short, general anesthesia; narcoanalysis, induction anesthesia before other anesthetics

Investigational uses: Increased intracranial pressure

Dosage and routes:

Induction

• *Adult:* IV 210-280 mg or 3-5 ml/kg

General anesthetic

• *Child:* IV 3-8 mg/kg then 1 mg/kg as needed

• *Adult:* IV 50-75 mg given at 20-40 sec intervals

Narcoanalysis

• *Adult:* IV 100 mg/min, not to exceed 50 ml/min

Sedation or narcosis

• *Adult:* RECT 12-20 mg/lb

Available forms: Powder for inj 2%, 2.5%

Side effects/adverse reactions:

RESP: **Respiratory depression, bronchospasm**

CNS: Retrograde amnesia, prolonged somnolence

CV: Tachycardia, hypotension, **myocardial depression, dysrhythmias**

EENT: Sneezing, coughing

INTEG: Chills, *shivering,* necrosis, pain at injection site

MS: Muscle irritability

Contraindications: Hypersensitivity, status asthmaticus, hepatic/intermittent porphyrias

Precautions: Severe cardiovascular disease, renal disease, hypotension, liver disease, myxedema, myasthenia gravis, asthma, increased intracranial pressure, pregnancy (C)

Pharmacokinetics:

IV: Onset 30-40 sec; half-life 11½ hr; crosses placenta

Interactions:

• Increased action: CNS depressants

 Increased CNS depression: kava kava

NURSING CONSIDERATIONS

Assess:

• VS q3-5min during IV administration, after dose, q4h postoperatively

• Extravasation; if it occurs, use nitroprusside or chloroprocaine to decrease pain, increase circulation

• Dysrhythmias or myocardial depression

Administer:

• Only with crash cart, resuscitative equipment nearby

IV

• After diluting 500 mg/20 ml sterile H_2O for inj; give each 25 mg or less/min, titrate to response

Additive compatibilities: Chloramphenicol, hydrocortisone sodium succinate, oxytocin, pentobarbital, phenobarbital, potassium chloride, sodium bicarbonate

Solution compatibilities: D_5/0.45% NaCl, D_5W, multiple electrolyte sol, 0.45% NaCl, 0.9% NaCl, 1/6 M sodium lactate

Syringe compatibilities: Aminophylline, hyaluronidase, hydrocortisone sodium succinate, neostigmine, pentobarbital, propofol, scopolamine, tubocurarine

---

 = Nursing alert   = Herb-drug interaction   🚫 = Do not crush

Y-site compatibilities: Doxacurium, fentanyl, heparin, milrinone, mivacurium, nitroglycerin, ranitidine

Evaluate:

• Therapeutic response: maintenance of anesthesia

---

thioridazine (℞)

(thye-or-rid'a-zeen)
Mellaril, Mellaril Concentrate, Mellaril-5, Novoridazine*, thioridazine HCl
Func. class.: Antipsychotic, neuroleptic
Chem. class.: Phenothiazine piperidine

Action: Depresses cerebral cortex, hypothalamus, limbic system, which control activity, aggression; blocks neurotransmission produced by dopamine at synapse; exhibits strong α-adrenergic, anticholinergic blocking action; mechanism for antipsychotic effects is unclear

Uses: Psychotic disorders, schizophrenia, behavioral problems in children, anxiety, major depressive disorders, organic brain syndrome

Dosage and routes:

Psychosis

• *Adult:* **PO** 25-100 mg tid, max dose 800 mg/day; dose is gradually increased to desired response, then reduced to minimum maintenance

Depression/behavioral problems/organic brain syndrome

• *Adult:* **PO** 25 mg tid, range from 10 mg bid-qid to 50 mg tid-qid; decreased dose in elderly

• *Geriatric:* **PO** 10-25 mg qd-bid, increase 4-7 days by 10-25 mg to desired dose

• *Child 2-12 yr:* **PO** 0.5-3 mg/kg/day in divided doses

Available forms: Tabs 10, 15, 25, 50, 100, 150, 200, 300 mg; conc 30, 100 mg/ml; susp 25, 100 mg/5 ml; syr 10 mg/15 ml

Side effects/adverse reactions:

RESP: **Laryngospasm,** dyspnea, **respiratory depression**

CNS: EPS (rare): *pseudoparkinsonism, akathisia, dystonia, tardive dyskinesia,* **seizures,** *headache,* confusion

HEMA: Anemia, **leukopenia, leukocytosis, agranulocytosis**

INTEG: Rash, photosensitivity, dermatitis

EENT: Blurred vision, glaucoma, dry eyes

GI: Dry mouth, nausea, vomiting, anorexia, constipation, diarrhea, jaundice, weight gain

GU: Urinary retention, urinary frequency, enuresis, impotence, amenorrhea, gynecomastia

CV: Orthostatic hypotension, **cardiac arrest,** ECG changes, **tachycardia**

Contraindications: Hypersensitivity, blood dyscrasias, coma, child <2 yr, brain damage, bone marrow depression

Precautions: Pregnancy (C), lactation, seizure disorders, hypertension, hepatic disease, cardiac disease

Pharmacokinetics:

PO: Onset erratic, peak 2-4 hr; metabolized by liver, excreted in urine, breast milk; crosses placenta, half-life 26-36 hr

Interactions:

• Oversedation: other CNS depressants, alcohol, barbiturate anesthetics

• Toxicity: epinephrine

• Decreased absorption: aluminum hydroxide, magnesium hydroxide antacids

• Decreased effects of lithium, levodopa

• Increased effects of both drugs: β-adrenergic blockers, alcohol

T

• Increased anticholinergic effects: anticholinergics

⚕ Increased CNS depression: kava kava

Lab test interferences:

Increase: Liver function tests, cardiac enzymes, cholesterol, blood glucose, prolactin, bilirubin, PBI, cholinesterase, ^{131}I

Decrease: Hormones (blood, urine)

False positive: Pregnancy test, PKU

False negative: Urinary steroid, pregnancy test

NURSING CONSIDERATIONS
Assess:

• Mental status before first dose

• Swallowing of PO medication; check for hoarding or giving of medication to other patients

• I&O ratio; palpate bladder if low urinary output occurs

• Bilirubin, CBC, liver function studies qmo

• Urinalysis is recommended before and during prolonged therapy

• Affect, orientation, LOC, reflexes, gait, coordination, sleep pattern disturbances

• B/P standing and lying; also include pulse and respirations q4h during initial treatment; establish baseline before starting treatment; report drops of 30 mm Hg

• Dizziness, faintness, palpitations, tachycardia on rising

• EPS including akathisia (inability to sit still, no pattern to movements), tardive dyskinesia (bizarre movements of jaw, mouth, tongue, extremities), pseudoparkinsonism (rigidity, tremors, pill rolling, shuffling gait)

◆ For neuroleptic malignant syndrome: altered mental status, muscle rigidity, increased CPK, hyperthermia

• Skin turgor qd

• Constipation, urinary retention qd; increase bulk, water in diet

Administer:

• Antiparkinsonian agent on order from prescriber for EPS

• Concentrate mixed in citrus juices or distilled or acidified tap water

• Decreased dose in elderly

Perform/provide:

• Decreased sensory input by dimming lights, avoiding loud noises

• Supervised ambulation until stabilized on medication if needed; do not involve in strenuous exercise program because fainting is possible; patient should not stand still for long periods

• Increased fluids to prevent constipation

• Sips of water, candy, gum for dry mouth

• Storage in tight, light-resistant container; avoid contact with skin

Evaluate:

• Therapeutic response: decrease in emotional excitement, hallucinations, delusions, paranoia, reorganization of patterns of thought, speech

Teach patient/family:

• That orthostatic hypotension occurs frequently, to rise from sitting or lying position gradually; to avoid hazardous activities until stabilized on medication

• To remain lying down after IM injection for at least 30 min

• To avoid hot tubs, hot showers, tub baths; hypotension may occur

• To avoid abrupt withdrawal of thioridazine, or EPS may result; drug should be withdrawn slowly

• To avoid OTC preparations (cough, hay fever, cold) unless approved by prescriber; serious drug interactions may occur; avoid use with alcohol, CNS depressants; increased drowsiness may occur

• To use a sunscreen

• About compliance with drug regimen

◆ = Nursing alert   *⚕* = Herb-drug interaction   ⊘ = Do not crush

• About the necessity for meticulous oral hygiene, since oral candidiasis may occur

• To report sore throat, malaise, fever, bleeding, mouth sores; if these occur, CBC should be drawn and drug discontinued

• That in hot weather, heat stroke may occur; take extra precautions to stay cool

Treatment of overdose: Lavage if orally ingested, provide an airway; do not induce vomiting

---

thiotepa (℞)

(thye-oh-tep'a)
Thioplex
Func class.: Antineoplastic
Chem. class.: Alkylating agent

Action: Responsible for crosslinking DNA strands leading to cell death; activity is not cell cycle phase specific

Uses: Hodgkin's disease, lymphomas; breast, ovarian, lung, bladder cancer; neoplastic effusions

Dosage and routes:
• *Adult:* **IV** 0.3-0.4 mg/kg at 1 4 wk intervals

Neoplastic effusions
• *Adult:* **INTRACAVITY** 0.6-0.8 mg/kg

Bladder cancer
• *Adult:* **INSTILL** 60 mg/30-60 ml water for inj instilled in bladder for 2 hr once weekly × 4 wk

Available forms: Powder for inj 15 mg

Side effects/adverse reactions:
CNS: Dizziness, headache
HEMA: ***Thrombocytopenia, leukopenia, pancytopenia***
GI: Nausea, vomiting, anorexia
GU: Hyperuricemia, ***hematuria, amenorrhea, azoospermia***
INTEG: Rash, pruritus

Contraindications: Hypersensitivity, pregnancy (D)

Precautions: Radiation therapy, bone marrow suppression, impaired renal or hepatic function

Pharmacokinetics: Onset slow, metabolized in liver, excreted in urine

Interactions:
• Increased apnea: neuromuscular blockers

NURSING CONSIDERATIONS
Assess:
• CBC, differential, platelet count qwk; withhold drug if WBC is <4000 or platelet count is <75,000; notify prescriber

• Renal function studies: BUN, serum uric acid, urine CrCl before, during therapy

• I&O ratio, report fall in urine output of 30 ml/hr

• Monitor temp q4h (may indicate beginning infection)

• Liver function tests before, during therapy (bilirubin, AST [SGOT], ALT [SGPT], LDH) as needed or monthly

• Bleeding: hematuria, guaiac, bruising or petechiae, mucosa or orifices q8h

• Food preferences; list likes, dislikes

• Yellow skin, sclera; dark urine, clay-colored stools, itchy skin, abdominal pain, fever, diarrhea

• Buccal cavity q8h for dryness, sores, ulceration, white patches, oral pain, bleeding, dysphagia

◆ Symptoms indicating severe allergic reaction: rash, pruritus, urticaria, itching, flushing

Administer:
• Antiemetic 30-60 min before giving drug to prevent vomiting

IV
• After diluting 15 mg/1.5 ml of sterile H$_2$O for inj; give over 1-3 min; may be further diluted in 50-

100 ml compatible sol, use a 0.22 μ filter

Y-site compatibilities: Acyclovir, allopurinol, amifostine, amikacin, aminophylline, amphotericin B, ampicillin, ampicillin/sulbactam, aztreonam, bleomycin, bumetanide, buprenorphine, butorphanol, calcium gluconate, carboplatin, carmustine, cefazolin, cefepime, cefoperazone, cefonicid, cefotaxime, cefotetan, cefoxitin, ceftazidime, ceftizoxime, ceftriaxone, cefuroxime, chlorpromazine, cimetidine, ciprofloxacin, clindamycin, cyclophosphamide, cytarabine, dacarbazine, dactinomycin, daunorubicin, diphenhydramine, dobutamine, dopamine, doxorubicin, doxycycline, droperidol, enalaprilat, etoposide, famotidine, floxuridine, fluconazole, fludarabine, fluorouracil, furosemide, gallium, ganciclovir, centamicin, granisetron, haloperidol, heparin, hydrocortisone, hydromorphone, hydroxyzine, idarubicin, ifosfamide, imipenem-cilastatin, leucovorin, lorazepam, magnesium sulfate, mannitol, melphalan, meperidine, mesna, methotrexate, methylprednisolone, metoclopramide, metronidazole, mezlocillin, miconazole, mitomycin, mitoxantrone, morphine, nalbuphine, netilmicin, ofloxacin, ondansetron, paclitaxel, piperacillin, piperacillin/tazobactam, plicamycin, potassium chloride, prochlorperazine, promethazine, ranitidine, sodium bicarbonate, streptozocin, teniposide, ticarcillin, ticarcillin/clavulanate, tobramycin, trimethoprim-sulfamethoxazole, vancomycin, vinblastine, vincristine, zidovudine

Perform/provide:
• Storage in light-resistant container; refrigerate
• Strict medical asepsis, protective isolation if WBC levels are low

• Increase fluid intake to 2-3 L/day to prevent urate deposits, calculi formation
• Warm compresses at injection site for inflammation

Evaluate:
• Therapeutic response: decreased tumor size, spread of malignancy

Teach patient/family:
• About protective isolation
• That azoospermia or amenorrhea can occur; reversible after discontinuing treatment; to use effective contraception during treatment
• To report any bleeding, white spots or ulcerations in mouth to prescriber; to examine mouth qd
• To report signs of infection: fever, sore throat, flu symptoms
• To report signs of anemia: fatigue, headache, faintness, shortness of breath, irritability
• To avoid use of razors, commercial mouthwash
• To avoid use of aspirin products, ibuprofen

---

thiothixene (℞)

(thye-oh-thix'een)
Navane, thiothixene
Func. class.: Antipsychotic, neuroleptic
Chem. class.: Thioxanthene

Action: Depresses cerebral cortex, hypothalamus, limbic system, which control activity, aggression; blocks neurotransmission produced by dopamine at synapse; exhibits strong α-adrenergic blocking action; mechanism for antipsychotic effects is unclear

Uses: Psychotic disorders, schizophrenia, acute agitation

Dosage and routes:
• *Adult:* **PO** 2-5 mg bid-qid depending on severity of condition; dose

---

 = Nursing alert   = Herb-drug interaction   ⊘ = Do not crush

gradually increased to 15-30 mg if needed; **IM** 4 mg bid-qid; max dose 30 mg qd; administer **PO** dose as soon as possible

• *Geriatric:* **PO** 1-2 mg qd-bid, increase by 1-2 mg q4-7 days to desired dose

Available forms: Caps 1, 2, 5, 10, 20 mg; conc 5 mg/ml; inj 2 mg/ml; powder for inj 5 mg/ml

Side effects/adverse reactions:
RESP: **Laryngospasm,** dyspnea, **respiratory depression**

CNS: EPS: pseudoparkinsonism, akathisia, dystonia, tardive dyskinesia; seizures, *headache*

HEMA: Anemia, **leukopenia, leukocytosis, agranulocytosis**

INTEG: Rash, photosensitivity, dermatitis

EENT: Blurred vision, glaucoma

GI: Dry mouth, nausea, vomiting, anorexia, constipation, diarrhea, jaundice, weight gain

GU: Urinary retention, urinary frequency, enuresis, impotence, amenorrhea, gynecomastia

CV: Orthostatic hypotension, hypertension, **cardiac arrest,** ECG changes, **tachycardia**

Contraindications. Hypersensitivity, blood dyscrasias, child <12 yr, bone marrow depression, circulatory collapse, CNS depression, coma, alcoholism, CV disease, hepatic disease, Reye's syndrome, narrow-angle glaucoma

Precautions: Pregnancy (C), lactation, seizure disorders, hypertension, hepatic disease, elderly

Pharmacokinetics:
PO: Onset slow, peak 2-8 hr, duration up to 12 hr

IM: Onset 15-30 min, peak 1-6 hr, duration up to 12 hr

Metabolized by liver, excreted in urine, breast milk; crosses placenta, half-life 34 hr

Interactions:
• Oversedation: other CNS depressants, alcohol, barbiturate anesthetics

• Toxicity: epinephrine

• Decreased absorption: aluminum hydroxide, magnesium hydroxide antacids

• Decreased effects of thiothixene: lithium, levodopa

• Increased effects of both drugs: β-adrenergic blockers, alcohol

• Increased anticholinergic effects: anticholinergics

🖉 Increased CNS depression: kava kava

Lab test interferences:
Increase: Liver function tests, cardiac enzymes, cholesterol, blood glucose, prolactin, bilirubin, PBI, cholinesterase, ^{131}I

Decrease: Uric acid

NURSING CONSIDERATIONS
Assess:

• For oculogyric crisis

• Mental status before initial administration

• Swallowing of PO medication; check for hoarding or giving of medication to other patients

• I&O ratio, palpate bladder if low urinary output occurs

• Bilirubin, CBC, liver function studies qmo

• Urinalysis is recommended before and during prolonged therapy

• Affect, orientation, LOC, reflexes, gait, coordination, sleep pattern disturbances

• B/P standing and lying; pulse and respirations q4h during initial treatment; establish baseline before starting treatment; report drops of 30 mm Hg

• Dizziness, faintness, palpitations, tachycardia on rising

• EPS including akathisia (inability to sit still, no pattern to movements), tardive dyskinesia (bizarre move-

T

ments of jaw, mouth, tongue, extremities), pseudoparkinsonism (rigidity, tremors, pill rolling, shuffling gait)

⬥ For neuroleptic malignant syndrome: muscle rigidity, altered mental status, increased CPK, hyperthermia

• Constipation, urinary retention daily; increase bulk, water in diet

Administer:

• Antiparkinsonian agent on order from prescriber for EPS

• Concentrate mixed in citrus juices or distilled or acidified tap water

• IM injection into large muscle mass

Syringe compatibilities: Benztropine, diphenhydramine, hydroxyzine

Perform/provide:

• Decreased sensory input by dimming lights, avoiding loud noises

• Supervised ambulation until stabilized on medication; do not involve in strenuous exercise program because fainting is possible; patient should not stand still for long periods

• Increased fluids to prevent constipation

• Sips of water, candy, gum for dry mouth

• Storage in tight, light-resistant container; keep reconstituted sol at room temp for up to 48 hr; avoid contact with skin

Evaluate:

• Therapeutic response: decrease in emotional excitement, hallucinations, delusions, paranoia, reorganization of patterns of thought, speech

Teach patient/family:

• That orthostatic hypotension occurs frequently, and to rise from sitting or lying position gradually; to

avoid hazardous activities until stabilized on medication

• To remain lying down after IM inj for at least 30 min

• To avoid hot tubs, hot showers, tub baths; hypotension may occur

• To avoid abrupt withdrawal of this drug, or EPS may result; drug should be withdrawn slowly

• To avoid OTC preparations (cough, hay fever, cold) unless approved by prescriber; serious drug interactions may occur; avoid use with alcohol, CNS depressants; increased drowsiness may occur

• To use a sunscreen

• About compliance with drug regimen

• About EPS

• The necessity for meticulous oral hygiene, since oral candidiasis may occur

• To report sore throat, malaise, fever, bleeding, mouth sores; if these occur, CBC should be drawn and drug discontinued

• That in hot weather, heat stroke may occur; take extra precautions to stay cool

Treatment of overdose: Lavage if orally ingested; provide an airway; do not induce vomiting

---

thrombin (℞)

Thrombinar, Thrombogen, Thrombostat

Func. class.: Hemostatic
Chem. class.: Bovine thrombin

Action: Converts fibrinogen to fibrin, promotes clotting

Uses: GI hemorrhage, bleeding in dental, plastic, nasal, laryngeal surgery, skin grafting

Dosage and routes:

• *Adult:* **TOP** apply 100 U/1 ml sterile isotonic NaCl or distilled H_2O in light to moderate bleeding, or 1000-

 = Nursing alert   ▰ = Herb-drug interaction   Ⓢ = Do not crush

2000 U/ml sterile isotonic NaCl in severe bleeding; dry area before applying

Available forms: Powder 1000, 5000, 10,000, 20,000, 50,000 U

Side effects/adverse reactions:

INTEG: Rash, allergic reactions

*HEMA: **Intravascular clotting when entering large blood vessels***

Contraindications: Hypersensitivity to bovine products

Precautions: Pregnancy (C), children

NURSING CONSIDERATIONS

Assess:

◆▶ For allergic reactions: fever, rash, itching, changes in VS; thrombosis formation

Administer:

• Only to area sponged free of blood
• After preparing with NS, isotonic saline
• With blood available for transfusion

Perform/provide:

• Storage in refrigerator; use reconstituted sol within 3 hr, some can be administered up to 48 hr after reconstitution if refrigerated or preferably frozen shortly after reconstituted; discard unused portion

Evaluate:

• Therapeutic response: control of bleeding

---

thyroid USP (desiccated) (℞)

(thye′roid)

Armour Thyroid, Cholaxin*, S-P-T, Thyrar, Thyroid Strong, Thyroid USP

Func. class.: Thyroid hormone

Chem. class.: Active thyroid hormone in natural state and ratio

---

Action: Increases metabolic rates, increases cardiac output, O_2 consumption, body temp, blood volume, growth, development at cellular level

Uses: Hypothyroidism, cretinism (juvenile hypothyroidism), myxedema

Dosage and routes:

Hypothyroidism

• *Adult:* **PO** 65 mg qd, increased by 65 mg q30d until desired response; maintenance dose 65-195 mg qd
• *Elderly:* **PO** 7.5-15 mg qd, double dose q6-8wk until desired response

Cretinism/juvenile hypothyroidism

• *Child over 1 yr:* **PO** up to 180 mg qd titrated to response
• *Child 4-12 mo:* **PO** 30-60 mg qd
• *Child 1-4 mo:* **PO** 15-30 mg qd; may increase q2wk; titrated to response; maintenance dose 30-45 mg qd

Myxedema

• *Adult:* **PO** 16 mg qd, double dose q2wk, maintenance 65-195 mg/day

Available forms: Tabs 16, 32, 65, 98, 130, 195, 260, 325 mg; tabs enteric coated 32, 65, 130 mg; sugar-coated tabs 32, 65, 130, 195 mg; caps 65, 130, 195, 325 mg

Side effects/adverse reactions:

CNS: Insomnia, tremors, headache, thyroid storm

CV: Tachycardia, palpitations, angina, dysrhythmias, hypertension, ***cardiac arrest***

GI: Nausea, diarrhea, increased or decreased appetite, cramps

MISC: Menstrual irregularities, weight loss, sweating, heat intolerance, fever

Contraindications: Adrenal insufficiency, MI, thyrotoxicosis

Precautions: Elderly, angina pectoris, hypertension, ischemia, cardiac disease, pregnancy (A), lactation

Pharmacokinetics:

PO: Peak 12-48 hr, half-life 6-7 days

Interactions:
• Decreased absorption of thyroid: cholestyramine
• Increased effects of anticoagulants, sympathomimetics, tricyclic antidepressants, catecholamines
• Decreased effects of digitalis drugs, insulin, hypoglycemics
• Decreased effects of thyroid: estrogens

Lab test interferences:
Increase: CPK, LDH, AST (SGOT), PBI, blood glucose
Decrease: TSH, ^{131}I uptake test, uric acid, triglycerides

NURSING CONSIDERATIONS
Assess:
• B/P, pulse before each dose
• I&O ratio
• Weight qd in same clothing, using same scale, at same time of day
• Height, growth rate of child
• T_3, T_4, which are decreased; radioimmunoassay of TSH, which is increased; radio uptake, which is decreased if dosage is too low
• Pro-time may require decreased anticoagulant; check for bleeding, bruising
• Increased nervousness, excitability, irritability; may indicate too high dose of medication, usually after 1-3 wk of treatment
• Cardiac status: angina, palpitation, chest pain, change in VS

Administer:
• In AM if possible as a single dose to decrease sleeplessness
• At same time each day to maintain drug level
• Only for hormone imbalances; not to be used for obesity, male infertility, menstrual disorders, lethargy
• Lowest dose that relieves symptoms

Perform/provide:
• Removal of medication 4 wk before RAIU test

Evaluate:
• Therapeutic response: absence of depression; increased weight loss, diuresis, pulse, appetite; absence of constipation, peripheral edema, cold intolerance; pale, cool, dry skin; brittle nails, alopecia, coarse hair, menorrhagia, night blindness, paresthesias, syncope, stupor, coma, rosy cheeks

Teach patient/family:
• That hair loss will occur in child, is temporary
• To report excitability, irritability, anxiety; indicates overdose
• Not to switch brands unless directed by prescriber
• That hypothyroid child will show almost immediate behavior/personality change
• That treatment drug is not to be taken to reduce weight
• To avoid OTC preparations with iodine; read labels
• To avoid iodine food, iodized salt, soybeans, tofu, turnips, some seafood, some bread

---

thyrotropin (thyroid-stimulating hormone, TSH) (R)
(thye-roe-troe′pin)
Thytropar
Func. class.: Thyroid hormone
Chem. class.: TSH

Action: Increases uptake of iodine by thyroid gland, production and release of thyroid hormone
Uses: Diagnosis and treatment of thyroid cancer, diagnosis of primary/secondary hypothyroidism
Dosage and routes:
Diagnosis of hypothyroidism
• *Adult:* **IM/SC** 10 IU qd × 1-3 days
Diagnosis of thyroid cancer
• *Adult:* **IM/SC** 10 IU qd × 3-7 days

⬥ = Nursing alert   🌿 = Herb-drug interaction   🚫 = Do not crush

Treatment of thyroid cancer
• *Adult:* **IM/SC** 10 IU qd × 3-8 days
Available forms: Powder for inj 10 IU/vial
Side effects/adverse reactions:
INTEG: Urticaria
CNS: Headache, fever
CV: Tachycardia, angina, *atrial fibrillation, CHF,* hypotension
GI: Nausea, vomiting
SYST: Anaphylactic reactions
Contraindications: Hypersensitivity, coronary thrombosis, untreated Addison's disease
Precautions: Angina pectoris, adrenal insufficiency, pregnancy (C), lactation, children
Pharmacokinetics:
IM/SC: Onset 8 hr, peak 24-48 hr
NURSING CONSIDERATIONS
Administer:
• After dilution with 2 ml sterile NS
• Three-day dose schedule for myxedema (pituitary)
• In combination with ^{131}I to treat thyroid cancer
Treatment of overdose: Discontinue drug, give supportive care

---

tiagabine (℞)
(tie-ah-ga'been)
Gabatril
Func. class.: Anticonvulsant

Action: Mechanism unknown; may increase seizure threshold; structurally similar to GABA; tiagabine binding sites in neocortex, hippocampus
Uses: Adjunct treatment of partial seizures
Dosage and routes:
• *Adult:* **PO** 4 mg qd, may increase by 4-8 mg qwk until desired response, max 32 mg/day
• *Child 12-18 yr:* **PO** 4 mg qd, may increase by 4 mg at beginning of wk

2; may increase by 4-8 mg qwk until desired response; max 32 mg/day
Available forms: Tabs 4, 12, 16, 20 mg
Side effects/adverse reactions:
CNS: Dizziness, anxiety, somnolence, ataxia, amnesia, unsteady gait, depression
CV: Vasodilation
GI: Nausea, vomiting, diarrhea
INTEG: Pruritus, rash
RESP: Pharyngitis, coughing
Contraindications: Hypersensitivity to this drug
Precautions: Hepatic disease, renal disease, pregnancy (C), lactation, child <12 yr, elderly
Pharmacokinetics: Absorption >95%, half-life 7-9 hrs
Interactions:
Unknown
NURSING CONSIDERATIONS
Assess:
• Renal studies: urinalysis, BUN, urine creatinine q3mo
• Hepatic studies: ALT (SGPT), AST (SGOT), bilirubin
• Description of seizures
• Mental status: mood, sensorium, affect, behavioral changes; if mental status changes, notify prescriber
• Eye problems, need for ophthalmic examinations before, during, after treatment (slit lamp, funduscopy, tonometry)
• Allergic reaction: purpura, red raised rash; if these occur, drug should be discontinued
Perform/provide:
• Storage at room temp away from heat and light
• Hard candy, frequent rinsing of mouth, gum for dry mouth
• Assistance with ambulation during early part of treatment; dizziness occurs
• Seizure precautions: padded side rails; move objects that may harm patient

T

• Increased fluids, bulk in diet for constipation

Evaluate:

• Therapeutic response: decreased seizure activity; document on patient's chart

Teach patient/family:

• To carry Medic Alert ID stating patient's name, drugs taken, condition, prescriber's name and phone number

• To avoid driving, other activities that require alertness

• Not to discontinue medication quickly after long-term use

Treatment of overdose: Lavage, VS

---

ticarcillin (R)

(tye-kar-sill'in)
Ticar
Func. class.: Broad-spectrum antiinfective
Chem. class.: Extended-spectrum penicillin

Action: Interferes with cell wall replication of susceptible organisms; osmotically unstable cell wall swells, bursts from osmotic pressure.

Uses: Respiratory, soft tissue, urinary tract infections, bacterial septicemia; effective for gram-positive cocci *(S. aureus, S. faecalis, S. pneumoniae)*, gram-negative cocci *(N. gonorrhoeae)*, gram-positive bacilli *(C. perfringens, C. tetani)*, gram-negative bacilli *(Bacteroides, F. nucleatum, E. coli, P. mirabilis, Salmonella, M. morganii, P. rettgeri, Enterobacter, P. aeruginosa, Serratia, Peptococcus, Peptostreptococcus, Eubacterium)*

Dosage and routes:

• Dosage reduction needed for renal impairment CrCl <30 ml/min

• *Adult:* **IV/IM** 4-24 g/day in divided doses q4-6h; infuse over ½-2 hr

• *Child:* **IV/IM** 50-300 mg/kg/day in divided doses q4-8h

• *Neonate:* **IV INF** 75-100 mg/kg/ 8-12 hr

Available forms: Inj 1, 3, 6, 20, 30 g

Side effects/adverse reactions:

HEMA: Anemia, increased bleeding time, *bone marrow depression, granulocytopenia*

GI: Nausea, vomiting, diarrhea; increased AST, ALT; abdominal pain, glossitis, colitis

GU: Oliguria, proteinuria, hematuria, *vaginitis, moniliasis, glomerulonephritis*

CNS: Lethargy, hallucinations, anxiety, depression, twitching, *coma, convulsions*

INTEG: Rash

META: Hypokalemia

Contraindications: Hypersensitivity to penicillins

Precautions: Hypersensitivity to cephalosporins, pregnancy (B), lactation, renal disease

Pharmacokinetics:

IM: Peak 1 hr, duration 4-6 hr

IV: Peak 30-45 min, duration 4 hr, half-life 70 min; small amount metabolized in liver; excreted in urine, breast milk

Interactions:

• Decreased antimicrobial effect of ticarcillin: tetracyclines, aminoglycosides IV

• Increased effect of: neuromuscular blockers, heparin

• Increased ticarcillin concentrations: aspirin, probenecid

Lab test interferences:

False positive: Urine glucose, urine protein

NURSING CONSIDERATIONS

Assess:

• I&O ratio; report hematuria, oliguria, since penicillin in high doses is nephrotoxic

---

◆ = Nursing alert   ▨ = Herb-drug interaction   ⃠ = Do not crush

◆ Any patient with compromised renal system, since drug is excreted slowly in poor renal system function; toxicity may occur rapidly

• Liver studies: AST (SGOT), ALT (SGPT)

• Blood studies: WBC, RBC, Hgb, Hct, bleeding time

• Renal studies: urinalysis, protein, blood, BUN, creatinine

• C&S before drug therapy; drug may be given as soon as culture is taken

• Bowel pattern before, during treatment

• Skin eruptions after administration of penicillin to 1 wk after discontinuing drug

• Respiratory status: rate, character, wheezing, tightness in chest

• Allergies before initiation of treatment, reaction of each medication; highlight allergies on chart

Administer:

• Drug after C&S has been completed

IV

• After diluting 1 g or less/4 ml sterile H₂O for inj; dilute further with 10-20 ml or more D₅W, NS, or sterile H₂O for inj sol; give 1 g or less/5 min or more or by intermittent inf over ½-2 hr or by continuous inf at prescribed rate

Additive compatibilities: Ranitidine, verapamil

Y-site compatibilities: Acyclovir, allopurinol, amifostine, aztreonam, cyclophosphamide, diltiazem, famotidine, filgrastim, fludarabine, granisetron, heparin, hydromorphone, IL-2, insulin (regular), magnesium sulfate, melphalan, meperidine, morphine, ondansetron, perphenazine, propofol, sargramostim, teniposide, theophylline, thiotepa, verapamil, vinorelbine

Perform/provide:

• Adrenalin, suction, tracheostomy set, endotracheal intubation equipment

• Adequate fluid intake (2 L) during diarrhea episodes

• Scratch test to assess allergy on order from prescriber; usually done when penicillin is only drug of choice

• Storage at room temp, reconstituted sol 72 hr at room temp

Evaluate:

• Therapeutic response: absence of fever, purulent drainage, redness, inflammation

Teach patient/family:

• That culture may be taken after completed course of medication

• To report sore throat, fever, fatigue (may indicate superinfection)

• To wear or carry Medic Alert ID if allergic to penicillins

• To notify nurse of diarrhea

Treatment of overdose: Withdraw drug, maintain airway, administer epinephrine, aminophylline, O₂, IV corticosteroids for anaphylaxis

---

ticarcillin/clavulanate (℞)

Timentin

Func. class.: Broad-spectrum antiinfective

Chem. class.: Extended-spectrum penicillin

Action: Interferes with cell wall replication of susceptible organisms; osmotically unstable cell wall swells, bursts from osmotic pressure

Uses: Respiratory, soft tissue, and urinary tract infections, bacterial septicemia; effective for gram-positive cocci (*S. aureus, S. faecalis, S. pneumoniae*), gram-negative cocci (*N. gonorrhoeae*), gram-positive bacilli

(C. perfringens, C. tetani), gram-negative bacilli *(Bacteroides, F. nucleatum, E. coli, P. mirabilis, Salmonella, M. morganii, P. rettgeri, Enterobacter, P. aeruginosa, Serratia, Peptococcus, Peptostreptococcus, Eubacterium)*

Dosage and routes:
• Dosage reduction indicated in renal impairment (CrCl <30 ml/min)
• *Adult:* IV INF 1 vial containing ticarcillin 3 g, clavulanate 0.1 g q4-6h, infuse over 30 min
• *Child <60 kg:* IV INF 200-300 mg ticarcillin/kg/day in divided doses q4-6h

Available forms: Inj 3 g ticarcillin, 0.1 g clavulanate; IV INF 3 g ticarcillin, 0.1 g clavulanate

Side effects/adverse reactions:
HEMA: Anemia, increased bleeding time, **bone marrow depression, granulocytopenia**
GI: Nausea, vomiting, diarrhea; increased AST, ALT; abdominal pain, glossitis, colitis
GU: Oliguria, proteinuria, hematuria, *vaginitis, moniliasis, **glomerulonephritis***
CNS: Lethargy, hallucinations, anxiety, depression, twitching, **coma, convulsions**
META: Hyperkalemia, hypokalemia, alkalosis, hypernatremia

Contraindications: Hypersensitivity to penicillins; neonates
Precautions: Hypersensitivity to cephalosporins, pregnancy (B), renal disease

Pharmacokinetics:
IV: Peak 30-45 min, duration 4 hr, half-life 64-68 min; excreted in urine
Interactions:
• Decreased antimicrobial effect of ticarcillin: tetracyclines, aminoglycosides IV
• Increased effect of: neuromuscular blockers, heparin
• Increased ticarcillin concentrations: aspirin, probenecid

Lab test interferences:
False positive: Urine glucose, urine protein, Coombs' test

NURSING CONSIDERATIONS
Assess:
• I&O ratio; report hematuria, oliguria, since penicillin in high doses is nephrotoxic
 Any patient with compromised renal system, since drug is excreted slowly in poor renal system function; toxicity may occur rapidly
• Liver studies: AST (SGOT), ALT (SGPT)
• Blood studies: WBC, RBC, Hct, Hgb, bleeding time
• Renal studies: urinalysis, protein, blood, BUN, creatinine
• C&S before drug therapy; drug may be given as soon as culture is taken
• Bowel pattern before, during treatment
• Skin eruptions after administration of penicillin to 1 wk after discontinuing drug
• Respiratory status: rate, character, wheezing, and tightness in chest
• Allergies before initiation of treatment, reaction of each medication; highlight allergies on chart

Administer:
• Drug after C&S
IV
• After diluting 3.1 g or less/13 ml of sterile H_2O or NaCl (200 mg/ml), shake; may further dilute in 50-100 ml or more NS, D_5W, or LR sol and run over ½ hr

Y-site compatibilities: Allopurinol, amifostine, aztreonam, cefepime, cyclophosphamide, diltiazem, famotidine, filgrastim, fluconazole, fludarabine, foscarnet, gallium, granisetron, heparin, insulin (regular) melphalan, meperidine, morphine, ondansetron, perphenazine, propofol, sargramostim, teniposide, theophylline, thiotepa, vinorelbine

Perform/provide:

• Adrenaline, suction, tracheostomy set, endotracheal intubation equipment

• Adequate fluid intake (2 L) during diarrhea episodes

• Scratch test to assess allergy on order from prescriber; usually done when penicillin is only drug of choice

• Storage at room temp, reconstituted sol 12-24 hr or 3-7 days refrigerated

Evaluate:

• Therapeutic response: absence of fever, purulent drainage, redness, inflammation

Teach patient/family:

• To report persistent diarrhea

• That culture may be taken after completed course of medication

• To report sore throat, fever, fatigue (may indicate superinfection)

• To wear or carry Medic Alert ID if allergic to penicillins

Treatment of overdose: Withdraw drug, maintain airway, administer epinephrine, O₂, IV corticosteroids for anaphylaxis

---

ticlopidine (℞)

(ly-**kloe**'pi-deen)

Ticlid

Func. class.: Platelet aggregation inhibitor

Action: Inhibits first and second phases of ADP-induced effects in platelet aggregation

Uses: Reducing the risk of stroke in high-risk patients

Dosage and routes:

• *Adult:* **PO** 250 mg bid with food

Available forms: Tabs 250 mg

Side effects/adverse reactions:

INTEG: Rash, pruritus

GI: Nausea, vomiting, *diarrhea,* GI discomfort, ***cholestatic jaundice, hepatitis,*** increased cholesterol, LDL, VLDL, TG

HEMA: ***Bleeding (epistaxis, hematuria, conjunctival hemorrhage, GI bleeding), agranulocytosis, neutropenia, thrombocytopenia***

CNS: Dizziness

Contraindications: Hypersensitivity, active liver disease, blood dyscrasias, active bleeding

Precautions: Past liver disease, renal disease, elderly, pregnancy (B), lactation, children, increased bleeding risk

Pharmacokinetics: Peak 1-3 hr, metabolized by liver, excreted in urine, feces; half-life increases with repeated dosing

Interactions:

• Increased bleeding tendencies: anticoagulants, aspirin

• Decreased plasma levels of ticlopidine: antacids

• Decreased plasma levels of digoxin

• Increased effects of ticlopidine: cimetidine

• Increased effects of theophylline

• Increased risk of bleeding: alfalfa, angelica

NURSING CONSIDERATIONS

Assess:

• Liver function studies: AST (SGOT), ALT (SGPT), bilirubin, creatinine (long-term therapy)

• Blood studies: CBC; CBC q2 wk × 3 mo, Hct, Hgb, pro-time (long-term therapy)

Administer:

• With food to decrease gastric symptoms

Evaluate:

• Therapeutic response: absence of stroke

Teach patient/family:

• That blood work will be necessary during treatment

- To report any unusual bleeding to prescriber
- To take with food or just after eating to minimize GI discomfort
- To report side effects such as diarrhea, skin rashes, subcutaneous bleeding, signs of cholestasis (yellow skin and sclera, dark urine, light-colored stools)

---

tiludronate (Rx)

(till-oo'droe-nate)
Skelid
Func. class.: Parathyroid agent (calcium regulator)
Chem. class.: Bisphosphonate

Action: Decreases bone resorption and new bone development

Uses: Paget's disease

Dosage and routes:
- *Adult:* **PO** 400 mg qd, with 8 oz water × 3 mo

Available forms: Tabs 240 mg (equal to 200/mg tiludronic acid)

Side effects/adverse reactions:
GI: Nausea, diarrhea, dry mouth, gastritis, vomiting, flatulence, gastric ulcers
RESP: Rhinitis, rales, sinusitis, URI
CNS: Headache, somnolence, dizziness, anxiety, vertigo, nervousness, involuntary movements
ENDO: Hyperparathyroidism
INTEG: Rash, epidermal necrosis, pruritus, sweating
GU: Nephrotoxicity, UTI
MS: Bone pain, decreased mineralization of nonaffected bones, pathological fractures

Contraindications: Hypersensitivity to bisphosphonates, pathologic fractures, children, colitis, severe renal disease with creatinine >5 mg/dl

Precautions: Pregnancy (C), renal disease, lactation, restricted vit D/Ca, GI disease

Pharmacokinetics:
Half-life 150 hr; duration 6 mo

Interactions:
- Decreased absorption of tiludronate: antacids, mineral supplements with magnesium, calcium, aluminum, aspirin
- Increased effect of tiludronate: indomethacin

NURSING CONSIDERATIONS
Assess:
- GI symptoms, polyuria, flushing, head swelling, tingling, headache—may indicate hypercalcemia; nervousness, irritability, twitching, seizures, spasm, paresthesia indicates hypocalcemia at start of treatment
- Nutritional status; evaluate diet for sources of vitamin D (milk, some seafood), calcium (dairy products, dark green vegetables), phosphates
- BUN, creatinine, uric acid, chloride, electrolytes, urine pH, urinary calcium, magnesium, phosphate, urinalysis (calcium should be kept at 9-10 mg/dl), albumin, alk phosphatase baseline and q3-6 mo; check urine sediment for casts throughout treatment
- For increased drug level—toxic reactions occur rapidly; have calcium chloride or gluconate on hand if calcium level drops too low; check for tetany

Administer:
- On empty stomach to improve absorption (2 hr ac), with 6-8 oz water

Evaluate:
- Therapeutic response: calcium levels 9-10 mg/dl; decreasing symptoms of Paget's disease

Teach patient/family:
- To notify prescriber of hypercalcemic relapse: renal calculi, nausea, vomiting, thirst, lethargy, deep bone or flank pain
- To follow a low-calcium diet as prescribed (Paget's disease, hypercalcemia)

◆ = Nursing alert   = Herb-drug interaction ⊘ = Do not crush

• To notify prescriber of diarrhea, nausea; dose may be divided to lessen these symptoms

---

timolol (℞)

(tye′moe-lole)

Blocadren, timolol maleate

Func. class.: Antihypertensive

Chem. class.: Nonselective β-blocker

Action: Competitively blocks stimulation of β-adrenergic receptor within vascular smooth muscle (decreases rate of SA node discharge, increases recovery time), slows conduction of AV node, decreases heart rate, which decreases O_2 consumption in myocardium; also decreases renin-aldosterone-angiotensin system, at high doses inhibits $β_2$-receptors in bronchial system

Uses: Mild to moderate hypertension, sinus tachycardia, persistent atrial extrasystoles, tachydysrhythmias, prophylaxis of angina pectoris, reduction of mortality after MI, migraine prevention

Investigational uses: Mitral valve prolapse, hypertrophic cardiomyopathy, thyrotoxicosis, tremors, anxiety, pheochromocytoma, tachydysrhythmias, angina pectoris

Dosage and routes:

Hypertension

• *Adult:* **PO** 10 mg bid, or 20 mg qd, may increase by 10 mg q2-3d, not to exceed 60 mg/day

Myocardial infarction

• *Adult:* **PO** 10 mg bid beginning 1-4 wks after MI

Migraine headache prevention

• *Adult:* **PO** 10 mg bid or 20 mg qd; may increase to 30 mg/day, 20 mg in AM, 10 mg in PM

Available forms: Tabs 5, 10, 20 mg

Side effects/adverse reactions:

CV: Hypotension, bradycardia, ***CHF,*** edema, chest pain, claudication

CNS: Insomnia, dizziness, hallucinations, anxiety

GI: Nausea, vomiting, ***ischemic colitis,*** diarrhea, *abdominal pain,* ***mesenteric arterial thrombosis***

INTEG: Rash, alopecia, pruritus, fever

HEMA: ***Agranulocytosis, thrombocytopenia, purpura***

EENT: Visual changes, sore throat, *double vision,* dry burning eyes

GU: Impotence, frequency

RESP: ***Bronchospasm,*** *dyspnea,* cough, rales

META: Hypoglycemia

MUSC: Joint pain, muscle pain

Contraindications: Hypersensitivity to β-blockers, cardiogenic shock, heart block (2nd or 3rd degree), sinus bradycardia, CHF, cardiac failure

Precautions: Major surgery, pregnancy (C), lactation, diabetes mellitus, renal disease, thyroid disease, COPD, well-compensated heart failure, CAD, nonallergic bronchospasm

Pharmacokinetics:

PO: Peak 2-4 hr; half-life 3-4 hr; excreted 30%-45% unchanged; 60%-65% metabolized by liver; excreted in urine, breast milk

Interactions:

• Increased hypotension, bradycardia: reserpine, hydralazine, methyldopa, prazosin, anticholinergics, alcohol, reserpine, nitrates

• Decreased antihypertensive effects: indomethacin, thyroid

• Increased hypoglycemic effects: insulin, sulfonylureas

• Decreased bronchodilation: theophyllines

Lab test interferences:

Increase: Liver function tests, renal function tests, K, uric acid

---

Decrease: Hct, Hgb, HDL

NURSING CONSIDERATIONS

Assess:

- I&O, weight qd
- B/P during initial treatment, periodically thereafter, pulse q4h; note rate, rhythm, quality
- Apical/radial pulse before administration; notify prescriber of any significant changes
- Baselines in renal, liver function tests before therapy begins
- Edema in feet, legs qd
- Skin turgor, dryness of mucous membranes for hydration status

Administer:

- PO ac, hs, tablet may be crushed or swallowed whole
- Reduced dosage in renal dysfunction

Perform/provide:

- Dry storage at room temp; do not freeze

Evaluate:

- Therapeutic response: decreased B/P after 1-2 wk

Teach patient/family:

- To take with or immediately after meals
- Not to discontinue drug abruptly; taper over 2 wk; may cause precipitate angina
- Not to use OTC products containing α-adrenergic stimulants (nasal decongestants, cold preparations) unless directed by prescriber
- To report bradycardia, dizziness, confusion, depression, fever, sore throat, shortness of breath to prescriber
- To take pulse at home; advise when to notify prescriber
- To avoid alcohol, smoking, sodium intake
- To comply with weight control, dietary adjustments, modified exercise program
- To carry Medic Alert ID to identify drug, allergies
- To avoid hazardous activities if dizziness is present
- To report symptoms of CHF: difficult breathing, especially on exertion or when lying down; night cough; swelling of extremities
- To take medication hs to minimize effect of orthostatic hypotension
- To wear support hose to minimize effects of orthostatic hypotension

Treatment of overdose: Lavage, IV atropine for bradycardia, IV theophylline for bronchospasm, digitalis, O_2, diuretic for cardiac failure, hemodialysis; administer vasopressor (norepinephrine)

---

tiopronin (℞)

(tye-o-pro′nen)
Thiola
Func. class.: Orphan drug
Chem. class.: Active reducing, complexing thiol compound

Action: Prevents cystine (kidney) stone formation by increasing amount of water-soluble cystine

Uses: Prevention of kidney stone formation in patients with severe homozygous cystinuria with urinary cystine greater than 500 mg/day, who are resistant to conservative treatment

Dosage and routes:

- *Adult:* **PO** 800-1000 mg/day, given in divided doses tid at least 1 hr before or 2 hr after meals
- *Child:* **PO** 15 mg/kg/day, given in divided doses tid at least 1 hr before or 2 hr after meals

Available forms: Tabs 100 mg

Side effects/adverse reactions:

MISC: Blunting of taste
INTEG: Erythema, maculopapular rash, wrinkling skin, lupuslike syn-

---

◆ = Nursing alert   ∥ = Herb-drug interaction   Ⓢ = Do not crush

drome (fever, arthralgia, lymphadenopathy), pruritus
CNS: Drug fever
META: Vit B$_6$ deficiency
Contraindications: History of agranulocytosis, thrombocytopenia, aplastic anemia
Precautions: Pregnancy (C), lactation, myasthenia gravis, Goodpasture's syndrome, children <9 yr
Pharmacokinetics: Reduction of urinary cystine of 250-500 mg on 1-2 g/day may be expected; excreted in urine 78% in 3 days
NURSING CONSIDERATIONS
Assess:
• I&O during treatment; check urine for stones; strain all urine, keep output at 2 L/day
• Diet for alkaline foods: dairy products; prevent overindulgence of Na, alkali foods, since hypercalcinuria results
• Urine pH; notify prescriber of pH over 7
• Urinary cystine 1 mo after treatment, q3mo thereafter
Administer:
PO
• After adequate hydration, conservative treatment: 3 L/day fluid, 16 oz fluid at meals and hs
Perform/provide:
• Storage at room temp
Evaluate:
• Therapeutic response: decrease in urinary cystine to <250 mg/L, absence of pain, hematuria
Teach patient/family:
• To watch for lupuslike syndrome: fever, joint pain, swollen lymph glands; drug may have to be discontinued

tizanidine
(ti-za'nih-deen)
Zanaflex
Func. class.: Skeletal muscle relaxant, α_2-adrenergic agonist
Chem. class.: Imidazoline

Action: Increases presynaptic inhibition of motor neurons and reduces spasticity by α_2-adrenergic agonism
Uses: Acute/intermittent management of increased muscle tone associated with spasticity
Dosage and routes:
• *Adult:* **PO** 4 mg, increase gradually by 2-4 mg increments, may repeat dose q6-8h, not to exceed 36 mg/24 hr
Available forms: Tabs 4 mg
Side effects/adverse reactions:
GI: Dry mouth, vomiting, increased ALT (SGPT), abnormal liver function studies, constipation
CNS: Somnolence, dizziness, speech disorder, dyskinesia, nervousness, hallucination, psychosis
OTHER: UTI, infection, blurred vision, urinary frequency, flu syndrome, pharyngitis, rhinitis
Contraindications: Hypersensitivity
Precautions: Hypotension, liver disease, pregnancy (C), lactation, elderly, children, renal disease
Pharmacokinetics: Completely absorbed, widely distributed; half-life 2.5 hr, peak 1½ hr; protein binding 30%; metabolized by liver, excreted in urine, feces
Interactions:
• Increased CNS depression: alcohol
• Decreased clearance of tizanidine: oral contraceptives

T

NURSING CONSIDERATIONS
Assess:
• For hypotension, gradual dosage increase should lessen hypotensive effects; have patient rise slowly from supine to upright; watch those patients receiving antihypertensives for increased effects
• For increased sedation, dizziness, hallucinations, psychosis; drug may need to be discontinued
• Vision by ophthalmic exam, corneal opacities may occur
• Liver function studies: 1, 3, 6 mo during treatment and periodically thereafter

Teach patient/family:
• To rise slowly from lying or sitting to upright position
• To ask for assistance if dizziness, sedation occur; to avoid drinking alcohol, to avoid operating machinery or driving until effects are known

---

tobramycin (℞)

(toe-bra-mye'sin)
Nebcin, tobramycin sulfate , Tobrax
Func. class.: Antiinfective
Chem. class.: Aminoglycoside

Action: Interferes with protein synthesis in bacterial cell by binding to ribosomal subunit, causing inaccurate peptide sequence to form in protein chain, causing bacterial death

Uses: Severe systemic infections of CNS, respiratory, GI, urinary tract, bone, skin, soft tissues caused by *P. aeruginosa, E. coli, Enterobacter, Providencia, Citrobacter, Staphylococcus, Proteus, Klebsiella, Serratia*

Dosage and routes:
• *Adult:* **IM/IV** 3 mg/kg/day in divided doses q8h; may give up to 5 mg/kg/day in divided doses q6-8h; once qd dosing is an option

• *Child:* **IM/IV** 6-7.5 mg/kg/day in 3-4 equal divided doses
• *Neonate <1 wk:* **IM** up to 4 mg/kg/day in divided doses q12h; **IV** up to 4 mg/kg/day in divided doses q12h diluted in 50-100 mg NS or D_5W; give over 30-60 min

Available forms: Inj 10, 40 mg/ml; powder for inj 1.2 g; inj 20 mg/2 ml

Side effects/adverse reactions:
GU: **Oliguria, hematuria, renal damage, azotemia, renal failure, nephrotoxicity**
CNS: Confusion, depression, numbness, tremors, **convulsions,** muscle twitching, **neurotoxicity,** dizziness, vertigo
EENT: **Ototoxicity,** deafness, visual disturbances, tinnitus
HEMA: **Agranulocytosis, thrombocytopenia, leukopenia, eosinophilia,** anemia
GI: Nausea, vomiting, anorexia; increased ALT (SGPT), AST (SGOT); bilirubin, hepatomegaly, **hepatic necrosis,** splenomegaly
CV: Hypotension, hypertension, palpitation
INTEG: Rash, burning, urticaria, dermatitis, alopecia

Contraindications: Severe renal disease, hypersensitivity to aminoglycosides

Precautions: Neonates, mild renal disease, pregnancy (C), myasthenia gravis, lactation, hearing deficits, Parkinson's disease, elderly

Pharmacokinetics:
IM: Onset rapid, peak 1 hr
IV: Onset immediate, peak 1 hr
Plasma half-life 2-3 hr prolonged in neonates; not metabolized, excreted unchanged in urine, crosses placental barrier, poor penetration into CSF

Interactions:
• Increased ototoxicity, neurotoxicity, nephrotoxicity: other aminoglycosides, amphotericin B, polymyxin, vancomycin, ethacrynic acid, furo-

---

semide, mannitol, methoxyflurane, cisplatin, cephalosporins, bacitracin, acyclovir, penicillins

NURSING CONSIDERATIONS
Assess:
• Weight before treatment; dosage is usually based on ideal body weight, but may be calculated on actual body weight
• I&O ratio, urinalysis qd for proteinuria, cells, casts; report sudden change in urine output
• VS during infusion; watch for hypotension, change in pulse
• IV site for thrombophlebitis, including pain, redness, swelling q30min; change site if needed; apply warm compresses to discontinued site
• Serum peak, drawn at 30-60 min after IV infusion or 60 min after IM injection, trough drawn just before next dose, peak 4-12 μg/ml, trough 1-2 μg/ml
• Urine pH if drug is used for UTI; urine should be kept alkaline
• Renal impairment by securing urine for CrCl testing, BUN, serum creatinine; lower dosage should be given in renal impairment (CrCl <80 ml/min); monitor electrolytes: potassium, sodium, chloride, magnesium monthly, if patient is on long-term therapy
• Deafness by audiometric testing; ringing, roaring in ears; vertigo; assess hearing before, during, after treatment
• Dehydration: high specific gravity, decrease in skin turgor, dry mucous membranes, dark urine
• Overgrowth of infection: fever, malaise, redness, pain, swelling, perineal itching, diarrhea, stomatitis, change in cough, sputum
• C&S before starting treatment to identify infecting organism

• Vestibular dysfunction: nausea, vomiting, dizziness, headache; drug should be discontinued if severe
• Inj sites for redness, swelling, abscesses; use warm compresses at site
Administer:
• IM inj in large muscle mass; rotate inj sites
• Drug in evenly spaced doses to maintain blood level; separate aminoglycosides and penicillins by ≥1 hr
• Bicarbonate to alkalinize urine if ordered in treating UTI, as drug is most active in an alkaline environment
IV
• Diluted in 50-100 ml NS or D$_5$W (adult), infuse over 20-60 min
Additive compatibilities: Aztreonam, bleomycin, calcium gluconate, cefoxitin, ciprofloxacin, clindamycin, furosemide, metronidazole, ofloxacin, ranitidine, verapamil
Syringe compatibilities: Doxapram
Y-site compatibilities: Acyclovir, amifostine, amiodarone, amsacrine, aztreonam, ciprofloxacin, cyclophosphamide, diltiazem, enalaprilat, esmolol, filgrastim, fluconazole, fludarabine, foscarnet, furosemide, granisetron, hydromorphone, IL-2, insulin (regular), labetalol, magnesium sulfate, melphalan, meperidine, midazolam, morphine, perphenazine, tacrolimus, teniposide, theophylline, thiotepa, tolazoline, vinorelbine, zidovudine
Perform/provide:
• Adequate fluids of 2-3 L/day unless contraindicated to prevent irritation of tubules
• Flush of IV line with NS or D$_5$W after infusion
• Supervised ambulation, other safety measures with vestibular dysfunction

T

Evaluate:
• Therapeutic response: absence of fever, draining wounds, negative C&S after treatment

Teach patient/family:
• To report headache, dizziness, symptoms of overgrowth of infection, renal impairment
• To report loss of hearing; ringing, roaring in ears; feeling of fullness in head

Treatment of overdose: Hemodialysis; monitor serum levels of drug

---

tocainide (R)

(toe-kay'nide)
Tonocard

Func. class.: Antidysrhythmic (Class Ib)
Chem. class.: Lidocaine analog

Action: Suppresses automaticity of tissue conduction and spontaneous depolarization of ventricles during diastole; does not affect heart rate

Uses: Life-threatening ventricular dysrhythmias (multifocal/unifocal PVCs), ventricular tachycardia

Dosage and routes:
• *Adult:* **PO** 600 mg loading dose, then 400 mg q8h

Available forms: Tabs 400, 600 mg

Side effects/adverse reactions:
CNS: Headache, dizziness, involuntary movement, confusion, psychosis, restlessness, irritability, paresthesias, tremors, *seizures*
EENT: Tinnitus, blurred vision, hearing loss
GI: Nausea, vomiting, anorexia, diarrhea, hepatitis
CV: Hypotension, bradycardia, angina, PVCs, *heart block, cardiovascular collapse, arrest, CHF,* chest pain, tachycardia, prodysrhythmia

RESP: Dyspnea, *respiratory depression, pulmonary fibrosis*
INTEG: Rash, urticaria, edema, swelling
HEMA: Blood dyscrasias: leukopenia, agranulocytosis, hypoplastic anemia, thrombocytopenia

Contraindications: Hypersensitivity to amides, severe heart block

Precautions: Pregnancy (C), lactation, children, renal disease, liver disease, CHF, respiratory depression, myasthenia gravis, blood dyscrasias

Pharmacokinetics:
PO: Peak 0.5-3 hr; half-life 10-17 hr; metabolized by liver, excreted in urine

Interactions:
• Increased effects: propranolol, quinidine, all other antidysrhythmics
• Decreased tocainide effects: cimetidine, rifampin
🥢 Potassium deficiency, antidysrhythmic action: aloe, buckthorn bark/berry, cascara sagrada bark, senna pod/leaf

Lab test interferences:
Increase: CPK
False positive: ANA titer

NURSING CONSIDERATIONS
Assess:
• Chest x-ray film, pulmonary function tests, liver enzymes during treatment
• CBC during beginning treatment
• I&O ratio; check for decreasing output
• Blood levels (therapeutic level 4-10 µg/ml)
• B/P continuously for fluctuations
• Lung fields; bilateral rales may occur in CHF patient
• Increased respiration, increased pulse; drug should be discontinued
• Toxicity: fine tremors, dizziness
• Blood dyscrasias: fatigue, sore throat, fever, bruising

◆ = Nursing alert   🥢 = Herb-drug interaction   🚫 = Do not crush

• Cardiac status, respiration: rate, rhythm, character
Evaluate:
• Therapeutic response: decreased dysrhythmia
Treatment of overdose: O_2, artificial ventilation, ECG; administer dopamine for circulatory depression, diazepam or thiopental for convulsions

---

tolazoline (℞)

(toe-laz′a-leen)
Priscoline
Func. class.: Peripheral vasodilator
Chem. class.: Imidazoline derivative

Action: Peripheral vasodilation occurs by direct relaxation on vascular smooth muscle; also has weak α- and β-adrenergic properties
Uses: Persistent pulmonary hypertension and hypoxic pulmonary hypertension of newborn
Dosage and routes:
• *Neonate:* **IV** 1-2 mg/kg via scalp vein; **IV INF** 1-2 mg/kg/hr
Available forms: Inj 25 mg/ml
Side effects/adverse reactions:
CV: Hypotension, tachycardia, dysrhythmias, hypertension, ***cardiovascular collapse***
*RESP: **Pulmonary hemorrhage***
GU: Edema, oliguria, hematuria
GI: Vomiting, diarrhea, peptic ulcer, ***GI hemorrhage, hepatitis***
INTEG: Flushing, tingling, rash, chills, sweating, increased pilomotor activity
*HEMA: **Thrombocytopenia, leukopenia***
Contraindications: Hypersensitivity, CVA, CAD
Precautions: Pregnancy (C), mitral stenosis

Pharmacokinetics:
IM/SC: Peak 30-60 min, duration 3-4 hr, excreted in urine, half-life 3-10 hr
Interactions:
• Increased effects with β-blockers, antihypertensives
• Decreased B/P, rebound hypertension: epinephrine
NURSING CONSIDERATIONS
Assess:
• ABGs, electrolytes, VS in newborn
• B/P, pulse during treatment until stable; take B/P lying; orthostatic hypotension is common
• Hepatic tests: AST, ALT, bilirubin; liver enzymes may increase
• Blood studies: CBC, platelets; watch for thrombocytopenia, agranulocytosis
• Hepatic involvement: vomiting, jaundice; drug should be discontinued
• For bleeding from GI tract: coffee grounds vomitus, increased pulse, pain in upper gastric area
• Affected areas for changes in temp, color
Administer:
IV
• Undiluted; give 10 mg or less over 1 min; in scalp vein may be diluted in D_5, D_5NS, LR, NS, ½NS, Ringer's sol; run over 1 hr
• Decreased dose for patients with low urine output (<1 ml/kg/h)
Additive compatibilities: Verapamil
Y-site compatibilities: Aminophylline, ampicillin, calcium gluconate, cefotaxime, cimetidine, dobutamine, dopamine, furosemide, gentamicin, phytonadione, sodium bicarbonate, tobramycin, vancomycin
Perform/provide:
• Dark storage at room temp
Evaluate:
• Therapeutic response: decrease in

T

---

pulmonary hypertension or pulse volume, increased temp in extremities

Teach patient/family:
• To report jaundice, dark urine, joint pain, fatigue, malaise, bruising, easy bleeding; may indicate blood dyscrasias

Treatment of overdose: Administer IV fluids, head-low position

---

tolbutamide (℞)

(tole-byoo′ta-mide)
Mobenol*, Novobutamide*, Orinase, tolbutamide, Tolbutone*

Func. class.: Antidiabetic
Chem. class.: Sulfonylurea (1st generation)

Action: Causes functioning β-cells in pancreas to release insulin, leading to drop in blood glucose levels; may improve binding to insulin receptors or increase the number of insulin receptors with prolonged administration; may also reduce basal hepatic secretion; not effective if patient lacks functioning β-cells

Uses: Type II (NIDDM) diabetes mellitus

Dosage and routes:
• *Adult:* **PO** 1-2 g/day in divided doses, titrated to patient response; **IV** 1 g (Fajans test)
• *Geriatric:* **PO** 250 mg qd-tid, titrate to desired dose

Available forms: Tabs 250, 500 mg scored; inj

Side effects/adverse reactions:
CNS: Headache, weakness, paresthesia, tinnitus, dizziness, vertigo
GI: Nausea, fullness, heartburn, *hepatotoxicity, cholestatic jaundice,* taste alteration, diarrhea
HEMA: Leukopenia, thrombocytopenia, agranulocytosis, aplastic anemia, increased AST (SGOT), ALT (SGPT), alk phosphatase
INTEG: Rash, allergic reactions, pruritus, urticaria, eczema, photosensitivity, erythema
ENDO: Hypoglycemia
MS: Joint pains

Contraindications: Hypersensitivity to sulfonylureas, juvenile or brittle diabetes

Precautions: Pregnancy (C), elderly, cardiac disease, thyroid disease, severe hypoglycemic reactions, renal disease, hepatic disease, lactation

Pharmacokinetics:
PO: Completely absorbed by GI route; onset 30-60 min, peak 3-5 hr, duration 6-12 hr; half-life 4-5 hr; metabolized in liver; excreted in urine (metabolites), breast milk; 90%-95% plasma protein bound

Interactions:
• Increased hypoglycemic reaction: oral anticoagulants, chloramphenicol, cimetidine, MAOIs, insulin, guanethidine, methyldopa, nonsteroidal antiinflammatories, salicylates, probenecid, sulfonamides, ranitidine
• Mask symptoms of hypoglycemia: β-blockers
• Decreased effects of both drugs: diazoxide
• Increased effects of tolbutamide: insulin, MAOIs
• Possible disulfiram-like reaction
• Decreased action of tolbutamide: calcium channel blockers, corticosteroids, oral contraceptives, thiazide diuretics, thyroid preparations, estrogens, phenobarbital, phenytoin, rifampin, phenothiazines, sympathomimetics

Lab test interferences:
Decrease: RAIU test
Interference: Urinary albumin

NURSING CONSIDERATIONS
Assess:
• Hypoglycemic, hyperglycemic reaction; can occur soon after meals
Administer:
PO
• Drug 30 min before meals
Perform/provide:
• Storage in tight container in cool environment
Evaluate:
• Therapeutic response: decrease in polyuria, polydipsia, polyphagia, clear sensorium, absence of dizziness, stable gait
Teach patient/family:
• To check for symptoms of cholestatic jaundice (dark urine, pruritus, yellow sclera); if these occur, prescriber should be notified
• To use a capillary blood glucose test while on this drug
• To test urine glucose levels with Chemstrip 3 × /day
• The symptoms of hypoglycemia, hyperglycemia, what to do about each; have glucagon emergency kit available
• That this drug must be taken daily; explain consequence of discontinuing drug abruptly
• To take drug in morning to prevent hypoglycemic reaction at night
• To avoid OTC medications and alcohol unless directed by prescriber; explain disulfiram-like reaction
• That diabetes is a lifelong illness; drug will not cure disease
• That all food in diet plan must be eaten to prevent hypoglycemia
• To carry a MedicAlert ID for emergency purposes
Treatment of overdose: 10%-50% glucose sol IV or 1 mg glucagon

---

tolmetin (℞)
(tole'met-in)
Tolectin DS, Tolectin 200, Tolectin 600, tolmetin sodium
Func. class.: Nonsteroidal antiinflammatory
Chem. class.: Pyrrole acetic acid derivative

Action: Inhibits prostaglandin synthesis by decreasing an enzyme needed for biosynthesis; analgesic, antiinflammatory, antipyretic
Uses: Mild to moderate pain, osteoarthritis, rheumatoid arthritis
Dosage and routes:
• *Adult:* **PO** 400 mg tid-qid, not to exceed 2 g/day
• *Child >2 yr:* **PO** 15-30 mg/kg/day in 3 or 4 divided doses
Available forms: Caps 400 mg; tabs 200, 600 mg
Side effects/adverse reactions:
GI: Nausea, anorexia, vomiting, diarrhea, jaundice, *cholestatic hepatitis,* constipation, flatulence, cramps, dry mouth, peptic ulcer, ulceration, bleeding, perforation
CNS: Dizziness, drowsiness, fatigue, tremors, confusion, insomnia, anxiety, depression, headache
CV: Tachycardia, peripheral edema, palpitations, dysrhythmias, hypertension
INTEG: Purpura, rash, pruritus, sweating
GU: Nephrotoxicity: dysuria, hematuria, oliguria, azotemia, pseudoproteinuria
HEMA: Blood dyscrasias
EENT: Tinnitus, hearing loss, blurred vision
Contraindications: Hypersensitivity, asthma, severe renal disease, severe hepatic disease, ulcer disease
Precautions: Pregnancy (B), lactation, children, bleeding disorders,

T

GI disorders, cardiac disorders, hypersensitivity to other antiinflammatory agents, peptic ulcer disease

Pharmacokinetics:
PO: Peak 2 hr, half-life 3-3½ hr; metabolized in liver, excreted in urine (metabolites), excreted in breast milk, 99% protein binding

Interactions:
• Increased action of warfarin, phenytoin, sulfonamides

NURSING CONSIDERATIONS
Assess:
• Renal, liver, blood studies: BUN, creatinine, AST (SGOT), ALT (SGPT), Hgb before treatment, periodically thereafter
• I&O ratio
• Audiometric, ophthalmic exam before, during, after treatment
• For eye, ear problems: blurred vision, tinnitus (may indicate toxicity)

Administer:
• With food to decrease GI symptoms; best to take on empty stomach to facilitate absorption; tab may be crushed

Perform/provide:
• Storage at room temp

Evaluate:
• Therapeutic response: decreased pain, stiffness, swelling in joints, ability to move more easily

Teach patient/family:
• To report blurred vision, ringing, roaring in ears (may indicate toxicity)
• To avoid driving, other hazardous activities if dizzy or drowsy
• To report change in urine pattern, weight increase, edema, pain increase in joints, fever, blood in urine (indicates nephrotoxicity)
• That therapeutic effects may take up to 1 mo
• To drink 8 glasses water daily
• About drug interactions

topiramate (℞)
(toh-pire'ah-mate)
Topamax
Func. class.: Anticonvulsant, miscellaneous
Chem. class.: Carbamate derivative

Action: Mechanism of action unknown; may prevent seizure spread as opposed to an elevation of seizure threshold

Uses: Partial seizures, with or without generalization in adults

Dosage and routes:
Renal dose
• CrCl <70 ml/min give ½ dose
Adjunctive therapy
• *Adult:* PO add 400 mg in 2 divided doses

Available forms: Tabs 25, 100, 200 mg

Side effects/adverse reactions:
RESP: URI, pharyngitis, sinusitis
EENT: Diplopia, vision abnormality
INTEG: Rash
MISC: Weight loss, leukopenia
CNS: Dizziness, fatigue, cognitive disorder, insomnia, anxiety, depression, paresthesia
ENDO: Weight loss
GI: Diarrhea, anorexia, nausea, dyspepsia, abdominal pain, constipation, dry mouth
GU: Breast pain, dysmenorrhea, menstrual disorder

Contraindications: Hypersensitivity

Precautions: Hepatic, renal, cardiac disease, elderly, lactation, children, pregnancy (C)

Pharmacokinetics: Well absorbed, terminal half-life 21 hr; excreted in urine (55%-97% unchanged), crosses placenta, excreted in breast milk, protein binding (9%-17%); steady state 4 days

Interactions:

- Decreased levels of: oral contraceptives, digoxin
- Increased levels of: alcohol, CNS depressants, carbonic anhydrase inhibitors
- Decreased levels of topiramate: food, phenytoin, carbamazepine, valproic acid

NURSING CONSIDERATIONS
Assess:

- Renal studies: urinalysis, BUN, urine creatinine q3mo
- Hepatic studies: ALT (SGPT), AST (SGOT), bilirubin
- CBC during long-term therapy
- Description of seizures
- Mental status: mood, sensorium, affect, behavioral changes; if mental status changes, notify prescriber
- Body weight, evidence of cognitive disorder

Administer:

- 🚫 Whole; do not break, crush, or chew tabs, very bitter
- May take with food

Perform/provide:

- Storage at room temp away from heat and light
- Assistance with ambulation during early part of treatment; dizziness occurs
- Seizure precautions: padded side rails, move objects that may harm patient

Evaluate:

- Therapeutic response: decreased seizure activity

Teach patient/family:

- To carry Medic Alert ID stating patient's name, drugs taken, condition, prescriber's name, phone number
- To avoid driving, other activities that require alertness
- Not to discontinue medication quickly after long-term use

Treatment of overdose: Lavage, VS

---

topotecan
(toh-poh-tee′kan)
Hycamtin
Func. class.: Antineoplastic hormone
Chem. class.: Semi-synthetic derivative of camptothecin (topoisomerase inhibitor)

Action: Antitumor drug with topoisomerase I-inhibitory activity topoisomerase I relieves torsional strain in DNA by causing single-strand breaks; causes double-strand DNA damage

Uses: Metastatic carcinoma of the ovary after failure of traditional chemotherapy

Dosage and routes:

- *Adult:* **IV INF** 1.5 mg/m^2 over 20 min qd × 5 days starting on day 1 of a 21-day course × 4 courses; may be reduced to 0.25 mg/m^2 for subsequent courses if severe neutropenia occurs

Available forms: Lyophilized powder for inj 4 mg (free base)

Side effects/adverse reactions:

HEMA: Neutropenia, leukopenia, thrombocytopenia, anemia, sepsis
GI: Abdominal pain, constipation, diarrhea, obstruction, nausea, stomatitis, vomiting; increased ALT, AST; anorexia
CNS: Arthralgia, asthenia, headache, myalgia, pain
RESP: Dyspnea
INTEG: Total alopecia

Contraindications: Hypersensitivity, lactation, severe bone marrow depression

Precautions: Children, pregnancy (C)

Interactions:

- Increased duration of neutropenia when used with: G-CSF

• Increased myelosuppression when used with: cisplatin

Pharmacokinetics: Rapidly and completely absorbed; excreted in urine and feces as metabolites; half-life 6 hr, geriatric half-life 8 hr; 94% bound to plasma proteins

NURSING CONSIDERATIONS
Assess:
• Liver function studies: AST (SGOT), ALT (SGPT), alk phosphatase, which may be elevated
• For CNS symptoms: drowsiness, confusion, depression, anxiety
• CBC, differential, platelet count weekly; withhold drug if WBC is <3500/mm^3 or platelet count is <100,000/mm^3; notify prescriber of these results; drug should be discontinued
• Buccal cavity q8h for dryness, sores or ulceration, white patches, oral pain, bleeding, dysphagia
• GI symptoms: frequency of stools, cramping
• Signs of dehydration: rapid respiration, poor skin turgor, decreased urine output, dry skin, restlessness, weakness

Perform/provide:
• Increased fluid intake to 2-3 L/day to prevent dehydration, unless contraindicated
• Changing of IV site q48h
• Rinsing of mouth tid-qid with water, club soda; brushing of teeth bid-tid with soft brush or cotton-tipped applicator for stomatitis; use unwaxed dental floss
• Nutritious diet with iron, vit K supplements, low fiber, few dairy products

Evaluate:
• Therapeutic response: decreased tumor size, spread of malignancy

Teach patient/family:
• To avoid foods with citric acid or hot or rough texture if stomatitis is present; to drink adequate fluids
• To report stomatitis; any bleeding, white spots, ulcerations in mouth; tell patient to examine mouth qd; report symptoms
• To report signs of anemia: fatigue, headache, faintness, shortness of breath, irritability
• To use contraception during therapy

---

toremifene (℞)
(tor-em'ih-feen)
Fareston
Func. class.: Antineoplastic
Chem. class.: Antiestrogen hormone

Action: Inhibits cell division by binding to cytoplasmic estrogen receptors; resembles normal cell complex but inhibits DNA synthesis and estrogen response of target tissue

Uses: Advanced breast carcinoma not responsive to other therapy in estrogen-receptor-positive patients (usually postmenopausal)

Dosage and routes:
• *Adult:* **PO** 60 mg qd
Available forms: Tabs 60 mg

Side effects/adverse reactions:
HEMA: **Thrombocytopenia, leukopenia**
GI: *Nausea, vomiting,* altered taste (anorexia)
GU: Vaginal bleeding, pruritus vulvae
INTEG: Rash, alopecia
CV: Chest pain
CNS: *Hot flashes, headache, lightheadedness,* depression
META: Hypercalcemia
EENT: Ocular lesions, retinopathy, corneal opacity, blurred vision (high doses)

Contraindications: Hypersensitivity, pregnancy (D)

◆ = Nursing alert   ✐ = Herb-drug interaction   ⊘ = Do not crush

Precautions: Leukopenia, thrombocytopenia, lactation, cataracts

Pharmacokinetics:

PO: Peak 3 hr, excreted primarily in feces

Lab test interferences:

Increase: Serum Ca

NURSING CONSIDERATIONS

Assess:

• CBC, differential, platelet count qwk; withhold drug if WBC is <3500 or platelet count is <100,000; notify prescriber

• Bleeding: hematuria, guaiac, bruising, petechiae, mucosa or orifices q8h

• Food preferences; list likes, dislikes

• Effects of alopecia on body image; discuss feelings about body changes

◆ Symptoms indicating severe allergic reactions: rash, pruritus, urticaria, purpuric skin lesions, itching, flushing

Administer:

• Antacid before oral agent; give drug after evening meal, before bedtime

• Antiemetic 30-60 min before giving drug to prevent vomiting

Perform/provide:

• Liquid diet, if needed, including cola, Jell-O; dry toast or crackers may be added if patient is not nauseated or vomiting

• Increase fluid intake to 2-3 L/day to prevent dehydration

• Nutritious diet with iron, vitamin supplements as ordered

• Storage in light-resistant container at room temp

Evaluate:

• Therapeutic response: decreased tumor size, spread of malignancy

Teach patient/family:

• To report any complaints, side effects to prescriber

• That vaginal bleeding, pruritus, hot flashes are reversible after discontinuing treatment

• To report immediately decreased visual acuity, which may be irreversible; stress need for routine eye exams; care providers should be told about tamoxifen therapy

• To report vaginal bleeding immediately

• That tumor flare—increase in size of tumor, increased bone pain—may occur and will subside rapidly; may take analgesics for pain

• That premenopausal women must use mechanical birth control because ovulation may be induced

• That hair may be lost during treatment; a wig or hairpiece may make patient feel better; new hair may be different in color, texture.

---

torsemide (℞)

(tor′suh-mide)

Demadex

Func. class.: Loop diuretic

Chem. class.: Sulfonamide derivative

Action: Acts on loop of Henle, proximal, distal tubule by inhibiting absorption of chloride, sodium, water

Uses: Treatment of hypertension and edema in CHF, hepatic disease, renal disease

Dosage and routes:

CHF

• *Adult:* **PO/IV** 10-20 mg/day, may increase as needed up to 200 mg/day

Chronic renal failure

• *Adult:* **PO/IV** 20 mg/day, may increase up to 200 mg/day

Hepatic cirrhosis

• *Adult:* **PO/IV** 5-10 mg/day may increase as needed up to 40 mg/day

Hypertension
• *Adult:* **PO** 5 mg/day may increase to 10 mg/day

Available forms: Tabs 5, 10, 20, 100 mg; 10 mg/ml vials of 2, 5 ml

Side effects/adverse reactions:

CNS: Headache, dizziness, asthenia, insomnia, nervousness

CV: Orthostatic hypotension, chest pain, ECG changes, *circulatory collapse,* ventricular tachycardia

EENT: Loss of hearing, ear pain, tinnitus, blurred vision

ENDO: Hyperglycemia, hyperuricemia

ELECT: Hypokalemia, hypochloremic alkalosis, hypomagnesemia, hypocalcemia, hyponatremia, metabolic alkalosis

GI: Nausea, diarrhea, dyspepsia, GI hemorrhage, rectal bleeding, cramps

GU: Polyuria, renal failure, glycosuria

INTEG: Rash, photosensitivity

MS: Cramps, stiffness

RESP: Rhinitis, cough increase

Contraindications: Hypersensitivity to sulfonamides, anuria, hypovolemia, infants, lactation, electrolyte depletion

Precautions: Diabetes mellitus, dehydration, severe renal disease, pregnancy (C)

Pharmacokinetics:

PO: Rapidly absorbed; duration 6 hr; excreted in urine, feces, breast milk; crosses placenta; half-life 2-4 hr, plasma protein binding 97%-99%

Interactions:
• Increased toxicity: lithium, nondepolarizing skeletal muscle relaxants, digitalis
• Increased action of antihypertensives, oral anticoagulants, nitrates
• Increased ototoxicity: aminoglycosides, cisplatin, vancomycin
• Decreased antihypertensive effect of torsemide: indomethacin, metolazone
• Incompatible with acidic sol, vit C, corticosteroids, diphenhydramine, dobutamine, esmolol, epinephrine, gentamicin, meperidine, milrinone, netilmicin, norepinephrine, reserpine, spironolactone, tetracyclines in sol
• Incompatible with any drug in syringe

Lab test interferences:
Interference: GTT

NURSING CONSIDERATIONS

Assess:
• Hearing when giving high doses
• Weight, I&O daily to determine fluid loss; effect of drug may be decreased if used qd
• Rate, depth, rhythm of respiration, effect of exertion
• B/P lying, standing; postural hypotension may occur
• Electrolytes: K, Na, Cl; include BUN, blood sugar, CBC, serum creatinine, blood pH, ABGs, uric acid, Ca, Mg
• Glucose in urine of diabetic
• Signs and symptoms of metabolic alkalosis: drowsiness, restlessness
• Signs and symptoms of hypokalemia: postural hypotension, malaise, fatigue, tachycardia, leg cramps, weakness
• Rashes, temp elevation qd
• Confusion, especially in elderly; take safety precautions if needed

Administer:
• In AM to avoid interference with sleep if using drug as a diuretic
• K replacement if K < 3 mg/dl
• With food if nausea occurs; absorption may be decreased slightly

Evaluate:
• Therapeutic response: improvement in edema of feet, legs, sacral area qd if medication is being used in CHF

 = Nursing alert   ⫸ = Herb-drug interaction   ⊘ = Do not crush

Teach patient/family:
• To rise slowly from lying, sitting position
• To recognize adverse reactions: muscle cramps, weakness, nausea, dizziness
• To take with food or milk for GI symptoms
• To take early in day to prevent nocturia

Treatment of overdose: Lavage if taken orally; monitor electrolytes, administer dextrose in saline; monitor hydration, CV, renal status

---

trace elements (R)

Concentrated Multiple Trace Elements, ConTE-PAK-4, M.T.E.-4, M.T.E.-4 Concentrated, M.T.E.-5, M.T.E.-5 Concentrated, M.T.E.-6, M.T.E.-6 Concentrated, M.T.E.-7, MulTE-PAK-4, MulTE-PAK-5, Multiple Trace Element, Multiple Trace Element Neonatal, Multiple Trace Element Pediatric, Neotrace 4, PedTE-PAK-4, Pedtrace-4, P.T.E.-4, P.T.E.-5

Func. class.: Mineral supplements

Action: Needed for adequate absorption and synthesis of amino acids
Uses: Prevention of trace element deficiency
Dosage and routes:
Usual dosage may be given in TPN sol
Chromium
• *Adult:* **IV** 10-15 µg qd
• *Child:* **IV** 0.14-0.20 µg/kg/day
Copper
• *Adult:* **IV** 0.5-1.5 mg/day
• *Child:* **IV** .05-0.2 mg/kg/day
Iodine
• *Adult:* **IV** 1 µg/kg/day

Manganese
• *Adult:* **IV** 1-3 mg/day
Selenium
• *Adult:* **IV** 40-120 µg/day
• *Child:* **IV** 3 µg/kg/day
Zinc
• *Adult:* **IV** 2-4 mg/day
• *Child:* **IV** 0.05 mg/kg/day
Available forms: Many forms available—see particular elements
Side effects/adverse reactions: Depends on element
Precautions: Liver, biliary disease, pregnancy (C), lactation, vomiting, diarrhea

NURSING CONSIDERATIONS
Assess:
• Trace element levels; notify prescriber if low; copper 0.07-0.15 mg/ml, zinc 0.05-0.15 mg/100 ml, manganese 4-20 µg/100 ml, selenium 0.1-0.19 µg/ml
• Trace element deficiency of patient receiving TPN for extended period
Administer:
• By IV infusion, often mixed with TPN solution
Evaluate:
• Therapeutic response: absence of element deficiency

---

tramadol (R)

(tram′a-dole)
Ultram
Func. class.: Central analgesic

T

Action: Not completely understood, binds to opioid receptors, inhibits reuptake of norepinephrine, serotonin; does not cause histamine release or affect heart rate
Uses: Management of moderate to severe pain
Dosage and routes:
Renal dose
• CrCl <30 ml/min give q12h, max 200 mg/day

• *Adult:* **PO** 50-100 mg prn q4-6h; not to exceed 400 mg/day
• *Elderly (>75 years):* **PO** <300 mg/day in divided doses
Hepatic impairment
• **PO** 50 mg q12h
Available forms: Tabs 50 mg
Side effects/adverse reactions:
CNS: Dizziness, CNS stimulation, somnolence, headache, anxiety, confusion, euphoria, *seizure,* hallucinations
GI: Nausea, constipation, vomiting, dry mouth, diarrhea, abdominal pain, anorexia, flatulence, *GI bleeding*
CV: Vasodilation, orthostatic hypotension, tachycardia, hypertension, abnormal ECG
INTEG: Pruritus, rash, urticaria, vesicles
GU: Urinary retention/frequency, menopausal symptoms, dysuria, menstrual disorder
Interactions:
• Decreased levels of tramadol: carbamazepine
• Inhibition of norepinephrine and serotonin reuptake: MAO inhibitors, use together with caution
• Increased CNS depression: alcohol, sedatives, hypnotics, opiates
⚘ Increased CNS depression: kava kava
Lab test interferences:
Increase: Creatinine, liver enzymes
Decrease: Hgb
Contraindications: Hypersensitivity, acute intoxication with any CNS depressant
Precautions: Seizure disorder, pregnancy (C), lactation, children, elderly, renal or hepatic disease, respiratory depression, head trauma, increased intracranial pressure, acute abdominal condition, drug abuse
Pharmacokinetics: Rapidly and almost completely absorbed, steady state 2 days, may cross blood-brain barrier, extensively metabolized, 30% excreted in the urine as unchanged drug

NURSING CONSIDERATIONS
Assess:
• Pain: location, type, character, give before pain becomes extreme
• I&O ratio: check for decreasing output; may indicate urinary retention
• Need for drug
• For constipation: increase fluids, bulk in diet
• CNS changes: dizziness, drowsiness, hallucinations, euphoria, LOC, pupil reaction
• Allergic reactions: rash, urticaria
Administer:
PO
• With antiemetic for nausea, vomiting
• When pain is beginning to return; determine dosage interval by patient response
Perform/provide:
• Storage in cool environment, protected from sunlight
• Assistance with ambulation
• Safety measures: side rails, nightlight, call bell within easy reach
Evaluate:
• Therapeutic response: decrease in pain
Teach patient/family:
• To report any symptoms of CNS changes, allergic reactions
• That drowsiness, dizziness, and confusion may occur, to call for assistance
• To make position changes slowly, orthostatic hypotension may occur
• To avoid OTC medications and alcohol unless approved by prescriber

---

➡ = Nursing alert   ⚘ = Herb-drug interaction   ⊘ = Do not crush

trandolapril (℞)
(tran-doe′la-prill)
Mavik
Func. class.: Antihypertensive
Chem. class.: Angiotension-converting enzyme inhibitor

Action: Selectively suppresses renin-angiotensin-aldosterone system; inhibits ACE; prevents conversion of angiotensin I to angiotensin II, dilates arterial and venous vessels, lowers B/P

Uses: Hypertension

Dosage and routes:
• *Adult:* PO 1 mg/day, 2 mg/day in African-Americans, make dosage adjustment ≥wk; up to 8 mg/day
Renal dose
• CrCl <30 ml/min give 0.5 mg/day, may increase gradually up to 4 mg/day

Available forms: Tabs 1, 2, 4 mg

Side effects/adverse reactions:
CV: Hypotension, MI, palpitations, angina, TIAs, ***stroke,*** bradycardia, dysrhythmias
CNS: Dizziness, paresthesias, headache, fatigue, drowsiness, depression, sleep disturbances
GI: Nausea, vomiting, cramps, diarrhea, constipation, ileus, pancreatitis, hepatitis
INTEG: Rash, purpura
*HEMA: **Agranulocytosis, neutropenia, leukopenia, anemia***
*GU: **Proteinuria, renal failure***
RESP: Dyspnea, cough
MISC: Hyperkalemia, hyponatremia, impotence

Contraindications: Hypersensitivity, history of angioedema, pregnancy (D) (2nd/3rd trimester)

Precautions: Renal disease, hyperkalemia, hepatic disease, bilateral renal stenosis, post kidney transplant, aorta/mitral value stenosis, cirrhosis, severe renal disease, untreated CHF, autoimmune disease, severe hypertension

Pharmacokinetics:
PO: Peak 4-10 hr; half-life 0.6-1.1 hr, 16-24 hr; metabolized by liver, excreted in urine

Interactions:
• Hypersensitivity: allopurinol
• Severe hypotension: diuretics, other antihypertensives
• Decreased effects of trandolapril: aspirin, antacids
• Increased K levels: salt substitutes, K-sparing diuretics, K supplements
• May increase effects of ergots, neuromuscular blocking agents, antihypertensives, hypoglycemics, barbiturates, reserpine, levodopa
• Effects may be increased by phenothiazines, diuretics, phenytoin, quinidine, nifedipine

NURSING CONSIDERATIONS
Assess:
• B/P, pulse q4h; note rate, rhythm, quality
• Electrolytes: K, Na, Cl
• Baselines in renal, liver function tests before therapy begins
• Edema in feet, legs daily
• Skin turgor, dryness of mucous membranes for hydration status
• Symptoms of CHF: edema, dyspnea, wet rales

Evaluate:
• Therapeutic response: decreased B/P

Teach patient/family:
• Not to use OTC (cough, cold, orallergy) products unless directed by prescriber
• To avoid sunlight or wear sunscreen for photosensitivity
• To comply with dosage schedule, even if feeling better
• To notify prescriber of mouth sores, sore throat, fever, swelling of

hands or feet, irregular heartbeat, chest pain, signs of angioedema
• That excessive perspiration, dehydration, vomiting, diarrhea may lead to fall in blood pressure; consult prescriber if these occur
• That drug may cause dizziness, fainting; light-headedness may occur during 1st few days of therapy
• That drug may cause skin rash or impaired perspiration
• Not to discontinue drug abruptly
• Not to use OTC products unless directed by prescriber
• To rise slowly to sitting or standing position to minimize orthostatic hypotension

---

tranylcypromine (℞)

(tran-ill-sip'roe-meen)
Parnate
Func. class.: Antidepressant-MAOI
Chem. class.: Nonhydrazine

Action: Increases concentrations of endogenous epinephrine, norepinephrine, serotonin, dopamine in storage sites in CNS by inhibition of MAO; increased concentration reduces depression

Uses: Depression, when uncontrolled by other means

Investigational uses: Bulimia, cocaine addiction, migraines, seasonal affective disorder, panic disorder

Dosage and routes:
• *Adult:* **PO** 10 mg bid; may increase to 30 mg/day after 2 wk; up to 60 mg/day

Available forms: Tabs 10 mg

Side effects/adverse reactions:
HEMA: Anemia
CNS: Dizziness, drowsiness, confusion, headache, anxiety, tremors, stimulation, weakness, hyperreflexia, mania, insomnia, fatigue, weight gain
GI: Constipation, dry mouth, nausea, vomiting, *anorexia,* diarrhea, weight gain
GU: Change in libido, urinary frequency
INTEG: Rash, flushing, increased perspiration
CV: Orthostatic hypotension, hypertension, dysrhythmias, hypertensive crisis
EENT: Blurred vision
*ENDO: **SIADH-like syndrome***
Contraindications: Hypersensitivity to MAOIs, elderly, hypertension, CHF, severe hepatic disease, pheochromocytoma, severe renal disease, severe cardiac disease
Precautions: Suicidal patients, convulsive disorders, severe depression, schizophrenia, hyperactivity, diabetes mellitus, pregnancy (C), lactation
Pharmacokinetics: Metabolized by liver, excreted by kidneys, crosses placenta, excreted in breast milk
Interactions:
• Increased pressor effects: guanethidine, clonidine, indirect-acting sympathomimetics (ephedrine), buspirone
• Increased effects of: direct-acting sympathomimetics (epinephrine), alcohol, barbiturates, benzodiazepines, CNS depressants, levodopa, beta blockers, antidiabetics, sulfonamide, rauwolfia alkaloids, methyldopa, L-tryptophan, thiazide diuretics, sumatriptan
• Serotonin-syndrome: fluoxetine, fluvoxamine, sertraline, paroxetine
• Hypertensive crisis: tricyclic antidepressants, meperidine, dibenzazepine agents, methylphenidate, dextromethorphan
🌿 Increased sympathomimetic action: ephedra
🌿 Increased B/P: Brewer's yeast

◆ = Nursing alert   🌿 = Herb-drug interaction   🚫 = Do not crush

NURSING CONSIDERATIONS
Assess:
• B/P (lying, standing), pulse; if systolic B/P drops 20 mm Hg, stop drug, notify prescriber
• Blood studies: CBC, leukocytes, cardiac enzymes (long-term therapy)
• Hepatic studies: ALT (SGPT), AST (SGOT), bilirubin; hepatotoxicity may occur
◆ Toxicity: increased headache, palpitation; discontinue drug immediately; prodromal signs of hypertensive crisis
• Mental status changes: mood, sensorium, affect, memory (long, short), increase in psychiatric symptoms
• Urinary retention, constipation, edema: take weight weekly
• Withdrawal symptoms: headache, nausea, vomiting, muscle pain, weakness

Administer:
• Increased fluids, bulk in diet if constipation occurs
• With food or milk for GI symptoms
• Crushed if patient is unable to swallow medication whole
• Dosage hs if oversedation occurs during day
• Gum, hard candy, frequent sips of water for dry mouth
• Phentolamine for severe hypertension

Perform/provide:
• Cool storage in tight container
• Assistance with ambulation during beginning therapy for drowsiness/dizziness
• Safety measures including side rails
• Checking to see if PO medication swallowed

Evaluate:
• Therapeutic response: decreased depression

Teach patient/family:
• That therapeutic effects may take 48 hr-3 wks
• To avoid driving, other activities requiring alertness
• To avoid alcohol ingestion, CNS depressants, OTC medications: cold, weight loss, hay fever, cough syrup
• Not to discontinue medication quickly after long-term use
• To avoid high-tyramine foods: cheese (aged), sour cream, yogurt, beer, wine, pickled products, liver, raisins, bananas, figs, avocados, meat tenderizers, chocolate, increased caffeine, ginseng
• To report headache, palpitation, neck stiffness

Treatment of overdose: Lavage, activated charcoal; monitor electrolytes, vital signs; diazepam IV, NaHCO₃

---

trazodone (℞)
(tray′zo-done)
Desyrel, Desyrel Dividose, trazodone HCl
Func. class.: Antidepressant, miscellaneous
Chem. class.: Triazolopyridine

Action: Selectively inhibits serotonin uptake by brain, potentiates behavorial changes

Uses: Depression

Investigational uses: Chronic pain syndromes

Dosage and routes:
• *Adult:* PO 150 mg/day in divided doses; may increase by 50 mg/day q3-4d, not to exceed 600 mg/day
• *Geriatric:* PO 25-50 mg hs, increase by 25-50 mg q3-7days to desired dose

Available forms: Tabs 50, 100, 150, 300 mg

Side effects/adverse reactions:

HEMA: **Agranulocytosis, thrombocytopenia, eosinophilia, leukopenia**

CNS: Dizziness, drowsiness, confusion, headache, anxiety, tremors, stimulation, weakness, insomnia, nightmares, EPS (elderly), increase in psychiatric symptoms

GI: Diarrhea, dry mouth, nausea, vomiting, **paralytic ileus,** increased appetite, cramps, epigastric distress, jaundice, **hepatitis,** stomatitis

GU: Retention, **acute renal failure, priapism**

INTEG: Rash, urticaria, sweating, pruritus, photosensitivity

CV: Orthostatic hypotension, ECG changes, tachycardia, **hypertension,** palpitations

EENT: Blurred vision, tinnitus, mydriasis

Contraindications: Hypersensitivity to tricyclic antidepressants, recovery phase of MI, convulsive disorders, prostatic hypertrophy

Precautions: Suicidal patients, severe depression, increased intraocular pressure, narrow-angle glaucoma, urinary retention, cardiac disease, hepatic disease, hyperthyroidism, electroshock therapy, elective surgery, pregnancy (C)

Pharmacokinetics: Metabolized by liver, excreted by kidneys, feces; half-life 4.4-7.5 hr

Interactions:

• Decreased effects of guanethidine, clonidine, indirect-acting sympathomimetics (ephedrine)

• Increased effects of direct-acting sympathomimetics (epinephrine), alcohol, barbiturates, benzodiazepines, CNS depressants

• Hyperpyretic crisis, convulsions, hypertensive episode: MAOI (pargyline [Eutonyl])

 Increased CNS depression: kava kava

Lab test interferences:

Increase: Serum bilirubin, blood glucose, alk phosphatase

False increase: Urinary catecholamines

Decrease: VMA, 5-HIAA

NURSING CONSIDERATIONS

Assess:

• B/P (lying, standing), pulse q4h; if systolic B/P drops 20 mm Hg, hold drug, notify prescriber; take vital signs q4h in patients with cardiovascular disease

• Blood studies: CBC, leukocytes, differential, cardiac enzymes if patient is receiving long-term therapy

• Hepatic studies: AST (SGOT), ALT (SGPT), bilirubin

• Weight qwk; appetite may increase with drug

• ECG for flattening of T wave, bundle branch block, AV block, dysrhythmias in cardiac patients

• EPS, primarily in elderly: rigidity, dystonia, akathisia

• Mental status changes: mood, sensorium, affect, suicidal tendencies, increase in psychiatric symptoms, depression, panic

• Urinary retention, constipation; constipation most likely in children

• Withdrawal symptoms: headache, nausea, vomiting, muscle pain, weakness; not usual unless drug discontinued abruptly

• Alcohol consumption; hold dose until morning

Administer:

• Increased fluids, bulk in diet if constipation occurs, especially in elderly

• With food, milk for GI symptoms

• Dosage hs for oversedation during day; may take entire dose hs; elderly may not tolerate qd dosing

• Gum, hard candy, frequent sips of water for dry mouth

◆ = Nursing alert   = Herb-drug interaction   ⃠ = Do not crush

Perform/provide:

• Storage in tight, light-resistant container at room temp

• Assistance with ambulation during beginning therapy for drowsiness/dizziness

• Safety measures, including side rails, primarily for elderly

• Checking to see if PO medication swallowed

Evaluate:

• Therapeutic response: decreased depression

Teach patient/family:

• That therapeutic effects may take 2-3 wk

• To use caution in driving, other activities requiring alertness because of drowsiness, dizziness, blurred vision

• To avoid alcohol ingestion, other CNS depressants

• Not to discontinue medication quickly after long-term use; may cause nausea, headache, malaise

• To wear sunscreen or large hat, since photosensitivity occurs

Treatment of overdose: ECG monitoring; induce emesis; lavage, activated charcoal; administer anticonvulsant

---

tretinoin (vit A acid, retinoic acid) (℞)

(tret'i-noyn)

Retin-A, Stievaa*, Vesanoid, Tretinoin LF, IV

Func. class.: Vit A acid, acne product; antineoplastic (misc.)

Chem. class.: Tretinoin derivative

Action: Decreases cohesiveness of follicular epithelium, decreases microcomedone formation (TOP); induces maturation of acute promyelocytic leukemia, exact action is unknown (PO)

Uses: Acne vulgaris (grades 1-3) (TOP); (PO) acute promyelocytic leukemia

Investigational uses: Skin cancer

Dosage and routes:

• *Adult and child:* **TOP** cleanse area, apply hs; cover lightly

Promyelocytic leukemia

• *Adult:* **PO** 45 mg/m^2/day given as 2 evenly divided doses until remission, discontinue treatment 30 days after remission or 90 days of treatment, whichever is first

Available forms: Cream 0.05%, 0.01%; gel 0.025%, 0.01%; liq 0.05%; caps 10 mg

Side effects/adverse reactions:

INTEG: (TOP) Rash, stinging, warmth, redness, erythema, blistering, crusting, peeling, contact dermatitis, hypopigmentation, hyperpigmentation

Oral

CNS: Headache, fever, sweating

*GI· Nausea, vomiting, **hemorrhage**, abdominal pain, diarrhea, constipation, dyspepsia, distention, hepatitis*

Contraindications: Hypersensitivity to retinoids or sensitivity to parabens, pregnancy (D)

Precautions: Lactation, eczema, sunburn

Pharmacokinetics:

TOP: Poor systemic absorption

Interactions:

• Increase peeling: medication containing agents such as sulfur, benzoyl peroxide, resorcinol, salicylic acid (top)

• Use with caution medicated, abrasive soaps, cleansers that have drying effect, products with high concentrations of alcohol astringents (top)

• Increased plasma concentrations of tretinoin: ketoconazole (oral)

NURSING CONSIDERATIONS
Assess:
Topical
• Area of body involved, what helps or aggravates condition; cysts, dryness, itching; lesions may worsen at beginning of treatment
Oral
• Liver function, coagulation, hematologic parameters, also cholesterol, triglyceride
Administer:
TOP
• Once daily before hs; cover area lightly using gauze; use gloves to apply
Perform/provide:
Topical
• Storage at room temp
• Hand washing after application
Evaluate:
• Therapeutic response: decrease in size and number of lesions
Teach patient/family:
Topical
• To avoid application on normal skin, getting cream in eyes, nose, other mucous membranes
• To avoid sunlight, sunlamps, or use protective clothing, sunscreen
• That treatment may cause warmth, stinging, dryness, peeling will occur
• That cosmetics may be used over drug; not to use shaving lotions
• That rash may occur during first 1-3 wk of therapy
• That drug does not cure condition; only relieves symptoms
• That therapeutic results may be seen in 2-3 wk but may not be optimal until after 6 wk

---

triamcinolone (℞)

(trye-am-sin′oh-lone)
Amcort, Aristocort, Aristocort Forte, Aristocort Intralesional, Aristospan Intra-Articular, Aristospan Intralesional, Articulose L.A., Atolone, Azmacort, Cenocort A-40, Cenocort Forte, Kenacort, Kenaject-40, Kenalog, Kenalog-10, Kenalog-40, Tac-3, Tac-40, Triam-A, triamcinolone, triamcinolone acetonide, Triam Forte, Triamolone 40, Triamonide 40, Tri-Kort, Trilog, Trilone, Trisoject

Func. class.: Corticosteroid
Chem. class.: Glucocorticoid, intermediate-acting

Action: Decreases inflammation by suppression of migration of polymorphonuclear leukocytes, fibroblasts, reversal to increase capillary permeability and lysosomal stabilization

Uses: Severe inflammation, immunosuppression, neoplasms, asthma (steroid dependent), collagen, respiratory, dermatologic disorders

Dosage and routes:
• *Adult:* **PO** 4-12 mg/day in divided doses qd-qid; **IM** 40 mg qwk (acetonide, or diacetate), 5-48 mg into neoplasms (diacetate, acetonide), 2-40 mg into joint or soft tissue (diacetate, acetonide), 0.5 mg/in^2 of affected intralesional skin (hexacetonide), 2-20 mg into joint or soft tissue (hexacetonide)
• *Child:* **PO** 117 µg/kg/day as a single or divided dose

Asthma
• *Adult:* **INH** 2 tid-qid, not to exceed 16 **INH**/day
• *Child 6-12 yr:* **INH** 1-2 tid-qid, not to exceed 12 **INH**/day

Available forms: Tabs 1, 2, 4, 8, 16

 = Nursing alert   = Herb-drug interaction   = Do not crush

mg; syr 2 mg/5 ml, 4.85 mg/5 ml; inj 25, 40 mg/ml diacetate; inj 3, 10, 40 mg/ml acetonide; inj 20, 5 mg/ml hexacetonide; aerosol actuation/100 μg (acetonide)

Side effects/adverse reactions:

INTEG: Acne, poor wound healing, ecchymosis, petcchiae

CNS: Depression, flushing, sweating, headache, mood changes

*CV: Hypertension, **circulatory collapse, thrombophlebitis, embolism,*** tachycardia, edema

*HEMA: **Thrombocytopenia***

MS: Fractures, osteoporosis, weakness

*GI: Diarrhea, nausea, abdominal distention, **GI hemorrhage,** increased appetite, **pancreatitis***

EENT: Fungal infections, increased intraocular pressure, blurred vision

Contraindications: Psychosis, hypersensitivity, idiopathic thrombocytopenia, acute glomerulonephritis, amebiasis, fungal infections, nonasthmatic bronchial disease, child <2 yr, AIDS, TB

Precautions: Pregnancy (C), diabetes mellitus, glaucoma, osteoporosis, seizure disorders, ulcerative colitis, CHF, myasthenia gravis, renal disease, esophagitis, peptic ulcer

Pharmacokinetics:

PO/IM: Peak 1-2 hr, half-life 2-5 hr

Interactions:

- Decreased action of triamcinolone: cholestyramine, colestipol, barbiturates, rifampin, ephedrine, phenytoin, theophylline
- Decreased effects of anticoagulants, anticonvulsants, antidiabetics, ambenonium, neostigmine, isoniazid, toxoids, vaccines, anticholinesterases, salicylates, somatrem
- Increased side effects: alcohol, salicylates, indomethacin, amphotericin B, digitalis, cyclosporine, diuretics

- Increased action of triamcinolone: salicylates, estrogens, indomethacin, oral contraceptives, ketoconazole, macrolide antibiotics

🖉 Increased potassium loss: aloe, buckthorn bark/berry, rhubarb root, senna leaf/fruits

Lab test interferences:

Increase: Cholesterol, Na, blood glucose, uric acid, Ca, urine glucose

Decrease: Ca, K, T_4, T_3, thyroid ^{131}I uptake test, urine 17-OHCS, 17-KS, PBI

False negative: Skin allergy tests

NURSING CONSIDERATIONS

Assess:

- K, blood sugar, urine glucose while on long-term therapy; hypokalemia and hyperglycemia
- Weight qd; notify prescriber if weekly gain >5 lb
- B/P q4h, pulse; notify prescriber if chest pain occurs
- I&O ratio; be alert for decreasing urinary output, increasing edema
- Plasma cortisol levels during long-term therapy (normal level: 138-635 nmol/L SI units when drawn at 8 AM)
- Infection: increased temp, WBC, even after withdrawal of medication; drug masks infection
- K depletion: paresthesias, fatigue, nausea, vomiting, depression, polyuria, dysrhythmias, weakness
- Edema, hypertension, cardiac symptoms
- Mental status: affect, mood, behavioral changes, aggression

Administer:

- After shaking susp (parenteral)
- Titrated dose; use lowest effective dose
- IM injection deep in large muscle mass; rotate sites; avoid deltoid; use 21G needle
- In one dose in AM to prevent adrenal suppression; avoid SC administration; may damage tissue

• With food or milk to decrease GI symptoms

Perform/provide:

• Assistance with ambulation for patient with bone tissue disease to prevent fractures

• Use of spacer device for elderly patients with inhaler

Evaluate:

• Therapeutic response: ease of respirations, decreased inflammation

Teach patient/family:

• That ID as steroid user should be carried

• To notify prescriber if therapeutic response decreases; dosage adjustment may be needed

• Not to discontinue abruptly; adrenal crisis can result

• To avoid OTC products: salicylates, alcohol in cough products, cold preparations unless directed by prescriber

• About cushingoid symptoms

• The symptoms of adrenal insufficiency: nausea, anorexia, fatigue, dizziness, dyspnea, weakness, joint pain

---

triamcinolone (topical-oral) (OTC)

(trye-am-sin'oh-lone)
Kenalog in Orabase, Oralone Dental

Func. class.: Topical anesthetic
Chem. class.: Synthetic fluorinated adrenal corticosteroid

Action: Inhibits nerve impulses from sensory nerves

Uses: Oral pain

Dosage and routes:

• *Adult and child:* **TOP** press ¼ inch into affected area until film appears, repeat bid-tid

Available forms: Paste 0.1%

Side effects/adverse reactions:
INTEG: Rash, irritation, sensitization

Contraindications: Hypersensitivity, infants <1 yr, application to large areas, presence of fungal, viral, or bacterial infections of mouth or throat

Precautions: Child <6 yr, sepsis, pregnancy (C), denuded skin

NURSING CONSIDERATIONS

Assess:

• Allergy: rash, irritation, reddening, swelling

• Infection: if affected area is infected, do not apply

Administer:

• After cleansing oral cavity

Evaluate:

• Therapeutic response: absence of pain in affected area

Teach patient/family:

• To report rash, irritation, redness, swelling

• How to apply paste

---

triamterene (℞)

(trye-am'ter-een)
Dyrenium

Func. class.: Potassium-sparing diuretic
Chem. class.: Pteridine derivative

Action: Acts on distal tubule to inhibit reabsorption of sodium, chloride; increase potassium retention

Uses: Edema, may be used with other diuretics; hypertension

Dosage and routes:

• *Adult:* **PO** 100 mg bid pc, not to exceed 300 mg/day

• *Geriatric:* **PO** 50 mg qd, max 100 mg/day

Available forms: Caps 50, 100 mg

Side effects/adverse reactions:
GI: Nausea, *diarrhea, vomiting,* dry mouth, jaundice, liver disease

---

ELECT: Hyperkalemia, hyponatremia, hypochloremia
CNS: Weakness, headache, dizziness, fatigue
INTEG: Photosensitivity, rash
HEMA: **Thrombocytopenia, megaloblastic anemia,** low folic acid levels
GU: **Azotemia, interstitial nephritis,** increased BUN, creatinine, renal stones, bluish discoloration of urine

Contraindications: Hypersensitivity, anuria, severe renal disease, severe hepatic disease, hyperkalemia, pregnancy (B), lactation

Precautions: Dehydration, hepatic disease, CHF, renal disease, cirrhosis

Pharmacokinetics:
PO: Onset 2 hr, peak 6-8 hr, duration 12-16 hr; half-life 3 hr; metabolized in liver, excreted in bile and urine

Interactions:
• Nephrotoxicity: indomethacin
• Enhanced action of antihypertensives, amantadine
• Increased hyperkalemia: other K-sparing diuretics, K products, ACE inhibitors, salt substitutes
• Decreased renal clearance of triamterene: cimetidine

Lab test interferences:
Interference: Quinidine serum levels, LDH

NURSING CONSIDERATIONS
Assess:
• Weight, I&O qd to determine fluid loss; effect of drug may be decreased if used qd
• Electrolytes: K, Na, Cl; include BUN, blood sugar, CBC, serum creatinine, blood pH, ABGs, liver function tests
• Improvement in CVP q8h
• Signs of metabolic acidosis: drowsiness, restlessness
• Rashes, temp qd

• Confusion, especially in elderly; take safety precautions if needed
• Hydration: skin turgor, thirst, dry mucous membranes

Administer:
• In AM to avoid interference with sleep
• With food if nausea occurs; absorption may be decreased slightly

Evaluate:
• Therapeutic response: improvement in edema of feet, legs, sacral area qd if medication is being used in CHF

Teach patient/family:
• To take medication after meals for GI upset
• To avoid prolonged exposure to sunlight; photosensitivity may occur; may turn urine blue
• To avoid foods high in K: oranges, bananas, salt substitutes, dried apricots, dates
• To notify prescriber of weakness, headache, nausea, vomiting, dry mouth, fever, sore throat, mouth sores, unusual bleeding or bruising

Treatment of overdose: Lavage if taken orally; monitor electrolytes; administer IV fluids, dialysis; monitor hydration, CV, renal status

---

triazolam (℞)

(trye-ay′zoe-lam)

Apo-Triazo*, Halcion, Novo-triolam*, Nu-Triazol*

Func. class.: Sedative-hypnotic
Chem. class.: Benzodiazepine

Controlled Substance Schedule IV (USA), Schedule F (Canada)

Action: Produces CNS depression at limbic, thalamic, hypothalamic levels of CNS; may be mediated by neurotransmitter γ-aminobutyric acid (GABA); results are sedation, hypnosis, skeletal muscle relaxation, anticonvulsant activity, anxiolytic action

Uses: Insomnia, sedative, hypnotic

Dosage and routes:

• *Adult:* PO 0.125-0.5 mg hs
• *Elderly:* PO 0.625-0.125 mg hs

Available forms: Tabs 0.125, 0.25 mg

Side effects/adverse reactions:

*HEMA: **Leukopenia, granulocytopenia** (rare)*

CNS: Headache, lethargy, drowsiness, daytime sedation, dizziness, confusion, light-headedness, anxiety, irritability, amnesia, poor coordination

GI: Nausea, vomiting, diarrhea, heartburn, abdominal pain, constipation

CV: Chest pain, pulse changes

Contraindications: Hypersensitivity to benzodiazepines, pregnancy (X), lactation, intermittent porphyria

Precautions: Anemia, hepatic disease, renal disease, suicidal individuals, drug abuse, elderly, psychosis, child <15 yr, acute narrow-angle glaucoma, seizure disorders

Pharmacokinetics:

PO: Onset 30-45 min, duration 6-8 hr; metabolized by liver, excreted by kidneys (inactive metabolites), crosses placenta, excreted in breast milk; half-life 2-3 hr

Interactions:

• Increased effects of cimetidine, disulfiram, erythromycin, macrolides, probenecid, isoniazid, oral contraceptives
• Increased action of both drugs: alcohol, CNS depressants
• Decreased effect of antacids, theophylline, rifampin, smoking
🌿 Increased CNS depression: kava kava

Lab test interferences:

Increase: ALT (SGPT), AST (SGOT), serum bilirubin

Decrease: RAI uptake

False increase: Urinary 17-OHCS

NURSING CONSIDERATIONS

Assess:

• Blood studies: Hct, Hgb, RBC if blood dyscrasias suspected (rare)
• Hepatic studies: AST (SGOT), ALT (SGPT), bilirubin if liver damage has occurred
• Mental status: mood, sensorium, affect, memory (long, short)
• Blood dyscrasias: fever, sore throat, bruising, rash, jaundice, epistaxis (rare)
• Type of sleep problem: falling asleep, staying asleep

Administer:

• After removal of cigarettes to prevent fires
• After trying conservative measures for insomnia
• ½ hr before hs for sleeplessness
• On empty stomach for fast onset, but may be taken with food if GI symptoms occur

Perform/provide:

• Assistance with ambulation after receiving dose
• Safety measures: side rails, night-light, call bell within easy reach
• Checking to see if PO medication has been swallowed
• Cool storage in tight container

Evaluate:

• Therapeutic response: ability to sleep at night, decreased amount of early morning awakening if taking drug for insomnia

Teach patient/family:

• That dependence is possible after long-term use
• To avoid driving, other activities requiring alertness until drug is stabilized
• To avoid alcohol ingestion, CNS depressants; serious CNS depression may result
• That effects may take 2 nights for

⬥ = Nursing alert   🌿 = Herb-drug interaction   🚫 = Do not crush

benefits to be noticed; for short-term use only

• Alternative measures to improve sleep: reading, exercise several hours before hs, warm bath, warm milk, TV, self-hypnosis, deep breathing

• That hangover is common in elderly but less common than with barbiturates; rebound insomnia may occur for 1-2 nights after discontinuing drug

Treatment of overdose: Lavage, activated charcoal; monitor electrolytes, VS

---

trientine (R)

(tri'en-teen)
Syprine

Func. class.: Heavy-metal antagonist

Chem. class.: Chelating agent (thiol compound)

Action: Binds with ions of lead, mercury, copper, iron, zinc to form a water-soluble complex excreted by kidneys

Uses: Wilson's disease

Dosage and routes:
• *Adult:* **PO** 750-2000 mg in divided doses bid-qid
• *Child:* **PO** 500-1500 mg in divided doses bid-qid

Available forms: Caps 125, 250 mg; tabs 250 mg

Side effects/adverse reactions:
HEMA: Anemia, *iron deficiency*
INTEG: Urticaria, fever
SYST: Hypersensitivity
GI: Epigastric distress, anorexia, heartburn

Contraindications: Hypersensitivity, cystinuria, rheumatoid arthritis, biliary cirrhosis

Precautions: Pregnancy (C), lactation, children, iron deficiency anemia

Pharmacokinetics:
PO: Peak 1 hr, metabolized in liver, excreted in urine

Interactions:
• Decreased action of trientine: mineral supplements

NURSING CONSIDERATIONS
Assess:
• Monitor hepatic, renal studies: ALT (SGPT), AST (SGOT), alk phosphatase, BUN, creatinine, serum copper level
• Monitor I&O
• For anemia: fatigue, Hct, Hgb
• Allergic reactions (rash, urticaria); drug should be discontinued

Administer:
• On an empty stomach, ½-1 hr before meals or 2 hr after meals
• Vit B$_6$ daily; depleted by this drug

Evaluate:
• Therapeutic response: improvement in neurologic, psychiatric symptoms

Teach patient/family:
• That therapeutic effect may take 1-3 mo or longer
• To report urticaria, fever, fatigue

---

trifluoperazine (R)

(trye-floo-oh-per'a-zeen)
Novoflurazine*, Solazine*, Stelazine, Suprazine, Terfluzine, trifluoperazine HCl, Triflurin

Func. class.: Antipsychotic, neuroleptic

Chem. class.: Phenothiazine, piperazine

Action: Depresses cerebral cortex, hypothalamus, limbic system, which control activity, aggression; blocks neurotransmission produced by dopamine at synapse; exhibits strong α-adrenergic, anticholinergic blocking action; mechanism for antipsychotic effects is unclear

Uses: Psychotic disorders, nonpsychotic anxiety, schizophrenia

Dosage and routes:

Psychotic disorders

• *Adult:* **PO** 2-5 mg bid, usual range 15-20 mg/day, may require 40 mg/day or more; **IM** 1-2 mg q4-6h

• *Geriatric:* **PO** 0.5-1 mg qd-bid, increase q4-7 days by 0.5-1 mg/day to desired dose

• *Child >6 yr:* **PO** 1 mg qd or bid; **IM** not recommended for children, but 1 mg may be given qd or bid

Nonpsychotic anxiety

• *Adult:* **PO** 1-2 mg bid, not to exceed 5 mg/day; do not give longer than 12 wk

Available forms: Tabs 1, 2, 5, 10 mg; conc 10 mg/ml; inj 2 mg/ml

Side effects/adverse reactions:

RESP: **Laryngospasm,** dyspnea, *respiratory depression*

CNS: EPS: pseudoparkinsonism, akathisia, dystonia, tardive dyskinesia, seizures, headache

HEMA: Anemia, **leukopenia, leukocytosis, agranulocytosis**

INTEG: Rash, photosensitivity, dermatitis

EENT: Blurred vision, glaucoma, dry eyes

GI: Dry mouth, nausea, vomiting, anorexia, constipation, diarrhea, jaundice, weight gain

GU: Urinary retention, urinary frequency, enuresis, impotence, amenorrhea, gynecomastia

CV: Orthostatic hypotension, hypertension, **cardiac arrest,** ECG changes, **tachycardia**

Contraindications: Hypersensitivity, cardiovascular disease, coma, blood dyscrasias, severe hepatic disease, child <6 yr, glaucoma

Precautions: Breast cancer, seizure disorders, pregnancy (C), lactation, diabetes mellitus, respiratory conditions, prostatic hypertrophy, elderly

Pharmacokinetics:

PO: Onset rapid, peak 2-3 hr, duration 12 hr

IM: Onset immediate, peak 1 hr, duration 12 hr

Metabolized by liver, excreted in urine, breast milk; crosses placenta

Interactions:

• Oversedation: other CNS depressants, alcohol, barbiturate anesthetics

• Toxicity: epinephrine

• Decreased absorption: aluminum hydroxide, magnesium hydroxide antacids

• Decreased effects of lithium, levodopa

• Increased effects of both drugs: β-adrenergic blockers, alcohol

• Increased anticholinergic effects: anticholinergics

�различ Increased CNS depression: kava kava

Lab test interferences:

Increase: Liver function tests, cardiac enzymes, cholesterol, blood glucose, prolactin, bilirubin, PBI, cholinesterase, ^{131}I

Decrease: Hormones (blood, urine)

False positive: Pregnancy tests, PKU

False negative: Urinary steroids, 17-OHCS, pregnancy tests

NURSING CONSIDERATIONS

Assess:

• Mental status before initial administration

• Swallowing of PO medication; check for hoarding or giving of medication to other patients

• I&O ratio; palpate bladder if low urinary output occurs

• Bilirubin, CBC, liver function studies qmo

• Urinalysis is recommended before and during prolonged therapy

---

➡ = Nursing alert   🌿 = Herb-drug interaction   🚫 = Do not crush

• Affect, orientation, LOC, reflexes, gait, coordination, sleep pattern disturbances

• For hypo-/hyperglycemia; appetite patterns

• B/P standing and lying; also include pulse, respirations q4h during initial treatment; establish baseline before starting treatment; report drops of 30 mm Hg

• Dizziness, faintness, palpitations, tachycardia on rising

• EPS including akathisia (inability to sit still, no pattern to movements), tardive dyskinesia (bizarre movements of jaw, mouth, tongue, extremities), pseudoparkinsonism (rigidity, tremors, pill rolling, shuffling gait)

• Skin turgor qd

• Constipation, urinary retention qd; if these occur increase bulk, water in diet

Administer:

• Reduced dose in elderly

• Antiparkinsonian agent on order from prescriber for EPS

PO

• Conc in 120 ml of tomato or fruit juice, milk, orange, carbonated beverage, coffee, tea, water, or semi-solid foods (soup, pudding)

Perform/provide:

• Decreased stimulus by dimming lights, avoiding loud noises

• Supervised ambulation until stabilized on medication if needed; do not involve in strenuous exercise program because fainting is possible; patient should not stand still for long periods

• Increased fluids and bulk in diet to prevent constipation

• Sips of water, candy, gum for dry mouth

• Storage in tight, light-resistant container, oral sol in amber bottles; slight yellowing of inj or conc is common, does not affect potency

Evaluate:

• Therapeutic response: decrease in emotional excitement, hallucinations, delusions, paranoia, reorganization of patterns of thought, speech

Teach patient/family:

• That orthostatic hypotension occurs frequently, and to rise from sitting or lying position gradually; avoid hazardous activities until stabilized on medication

• To remain lying down after IM injection for at least 30 min

• To avoid hot tubs, hot showers, tub baths; hypotension may occur

• To avoid abrupt withdrawal of this drug, or EPS may result; drug should be withdrawn slowly

• To avoid OTC preparations (cough, hay fever, cold) unless approved by prescriber, since serious drug interactions may occur; avoid use with alcohol, CNS depressants; increased drowsiness may occur

• To use a sunscreen

• About compliance with drug regimen

• About the necessity for meticulous oral hygiene; oral candidiasis may occur

• To report sore throat, malaise, fever, bleeding, mouth sores; CBC should be drawn and drug discontinued

• That in hot weather, heat stroke may occur; take extra precautions to stay cool

Treatment of overdose: Lavage if orally ingested; provide an airway; do not induce vomiting

T

---

triflupromazine (R_X)
(trye-floo-proe'ma-zeen)
Vesprin
Func. class.: Antipsychotic, neuroleptic
Chem. class.: Phenothiazine, aliphatic

Action: Depresses cerebral cortex, hypothalamus, limbic system, which control activity, aggression; blocks neurotransmission produced by dopamine at synapse; exhibits strong α-adrenergic, anticholinergic blocking action; mechanism for antipsychotic effects is unclear

Uses: Psychotic disorders, schizophrenia, acute agitation, nausea, vomiting

Dosage and routes:
Psychosis
• *Adult:* **PO** 10-50 mg bid-tid depending on severity of condition; dose is gradually increased to desired dose; **IM** 60 mg; not to exceed 150 mg/day
• *Child >2 yr:* **PO** 0.5-2 mg/kg/day in 3 divided doses; may increase to 10 mg if needed; **IM** 0.2 to 0.25 mg/kg to a maximum total dose of 10 mg/day
Nausea/vomiting
• *Adult:* **PO** 20-30 mg qd; **IV** 1-3 mg; **IM** 5-15 mg, q4h, max 60 mg qd
• *Child >2 yr:* **PO/IM** 0.2 mg/kg, max 10 mg qd
Acute agitation
• *Adult:* **IM** 60-150 mg/day in 3 divided doses
• *Child >2 yr:* **IM** 0.2-0.25 mg/kg/day in divided doses, max 10 mg qd
Available forms: Tabs 10, 25, 50 mg*; inj 10, 20 mg/ml

Side effects/adverse reactions:
RESP: ***Laryngospasm,*** dyspnea, *respiratory depression*

*CNS: EPS: pseudoparkinsonism, akathisia, dystonia, tardive dyskinesia; drowsiness, headache, **seizures***
HEMA: Anemia, ***leukopenia, leukocytosis, agranulocytosis***
INTEG: Rash, photosensitivity, dermatitis
EENT: Blurred vision, glaucoma
GI: Dry mouth, nausea, vomiting, anorexia, constipation, diarrhea, jaundice, weight gain
GU: Urinary retention, urinary frequency, enuresis, impotence, amenorrhea, gynecomastia
CV: Orthostatic hypotension, hypertension, ***cardiac arrest,*** ECG changes, ***tachycardia***

Contraindications: Hypersensitivity, blood dyscrasias, coma, child <2½ yr, brain damage, bone marrow depression

Precautions: Pregnancy (C), lactation, seizure disorders, hepatic disease, cardiac disease

Pharmacokinetics:
PO: Onset erratic, peak 2-4 hr, duration 4-6 hr
IM: Onset 15-30 min, peak 1 hr, duration 4-6 hr
Metabolized by liver, excreted in urine, breast milk; feces, crosses placenta

Interactions:
• Oversedation: other CNS depressants, alcohol, barbiturate anesthetics
• Toxicity: epinephrine
• Decreased absorption: aluminum hydroxide, magnesium hydroxide antacids
• Decreased effects of lithium, levodopa
• Increased effects of both drugs: β-adrenergic blockers, alcohol
• Increased anticholinergic effects: anticholinergics
 Increased CNS depression: kava kava

 = Nursing alert 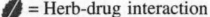 = Herb-drug interaction ⊘ = Do not crush

Lab test interferences:

Increase: Liver function tests, cardiac enzymes, cholesterol, blood glucose, prolactin, bilirubin, PBI, cholinesterase, ^{131}I

Decrease: Hormones (blood, urine)

False positive: Pregnancy tests, PKU

False negative: Urinary steroids, pregnancy tests

NURSING CONSIDERATIONS

Assess:

• Swallowing of PO medication; check for hoarding or giving of medication to other patients

• I&O ratio; palpate bladder if low urinary output occurs

• Bilirubin, CBC, liver function studies qmo

• Urinalysis is recommended before and during prolonged therapy

• Affect, orientation, LOC, reflexes, gait, coordination, sleep pattern disturbances

• B/P standing and lying; pulse, respirations q4h during initial treatment; establish baseline before starting treatment; report drops of 30 mm Hg

• For neuroleptic malignant syndrome: altered mental status, muscle rigidity, increased CPK, hyperthermia

• Dizziness, faintness, palpitations, tachycardia on rising

• EPS, including akathisia (inability to sit still, no pattern to movements), tardive dyskinesia (bizarre movements of jaw, mouth, tongue, extremities), pseudoparkinsonism (rigidity, tremors, pill rolling, shuffling gait)

• Assess for hypo-/hyperglycemia; appetite patterns

• Constipation, urinary retention qd; if these occur, increase bulk, water in the diet

Administer:

• Reduced dose to elderly

• Antiparkinsonian agent on order from prescriber for EPS

• IM inj into large muscle mass; avoid contact with skin

IV

• IV after diluting 10 mg/9 ml of NS; give 1 mg or less/2 min

Additive compatibilities: Meperidine, netilmicin

Syringe compatibilities: Glycopyrrolate

Perform/provide:

• Decreased stimulus by dimming lights, avoiding loud noises

• Supervised ambulation until stabilized on medication; do not involve in strenuous exercise program because fainting is possible; patient should not stand still for long periods

• Increased fluids to prevent constipation

• Sips of water, candy, gum for dry mouth

• Storage in tight, light-resistant container

Evaluate:

• Therapeutic response: decrease in emotional excitement, hallucinations, delusions, paranoia, reorganization of patterns of thought, speech

Teach patient/family:

• That orthostatic hypotension occurs frequently, and to rise from sitting or lying position gradually; to avoid hazardous activities until stabilized on medication

• To remain lying down for at least 30 min after IM inj

• To avoid hot tubs, hot showers, tub baths; hypotension may occur

• To avoid abrupt withdrawal; or EPS may result; drug should be withdrawn slowly

• To avoid OTC preparations (cough, hay fever, cold) unless approved by prescriber; serious drug interactions may occur; avoid use with alcohol,

T

CNS depressants; increased drowsiness may occur
• To use sunscreen
• About compliance with drug regimen
• About the necessity for meticulous oral hygiene, since oral candidiasis may occur
• To report sore throat, malaise, fever, bleeding, mouth sores; if these occur, CBC should be drawn and drug discontinued
• That in hot weather, heat stroke may occur; take extra precautions to stay cool

Treatment of overdose: Lavage if orally ingested; provide an airway; *do not induce vomiting*

---

trihexyphenidyl (℞)
(trye-hex-ee-fen'i-dill)
Artane, Artane Sequels, Novohexidyl*, Trihexane, Trihexy-2, Trihexy-5, trihexyphenidyl HCl
Func. class.: Cholinergic blocker
Chem. class.: Synthetic tertiary amine

Action: Blocks central muscarinic receptors, which decreases involuntary movements, sweating, salivation

Uses: Parkinson symptoms, drug-induced EPS

Dosage and routes:
Parkinson symptoms
• *Adult:* **PO** 1 mg, increased by 2 mg q3-5d to a total of 6-10 mg/day
Drug-induced EPS
• *Adult:* **PO** 1 mg/day; usual dose 5-15 mg/day
Available forms: Tabs 2, 5 mg; caps sus-rel 5 mg; elix 2 mg/5 ml

Side effects/adverse reactions:
CNS: Confusion, anxiety, restlessness, irritability, delusions, hallucinations, headache, sedation, depression, incoherence, dizziness, flushing, weakness
EENT: Blurred vision, photophobia, dilated pupils, difficulty swallowing, dry eyes, increased intraocular tension, angle-closure glaucoma
CV: Palpitations, tachycardia, postural hypotension
INTEG: Urticaria, rash
MISC: Suppression of lactation, nasal congestion, decreased sweating, increased temp, hyperthermia, heat stroke, numbness of fingers
MS: Weakness, cramping
GI: Dryness of mouth, constipation, nausea, vomiting, abdominal distress, ***paralytic ileus***
GU: Hesitancy, retention, dysuria

Contraindications: Hypersensitivity, narrow-angle glaucoma, myasthenia gravis, GI/GU obstruction, tachycardia, myocardial ischemia, unstable CV disease, prostatic hypertrophy

Precautions: Pregnancy (C), elderly, lactation, tachycardia, abdominal obstruction, infection, children, gastric ulcer

Pharmacokinetics:
PO: Onset 1 hr, peak 2-3 hr, duration 6-12 hr, excreted in urine

Interactions:
• Increased anticholinergic effects: antihistamines, phenothiazines, amantadine
• Decreased action of haloperidol

NURSING CONSIDERATIONS
Assess:
• I&O ratio; retention commonly causes decreased urinary output
• B/P, pulse frequently while dose is being determined
• Urinary hesitancy, retention; palpate bladder if retention occurs
• Constipation; increase fluids, bulk, exercise
• For tolerance over long-term therapy; dosage may have to be increased or medication changed

◆ = Nursing alert   ⏺ = Herb-drug interaction   ⊘ = Do not crush

- Mental status: affect, mood, CNS depression, worsening of mental symptoms during early therapy

Administer:
- With or after meals for GI upset; may give with fluids other than water
- At hs to avoid daytime drowsiness in patient with parkinsonism

Perform/provide:
- Storage at room temp in light-resistant container
- Hard candy, frequent drinks, sugarless gum to relieve dry mouth

Evaluate:
- Therapeutic response: parkinsonism: shuffling gait, muscle rigidity, involuntary movements

Teach patient/family:
- Not to discontinue this drug abruptly; to taper off over 1 wk
- To avoid driving, other hazardous activities; drowsiness may occur
- To avoid OTC medications: cough, cold preparations with alcohol, antihistamines unless directed by prescriber
- To avoid sudden position changes
- To avoid hot climates; overheating may occur

---

trimeprazine (℞)

(trye-mep'ra-zeen)

Panectyl*, Temaril

Func. class.: Antihistamine

Chem. class.: Phenothiazine analog, H₁-receptor antagonist

Action: Acts on blood vessels, GI, respiratory system by competing with histamine for H₁-receptor site; decreases allergic response by blocking histamine

Uses: Pruritus

Dosage and routes:
- *Adult:* PO 2.5 mg qid; **TIME-REL** 5 mg bid
- *Geriatric:* PO 2.5 mg bid
- *Child 3-12 yr:* PO 2.5 mg tid or hs
- *Child 6 mo-1 yr:* PO 1.25 mg tid or hs

Available forms: Tabs 2.5 mg; timerel spanules 5 mg; syr 2.5 mg/5 ml

Side effects/adverse reactions:

CNS: Dizziness, drowsiness, fatigue, anxiety, euphoria, confusion, paresthesia, neuritis, EPS (high doses)

CV: Hypotension, palpitations, tachycardia

RESP: Increased thick secretions, wheezing, chest tightness

HEMA: **Thrombocytopenia, agranulocytosis, hemolytic anemia**

GI: Dry mouth, nausea, vomiting, anorexia, constipation, diarrhea

INTEG: Rash, urticaria, photosensitivity

GU: Retention, dysuria, frequency

EENT: Blurred vision, dilated pupils, tinnitus, nasal stuffiness, dry nose, throat, mouth

Contraindications: Hypersensitivity to H₁-receptor antagonist, acute asthma attack, lower respiratory tract disease

Precautions: Increased intraocular pressure, renal disease, cardiac disease, hypertension, bronchial asthma, seizure disorder, stenosed peptic ulcers, hyperthyroidism, prostatic hypertrophy, bladder neck obstruction, pregnancy (C)

Interactions:
- Increased CNS depression: barbiturates, narcotics, hypnotics, tricyclic antidepressants, alcohol
- Decreased effect of oral anticoagulants, heparin
- Increased effect of trimeprazine: MAOIs
- Increased anticholinergic effect: henbane leaf

Lab test interferences:
False negative: Skin allergy tests

NURSING CONSIDERATIONS
Assess:

• I&O ratio; be alert for urinary retention, frequency, dysuria; drug should be discontinued

• CBC during long-term therapy; blood dyscrasias

• Respiratory status: rate, rhythm, increase in bronchial secretions, wheezing, chest tightness

• Cardiac status: palpitations, increased pulse, hypotension

• Mental status in elderly

Administer:

• Coffee, tea, cola (caffeine) to decrease drowsiness

• With meals for GI symptoms; absorption may slightly decrease

• Sus-rel formulation only to adults

Perform/provide:

• Hard candy, gum, frequent rinsing of mouth for dryness

• Storage in tight container at room temp

Evaluate:

• Therapeutic response: decreased itching associated with pruritus

Teach patient/family:

• To notify prescriber of confusion, sedation, hypotension

• To avoid driving, other hazardous activity if drowsiness occurs

• To avoid concurrent use of alcohol, other CNS depressants

Treatment of overdose: Administer ipecac syrup or lavage, diazepam, vasopressors, barbiturates (short-acting)

---

trimethadione (Ŗ)
(trye-meth-a-dye′one)
Tridione
Func. class.: Anticonvulsant
Chem. class.: Oxazolidinedione

Action: Decreases seizures in cortex, basal ganglia; decreases synaptic stimulation to low-frequency impulses

Uses: Refractory absence (petit mal) seizures

Dosage and routes:

• *Adult:* PO 300 mg tid, may increase by 300 mg/wk, not to exceed 600 mg qid

• *Child:* PO 20-50 mg/kg/day, in 3-4 divided doses

Available forms: Caps 300 mg; chew tabs 150 mg; sol 200 mg/5 ml; oral sol 40 mg/ml

Side effects/adverse reactions:

*HEMA: **Thrombocytopenia, agranulocytosis, leukopenia, neutropenia, hemolytic anemia,** increased protime, **eosinophilia, aplastic anemia***

CNS: Drowsiness, dizziness, fatigue, paresthesia, irritability, headache, insomnia, myasthenia gravis-like syndrome, precipitate tonic-clonic seizures

GU: Albuminuria, ***nephrosis,*** abdominal pain, weight loss

GI: Nausea, vomiting, bleeding gums, abnormal liver function tests

*INTEG: **Exfoliative dermatitis,*** rash, alopecia, petechiae, erythema

EENT: Photophobia, diplopia, epistaxis, retinal hemorrhage

CV: Hypertension, hypotension

Contraindications: Hypersensitivity, blood dyscrasias, pregnancy (D)

Precautions: Hepatic disease, renal disease

Pharmacokinetics:

PO: Peak 30 min-2 hr, excreted by kidneys, half-life 6-13 days

NURSING CONSIDERATIONS
Assess:

• Blood studies: Hct, Hgb, RBC, serum folate, vit D; hepatic studies: AST (SGOT), ALT (SGPT), bilirubin, creatinine; drug should be stopped if neutrophil count falls below 2500/mm^3 on long-term therapy

• Mental status: mood, sensorium, affect, memory (long, short)

- Rash, alopecia, convulsions; discontinue drug if these occur

Administer:
- After diluting oral sol with H_2O, give slowly through lavage needle
- Oral with juice or milk to cover taste/smell; decreases GI symptoms

Perform/provide:
- Ventilation of room

Evaluate:
- Therapeutic response: decreased seizures

Teach patient/family:
- To notify prescriber of skin rash, alopecia, sore throat, fever, bruising, epistaxis, or visual disturbances, particularly day blindness
- That physical dependency may result from extended use
- To avoid driving, other activities that require alertness
- Not to discontinue medication quickly after long-term use; convulsions may result
- That drug may take 1-4 wk to work; patient may still have seizures
- To report symptoms of renal damage: edema, urinary frequency, burning, cloudy urine

---

trimethobenzamide (℞)

(trye-meth-oh-ben′za-mide)
Arrestin, Benzacot, Brogan, Stemetic, T-Gen, Tebamide, Ticon, Tigan, Tiject-20, Triban, Trimazide, Trimethobenzamide, trimethobenzamide HCl

Func. class.: Antiemetic, anticholinergic

Chem. class.: Ethanolamine derivative

Action: Acts centrally by blocking chemoreceptor trigger zone, which in turn acts on vomiting center

Uses: Nausea, vomiting, prevention of postoperative vomiting

Dosage and routes:
Postoperative vomiting
- *Adult:* **IM/RECT** 200 mg before or during surgery; may repeat 3 hr after

Discontinuing anesthesia
- *Child 13-40 kg:* **PO/RECT** 100-200 mg tid-qid
- *Child <13 kg:* **PO/RECT** 100 mg tid-qid

Nausea/vomiting
- *Adult:* **PO** 250 mg tid-qid; **IM/RECT** 200 mg tid-qid

Available forms: Caps 100, 250 mg; supp 100, 200 mg; inj 100 mg/ml

Side effects/adverse reactions:
CNS: Drowsiness, restlessness, headache, dizziness, insomnia, confusion, nervousness, tingling, *vertigo,* EPS
GI: Nausea, anorexia, diarrhea, vomiting, constipation
CV: Hypertension, hypotension, palpitation
INTEG: Rash, urticaria, fever, chills, flushing
EENT: Dry mouth, blurred vision, diplopia, nasal congestion, photosensitivity

Contraindications: Hypersensitivity to narcotics, shock, children (parenterally)

Precautions: Children, cardiac dysrhythmias, elderly, asthma, pregnancy (C), prostatic hypertrophy, bladder-neck obstruction, narrow-angle glaucoma, stenosing peptic ulcer, pyloroduodenal obstruction

Pharmacokinetics:
PO: Onset 20-40 min, duration 3-4 hr
IM: Onset 15 min, duration 2-3 hr
Metabolized by liver, excreted by kidneys

Interactions:
- Increased effect: CNS depressants

T

• May mask ototoxic symptoms associated with antibiotics

NURSING CONSIDERATIONS
Assess:
• For nausea, vomiting before, after treatment
• VS, B/P; check patients with cardiac disease more often
• Signs of toxicity of other drugs or masking of symptoms of disease: brain tumor, intestinal obstruction
• Observe for drowsiness, dizziness

Administer:
• IM inj in large muscle mass; aspirate to avoid IV administration
• Tablets may be swallowed whole, chewed, allowed to dissolve

Syringe compatibilities: Glycopyrrolate, hydromorphone, midazolam, nalbuphine

Y-site compatibilities: Heparin, hydrocortisone, potassium chloride, vit B/C

Evaluate:
• Therapeutic response: decreased nausea, vomiting

Teach patient/family:
• To avoid hazardous activities, activities requiring alertness; dizziness may occur; to request assistance with ambulation
• To avoid alcohol, other depressants
• To keep out of children's reach

---

trimethoprim (℞)
(trye-meth′oh-prim)
Proloprim, Trimethoprim, Trimpex
Func. class.: Urinary antiinfective
Chem. class.: Folate antagonist

Action: Prevents bacterial synthesis by blocking enzyme reduction of dihydrofolic acid

Uses: *E.coli, P. mirabilis, Klebsiella, Enterobacter* UTIs

Dosage and routes:
Renal dose
• CrCl 15-30 ml/min 50 mg q12h; CrCl <15 ml/min avoid use
• *Adult:* **PO** 100 mg q12h × 10 days
• *Child:* 4 mg/kg/day divided q12h
Available forms: Tabs 100, 200 mg

Side effects/adverse reactions:
INTEG: **Exfoliative dermatitis,** pruritus, rash
HEMA: **Thrombocytopenia, leukopenia, neutropenia, megaloblastic anemia** (rare)
GI: Nausea, vomiting, abdominal pain, abnormal taste, increased AST (SGOT), ALT (SGPT), bilirubin, creatinine
CNS: Fever

Contraindications: Hypersensitivity, CrCl <15 ml/min, megaloblastic anemia

Precautions: Folate deficiency, pregnancy (C), lactation, fragile X chromosome, child <12 yr old, renal disease, hepatic disease

Pharmacokinetics:
PO: Peak 1-4 hr, half-life 8-11 hr; metabolized in liver, excreted in urine (unchanged 60%), breast milk; crosses placenta

Interactions:
• Increased action of phenytoin

NURSING CONSIDERATIONS
Assess:
• Nocturia; may indicate drug resistance
• Signs of infection, anemia
• AST (SGOT), ALT (SGPT), BUN, bilirubin, creatinine, urine cultures
• C&S; drug may be given as soon as culture is obtained
• Skin eruptions

Administer:
• With full glass of water

Perform/provide:
• Storage in tight, light-resistant container

◆ = Nursing alert   ⫽ = Herb-drug interaction   🚫 = Do not crush

- Adequate intake of fluids (2 L) to decrease bacteria in bladder

Evaluate:
- Therapeutic response: absence of pain in bladder area, negative C&S

Teach patient/family:
- All aspects of drug therapy: need to complete entire course of medication to ensure organism death (10-14 days); culture may be taken after completed course of medication
- That drug must be taken in equal intervals around clock to maintain blood levels
- To notify nurse of nausea, vomiting, rash, severe fatigue, sore throat

---

trimethoprim/ sulfamethoxazole (℞)

(trye-meth'oh prim)/sul-fa meth-ox'a-zole [ko-trye-mox'a-zole])
Apo-Sulfatrim*, Bactrim*, Bethaprim, Comoxol, Cotrim, Septra, Sulfatrim

Func. class.: Antiinfective
Chem. class.: Miscellaneous sulfonamide

Action: Sulfamethoxazole (SMZ) interferes with bacterial biosynthesis of proteins by competitive antagonism of PABA when adequate levels are maintained; trimethoprim (TMP) blocks synthesis of tetrahydrofolic acid; combination blocks 2 consecutive steps in bacterial synthesis of essential nucleic acids, protein

Uses: UTI, otitis media, acute and chronic prostatitis, shigellosis, *P. carinii* pneumonitis, chronic bronchitis, chancroid, traveler's diarrhea

Dosage and routes: Based on TMP content

UTI
- *Adult:* **PO** 160 mg TMP q12h × 10-14 days
- *Child:* **PO** 8 mg/kg TMP qd in 2 divided doses q12h

Otitis media
- *Child:* **PO** 8 mg/kg TMP qd in 2 divided doses q12h × 10 days

Chronic bronchitis
- *Adult:* **PO** 160 mg TMP q12h × 14 days

Pneumocystis carinii pneumonitis
- *Adult and child:* **PO** 20 mg/kg TMP qd in 4 divided doses q6h × 14 days; **IV** 15-20 mg/kg/day (based on TMP) in 3-4 divided doses for up to 14 days
- Dosage reduction necessary in moderate to severe renal impairment (CrCl <30 ml/min)

Available forms: Tabs 80 mg trimethoprim/400 mg sulfamethoxazole, 160 mg trimethoprim/800 mg sulfamethoxazole; susp 40 mg/200 mg/5 ml; IV 16 mg/80 mg/ml

Side effects/adverse reactions:
CNS: Headache, insomnia, hallucinations, depression, vertigo, fatigue, anxiety, convulsions, drug fever, chills, aseptic meningitis
CV: **Allergic myocarditis**
GI: *Nausea, vomiting, abdominal pain,* stomatitis, **hepatitis,** glossitis, pancreatitis, diarrhea, **enterocolitis,** anorexia
GU: **Renal failure, toxic nephrosis;** increased BUN, creatinine; crystalluria
HEMA: **Leukopenia, neutropenia, thrombocytopenia, agranulocytosis, hemolytic anemia, hypoprothrombinemia, Henoch-Schönlein purpura, methemoglobinemia, eosinophilia I**
INTEG: Rash, dermatitis, urticaria, **Stevens-Johnson syndrome,** erythema, photosensitivity, pain, inflammation at injection site

---

RESP: Cough, shortness of breath
SYST: **Anaphylaxis, SLE**

Contraindications: Hypersensitivity to trimethoprim or sulfonamides, pregnancy at term, megaloblastic anemia, infants <2 mo, CrCl <15 ml/min, lactation, porphyria

Precautions: Pregnancy (C), renal disease, elderly, G6PD deficiency, impaired hepatic/renal function, possible folate deficiency, severe allergy, bronchial asthma

Pharmacokinetics:

PO: Rapidly absorbed, peak 1-4 hr; half-life 8-13 hr, excreted in urine (metabolites and unchanged), breast milk; crosses placenta; 68% bound to plasma proteins; TMP achieves high levels in prostatic tissue and fluid

Interactions:

• Increased hypoglycemic response: sulfonylurea agents
• Increased anticoagulant effects: oral anticoagulants
• Decreased hepatic clearance of phenytoin
• Decreased response: cyclosporine
• Increased bone marrow depressant effects: methotrexate
• Thrombocytopenia: thiazide diuretics

Lab test interferences:

Increase: Alk phosphatase, creatinine, bilirubin

False positive: Urinary glucose test

NURSING CONSIDERATIONS

Assess:

• Allergic reactions: rash, fever (AIDS patients more susceptible)
• I&O ratio; note color, character, pH of urine if drug administered for UTI; output should be 800 ml less than intake; if urine is highly acidic, alkalization may be needed
• Kidney function studies: BUN, creatinine, urinalysis (long-term therapy)

• Type of infection; obtain C&S before starting therapy
• Blood dyscrasias, skin rash, fever, sore throat, bruising, bleeding, fatigue, joint pain
• Allergic reaction: rash, dermatitis, urticaria, pruritus, dyspnea, bronchospasm

Administer:

• With full glass of water to maintain adequate hydration; increase fluids to 2 L/day to decrease crystallization in kidneys
• Medication after C&S; repeat C&S after full course of medication
• After diluting 5 ml of drug/125 ml D_5W, run over 1-1½ hr
• With resuscitative equipment, epinephrine available; severe allergic reactions may occur

Syringe compatibilities: Heparin

Y-site compatibilities: Acyclovir, aldesleukin, allopurinol, amifostine, atracurium, aztreonam, cefepime, cyclophosphamide, diltiazem, enalaprilat, esmolol, filgrastim, fludarabine, gallium, granisetron, hydromorphone, labetalol, lorazepam, magnesium sulfate, melphalan, meperidine, morphine, pancuronium, perphenazine, piperacillin/tazobactam, sargramostim, tacrolimus, teniposide, thiotepa, vecuronium, zidovudine

Perform/provide:

• Storage in tight, light-resistant container at room temp

Evaluate:

• Therapeutic response: absence of pain, fever, C&S negative

Teach patient/family:

• To take each oral dose with full glass of water to prevent crystalluria; drink 8-10 glasses of water/day; to take on an empty stomach 1 hr ac, 2 hr pc
• To complete full course of treatment to prevent superinfection

---

◆ = Nursing alert   🖋 = Herb-drug interaction   🚫 = Do not crush

• To avoid sunlight or use sunscreen to prevent burns
• To avoid OTC medications (aspirin, vit C) unless directed by prescriber
• If diabetic, to use Clinistix or Tes-Tape
• To use alternative contraceptive measures; decreased effectiveness of oral contraceptives may result
• To notify prescriber if skin rash, sore throat, fever, mouth sores, unusual bruising, bleeding occur

---

trimetrexate (℞)

(tri-me-trex′ate)
Neutrexin
Func. class.: Antiinfective-misc.
Chem. class.: Nonclassical folic acid antagonist

Action: Inhibits an enzyme that reduces folic acid, which is needed for purine biosynthesis in all cells; result is disruption of RNA, DNA, cell death; leucovorin usually transported into cells by active, carrier-mediated process; however, *Pneumocystis carinii* organisms lack carrier system; trimetrexate must be given with leucovorin to protect normal cells

Uses: Moderate to severe *P. carinii* pneumonia as an alternative to TMP/SMZ; may be useful in treating non–small cell lung, prostate, colorectal cancer

Dosage and routes:

Leucovorin must be given concurrently and for 72 hr past last trimetrexate dose
• *Adult:* **IV** 45 mg/m² qd over 60-90 min; with leucovorin **IV** 20 mg/m² over 5-10 min q6h for a daily dose of 80 mg/m² or **PO** qid 20 mg/m² evenly spaced during the day; **PO** dose should be rounded to the next

higher 25 mg; course is trimetrexate 21 days, leucovorin 24 days; modifications in dose must be based on hematologic toxicity
Available forms: Powder for inj lyophilized 25 mg

Side effects/adverse reactions:
CNS: Confusion, fatigue, fever
GI: Nausea, vomiting, **hepatotoxicity,** ulcer, stomatitis
GU: Increased serum creatinine
HEMA: **Thrombocytopenia, anemia**
INTEG: Rash, pruritus
META: Hyponatremia, hypocalcemia

Contraindications: Hypersensitivity to trimetrexate, leucovorin, methotrexate, thrombocytopenia (<25,000/mm³), severe anemia, neutropenia (<500/mm³), pregnancy (D)

Precautions: Renal disease, hepatic disease, lactation, children, seizures

Pharmacokinetics

Terminal half-life 7-15 hr; may be 95%-98% protein bound

Interactions:
Specific interactions not known; these interactions may occur:
• Increased toxicity: aspirin, sulfa drugs, other antineoplastics, radiation
• Decreased effect of trimetrexate: erythromycin, ketoconazole, fluconazole, rifampin, rifabutin, cimetidine

NURSING CONSIDERATIONS
Assess:
• CBC, differential, platelet count qwk; withhold drug if neutrophils <500/mm³ or platelet count <25,000/mm³; notify prescriber; drug should be discontinued; hematologic toxicity should be graded 1-4, 4 most severe
• Renal function studies: BUN, serum uric acid, urine CrCl, electrolytes before, during therapy; treatment should be interrupted when creatinine >2.5 mg/dl

• I&O ratio; report urine output <30 ml/hr

• Monitor temp q4h; fever may indicate beginning infection; no rectal temps

• Liver function tests before, during therapy: bilirubin, alk phosphatase, AST (SGOT), ALT (SGPT); treatment should be interrupted when alk phosphatase or transaminase >5 × upper normal limit

• Bleeding time, coagulation time during treatment

Administer:

• Antiemetic 30-60 min before giving drug to prevent vomiting

• Topical or systemic analgesics for pain

• Transfusion for anemia

IV

• Reconstitute with 2 ml D_5 or sterile H_2O (12.5 mg/ml) filter 0.22 μ prior to dilution; dilute reconstituted sol with D_5 for concentration of 0.25-2 mg/ml; give over 60 min; flush IV line thoroughly with 10 ml D_5 before, after dose

• Trimetrexate and leucovorin sol separately; leucovorin may be given before or after trimetrexate; IV line must be flushed between infusions

• If trimetrexate comes in contact with skin, wash with soap, water immediately

Y-site compatibilities: Amifostine, zidovudine

Perform/provide:

• Strict medical asepsis and protective isolation if WBC levels low

• Liquid diet: carbonated beverage, Jell-O; dry toast, crackers may be added when patient is not nauseated or vomiting

• Rinsing of mouth tid-qid with water, club soda; brushing of teeth bid-tid with soft brush or cotton-tipped applicators for stomatitis; use unwaxed dental floss

• Nutritious diet with iron, vitamin supplements

• Storage after reconstitution up to 24 hr refrigerated; do not freeze reconstituted sol; discard after 24 hr

Evaluate:

• Therapeutic response: decreased symptoms of pneumocystis

• Bleeding: hematuria, guaiac, bruising or petechiae, mucosa or orifices q8h

• Food preferences; list likes, dislikes

• Hepatotoxicity: yellow skin, sclera; dark urine, clay-colored stools, pruritus, abdominal pain, fever, diarrhea

• Buccal cavity q8h for dryness, sores, ulceration, white patches, oral pain, bleeding, dysphagia

• Symptoms of severe allergic reaction: rash, urticaria, itching, flushing

Teach patient/family:

• About protective isolation

• To report any complaints, side effects to nurse or prescriber: black, tarry stools; chills, fever, sore throat, bleeding, bruising, cough, shortness of breath, dark or bloody urine

• To avoid foods with citric acid, hot or rough texture if stomatitis is present

• To report to prescriber stomatitis: any bleeding, white spots, ulcerations in mouth; to examine mouth qd, report symptoms to nurse

• To drink 10-12 glasses of fluid/day

• To avoid alcohol, salicylates

• To avoid use of razors, commercial mouthwash

◆ = Nursing alert   🖉 = Herb-drug interaction   ⊘ = Do not crush

trimipramine (℞)

(tri-mip'ra-meen)
Surmontil, Trimipramine Maleate, Trisoralen
Func. class.: Antidepressant—tricyclic
Chem. class.: Tertiary amine

Action: Selectively inhibits serotonin uptake by brain; potentiates behavioral changes

Uses: Depression, enuresis in children

Dosage and routes:
• *Adult:* **PO** 75 mg/day in divided doses, may be increased to 200 mg/day
• *Geriatric:* **PO** 25 mg hs, increase by 25 mg q3-7 days, max 100 mg/day
• *Child >6 yr:* 25 mg hs, may increase to 50 mg in child <12 yr or 75 mg in child >12 yr

Available forms: Caps 25, 50, 100 mg

Side effects/adverse reactions:
HEMA: Agranulocytosis, thrombocytopenia, eosinophilia, leukopenia
CNS: Dizziness, drowsiness, confusion, headache, anxiety, tremors, stimulation, weakness, insomnia, nightmares, EPS (elderly), increase in psychiatric symptoms
GI: Diarrhea, *dry mouth,* nausea, vomiting, *paralytic ileus,* increased appetite, cramps, epigastric distress, jaundice, *hepatitis,* stomatitis, *constipation*
GU: Retention, acute renal failure
INTEG: Rash, urticaria, sweating, pruritus, photosensitivity
CV: Orthostatic hypotension, ECG changes, tachycardia, hypertension, palpitations
EENT: Blurred vision, tinnitus, mydriasis

Contraindications: Hypersensitivity to tricyclic antidepressants, recovery phase of MI, convulsive disorders, prostatic hypertrophy
Precautions: Suicidal patients, severe depression, increased intraocular pressure, narrow-angle glaucoma, urinary retention, cardiac disease, hepatic disease, hyperthyroidism, electroshock therapy, elective surgery, pregnancy (C), elderly
Pharmacokinetics: Metabolized by liver, excreted by kidneys, steady state 2-6 days; half-life 7-30 hr
Interactions:
• Decreased effects of: guanethidine, clonidine, indirect-acting sympathomimetics (ephedrine)
• Increased effects of direct-acting sympathomimetics (epinephrine), alcohol, barbiturates, benzodiazepines, CNS depressants
• Hyperpyretic crisis, convulsions, hypertensive episode: MAOI (pargyline [Eutonyl])
⬤ Increased anticholinergic effect: belladonna leaf/root, henbane leaf
⬤ Increased antidepressant action: scopolia root

Lab test interferences:
Increase: Serum bilirubin, blood glucose, alk phosphatase
False increase: Urinary catecholamines
Decrease: VMA, 5-HIAA

NURSING CONSIDERATIONS
Assess:
• B/P (lying, standing), pulse q4h; if systolic B/P drops 20 mm Hg, hold drug, notify prescriber; take vital signs q4h in patients with cardiovascular disease
• Blood studies: CBC, leukocytes, differential, cardiac enzymes if patient is receiving long-term therapy
• Hepatic studies: AST (SGOT), ALT (SGPT), bilirubin, creatinine
• Weight qwk; appetite may increase with drug

T

• ECG for flattening of T wave, bundle branch block, AV block, dysrhythmias in cardiac patients
• EPS primarily in elderly: rigidity, dystonia, akathisia
• Mental status changes: mood, sensorium, affect, suicidal tendencies, increase in psychiatric symptoms, depression, panic
• Urinary retention, constipation; constipation is more likely to occur in children, elderly
• Withdrawal symptoms: headache, nausea, vomiting, muscle pain, weakness; not usual unless drug is discontinued abruptly
• Alcohol consumption; hold dose until morning

Administer:
• Increased fluids, bulk in diet for constipation, urinary retention
• With food, milk for GI symptoms
• Dosage hs for oversedation during day; may take entire dose hs; elderly may not tolerate once/day dosing
• Gum, hard candy, or frequent sips of water for dry mouth

Perform/provide:
• Storage in tight, light-resistant container at room temp
• Assistance with ambulation during beginning therapy for drowsiness/dizziness
• Safety measures, including side rails, primarily for elderly
• Checking to see if PO medication swallowed

Evaluate:
• Therapeutic response: decreased depression or enuresis

Teach patient/family:
• That therapeutic effects may take 2-3 wk
• To use caution in driving, other activities requiring alertness because of drowsiness, dizziness, blurred vision

• To avoid alcohol ingestion, other CNS depressants
• Not to discontinue medication quickly after long-term use; may cause nausea, headache, malaise
• To wear sunscreen or large hat, since photosensitivity occurs

Treatment of overdose: ECG monitoring; induce emesis; lavage, activated charcoal; administer anticonvulsant

---

tripelennamine (R)

(tri-pel-enn'a-meen)
PBZ, PBZ-SR, Pelamine, tripelennamine HCl
Func. class.: Antihistamine
Chem. class.: Ethylenediamine derivative

Action: Acts on blood vessels, GI, respiratory system by competing with histamine for H_1-receptor site; decreases allergic response by blocking histamine

Uses: Rhinitis, allergy symptoms

Dosage and routes:
• *Adult:* **PO** 25-50 mg q4-6h, not to exceed 600 mg/day; **TIME-REL** 100 mg bid-tid, not to exceed 600 mg/day
• *Child >5 yr:* **PO TIME-REL** 50 mg q8-12h, not to exceed 300 mg/day
• *Child <5 yr:* **PO** 5 mg/kg/day in 4-6 divided doses, not to exceed 300 mg/day

Available forms: Tabs 25, 50 mg; time-rel tabs 100 mg; elix 37.5 mg/5 ml

Side effects/adverse reactions:
CNS: Dizziness, drowsiness, poor coordination, fatigue, anxiety, euphoria, confusion, paresthesia, neuritis
CV: Hypotension, palpitations, tachycardia
RESP: Increased thick secretions, wheezing, chest tightness

◆ = Nursing alert   ✿ = Herb-drug interaction   ⊘ = Do not crush

*HEMA: **Thrombocytopenia, agranulocytosis, hemolytic anemia***
GI: Constipation, dry mouth, nausea, vomiting, anorexia, diarrhea
INTEG: Rash, urticaria, photosensitivity
GU: Retention, dysuria, frequency
EENT: Blurred vision, dilated pupils, tinnitus, nasal stuffiness, dry nose, throat, mouth
Contraindications: Hypersensitivity to H$_1$-receptor antagonist, acute asthma attack, lower respiratory tract disease
Precautions: Increased intraocular pressure, renal disease, cardiac disease, hypertension, bronchial asthma, seizure disorder, stenosed peptic ulcers, hyperthyroidism, prostatic hypertrophy, bladder neck obstruction, pregnancy (C)
Pharmacokinetics:
PO: Onset 15-30 min, duration 4-6 hr; detoxified in liver, excreted by kidneys
Interactions:
• Increased CNS depressants: barbiturates, narcotics, hypnotics, tricyclic antidepressants, alcohol
• Decreased effect of oral anticoagulants, heparin
• Increased effect of tripelennamine: MAOIs
⚫ Increased anticholinergic effect: henbane leaf
Lab test interferences:
False negative: Skin allergy test
False positive: Urine pregnancy tests
NURSING CONSIDERATIONS
Assess:
• I&O ratio; be alert for urinary retention, frequency, dysuria; drug should be discontinued
• CBC during long-term therapy; blood dyscrasias
• Respiratory status: rate, rhythm, increase in bronchial secretions, wheezing, chest tightness

• Cardiac status: palpitations, increased pulse, hypotension
Administer:
• With meals for GI symptoms; absorption may slightly decrease
Perform/provide:
• Hard candy, gum, frequent rinsing of mouth for dryness
• Storage in tight container at room temp
Evaluate:
• Therapeutic response: decrease in itching associated with pruritus
Teach patient/family:
• All aspects of drug use; to notify prescriber of confusion, sedation, hypotension
• To avoid driving, other hazardous activity if drowsiness occurs
• To avoid concurrent use of alcohol, other CNS depressants
Treatment of overdose: Administer ipecac syrup or lavage, diazepam, vasopressors, barbiturates (short-acting)

---

triprolidine (OTC, ℞)
(trye-proe'li-deen)
Actidil, Alleract, Myidil, triprolidine HCl
Func. class.: Antihistamine
Chem. class.: Alkylamine, H$_1$-receptor antagonist

Action: Acts on blood vessels, GI, respiratory system by competing with histamine for H$_1$-receptor site; decreases allergic response by blocking histamine
Uses: Rhinitis, allergy symptoms
Dosage and routes:
• *Adult:* **PO** 2.5 mg tid-qid
• *Child >6 yr:* **PO** 1.25 mg tid-qid
• *Child 4-6 yr:* **PO** 0.9 mg tid-qid
• *Child 2-4 yr:* **PO** 0.6 mg tid-qid
• *Child 4 mo-2 yr:* **PO** 0.3 mg tid-qid

Available forms: Tabs 2.5 mg; syr 1.25 mg/5 ml

Side effects/adverse reactions:

CNS: Dizziness, drowsiness, poor coordination, fatigue, anxiety, euphoria, confusion, paresthesia, neuritis

CV: Hypotension, palpitations, tachycardia

RESP: Increased thick secretions, wheezing, chest tightness

HEMA: Thrombocytopenia, agranulocytosis, hemolytic anemia

GI: Constipation, dry mouth, nausea, vomiting, anorexia, diarrhea

INTEG: Rash, urticaria, photosensitivity

GU: Retention, dysuria, frequency

EENT: Blurred vision, dilated pupils, tinnitus, nasal stuffiness, dry nose, throat, mouth

Contraindications: Hypersensitivity to H_1-receptor antagonist, acute asthma attack, lower respiratory tract disease

Precautions: Increased intraocular pressure, renal disease, cardiac disease, hypertension, bronchial asthma, seizure disorder, stenosed peptic ulcers, hyperthyroidism, prostatic hypertrophy, bladder neck obstruction, pregnancy (C)

Pharmacokinetics:

PO: Onset 20-60 min, duration 8-12 hr; detoxified in liver, excreted by kidneys (metabolites/free drug), half-life 20-24 hr

Interactions:

• Increased CNS depressants: barbiturates, narcotics, hypnotics, tricyclic antidepressants, alcohol

• Decreased effect of oral anticoagulants, heparin

• Increased effect of triprolidine: MAOIs

◗ Increased anticholinergic effect: henbane leaf

Lab test interferences:

False negative: Skin allergy tests

NURSING CONSIDERATIONS

Assess:

• I&O ratio; be alert for urinary retention, frequency, dysuria; drug should be discontinued

• CBC during long-term therapy; blood dyscrasias

• Respiratory status: rate, rhythm, increase in bronchial secretions, wheezing, chest tightness

• Cardiac status: palpitations, increased pulse, hypotension

Administer:

• With meals for GI symptoms; absorption may slightly decrease

Perform/provide:

• Hard candy, gum, frequent rinsing of mouth for dryness

• Storage in tight container at room temp

Evaluate:

• Therapeutic response: decreased itching associated with pruritus

Teach patient/family:

• All aspects of drug use; to notify prescriber of confusion, sedation, hypotension

• To avoid driving, other hazardous activity if drowsiness occurs

• To avoid concurrent use of alcohol, other CNS depressants

Treatment of overdose: Administer ipecac syrup or lavage, diazepam, vasopressors, barbiturates (short-acting)

---

troglitazone (℞)

(troh´glit-ah-zone)

Rezulin

Func. class.: Antidiabetic, oral

Chem. class.: Thiazolidinedione

Action: Improves insulin resistance

Uses: Stable adult-onset diabetes mellitus (type II) NIDDM, nondiabetic obese patients, polycystic ovary syndrome, Werner's syndrome

---

◆ = Nursing alert   ◗ = Herb-drug interaction   ⊘ = Do not crush

Dosage and routes:
• *Adult:* **PO** 200 mg bid
Available forms: Tabs 200, 300, 400 mg
Side effects/adverse reactions:
CV: Palpitations; increased LDH
GI: Nausea, vomiting, diarrhea, anorexia
HEMA: Decreased RBC, Hct, Hgb
INTEG: Rash
Contraindications: Hypersensitivity, diabetic ketoacidosis
Precautions: Pregnancy (C), elderly, thyroid disease, hepatic, renal disease
Pharmacokinetics: Maximal reductions in FBS after 6-12 wk
NURSING CONSIDERATIONS
Assess:
• For hypoglycemic reactions (sweating, weakness, dizziness, anxiety, tremors, hunger), hyperglycemic reactions soon after meals
• CBC (baseline, q3mo) during treatment; check liver function tests periodically AST (SGOT), LDH, renal studies: BUN, creatinine, urinary glucose
• FBS, glycosylated Hgb, fasting plasma insulin, plasma lipids/lipoproteins, B/P, body weight during treatment
Administer:
• Twice a day give with meals to decrease GI upset and provide best absorption
• Tabs crushed and mixed with food or fluids for patients with difficulty swallowing
Perform/provide:
• Conversion from other oral hypoglycemic agents; change may be made without gradual dosage change; monitor serum or urine glucose and ketones tid during conversion
• Storage in tight container in cool environment

Teach patient/family:
• To use capillary blood glucose test or Chemstrip tid; that periodic liver function testing is mandatory
• The symptoms of hypo/hyperglycemia, what to do about each
• That the drug must be continued on daily basis; explain consequence of discontinuing drug abruptly
• To avoid OTC medications unless approved by prescriber
• That diabetes is lifelong illness; that this drug is not a cure; only controls symptoms
• That all food included in diet plan must be eaten to prevent hypoglycemia
• To carry Medic Alert ID and glucagon emergency kit for emergencies
Evaluate:
• Therapeutic response: Decrease in polyuria, polydipsia, polyphagia, clear sensorium; absence of dizziness; stable gait, blood glucose at normal level

tromethamine (℞)
(troe-meth'a-meen)
Tham, Tham-E
Func. class.: Alkalinizer
Chem. class.: Amine

Action: Proton acceptor that corrects acidosis by combining with hydrogen ions to form bicarbonate and buffer; acts as diuretic (osmotic)
Uses: Acidosis (metabolic) associated with cardiac disease, COPD
Dosage and routes:
• *Adult:* **IV** 0.3 M required = kg of weight × HCO_3 deficit (mEq/L)
• *Child:* **IV** same as above given over 3-6 hr, not to exceed 40 ml/kg
Available forms: Inj 36 mg/ml, powder for inj 36 g

Side effects/adverse reactions:
CV: Irregular pulse, ***cardiac arrest***
META: Alkalosis, hypoglycemia
RESP: Shallow, slow respirations, cyanosis, ***apnea***
*GI: **Hepatic necrosis***
INTEG: Infection at injection site, extravasation, phlebitis
Contraindications: Hypersensitivity, anuria, uremia
Precautions: Severe respiratory disease/respiratory depression, pregnancy (C), cardiac edema, renal disease, infants
Pharmacokinetics:
IV: Excreted in urine
Interactions:
🍃 Decreased alkaline effect: oak bark
NURSING CONSIDERATIONS
Assess:
• Respiratory rate, rhythm, depth; notify prescriber of abnormalities that may indicate acidosis
• Electrolytes, blood glucose, chloride; CO_2, before, during treatment
• Urine pH, urinary output, urine glucose during beginning treatment
• I&O ratio, report large increase or decrease
• IV site for extravasation, phlebitis, thrombosis
• For signs of K^+ depletion
Administer:
• IV slowly to avoid pain at infusion site and toxicity
• IV undiluted as inf or added to priming fluid or ACD blood; give 5 ml or less/min
Evaluate:
• Therapeutic response: decreased metabolic acidosis
Teach patient/family:
• To increase K^+ in diet: bananas, oranges, cantaloupe, honeydew, spinach, potatoes, dried fruit

tubocurarine (℞)
(too-boe-kyoor-ar'een)
Tubarine*, Tubocuraine
Func. class.: Neuromuscular blocker
Chem. class.: Curare alkaloid

Action: Inhibits transmission of nerve impulses by binding with cholinergic receptor sites, antagonizing action of acetylcholine
Uses: Facilitation of endotracheal intubation, skeletal muscle relaxation during mechanical ventilation, surgery, or general anesthesia
Dosage and routes:
• *Adult:* **IV BOL** 0.4-0.5 mg/kg, then 0.08-0.10 mg/kg 20-45 min after 1st dose if needed for long procedures
Available forms: Inj 3 mg/ml, 20 U/ml
Side effects/adverse reactions:
CV: Bradycardia, tachycardia, increased, decreased B/P
*RESP: **Prolonged apnea, bronchospasm, cyanosis, respiratory depression***
EENT: Increased secretions
INTEG: Rash, flushing, pruritus, urticaria
Contraindications: Hypersensitivity
Precautions: Pregnancy (C), cardiac disease, lactation, children <2 yr, electrolyte imbalances, dehydration, neuromuscular disease, respiratory disease
Pharmacokinetics:
IV: Onset 15 sec, peak 2-3 min, duration ½-1½ hr; half-life 1-3 hr; degraded in liver, kidney (minimally); excreted in urine (unchanged) crosses placenta
Interactions:
• Increased neuromuscular blockade: aminoglycosides, clindamy-

---

◆ = Nursing alert   🍃 = Herb-drug interaction   🚫 = Do not crush

cin, lincomycin, quinidine, local anesthetics, polymyxin antibiotics, lithium, narcotic analgesics, thiazides, enflurane, isoflurane, trimethaphan, magnesium salts
• Dysrhythmias: theophylline

NURSING CONSIDERATIONS
Assess:
• For electrolyte imbalances (K, Mg); may lead to increased action of this drug
• Vital signs (B/P, pulse, respirations, airway) q15min until fully recovered; rate, depth, pattern of respirations, strength of hand grip
• I&O ratio; check for urinary retention, frequency, hesitancy
• Recovery: decreased paralysis of face, diaphragm, leg, arm, rest of body; allow to recover fully before completing neurologic assessment
• Allergic reactions: rash, fever, respiratory distress, pruritus; drug should be discontinued

Administer:
• With diazepam or morphine when used for therapeutic paralysis; provides no sedation alone
• Using nerve stimulator by anesthesiologist to determine neuromuscular blockade
• Anticholinesterase to reverse neuromuscular blockade
• IV undiluted 3 mg/ml; give single dose over 1-1½ sec by qualified person; diluted to 4 ml in NS given 0.5 ml/2 min for myasthenia testing

Solution compatibilities: D_5, $D_{10}W$, 0.9% NaCl, 0.45% NaCl, Ringer's, LR, dextrose/Ringer's or dextrose/LR combinations

Syringe compatibilities: Pentobarbital, thiopental

Perform/provide:
• Storage in light-resistant area; use only fresh sol
• Reassurance if communication is difficult during recovery from neuromuscular blockade

Evaluate:
• Therapeutic response: paralysis of jaw, eyelid, head, neck, rest of body
Treatment of overdose: Edrophonium or neostigmine, atropine, monitor VS; may require mechanical ventilation

---

urea (℞)
(yoor-ee′a)
Ureaphil, Carbamex*
Func. class.: Diuretic, osmotic
Chem. class.: Carbonic acid diamide salt

Action: Elevates plasma osmolality, increasing flow of water into plasma from ocular and cranial fluids
Uses: To decrease intracranial pressure, intraocular pressure
Dosage and routes:
• *Adult:* **IV** 1-1.5 g/kg of 30% sol over 1-3 hr, not to exceed 4 ml/min; do not exceed 120 g/day
• *Child >2 yr:* **IV** 0.5-1.5 g/kg, not to exceed 4 ml/min
• *Child <2 yr:* **IV** 0.1 g/kg, not to exceed 4 ml/min
Available forms: Inj 40 g/150 ml
Side effects/adverse reactions:
CNS: Dizziness, disorientation, fever, syncope, *headache*
GI: Nausea, vomiting
INTEG: Venous thrombosis, phlebitis, extravasation
Contraindications: Severe renal disease, active intracranial bleeding, marked dehydration, liver failure
Precautions: Hepatic disease, renal disease, pregnancy (C), electrolyte imbalances, lactation
Pharmacokinetics:
IV: Onset ½-1 hr, peak 1 hr, duration 3-10 hr (diuresis), 5-6 hr (intraocu-

U

lar pressure); half-life 1 hr; excreted in urine, breast milk; crosses placenta

Interactions:
• Incompatible with whole blood, alkalies in sol or syringe
• Increased renal excretion of lithium

NURSING CONSIDERATIONS

Assess:
• Weight, I&O qd to determine fluid loss; effect of drug may be decreased if used qd; for hourly urinary output
• Rate, depth, rhythm of respiration, effect of exertion
• B/P lying, standing, postural hypotension may occur
• Electrolytes: K, Na, Cl; include BUN, blood sugar, CBC, serum creatinine, blood pH, ABGs, liver function tests
• Fever, signs of extravasation
• Confusion, especially in elderly; take safety precautions if needed
• Hydration: skin turgor, thirst, dry mucous membranes

Administer:
• IV after diluting 30 g/100 ml diluent with D$_5$, D$_{10}$; run 30% sol over 1-2 hr; check for extravasation; do not exceed 4 ml/min; may cause bleeding; use IV filter
• Within minutes of reconstitution; sol becomes ammonia on standing

Evaluate:
• Therapeutic response: improvement in edema of feet, legs, sacral area daily in CHF

Teach patient/family:
• That drug will cause diuresis in ½ hr

Treatment of overdose: Lavage if taken orally; monitor electrolytes, administer IV fluids, monitor BUN, hydration, CV status

---

urofollitropin (R)
(yoor-o-foll'ee-troh-pin)
Fertinex, Metrodin
Func. class.: Ovulation stimulant
Chem. class.: Gonadotropin

Action: Stimulates ovarian follicular growth in primary ovarian failure

Uses: Induction of ovulation in polycystic ovarian disease in those who have elevated LH/FSH ratios and do not respond to other treatment, assisted reproductive technologies (in vitro fertilization)

Dosage and routes:
• *Adult:* **IM** 75 IU/day × 7-12 days, then 5000-10,000 U HCG 1 day after last urofollitropin if pregnancy does not occur; may repeat for 2 courses before increasing dose to 150 IU/day 7-12 days then 5000-10,000 U HCG 1 day after last urofollitropin; may repeat for 2 more courses
• *Adult:* **SC** (Fertinex) used in combination with HCG

Available forms: Powder for injection 0.83 mg (76 IU FSH)/ampule, 1.66 mg (150 IU FSH)/ampule

Side effects/adverse reactions:
CNS: Malaise
GI: Nausea, vomiting, constipation, increased appetite, abdominal pain
INTEG: Rash, dermatitis, urticaria, alopecia
GU: Polyuria, frequency, birth defects, spontaneous abortions, multiple ovulation, breast pain

Contraindications: Hypersensitivity, pregnancy (X), undiagnosed vaginal bleeding, intracranial lesion, ovarian cyst not caused by polycystic ovarian disease

Precautions: Lactation, arterial thromboembolism

 = Nursing alert   = Herb-drug interaction   = Do not crush

Pharmacokinetics: Detoxified in liver, excreted in feces, stored in fat

NURSING CONSIDERATIONS

Assess:

• At same time qd to maintain drug level

Administer:

• After dissolving contents of ampule in 1-2 ml of sterile saline, give immediately, discard unused portion

Evaluate:

• Therapeutic response: ovulation, pregnancy

Teach patient/family:

• That multiple births are common after taking this drug

• To notify prescriber of low abdominal pain; may indicate ovarian cyst, cyst rupture

• The correct method of taking, recording basal body temp to determine whether ovulation has occurred

• That if ovulation can be determined (there is a slight decrease, then a sharp increase for ovulation), to attempt coitus 3 days before and qod until after ovulation

• That if pregnancy is suspected, notify prescriber immediately

---

urokinase (℞)

(yoor-oh-kin'ase)

Abbokinase, Abbokinase Open-Cath

Func. class.: Thrombolytic enzyme

Chem. class.: β-Hemolytic streptococcus filtrate (purified)

Action: Promotes thrombolysis by directly converting plasminogen to plasmin

Uses: Venous thrombosis, pulmonary embolism, arterial thrombosis, arterial embolism, arteriovenous cannula occlusion, lysis of coronary artery thrombi after MI

Dosage and routes:

Lysis of pulmonary emboli

• *Adult and child:* IV 4400 IU/kg/hr × 12-24 hr, not to exceed 200 ml; then IV heparin, then anticoagulants

Coronary artery thrombosis

• *Adult:* INSTILL 6000 IU/min into occluded artery for 1-2 hr after giving IV BOL of heparin 2500-10,000 U

• May also give as IV INF 2 million-3 million U over 45-90 min

Venous catheter occlusion

• *Adult and child:* INSTILL 5000 IU into line, wait 5 min, then aspirate, repeat aspiration attempts q5min × ½ hr; if occlusion has not been removed, cap line and wait ½-1 hr, then aspirate; may need 2nd dose if still occluded

Available forms: Powder for inj, lyophilized; 250,000 IU/vial; powder for catheter clearance

Side effects/adverse reactions:

HEMA: Decreased Hct, **bleeding**

INTEG: Rash, urticaria, phlebitis at IV infusion site, itching, flushing

CNS: Headache, fever

GI: Nausea, vomiting

RESP: Altered respirations, SOB, **bronchospasm,** cyanosis

MS: Low back pain

CV: Hypertension, dysrhythmias

EENT: Periorbital edema

SYST: **GI, GU, intracranial, retroperitoneal bleeding,** surface bleeding, **anaphylaxis** (rare)

Contraindications: Hypersensitivity, active bleeding, intraspinal surgery, neoplasms of CNS, ulcerative colitis/enteritis, severe hypertension, renal disease, hepatic disease, hypocoagulation, COPD, subacute bacterial endocarditis, rheumatic valvular disease, cerebral embolism/thrombosis/hemorrhage, intraarterial diagnostic procedure or surgery (10 days), recent major surgery

U

Precautions: Arterial emboli from left side of heart, pregnancy (B)

Pharmacokinetics:

IV: Half-life 10-20 min; small amounts excreted in urine

Interactions:

• Bleeding potential: aspirin, indomethacin, phenylbutazone, anticoagulants

Lab test interferences:

Increase: PT, APTT, TT

NURSING CONSIDERATIONS
Assess:

• VS, B/P, pulse, resp, neurologic signs, temp at least q4h; temp >104° F (40° C) is an indicator of internal bleeding; cardiac rhythm following intracoronary administration

• For neurologic changes that may indicate intracranial bleeding

• Retroperitoneal bleeding: back pain, leg weakness, diminished pulses

• Peripheral pulses, lung sounds, respiratory function

• Allergy: fever, rash, itching, chills; mild reaction may be treated with antihistamines

• Bleeding during 1st hr of treatment (hematuria, hematemesis, bleeding from mucous membranes, epistaxis, ecchymosis)

• Blood studies (Hct, platelets, PTT, PT, TT, APTT) before starting therapy; PT or APTT must be less than 2 × control before starting therapy TT; or PT q3-4h during treatment

Administer:

IV

• Using infusion pump, terminal filter (0.45 μm or smaller)

• Reconstituting only with 5.2 ml sterile water for inj (not bacteriostatic water), and roll (not shake) to enhance reconstitution; further dilute with 190 ml; give as intermittent inf or give to clear cannula by using 1 ml of diluted drug; inject into cannula slowly, clamp 5 min, aspirate clot; avoid excessive pressure when urokinase is injected into catheter; force could rupture catheter or expel clot into circulation

• As soon as thrombi identified; not useful for thrombi over 1 wk old

• Cryoprecipitate or fresh frozen plasma if bleeding occurs

• Loading dose at beginning of therapy; may require increased loading doses

• Heparin therapy after thrombolytic therapy is discontinued, TT or APTT less than 2 × control (about 3-4 hr)

Y-site compatibilities: TPN 55, 56

Perform/provide:

• Storage in refrigerator; use immediately after reconstitution

• Bed rest during entire course of treatment; use caution in handling patients

• Avoidance of venous, arterial puncture procedures, inj, rectal temp

• Treatment of fever with acetaminophen or aspirin

• Placement of sign above patient's bed stating urokinase therapy

• Pressure for 30 sec to minor bleeding sites; 30 min to sites of arterial puncture followed by pressure dressing; inform prescriber if hemostasis not attained, apply pressure dressing

Evaluate:

• Therapeutic response: decreased clotting, thrombosis, embolism

 = Nursing alert   = Herb-drug interaction   = Do not crush

ursodiol (℞)

(ur-soh-die'-ohl)
Actigall
Func. class.: Gallstone solubilizing agent
Chem. class.: Ursodeoxycholic acid

Action: Suppresses hepatic synthesis, secretion of cholesterol; inhibits intestinal absorption of cholesterol

Uses: Dissolution of radiolucent, noncalcified gallbladder stones (less than 20 mm in diameter) in which surgery is not indicated

Dosage and routes:
• *Adult:* **PO** 8-10 mg/kg/day in 2-3 divided doses using gallbladder ultrasound q6mo; determine if stones have dissolved, if so, continue therapy, repeat ultrasound within 1-3 mo

Available forms: Caps 300 mg

Side effects/adverse reactions:
GI: Diarrhea, nausea, vomiting, abdominal pain, constipation, stomatitis, flatulence, dyspepsia, biliary pain
INTEG: Pruritus, rash, urticaria, dry skin, sweating, alopecia
CNS: Headache, anxiety, depression, insomnia, fatigue
MS: Arthralgia, myalgia, back pain
OTHER: Cough, rhinitis

Contraindications: Calcified cholesterol stones, radiopaque stones, radiolucent bile pigment stones, chronic liver disease, hypersensitivity

Precautions: Pregnancy (B), lactation, children

Pharmacokinetics: 80% excreted in feces, 20% metabolized, excreted into bile, lost in feces

Interactions:
• Reduced action of ursodiol: cholestyramine, colestipol, aluminum-based antacids
• Increased risk of stone formation: clofibrate, gemfibrozil, estrogens, oral contraceptives

NURSING CONSIDERATIONS
Assess:
• GI status: diarrhea, abdominal pain, nausea, vomiting; drug may have to be discontinued if side effects are severe
• Skin for pruritus, rash, urticaria, dry skin; provide soothing lotion to lesions
• Musculoskeletal status: aches or stiffness in joints

Administer:
• For up to 9-12 mo; if no improvement is seen, discontinue drug

Evaluate:
• Therapeutic response: decreasing size of stones on ultrasound

Teach patient/family:
• That anxiety, depression, insomnia are side effects and are reversible after discontinuing drug

valacyclovir (℞)

(val-a-sye'kloh-vir)
Valtrex
Func. class.: Antiviral
Chem. class.: Acyclic purine nucleoside analog

Action: Interferes with DNA synthesis by conversion to acyclovir, causing decreased viral replication, time of lesional healing

Uses: Herpes zoster (not immunosuppressed), recurrent genital herpes (not immunosuppressed)

Dosage and routes:
Genital herpes
• *Adult:* **PO** 1 g bid × 10 days initially; 1 g qd or 500 mg bid in those with <10 recurrences/yr
Herpes zoster
• *Adult:* **PO** 1 g tid × 1 wk

Available forms: Tabs 500 mg
Side effects/adverse reactions:
CNS: Tremors, lethargy, *dizziness, headache,* weakness
GI: Nausea, vomiting, diarrhea, abdominal pain, constipation
INTEG: Rash
Contraindications: Hypersensitivity to this drug or acyclovir
Precautions: Lactation, hepatic disease, renal diseae, electrolyte imbalance, dehydration, pregnancy (B)
Pharmacokinetics:
PO: Onset unknown, terminal half-life 2½-3½ hr; converted to acyclovir that crosses placenta and enters breast milk
Interactions:
• Increased blood levels of valacyclovir: cimetidine, probenecid
NURSING CONSIDERATIONS
Assess:
• Signs of infection; characteristics of lesions
• C&S before drug therapy; drug may be taken as soon as culture is taken; repeat C&S after treatement; determine the presence of other sexually transmitted diseases
• Bowel pattern before, during treatment
• Skin eruptions: rash
• Allergies before treatment, reaction of each medication; place allergies on chart in bright red letters
Evaluate:
• Therapeutic response: absence of itching, painful lesions; crusting and healed lesions
Teach patient/family:
• To take as prescribed; if dose is missed, take as soon as remembered up to 1 hr before next dose; do not double dose
• That drug may be taken orally before infection occurs; drug should be taken when itching or pain occurs, usually before eruptions

• That partners need to be told that patient has herpes; they can become infected; condoms must be worn to prevent reinfections
• That drug does not cure infection. just controls symptoms and does not prevent infection to others
Treatment of overdose: Discontinue drug, hemodialysis, resuscitate if needed

---

valproate
(val'proh-ate)
Depacon
valproic acid
(val'proh-ik)
Depakene, Myproic acid
divalproex sodium
(dye-val'proh-ex)
Depakote, Epival*
Func. class: Anticonvulsant
Chem. class: Carboxylic acid derivative

Action: Increases levels of γ-aminobutyric acid (GABA) in brain, which decreases seizure activity
Uses: Simple (petit mal), complex (petit mal) absence, mixed, manic episodes associated with bipolar disorder, migraine
Investigational uses: Tonic-clonic (grand mal), myoclonic seizures, migraines
Dosage and routes:
Epilepsy
• *Adult and child:* PO 15 mg/kg/day divided in 2-3 doses, may increase by 5-10 mg/kg/day qwk, not to exceed 60 mg/kg/day in 2-3 divided doses; **IV** ≤20 mg/min over 1 hr
Mania (divalproex sodium)
• *Adult:* PO 750 mg qd in divided doses, max 60 mg/kg/day

 = Nursing alert   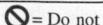 = Herb-drug interaction   ⊘ = Do not crush

Migraine
• *Adult:* **PO** 250 mg bid, may increase to 1000 mg/day if needed
Available forms: Valproic acid: caps 250 mg; divalproex: tabs delayed rel 125, 250, 500 mg; 125 mg sprinkle cap; valproate: syr 250 mg/5 ml; inj: 5 ml

Side effects/adverse reactions:
HEMA: ***Thrombocytopenia, leukopenia, lymphocytosis,*** increased pro-time
CNS: Sedation, drowsiness, dizziness, headache, incoordination, paresthesia, depression, hallucinations, behavioral changes, tremors, aggression, weakness
GI: Nausea, vomiting, constipation, diarrhea, heartburn, anorexia, cramps, ***hepatic failure, pancreatitis, toxic hepatitis,*** stomatitis
INTEG: Rash, alopecia, bruising
GU: Enuresis, irregular menses
EENT: Visual disturbances

Contraindications: Hypersensitivity, pregnancy (D), hepatic disease
Precautions: Lactation, child <2 yr
Pharmacokinetics:
PO: Onset 15-30 min, peak 1-4 hr, duration 4-6 hr
Metabolized by liver; excreted by kidneys; breast milk; crosses placenta; half-life 9-16 hr

Interactions:
• Increased effects: CNS depressants
• Increased toxicity of valproic acid: salicylates
• Increased toxicity of: warfarin
• Increased action of phenytoin
• Increased CNS effects of: phenobarbital, primadone
• Increased sedation: benzodiazepines
• Decreased metabolism of valproic acid: cimetidine
Lab test interferences:
False positive: Ketones
Interference: Thyroid function tests

NURSING CONSIDERATIONS
Assess:
• Blood studies: Hct, Hgb, RBC, serum folate, pro-time, platelets, vit D if on long-term therapy
• Hepatic studies: AST (SGOT), ALT (SGPT), bilirubin, creatinine, failure
• Blood levels: therapeutic level 50-100 µg/ml
• Mental status: mood, sensorium, affect, memory (long, short)
• Respiratory dysfunction: respiratory depression, character, rate, rhythm; hold drug if respirations are <12/min or if pupils are dilated
Administer:
PO
🚫 Tablets or capsules whole; do not break, crush, or chew
• Elixir alone; do not dilute with carbonated beverage; do not give syrup to patients on sodium restriction
• Give with food or milk to decrease GI symptoms
Evaluate:
• Therapeutic response: decreased seizures
Teach patient/family:
• That physical dependency may result from extended use
• To avoid driving, other activities that require alertness
• Not to discontinue medication quickly after long term use; convulsions may result
• To report visual disturbances, rash, diarrhea, light-colored stools, jaundice, protracted vomiting to prescriber

valsartan (℞)

(val'sahr-tan)
Diovan
Func. class.: Antihypertensive
Chem. class.: Angiotensin II receptor (Type AT_1)

Action: Blocks the vasoconstrictor and aldosterone-secreting effects of angiotensin II; selectively blocks the binding of angiotensin II to the AT_1 receptor found in tissues

Uses: Hypertension, alone or in combination

Dosage and routes:
• *Adult:* **PO** 80-160 mg qd alone or in combination with other antihypertensives

Available forms: Tabs 80, 160 mg

Side effects/adverse reactions:

CNS: Dizziness, insomnia, depression, drowsiness, vertigo

CV: Angina pectoris, 2nd degree AV block, *cerebrovascular accident,* hypotension, *myocardial infarction, dysrhythmias*

EENT: Conjunctivitis

GI: Diarrhea, abdominal pain, nausea, *hepatotoxicity*

GU: Impotence, *nephrotoxicity*

HEMA: Anemia, neutropenia

MS: Cramps, myalgia, pain, stiffness

RESP: Cough

Contraindications: Hypersensitivity, pregnancy, severe hepatic disease, bilateral renal artery stenosis

Precautions: Hypersensitivity to ACE inhibitors: congestive heart failure, hypertrophic cardiomyopathy aortic/mitral valve stenosis, CAD; lactation, children, elderly

Pharmacokinetics:
Peak 2 hr, duration >24 hr, extensively metabolized, half-life 9 hr; excreted in feces, urine, breast milk

NURSING CONSIDERATIONS
Assess:
• B/P, pulse q4h; note rate, rhythm, quality
• Blood studies: BUN, creatinine, LFTs before treatment
• Electrolytes: K, Na, Cl, total CO_2
• Baselines in renal, liver function tests before therapy begins
• Edema in feet, legs qd
• Skin turgor, dryness of mucous membranes for hydration status

Administer:
PO
• Without regard to meals

Evaluate:
• Therapeutic response: decreased B/P

Teach patient/family:
• To comply with dosage schedule, even if feeling better
• To notify prescriber of fever, swelling of hands or feet, irregular heartbeat, chest pain
• That excessive perspiration, dehydration, diarrhea may lead to fall in blood pressure; consult prescriber if these occur
• That drug may cause dizziness, fainting; light-headedness may occur
• To rise slowly to sitting or standing position to minimize orthostatic hypotension
• Not to take this medication if pregnant or breastfeeding, or have had an allergic reaction to this drug
• That if a dose is missed, to take it as soon as possible, unless it is within an hour before next dose

---

 = Nursing alert   = Herb-drug interaction   = Do not crush

vancomycin (℞)

(van-koe-mye'sin)
Lyphocin, Vancocin, Vancoled,
vancomycin HCl
Func. class.: Antiinfective-misc.
Chem. class.: Tricyclic glyco-
peptide

Action: Inhibits bacterial cell wall
synthesis

Uses: Resistant staphylococcal infections, pseudomembranous colitis, staphylococcal enterocolitis, endocarditis prophylaxis for dental procedures

Dosage and routes:
Serious staphylococcal infections
• *Adult:* IV 500 mg q6h or 1 g q12h
• *Child:* IV 40 mg/kg/day divided
q6-8h
• *Neonate:* IV 15 mg/kg initially
followed by 10 mg/kg q8-24h
*Pseudomembranous/staphylococ-
cal enterocolitis*
• *Adult:* PO 500 mg/day in divided
doses for 7-10 days
• *Child:* PO 40 mg/kg/day divided
q6h, not to exceed 2 g/day
Endocarditis prophylaxis
• *Adult:* IV 1 g over 1 hr, 1 hr before
dental procedure
Available forms: Pulvules 125, 250
mg; powder for oral sol 1, 10 g;
powder for inj 500 mg, 1 g

Side effects/adverse reactions:
*CV: **Cardiac arrest, vascular col-
lapse** (rare)*
*EENT: **Ototoxicity, permanent deaf-
ness,** tinnitus*
*HEMA: **Leukopenia, eosinophilia,
neutropenia***
*GI: **Nausea***
RESP: Wheezing, dyspnea
*SYST: **Anaphylaxis***
*GU: **Nephrotoxicity,** increased BUN,
creatinine, albumin, **fatal uremia***
INTEG: Chills, fever, rash, throm-
bophlebitis at injection site, urti-
caria, pruritus, necrosis (Red Man's
syndrome)

Contraindications: Hypersensitivity, previous hearing loss

Precautions: Renal disease, pregnancy (C), lactation, elderly, neonates

Pharmacokinetics:
IV: Peak 5 min; half-life 4-8 hr; excreted in urine (active form); IV,
feces PO crosses placenta
PO: Absorption: poor

Interactions:
• Ototoxicity or nephrotoxicity: aminoglycosides, cephalosporins, colistin, polymyxin, bacitracin, cisplatin,
amphotericin B, nondepolarizing
muscle relaxants

NURSING CONSIDERATIONS
Assess:
• I&O ratio; report hematuria, oliguria; nephrotoxicity may occur
• Any patient with compromised renal system; drug is excreted slowly
in poor renal system function; toxicity may occur rapidly; BUN, creatinine
• Blood studies: WBC
• Serum levels: peak 1 hr after 1 hr
inf 25-40 mg/ml, trough prior to
next dose 5-10 mg/ml
• C&S; drug may be given as soon
as culture is taken
• Auditory function during, after
treatment
• B/P during administration; sudden drop may indicate Red Man's
syndrome
• Signs of infection
• Hearing loss, ringing, roaring in
ears; drug should be discontinued
• Skin eruptions
• Respiratory status: rate, character,
wheezing, tightness in chest
• Allergies before treatment, reaction of each medication; place allergies on chart in bright red letters;
notify all people giving drugs

Administer:

• Antihistamine if Red Man's syndrome occurs: decreased B/P, flushing of neck, face

• Dose based on serum concentration

IV

• After reconstitution with 10 ml sterile water for injection (500 mg/10 ml); further dilution is needed for IV, 500 mg/100 ml NS, D₅W given as int inf over 1 hr; decrease rate of infusion if Red Man's syndrome occurs

Additive compatibilities: Amikacin, atracurium, calcium gluconate, cefepime, cimetidine, corticotropin, dimenhydrinate, hydrocortisone, meropenem, ofloxacin, potassium chloride, ranitidine, verapamil, vit B/C

Y-site compatibilities: Acyclovir, allopurinol, amifostine, amiodarone, amsacrine, atracurium, cyclophosphamide, diltiazem, enalaprilat, esmolol, filgrastim, fluconazole, fludarabine, gallium, granisetron, hydromorphone, insulin (regular), labetalol, lorazepam, magnesium sulfate, melphalan, meperidine, meropenem, midazolam, morphine, ondansetron, paclitaxel, pancuronium, perphenazine, propofol, sodium bicarbonate, tacrolimus, teniposide, theophylline, thiotepa, tolazoline, vecuronium, vinorelbine, warfarin, zidovudine

Perform/provide:

• Storage at room temp for up to 2 wk after reconstitution

• Adrenaline, suction, tracheostomy set, endotracheal intubation equipment on unit; anaphylaxis may occur

• Adequate intake of fluids (2 L) to prevent nephrotoxicity

Evaluate:

• Therapeutic response: absence of fever, sore throat; neg culture

Teach patient/family:

• All aspects of drug therapy: need to complete entire course of medication to ensure organism death (7-10 days); culture may be taken after completed course of medication

• To report sore throat, fever, fatigue; could indicate superinfection

• That drug must be taken in equal intervals around clock to maintain blood levels

---

vecuronium (℞)

(vek-yoo-roe'nee-um)

Norcuron

Func. class.: Neuromuscular blocker

Chem. class.: Monoquaternary analog of pancuronium

Action: Inhibits transmission of nerve impulses by binding with cholinergic receptor sites, antagonizing action of acetylcholine

Uses: Facilitation of endotracheal intubation, skeletal muscle relaxation during mechanical ventilation, surgery, general anesthesia

Dosage and routes:

• *Adult and child >9 yr:* **IV BOL** 0.08-0.10 mg/kg, then 0.01-0.015 mg/kg for prolonged procedures

Available forms: 10 mg/5 ml vial

Side effects/adverse reactions:

CNS: Skeletal muscle weakness or paralysis (rare)

RESP: **Prolonged apnea, possible respiratory paralysis**

Contraindications: Hypersensitivity

Precautions: Pregnancy (C), cardiac disease, lactation, children <2 yr, electrolyte imbalances, dehydration, neuromuscular disease, respiratory disease, hepatic disease

---

◆ = Nursing alert   ▰ = Herb-drug interaction   ⊘ = Do not crush

Pharmacokinetics:
IV: Onset 15 min, peak 3-5 min, duration 45-60 min; half-life 65-75 min; not metabolized; excreted in feces; crosses placenta

Interactions:
• Increased neuromuscular blockade: aminoglycosides, clindamycin, lincomycin, quinidine, local anesthetics, polymyxin antibiotics, lithium, narcotic analgesics, thiazides, enflurane, isoflurane, succinylcholine
• Dysrhythmias: theophylline

NURSING CONSIDERATIONS
Assess:
• For electrolyte imbalances (K, Mg); may lead to increased action of this drug
• Vital signs (B/P, pulse, respirations, airway) q15min until fully recovered; rate, depth, pattern of respirations, strength of hand grip
• I&O ratio; check for urinary retention, frequency, hesitancy
• Recovery: decreased paralysis of face, diaphragm, leg, arm, rest of body; allow to recover fully before completing neurologic assessment
• Allergic reactions: rash, fever, respiratory distress, pruritus; drug should be discontinued

Administer:
• With diazepam or morphine when used for therapeutic paralysis; provides no sedation alone
• Using nerve stimulator by anesthesiologist to determine neuromuscular blockade
• Anticholinesterase to reverse neuromuscular blockade
• IV after diluting with diluent provided; give by direct IV over 1 min; may give as continuous inf 10-20 mg/100 ml; titrate to patient response (only by qualified person)

Y-site compatibilities: Aminophylline, cefazolin, cefuroxime, cimetidine, diltiazem, dobutamine, dopamine, epinephrine, esmolol, fentanyl, fluconazole, gentamicin, heparin, hydrocortisone, hydromorphone, isoproterenol, labetalol, lorazepam, midazolam, milrinone, morphine, nicardipine, nitroglycerin, norepinephrine, propofol, ranitidine, sodium nitroprusside, trimethoprim/sulfamethoxazole, vancomycin

Perform/provide:
• Storage in refrigerator; discard in 24 hr
• Reassurance if communication is difficult during recovery from neuromuscular blockade

Evaluate:
• Therapeutic response: paralysis of jaw, eyelid, head, neck, rest of body

Treatment of overdose: Edrophonium or neostigmine, atropine, monitor VS; may require mechanical ventilation

---

venlafaxine (℞)

(ven-la-fax'een)

Effexor

Func. class.: Second-generation antidepressant (misc)

Action: Potent inhibitor of neuronal serotonin and norepinephrine uptake, weak inhibitor of dopamine; no muscarinic, histaminergic, or α-adrenergic receptors in vitro

Uses: Depression

Dosage and routes:
Renal dose
• Mild-moderate impairment, 75% of dose

Hepatic dose
• Moderate impairment, 50% of dose
• *Adult:* **PO** 75 mg/day in 2 or 3 divided doses; taken with food, may be increased to 150 mg/day; if needed, may be further increased to 225 mg/day; increments of 75 mg/

day at intervals of no less than 4 days; some hospitalized patients may require up to 375 mg/day in 3 divided doses

Available forms: Tabs scored 25, 37.5, 50, 75, 100 mg

Side effects/adverse reactions:

CNS: Emotional lability, vertigo, apathy, ataxia, CNS stimulation, euphoria, hallucinations, hostility, increased libido, hypertonia, hypotonia, psychosis

CV: Migraine, angina pectoris, hypertension, extrasystoles, postural hypotension, syncope, thrombophlebitis

EENT: Abnormal vision, ear pain, cataract, conjunctivitis, corneal lesions, dry eyes, otitis media, photophobia

GI: Dysphagia, eructation, colitis, gastritis, gingivitis, rectal hemorrhage, stomatitis, stomach and mouth ulceration

GU: Anorgasmia, dysuria, hematuria, metrorrhagia, vaginitis, impaired urination, albuminuria, amenorrhea, kidney calculus, cystitis, nocturia, breast and bladder pain, polyuria, uterine hemorrhage, vaginal hemorrhage, moniliasis

INTEG: Ecchymosis, acne, alopecia, brittle nails, dry skin, photosensitivity

META: Peripheral edema, weight gain, diabetes mellitus, edema, glycosuria, hyperlipemia, hypokalemia

MS: Arthritis, bone pain, bursitis, myasthenia tenosynovitis

RESP: Bronchitis, dyspnea, asthma, chest congestion, epistaxis, hyperventilation, laryngitis

SYST: Accidental injury, malaise, neck pain, enlarged abdomen, cyst, facial edema, hangover, hernia

Contraindications: Hypersensitivity

Precautions: Mania, pregnancy (C), lactation, children, elderly, hypertension, seizure disorder

Pharmacokinetics: Well absorbed, extensively metabolized in the liver to an active metabolite; 87% of drug recovered in urine; 27% protein binding; half-life 5-7, 11-13 hr respectively

Interactions:

• Hyperthermia, rigidity, rapid fluctuations of vital signs, mental status changes: MAOIs

NURSING CONSIDERATIONS
Assess:

• B/P lying, standing; pulse q/4 h; if systolic B/P drops 20 mm Hg, hold drug, notify prescriber; take VS q4h in patients with cardiovascular disease

• Blood studies: CBC, leukocytes, differential cardiac enzymes if patient is receiving long-term therapy

• Hepatic studies: AST (SGOT), ALT (SGPT), bilirubin

• Weight qwk; appetite may increase with drug

• With food, milk for GI symptoms

• Gum, hard candy, frequent sips of water for dry mouth

• Mental status: mood, sensorium, affect, suicidal tendencies, increase in psychiatric symptoms; depression, panic

• Withdrawal symptoms: headache, nausea, vomiting, muscle pain, weakness; not usual unless drug is discontinued abruptly

Perform/provide:

• Storage in tight container at room temp; do not freeze

• Assistance with ambulation during beginning therapy, since drowsiness, dizziness occur

• Checking to see if PO medication swallowed

Evaluate:

• Therapeutic response; decreased depression

 = Nursing alert   ◢ = Herb-drug interaction   ⊗ = Do not crush

Teach patient/family:

• To dispense in small amounts because of suicide potential, especially in the beginning of therapy

• To use with caution when driving or other activities requiring alertness because of drowsiness, dizziness, blurred vision

• To avoid alcohol ingestion, other CNS depressants

• Not to discontinue medication quickly after long-term use; may cause nausea, headache, malaise

• To wear sunscreen or large hat, since photosensitivity occurs

Treatment of overdose: ECG monitoring; induce emesis; lavage, activated charcoal; administer anticonvulsant

---

verapamil (R̶x̶)

(ver-ap′a-mill)

Calan, Calan SR, Isoptin, Isoptin SR , verapamil HCl, verapamil HCl SR, Verelan

Func. class.: Calcium channel blocker; antihypertensive; antianginal

Chem. class.: Phenylalkylamine

Action: Inhibits calcium ion influx across cell membrane during cardiac depolarization; produces relaxation of coronary vascular smooth muscle; dilates coronary arteries; decreases SA/AV node conduction; dilates peripheral arteries

Uses: Chronic stable angina pectoris, vasospastic angina, dysrhythmias, hypertension

Investigational uses: Prevention of migraine headaches, ventricular outflow obstruction in hypertrophic cardiomyopathy

Dosage and routes:

• *Adult:* **PO** 80 mg tid or qid, increase qwk; **IV BOL** 5-10 mg >2 min, repeat if necessary in 30 min

• *Child 1-15 yr:* **IV BOL** 0.1-0.3 mg/kg >2 min, repeat in 30 min, not to exceed 10 mg in a single dose

Available forms: Tabs 40, 80, 120 mg; sus rel tabs 120, 180, 240 mg; inj 5 mg/ml; sus rel caps 120, 180, 240, 360 mg

Side effects/adverse reactions:

CV: Edema, **CHF,** bradycardia, hypotension, palpitations, AV block

GI: Nausea, diarrhea, gastric upset, *constipation,* increased liver function studies

GU: Nocturia, polyuria

CNS: Headache, drowsiness, dizziness, anxiety, depression, weakness, insomnia, confusion, light-headedness

Contraindications: Sick sinus syndrome, 2nd- or 3rd-degree heart block, hypotension less than 90 mm Hg systolic, cardiogenic shock, severe CHF

Precautions: CHF, hypotension, hepatic injury, pregnancy (C), lactation, children, renal disease, concomitant β-blocker therapy

Pharmacokinetics:

IV: Onset 3 min, peak 3-5 min, duration 10-20 min

PO: Onset variable, peak 3-4 hr, duration 17-24 hr, half-life (biphasic) 4 min, 3-7 hr (terminal)

Metabolized by liver, excreted in urine (96% as metabolites)

Interactions:

• Increased hypotension: prazosin, quinidine

• Increased effects: β-blockers, antihypertensives, cimetidine, digoxin

• Decreased effects of lithium

• Increased levels of digoxin, theophylline, cyclosporine, carbamazepine, nondepolarizing muscle relaxants

Lab test interferences:

Increase: Liver function tests

V

NURSING CONSIDERATIONS
Assess:
• Cardiac status: B/P, pulse, respiration, ECG intervals (PR, QRS, QT)
Administer:
• Before meals, hs; sus rel give with food
IV
• Undiluted through Y-tube or 3-way stopcock of compatible sol; give over 2 min, or 3 min elderly
Additive compatibilities: Amikacin, amiodarone, ascorbic acid, atropine, bretylium, calcium chloride, calcium gluconate, cefamandole, cefazolin, cefotaxime, cefoxitin, cephapirin, chloramphenicol, cimetidine, clindamycin, dexamethasone, diazepam, digoxin, dopamine, epinephrine, erythromycin, gentamicin, heparin, hydrocortisone sodium phosphate, hydrocortisone, hydromorphone, insulin (regular), isoproterenol, lidocaine, magnesium sulfate, mannitol, meperidine, metaraminol, methicillin, methyldopate, methylprednisolone, metoclopramide, mezlocillin, morphine, moxalactam, multivitamins, naloxone, nitroglycerin, norepinephrine, oxytocin, pancuronium, penicillin G potassium, penicillin G sodium, pentobarbital, phenobarbital, phentolamine, phenytoin, piperacillin, potassium chloride, potassium phosphates, procainamide, propranolol, protamine, quinidine, sodium bicarbonate, sodium nitroprusside, theophylline, ticarcillin, tobramycin, tolazoline, vancomycin, vasopressin, vit B/C
Syringe compatibilities: Amrinone, heparin, milrinone
Y-site compatibilities: Amrinone, ciprofloxacin, dobutamine, dopamine, famotidine, hydralazine, meperidine, methicillin, milrinone, penicillin G potassium, piperacillin, propofol, ticarcillin

Evaluate:
• Therapeutic response: decreased anginal pain, decreased B/P, dysrhythmias
Teach patient/family:
• To increase fluids/fiber to counteract constipation
• How to take pulse before taking drug; to keep record or graph
• To avoid hazardous activities until stabilized on drug, dizziness no longer a problem
• To limit caffeine consumption; no alcohol products
• To avoid OTC drugs unless directed by prescriber
• To comply with all areas of medical regimen: diet, exercise, stress reduction, drug therapy
• To change positions slowly to prevent syncope
Treatment of overdose: Defibrillation, atropine for AV block, vasopressor for hypotension

---

vidarabine (℞)
(vih-dar′ah-bean)
Vira-A
Func. class.: Antibacterial, antiviral
Chem. class.: Purine nucleoside

Action: Inhibits bacterial/viral replication by preventing DNA synthesis
Uses: Herpes simplex virus encephalitis, varicella-zoster encephalomyelitis, herpes zoster in immunosuppressed
Dosage and routes:
Herpes simplex encephalitis
• *Adult and child:* **IV INF** 15 mg/kg/day × 10 days; infuse over 12-24 hr
Herpes zoster in immunocompromised patients
• *Adult and child:* **IV** 10 mg/kg/day × 5 day

 = Nursing alert   = Herb-drug interaction   = Do not crush

Herpes simplex
• *Neonate:* **IV** 15 mg/kg/day × 10 days
Available forms: Susp for inj 200 mg/ml
Side effects/adverse reactions:
CNS: Psychosis, hallucinations, dizziness, weakness, tremors, *fatal metabolic encephalopathy,* confusion, malaise, headache
META: SIADH
*HEMA: **Anemia, thrombocytopenia, neutropenia***
GI: Nausea, vomiting, anorexia, diarrhea, weight loss
INTEG: Pain, thrombophlebitis at injection site
Contraindications: Hypersensitivity
Precautions: Renal disease, liver disease, lactation, pregnancy (C)
Pharmacokinetics: Crosses blood-brain barrier, excreted by kidneys (metabolites), crosses placenta, half-life 1½-3 hr
Interactions:
• Increased neurologic side effects: allopurinol
• Incompatible with blood, protein products
NURSING CONSIDERATIONS
Assess:
• Liver studies: AST (SGOT), ALT (SGPT)
• Blood studies: WBC, differential, RBC, Hct, Hgb, platelets
• Renal studies: urinalysis, protein, blood
• C&S; drug may be given as soon as culture is taken; C&S may be taken after therapy
• Bowel pattern before, during treatment
• Fluid overload; drug requires large volume to stay in sol
• Weakness, tremors, confusion, dizziness, psychosis; drug may have to be decreased or discontinued

Administer:
• Shake sol; dilute to 450 mg/L IV; give fluid at constant rate over 12-24 hr, using in-line filter with mean pore diameter of 0.45 mm or less
Evaluate:
• Therapeutic response: decreased infection

---

vinblastine (VLB) (℞)
(vin-blast′een)
Velban, Velbe*, vinblastine sulfate
Func. class.: Antineoplastic
Chem. class.: Vinca rosea alkaloid

Action: Inhibits mitotic activity, arrests cell cycle at metaphase; inhibits RNA synthesis, blocks cellular use of glutamic acid needed for purine synthesis; a vesicant
Uses: Breast, testicular cancer, lymphomas, neuroblastoma; Hodgkin's, non-Hodgkin's lymphomas; mycosis fungoides, histiocytosis, Kaposi's sarcoma
Dosage and routes:
• *Adult:* **IV** 0.1 mg/kg or 3.7 mg/m² qwk or q2wk, not to exceed 0.5 mg/kg or 18.5 mg/m² qwk
• *Child:* 2.5 mg/m² then 3.75, 5, 6.25, 7.5 at 7-day intervals
Available forms: Inj, powder 10 mg for 10 ml IV
Side effects/adverse reactions:
*HEMA: **Thrombocytopenia, leukopenia, myelosuppression***
GI: Nausea, vomiting, ileus, anorexia, stomatitis, constipation, abdominal pain, GI, rectal bleeding, ***hepatotoxicity,*** pharyngitis
GU: Urinary retention, ***renal failure***
INTEG: Rash, alopecia, photosensitivity
*RESP: **Fibrosis, pulmonary infiltrate***

V

Side effects: *italics* = common; ***bold italics*** = life-threatening

CV: Tachycardia, orthostatic hypotension

CNS: Paresthesias, peripheral neuropathy, depression, headache, ***convulsions***

META: SIADH

Contraindications: Hypersensitivity, infants, pregnancy (D)

Precautions: Renal disease, hepatic disease

Pharmacokinetics: Half-life (triphasic) 35 min, 53 min, 19 hr; metabolized in liver, excreted in urine, feces; crosses blood-brain barrier

Interactions:
- Increased action of methotrexate
- Do not use with radiation
- Synergism: bleomycin
- Decreased phenytoin level: phenytoin
- Bronchospasm: mitomycin

NURSING CONSIDERATIONS
Assess:
- CBC, differential, platelet count qwk; withhold drug if WBC is <4000 or platelet count is <75,000; notify prescriber
- Pulmonary function tests, chest x-ray studies before, during therapy; chest x-ray film should be obtained q2wk during treatment
- Neurologic status: sensory-vibratory evaluation if side effects occur
- Renal function studies: BUN, serum uric acid, urine CrCl, electrolytes before, during therapy
- I&O ratio; report fall in urine output of 30 ml/hr
- Monitor temp q4h; may indicate beginning infection
- Liver function tests before, during therapy (bilirubin, AST [SGOT], ALT [SGPT], LDH) as needed or qmo
- RBC, Hct, Hgb, since these may be decreased

- Bleeding: hematuria, guaiac, bruising or petechiae, mucosa of orifices q8h
- Dyspnea, rales, unproductive cough, chest pain, tachypnea, fatigue, increased pulse, pallor, lethargy
- Food preferences; list likes, dislikes
- Effects of alopecia on body image; discuss feelings about body changes
- Sensitivity of feet/hands, which precedes neuropathy
- Inflammation of mucosa, breaks in skin
- Yellow skin, sclera; dark urine, clay-colored stools, itchy skin, abdominal pain, fever, diarrhea
- Buccal cavity q8h for dryness, sores or ulceration, white patches, oral pain, bleeding, dysphagia
- Local irritation, pain, burning, discoloration at injection site
- Symptoms indicating severe allergic reaction: rash, pruritus, urticaria, purpuric skin lesions, itching, flushing
- Frequency of stools and characteristics: cramping; acidosis; signs of dehydration: rapid respirations, poor skin turgor, decreased urine output, dry skin, restlessness, weakness

Administer:
- Antiemetic 30-60 min before giving drug and prn to prevent vomiting
- Local or systemic drugs for infection
- Transfusion for anemia
- Antispasmodic for GI symptoms
IV
- After diluting 10 mg/10 ml NaCl; give through Y-tube or 3-way stopcock or directly over 1 min
- Hyaluronidase 150 U/ml in 1 ml

◆ = Nursing alert   ⫸ = Herb-drug interaction   ⊘ = Do not crush

NaCl, warm compress for extravasation for vesicant activity treatment

Additive compatibilities: Bleomycin

Syringe compatibilities: Bleomycin, cisplatin, cyclophosphamide, droperidol, fluorouracil, leucovorin, methotrexate, metoclopramide, mitomycin, vincristine

Y-site compatibilities: Allopurinol, amifostine, aztreonam, bleomycin, cisplatin, cyclophosphamide, doxorubicin, droperidol, filgrastim, fludarabine, fluorouracil, granisetron, heparin, leucovorin, melphalan, methotrexate, metoclopramide, mitomycin, ondansetron, paclitaxel, piperacillin/tazobactam, sargramostim, teniposide, thiotepa, vincristine, vinorelbine

Perform/provide:
• Deep-breathing exercises with patient 3-4 ×/day; place in semi-Fowler's position
• Liquid diet: cola, Jell-O; dry toast or crackers may be added if patient is not nauseated or vomiting
• Increase fluid intake to 2-3 L/day to prevent urate deposits, calculi formation
• Rinsing of mouth tid-qid with water
• Brushing of teeth bid-tid with soft brush or cotton-tipped applicators for stomatitis; use unwaxed dental floss
• Nutritious diet with iron, vitamin supplements
• HOB raised to facilitate breathing

Evaluate:
• Therapeutic response: decreased tumor size, spread of malignancy

Teach patient/family:
• To report any complaints or side effects to nurse or prescriber
• To report any changes in breathing or coughing
• That hair may be lost during treatment, a wig or hairpiece may make patient feel better; tell patient that new hair may be different in color, texture
• To report change in gait or numbness in extremities; may indicate neuropathy
• To avoid foods with citric acid, hot or rough texture
• To report any bleeding, white spots or ulcerations in mouth to prescriber; to examine mouth qd

---

vincristine (VCR) (℞)
(vin-kris'teen)
Oncovin, Vincasar PFS, vincristine sulfate
Func. class.: Antineoplastic-misc
Chem. class.: Vinca alkaloid

Action: Inhibits mitotic activity, arrests cell cycle at metaphase; inhibits RNA synthesis, blocks cellular use of glutamic acid needed for purine synthesis; a vesicant

Uses: Breast, lung cancer, lymphomas, neuroblastoma, Hodgkin's disease, acute lymphoblastic and other leukemias, rhabdomyosarcoma, Wilms' tumor, osteogenic and other sarcomas

Dosage and routes:
• *Adult:* IV 1-2 mg/m²/wk, not to exceed 2 mg
• *Child:* IV 1.5-2 mg/m²/wk, not to exceed 2 mg
Available forms: Inj 1 mg/ml

Side effects/adverse reactions:
INTEG: Alopecia
HEMA: ***Thrombocytopenia, leukopenia, myelosuppression, anemia***
GI: Nausea, vomiting, anorexia, stomatitis, constipation, ***paralytic ileus***, abdominal pain, ***hepatotoxicity***

CV: Orthostatic hypotension

CNS: Decreased reflexes, numbness, weakness, motor difficulties, CNS depression, cranial nerve paralysis, *seizures*

Contraindications: Hypersensitivity, infants, pregnancy (D)

Precautions: Renal disease, hepatic disease, hypertension, neuromuscular disease

Pharmacokinetics: Half-life (triphasic) 0.85 min, 7.4 min, 164 min; metabolized in liver; excreted in bile, feces; crosses placental barrier, blood-brain barrier

Interactions:
• Increased action of methotrexate, anticoagulants
• Do not use with radiation
• Neurotoxicity: peripheral nervous system drugs
• Decreased digoxin level: digoxin
• Decreased action of vincristine: L-asparaginase
• Acute pulmonary reactions: mitomycin-c

NURSING CONSIDERATIONS
Assess:
• CBC, differential, platelet count qwk; withhold drug if WBC is <4000 or platelet count is <75,000; notify prescriber
• Renal function studies: BUN, serum uric acid, urine CrCl, electrolytes before, during therapy
• I&O ratio, report fall in urine output of 30 ml/hr
• Monitor temp q4h; may indicate beginning infection
• Liver function tests before, during therapy (bilirubin, AST [SGOT], ALT [SGPT], LDH) as needed or monthly
• RBC, Hct, Hgb; may be decreased
• Deep tendon reflexes; drug is neurotoxic
• Sensitivity of feet/hands, which precedes neuropathy
• Bleeding: hematuria, guaiac, bruising or petechiae, mucosa of orifices q8h
• Food preferences; list likes, dislikes
• Effects of alopecia on body image, discuss feelings about body changes
• Inflammation of mucosa, breaks in skin
• Yellow skin, sclera; dark urine, clay-colored stools, itchy skin, abdominal pain, fever, diarrhea
• Buccal cavity q8h for dryness, sores or ulceration, white patches, oral pain, bleeding, dysphagia
• Symptoms indicating severe allergic reaction: rash, pruritus, urticaria, purpuric skin lesions, itching, flushing
• Frequency of stools, characteristics: cramping, acidosis; signs of dehydration: rapid respirations, poor skin turgor, decreased urine output, dry skin, restlessness, weakness

Administer:
• Agents to prevent constipation
• Antiemetic 30-60 min before giving drug and prn
• Transfusion for anemia
• Antispasmodic for GI symptoms

IV
• After diluting with diluent provided or 1 mg/10 ml of sterile H_2O or NaCl; give through Y-tube or 3-way stopcock or directly over 1 min
• Hyaluronidase 150 U/ml in 1 ml NaCl; apply warm compress for extravasation

Additive compatibilities: Bleomycin, cytarabine, fluorouracil, methotrexate

Syringe compatibilities: Bleomycin, cisplatin, cyclophosphamide, doxapram, doxorubicin, droperidol, fluorouracil, heparin, leucovorin, methotrexate, metoclopramide, mitomycin, vinblastine

Y-site compatibilities: Allopurinol, amifostine, aztreonam, bleomycin, cisplatin, cladribine, cyclophosphamide, doxorubicin, droperidol, filgrastim, fludarabine, fluorouracil, granisetron, heparin, leucovorin, melphalan, methotrexate, metoclopramide, mitomycin, ondansetron, paclitaxel, piperacillin/tazobactam, sargramostim, teniposide, thiotepa, vinblastine, vinorelbine

Perform/provide:

• Liquid diet: cola, Jell-O; dry toast or crackers may be added if patient is not nauseated or vomiting

• Rinsing of mouth tid-qid with water

• Brushing of teeth bid-tid with soft brush or cotton-tipped applicators for stomatitis; use unwaxed dental floss

• Nutritious diet with iron, vitamin supplements

Evaluate:

• Therapeutic response: decreased tumor size, spread of malignancy

Teach patient/family:

• To report change in gait or numbness in extremities; may indicate neuropathy

• To report any complaints or side effects to nurse or prescriber

• To report any bleeding, white spots or ulcerations in mouth to prescriber; to examine mouth qd

---

vinorelbine (℞)

(vi-nor′el-bine)

Navelbine

Func. class.: Antineoplastic-misc

Chem. class.: Semisynthetic vinca alkaloid

Action: Inhibits mitotic activity, arrests cell cycle at metaphase; inhibits RNA synthesis, blocks cellular use of glutamic acid needed for purine synthesis; a vesicant

Uses: Unresectable advanced non-small cell lung cancer (NSCLC) stage IV; may be used alone or in combination with cisplatin for stage III or IV NSCLC breast cancer

Dosage and routes:

• *Adult:* **IV** 30 mg/m^2 qwk

Available forms: Powder 10 mg for 10 ml inj

Side effects/adverse reactions:

CV: Chest pain

RESP: Shortness of breath

HEMA: **Neutropenia, anemia, thrombocytopenia, granulocytopenia**

GI: Nausea, vomiting, ileus, *anorexia, stomatitis,* constipation, abdominal pain, diarrhea, ***hepatotoxicity***

INTEG: Rash, alopecia, photosensitivlty

CNS: Paresthesias, peripheral neuropathy, depression, headache, ***convulsions,*** weakness, jaw pain

META: **SIADH**

MS: Myalgia

Contraindications: Hypersensitivity, infants, pregnancy (D), granulocyte count <1000 cells/mm^3 pretreatment

Precautions: Renal, hepatic disease, elderly, lactation, children

Pharmacokinetics: Half-life 27-43 hr, peak 1-2 hr

Interactions:

• Possible increased toxicity: fluorouracil

NURSING CONSIDERATIONS

Assess:

• B/P, (baseline and q15min) during administration

• CBC, differential, platelet count weekly; withhold drug if WBC is <4000/mm^3 or platelet count is <75,000/mm^3; notify prescriber of results, recovery will take 3 wk

V

Side effects: *italics* = common; ***bold italics*** = life-threatening

• For dyspnea, rales, unproductive cough, chest pain, tachypnea
• Renal function studies: BUN, serum uric acid, urine CrCl before, during therapy; I&O ratio; report fall in urine output of 30 ml/hr; for decreased hyperuricemia
• For cold, fever, sore throat (may indicate beginning infection); notify prescriber if these occur
• For bleeding: hematuria, guaiac, bruising or petechiae, mucosa or orifices q8h, no rectal temps; avoid IM injections; use pressure to venipuncture sites
• Nutritional status: an antiemetic may be needed
• For symptoms of severe allergic reactions: rash, pruritus, urticaria, itching, flushing, bronchospasm, hypotension, epinephrine and crash cart should be nearby

Administer:
• Antiemetic 30-60 min before giving drug and prn to prevent vomiting

IV
• Hyaluronidase 150 U/ml in 1 ml NaCl, warm compress for extravasation for vesicant activity treatment
• By cont inf: 40 mg/m^2 q3wk after an IV bol of 8 mg/m^2; may be given in combination with doxorubicin, fluorouracil, cisplatin

Y-site compatibilities: Amikacin, aztreonam, bleomycin, bumetanide, buprenorphine, butorphanol, calcium gluconate, carboplatin, carmustine, cefotaxime, ceftazidime, ceftizoxime, chlorpromazine, cimetidine, cisplatin, clindamycin, cyclophosphamide, cytarabine, dacarbazine, dactinomycin, daunorubicin, dexamethasone, diphenhydramine, doxorubicin, doxycycline, droperidol, enalaprilat, etoposide, famotidine, filgrastim, floxuridine, fluconazole, fludarabine, gallium, genta-

micin, granisetron, haloperidol, heparin, hydrocortisone, hydromorphone, hydroxyzine, idarubicin, ifosfamide, imipenem-cilastatin, lorazepam, mannitol, mechlorethamine, melphalan, meperidine, mesna, methotrexate, metoclopramide, metronidazole, minocycline, mitoxantrone, morphine, nalbuphine, netilmicin, ondansetron, plicamycin, streptozocin, teniposide, ticarcillin, ticarcillin/clavulanate, tobramycin, vancomycin, vinblastine, vincristine, zidovudine

Perform/provide:
• Liquid diet: cola, Jell-O; dry toast or crackers if patient not nauseated or vomiting
• Brushing of teeth bid-tid with soft brush or cotton-tipped applicators for stomatitis; unwaxed dental floss
• Nutritious diet with iron, vitamin supplements

Evaluate:
• Therapeutic response: decreased tumor size, spread of malignancy

Teach patient/family:
• To report change in gait or numbness in extremities; may indicate neuropathy
• To report any complaints or side effects to nurse or prescriber
• To examine mouth qd for bleeding, white spots, ulcerations; notify prescriber

---

vitamin A (℞, OTC)

Aquasol A, Del-Vi-A, Vitamin A
Func. class.: Vitamin, fat soluble
Chem. class.: Retinol

Action: Needed for normal bone, tooth development, visual dark adaptation, skin disease, mucosa tissue repair, assists in production of adrenal steroids, cholesterol, RNA
Uses: Vit A deficiency

 = Nursing alert   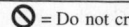 = Herb-drug interaction   🚫 = Do not crush

Dosage and routes:
• *Adult and child >8 yr:* **PO** 100,000-500,000 IU qd × 3 days, then 50,000 qd × 2 wk; dose based on severity of deficiency; maintenance 10,000-20,000 IU for 2 mo
• *Child 1-8 yr:* **IM** 5000-15,000 IU qd × 10 days
• *Infant <1 yr:* **IM** 5000-15,000 IU × 10 days
Maintenance
• *Child 4-8 yr:* **IM** 15,000 IU qd × 2 mo
• *Child <4 yr:* **IM** 10,000 IU qd × 2 mo
Available forms: Caps 10,000, 25,000, 50,000 IU; drops 5000 IU; inj 50,000 IU/ml; tabs 10,000, 25,000, 50,000 IU

Side effects/adverse reactions:
GI: Nausea, vomiting, anorexia, abdominal pain, ***jaundice***
CNS: Headache, ***increased intracranial pressure, intracranial hypertension,*** lethargy, malaise
EENT: Gingivitis, papilledema, exophthalmos, inflammation of tongue and lips
INTEG: Drying of skin, pruritus, increased pigmentation, night sweats, alopecia
MS: Arthralgia, retarded growth, hard areas on bone
META: Hypomenorrhea, hypercalcemia

Contraindications: Hypersensitivity to vit A, malabsorption syndrome (PO)
Precautions: Lactation, impaired renal function, pregnancy (A)
Pharmacokinetics: Stored in liver, kidneys, fat; excreted (metabolites) in urine, feces
Interactions:
• Decreased absorption of vit A: mineral oil, cholestyramine, colestipol
• Increased levels of vit A: corticosteroids, oral contraceptives

• Do not administer IV because of risk of anaphylactic shock
Lab test interferences:
False increase: Bilirubin, serum cholesterol

NURSING CONSIDERATIONS
Assess:
• Nutritional status: yellow and dark green vegetables, yellow/orange fruits, A-fortified foods, liver, egg yolks
• Vit A deficiency: decreased growth, night blindness, dry, brittle nails, hair loss, urinary stones, increased infection, hyperkeratosis of skin, drying of cornea
Administer:
PO
• With food (PO) for better absorption
Perform/provide:
• Storage in tight, light-resistant container
Evaluate:
• Therapeutic response: increased growth rate, weight; absence of dry skin and mucous membranes, night blindness
Teach patient/family:
• That if dose is missed, it should be omitted
• That ophthalmic exams may be required periodically throughout therapy
• Not to use mineral oil while taking this drug
• To notify prescriber of nausea, vomiting, lip cracking, loss of hair, headache
• Not to take more than the prescribed amount
Treatment of overdose: Discontinue drug

vitamin D (chole-calciferol, vitamin D₃ or ergocalciferol, vitamin D₂) (℞, OTC)

Calciferol, Drisdol, Radiostol*, Radiostol Forte*, Delta-D, Vitamin D, Vitamin D₃

Func. class.: Vit D
Chem. class.: Fat soluble

Action: Needed for regulation of calcium, phosphate levels, normal bone development, parathyroid activity, neuromuscular functioning

Uses: Vit D deficiency, rickets, renal osteodystrophy, hypoparathyroidism, hypophosphatemia, psoriasis, rheumatoid arthritis

Dosage and routes:
Deficiency
• *Adult:* **PO/IM** 12,000 IU qd, then increased to 500,000 IU/day
• *Child:* **PO/IM** 1500-5000 IU qd × 2-4 wk, may repeat after 2 wk or 600,000 IU as single dose

Hypoparathyroidism
• *Adult and child:* **PO/IM** 200,000 IU given with 4 g Ca tab

Available forms: Tabs 400, 1000, 50,000 IU; caps 25,000, 50,000 IU; liq 8000 IU/ml; inj 500,000 IU/ml, 500,000 IU/5 ml

Side effects/adverse reactions:
GI: Nausea, vomiting, anorexia, cramps, diarrhea, constipation, metallic taste, dry mouth, decreased libido
CNS: Fatigue, weakness, drowsiness, **convulsions,** headache, psychosis
GU: Polyuria, nocturia, **hematuria, albuminuria, renal failure**
CV: Hypertension, dysrhythmias
MS: Decreased bone growth, early joint pain, early muscle pain
INTEG: Pruritus, photophobia

Contraindications: Hypersensitivity, hypercalcemia, renal dysfunction, hyperphosphatemia
Precautions: Cardiovascular disease, renal calculi, pregnancy (A)
Pharmacokinetics: Half-life 7-12 hr; stored in liver, duration 2 mo; excreted in bile (metabolites) and urine

Interactions:
• Decreased effects of vit D: cholestyramine, colestipol, phenobarbital, phenytoin
• Increased toxicity: diuretics (thiazides), antacids, verapamil

NURSING CONSIDERATIONS
Assess:
• Vit D levels q2wk during treatment
• Ca, PO₄, Mg, BUN, alk phosphatase, urine Ca, creatinine
• In children, monitor height and weight
• Nutritional status: egg yolk, fortified dairy products, cod, halibut, salmon, sardines

Administer:
• IM inj deep in large muscle mass; administer slowly; aspirate carefully; rotate inj sites; avoid IV administration

Evaluate:
• Therapeutic response: absence of rickets/osteomalacia, adequate Ca/phosphate levels, decrease in bone pain

Teach patient/family:
• That if dose is missed, to omit
• The necessary foods in diet
• To avoid vitamin supplements unless directed by prescriber
• To keep appointments with health care providers; line between therapeutic and toxic doses is narrow
• To report weakness, lethargy, headache, anorexia, loss of weight
• To report nausea, vomiting, abdominal cramps, diarrhea, consti-

pation, excessive thirst, polyuria, muscle and bone pain
• To decrease intake of antacids and laxatives containing Mg

---

vitamin E (OTC)

Amino-Opti-E, Aquasol E, Daltose*, E-Complex-600, E-Ferol, E-Vitamin Succinate, E-200 I.U. Softgels, Gordo-Vite E, Tocopherol, Vitamin E, Vita-Plus E Softgells, Vitec

Func. class.: Vit E
Chem. class.: Fat soluble

Action: Needed for digestion and metabolism of polyunsaturated fats, decreases platelet aggregation, decreases blood clot formation, promotes normal growth and development of muscle tissue, prostaglandin synthesis

Uses: Vit E deficiency, impaired fat absorption, hemolytic anemia in premature neonates, prevention of retrolental fibroplasia, sickle cell anemia, supplement in malabsorption syndrome

Dosage and routes:
Deficiency
• *Adult:* PO 60-75 IU qd
• *Child:* PO 1 mg/0.6 g of dietary fat
Prevention of deficiency
• *Adult:* PO 30 IU/day; **TOP** apply to affected areas
• *Infants:* PO 5 IU/day
Available forms: Caps 100, 200, 400, 500, 600, 1000 IU; tabs 100, 200, 400 IU; drops 50 mg/ml; chew tabs 400 U; ointment, cream, lotion, oil

Side effects/adverse reactions:
META: Altered metabolism of hormones: thyroid, pituitary, adrenal; altered immunity
MS: Weakness
CNS: Headache, fatigue
GI: Nausea, cramps, diarrhea

GU: Gonadal dysfunction
CV: Increased risk of thrombophlebitis
EENT: Blurred vision
INTEG: Sterile abscess, contact dermatitis

Contraindications: None significant
Precautions: Pregnancy (A)
Pharmacokinetics:
PO: Metabolized in liver, excreted in bile
Interactions:
• Increased action of oral anticoagulants
• Decreased absorption: cholestyramine, colestipol, mineral oil, sucralfate

NURSING CONSIDERATIONS
Assess:
• Vit E levels during treatment
• Nutritional status: wheat germ, dark green leafy vegetables, nuts, eggs, liver, vegetable oils, dairy products, cereals
Administer:
PO
• Administer with or after meals
• *Chewable tabs:* Chew well
• *Sol:* May be dropped in mouth or mixed with food
TOP
• To moisturize dry skin
Perform/provide:
• Storage in tight, light-resistant container
Evaluate:
• Therapeutic response: absence of hemolytic anemia, adequate vit E levels, improvement in skin lesions, decreased edema
Teach patient/family:
• The necessary foods in diet
• To omit if dose is missed
• To avoid vitamin supplements unless directed by prescriber

V

warfarin (℞)

(war'far-in)

Coumadin, Sofarin, warfarin sodium, Warfilone Sodium*

Func. class.: Anticoagulant

Action: Interferes with blood clotting by indirect means; depresses hepatic synthesis of vit K-dependent coagulation factors (II, VII, IX, X)

Uses: Pulmonary emboli, deep-vein thrombosis, MI, atrial dysrhythmias, postcardiac valve replacement

Dosage and routes:

• *Adult:* **PO/IV** 10-15 mg/day × 3 days, then titrated to prothrombin time qd

• *Child:* 0.1 mg/kg/day titrated to INR

Available forms: Tabs 1, 2, 2.5, 5, 7.5, 10 mg; inj 50 mg/2 ml

Side effects/adverse reactions:

GI: Diarrhea, nausea, vomiting, anorexia, stomatitis, cramps, *hepatitis*

GU: Hematuria

INTEG: Rash, dermatitis, urticaria, alopecia, pruritus

CNS: Fever

HEMA: Hemorrhage, agranulocytosis, leukopenia, eosinophilia

Contraindications: Hypersensitivity, hemophilia, leukemia with bleeding, peptic ulcer disease, thrombocytopenic purpura, hepatic disease (severe), severe hypertension, subacute bacterial endocarditis, acute nephritis, blood dyscrasias, pregnancy (D), eclampsia, preeclampsia, lactation

Precautions: Alcoholism, elderly

Pharmacokinetics:

PO: Onset 12-24 hr, peak 1½-3 days, duration 3-5 days, half-life 1½-2½ days; metabolized in liver, excreted in urine/feces (active/inactive metabolites), crosses placenta, 99% bound to plasma proteins

Interactions:

• Increased action of warfarin: allopurinol, chloramphenicol, amiodarone, diflunisal, heparin, steroids, cimetidine, disulfiram, thyroid, glucagon, metronidazole, quinidine, sulindac, sulfinpyrazone, sulfonamides, clofibrate, salicylates, ethacrynic acids, indomethacin, mefenamic acid, oxyphenbutazones, phenylbutazone, cefamandole, chloral hydrate, cotrimoxazole, erythromycin, quinolone antibiotics, isoniazid, thrombolytic agents, tricyclic antidepressants

• Decreased action of warfarin: barbiturates, griseofulvin, ethchlorvynol, carbamazepine, rifampin, oral contraceptives, phenytoin, estrogens, vit K, cholestyramine, corticosteroids, mercaptopurine, sucralfate, vit K foods, vit supplements

• Increased toxicity: oral sulfonylureas, phenytoin

 Increased risk of bleeding: bromelain, cinchona bark

Lab test interferences:

Increase: T_3 uptake

Decrease: Uric acid

NURSING CONSIDERATIONS

Assess:

• Blood studies (Hct, platelets, occult blood in stools) q3mo

• Prothrombin time, which should be 1½-2 × control, PT; often done qd initially or INR (international normalized ratio)

• Bleeding gums, petechiae, ecchymosis, black tarry stools, hematuria

• Fever, skin rash, urticaria

• Needed dosage change q1-2wk; when stable, PT q3wk

Administer:

• At same time each day to maintain steady blood levels

• Tabs whole or crushed

 = Nursing alert   = Herb-drug interaction   🚫 = Do not crush

• Avoiding all IM injections that may cause bleeding

IV

• After diluting with diluent provided (50 mg/2 ml); rotate vial, give through Y-tube or 3-way stopcock at [dH]25 mg/min

Y-site compatibilities: Amikacin, ascorbic acid, cefazolin, cephapirin, dopamine, epinephrine, heparin, lidocaine, metaraminol, morphine, nitroglycerin, oxytocin, ranitidine

Perform/provide:

• Storage in tight container

Evaluate:

• Therapeutic response: decrease of deep-vein thrombosis

Teach patient/family:

• To avoid OTC preparations that may cause serious drug interactions unless directed by prescriber

• To use soft-bristle toothbrush to avoid bleeding gums, and to use electric razor

• To carry a Medic Alert ID identifying drug taken

• The importance of compliance

• To report any signs of bleeding: gums, under skin, urine, stools

• To avoid hazardous activities (football, hockey, skiing), dangerous work

• The importance of avoiding unusual changes in vitamin intake, diet or life-style

• To inform dentists and other physicians of anticoagulant intake

• That smoking increases dose requirements

• To limit foods high in vit K

Treatment of overdose: Administer vit K

zafirlukast (℞)
(za-feer′loo-cast)
Accolate
Func. class.: Misc. respiratory drug
Chem class: Leukotriene receptor antagonist

Action: Antagonizes the contractile action of leukotrienes (LTC_4, LTD_4, LTE_4) in airway smooth muscle; inhibits bronchoconstriction caused by antigens

Uses: Prophylaxis and chronic treatment of asthma in adults/children >12 yr

Dosage and routes:

• *Adult:* **PO** 20 mg bid, take 1 hr ac or 2 hr pc

Available forms: Tabs 20 mg

Contraindications: Hypersensitivity

Precautions: Pregnancy (B), elderly, lactation, children, hepatic disease

Interactions:

• Increased plasma levels of zafirlukast: aspirin

• Decreased plasma levels of zafirlukast: erythromycin, terfenadine, theophylline

• Increased pro-time: warfarin

• Drug/food: decreased bioavailability

Side effects/adverse reactions:

CNS: Headache, dizziness

GI: Nausea, diarrhea, abdominal pain, vomiting

OTHER: Infections, pain, asthenia, myalgia, fever, dyspepsia, increased ALT

Pharmacokinetics: Unknown

NURSING CONSIDERATIONS

Assess:

◆Adult patients carefully for symptoms of Churg-Strauss syndrome (rare), including eosinophilia, vasculitic rash, worsening pulmonary symptoms, cardiac complications, and/or neuropathy

• Respiratory rate, rhythm, depth; auscultate lung fields bilaterally; notify prescriber of abnormalities

Administer:

• PO after meals for GI symptoms; absorption may be affected

Evaluate:

• Therapeutic response: ability to breathe more easily

Teach patient/family:

• To check OTC medications, current prescription medications, which will increase stimulation

• To avoid hazardous activities; dizziness may occur

• That if GI upset occurs, to take drug with 8 oz water; avoid food if possible, absorption may be decreased

• To notify prescriber of nausea, vomiting, diarrhea, abdominal pain

---

zalcitabine (℞)

(zal-sit'a-bin)
ddC, dideoxycytidine HIVID
Func. class.: Antiviral
Chem. class.: Synthetic pyrimidine nucleoside analog of 2'-deoxycytidine

Action: Inhibits HIV replication by the conversion of this drug by cellular enzymes to an active antiviral metabolite

Uses: Advanced HIV infections in adults, children >13 yr who cannot use zidovudine or who do not respond to treatment

Dosage and routes:

• *Adult:* **PO** combined with zidovudine in advanced HIV infection: 0.75 mg concomitantly with 200 mg zidovudine q8h; dosage reduction not necessary for patients weighing >30 kg; in presence of peripheral neuropathy initiate dose at 0.375 mg q8h of zalcitabine

Renal dose

• CrCl <40 ml/min

Available forms: Tabs 0.375, 0.75 mg

Side effects/adverse reactions:

GI: Pancreatitis, *diarrhea, nausea, vomiting,* abdominal pain, constipation, stomatitis, dysplasia, liver abnormalities, *oral ulcers,* flatulence, taste perversion, dry mouth, oral thrush, melena, *increased ALT (SGPT), AST (SGOT), alk phosphatase, amylase*

GU: Uric acid, **toxic nephropathy,** polyuria

CNS: Headache, peripheral neuropathy, seizures, confusion, anxiety, hypertonia, abnormal thinking, asthenia, insomnia, CNS depression, pain, *dizziness,* chills, *fever*

RESP: Cough, pneumonia, dyspnea, asthma, hypoventilation

ENDO: Hypoglycemia, hyponatremia, hyperbilirubinemia, hyperglycemia

INTEG: Rash, pruritus, alopecia, sweating, acne

MS: Myalgia, arthritis, myopathy, muscular atrophy

CV: Hypertension, vasodilation, dysrhythmia, syncope, palpitation, tachycardia

EENT: Ear pain, otitis, photophobia, visual impairment

*HEMA: **Leukopenia, granulocytopenia, thrombocytopenia,*** anemia

Contraindications: Hypersensitivity

Precautions: Renal, hepatic disease, pregnancy (C), lactation, child <13 yr, peripheral neuropathy, heart failure

Pharmacokinetics:

PO: Elimination half-life 1.62 hr; administration within 5 min of food

---

 = Nursing alert   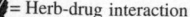 = Herb-drug interaction   ◯ = Do not crush will decrease absorption; elimination via kidneys

Interactions:

• Increased risk of pancreatitis with agents that can cause pancreatitis

• Increased risk of peripheral neuropathy with other agents that can cause peripheral neuropathy: aminoglycosides, amphotericin B, chloramphenicol, cimetidine, cisplatin, dapsone, disulfiram, ethionamide, foscarnet, glutethimide, gold, hydralazine, iodoquinol, isoniazid, metronidazole, nitrofurantoin, phenytoin, probenecid, ribavirin, vincristine; use with didanosine is not recommended

• Decreased absorption: ketoconazole, dapsone, food, antacids, metoclopramide

• Do not administer with tetracyclines

• Decreased concentrations of fluoroquinolone antibiotics

NURSING CONSIDERATIONS

Assess:

• Neuropathy: tingling or pain in hands and feet, distal numbness

• Pancreatitis: abdominal pain, nausea, vomiting, elevated liver enzymes; drug should be discontinued, since condition can be fatal

• Children by dilated retinal examination q6mo to rule out retinal depigmentation

• CBC, differential, platelet count qwk; withhold drug if WBC is <4000/mm^3 or platelet count is <75,000/mm^3; notify prescriber

• Renal function studies: BUN, serum uric acid, urine CrCl before, during therapy

• Temp q4h; may indicate beginning infection

• Liver function tests before, during therapy (bilirubin, AST [SGOT], ALT [SGPT]), triglycerides, amylase prn or qmo

Administer:

• Antibiotics: for prophylaxis of infection

Perform/provide:

• Strict medical asepsis, protective isolation if WBC levels are low

Evaluate:

• Therapeutic response: absence of infection; symptoms of HIV

Teach patient/family:

• To report signs of infection: fever, sore throat, flu symptoms

• To report signs of anemia: fatigue, headache, faintness, shortness of breath, irritability

• To report bleeding; avoid use of razors, commercial mouthwash

• That hair may be lost during therapy; a wig or hairpiece may make patient feel better

---

zidovudine (℞)

(zye-doe'-vue-deen)

Apo-Zidovudine*, Azidothymidine, AZT, Novo-AZT*, Retrovir

Func. class.: Antiviral

Chem. class.: Thymidine analog

Action: Inhibits replication of HIV virus by incorporating into cellular DNA by viral reverse transcriptase, thereby terminating the cellular DNA chain

Uses: Symptomatic/asymptomatic HIV infections (AIDS, ARC), confirmed *P. carinii* pneumonia, absolute CD4 lymphocytes of <200/mm^3, prevention of maternal-fetal HIV transmission

Dosage and routes:

• *Adult:* **PO** 200 mg q4h; may have to stop treatment if severe bone marrow depression occurs, and restart after bone marrow recovery; **IV** 1-2 mg/kg q4h, initiate **PO** as soon as possible

z

- *Child:* **PO** 90-180 mg/m^2/dose q6h; **IV** same as adult
- *Neonates:* **PO** 2-3 mg/kg/dose q6h; **IV** same as adult

Prevention of maternal-fetal HIV transmission

- *Neonatal:* **PO** 2 mg/kg/dose q6h × 6 wk beginning 8-12 hr after birth; **IV** 1.5 mg/kg/dose over 30 min q6h until able to take **PO**
- *Maternal (>14 wk gestation):* **PO** 100 mg 5×/day until start of labor, then **IV** 2 mg/kg over 1 hr followed by **IV INF** 1 mg/kg/hr until umbilical cord clamped

Asymptomatic HIV infection

- *Child 3 mo to 12 yr:* **PO** 90-180 mg/m^2 q6h (max 200 mg q6h); **IV** 1-2 mg/kg over 1 hr q4h
- *Adult:* **PO** 100 mg q4h while awake (5×/day)

Symptomatic HIV infection

- *Child 3 mo to 12 yr:* **PO** 90-180 mg/m^2 q6h (max 200 mg q6h); **IV** 1-2 mg/kg over 1 hr q4h
- *Adult:* **PO** 100 mg q4h; **IV** 1-2 mg/kg over 1 hr q4h

Prevention of HIV following needlestick

- *Adult:* **PO** 200 mg tid plus lamivudine 150 mg bid, plus a protease inhibitor for high-risk exposure; begin within 2 hr of exposure

Available forms: Caps 100 mg; inj 200 mg/20 ml; oral syr 50 mg/5 ml

Side effects/adverse reactions:

HEMA: **Granulocytopenia, anemia**
CNS: Fever, headache, malaise, diaphoresis, *dizziness, insomnia,* paresthesia, somnolence, chills, tremor, twitching, anxiety, confusion, depression, lability, vertigo, loss of mental acuity
GI: Nausea, vomiting, diarrhea, anorexia, cramps, *dyspepsia,* constipation, dysphagia, *flatulence,* rectal bleeding, mouth ulcer
RESP: Dyspnea

EENT: Taste change, hearing loss, photophobia
INTEG: Rash, acne, pruritus, urticaria
MS: Myalgia, arthralgia, muscle spasm
GU: Dysuria, polyuria, frequency, hesitancy

Contraindications: Hypersensitivity

Precautions: Granulocyte count <1000/mm^3 or Hgb <9.5 g/dl, pregnancy (C), lactation, child, severe renal disease, impaired hepatic disease

Pharmacokinetics:

PO: Rapidly absorbed from GI tract, peak ½-1½ hr, metabolized in liver (inactive metabolites), excreted by kidneys

Interactions:

- Toxicity: amphotericin B, dapsone, flucytosine, adriamycin, interferon, vincristine, vinblastine, pentamidine, probenecid, experimental nucleoside analogs, benzodiazepines, cimetidine, morphine, sulfonamides, acyclovir, ganciclovir, doxorubicin, acetaminophen, indomethacin, fluconazole, phenytoin, trimethoprim
- Granulocytopenia: acetaminophen, aspirin, indomethacin

NURSING CONSIDERATIONS
Assess:

- Blood counts q2wk; watch for decreasing granulocytes, Hgb; if low, therapy may have to be discontinued and restarted after hematologic recovery; blood transfusions may be required

Administer:

- By mouth; capsules should be swallowed whole
- Trimethoprim/sulfamethoxazole, pyrimethamine, or acyclovir as ordered to prevent opportunistic infections; if these drugs are given, watch for neurotoxicity

---

 = Nursing alert   ▰ = Herb-drug interaction   ⊘ = Do not crush

IV
• After diluting each 1 mg/0.25 ml or more D₅W to 4 mg/ml or less; give over 1 hr
Y-site compatibilities: Acyclovir, allopurinol, amifostine, amikacin, amphotericin B, aztreonam, cefepime, ceftazidime, ceftriaxone, cimetidine, clindamycin, dexamethasone, dobutamine, dopamine, erythromycin, filgrastim, fluconazole, fludarabine, gentamicin, granisetron, heparin, imipenem/cilastatin, lorazepam, melphalan, metoclopramide, morphine, nafcillin, ondansetron, oxacillin, paclitaxel, pentamidine, phenylephrine, piperacillin, piperacillin/tazobactam, potassium chloride, ranitidine, sargramostim, teniposide, thiotepa, tobramycin, trimethoprim/sulfamethoxazole, trimetrexate, vancomycin, vinorelbine
Perform/provide:
• Storage in cool environment; protect from light
Evaluate:
• Blood dyscrasias (anemia, granulocytopenia): bruising, fatigue, bleeding, poor healing
Teach patient/family:
• That GI complaints and insomnia resolve after 3-4 wk of treatment
• That drug is not cure for AIDS but will control symptoms
• To notify prescriber of sore throat, swollen lymph nodes, malaise, fever; other infections may occur
• That patient is still infective, may pass AIDS virus on to others
• That follow-up visits must be continued since serious toxicity may occur; blood counts must be done q2wk
• That drug must be taken q4h around clock, even during night; to take 30 min ac or in pc
• That serious drug interactions may occur if OTC products are ingested; check with prescriber before taking aspirin, acetaminophen, indomethacin
• That other drugs may be necessary to prevent other infections
• That drug may cause fainting or dizziness

---

zileuton (R)
(zye'loo-tahn)
Zyflo
Func. class.: Leukotriene pathway inhibitor
Chem. class.: 5-1: poxygenase inhibitor

Action: Inhibits leukotriene (LT) formation; leukotrienes exert their effects by increasing neutrophil, eosinophil migration; aggregation of neutrophils, monocytes; smooth muscle contraction, capillary permeability; these actions further lead to bronchoconstriction, inflammation, edema
Uses: Allergic rhinitis, asthma
Investigational uses: Ulcerative colitis, rheumatoid arthritis
Dosage and routes:
Asthma
• *Adult and child:* 12 yr: **PO** 600 mg qid, may be given with meal & hs
Ulcerative colitis
• *Adult:* **PO** 600 mg bid
Available forms: Tabs 600 mg
Side effects/adverse reactions:
CNS: Dizziness, insomnia, fatigue, paresthesias, headache
GI: Nausea, abdominal pain, dyspepsia, diarrhea, LFTs abnormalities
INTEG: Hives
MS: Myalgia, asthenia
Contraindications: Hepatic disease, elevations in LFTs 3× upper limits, hypersensitivity

Z

Precautions: Acute attacks of asthma, alcohol consumption, pregnancy (C)

Pharmacokinetics:

PO: Rapidly absorbed, peak 1-3 hr, half-life 2.1-2.5 hr, protein binding 93% (albumin); metabolized by liver, excretion in urine

Interactions:

• Increased action of zilenton: theophylline, propranolol

• May increase effects of anticoagulants

NURSING CONSIDERATIONS
Assess:

• CBC, blood chemistry during treatment

• LFTs before and qmo × 3 mo, then q2-3mo during treatment

• Respiratory rate, rhythm, depth; auscultate lung fields bilaterally; notify prescriber of abnormalities

• Allergic reactions: rash, urticaria; drug should be discontinued

Administer:
PO

• After meals for GI symptoms; absorption may be affected

Evaluate:

• Therapeutic response: ability to breathe more easily

Teach patient/family:

• To check OTC medications, current prescription medications for ephedrine, which will increase stimulation; to avoid alcohol

• To avoid hazardous activities; dizziness may occur

• That if GI upset occurs to take drug with 8 oz water or food; absorption may be decreased slightly

• To notify prescriber of nausea, vomiting, anxiety, insomnia

---

zinc (℞, OTC)

Orazinc, PMS Egozine*, Verazinc, Zinca-Pak, Zincate, Zinc 15, Zinc-220, zinc sulfate

Func. class.: Trace element; nutritional supplement

Action: Needed for adequate healing, bone and joint development (23% zinc)

Uses: Prevention of zinc deficiency, adjunct to vit A therapy

Investigational uses: Wound healing

Dosage and routes:

Dietary supplement

• *Adult:* PO 25-50 mg/day

Nutritional supplement (IV)

• *Adult:* IV 2.5-4 mg/day; may increase by 2 mg/day if needed

• *Child 1-5 yr:* IV 100 μg/kg/day

• *Infant <1.5-3 kg:* IV 300 μg/kg/day

Available forms: Tabs 66, 110 mg; caps 220 mg; inj 1 mg, 5 mg/ml

Side effects/adverse reactions:

GI: Nausea, vomiting, cramps, heartburn, ulcer formation

Overdose: Diarrhea, rash, dehydration, restlessness

Precautions: Pregnancy (A)

Interactions:

• Decreased absorption of other covalent cations

NURSING CONSIDERATIONS
Assess:

• Zinc levels during treatment

Administer:

• With meals to decrease gastric upset; to avoid dairy products

Evaluate:

• Therapeutic response: absence of zinc deficiency

Teach patient/family:

• That element must be taken for 2 mo to be effective

 = Nursing alert   /// = Herb-drug interaction   ⊘ = Do not crush

• To report immediately nausea, diarrhea, rash, severe vomiting, restlessness, abdominal pain, tarry stools

---

zolpidem (℞)

(zole'pih-dem)
Ambien
Func. class.: Sedative-hypnotic
Chem. class.: Nonbenzodiazepine of imidazopyridine class

Action: Produces CNS depression at limbic, thalamic, hypothalamic levels of CNS; may be mediated by neurotransmitter-aminobutyric acid (GABA); results are sedation, hypnosis, skeletal muscle relaxation, anticonvulsant activity, anxiolytic action

Uses: Insomnia, short-term treatment

Dosage and routes:
• *Adult:* **PO** 10 mg hs × 7-10 days only; total dose should not exceed 10 mg
• *Geriatric:* **PO** 5 mg hs
Available forms: Tabs 5, 10 mg

Side effects/adverse reactions:
HEMA: **Leukopenia, granulocytopenia** (rare)
CNS: Headache, lethargy, drowsiness, daytime sedation, dizziness, confusion, light-headedness, anxiety, irritability, amnesia, poor coordination
GI: Nausea, vomiting, diarrhea, heartburn, abdominal pain, constipation
CV: Chest pain, palpitation

Contraindications: Hypersensitivity to benzodiazepines

Precautions: Anemia, hepatic disease, renal disease, suicidal individuals, drug abuse, elderly, psychosis, child <18 yr, seizure disorders, pregnancy (B), lactation

Pharmacokinetics:
PO: Onset 1.5 hr, metabolized by liver, excreted by kidneys (inactive metabolites), crosses placenta, excreted in breast milk; half-life 2-3 hr

Interactions:
• Increased action of both drugs: alcohol, CNS depressants
🖋 Increased CNS depression: kava kava

Lab test interferences:
• *Increase:* ALT (SGPT), AST (SGOT), serum bilirubin
• *Decrease:* RAI uptake
• *False increase:* Urinary 17-OHCS

NURSING CONSIDERATIONS
Assess:
• Blood studies: Hct, Hgb, RBC, if blood dyscrasias are suspected (rare)
• Hepatic studies: AST (SGOT), ALT (SGPT), bilirubin if liver damage has occurred
• Mental status: mood, sensorium, affect, memory (long, short)
• Blood dyscrasias: fever, sore throat, bruising, rash, jaundice, epistaxis (rare)
• Type of sleep problem: falling asleep, staying asleep

Administer:
• After removal of cigarettes to prevent fires
• After trying conservative measures for insomnia
• ½-1 hr before hs for sleeplessness
• On empty stomach for fast onset but may be taken with food if GI symptoms occur

Perform/provide:
• Assistance with ambulation after receiving dose
• Safety measures: side rails, nightlight, call bell within easy reach
• Checking to see if PO medication has been swallowed
• Storage in tight container in cool environment

Z

Evaluate:
• Therapeutic response: ability to sleep at night, decreased amount of early morning awakening if taking drug for insomnia

Teach patient/family:
• That dependence is possible after long-term use
• To avoid driving or other activities requiring alertness until drug is stabilized
• To avoid alcohol ingestion, CNS depressants; serious CNS depression may result

• That effects may take 2 nights for benefits to be noticed
• Alternative measures to improve sleep: reading, exercise several hours before hs, warm bath, warm milk, TV, self-hypnosis, deep breathing
• That hangover is common in elderly but less common than with barbiturates; rebound insomnia may occur for 1-2 nights after discontinuing drug

Treatment of overdose: Lavage, activated charcoal; monitor electrolytes, vital signs

Appendix a

Selected new drugs

alatrofloxacin/ trovafloxacin (℞)

(ah-lat-troh-floks'ah-sin/troh-vah-floks'a-sin)

Trovan

Func. class.: Antiinfective
Chem. class.: Fluoroquinolone

Action: Interferes with conversion of intermediate DNA fragments into high-molecular-weight DNA in bacteria; DNA gyrase inhibitor

Uses: Nosocomial pneumonia; *E. coli, P. aeruginosa, H. influenzae, S. aureus*; community-acquired pneumonia: *S. pneumoniae, H. influenzae, S. aureus, K. pneumoniae, M. pneumoniae, M. catarrhalis, L. pneumophilia, C. pneumoniae*; chronic bronchitis, acute sinusitis, complicated intraabdominal infections, gyn/pelvic infection, skin/skin structure infections, UTIs, chronic bacterial prostatitis, urethral gonorrhea in males, PID, cervicitis caused by susceptible organisms

Dosage and routes:
• *Adult:* **IV/PO** 200-300 mg qd for 7-14 days, depending on infection
Available forms: Sol for inj 5 mg/ml (alatrofloxacin); tabs 100, 200 mg (trovafloxacin)

Side effects/adverse reactions:
CNS: Headache, dizziness, insomnia, anxiety
GI: Nausea, flatulence, vomiting, diarrhea, abdominal pain, ***pseudomembranous colitis***

GU: Vaginitis, crystalluria
INTEG: Rash, pruritus, photosensitivity

Contraindications: Hypersensitivity to quinolones, seizure disorders, cerebral atherosclerosis, photosensitivity

Precautions: Pregnancy (C), lactation, children

Pharmacokinetics: Metabolized in liver, excreted in urine unchanged

Interactions:
• Do not use with magnesium in the same IV line

Solution compatibilities: D_5, ½NaCl, D_5 ½NaCl, D_5/0.2% NaCl, LR

Lab test interferences: *Decrease:* Glucose, lymphocytes

NURSING CONSIDERATIONS
Assess:
• For previous sensitivity reaction to fluoroquinolones
• For signs and symptoms of infection: characteristics of sputum, WBC >10,000, fever; obtain baseline information before and during treatment
• C&S before beginning drug therapy to identify if correct treatment has been initiated
• For allergic reactions: rash, urticaria, pruritus, chills, fever, joint pain; may occur a few days after therapy begins; epinephrine and resuscitation equipment should be available for anaphylactic reaction
• Bowel pattern qd; if severe diarrhea occurs, drug should be discontinued

---

• For overgrowth of infection, perineal itching, fever, malaise, redness, pain, swelling, drainage, rash, diarrhea, change in cough, sputum
Evaluate:
• Therapeutic response: absence of signs/symptoms of infection (WBC <10,000/mm^3, temp WNL)
Teach patient/family:
• To contact prescriber if vaginal itching, loose foul-smelling stools, or furry tongue occurs (may indicate superinfection); to report itching, rash, pruritus, urticaria, tendon pain
• To notify prescriber of diarrhea with blood or pus

---

basiliximab (℞)

(bas-ih-liks'ih-mab)
Simulect
Func. class.: Immunosuppressive
Chem. class.: Murine/human monoclonal antibody (Interleukin-2) receptor antagonist

Action: Binds to and blocks the IL-2 receptor, which is selectively expressed on the surface of activated T-lymphocytes; impairs the immune system to antigenic challenges
Uses: Acute allograft rejection in renal transplant patients when used with cyclosporine and corticosteroids
Dosage and routes:
• *Adult:* **IV** 20 mg × 2 doses; 1st dose within 2 hr before transplant surgery; 2nd dose given 4 days after transplantation
• *Child 2-15 yr:* 12 mg/m^2 × 2 doses; 1st dose within 2 hr before transplant surgery; 2nd dose given 4 days after transplantation
Available forms: Powder for inj 20 mg

Side effects/adverse reactions:
CNS: Pyrexia, chills, tremors, headache, insomnia
RESP: Dyspnea, wheezing, **pulmonary edema**
CV: Chest pain, angina, **cardiac failure,** hypotension
MS: Arthralgia, myalgia
GI: Vomiting, nausea, diarrhea, constipation, abdominal pain
MISC: Infection, moniliasis
Contraindications: Hypersensitivity
Precautions: Pregnancy (B), infections, elderly, lactation, children
NURSING CONSIDERATIONS
Assess:
• Blood studies: Hgb, WBC, platelets during treatment qmo; if leukocytes are <3000/mm^3, drug should be discontinued
• Liver function studies: alk phosphatase, AST (SGOT), ALT (SGPT), bilirubin
• Hepatotoxicity: dark urine, jaundice, itching, light-colored stools; drug should be discontinued
Administer:
• All medications PO if possible; avoid IM injection, since infection may occur
IV
• After adding 5 ml sterile water for inj, shake gently to dissolve, reconstitute to a vol of 50 ml with 0.9% NaCl or D$_5$, gently invert bag, do not shake
Evaluate:
• Therapeutic response: absence of graft rejection
Teach patient/family:
• To report fever, chills, sore throat, fatigue, since serious infection may occur

---

 = Nursing alert   = Herb-drug interaction   🚫 = Do not crush

calfactant (℞)

(cal-fak'tant)
Infasurf
Func. class.: Natural lung surfactant extract

Action: Replenishes surfactant and restores surface activity to the lungs in premature infants

Uses: Prevention and treatment (rescue) of respiratory distress syndrome in premature infants

Dosage and routes:
• **INTRATRACHEAL INSTILL:** 3 ml/kg of birth wt, given as 2 doses of 1.5 ml/kg, repeat doses of 3 ml/kg of birth wt until up to 3 doses 12 hr apart have been given

Available forms: Susp 35 mg phospholipids/ml in 0.9% NaCl with 0.65 mg proteins in single-use vials containing 6 ml susp

Side effects/adverse reactions:
Concurrent illnesses that have occurred during treatment are in bold

RESP: **Pulmonary air leaks, pulmonary interstitial emphysema, apnea, pulmonary hemorrhage**

SYST· **Patent ductus arteriosus, intracranial hemorrhage, severe intracranial hemorrhage, necrotizing enterocolitis, posttreatment sepsis, posttreatment infection**, bradycardia, oxygen desaturation, pallor, vasoconstriction, hypotension, hypertension

Precautions: Bradycardia, rales, infections

Pharmacokinetics: Becomes lung associated within hours of administration

NURSING CONSIDERATIONS
Assess:
• Respiratory rate, rhythm, character, chest expansion, color, transcutaneous saturation, ABGs

• Endotracheal tube placement before dosing; for apnea after endotracheal administration

• Reflux of drug into the endotracheal tube during administration; stop drug if this occurs, and if needed, increase peak inspiratory pressure on the ventilator by 4-5 cm H_2O until tube is cleared

• Infant for repeat dosing using radiographic confirmation of RDS; repeat doses should be given as above; ventilator settings for repeat doses FIo_2 were decreased by 0.2 or amount to prevent cyanosis; ventilator rate of 30/min; inspiratory time <1 sec; if infant's pretreatment rate was >30, it was left unchanged during dosing; resume usual ventilator management after dosing

Administer:
• After suctioning
• By endotracheal administration only by persons trained in neonatal intubation and ventilation
• After using a No. 5 Fr end-hole catheter inserted into the endotracheal tube with the tip protruding just beyond the end of the endotracheal tube; shorten the catheter before insertion; do not insert the drug into the mainstem bronchus
• Divide doses and administer with infant in different positions
• Determine dosing by weight of infant; slowly withdraw contents into plastic syringe through 20G needle; do not filter or shake; attach premeasured No. 5 Fr catheter to syringe; fill with drug and discard excess through catheter so only dose to be given remains in syringe
• For prevention dosing, stabilize, weigh, and intubate infant; give drug within 15 min of birth if possible; position infant and inject first dose through catheter over 2-3 sec; remove catheter and manually venti-

late with O_2 to prevent cyanosis (60 bpm) and sufficient positive pressure to promote adequate air exchange and chest wall excursion
• For rescue dosing, give dosing as soon as infant is placed on ventilator after birth; immediately before administering dose, change ventilator settings to 60/min, inspiratory time 0.5 sec, FIo_2 1; position infant and inject first dose through catheter over 2-3 sec; remove catheter; return to mechanical ventilator
• Ventilate infant for >30 sec or until stable after prevention or rescue strategy; reposition for next dose; same procedure for subsequent dosing; do not suction for at least 1 hr after dosing unless airway obstruction is evident; resume ventilator therapy after dosing

Perform/provide:
• Reduction in peak ventilator inspiratory pressures immediately if chest expansion improves substantially after dose
• Reduction in FIo_2 in small, repeated steps when infant becomes pink and transcutaneous oxygen saturation is in excess of 95%; oxygen saturation should remain between 90% and 95%
• Suctioning of all infants before administration to prevent mucus plugging; if endotracheal tube obstruction is suspected, remove obstruction and replace tube immediately
• Storage in refrigeration; protect from light; warm to room temperature for >20 min or warm in hand >8 min before giving; do not use artificial warming methods; enter a vial only once; unopened, unused vials that have been warmed to room temperature may be rerefrigerated within 8 hr of warming; do not warm and return to refrigerator more than once

Evaluate:
• Therapeutic response: significant improvement in respiratory status

---

candesartan (℞)
(can-deh-sar′tan)
Atacand
Func. class.: Antihypertensive
Chem. class.: Angiotensin II receptor (Type AT_1)

Action: Blocks the vasoconstrictor and aldosterone-secreting effects of angiotensin II; selectively blocks the binding of angiotensin II to the AT_1 receptor found in tissues
Uses: Hypertension, alone or in combination
Dosage and routes:
• *Adult:* **PO** 16 mg qd initially in patients who are not volume depleted, range 8-32 mg/day; may be given with a diuretic
Available forms: Tabs 4, 8, 16, 32
Side effects/adverse reactions:
CNS: Dizziness, fatigue, headache
GI: Diarrhea, nausea
MS: Arthralgia, pain
RESP: Cough, upper respiratory infection
SYST: Angioedema
Contraindications: Hypersensitivity
Precautions: Hypersensitivity to ACE inhibitors; pregnancy (C) 1st trimester, (D) 2nd and 3rd trimesters; lactation; children; elderly
Pharmacokinetics: Extensively metabolized, excreted in urine and feces

NURSING CONSIDERATIONS
Assess:
• B/P, pulse q4h; note rate, rhythm, quality
• Electrolytes: K, Na, Cl
• Baselines in renal, liver function tests before therapy begins
• Edema in feet, legs qd

◆ = Nursing alert   ▮ = Herb-drug interaction   ⊘ = Do not crush

• Skin turgor, dryness of mucous membranes for hydration status; for angioedema

Administer:

• Without regard to meals

Evaluate:

• Therapeutic response: decreased B/P

Teach patient/family:

• To comply with dosage schedule, even if feeling better

• To notify prescriber of mouth sores, fever, swelling of hands or feet, irregular heartbeat, chest pain

• That excessive perspiration, dehydration, vomiting, diarrhea may lead to fall in blood pressure; to consult prescriber if these occur

• That drug may cause dizziness, fainting; light-headedness may occur

• To rise slowly to sitting or standing position to minimize orthostatic hypotension

---

capecitabine (℞)

(cap-eh-sit'ah-been)
Xeloda
Func. class.: Antineoplastic, antimetabolite
Chem. class.: Fluoropyrimidine carbamate

Action: Competes with physiologic substrate of DNA synthesis, thus interfering with cell replication in the S phase of cell cycle (before mitosis)

Uses: Metastatic breast cancer

Dosage and routes:

• *Adult:* PO 2500 mg/m^2/day in 2 divided doses q12h at end of meal × 2 wk, then 1 wk rest period; given in 3 wk cycles

Available forms: Tabs 150, 500 mg

Side effects/adverse reactions:

*HEMA: **Neutropenia, lymphopenia, thrombocytopenia, myelosuppression,** anemia*

GI: Nausea, vomiting, anorexia, diarrhea, stomatitis, abdominal pain

OTHER: Hyperbilirubinemia, eye irritation, pyrexia, edema, myalgia, limb pain

INTEG: Hand and foot syndrome, dermatitis, nail disorder

CNS: Dizziness, headache, paresthesia, fatigue, insomnia

Contraindications: Hypersensitivity to 5-fluorouracil, infants, pregnancy (D)

Precautions: Renal disease, hepatic disease, lactation, children, elderly

Pharmacokinetics: Readily absorbed, peak 1½ hr; food decreases absorption; extensively metabolized in the liver; elimination half-life 45 min

Interactions:

• Increased toxicity: leucovorin

• Increased capecitabine levels: antacid

NURSING CONSIDERATIONS

Assess:

• CBC (RBC, Hct, Hgb), differential, platelet count weekly; withhold drug if WBC is <4000/mm^3, platelet count is <75,000/mm^3, or RBC, Hct, Hgb low; notify prescriber of these results

• Renal function studies: BUN, serum uric acid, urine creatinine clearance, electrolytes before and during therapy

• Monitor temperature q4h; fever may indicate beginning infection; no rectal temperatures

• Liver function tests before and during therapy: bilirubin, ALT (SGPT), AST (SGOT), alk phosphatase, as needed or monthly

• Bleeding: hematuria, hemepositive stools, bruising or petechiae, mucosa or orifices q8h

---

• Dyspnea, rales, unproductive cough, chest pain, tachypnea, fatigue, increased pulse, pallor, lethargy; personality changes, with high doses
• Edema in feet, joint pain, stomach pain, shaking
• Inflammation of mucosa, breaks in skin
• Yellowing of skin, sclera; dark urine; clay-colored stools; itchy skin; abdominal pain; fever; diarrhea
• Buccal cavity q8h for dryness, sores or ulceration, white patches, oral pain, bleeding, dysphagia
• Local irritation, pain, burning, discoloration at injection site
• GI symptoms: frequency of stools, cramping
• Acidosis, signs of dehydration: rapid respirations, poor skin turgor, decreased urine output, dry skin, restlessness, weakness

Administer:
• Antiemetic 30-60 min before giving drug and prn

Perform/provide:
• Strict medical asepsis and protective isolation if WBC levels are low
• Rinsing of mouth tid-qid with water, club soda; brushing of teeth bid-tid with soft brush or cotton-tipped applicators for stomatitis; use unwaxed dental floss
• HOB raised to facilitate breathing if dyspnea or pneumonia

Evaluate:
• Therapeutic response: decreased tumor size, spread of malignancy

Teach patient/family:
• Why protective isolation is necessary
• To report any coughing, chest pain, changes in breathing; may indicate beginning of pneumonia
• To avoid foods with citric acid, hot or rough texture if stomatitis is present

• To report stomatitis: any bleeding, white spots, ulcerations in mouth; to examine mouth qd and report any symptoms
• To report signs of infection: increased temperature, sore throat, flu symptoms
• To report signs of anemia: fatigue, headache, faintness, shortness of breath, irritability
• To report bleeding; to avoid use of razors, commercial mouthwash

---

cefdinir (℞)

(sef'dih-ner)
Omnicef
Func. class.: Antibiotic, broad-spectrum
Chem. class.: Cephalosporin (3rd generation)

Action: Inhibits bacterial cell wall synthesis, rendering cell wall osmotically unstable, leading to cell death

Uses: *H. influenzae, H. parainfluenzae, M. catarrhalis, S. pneumoniae, S. pyogenes, S. aureus*

Dosage and routes:
Uncomplicated skin and skin structure/infections/community-acquired pneumonia
• *Adult and child ≥ 13 yr:* **PO** 300 mg q12h × 10 days
Acute exacerbations of chronic bronchitis/acute maxillary sinusitis
• *Adult and child ≥ 13 yr:* **PO** 300 mg q12h or 600 mg q24h × 10 days
Pharyngitis/tonsillitis
• *Adult and child ≥ 13 yr:* **PO** 300 mg q12h or 600 mg q24h × 10 days
Available forms: Caps 300 mg, oral susp 125 mg/ml

Side effects/adverse reactions:
CNS: Headache, dizziness, weakness, paresthesia, fever, chills

---

⬥ = Nursing alert   🖋 = Herb-drug interaction   ⊘ = Do not crush

GI: Nausea, vomiting, diarrhea, anorexia, pain, glossitis, bleeding; increased AST (SGOT), ALT (SGPT), bilirubin, LDH, alk phosphatase; abdominal pain
GU: Proteinuria, vaginitis, pruritus, candidiasis, increased BUN, *nephrotoxicity, renal failure*
HEMA: Leukopenia, thrombocytopenia, agranulocytosis, anemia, *neutropenia, lymphocytosis, eosinophilia, pancytopenia, hemolytic anemia (rare)*
INTEG: Rash, urticaria, dermatitis, thrombophlebitis
SYST: Anaphylaxis
Contraindications: Hypersensitivity to cephalosporins; infants <1 mo
Precautions: Hypersensitivity to penicillins, pregnancy (B), lactation, renal disease
Pharmacokinetics: Unchanged in urine; crosses placenta, blood-brain barrier; eliminated in breast milk; not metabolized
Interactions:
• Increased toxicity: aminoglycosides, furosemide, colistin, ethacrynic acid, vancomycin
• Increased risk for bleeding: anticoagulants
Lab test interferences:
• *False increase:* Creatinine (serum urine), urinary 17-KS
• *False positive:* Urinary protein, direct Coombs' test, urine glucose
• *Interference:* Cross-matching
NURSING CONSIDERATIONS
Assess:
• Sensitivity to penicillin, other cephalosporins
• Nephrotoxicity: increased BUN, creatinine
• Blood studies: AST (SGOT), ALT (SGPT), CBC, Hct, bilirubin, LDH, alk phosphatase, Coombs' test monthly if patient is on long-term therapy

• Electrolytes: K, Na, Cl monthly if patient is on long-term therapy
• Bowel pattern qd; if severe diarrhea occurs, drug should be discontinued (may indicate pseudomembranous colitis)
• Urine output: if decreasing, notify prescriber, may indicate nephrotoxicity
• Allergic reactions: rash, urticaria, pruritus, chills, fever, joint pain, angioedema, may occur a few days after therapy begins
• Bleeding: ecchymosis, bleeding gums, hematuria, stool guaiac
• Overgrowth of infection: perineal itching, fever, malaise, redness, pain, swelling, drainage, rash, diarrhea, change in cough, sputum
Administer:
• Oral suspension after adding 39 ml water to the 60 ml bottle; 65 ml water to the 120 ml bottle; discard unused portion after 10 days
• After C&S completed
Evaluate:
• Therapeutic response: decreased symptoms of infection
Teach patient/family:
• If diabetic, to check blood glucose level
• To report severe diarrhea; may indicate pseudomembranous colitis
• To report sore throat, bruising, bleeding, joint pain; may indicate blood dyscrasias (rare)
Treatment of anaphylaxis: Epinephrine, antihistamines; resuscitate if needed

---

* = Canada only   Side effects: *italics* = common; ***bold italics*** = life-threatening

citalopram (℞)

(sigh-tal'oh-pram)
Celexa
Func. class.: Antidepressant
Chem. class.: Selective serotonin reuptake inhibitor (SSRI)

Action: Inhibits CNS neuron uptake of serotonin but not of norepinephrine

Uses: Major depressive disorder

Dosage and routes:

• *Adult:* **PO** 20 mg qd AM or PM, may increase if needed to 40 mg/day after 1 wk; maintenance: after 6-8 wk of initial treatment, continue for 24 wk (32 wk total), reevaluate long-term usefulness

Available forms: Tabs 20, 40 mg

Side effects/adverse reactions:

CNS: Headache, nervousness, insomnia, drowsiness, anxiety, tremor, dizziness, fatigue, sedation, poor concentration, abnormal dreams, agitation, **convulsions,** apathy, euphoria, hallucinations, delusions, psychosis

GI: Nausea, diarrhea, dry mouth, anorexia, dyspepsia, constipation, cramps, vomiting, taste changes, flatulence, decreased appetite

INTEG: Sweating, rash, pruritus, acne, alopecia, urticaria

RESP: Infection, pharyngitis, nasal congestion, sinus headache, sinusitis, cough, dyspnea, bronchitis, asthma, hyperventilation, pneumonia

CV: Hot flashes, palpitations, angina pectoris, **hemorrhage,** hypertension, tachycardia, first-degree AV block, bradycardia, *MI,* thrombophlebitis

MS: Pain, arthritis, twitching

GU: Dysmenorrhea, decreased libido, urinary frequency, UTI, amenorrhea, cystitis, impotence, urine retention

EENT: Visual changes, ear/eye pain, photophobia, tinnitus

SYST: Asthenia, viral infection, fever, allergy, chills

Contraindications: Hypersensitivity

Precautions: Pregnancy (B), lactation, children, elderly, diabetes mellitus

Pharmacokinetics:

PO: Metabolized in liver; excreted in urine; steady state 28-35 days

Interactions:

• Do not use with MAOIs

• Increased citalopram levels: macrolides, azole antifungals

• Increased plasma levels of: β-blockers

• Decreased citalopram levels; carbamazepine

• Increased serotonergic effects: lithium

 Avoid use with St. John's wort

Lab test interferences:

• *Increase:* Serum bilirubin, blood glucose, alk phosphatase

• *Decrease:* VMA, 5-HIAA

• *False increase:* Urinary catecholamines

NURSING CONSIDERATIONS

Assess:

• Mental status: mood, sensorium, affect, suicidal tendencies, increase in psychiatric symptoms, depression, panic

• B/P (lying/standing), pulse q4h; if systolic B/P drops 20 mm Hg, hold drug, notify prescriber; take vital signs q4h in patients with cardiovascular disease

• Blood studies: CBC, leukocytes, differential, cardiac enzymes if patient is receiving long-term therapy; check platelets; bleeding can occur

• Hepatic studies: AST (SGOT), ALT (SGPT), bilirubin, creatinine

---

◆ = Nursing alert   = Herb-drug interaction   🚫 = Do not crush

• Weight qwk; appetite may decrease with drug
• ECG for flattening of T wave, bundle branch, AV block, dysrhythmias in cardiac patients
• EPS primarily in elderly: rigidity, dystonia, akathisia
• Urinary retention, constipation
⬥Withdrawal symptoms: headache, nausea, vomiting, muscle pain, weakness; not usual unless drug discontinued abruptly
• Alcohol consumption; if alcohol is consumed, hold dose until AM

Administer:
• Increased fluids, bulk in diet if constipation, urinary retention occur
• With food or milk for GI symptoms
• Crushed if patient is unable to swallow medication whole
• Dosage hs if oversedation occurs during the day; may take entire dose hs
• Gum, hard candy, frequent sips of water for dry mouth

Perform/provide:
• Storage at room temp; do not freeze
• Assistance with ambulation during therapy, since drowsiness, dizziness occur
• Safety measures primarily in elderly
• Checking to see if PO medication swallowed

Evaluate:
• Therapeutic response: decreased depression

Teach patient/family:
• That therapeutic effect may take 2-3 wk
• To use caution in driving, other activities requiring alertness because of drowsiness, dizziness, blurred vision
• Not to discontinue medication quickly after long-term use; may cause nausea, headache, malaise

• To avoid alcohol ingestion, other CNS depressants
• To notify prescriber if pregnant or plan to become pregnant or breastfeed

---

daclizumab (℞)
(dah-kliz'uh-mab)
Zenapax
Func. class.: Immunosuppressive
Chem. class.: Humanized IgG1 monoclonal antibody

Action: Binds to the IL-2 (interleukin-2) receptor antagonist
Uses: Acute allograft rejection in renal transplant patients
Dosage and routes:
• *Adult:* **IV** 1 mg/kg as part of a regimen that includes cyclosporine and corticosteroids, mix calculated vol with 50 ml of 0.9% NaCl and give via peripheral/central vein over 15 min
Available forms: Inj conc 25 mg/ml
Side effects/adverse reactions:
CNS: Chills, tremors, headache, prickly sensation
RESP: Dyspnea, wheezing, **pulmonary edema,** coughing, atelectasis, congestion
GI: Vomiting, nausea, diarrhea, constipation, abdominal pain, pyrosis
CV: Hypertension, **tachycardia, thrombosis,** bleeding
GU: Oliguria, dysuria, **renal tubular necrosis,** renal damage, **hydronephrosis**
INTEG: Impaired wound healing
Contraindications: Hypersensitivity
Precautions: Pregnancy (C), child <2 yr, lactation, elderly
NURSING CONSIDERATIONS
Assess:
• Blood studies: Hgb, WBC, plate-

lets during treatment qmo; if leukocytes are <3000/mm^3, drug should be discontinued

• Liver function studies: alk phosphatase, AST (SGOT), ALT (SGPT), bilirubin

• Hepatotoxicity: dark urine, jaundice, itching, light-colored stools; drug should be discontinued

Administer:

• All other medications PO if possible

• Avoid IM injection, since infection may occur

Solution compatibilities: 0.9% NaCl

Evaluate:

• Therapeutic response: absence of graft rejection

Teach patient/family:

• To report fever, chills, sore throat, fatigue, since serious infection may occur

---

efavirenz (R)

(ef-ah-veer'enz)

Sustiva

Func. class.: Antiviral

Chem. class.: Non-nucleoside reverse transcriptase inhibitor (NNRTI)

Action: Binds directly to reverse transcriptase and blocks RNA, DNA causing a disruption of the enzyme's site

Uses: HIV-1 in combination with other antiretrovirals

Dosage and routes:

• *Adult:* **PO** 600 mg qd hs in combination with protease inhibitor or nucleoside analog reverse transcriptase inhibitors (NRTIs)

• *Child: 10-<15 kg:* **PO** 200 mg qd hs

• *Child: 15-<20 kg:* **PO** 250 mg qd hs

• *Child: 20-<25 kg:* **PO** 300 mg qd hs

• *Child: 25-<32.5 kg:* **PO** 350 mg qd hs

• *Child: 32.5-<40 kg:* **PO** 400 mg qd hs

• *Child: ≥ 40 kg:* Adult dose

Available forms: Caps 50, 100, 200 mg

Side effects/adverse reactions:

GI: Diarrhea, abdominal pain, *nausea*

CNS: Headache

INTEG: Rash, dizziness, fatigue, impaired concentration, insomnia, abnormal dreams, depression

Contraindications: Hypersensitivity

Precautions: Liver disease, pregnancy (C), lactation, children <3 yr, renal disease, myelosuppression

Pharmacokinetics: Well absorbed, metabolized by liver, terminal half-life 52-76 hr

Interactions:

• Decreased efavirenz levels: rifamycins

• Do not give together with astemizole, benzodiazepines, ergots, cisapride

• Decreased levels of: indinavir, saquinavir

• Increased levels of both drugs: ritonavir

• Increased levels of: warfarin

NURSING CONSIDERATIONS

Assess:

• Signs of infection, anemia

• Liver studies: ALT, AST: renal studies

• C&S before drug therapy; drug may be taken as soon as culture is taken; repeat C&S after treatment; determine the presence of other sexually transmitted disease

• Bowel pattern before, during treatment; if severe abdominal pain with bleeding occurs, drug should be discontinued; monitor hydration

---

◆ = Nursing alert   🖉 = Herb-drug interaction   🚫 = Do not crush

• Skin eruptions; rash, urticaria, itching

• Allergies before treatment, reaction to each medication; place allergies on chart

• CBC, blood chemistry, plasma HIV RNA, absolute CD4+/CD8+ cell counts/%, serum beta-2 microglobulin, serum ICD+24 antigen levels, cholesterol, hepatic enzymes

• Signs of toxicity: severe nausea/vomiting, maculopapular rash

Teach patient/family:

• To take as prescribed; if dose is missed, take as soon as remembered; do not double dose

• To make sure health-care provider knows all the medications being taken

• That if severe rash occurs, to notify health-care provider

• Not to breastfeed if taking this drug

---

eptifibatide

(ep-tih-fib'ah-tide)
Integrilin
Func. class.: Antiplatelet agent
Chem. class.: Glycoprotein IIb/IIIa inhibitor

Action: Platelet glycoprotein antagonist. This agent reversibly prevents fibrinogen, von Willebrand's factor from binding to the glycoprotein IIb/IIIa receptor, inhibiting platelet aggregation

Uses: Acute coronary syndrome including those with PCI (percutaneous coronary intervention)

Dosage and routes:

Acute coronary syndrome

• *Adult:* IV BOL 180 µg/kg as soon as diagnosed, then IV CONT 2 µg/kg/min until discharge or CABG up to 72 hr; may decrease inf rate to 0.5 µg/kg/min if undergoing PCI; continue inf for 20-24 hr postprocedure, allowing up to 96 hr of treatment

PCI in patients without acute coronary syndrome

• *Adult:* IV BOL 135 µg/kg given immediately before PCI; then 0.5 µg/kg/min × 20-24 hr

Side effects/adverse reactions:

CV: ***Stroke,*** hypotension
SYST: ***Bleeding***

Contraindications: Hypersensitivity, active internal bleeding; history of bleeding, stroke within 1 mo; major surgery with severe trauma, severe hypotension, history of intracranial bleeding, intracranial neoplasm, arteriovenous malformation/aneurysm, aortic dissection, dependence on renal dialysis

Precautions: Bleeding, pregnancy (B), lactation, children, elderly, renal function impairment

Interactions:

• Increased bleeding: aspirin, heparin

Pharmacokinetics: Half-life 2.5 hr, steady state 4-6 hr, metabolism limited, excretion via kidneys

NURSING CONSIDERATIONS

Assess:

• Platelets, Hgb, Hct, creatinine, PT/APTT baseline, within 6 hr of loading dose and qd thereafter, patients undergoing PCI should have ACT monitored; maintain APTT 50-70 sec unless PCI is to be performed, during PCI, ACT should be 300-350 sec; if platelets drop <100,000/mm³, obtain additional platelet counts; if thrombocytopenia is confirmed, discontinue drug

• Monitor ECG continuously

Administer:

IV

• After withdrawing bolus dose from 10 ml vial, give IV push over 1-2 min; follow bolus dose with continuous inf using inf pump, give drug

---

undiluted directly from 100 ml vial, spike 100 ml vial with vented infusion set, use caution when centering spike on circle of stopper top

Perform/provide:
• Discontinuing drug prior to CABG

etanercept (℞)
(eh-tan′er-sept)
Enbrel
Func. class.: Biological

Uses: Acute, chronic rheumatoid arthritis that has not responded to other treatment

Dosage and routes:
• *Adult:* SC 25 mg 2×/wk, may be given with other drugs for rheumatoid arthritis
• *Child 4-17 yr:* SC 0.4 mg/kg, max 25 mg, 2×/wk

Available forms: Powder for inj: 25 mg

Side effects/adverse reactions:
GI: Abdominal pain, dyspepsia
CNS: Headache, asthenia, dizziness
INTEG: Rash, inj site reaction
RESP: Pharyngitis, cough, URI, non-URI, sinusitis, *rhinitis*

Contraindications: Hypersensitivity, sepsis

Precautions: Pregnancy (B), lactation, children <4 yr

Pharmacokinetics: Elimination half-life 115 hr

Interactions:
• Do not give concurrently with vaccines, immunizations should be brought up to date before treatment

NURSING CONSIDERATIONS
Assess:
• Pain, stiffness, swelling of joints during treatment

Administer:
• After reconstituting 1 ml of supplied diluent, slowly inject diluent into vial, swirl contents, do not shake, sol should be clear/colorless, do not use if cloudy or discolored
• Do not admix with other sol or medications, do not use filter

Evaluate:
• Therapeutic response: decreased inflammation, pain in joints

Teach patient/family:
• That drug must be continued for prescribed time to be effective
• To use caution when driving; dizziness may occur
• About self-administration if appropriate: inj should be made in thigh, abdomen, upper arm; rotate sites at least 1 in from old site

fenoldopam (℞)
(feh-nahl′doh-pam)
Corlopam
Func. class.: Antihypertensive
Chem. class.: Vasodilator

Action: Antagonizes D_1-like dopamine receptors; binds to α_2-adrenoceptors; increases renal blood flow

Uses: Hypertensive crisis when urgent decrease of pressure required; including malignant hypertension

Dosage and routes:
• *Adult:* CONT IV titrate initial dose upward or downward no more frequently than q15 min; increments should range between 0.05-0.1 µg/kg/min; initial doses of 0.03-0.1 µg/kg/min titrated slowly result in less reflex tachycardia

Available forms: Inj conc 10 mg/ml

Side effects/adverse reactions:
CNS: Headache, anxiety, dizziness
CV: Hypotension, ST-T-wave changes, angina pectoris, palpitations, *MI, ischemic heart disease*
GI: Nausea, vomiting, constipation, diarrhea
HEMA: Leukocytosis, bleeding
META: Increased BUN, glucose,

◆ = Nursing alert   = Herb-drug interaction   ⊘ = Do not crush

LDH, creatinine, hypokalemia
Contraindications: Hypersensitivity, sulfite sensitivity
Precautions: Tachycardia, pregnancy (B), lactation, children, intraocular pressure, hypokalemia
Pharmacokinetics: Elimination half-life 5 min, steady state 20 min
Interactions:
• Avoid use with β-blockers
NURSING CONSIDERATIONS
Assess:
• B/P q5min until stabilized, then qlh × 2 hr, then q4h
• Pulse, jugular venous distension q4h
• Electrolytes, blood studies: K, Na, Cl, CO_2, CBC, serum glucose
• Weight daily, I&O
• Edema in feet, legs daily
• Skin turgor, dryness of mucous membranes for hydration status
• Rales, dyspnea, orthopnea
• IV site for extravasation, rate
• Postural hypotension, take B/P sitting, standing
Administer:
IV
• After diluting contents of ampules in 0.9% NaCl, or 5% dextrose inj (40 µg/ml); then add 4 ml of conc (40 mg of drug/1000 ml); 2 ml of conc (20 mg of drug/500 ml); 1 ml of conc (10 mg of drug/250 ml)
• To patient in recumbent position; keep in that position for 1 hr after administration
Perform/provide:
• Diluted sol is stable in normal light/temp for 24 hr
Evaluate:
• Therapeutic response: decreased B/P

halofantrine (℞)
(hay-loh-fan'trin)
Halfan
Func. class.: Antimalarial
Chem. class.: Phenanthrene-methanol

Action: Inhibits parasite replications, transcription of DNA to RNA by forming complexes with DNA of parasite
Uses: Mild to moderate malaria
Dosage and routes:
• *Adult:* **PO** 500 mg q6h × 3 doses; may need to repeat after 1 wk
Available forms: Tabs 250 mg
Side effects/adverse reactions:
GI: Nausea, vomiting, anorexia, diarrhea
CV: Dysrhythmias
Contraindications: Hypersensitivity
Precautions: Severe GI disease, severe hepatic disease, cardiac dysrhythmias
Pharmacokinetics:
PO: Metabolized in liver, excreted in urine
NURSING CONSIDERATIONS
Assess:
• B/P, pulse, watch for tachycardia
• Liver studies qwk: ALT (SGPT), AST (SGOT), bilirubin
Administer:
PO
• 1 hr before or 2 hr after meals at same time each day to maintain level
Perform/provide:
• Storage in tight, light-resistant container
Evaluate:
• Therapeutic response: decreased symptoms of malaria
Teach patient/family:
• To take exactly as prescribed, to take full course that is prescribed

---

infliximab

(in-fliks'ih-mab)

Remicade

Func. class.: Monoclonal antibody

Action: Monoclonal antibody that neutralizes the activity of tumor necrosis factor alpha (TNF α) found in Crohn's disease; decreased infiltration of inflammatory cells

Uses: Crohn's disease, fistulizing; moderate-severe

Dosage and routes:

Crohn's disease (moderate-severe)
• *Adult:* IV INF 5 mg/kg

Crohn's disease (fistulizing)
• *Adult:* IV INF 5 mg/kg initially, then repeat dose 2 wk, 6 wk after 1st dose

Available forms: Powder for inj 100 mg

Side effects/adverse reactions:

SYST: Anaphylaxis

GI: Nausea, vomiting, abdominal pain, stomatitis, constipation, dyspepsia, flatulence

CNS: Headache, dizziness, depression, vertigo, fatigue, anxiety, fever

HEMA: Anemia

INTEG: Rash, dermatitis, urticaria, dry skin, sweating, flushing, hematoma, pruritus

RESP: URI, pharyngitis, bronchitis, cough, dyspnea, sinusitis

MS: Myalgia, back pain, arthralgia

GU: Dysuria, frequency

CV: Chest pain, hyper- and hypotension, *tachycardia*

Contraindications: Hypersensitivity to murines

Precautions: Pregnancy (C), lactation, children, elderly

Pharmacokinetics: Distributed to vascular compartment, half-life 9.5 days

NURSING CONSIDERATIONS

Assess:
• GI symptoms: nausea, vomiting, abdominal pain
• Take periodic blood counts (CBC)
• CV status: B/P, pulse, chest pain
• Allergic reaction: rash, dermatitis, urticaria, dyspnea, hypotension; discontinue if severe

Administer:

IV INF
• Immediately after reconstitution; reconstitute with 10 ml of sterile water for inj, further dilute total dose/250 ml 0.9% NaCl inj to a total conc. of between 0.4 and 4 mg/ml; use 21G or smaller needle for reconstitution, direct sterile water at glass wall of vial, gently swirl
• Give over ≥2 hr, use polyethylene-lined infusion with in-line, sterile, low-protein-bind filter

Perform/provide:
• Refrigerated storage, do not freeze

Evaluate:
• Therapeutic response: absence of fever, mucus in stools

leflunomide (℞)

(leh-floo'noh-mide)

Arava

Chem. class.: Pyrimidine synthesis inhibitor

Action: Inhibits an enzyme involved in pyrimidine synthesis and has antiproliferative effect

Uses: Rheumatoid arthritis

Dosage and routes:
• *Adult:* PO loading dose 100 mg/day × 3 days, maintenance 20 mg/day, may be decreased to 10 mg/day if not well tolerated

Available forms: Tabs 10, 20, 100 mg

Side effects/adverse reactions:

GI: Nausea, anorexia, vomiting, constipation, flatulence

◆ = Nursing alert   ∥ = Herb-drug interaction   ⊘ = Do not crush

CNS: Dizziness, insomnia, depression, paresthesia
CV: Palpitations, hypertension, chest pain, angina pectoris, migraine
INTEG: Rash, pruritus
RESP: Pharyngitis, rhinitis, bronchitis, cough, respiratory infection, pneumonia, sinusitis
Contraindications: Hypersensitivity, pregnancy (X), lactation
Precautions: Hepatic, renal disorders
Pharmacokinetics:
PO: Metabolized in liver to metabolite, excreted in urine
Interactions:
• Increased NSAIDs effect: NSAIDs
• Increased side effects of leflunomide: hepatotoxic agents
• Increased rifampin levels: rifampin
• Decreased effect of leflunomide: charcoal, cholestyramine
NURSING CONSIDERATIONS
Assess:
• Liver function studies: if ALT elevations are >twofold ULN, reduce dose to 10 mg/day
Administer:
PO
• With food for GI upset
Evaluate:
• Therapeutic response: decreased inflammation, pain in joints
Teach patient/family:
• That drug must be continued for prescribed time to be effective
• To take with food, milk, or antacids to avoid GI upset
• To use caution when driving; drowsiness, dizziness may occur
• To take with a full glass of water to enhance absorption
• To avoid pregnancy while taking this drug

lepirudin (℞)
(lep-ih-roo′din)
Refludan
Func. class.: Anticoagulant
Chem. class.: Hirudin

Action: Direct inhibitor of thrombin that is highly specific
Uses: Heparin-induced thrombocytopenia and other thromboembolic conditions
Dosage and routes:
• *Adult:* **IV** 0.4 mg/kg (≤110 kg) over 15-20 sec; then 0.15 mg/kg (≤110 kg/hr) as a cont inf for 2-10 days or longer
Available forms: Powder for inj 50 mg
Side effects/adverse reactions:
*CV: **Heart failure, pericardial effusion, ventricular fibrillation***
*SYST: **Multiorgan failure,** sepsis*
CNS: Fever
GI: GI bleeding, abnormal LFTs
*GU: **Hematuria,** abnormal kidney function*
*HEMA: **Hemorrhage, thrombocytopenia***
RESP: Pneumonia
INTEG: Allergic skin reactions
Contraindications: Hypersensitivity to hirudins
Precautions: Intracranial bleeding, renal function impairment, lactation, children, hepatic disease, pregnancy (B)
Pharmacokinetics: May be metabolized by the release of amino acids during catabolism; 50% unchanged in urine
Interactions:
• Increased risk of bleeding: coumadin derivatives
• Increased action of lepirudin: thrombolytics
◆ Bleeding gums, petechiae, ecchymosis, black tarry stools, he-

maturia, epistaxis, decrease in BP indicate bleeding and possible hemorrhage

NURSING CONSIDERATIONS
Assess:
• Obtain baseline in APTT before treatment; do not start treatment if APTT ratio ≥ 2.5, then APTT 4 hr after initiation of treatment and at least qd thereafter, if APTT above target, stop inf for 2 hr, then restart at 50%, take APTT in 4 hr; if below target, increase inf rate by 20%, take APTT in 4 hr, do not exceed inf rate of 0.21 mg/kg/hr without checking for coagulation abnormalities
• APTT, which should be 1.5-2.5 × control

 Bleeding gums, petechiae, ecchymosis, black tarry stools, hematuria/epistaxis, B/P, vaginal bleeding, puncture sites; indicate bleeding and possible hemorrhage
• Fever, skin rash, urticaria

Administer:
• Avoiding all IM injections that may cause bleeding
• After reconstitution and further dilution under sterile conditions; use water for inj or 0.9% NaCl; for further dilution 0.9% NaCl or D₅; for rapid and complete reconstitution, inject 1 ml of diluent into vial and shake gently, use immediately, warm to room temp before use

IV BOL
• Use sol with conc. of 5 mg/ml, reconstitute 5 mg (1 vial)/1 ml of water for inj or 0.9% NaCl, use body wt for correct calculation as to weight

IV INF
• Use sol with a conc. of 0.2 or 0.4 mg/ml; reconstitute 100 mg (2 vials) with 1 ml each (2 ml) water for inj or 0.9% NaCl, transfer to inf bag with either 500 or 250 ml of 0.9% NaCl or D₅

Evaluate:
• Therapeutic response
Teach patient/family:
• To use soft-bristle toothbrush to avoid bleeding gums, avoid contact sports, use electric razor, avoid IM injection
• To report any signs of bleeding: gums, under skin, urine, stools

---

montelukast (℞)
(mon-teh-loo'kast)
Singulair
Func. class.: Leukotriene receptor
Chem. class.: Cysteinyl

Action: Inhibits leukotriene (LTD₄) formation; leukotrienes exert their effects by increasing neutrophil, eosinophil migration; aggregation of neutrophils, monocytes; smooth muscle contraction, capillary permeability; these actions further lead to bronchoconstriction, inflammation, edema

Uses: Chronic asthma

Dosage and routes:
Asthma
• *Adult and child ≥ 15 yr:* **PO** 10 mg qd PM
• *Child 6-14 yr:* **PO** 5 mg chew tab qd PM

Available forms: Tabs 10 mg; tabs, chew 5 mg

Side effects/adverse reactions:
CNS: Dizziness, fatigue, headache
GI: Abdominal pain, dyspepsia, LFT abnormalities
INTEG: Rash
MS: Asthenia
RESP: Influenza, cough, nasal congestion

Contraindications: Hypersensitivity

Precautions: Acute attacks of

asthma, alcohol consumption, pregnancy (B), lactation, child <6 yr, aspirin sensitivity

Pharmacokinetics: Rapidly absorbed, peak 3-4 hr, half-life 2.7-5.5 hr; protein binding 99%; metabolized by liver, excreted via bile

Interactions:

• Decreased montelukast levels: phenobarbital, rifampin

NURSING CONSIDERATIONS

Assess:

➡️Adult patients carefully for symptoms of Churg-Strauss syndrome (rare), including eosinophilia, vasculitic rash, worsening pulmonary symptoms, cardiac complications, and/or neuropathy

• CBC, blood chemistry, during treatment

• LFTs before and qmo × 3 mo, then q2-3mo during treatment (ALT; AST)

• Respiratory rate, rhythm, depth; auscultate lung fields bilaterally; notify prescriber of abnormalities

• Allergic reactions: rash, urticaria; drug should be discontinued

Administer:

PO

• In PM qd

Evaluate:

• Therapeutic response: ability to breathe more easily

Teach patient/family:

• To check OTC medications, current prescription medications for ephedrine, which will increase stimulation; to avoid alcohol

• To avoid hazardous activities; dizziness may occur

• That drug is not to be used for acute asthma attacks

naratriptan (℞)

(nair'ah-trip-tan)

Amerge

Func. class.: Migraine agent

Chem. class.: 5-HT$_1$-like receptor agonist

Action: Binds selectively to the vascular 5-HT$_1$ receptor subtype, exerts antimigraine effect; causes vasoconstriction in cranial arteries

Uses: Acute treatment of migraine with or without aura

Dosage and routes:

• *Adult:* **PO** 1 or 2.5 mg with fluids, if headache returns, repeat once after 4 hr, max 5 mg/24 hr

Available forms: Tab 1, 2.5 mg

Side effects/adverse reactions:

GI: Nausea

MS: Weakness, neck stiffness, myalgia

CNS: Dizziness, sedation, fatigue

Contraindications: Angina pectoris, history of MI, documented silent ischemia, ischemic heart disease, concurrent ergotamine-containing preparations, uncontrolled hypertension, hypersensitivity, severe renal disease (CrCl <15 ml/min); severe hepatic disease (child-Pugh grade C)

Precautions: Postmenopausal women, men >40 yr, risk factors for CAD, hypercholesterolemia, obesity, diabetes, impaired hepatic or renal function, pregnancy (C), lactation, children, elderly, peripheral vascular disease

Pharmacokinetics: Peak 30 min, 28%-31% plasma protein binding, half-life 6 hr, metabolized in the liver (metabolite), excreted in urine, feces; may be excreted in breast milk

Interactions:

• Extended vasopastic effects: ergot, ergot derivatives

• Weakness, hyperreflexia, incoordination: SSRIs (fluoxetine, fluvoxamine, paroxetine, sertraline)
• Smoking: Increases the clearance of naratriptan

NURSING CONSIDERATIONS
Assess:
• For stress level, activity, recreation, coping mechanisms
• Neurologic status: LOC blurred vision, nausea, vomiting, tingling in extremities preceding headache
Administer:
• With fluids
Perform/provide:
• Quiet, calm environment with decreased stimulation for noise, bright light, excessive talking
Evaluate:
• Therapeutic response: decrease in frequency, severity of headache
Teach patient/family:
• To report any side effects to prescriber
• Not to use if another 5-HT agonist or an ergot preparation has been used in the past 24 hr

---

palivizumab (℞)
(pal-ih-viz'uh-mab)
Synagis
Func. class.: Monoclonal antibody

Action: A humanized monoclonal antibody that exhibits neutralizing and fusion-inhibitory activity against respiratory syncytial virus (RSV)
Uses: Prevention of serious lower respiratory tract disease caused by RSV in pediatric patients
Dosage and routes:
• *Child:* IM 15 mg/kg, those patients who develop RSV should receive monthly doses during RSV season

Available forms: Lyophilized inj 100 mg
Side effects/adverse reactions:
GI: Nausea, vomiting, diarrhea, increased AST
RESP: URI
EENT: Otitis media, rhinitis, pharyngitis
INTEG: Rash, inj site reaction
Contraindications: Hypersensitivity, adults, cyanotic congenital heart disease
Precautions: Thrombocytopenia, coagulation disorders, established RSV, congenital heart disease, chronic lung disease, systemic allergic reactions
Pharmacokinetics: Mean half-life 20 days

NURSING CONSIDERATIONS
Assess:
• For presence of RSV infection, drug is given to prevent infection
• For side effects; report if allergic reaction is evident
Administer:
• IM only
• After adding 1 ml of sterile water for inj per 100 mg vial, gently swirl, let stand at room temp for 20 min until sol clarifies; given within 6 hr of reconstitution
Teach patient/family:
• To report upper respiratory infections, earaches, rash, sore throat

---

paricalcitol (℞)
(par-ih-cal'sih-tol)
Zemplar
Func. class.: Vit D analog
Chem. class.: Fat-soluble vitamin

Action: Reduces parathyroid hormone (PTH) levels; suppresses PTH levels in patients with chronic renal

---

 = Nursing alert   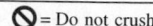 = Herb-drug interaction   🚫 = Do not crush

failure with absence of hypercalcemia/hyperphosphatemia. Serum PO_4, Ca, CaXP may increase
Uses: Hypoparathyroidism
Dosage and routes:
• *Adult:* **IV BOL** 0.04-0.1 µg/kg (2.8-7 µg) no more than qod during dialysis; may increase by 2-4 µg q2-4wk
Available forms: Inj 5 µg/ml
Side effects/adverse reactions:
GI: Nausea, vomiting, anorexia, dry mouth
CNS: Lightheadedness
CV: Palpitations
OTHER: Pneumonia, edema, chills, fever, flu, *sepsis*
Contraindications: Hypersensitivity, hypercalcemia
Precautions: Cardiovascular disease, renal calculi, pregnancy (C), elderly, lactation, children
Interactions:
• Digitalis toxicity: digitalis
NURSING CONSIDERATIONS
Assess:
• Ca, PO_4, q2×/wk during initial therapy; after dose is established take calcium and phosphorus qmo
Administer:
IV
• By IV bolus only
Evaluate:
• Decreased hypoparathyroidism in chronic renal disease
Teach patient/family:
• To report weakness, lethargy, headache, anorexia, loss of weight
• To report nausea, vomiting, palpitations

---

raloxifene (℞)

(ral-ox'ih-feen)
Evista
Func. class.: Selective estrogen receptor modulator (SERM)
Chem. class.: Benzthiophene

Action: Reduces resorption of bone and decreases bone turnover; mediated through estrogen receptor binding
Uses: Prevention of osteoporosis in postmenopausal women
Dosage and routes:
• *Adult:* **PO** 60 mg qd
Available forms: Tabs 60 mg
Side effects/adverse reactions:
CNS: Insomnia, migraines, depression
CV: Hot flashes
GI: Nausea, vomiting, diarrhea, anorexia, cramps
GU: Vaginitis, UTI, leukorrhea, endometrial disorder, breast pain
INTEG: Rash, sweating
META: Weight gain, peripheral edema
MS: Arthralgia, myalgia, leg cramps, arthritis
RESP: Sinusitis, pharyngitis, increased cough, pneumonia, laryngitis
Contraindications: Hypersensitivity, pregnancy (X), lactation
Precautions: Lactation, venous thromboembolic events, hepatic disease
Pharmacokinetics: Elimination half-life 28 hr; excreted in feces; excreted in breast milk; highly bound to plasma proteins
Interactions:
• Decreased action of anticoagulants
• Decreased action of raloxifene: ampicillin, cholestyramine

Side effects: *italics* = common; ***bold italics*** = life-threatening

• Administer cautiously with other highly protein-bound drugs

Lab test interferences:

• *Increase:* Apolipoprotein A_1, B, lipoprotein, fibrinogen, LDL cholesterol, total cholesterol, corticosteroid-binding globulin, thyroxine-binding globulin (TBG)

• *Decrease:* Calcium, total protein, albumin, platelets

NURSING CONSIDERATIONS

Assess:

• Blood glucose of diabetic patient

• Weight daily, notify prescriber of weekly weight gain >5 lb

• B/P q4h, watch for increase caused by H_2O and Na retention

• I&O ratio; decreasing urinary output, increasing edema

• Liver function studies, including AST (SGOT), ALT (SGPT), bilirubin, alk phosphatase

Administer:

PO

• Without regard to meals

Evaluate:

• Therapeutic response: prevention of osteoporosis

Teach patient/family:

• To weigh weekly, report gain >5 lb

• To discontinue 72 hr before prolonged bedrest; advise to avoid one position for long periods

• To take calcium supplements, vit D if intake is inadequate

• To increase exercise using weights

• To stop smoking and to decrease alcohol consumption

• That this drug does not help control hot flashes

• To report fever, acute migraine, insomnia, emotional distress; urinary tract infection, or vaginal burning/itching; swelling, warmth, or pain in calves

---

repaglinide (R)
(re-pag'lih-nide)
Prandin
Func. class.: Antidiabetic
Chem. class.: Meglitinides

Action: Causes functioning β-cells in pancreas to release insulin, leading to drop in blood glucose levels; closes ATP-dependent potassium channels in the β-cell membrane; this leads to opening of calcium channels; increased calcium influx induces insulin secretion

Uses: Stable adult-onset diabetes mellitus (type II) NIDDM

Dosage and routes:

• *Adult:* PO 0.5-4 mg

Available forms: Tabs 0.5, 1, 2 mg

Side effects/adverse reactions:

CNS: Headache, weakness, paresthesia

ENDO: Hypoglycemia

GI: Nausea, vomiting, diarrhea, constipation, dyspepsia

INTEG: Rash, allergic reactions

MS: Back pains, arthralgia

RESP: URI, sinusitis, rhinitis, bronchitis

Contraindications: Hypersensitivity to meglitinides, diabetic ketoacidosis, type I diabetes

Precautions: Pregnancy (C), elderly, cardiac disease, severe renal disease, severe hepatic disease, thyroid disease, severe hypoglycemic reactions, lactation, children

Pharmacokinetics:

PO: Completely absorbed by GI route; onset 2-4 hr, peak 2-8 hr, duration 24 hr; half-life 1 hr; metabolized in liver; excreted in urine, feces (metabolites); crosses placenta; 98% plasma protein bound

Interactions:

• Increased repaglinide metabolism:

  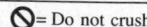

troglitazone, rifampin, barbiturates, carbamazepine
• Decreased repaglinide metabolism: antifungals (ketoconazole, miconazole), erythromycin
• Increased effect of repaglinide: NSAIDs, salicylates, sulfonamides, chloramphenicol, MAOIs, coumarins, β-blockers, probenecid
• Decreased action of repaglinide: calcium channel blockers, corticosteroids, oral contraceptives, thiazide diuretics, thyroid preparations, estrogens, phenothiazines, phenytoin, rifampin, isoniazid, phenobarbital, sympathomimetics
NURSING CONSIDERATIONS
Assess:
• Hypo/hyperglycemic reaction that can occur soon after meals
Administer:
• 15 min before meals; 2, 3, or 4×/day preprandially
• Skip dose if meal is skipped; add dose if meal is added
Perform/provide:
• Storage in tight container in cool environment
Evaluate:
• Therapeutic response: decrease in polyuria, polydipsia, polyphagia, clear sensorium, absence of dizziness, stable gait
Teach patient/family:
• To avoid alcohol; explain disulfiram reaction
• To use a capillary blood glucose test while on this drug
• The symptoms of hypo/hyperglycemia; what to do about each
• That drug must be continued on daily basis; explain consequences of discontinuing drug abruptly
• To avoid OTC medications unless ordered by prescriber
• That diabetes is a lifelong illness; drug will not cure disease

• That all food included in diet plan must be eaten to prevent hypoglycemia; to have glucagon emergency kit available
• To carry a Medic Alert ID for emergency purposes
Treatment of overdose: Glucose 25 g IV via dextrose 50% solution, 50 ml or 1 mg glucagon

---

rifapentine (R̞)
(riff'ah-pen-teen)
Priftin
Func. class.: Antitubercular
Chem. class.: Rifamycin derivative

Action: Inhibits DNA-dependent polymerase, decreases tubercle bacilli replication
Uses: Pulmonary tuberculosis, must be used with at least one other antitubercular
Dosage and routes:
Intensive phase
• *Adult:* PO 600 mg (four 150 mg tabs 2×/wk), with an interval of 72 hr between doses × 2 mo; must be given with at least one other antitubercular
Continuation phase
• *Adult:* PO continue with 1×/wk × 4 mo in combination with isoniazid or other appropriate antitubercular
Available forms: Tabs 150 mg
Side effects/adverse reactions:
INTEG: Rash, pruritus, urticaria, acne
EENT: Visual disturbances
MS: Gout, arthrosis
MISC: Edema, aggressive reaction
GI: Nausea, vomiting, anorexia, diarrhea, bilirubinemia, hepatitis, increased ALT, AST, *heartburn, **pancreatitis***
GU: ***Hematuria,*** pyuria, ***proteinuria,*** urinary casts

---

* = Canada only   Side effects: *italics* = common; ***bold italics*** = life-threatening

CNS: Headache, fatigue, anxiety, dizziness

HEMA: **_Thrombocytopenia, leukopenia, neutropenia, lymphopenia,_** anemia, **_leukocytosis,_** purpura, hematoma

Contraindications: Hypersensitivity to rifamycins

Precautions: Pregnancy (C), lactation, hepatic disease, blood dyscrasias, children <12 yr

Pharmacokinetics:
PO: Peak 5-6 hr, half-life 13 hr; metabolized in liver (active/inactive metabolites), excreted in urine and feces, excreted in breast milk, protein binding 97%, steady state 10 days

Interactions:
• Use with extreme caution with protease inhibitors
• Decreased action of: amitriptyline, anticoagulants, antidiabetics, barbiturates, chloramphenicol, clarithromycin, clofibrate, corticosteroids, cyclosporine, dapsone, delavirdine, diazepam, digoxin, diltiazem, disopyramide, doxycycline, fluconazole, fluoroquinolones, haloperidol, indinavir, itraconazole, ketoconazole, methadone, mexiletine, nelfinavir, nifedipine, nortriptyline, oral contraceptives, phenytoin, progestins, quinidine, quinine, ritonavir, saquinavir, sildenafil, tacrolimus, theophylline, thyroid preparations, tocainide, verapamil, zidovudine

Lab test interferences:
• *Interference:* Folate level, vit B_{12}

NURSING CONSIDERATIONS
Assess:
• Baselines in CBC, AST, ALT, bilirubin, platelets
• For infection: sputum culture, lung sounds
• Signs of anemia: Hct, Hgb, fatigue

• Liver studies qmo: ALT (SGPT), AST (SGOT), bilirubin
• Renal status qmo: BUN, creatinine, output, specific gravity, urinalysis
• Hepatic status: decreased appetite, jaundice, dark urine, fatigue

Administer:
PO
• May give with food for GI upset
• Antiemetic if vomiting occurs
• After C&S is completed; qmo to detect resistance

Evaluate:
• Therapeutic response: decreased symptoms of TB, culture negative

Teach patient/family:
• That compliance with dosage schedule, duration is necessary
• That scheduled appointments must be kept; relapse may occur
• That urine, feces, saliva, sputum, sweat, tears may be colored redorange; soft contact lenses may be permanently stained
• To use alternate method of contraception, oral contraceptive action may be decreased
• To report flulike symptoms: excessive fatigue, anorexia, vomiting, sore throat; unusual bleeding, yellowish discoloration of skin, eyes

---

risedronate (℞)
(rih-sed′roh-nate)
Actonel
Func. class.: Bone-resorption inhibitor
Chem. class.: Biphosphonate

Action: Absorbs calcium phosphate crystal in bone and may directly block dissolution of hydroxyapatite crystals of bone; inhibits bone resorption, apparently without inhibiting bone formation, mineralization

---

◆ = Nursing alert   ⓟ = Herb-drug interaction   🚫 = Do not crush

Uses: Paget's disease
Investigational uses: Osteoporosis in postmenopausal women
Dosage and routes:
• *Adult:* **PO** 30 mg qd × 2 mo; patients with Paget's disease should receive calcium and vit D if dietary intake is lacking; if relapse occurs, retreatment is advised
Available forms: Tabs 30 mg
Side effects/adverse reactions:
CNS: Dizziness, headache
GI: Abdominal pain, anorexia, diarrhea, nausea
MS: Bone pain, arthralgia
CV: Chest pain
Contraindications: Hypersensitivity to biphosphonates
Precautions: Children, lactation, pregnancy (C), renal disease
Pharmacokinetics: Rapidly cleared from circulation, taken up mainly by bones, eliminated primarily through kidneys
Interactions:
• Decreased absorption of risedronate: calcium supplements, antacids
Drug/food:
• Decreased bioavailability: take ½ hr before food or drinks
NURSING CONSIDERATIONS
Assess:
• Electrolytes: renal function studies; Ca, P, Mg, K
• For hypercalcemia: paresthesia, twitching, laryngospasm, Chvostek's, Trousseau's signs
Administer:
• PO for 2 months to be effective in Paget's disease
• With a full glass of water, patient should be in upright position
• Supplemental calcium and vit D in Paget's disease
Perform/provide:
• Storage in cool environment, out of direct sunlight

Evaluate:
• Therapeutic response: increased bone mass, absence of fractures

---

rituximab
(rih-tuks'ih-mab)
Rituxan
Func. class.: Misc. antineoplastic
Chem. class.: Murine/human monoclonal antibody

Action: Directed against the CD20 antigen that is found on malignant B lymphocytes; CD20 regulates a portion of cell-cycle initiation/differentiation
Uses: Non-Hodgkin's lymphoma (CD20 positive, B-cell)
Dosage and routes:
• *Adult:* **IV INF** 375 mg/m^2 qwk × 4 doses; give at 50 mg/hr for 1st inf; if hypersensitivity does not occur, increase rate by 50 mg/hr q½h, max 400 mg/hr; slow/interrupt inf if hypersensitivity occurs; other inf can be given at 100 mg/hr and increased by 100 mg/hr, max 400 mg/hr
Available forms: Inj 10 mg/ml
Side effects/adverse reactions:
GI: Nausea, vomiting, anorexia
INTEG: Irritation at site, rash
*HEMA: **Leukopenia, neutropenia, thrombocytopenia***
OTHER: Fever, chills, asthenia, headache, angioedema, hypotension, myalgia, ***bronchospasm***
Contraindications: Hypersensitivity, murine proteins
Precautions: Lactation, children, elderly, pregnancy (C)
Pharmacokinetics: Half-life 42-79 min
NURSING CONSIDERATIONS
Assess:
• CBC, differential, platelet count weekly; withhold drug if WBC is <3500/mm^3, or platelet count

---

<100,000/mm³; notify prescriber of these results; drug should be discontinued
• Food preferences: list likes, dislikes
• GI symptoms: frequency of stools
• Signs of dehydration: rapid respirations, poor skin turgor, decreased urine output, dry skin, restlessness, weakness

Administer:
IV inf
• After diluting to a final conc. of 1-4 mg/ml; use 0.9% NaCl, D₅W, gently invert bag to mix; do not mix with other drugs

Perform/provide:
• Increased fluid intake to 2-3 L/day to prevent dehydration, unless contraindicated
• Changing of IV site q48h
• Nutritious diet with iron, vitamin supplement, low fiber, few dairy products
• Storage of vials at 36°-40° F, protects vials from direct sunlight, inf sol is stable at 36°-46° F × 24 hr and room temp for another 12 hr

Evaluate:
• Therapeutic response: decrease in tumor size, decrease in spread of cancer

Teach patient/family:
• To report adverse reactions

---

rizatriptan (℞)
(rye-zah-trip′tan)
Maxalt, Maxalt-MLT
Func. class.: Migraine agent
Chem. class.: 5-HT₁-like receptor agonist

Action: Binds selectively to the vascular 5-HT₁ receptor subtype, exerts antimigraine effect; causes vasoconstriction in cranial arteries
Uses: Acute treatment of migraine

Dosage and routes:
• *Adult:* **PO** 5-10 mg single dose, redosing separate by 2 hr or more; max 30 mg/24 hr
Available forms: Maxalt: Tabs 5, 10 mg; Maxalt-MLT: Tabs, orally disintegrating 5, 10 mg

Side effects/adverse reactions:
CNS: Dizziness, headache, fatigue
RESP: Chest tightness, pressure
GI: Nausea, dry mouth

Contraindications: Angina pectoris, history of MI, documented silent ischemia, Prinzmetal's angina, ischemic heart disease, concurrent ergotamine-containing preparations, uncontrolled hypertension, hypersensitivity, basilar or hemiplegic migraine

Precautions: Postmenopausal women, men >40 yr, risk factors for CAD, hypercholesterolemia, obesity, diabetes, impaired hepatic or renal function, pregnancy (C), lactation, children, elderly

Pharmacokinetics: Onset of pain relief 10 min-2 hr, 14% plasma protein binding, metabolized in the liver (metabolite), excreted in urine, feces, half-life 2-3 hr

Interactions:
• Extended vasospastic effects: ergot, ergot derivatives
• Increased action of rizatriptan: cimetidine, oral contraceptives, MAOIs, propranolol

NURSING CONSIDERATIONS
Assess:
• Tingling, hot sensation, burning, feeling of pressure, numbness, flushing, injection site reaction
• For stress level, activity, recreation, coping mechanisms
• Neurologic status: LOC, blurring vision, nausea, vomiting, tingling in extremities preceding headache
• Ingestion of tyramine foods (pickled products, beer, wine, aged cheese), food additives, preserva-

---

 = Nursing alert   = Herb-drug interaction   = Do not crush

tives, colorings, artificial sweeteners, chocolate, caffeine, which may precipitate these types of headaches
Perform/provide:
• Quiet, calm environment with decreased stimulation for noise, bright light, excessive talking
Evaluate:
• Therapeutic response: decrease in frequency, severity of headache
Teach patient/family:
• Use of orally disintegrating tab: instruct patient not to open blister until use, to peel blister open with dry hands, to place tab on tongue, where it will dissolve, and to swallow with saliva (contains phenylalanine)
• To report any side effects to prescriber
• To use alternate contraception while taking drug if oral contraceptives are being used

---

sibutramine
(si-byoo'tra-meen)
Meridia
Func. class.: Appetite suppressant

Action: Inhibits reuptake of serotonin, norepinephrine, dopamine
Uses: Obesity in conjunction with other treatments
Dosage and routes:
• *Adult:* **PO** 10 mg qd; may be increased to 15 mg qd after 4 wk, or lowered to 5 mg qd depending on response
Available forms: Caps 5, 10, 15 mg
Side effects/adverse reactions:
CNS: Headache, insomnia, seizures, stimulation, drowsiness, dizziness, nervousness, emotional lability
CV: Hypotension, palpitations, vasodilation, *tachycardia*
GI: Anorexia, constipation, dry

mouth, taste aberration, nausea, increased appetite
GU: Dysmenorrhea
EENT: Laryngitis, pharyngitis, rhinitis, sinusitis
INTEG: Rash, sweating
Contraindications: Hypersensitivity, hypothyroidism, anorexia nervosa, severe hepatic/renal disease, uncontrolled hypertension, history of CAD, CHF, dysrhythmias, pregnancy, lactation, CVA
Precautions: History of seizures, elderly, children <16 yr, narrowangle glaucoma
Interactions:
• Fatal serotonin syndrome: MAOIs, SSRIs, naratriptan, zolmitriptan, sumatriptan, dihydroergotamine, dextromethorphan, lithium, pentazocine, meperidine, fentanyl, tryptophan, or other centrally acting appetite suppressants; do not use together
• Hypertension: decongestants
• Increased levels of sibutramine: ketoconazole
Pharmacokinetics: Extensively metabolized, widely distributed, half-life metabolites-14 hr, 16 hr
NURSING CONSIDERATIONS
Assess:
• B/P, pulse during treatment; if B/P or pulse rises or if palpitations, tachycardia occur, drug may need to be discontinued
• Patient's current dosage of antihypertensives, antidiabetics; these may need to be adjusted
• Need for medication and results when combined with other weight-loss strategies
Administer:
• PO with or without meals qd
Evaluate:
• Therapeutic response: decrease in weight over time

Teach patient/family:
• To discuss all other medications taken (including OTC) with health care provider; serious—even fatal—interactions can occur
• To take exactly as prescribed, and not to exceed recommended dose

---

telmisartan (℞)

(tel-mih-sar'tan)
Micardis
Func. class.: Antihypertensive
Chem. class.: Angiotensin II receptor (Type AT_1)

Action: Blocks the vasoconstrictor and aldosterone-secreting effects of angiotensin II; selectively blocks the binding of angiotensin II to the AT_1 receptor found in tissues
Uses: Hypertension, alone or in combination
Investigational uses: Heart failure
Dosage and routes:
• *Adult:* **PO** 40 mg qd; range 20-80 mg
Available forms: Tabs 40, 80 mg
Side effects/adverse reactions:
CNS: Dizziness, insomnia, *anxiety*
GI: Diarrhea, dyspepsia, *anorexia, vomiting*
MS: Myalgia, pain
RESP: Cough, *upper respiratory infection*
Contraindications: Hypersensitivity
Precautions: Hypersensitivity to ACE inhibitors: pregnancy (C) 1st trimester, (D) 2nd and 3rd trimesters; lactation, children, elderly
Pharmacokinetics: Extensively metabolized, terminal half-life 24 hr, highly bound to plasma proteins, excreted in urine and feces
Interactions:
• Increased digoxin peak concentrations, and in trough concentrations: digoxin

NURSING CONSIDERATIONS
Assess:
• B/P, pulse q4h; note rate, rhythm, quality
• Electrolytes: K, Na, Cl
• Baselines in renal, liver function tests before therapy begins
• Edema in feet, legs qd
• Skin turgor, dryness of mucous membranes for hydration status
Administer:
• Without regard to meals
• Increased dose to black patients, B/P response may be reduced
Evaluate:
• Therapeutic response: decreased B/P
Teach patient/family:
• To comply with dosage schedule, even if feeling better
• To notify prescriber of mouth sores, fever, swelling of hands or feet, irregular heartbeat, chest pain
• That excessive perspiration, dehydration, vomiting, diarrhea may lead to fall in blood pressure; consult prescriber if these occur
• That drug may cause dizziness, fainting; light-headedness may occur

---

tirofiban (℞)

(tie-roh-fee'ban)
Aggrastat
Func. class.: Antiplatelet
Chem. class.: Nonpeptide antagonist

Action: Activation of platelet glycoprotein (GP) IIb/IIIa receptor that leads to binding of fibrinogen and von Willebrand's factor, which causes platelet aggregation
Uses: Acute coronary syndrome
Dosage and routes:
• *Adult:* **IV** 0.4 µg/kg/min × 30 min,

---

then 0.1 µg/kg/min; give ½ dose in renal disease

Available forms: Inj for sol 250 µg/ml, inj 50 µg/ml

Side effects/adverse reactions:

CV: Bradycardia

CNS: Dizziness

INTEG: Rash

*HEMA: **Bleeding***

OTHER: Dissection, coronary artery edema, pain in legs/pelvis, sweating

Contraindications: Hypersensitivity, active internal bleeding, stroke, major surgery, severe trauma, intracranial neoplasm, aneurysm, hemorrhage

Precautions: Pregnancy (B), lactation, elderly, renal disease, bleeding tendencies

Pharmacokinetics: Half-life 2 hr, excretion via urine/feces; plasma clearance 20%-25% lower in elderly; renal insufficiency decreases plasma clearance

Interactions:

• Increased bleeding: aspirin, heparin

• Increased clearance of tirofiban: levothyroxine, omeprazole

NURSING CONSIDERATIONS

Assess:

• B/P pulse during treatment until stable; take B/P lying, standing; orthostatic hypotension is common

• Platelet counts, Hct, Hgb, prior to treatment, within 6 hr of loading dose and at least qd thereafter

Administer:

• IV: Give ½ dose in renal disease

• Dilute inj: withdraw and discard 100 ml from a 500 ml bag of sterile 0.9% NaCl or D_5W and replace this vol with 50 ml of tirofiban inj from one vial

• Tirofiban inj for sol is premixed in containers of 500 ml 0.9% NaCl (50 mg/ml)

• Minimize other arterial/venous punctures; IM inj, catheter use, intubation, to reduce bleeding risks

Evaluate:

• Therapeutic response: decreased platelet count

Teach patient/family:

• That it is necessary to quit smoking to prevent excessive vasoconstriction

• To avoid hazardous activities; dizziness may occur

---

tolcapone (℞)

(toll'cah-pone)

Tasmar

Func. class.: Antiparkinson agent

Chem. class.: Catecholamine inhibitor

Action: Selective, reversible inhibitor of catecholamine; used as adjunct to levodopa/carbidopa therapy

Uses: Parkinsonism

Dosage and routes:

• *Adult:* **PO** 100-200 mg tid, with levodopa/carbidopa therapy; max 600 mg/day

Available forms: Tabs 100, 200 mg

Side effects/adverse reactions:

CNS: Dystonia, dyskinesia, dreaming, *fatigue, headache, confusion, psychosis,* hallucination, dizziness

CV: Orthostatic hypotension, chest pain, hypotension

EENT: Cataract, eye inflammation

GI: Nausea, vomiting, anorexia, abdominal distress, diarrhea, constipation

GU: UTI, urine discoloration, uterine tumor, micturition disorder

*HEMA: **Hemolytic anemia, leukopenia, agranulocytosis***

INTEG: Sweating, alopecia

Contraindications: Hypersensitivity

---

* = Canada only   Side effects: *italics* = common; ***bold italics*** = life-threatening

Precautions: Renal disease, cardiac disease, hepatic disease, hypertension, pregnancy (C), asthma, lactation

Pharmacokinetics: Rapidly absorbed, protein binding 99%, extensively metabolized, half-life 2-3 hr, excreted in urine (60%), feces (40%)

Interactions:

• Inhibition of normal catecholamine metabolism: MAOIs, MAO-B inhibitor may be used

• May influence pharmacokinetics of: α-methyldopa, dobutamine, apomorphine, isoproterenol

NURSING CONSIDERATIONS

Assess:

• Liver function enzymes: AST (SGOT), ALT (SGPT), alk phosphatase, LDH, bilirubin, CBC

• Involuntary movements in parkinsonism: akinesia, tremors, staggering gait, muscle rigidity, drooling

• B/P, respiration during initial treatment; hypo/hypertension should be reported

• Mental status: affect, mood, behavioral changes

Administer:

• PO tid with levodopa/carbidopa therapy

Perform/provide:

• Assistance with ambulation during beginning therapy

Evaluate:

• Therapeutic response: decrease in akathisia, increased mood

Teach patient/family:

• To change positions slowly to prevent orthostatic hypotension

• That urine, sweat may change color

• That food taken within 1 hr ac or 2 hr pc increases action of drug by 20%

• To report nausea, vomiting, anorexia

---

tolterodine (℞)
(toll-tehr'oh-deen)
Detrol
Func. class.: Overactive bladder product
Chem. class.: Muscarinic receptor antagonist

Action: Relaxes smooth muscles in urinary tract by inhibiting acetylcholine at postganglionic sites

Uses: Overactive bladder (frequency, urgency)

Dosage and routes:

• *Adult:* **PO** 2 mg bid, hepatic disease 1 mg bid

Available forms: Tabs 1, 2 mg

Side effects/adverse reactions:

CNS: Anxiety, paresthesia, fatigue, *dizziness,* headache

CV: Chest pain, hypertension

EENT: Vision abnormalities, xerophthalmia

GI: Nausea, vomiting, anorexia, abdominal pain, constipation, dry mouth, dyspepsia

GU: Dysuria, retention, frequency, UTI

INTEG: Rash, pruritus

RESP: Bronchitis, cough, pharyngitis, URI

Contraindications: Hypersensitivity, uncontrolled narrow-angle glaucoma, urinary retention, gastric retention

Precautions: Pregnancy (C), lactation, children, renal/hepatic disease, controlled narrow-angle glaucoma

Pharmacokinetics: Rapidly absorbed, highly protein bound, extensively metabolized, excreted in urine/feces

Interactions:

• Increased action of tolterodine: macrolide antibiotics, antifungals

• Food increases the bioavailability of tolterodine

◆ = Nursing alert   ∥ = Herb-drug interaction   Ⓢ = Do not crush

NURSING CONSIDERATIONS
Assess:
• Urinary patterns: distention, nocturia, frequency, urgency, incontinence
• Allergic reactions: rash; if this occurs, drug should be discontinued
Evaluate:
• Urinary status: dysuria, frequency, nocturia, incontinence
Teach patient/family:
• To avoid hazardous activities; dizziness may occur

---

trastuzumab (℞)

(tras-tuz′uh-mab)
Herceptin
Func. class.: Miscellaneous antineoplastic
Chem. class.: Humanized monoclonal antibody

Action: DNA-derived monoclonal antibody selectively binds to extracellular portion of human epidermal growth factor receptor 2; it inhibits proliferation of cancer cells
Uses: Breast cancer; metastatic with overexpression of HER2
Dosage and routes:
• *Adult:* IV 4 mg/kg given over 90 min, then maintenance 2 mg/kg given over 30 min; do not give as IV push or BOL
Available forms: Lyophilized powder 440 mg
Side effects/adverse reactions:
CNS: Dizziness, numbness, paresthesias, depression, insomnia, neuropathy, peripheral neuritis
*CV: **Tachycardia, CHF***
INTEG: Rash, acne, herpes simplex
GI: Nausea, vomiting, anorexia, diarrhea
MISC: Flulike syndrome; fever, headache, chills
HEMA: Anemia, *leukopenia*
MS: Arthralgia, bone pain

META: Edema, peripheral edema
RESP: Cough, dyspnea, pharyngitis, rhinitis, sinusitis
Contraindications: Hypersensitivity to this drug, Chinese hamster ovary cell protein
Precautions: Pregnancy (B), lactation, children, elderly, cardiac disease, anemia, leukopenia
Pharmacokinetics: Half-life 1.7-12 days

NURSING CONSIDERATIONS
Assess:
• For symptoms of infection; may be masked by drug
• CNS reaction: LOC, mental status, dizziness, confusion
Administer:
• Acetaminophen as ordered to alleviate fever and headache
IV
• After reconstituting vial with 20 ml bacteriostatic water for inj, 1.1% benzyl alcohol preserved (supplied) to yield 21 mg/ml, mark date on vial 28 days from reconstitution date, if pt is allergic to benzyl alcohol, reconstitute with sterile water for inj–use immediately
• Do not mix or dilute with other drugs or dextrose sol
Perform/provide:
• Increased fluid intake to 2-3 L/day
Evaluate:
• Therapeutic response: decrease in size of tumors
Teach patient/family:
• To take acetaminophen for fever
• To avoid hazardous tasks, since confusion, dizziness may occur
• To report signs of infection: sore throat, fever, diarrhea, vomiting
• Emotional lability is common; notify prescriber if severe or incapacitating

---

valrubicin (R)

(val-roo'bih-sin)
Valstar

Func. class.: Antineoplastic, antibiotic

Chem. class.: Anthracycline glycoside

Action: A semisynthetic analog of doxorubicin that inhibits DNA synthesis primarily; replication is decreased by binding to DNA, which causes strand splitting; active throughout entire cell cycle; a vesicant

Uses: Bladder cancer

Dosage and routes:

• *Adult:* Intravesically 800 mg qwk ×6 wk, delay administration ≥2 wks after transurethral resection or fulguration

Available forms: Sol for intravesical instillation: 40 mg/ml

Side effects/adverse reactions:

*HEMA: **Thrombocytopenia, leukopenia,** anemia*

GI: Nausea, vomiting, anorexia, diarrhea

GU: UTI, urinary retention, hematuria

INTEG: Rash

CV: Chest pain

Contraindications: Hypersensitivity to anthracyclines or Cremophor El, urinary tract infection, small bladder

Precautions: Pregnancy (C), lactation, children

Pharmacokinetics: Penetrates into bladder wall, not metabolized

NURSING CONSIDERATIONS

Assess:

• I&O ratio; report fall in urine output to <30 ml/hr

• Monitor temperature q4h; fever may indicate beginning infection

• Local irritation, pain, burning at injection site

Administer:

• After urinary catheter is inserted under aseptic conditions, drain bladder and instill the diluted 75 ml valrubicin by gravity for several min, withdraw catheter, drug should be retained for 2 hr, then void

• Use procedure for handling and disposal of cytotoxic agents

• Do not use polyvinyl chloride (PVC) or IV tubing

• Prepare/store valrubicin sol in glass, polypropylene, or polyolefin tubing/containers

• For instillation, 5 ml vials (200 mg valrubicin/5 ml/vial) should be warmed to room temp, withdraw 20 ml from the 4 vials and dilute with 55 ml 0.9% NaCl inj to 75 ml of diluted valrubicin sol

• Valrubicin sol is clear red, at lower temps a waxy precipitate may form, warm in hand until sol is clear

Perform/provide:

• Strict hand-washing technique, gloves, protective clothing

• Increased fluid intake to 2-3 L/day to prevent urate, calculi formation

• Storage at room temperature for 12 hr after reconstituting

Evaluate:

• Therapeutic response: decreased tumor size, spread of malignancy

Teach patient/family:

• To report any complaints, side effects to nurse or prescriber

• That urine and other body fluids may be red-orange for 48 hr

• That contraceptive measures are recommended during therapy

◆ = Nursing alert   ✒ = Herb-drug interaction   ⊘ = Do not crush

Appendix c

Ophthalmic, otic, nasal, and topical products

OPHTHALMIC PRODUCTS

α-ADRENERGIC BLOCKER
dapiprazole (R)
(da-pip'ra-zole)
Rev-Eyes

ANESTHETICS
proparacaine (R)
(proe-par'a-kane)
AK-Taine, Alcaine, Diocane*, Ocu-Caine, Ophthaine, Ophthestic, Spectro-Caine
tetracaine (R)
(tet'ra-kane)
Minims Tetracaine, Pontocaine Eye, Pontocaine HCl, tetracaine

ANTIINFECTIVES
bacitracin (R)
(bass-l-tray'sin)
AK-Tracin, Bacitracin Ophthalmic
brimonidine (R)
(bri-moe'ni-deen)
Alphagan
chloramphenicol (R)
(klor-am-fen'i-kole)
AK-Chlor, Chloramphenicol, Chloramphenicol Ophthalmic, Chloromycetin Ophthalmic, Chloroptic, Chloroptic S.O.P., Fenicol*, Isopto Fenical*, Pentamycin*

ciprofloxacin (R)
(sip-ro-floks'a-sin)
Ciloxan
erythromycin (R)
(er-ith-roe-mye'sin)
AK-Mycin, Erythromycin, Ilotycin
gentamicin (R)
(jen-ta-mye'sin)
Garamycin Ophthalmic, Genoptic Ophthalmic, Genoptic S.O.P., Gentacidin, Gent-AK, gentamicin, Gentamicin Ophthalmic Liquifilm, Gentak
idoxuridine-IDU (R)
(eye-dox-yoor'i-deen)
Herplex, Stoxil
natamycin (R)
(nat-a-mye'sin)
Natacyn
norfloxacin (R)
(nor-floks'a-sin)
Chibroxin, Ofloxacin, Ocuflox
ofloxacin (R)
(oh-flox'a-sin)
Ocuflox
polymyxin B (R)
(pol-ee-mix'in)
Aerosporin, polymyxin B sulfate
silver nitrate 1% (R)
sulfacetamide sodium (R)
(sul-fa-seet'a-mide)

---

* = Canada only   Side effects: *italics* = common; ***bold italics*** = life-threatening

AK-Sulf, Bleph-10 Liquifilm, Bleph-10 S.O.P., Isopto Cetamide, Ophthacet, Sodium Sulamyd, sodium sulfacetamide 10%, sodium sulfacetamide 15%, sodium sulfacetamide 30%, SOSS-10, Sulfair 15

tetracycline (R_x)

(tet-ra-sye'kleen)

Achromycin Ophthalmic

tobramycin (R_x)

(toe-bra-mye'sin)

Tobrex

trifluridine (R_x)

(trye-floor'i-deen)

Viroptic

vidarabine (R_x)

(vye-dare'a-been)

Vira-A

β-ADRENERGIC BLOCKERS

betaxolol (R_x)

(beh-tax'oh-lole)

Betoptic, Betoptic 5

carteolol (R_x)

(kar-tee'oh-lole)

Ocupress

levobunolol (R_x)

(lee-voe-byoo'no-lole)

Betagen

metipranolol (R_x)

(met-ee-pran'oh-lole)

Optipranolol

timolol (R_x)

(tye'moe-lole)

Apo-Timop*, Betimol, Timoptic

**CHOLINERGICS
(Direct-acting)**

carbachol (R_x)

(kar'ba-kole)

Iosopto Carbachol, Miostat

pilocarpine (R_x)

(pye-loe-kar'peen)

Adsorbocarpine, Akarpine, Isopto Carpine, Ocu-Carpine, Ocusert-Pilo, Pilagan, Pilocar, pilocarpine, Pilopine HS, Piloptic-1, Piloptic-2, Pilostat, Pilopto-Carpine

CHOLINESTERASE INHIBITORS

demecarium (R_x)

(dem-e-kare'ee-um)

Humorsol

ecothiophate (R_x)

(ek-oh-thye'eh-fate)

Ecostigmine Iodide, Phospholine Iodide

isoflurophate (R_x)

(eye-soe-floor'oh-fate)

Floropryl

physostigmine (R_x)

(fi-zoe-stig'meen)

Eserine Salicylate, Isopto Eserin

CYCLOPLEGIC MYDRIATICS

atropine (R_x)

(a'troe-peen)

Atropine-1, Atropine Care Ophthalmic, Atropine Sulfate Ophthalmic, Atropine Sulfate S.O.P., Atropisol, Isopto Atropine

cyclopentolate (R_x)

(sye-kloe-pen'toe-late)

AK-Pentolate, Cyclogly, I-Pentolate

homatropine (R_x)

(home-a'troe-peen)

AK-Homatropine, I-Homatrine, Isopto Homatropine, Minims Homatropine*, Spectro-Homatropine

physostigmine (℞)
(fi-zoe-stig'meen)
Fisostin, Isopto Eserine Solution/Eserine Sulfate Ointment

scopolamine (℞)
(skoe-pol'a-meen)
Isopto-Hyoscine

tropicamide (℞)
(troe-pik'a-mide)
Mydriacyl, Tropicacyl, I-Piramide

GLUCOCORTICOIDS
dexamethasone (℞)
(dex-a-meth'a-sone)
AK-Dex, Decadron Phosphate, Dexamethasone Ophthalmic Suspension, Maxidex

fluorometholone (℞)
(flure-oh-meth'oh-lone)
Flarex, Fluor-Op, FML, FML Forte, FML Liquifilm

medrysone (℞)
(me'dri-sone)
HMS

prednisolone (℞)
(pred niss'oh-lone)
Econopred, Econopred Plus, AK-Pred, Inflamase Forte, Inflamase Mild Ophthalmic, Metreton Ophthalmic, Pred-Forte, Pred-Mild

rimexolone (℞)
(ri-mex'o lone)
Vexol

NONSTEROIDAL ANTIINFLAMMATORIES
diclofenac (℞)
(dye-kloe'fen-ak)
Voltaran

flurbiprofen (℞)
(flure-bih-proh'fen)
Ocufen

ketorolac (℞)
(kee-toe'role-ak)
Acular

suprofen (℞)
(soo-proe'fen)
Profenal

SYMPATHOMIMETICS
apraclonidine (℞)
(a-pra-klon'i-deen)
Lopidine

brimonidine (℞)
(brih-moh'nih-deen)
Alphagan

dipivefrin (℞)
(dye pi'vef-rin)
Propine

epinephrine bitartrate/epinephrine HCl/epinephryl borate (℞)
(ep-i-nef'rin)
Epitrate, Mytrate/Epifrin, Glaucon/Epinal, Eppy*

OPHTHALMIC DECONGESTANTS/ VASOCONSTRICTORS
naphazoline (OTC, ℞)
(naf-az'oh-leen)
AK-Con Ophthalmic, Albalon Liquifilm Ophthalmic, Allerest Eye Drops, Clear Eyes, Comfort Eye Drops, Degest 2, Nafazair, naphazoline HCl, Naphcon, Naphcon Forte, Opcon, Vasoclear, Vasocon Regular, Estivin II

oxymetazoline (℞)
(ox-i-meth'oh-lone)
OcuClear, Visine, LR

phenylephrine (OTC)

(fen-ill-ef'rin)

AK-Dilate Ophthalmic, AK-Nefrin Ophthalmic, Isopto Frin, Neo-Synephrine 2.5%, Neo-Synephrine 10% Plain, Neo-Synephrine Viscous, phenylephrine HCl, 2.5% Mydfrin Ophthalmic, Phenoptic Relief, Prefrin

tetrahydrozoline (OTC)

(tet-ra-hye-dro'zoe-leen)

Collyrium Fresh Eye Drops, Eyesine, Murine Plus Eye Drops, Optigene 3 Eye Drops, Soothe Eye Drops, tetrahydrozoline HCl, Tyzine HCl, Tyzine Pediatric, Visine Eye Drops

MISCELLANEOUS OPHTHALMICS

latanoprost

(la-tan'oh-proest)

Xalatan

dorzolamide (℞)

(dor-zol'a-mide)

Trusopt

Pregnancy categories: Demecarium, isoflurophate (X); apraclonidine, cyclopentolate, ecothiophate, glucocorticoids, levobunalol, metipranolol, pilocarpine, proparacaine, suprofen, tetracaine (C); dapiprazole, dipivefrin (B)

β-Adrenergic blockers
Action: Reduces production of aqueous humor by unknown mechanism
Uses: Ocular hypertension, chronic open-angle glaucoma

Anesthetics
Action: Decreases ion permeability by stabilizing neuronal membrane
Uses: Cataract extraction, tonometry, gonioscopy, removal of foreign objects, corneal suture removal, glaucoma surgery (ophth); pruritus, sunburn, toothache, sore throat, cold sores, oral pain, rectal pain and irritation, control of gagging (top)

Antiinfectives
Action: Inhibits folic acid synthesis by preventing PABA use, which is necessary for bacterial growth
Uses: Conjunctivitis, superficial eye infections, corneal ulcers, prophylaxis against infection after removal of foreign matter from the eye

Antiinflammatories
Action: Decreases inflammation, resulting in decreased pain, photophobia, hyperemia, cellular infiltration
Uses: Inflammation of eye, eyelids, conjunctiva, cornea; uveitis, iridocyclitis, allergic conditions, burns, foreign bodies, postoperatively in cataract

Carbonic anhydrase inhibitor
Action: Converted to epinephrine, which decreases aqueous production and increases outflow
Uses: Open-angle glaucoma, ocular hypertension

Direct-acting miotic
Action: Acts directly on cholinergic receptor sites; induces miosis, spasm of accommodation, fall in intraocular pressure, caused by stimulation of ciliary, pupillary sphincter muscles, which leads to pulling away of iris from filtration angle, resulting in increased outflow of aqueous humor
Uses: Primary glaucoma, early stages of wide-angle glaucoma (less useful in advanced stages), chronic open-angle glaucoma, acute narrow-angle glaucoma before emergency surgery; also neutralizes mydriatics used during eye exam; may be

---

◆ = Nursing alert   ∥ = Herb-drug interaction   ⊘ = Do not crush

used alternately with mydriatics to break adhesions between iris and lens

---

Side effects/adverse reactions:
CNS: Headache
CV: Hypertension, tachycardia, dysrhythmias
EENT: Burning, stinging
GI: Bitter taste
Contraindications: Hypersensitivity
Precautions: Pregnancy, lactation, children, aphakia, hypersensitivity to carbonic anhydrase inhibitors, sulfonamides, thiazide diuretics, ocular inhibitors, hepatic and renal insufficiency
NURSING CONSIDERATIONS
Assess:
• Ophth exams and intraocular pressure readings
• Blood counts; liver, renal function tests and serum electrolytes during long-term treatment
Perform/provide:
• Storage at room temp away from light
Evaluate:
• Positive therapeutic response
• Absence of increased intraocular pressure
Teach patient/family:
• How to instill drops
• That drug may cause burning, itching, blurring, dryness of eye area

NASAL AGENTS

NASAL DECONGESTANTS
azelastine (℞)
(ay-zell'ah-steen)
Astelin

desoxyephedrine (OTC)
(des-oxy-e-fed'rin)
Vicks Inhaler

ephedrine (OTC)
(e-fed'rin)
Kondon's Nasal Jelly, Pretz-D, Vicks Vatronol
epinephrine (OTC)
(ep-i-neff'rin)
Adrenalin
naphazoline (OTC)
(naff-a-zoe'leen)
Privine
oxymetazoline (OTC)
(ox-i-met-az'oh-leen)
Afrin, Afrin Children's Nose Drops, Allerest 12-Hour Nasal, Afrin, Afrin Children's Nose Drops, Allerest 12-Hour Nasal, Chlorphed-LA, Coricidin Nasal Mist, Dristan Long Lasting, Duramist Plus, Duration, Genasal, NTZ Long-Acting Nasal, Nafrine*, Neo-Synephrine 12 Hour, Nostrilla, oxymetazoline HCl, Sinarest 12-Hour, Sinex Long-Acting, Twice-A-Day Nasal, 4-Way Long Acting Nasal
phenylephrine (OTC)
(fen-ill-eff'rin)
Alconefrin 12, Children's Nostril, Neo-Synephrine, Sinex
propylhexadrine (OTC)
(proe-pil-hex'a-dreen)
Benzedrex Inhaler
tetrahydrozoline (OTC)
(tet-ra-hye-dro'zoe-leen)
Tyzine
xylometazoline (OTC)
(zye-loh-meh-tazz'oh-leen)
Otrivin, Otrivin Pediatric Nasal Drops, xylometazoline HCl

NASAL STEROIDS
beclomethasone (℞)
(be-kloe-meth'a-sone)

Beconase AQ Nasal, Beconase Inhalation, Vancenase AQ Nasal, Vancenase Nasal

dexamethasone (R)

(dex-a-meth'a-sone)
Decadron Phosphate Turbinaire

Pregnancy category: C
Action: Produces vasoconstriction (rapid, long acting) of arterioles, thereby decreasing fluid exudation, mucosal engorgement by stimulation of α-adrenergic receptors in vascular smooth muscle
Uses: Nasal congestion
Dosage and routes:
Desoxyephedrine
• *Adult and child >6 yr:* 1-2 **INH** in each nostril q2h or less
Ephedrine
• *Adult:* Fill dropper to the level marked, then use in each nostril q4h or less
Epinephrine
• *Adult and child >6 yr:* Apply with swab, drops, spray prn
Naphazoline
• *Adult and child >6 yr:* 1-2 drops/spray q6h or less
Oxymetazoline
• *Adult and child >6 yr:* **INSTILL** 2-3 gtt or sprays to each nostril bid
• *Child 2-6 yr:* **INSTILL** 2-3 gtt or sprays 0.025 sol bid, not to exceed 3 days
Phenylephrine
• *Adult and child >12 yr:* 2-3 drops/spray (0.25-0.5) in each nostril q3-4h or less; or 2-3 drops/spray (1%) in each nostril q4h or less
• *Child 6-12 yr:* 2-3 drops/spray (0.25%) in each nostril q3-4h
• *Infant >6 mo:* 1-2 drops (0.16%) in each nostril q3h
Propylhexadrine
• *Adult and child >6 yr:* 1-2 **INH** in each nostril q2h or less

Tetrahydrozoline
• *Adult and child >6 yr:* 2-4 drops (0.1%) q3-4h prn or 3-4 sprays in each nostril q4h prn
• *Child 2-6 yr:* 2-3 drops (0.05%) in each nostril q4-6h prn
Xylometazoline
• *Adult and child >12 yr:* 2-3 drops/spray (0.1%) in each nostril q8-10h
• *Child 2-12 yr:* 2-3 drops (0.05%) in each nostril q8-10h
Available forms: Nasal sol 0.025%, 0.05%
Side effects/adverse reactions:
CNS: Anxiety, restlessness, tremors, weakness, insomnia, dizziness, fever, headache
EENT: Irritation, burning, sneezing, stinging, dryness, rebound congestion
GI: Nausea, vomiting, anorexia
INTEG: Contact dermatitis
Contraindications: Hypersensitivity to sympathomimetic amines
Precautions: Child <6 yr, elderly, diabetes, cardiovascular disease, hypertension, hyperthyroidism, increased intracranial pressure, prostatic hypertrophy, pregnancy (C), glaucoma
NURSING CONSIDERATIONS
Assess:
• For redness, swelling, pain in nasal passages before and during treatment
• For syst absorption; hypertension, tachycardia; notify prescriber; syst absorption occurs at high doses or after prolonged use
Administer:
• Having patient tilt head back, squeeze bulb to create a vacuum, and draw correct amount of sol into dropper; insert 2 gtt of sol into nostril; repeat in other nostril
• Store in light-resistant container; do not expose to high temp or let sol come into contact with aluminum
• For <4 consecutive days

◆= Nursing alert   ✔= Herb-drug interaction   ⊘= Do not crush

• Environmental humidification to decrease nasal congestion, dryness
Evaluate:
• Therapeutic response: decreased nasal congestion
Teach patient/family:
• That stinging may occur for several applications; drying of mucosa may be decreased by environmental humidification
• To notify prescriber if irregular pulse, insomnia, dizziness, or tremors occur
• Proper administration to avoid syst absorption
• To rinse dropper with very hot water to prevent contamination

TOPICAL GLUCOCORTICOIDS

alclometasone (℞)
(al-kloe-met′a-sone)
Adovate

amcinonide (℞)
(am-sin′oh-nide)
Cyclocort

betamethasone (℞)
(bay-ta-meth′a-sone)
Alphatrex, Beben*, Betacort*, Betaderm, Betatrex, Beta-Val, Bethovate*, Betmethacort, Celestoderm*, Dermabet, Diprolene, Diprosone, Ectosonel*, Maxivate, Metaderm*, Novobetamet, Psorion, Uticort, Valisone, Valnac

clobetasol (℞)
(kloe-bay′ta-sol)
Dermovate*, Temovate

clocortolone (℞)
(kloe-kore′toe-lone)
Cloderm

desonide (℞)
(dess′oh-nide)
Des Owen, Tridesilon

desoximetasone (℞)
(dess-ox-i-met′a-sone)
Topicort

dexamethasone (℞)
(dex-a-meth′a-sone)
Aeroseb-Dex, Decaderm, Decaspray

diflorasone (℞)
(dye-flor′a-sone)
Florone, Maxiflor, Psorcon

fluocinolone (℞)
(floo-oh-sin′oh-lone)
Fluocin, Licon, Lidemol*, Lidex, Lyderm*, Topsyn*, Vasoderm

flurandrenolide (℞)
(flure-an-dren′oh-lide)
Cordran, Cordran SP, Cordran Tape, Drenison 1/4*, Drenison Tape*

fluticasone (℞)
(floo-tik′a-sone)
Cutivate

halcinonide (℞)
(hal-sin′oh-nide)
Halog, Halog-E

halobetasol (℞)
(hal-oh-bay′ta-sol)
Ultravate

hydrocortisone (℞)
(hye-droe-kor′ti-sone)
Actiocort, Aeroseb-HC, Ala-Cort, Allercort, Alphaderm, Anusol HC, Bactine, Barriere-HC*, Calde-CORT Anti-Itch, Carmol HC, Cetacort, Cortacet*, Cortaid, Cortate*, Cort-Dome, Cortef*, Corticaine, Corticreme*, Cortifair, Cortizone, Cortoderm*, Cortril, Delcort, Dermacort, DemiCort, Derm-

tex HC, Emo-Cort, Epifoam, FoilleCort, Gly-Cort, Gynecort, Hi-Cor, Hycort, Hyderm*, Hydro-Tex, Hytone, Lacti-Care-HC, Lanacort, Lemoderm, Locoid, My Cort, Novoehydrocort*, Nutracort Pharm, Pharmacort, Pentacort, Rederm, Rhulicort S-T Cort, Synacort, Sarna HC*, Texa-Cort, Unicort*, Westcort

methylprednisolone (℞)
(meth-ill-pred-niss′oh-lone)
Depo-Medrol

mometasone (℞)
(moe-met′a-sone)
Elocon

prednicarbate (℞)
(pred-ni-kar′bate)
Dermatop

triamcinolone (℞)
(trye-am-sin′oh-lone)
Aristocort, Flutex, Kenac, Kenalog, Kenonel, Triaderm*, Trianide*, Triderm, Trymex

Pregnancy category: C
Action: Antipruritic, antiinflammatory
Uses: Psoriasis, eczema, contact dermatitis, pruritus; usually reserved for severe dermatoses that have not responded to less potent formulation
Dosage and routes:
• *Adult and child:* Apply to affected area
Side effects/adverse reactions:
INTEG: Acne, atrophy, epidermal thinning, purpura, striae
Contraindications: Hypersensitivity, viral infections, fungal infections
Precautions: Pregnancy (C)

NURSING CONSIDERATIONS
Assess:
• Temp; if fever develops, drug should be discontinued
• For systemic absorption, increased temp, inflammation, irritation
Administer:
• Only to affected areas; do not get in eyes
• Leaving site uncovered or lightly covered; occlusive dressing is not recommended—systemic absorption may occur
• Use only on dermatoses; do not use on weeping, denuded, or infected area
• Cleansing before application of drug
• Continuing treatment for a few days after area has cleared
• Store at room temp
Evaluate:
• Therapeutic response: absence of severe itching, patches on skin, flaking
Teach patient/family:
• To avoid sunlight on affected area, burns may occur
• To limit treatment to 14 days

TOPICAL ANTIFUNGALS

amphotericin B (OTC)
(am-foe-ter′i-sin)
Fungizone

butenafine (℞)
(byoo-tin′a-feen)
Mentex

ciclopirox (OTC)
(sye-kloe-peer′ox)
Loprox

clioquinol (OTC)
(klye-oh-kwin′ole)
Vioform

 = Nursing alert   = Herb-drug interaction   = Do not crush

clotrimazole (OTC)

(kloe-trye'ma-zole)
Canestew*, Clotrimaderm*, Lotrimin, Lotrimin AF, Mycelex, Mycelex OTC, Myclo*, Neozol*

econazole (OTC)

(ee-kon'a-zole)
Spectazole

haloprogin (OTC)

(hal-oh-proe'jin)
Halotex

ketoconazole (OTC)

(kee-toe-kon'a-zole)
Nizoral

miconazole (OTC)

(mye-kon'a-zole)
Micatin, Monistat-Derm

naftifine (OTC)

(naff'ti-feen)
Naftin

nystatin (OTC)

(nye-stat'in)
Mycostatin, Nodostine*, Nilstat, Nyoderm*, Nystex

oxiconazole (OTC)

(ox-i-kon'a zole)
Oxistat

selenium (OTC)

(see-leen'ee-um)
Exsel, Head and Shoulders Intensive Treatment, Selenium Sulfide, Selsun, Selsun Blue

terbinafine (OTC)

(ter bin'a-feen)
Lamisil

tolnaftate (OTC)

(tole-naf'tate)
Absorbine Antifungal, Absorbine Jock Itch, Absorbine Jr. Antifungal, Aftate For Athlete's Foot, Aftate for Jock Itch, Desenex Spray, Genaspor, NP-27, Quinsana Plus, Tinactin, Ting, tolnaftate, Zeasorb-AF

undecylenic acid (OTC)

(un-deh-sih-len'ik)
Caldesene, Cruex, Decylenes, Desenex, Desenex Maximum Strength, Protectol

Pregnancy category: B
Action: Interferes with fungal cell membrane permeability
Uses: Tinea cruris, tinea pedis, diaper rash, minor skin irritations; amphotericin B is used for *Candida* infections
Dosage and routes:
• Massage into affected area, surrounding area qd or bid, continue for 7-14 days, not to exceed 4 wk
Side effects/adverse reactions:
INTEG: Burning, stinging, dryness, itching, local irritation
Contraindications: Hypersensitivity
Precautions: Pregnancy (B), lactation, children
Interactions: None
NURSING CONSIDERATIONS
Assess:
• Skin for fungal infections; peeling, dryness, itching before and throughout treatment
• For continuing infection; increased size, number of lesions
Administer:
Topical route
• To affected area, surrounding area; do not cover with occlusive dressings
• Store below 30° C (86° F)
Evaluate:
• Therapeutic response: decrease in size, number of lesions
Teach patient/family:
• To apply with glove to prevent further infection; not to cover with occlusive dressings

• That long-term therapy may be needed to clear infection (2 wk-6 mo depending on organism); compliance is needed even after feeling better

• Proper hygiene; hand-washing technique, nail care, use of concomitant top agents if prescribed

• To avoid use of OTC creams, ointments, lotions unless directed by prescriber

• To use medical asepsis (hand washing) before, after each application; to change socks and shoes once a day during treatment of tinea pedis

• To report to health care prescriber if infection persists or recurs; if blisters, burning, oozing, swelling occur

• To avoid alcohol because nausea, vomiting, hypertension may occur

• To use sunscreen or avoid direct sunlight to prevent photosensitivity

• To notify health-care prescriber of sore throat, fever, skin rash, which may indicate overgrowth of organisms

TOPICAL ANTIINFECTIVES

bacitracin (OTC)
(bass-i-tray'sin)
Baciguent, Bacitin*, Bacitracin

chloramphenicol (Ŗ)
(klor-am-fen'i-kole)
Chloromycetin

erythromycin (OTC)
(er-ith-roe-mye'sin)
A/T/S, Akne-Mycin, C-Solve 2, Erycette, Eryderm, Erygel, Erymax, Erythromycin, E-Solve 2, ETS-2%, Staticin, Theramycin Z, T-Statd

gentamicin (Ŗ)
(jen-ta-mye'sin)
G-Myticin, Garamycin, gentamicin

mafenide (Ŗ)
(ma'fe-nide)
Sulfamylon

mupirocin (Ŗ)
(myoo-peer'oh-sin)
Bactroban, Pseudomonic Acid A

neomycin (OTC)
(nee-oh-mye'sin)
Myciguent, Neomycin Sulfate

nitrofurazone (Ŗ)
(nye-troe-fyoor'a-zone)
Furacin, Nitrofurazone

silver sulfadiazine (Ŗ)
(sul-fa-dye'a-zeen)
Flamazine*, Silvadene, SSD, SSD AF, Thermazene

sodium sulfacetamide lotion 10% (Ŗ)
(sul-fa-see'ta-mide)
Klaron

tetracycline (Ŗ)
(tet-ra-sye'kleen)
Achromycin, Topicycline

Pregnancy category: C
Action: Interferes with bacterial protein synthesis
Uses: Skin infections, minor burns, wounds, skin grafts, primary pyodermas, otitis externa
Side effects/adverse reactions:
INTEG: Rash, urticaria, scaling, redness
Contraindications: Hypersensitivity, large areas, burns, ulcerations
Precautions: Pregnancy (C), lactation, impaired renal function, external ear or perforated eardrum

---

 = Nursing alert   = Herb-drug interaction   = Do not crush

NURSING CONSIDERATIONS
Assess:
• Allergic reaction: burning, stinging, swelling, redness
• For signs of nephrotoxicity or ototoxicity
Administer:
• Enough medication to cover lesions completely
• After cleansing with soap, water before each application; dry well
• To less than 20% of body surface area when patient has impaired renal function
Perform/provide:
• Storage at room temp in dry place
Evaluate:
• Therapeutic response: decrease in size, number of lesions

TOPICAL ANTIVIRALS

acyclovir (℞)
(ay-sye'kloe-ver)
Zovirax
penciclovir (℞)
(pen-sye'kloe-ver)
Denavir

Pregnancy category: C
Action: Interferes with viral DNA replication
Uses: Simple mucocutaneous herpes simplex, in immunocompromised clients with initial herpes genitalis
Side effects/adverse reactions:
INTEG: Rash, urticaria, stinging, burning, pruritus, vulvitis
Contraindications: Hypersensitivity
Precautions: Pregnancy (C), lactation
NURSING CONSIDERATIONS
Assess:
• Allergic reaction: burning, stinging, swelling, redness, rash, vulvitis, pruritus

Administer:
• Using finger cot or rubber glove to prevent further infection
• Enough medication to cover lesions completely
• After cleansing with soap, water before each application; dry well
Perform/provide:
• Storage at room temp in dry place
Evaluate:
• Therapeutic response: decrease in size, number of lesions
Teach patient/family:
• Not to use in eyes or when there is no evidence of infection
• To apply with glove to prevent further infection
• To avoid use of OTC creams, ointments, lotions unless directed by prescriber
• To use medical asepsis (hand washing) before, after each application and avoid contact with eyes
• To adhere strictly to prescribed regimen to maximize successful treatment outcome
• To begin taking drug when symptoms arise

TOPICAL ANESTHETICS

benzocaine (OTC)
(ben'zoe-kane)
Anbesol Maximum Strength, Baby Anbesol, Children's Chloraseptic, Medamint, Orabase Baby, Oracin, Ora-Jel, Oratect, Spec-T Anesthetic, T-Caine, Tyrobenz
dibucaine (OTC)
(dye'byoo-kane)
dibucaine, Nupercainal
lidocaine (OTC, ℞)
(lye'doe-kane)
Aloe Extra, Anestacon, Burn Relief, Derma Flex, lidocaine HCl

topical, lidocaine viscous, So-larcaine, Xylocaine, Xylocaine Viscous, Zilactin-L

pramoxine (OTC)
(pra-mox'een)
Fleet Relief, Prax, ProctoFoam, Tronolane, Tronothane

tetracaine (OTC)
(tet'ra-cane)
Pontocaine

Pregnancy category: C

Action: Inhibits conduction of nerve impulses from sensory nerves

Uses: Oral irritation, sore throat, toothache, cold sore, canker sore, sunburn, minor cuts, insect bites, pain, itching

Dosage and routes:
• *Adult and child:* **TOP** apply qid as needed; **RECT** insert tid and after each BM

Side effects/adverse reactions:
INTEG: Rash, irritation, sensitization

Contraindications: Hypersensitivity, infants <1 yr, application to large areas

Precautions: Child <6 yr, sepsis, pregnancy (C), denuded skin

NURSING CONSIDERATIONS

Assess:
• Pain: location, duration, characteristics before and after administration
• For infection: redness, drainage, inflammation; this drug should not be used until infection is treated

Perform/provide:
• Storage in tight, light-resistant container; do not freeze, puncture, or incinerate aerosol container

Evaluate:
• Therapeutic response: decreased redness, swelling, pain

Teach patient/family:
• To avoid contact with eyes
• Not to use for prolonged periods: use for <1 wk; if condition remains, prescriber should be contacted

VAGINAL ANTIFUNGALS

butoconazole (OTC)
(byoo-toh-kone'ah-zole)
Femstat

clotrimazole (OTC)
(kloe-trye'ma-zole)
Canesten*, Gyne-Lotrimin, Mycelex G, Mycelex Twin Pak, Myclo*

miconazole (OTC)
(mye-kon'a-zole)
Monistat, Monistat 3, Monistat 7, Monistat Dual Pak

nystatin (OTC)
(nye-stat'in)
mycostatin, Nilstat, Nadostine*, Nyoderm*, O-V Statin

terconazole (OTC)
(ter-kone'ah-zole)
Terazol

tioconazole (OTC)
(tye-oh-kone'ah-zole)
Gyne-Trosyd*, Vagistat

Pregnancy category: Nystatin (A); clotrimazole (B); butoconazole, terconazole (C)

Action: Interferes with fungal DNA replication; binds sterols in fungal cell membranes, which increases permeability, leaking of nutrients

Uses: Vaginal, vulval, vulvovaginal candidiasis (moniliasis)

Dosage and routes:
Butoconazole
• *Adult:* **VAG** 5 g (1 applicator) hs × 3-6 days
Clotrimazole
• *Adult:* 100 mg (1 vag tab, 100 mg) hs × 1 wk, or 200 mg (2 vag tab, 100 mg) hs × 3 nights, or 500 mg (1 vag

tab, 500 mg); or 5 g (1 applicator) hs × 1-2 wks

Miconazole
• *Adult:* 200 mg supp hs × 3 days or 100 mg supp × 1 wk
Nystatin
• *Adult:* 100,000 U qd × 2 wk
Terconazole
• *Adult:* **VAG** 5 g (1 applicator) hs × 7 days
Tioconazole
• *Adult:* 1 applicator hs × 1 wk

Side effects/adverse reactions:
GU: Vulvovaginal burning, itching, pelvic cramps
INTEG: Rash, urticaria, stinging, burning
MISC: Headache, body pain
Contraindications: Hypersensitivity
Precautions: Children <2 yr, pregnancy, lactation
Interactions: None

NURSING CONSIDERATIONS
Assess:
• For allergic reaction: burning, stinging, itching, discharge, soreness
Administer:
Topical route
• One full applicator every night high into the vagina
• Store at room temp in dry place
Evaluate:
• Therapeutic outcome: decrease in itching or white discharge (vaginal)
Teach patient/family:
• About asepsis (hand washing) before, after each application
• To apply with applicator only; to avoid use of any other vaginal product unless directed by prescriber; sanitary napkin may prevent soiling of undergarments
• To abstain from sexual intercourse until treatment is completed; reinfection and irritation may occur
• To notify prescriber if symptoms persist

OTIC STEROIDS

hydrocortisone
(hye-droe-kor′ti-sone)
Cortamed*, Otall (Ⓡ)

Pregnancy category: C
Action: Antiinflammatory, antipruritic
Uses: Ear canal inflammation
Side effects/adverse reactions:
EENT: Itching, irritation in ear
INTEG: Rash, urticaria
Contraindications: Hypersensitivity, perforated eardrum
Precautions: Pregnancy (C)

NURSING CONSIDERATIONS
Assess:
• For redness, swelling, fever, pain in ear, which indicates infection
Administer:
• After removing impacted cerumen by irrigation
• After cleaning stopper with alcohol
• After restraining child if necessary
• After warming sol to body temp
Evaluate:
• Therapeutic response: decreased ear pain, inflammation
Teach patient/family:
• The correct method of instillation using aseptic technique, including not touching dropper to ear
• That dizziness may occur after instillation

OTIC ANTIINFECTIVES

---

chloramphenicol (R)
(klor-am-fen′i-kole)
Chloromycetin Otic, Sopa-
mycetin*
neomycin (R)
(nee-oh-mye′sin)
Drotic, Otocort

Pregnancy category: C
Action: Inhibits protein synthesis
in susceptible microorganisms
Uses: Ear infection (external), short-
term use
Side effects/adverse reactions:
EENT: Itching, irritation in ear
INTEG: Rash, urticaria
Contraindications: Hypersensitiv-
ity, perforated eardrum
Precautions: Pregnancy (C)
NURSING CONSIDERATIONS
Assess:
• For redness, swelling, fever, pain
in ear, which indicates superinfec-
tion
Administer:
• After removing impacted ceru-
men by irrigation
• After cleaning stopper with alco-
hol
• After restraining child if neces-
sary
• After warming sol to body temp
Evaluate:
• Therapeutic response: decreased
ear pain
Teach patient/family:
• The correct method of instillation
using aseptic technique, including
not touching dropper to ear
• That dizziness may occur after in-
stillation

Appendix d

Combination products

A-200 Shampoo:
0.33% pyrethrins
4% piperonyl butoxide
Uses: Scabicide, pediculicide
Acid-X:
acetaminophen 500 mg
calcium carbonate 250 mg
Uses: Analgesic, antacid
Actifed:
pseudoephedrine 60 mg
triprolidine 2.5 mg
Uses: Decongestant
Actifed, Allergy, Nighttime:
pseudoephedrine 30 mg
diphenhydramine 25 mg
Uses: Decongestant, antihistamine
Actifed Plus:
pseudoephedrine 30 mg
triprolidine 1.25 mg
acetaminophen 500 mg
Uses: Decongestant, antihistamine
Actifed Sinus Daytime:
pseudoephedrine 30 mg
acetaminophen 500 mg
Uses: Decongestant
Actifed Sinus Nighttime:
pseudoephedrine 30 mg
diphenhydramine 25 mg
acetaminophen 500 mg
Uses: Decongestant, antihistamine
Advil Cold & Sinus Caplets:
pseudoephedrine 30 mg
ibuprofen 200 mg
Uses: Decongestant
**AK-Cide Ophthalmic Suspension/
Ointment:**
10% sulfacetamide sodium
0.5% prednisolone acetate

Uses: Ophth antiinfective, antiinflammatory
Aldactazide 25/25:
spironolactone 25 mg
hydrochlorothiazide 25 mg
Uses: Diuretic
Aldactazide 50/50:
spironolactone 50 mg
hydrochlorothiazide 50 mg
Uses: Diuretic
Aldoclor-150:
methyldopa 250 mg
chlorothiazide 150 mg
Uses: Antihypertensive
Aldoclor-250:
methyldopa 250 mg
chlorothiazide 250 mg
Uses: Antihypertensive
Aldoril-15:
methyldopa 250 mg
hydrochlorothiazide 15 mg
Uses: Antihypertensive
Aldoril-25:
methyldopa 250 mg
hydrochlorothiazide 25 mg
Uses: Antihypertensive
Alka-Seltzer Effervescent, Original:
sodium bicarbonate 1916 mg
citric acid 1000 mg
aspirin 325 mg
Uses: Antacid, adsorbent, antiflatulent
**Alka-Seltzer Plus Allergy Liqui-
Gels:**
pseudoephedrine 30 mg
chlorpheniramine 2 mg
acetaminophen 325 mg
Uses: Decongestant, antihistamine

Alka-Seltzer Plus Night-Time Cold Liqui-Gels:
doxylamine 6.25 mg
dextromethorphan 10 mg
pseudoephedrine 30 mg
acetaminophen 250 mg
Uses: Antitussive, decongestant

Alka-Seltzer Plus Cold & Cough Liqui-Gels:
dextromethorphan 10 mg
pseudoephedrine 30 mg
chlorpheniramine 2 mg
acetaminophen 250 mg
Uses: Antitussive, decongestant

Alka-Seltzer Plus Cold & Cough:
phenylpropanolamine 20 mg
chlorpheniramine 2 mg
dextromethorphan 10 mg
aspirin 325 mg
Uses: Antitussive, decongestant

Alka-Seltzer Plus Cold Liqui-Gels:
pseudoephedrine 30 mg
chlorpheniramine 2 mg
acetaminophen 250 mg
Uses: Decongestant, antihistamine

Alka-Seltzer Plus Cold Medicine:
chlorpheniramine 2 mg
phenylpropanolamine 20 mg
aspirin 325 mg
Uses: Antihistamine, analgesic

Alka-Seltzer Plus Flu & Body Aches Non-Drowsy Liqui-Gels:
pseudoephedrine 30 mg
dextromethorphan 10 mg
acetaminophen 250 mg
Uses: Decongestant, antitussive, analgesic

Alka-Seltzer Plus Night-Time Cold:
phenylpropanolamine 20 mg
doxylamine 6.25 mg
dextromethorphan 15 mg
aspirin 500 mg
Uses: Antitussive, analgesic

Alka-Seltzer Plus Sinus:
phenylpropanolamine 20 mg

aspirin 325 mg
Uses: Analgesic

Allerest Headache Strength Advanced Formula:
pseudoephedrine 30 mg
chlorpheniramine 2 mg
acetaminophen 325 mg
Uses: Decongestant, antihistamine

Allerest Maximum Strength Caplets:
pseudoephedrine 30 mg
chlorpheniramine 2 mg
Uses: Decongestant, antihistamine

Allerest Maximum Strength 12 Hour Caplets:
phenylpropanolamine 75 mg
chlorpheniramine 12 mg
Uses: Antihistamine

Allerest No-Drowsiness:
pseudoephedrine 30 mg
acetaminophen 325 mg
Uses: Decongestant, analgesic

Allerest Sinus Pain Formula:
pseudoephedrine 30 mg
chlorpheniramine 2 mg
acetaminophen 500 mg
Uses: Decongestant, antihistamine, analgesic

All-Nite Cold Formula Liquid:
Per 5 ml:
pseudoephedrine 10 mg
doxylamine 1.25 mg
dextromethorphan 5 mg
acetaminophen 167 mg
Uses: Decongestant, antihistamine, analgesic

Alor 5/500:
hydrocodone 5 mg
aspirin 500 mg
Uses: Analgesic

Amaphen:
acetaminophen 325 mg
butalbital 50 mg
caffeine 40 mg
Uses: Analgesic, barbiturates

◆ = Nursing alert　　 ∥ = Herb-drug interaction　　 ⊘ = Do not crush

Ambenyl Cough Syrup:
Per 5 ml:
bromodiphenhydramine 12.5 mg
codeine 10 mg
5% alcohol
Uses: Antihistamine, opioid analgesic

Anacin:
aspirin 400 mg
caffeine 32 mg
Uses: Analgesic

Anacin Maximum Strength:
aspirin 500 mg
caffeine 32 mg
Uses: Analgesic

Anacin PM (Aspirin Free):
diphenhydramine 25 mg
acetaminophen 500 mg
Uses: Analgesic

Anaplex HD Syrup:
Per 5 ml:
hydrocodone 1.7 mg
phenylephrine 5 mg
chlorpheniramine 2 mg
Uses: Analgesic, adrenergic, antihistamine

Anaplex Liquid:
Per 5 ml:
chlorpheniramine 2 mg
pseudoephedrine 30 mg
Uses: Antihistamine, decongestant

Anatuss:
guaifenesin 100 mg
dextromethorphan 15 mg
phenylpropanolamine 25 mg
acetaminophen 325 mg
Uses: Antitussive, expectorant, analgesic

Anatuss DM:
guaifenesin 400 mg
pseudoephedrine 60 mg
dextromethorphan 20 mg
Uses: Expectorant, adrenergic, antitussive

Anatuss DM Syrup:
Per 5 ml:
guaifenesin 100 mg
pseudoephedrine 30 mg
dextromethorphan 10 mg
Uses: Expectorant, adrenergic, antitussive

Anatuss LA:
pseudoephedrine 120 mg
guaifenesin 400 mg
Uses: Adrenergic, expectorant

Anatuss Syrup:
Per 5 ml:
guaifenesin 100 mg
dextromethorphan 15 mg
phenylpropanolamine 25 mg
Uses: Expectorant, antitussive

Anexsia 5/500:
hydrocodone 5 mg
acetaminophen 500 mg
Uses: Analgesic

Anexsia 7.5/650:
hydrocodone 7.5 mg
acetaminophen 650 mg
Uses: Analgesic

Anexsia 10/660:
hydrocodone 10 mg
acetaminophen 660 mg
Uses: Analgesic

Antihist-D:
clemastine 1.34 mg
phenylpropanolamine 75 mg
Uses: Antihistamine

Antrocol Elixir:
Per 5 ml:
atropine 0.195 mg
phenobarbital 16 mg
alcohol 20%
Uses: Anticholinergic, barbiturate

Apresazide 25/25:
hydralazine 25 mg
hydrochlorothiazide 25 mg
Uses: Antihypertensive

Aprodine w/Codeine Syrup:
Per 5 ml:
pseudoephedrine 30 mg
triprolidine 1.25 mg
codeine 10 mg
Uses: Adrenergic, analgesic

---

* = Canada only   Side effects: *italics* = common; ***bold italics*** = life-threatening

Aprodine Syrup:
Per 5 ml:
pseudoephedrine 30 mg
triprolidine 1.25 mg
Uses: Adrenergic, analgesic

A.R.M.:
phenylpropanolamine 25 mg
chlorpheniramine 4 mg
Uses: Antihistamine

Arthritis Pain Formula:
aspirin 500 mg
aluminum hydroxide 27 mg
magnesium hydroxide 100 mg
Uses: Analgesic, antacid

Arthrotec:
diclofenac 50 or 75 mg
misoprostol 200 µg
Uses: NSAID, gastric protectant

Asbron G Elixir:
theophylline 150 mg
guaifenesin 100 mg
alcohol 15%
Uses: Bronchodilator, expectorant

Asbron G Inlay:
theophylline 150 mg
guaifenesin 100 mg
sucrose
Uses: Bronchodilator, expectorant

Ascriptin A/D:
aspirin 325 mg
aluminum hydroxide 75 mg
magnesium hydroxide 75 mg
calcium carbonate 75 mg
Uses: Analgesic

Aspirin-Free Bayer Select Allergy Sinus:
pseudoephedrine 30 mg
chlorpheniramine 2 mg
acetaminophen 500 mg
Uses: Adrenergic, antihistamine, analgesic

Aspirin-Free Bayer Select Head & Chest Cold:
pseudoephedrine 30 mg
guaifenesin 100 mg
dextromethorphan 10 mg
acetaminophen 325 mg
Uses: Adrenergic, antitussive, expectorant, analgesic

Aspirin Free Excedrin:
acetaminophen 500 mg
caffeine 65 mg
Uses: Analgesic

Aspirin Free Excedrin Dual:
acetaminophen 500 mg
calcium carbonate 111 mg
magnesium carbonate 64 mg
magnesium oxide 30 mg
Uses: Analgesic, antacid

Augmentin 250:
amoxicillin 250 mg
clavulanic acid 125 mg
Uses: Antiinfective

Augmentin 500:
amoxicillin 500 mg
clavulanic acid 125 mg
Uses: Antiinfective

Augmentin 875:
amoxicillin 875 mg
clavulanic acid 125 mg
Uses: Antiinfective

Augmentin 125 Chewable:
amoxicillin 125 mg
clavulanic acid 31.25 mg
Uses: Antiinfective

Augmentin 250 Chewable:
amoxicillin 250 mg
clavulanic acid 62.5 mg
Uses: Antiinfective

Augmentin 125 mg/5 ml Suspension:
Per 5 ml:
amoxicillin 125 mg
clavulanic acid 31.25 mg
Uses: Antiinfective

Augmentin 250 mg/5 ml Suspension:
Per 5 ml:
amoxicillin 250 mg
clavulanic acid 62.5 mg
Uses: Antiinfective

◆ = Nursing alert   ⫸ = Herb-drug interaction   ⊘ = Do not crush

Auralgan Otic Solution:
5.4% antipyrine
1.4% benzocaine
Uses: Otic analgesic

B&O Supprettes No. 15A Supps:
belladonna extract 15 mg
opium 30 mg
Uses: Anticholinergic, narcotic analgesic

B&O Supprettes No. 16A Supps:
belladonna extract 16.2 mg
opium 60 mg
Uses: Anticholinergic, narcotic analgesic

Bactrim:
trimethoprim 80 mg
sulfamethoxazole 400 mg
Uses: Antiinfective

Bactrim DS:
trimethoprim 160 mg
sulfamethoxazole 800 mg
Uses: Antiinfective

Bactrim I.V.:
trimethoprim 80 mg
sulfamethoxazole 400 mg
Uses: Antiinfective

Bancap HC:
acetaminophen 500 mg
hydrocodone 5 mg
Uses: Analgesic

Bayer Plus, Extra Strength:
aspirin 500 mg
calcium carbonate
magnesium carbonate
magnesium oxide
Uses: Analgesic, antacid

Bayer Select Chest Cold:
dextromethorphan 15 mg
acetaminophen 500 mg
Uses: Antitussive, analgesic

Bayer Select Flu Relief:
acetaminophen 500 mg
pseudoephedrine 30 mg
dextromethorphan 15 mg
chlorpheniramine 2 mg

Uses: Analgesic, adrenergic, antitussive, antihistamine

Bayer Select Head & Chest Cold, Aspirin Free Caplets:
pseudoephedrine 30 mg
dextromethorphan 10 mg
guaifenesin 100 mg
acetaminophen 325 mg
Uses: Adrenergic, antitussive, expectorant, analgesic

Bayer Select Head Cold:
pseudoephedrine 30 mg
acetaminophen 500 mg
Uses: Adrenergic, analgesic

Bayer Select Maximum Strength Headache:
acetaminophen 500 mg
caffeine 65 mg
Uses: Nonnarcotic analgesic

Bayer Select Maximum Strength Menstrual:
acetaminophen 500 mg
pamabrom 25 mg
Uses: Nonnarcotic analgesic

Bayer Select Maximum Strength Night-Time Pain Relief:
acetaminophen 500 mg
diphenhydramine 25 mg
Uses: Analgesic, antihistamine

Bayer Select Maximum Strength Sinus Pain Relief:
acetaminophen 500 mg
pseudoephedrine 30 mg
Uses: Analgesic, adrenergic

Bayer Select Night Time Cold:
acetaminophen 500 mg
pseudoephedrine 30 mg
dextromethorphan 15 mg
triprolidine 1.25 mg
Uses: Analgesic, adrenergic, antitussive, antihistamine

Bellatal:
phenobarbital 16.2 mg
hyoscyamine sulfate 0.1037 mg
atropine sulfate 0.0194 mg

scopolamine hydrobromide 0.0065 mg
Uses: Barbiturate, anticholinergic
Bellergal-S:
ergotamine 0.6 mg
belladonna alkaloids 0.2 mg
phenobarbital 40 mg
Uses: α-Adrenergic blocker, anticholinergic, barbiturate
Bel-Phen-Ergot-SR:
phenobarbital 40 mg
ergotamine tartrate 0.6 mg
belladonna alkaloids 0.2 mg
Uses: α-Adrenergic blocker, anticholinergic, barbiturate
Benadryl Allergy Decongestant Liquid:
Per 5 ml:
diphenhydramine 12.5 mg
pseudoephedrine 30 mg
Uses: Antihistamine, adrenergic
Benadryl Allergy/Sinus Headache Caplets:
diphenhydramine 12.5 mg
pseudoephedrine 30 mg
acetaminophen 500 mg
Uses: Antihistamine, adrenergic, analgesic
Benadryl Decongestant Allergy:
pseudoephedrine 60 mg
diphenhydramine 25 mg
Uses: Adrenergic, antihistamine
Benylin Expectorant Liquid:
Per 5 ml:
dextromethorphan 5 mg
guaifenesin 100 mg
5% alcohol
Uses: Expectorant, antitussive
Benylin Multi-Symptom Liquid:
Per 5 ml:
dextromethorphan 5 mg
pseudoephedrine 15 mg
guaifenesin 100 mg
Uses: Antitussive, adrenergic, expectorant
Betoptic-Pilo:
0.25% betaxolol

1.75% pilocarpine
Uses: Ophthalmic
Biohist-LA Tablets:
pseudoephedrine 120 mg
carbinoxamine 8 mg
Uses: Adrenergic
Blephamide Ophthalmic Suspension/Ointment:
0.2% prednisolone
10% sodium sulfacetamide
Uses: Ophthalmic antiinfective, antiinflammatory
Bromatapp Tablets:
phenylpropanolamine 75 mg
brompheniramine 12 mg
Uses: Decongestant, antihistamine
Bromfed Capsules:
pseudoephedrine 120 mg
brompheniramine 12 mg
Uses: Antihistamine, adrenergic
Bromfed-PD Capsules:
pseudoephedrine 60 mg
brompheniramine 6 mg
Uses: Adrenergic, antihistamine
Bromfed Tablets:
pseudoephedrine 60 mg
brompheniramine 4 mg
Uses: Antihistamine, adrenergic
Bromfenex:
brompheniramine 12 mg
pseudoephedrine 120 mg
Uses: Antihistamine, adrenergic
Bromfenex PD:
brompheniramine 6 mg
pseudoephedrine 60 mg
Uses: Antihistamine, adrenergic
Bromo-Seltzer:
sodium bicarb 2781 mg
acetaminophen 325 mg
citric acid 2224 mg
Uses: Antacid, analgesic
Bromophen T.D.:
phenylephrine 15 mg
phenylpropanolamine 15 mg
brompheniramine 12 mg
Uses: Antihistamine, decongestant

 = Nursing alert   = Herb-drug interaction   = Do not crush

Brondelate Elixir:
theophylline 192 mg
guaifenesin 150 mg
Uses: Bronchodilator, expectorant
Brontex:
codeine 10 mg
guaifenesin 300 mg
Uses: Analgesic, expectorant
Bufferin:
aspirin 325 mg
calcium carbonate 158 mg
magnesium oxide 63 mg
magnesium carbonate 34 mg
Uses: Analgesic, antacid
Bufferin AF Nite-Time:
acetaminophen 500 mg
diphenhydramine 38 mg
Uses: Analgesic, antihistamine
Butibel:
belladonna extract 15 mg
butabarbital 15 mg
Uses: Anticholinergic, barbiturate
Cafatine PB:
ergotamine 1 mg
caffeine 100 mg
belladonna alkaloids 0.125 mg
pentobarbital 30 mg
Uses: Migraine agent
Cafergot:
ergotamine 1 mg
caffeine 100 mg
Uses: Adrenergic blocker
Cafergot Suppositories:
ergotamine 2 mg
caffeine 100 mg
Uses: Adrenergic blocker
Caladryl:
8% calamine, camphor
2.2% alcohol
1% pramoxine
Uses: Top antihistamine
Caladryl Clear:
1% pramoxine
0.1% zinc acetate
2% alcohol

camphor
Uses: Top antihistamine
Calcet:
calcium 152.8 mg
vitamin D 100 IU
Uses: Supplement
Calcidrine Syrup:
Per 5 ml:
codeine 8.4 mg
calcium iodide 152 mg
Uses: Analgesic
Caltrate 600+D:
vitamin D 200 IU
calcium 600 mg
Uses: Supplement
Cama Arthritis Pain Reliever:
aspirin 500 mg
magnesium oxide 150 mg
aluminum hydroxide 125 mg
Uses: Nonnarcotic analgesic, antacid
Capozide 25/15:
captopril 25 mg
hydrochlorothiazide 15 mg
Uses: Antihypertensive
Capozide 25/25:
captopril 25 mg
hydrochorothiazide 25 mg
Uses: Antihypertensive
Capozide 50/15:
captopril 50 mg
hydrochlorothiazide 15 mg
Uses: Antihypertensive
Capozide 50/25:
captopril 50 mg
hydrochlorothiazide 25 mg
Uses: Antihypertensive
Cardec DM Syrup:
Per 5 ml:
pseudoephedrine 60 mg
carbinoxamine 4 mg
dextromethorphan 15 mg
Uses: Adrenergic, antitussive
Cetacaine Topical:
14% benzocaine
2% tetracaine
0.5% benzalkonium chloride

0.005% cetyl dimethyl ethyl ammonium bromide
Uses: Local analgesic

Ceta Plus:
hydrocodone 5 mg
acetaminophen 500 mg
Uses: Analgesic

Cetapred Ophthalmic Ointment:
0.25% prednisolone
10% sodium sulfacetamide
Uses: Ophthalmic antiinfective, antiinflammatory

Cheracol Syrup:
Per 5 ml:
codeine 10 mg
guaifenesin 100 mg
Uses: Analgesic, expectorant

Cheracol Plus Liquid:
Per 5 ml:
phenylpropanolamine 8.3 mg
chlorpheniramine 1.3 mg
dextromethorphan 6.7 mg
8% alcohol
Uses: Antihistamine, antitussive

Children's Cepacol Liquid:
Per 5 ml:
acetaminophen 160 mg
pseudoephedrine 15 mg
Uses: Analgesic, adrenergic

Chlor-Trimeton Allergy-Sinus Caplets:
phenylpropanolamine 12.5 mg
chlorpheniramine 2 mg
acetaminophen 500 mg
Uses: Antihistamine, analgesic

Chlor-Trimeton 4 Hour Relief:
pseudoephedrine 60 mg
chlorpheniramine 4 mg
Uses: Antihistamine, adrenergic

Chlor-Trimeton 12 Hour Relief:
pseudoephedrine 120 mg
chlorpheniramine 8 mg
Uses: Antihistamine, adrenergic

Chromagen:
ferrous fumarate 66 mg

vitamin B_{12} 10 μg
vitamin C 250 mg
intrinsic factor 100 mg
Uses: Supplement

Claritin-D:
loratidine 5 mg
pseudoephedrine 120 mg
Uses: Antihistamine, adrenergic

Claritin-D 24-Hour:
loratidine 10 mg
pseudoephedrine 240 mg
Uses: Antihistamine, adrenergic

Clindex:
chlordiazepoxide 5 mg
clidinium 2.5 mg
Uses: Antianxiety, anticholinergic

Clomycin Ointment:
bacitracin 500 U
neomycin sulfate 3.5 g
polymyxin B sulfate 500 U
lidocaine 40 mg
Uses: Antiinfective, local anesthetic

Co-Apap:
pseudoephedrine 30 mg
chlorpheniramine 2 mg
dextromethorphan 15 mg
acetaminophen 325 mg
Uses: Adrenergic, antihistamine, antitussive, analgesic

Co-Gesic:
acetaminophen 500 mg
hydrocodone 5 mg
Uses: Analgesic

Codamine Syrup:
Per 5 ml:
hydrocodone 5 mg
phenylpropanolamine 25 mg
Uses: Analgesic

Codehist DH Elixir:
Per 5 ml:
pseudoephedrine 30 mg
chlorpheniramine 2 mg
codeine 10 mg
Uses: Adrenergic, antihistamine, analgesic

◆ = Nursing alert   ∥ = Herb-drug interaction   ⊘ = Do not crush

Codiclear DH Syrup:
Per 5 ml:
hydrocodone 5 mg
guaifenesin 100 mg
Uses: Analgesic, expectorant

Codimal:
pseudoephedrine 30 mg
chlorpheniramine 2 mg
acetaminophen 500 mg
Uses: Adrenergic, antihistamine, an
   algesic

Codimal DH Syrup:
Per 5 ml:
hydrocodone 1.66 mg
phenylephrine 5 mg
pyrilamine 8.33 mg
Uses: Analgesic, adrenergic

Codimal DM Syrup:
Per 5 ml:
phenylephrine 5 mg
pyrilamine 8.33 mg
dextromethorphan 10 mg
Uses: Adrenergic, antitussive

Codimal LA:
chlorpheniramine 8 mg
pseudoephedrine 120 mg
Uses: Antihistamine, adrenergic

Codimal PH Syrup:
Per 5 ml:
codeine 10 mg
phenylephrine 5 mg
pyrilamine 8.33 mg
Uses: Analgesic, adrenergic

Col-Probenecid:
probenecid 500 mg
colchicine 0.5 mg
Uses: Antigout agent

ColBenemid:
probenecid 500 mg
colchicine 0.5 mg
Uses: Antigout agent

Coldrine:
pseudoephedrine 30 mg
acetaminophen 500 mg
Uses: Decongestant, nonnarcotic analgesic

Coly-Mycin S Otic Suspension:
1% hydrocortisone
neomycin base 3.3 mg/ml
colistin 3 mg/ml
0.05% thonzonium bromide
Uses: Otic antiinfective

Combipres 0.1:
chlorthalidone 15 mg
clonidine 0.1 mg
Uses: Antihypertensive

Combipres 0.2:
chlorthalidone 15 mg
clonidine 0.2 mg
Uses: Antihypertensive

Combipres 0.3:
chlorthalidone 15 mg
clonidine 0.3 mg
Uses: Antihypertensive

Combivent:
ipratropium bromide 18 µg
albuterol 103 µg/actuation
Uses: Bronchodilator

Combivir:
lamivudine 150 mg
zidovudine 300 mg
Uses: Antiviral

Comhist Tablets:
phenylephrine 10 mg
chlorpheniramine 2 mg
phenyltoloxamine 25 mg
Uses: Adrenergic, antihistamine

Comhist LA:
phenylephrine 20 mg
chlorpheniramine 4 mg
phenyltoloxamine 50 mg
Uses: Adrenergic, antihistamine

Comtrex Liquid:
Per 5 ml:
chlorpheniramine 0.67 mg
acetaminophen 108.3 mg
dextromethorphan 3.3 mg
pseudoephedrine 10 mg
Uses: Antihistamine, analgesic, antitussive, decongestant

Comtrex Allergy-Sinus:
chlorpheniramine 2 mg

---

acetaminophen 500 mg
pseudoephedrine 30 mg
Uses: Antihistamine, analgesic, decongestant

Comtrex Liqui-Gels:
acetaminophen 325 mg
phenylpropanolamine 12.5 mg
chlorpheniramine 2 mg
dextromethorphan 10 mg
Uses: Analgesic, decongestant, antihistamine, antitussive

Comtrex Maximum Strength Caplets:
acetaminophen 500 mg
pseudoephedrine 30 mg
chlorpheniramine 2 mg
dextromethorphan 15 mg
Uses: Analgesic, decongestant, antihistamine, antitussive

Comtrex Maximum Strength Liqui-Gels:
acetaminophen 500 mg
phenylpropanolamine 12.5 mg
chlorpheniramine 2 mg
dextromethorphan 15 mg
Uses: Analgesic, decongestant, antihistamine, antitussive

Comtrex Maximum Strength Multi-Symptoms Cold, Flu Relief:
pseudoephedrine 30 mg
dextromethorphan 15 mg
chlorpheniramine 2 mg
acetaminophen 500 mg
Uses: Analgesic, decongestant, antihistamine, antitussive

Comtrex Maximum Strength Multi-Symptom Cold & Flu Relief Liqui-Gels:
acetaminophen 500 mg
phenylpropanolamine 12.5 mg
chlorpheniramine 2 mg
dextromethorphan 15 mg
Uses: Analgesic, decongestant, antihistamine, antitussive

Comtrex Maximum Strength Non-Drowsy Caplets:
acetaminophen 500 mg
pseudoephedrine 30 mg
dextromethorphan 15 mg
Uses: Analagesic, decongestant, antitussive

Congess SR:
guaifenesin 250 mg
pseudoephedrine 120 mg
Uses: Expectorant, decongestant

Congestac:
guaifenesin 400 mg
pseudoephedrine 60 mg
Uses: Expectorant, decongestant

Contac Cough & Chest Cold Liquid:
Per 5 ml:
pseudoephedrine 15 mg
dextromethorphan 5 mg
guaifenesin 50 mg
acetaminophen 125 mg
Uses: Decongestant, antitussive, expectorant, analgesic

Contac Cough & Sore Throat Liquid:
Per 5 ml:
dextromethorphan 5 mg
acetaminophen 125 mg
Uses: Antitussive, analgesic

Contac Day Allergy/Sinus:
pseudoephedrine 60 mg
acetaminophen 650 mg
Uses: Decongestant, analgesic

Contac Day Cold and Flu:
pseudoephedrine 60 mg
dextromethorphan 30 mg
acetaminophen 650 mg
Uses: Decongestant, antitussive, analgesic

Contac 12 Hour Capsules:
phenylpropanolamine 75 mg
chlorpheniramine 8 mg
Uses: Antihistamine

◆ = Nursing alert   ∥ = Herb-drug interaction   ⊘ = Do not crush

Contac Maximum Strength 12 Hour:
phenylpropanolamine 75 mg
chlorpheniramine 12 mg
Uses: Antihistamine
Contac Night Allergy Sinus:
pseudoephedrine 60 mg
diphenhydramine 50 mg
acetaminophen 650 mg
Uses: Decongestant, antihistamine, analgesic
Contac Night Cold and Flu Caplets:
pseudoephedrine 60 mg
diphenhydramine 50 mg
acetaminophen 650 mg
Uses: Decongestant, antihistamine, antitussive, analgesic
Contac Severe Cold & Flu Nighttime Liquid:
Per 5 ml:
pseudoephedrine 10 mg
chlorpheniramine 0.67 mg
dextromethorphan 5 mg
acetaminophen 167 mg
18.5% alcohol
Uses: Decongestant, antihistamine, antitussive, analgesic
Contuss Liquid:
Per 5 ml:
phenylpropanolamine 20 mg
phenylephrine 5 mg
guaifenesin 100 mg
Uses: Adrenergic, expectorant
Coricidin:
chlorpheniramine 2 mg
acetaminophen 325 mg
Uses: Antihistamine, analgesic
Coricidin 'D':
phenylpropanolamine 12.5 mg
chlorpheniramine 2 mg
acetaminophen 325 mg
Uses: Antihistamine, analgesic
Coricidin Maximum Strength Sinus Headache Caplets:
phenylpropanolamine 12.5 mg
chlorpheniramine 2 mg

acetaminophen 500 mg
Uses: Antihistamine, analgesic
Cortisporin Ophthalmic/Otic Suspension:
0.35% neomycin polymyxin B 10,000 U/ml
1% hydrocortisone
Uses: Ophthalmic antiinfective, antiinflammatory
Cortisporin Ophthalmic Ointment:
0.35% neomycin base
bacitracin 400 U
polymyxin B 10,000 U
hydrocortisone 1%
Uses: Ophthalmic antiinfective
Cortisporin Topical Cream:
0.5% neomycin sulfate
polymyxin B 10,000 U
0.5% hydrocortisone
Uses: Topical antiinfective
Cortisporin Topical Ointment:
0.5% neomycin sulfate
bacitracin 400 U
polymyxin B 5,000 U
1% hydrocortisone
Uses: Topical antiinfective
Corzide 40/5:
nadolol 40 mg
bendroflumethiazide 5 mg
Uses: Antihypertensive
Cough-X:
dextromethorphan 5 mg
benzocaine 2 mg
Uses: Antitussive, local anesthetic
Creon:
lipase 8,000 U
amylase 30,000 U
protease 13,000 U
pancreatin 300 mg
Uses: Digestive enzyme
Cyclomydril Ophthalmic Solution:
0.2% cyclopentolate
1% phenylephrine
Uses: Mydriatic
Dallergy Caplets:
chlorpheniramine 8 mg

phenylephrine 20 mg
methscopolamine 2.5 mg
Uses: Antihistamine, adrenergic
Dallergy Syrup:
Per 5 ml:
chlorpheniramine 2 mg
phenylephrine 10 mg
methscopolamine 0.625 mg
Uses: Antihistamine, adrenergic
Dallergy Tablets:
chlorpheniramine 4 mg
phenylephrine 10 mg
methscopolamine 1.25 mg
Uses: Antihistamine, adrenergic
Dallergy-D Syrup:
Per 5 ml:
phenylephrine 5 mg
chlorpheniramine 2 mg
Uses: Antihistamine, adrenergic
Damason-P:
hydrocodone 5 mg
aspirin 500 mg
Uses: Analgesic
Darvocet-N 100:
propoxyphene-N 100 mg
acetaminophen 650 mg
Uses: Analgesic
Darvon Compound-65:
propoxyphene 65 mg
aspirin 389 mg
caffeine 32.4 mg
Uses: Analgesic
Deconamine:
pseudoephedrine 60 mg
chlorpheniramine 4 mg
Uses: Antihistamine, decongestant
Deconamine CX:
hydrocodone 5 mg
pseudoephedrine 30 mg
guaifenesin 300 mg
Uses: Analgesic, decongestant, expectorant
Deconamine SR:
pseudoephedrine 120 mg
chlorpheniramine 8 mg
Uses: Antihistamine, decongestant

Deconamine Syrup:
Per 5 ml:
pseudoephedrine 30 mg
chlorpheniramine 2 mg
Uses: Antihistamine, decongestant
Defen-LA:
pseudoephedrine 60 mg
guaifenesin 600 mg
Uses: Decongestant, expectorant
Demazin:
phenylpropanolamine 25 mg
chlorpheniramine 4 mg
Uses: Antihistamine
Demi-Regroton:
chlorthalidone 25 mg
reserpine 0.125 mg
Uses: Antihypertensive
Demulen 1/50:
ethinyl estradiol 50 μg
ethynodiol diacetate 1 mg
Uses: Oral contraceptive
Dexacidin Ophthalmic Ointment/ Suspension:
Per ml:
0.1% dexamethasone
0.35% neomycin
polymyxin B 10,000 U/g
Uses: Ophth, antiinfective/antiinflammatory
Dexasporin Ophthalmic Ointment:
Per gram:
0.1% dexamethasone
0.35% neomycin
polymyxin B 10,000 U
Uses: Ophth, antiinfective/antiinflammatory
DHC Plus:
dihydrocodeine 16 mg
acetaminophen 356.4 mg
caffeine 30 mg
Uses: Analgesic
Dialose Plus:
docusate sodium 100 mg
yellow phenolphthalein 65 mg
Uses: Laxative

◆ = Nursing alert   ⬥ = Herb-drug interaction   ⊘ = Do not crush

Dieutrim T.D.:
benzocaine 9 mg
phenylpropanolamine 75 mg
carboxymethylcellulose 75 mg
Uses: Top anesthetic

Di-Gel Advanced Formula:
magnesium hydroxide 128 mg
calcium carbonate 280 mg
simethicone 20 mg
Uses: Antacid, adsorbent, antiflatulent

Di-Gel Liquid:
Per 5 ml:
aluminum hydroxide 200 mg
magnesium hydroxide 200 mg
simethicone 20 mg
Uses: Antacid, adsorbent, antiflatulent

Dihistine DH Liquid:
Per 5 ml:
pseudoephedrine 30 mg
chlorpheniramine 2 mg
codeine 10 mg
Uses: Decongestant, antihistamine, analgesic

Dilaudid Cough Syrup:
Per 5 ml:
guaifenesin 100 mg
hydromorphone 1 mg
5% alcohol
Uses: Expectorant, analgesic

Dilor-G Liquid:
dyphylline 300 mg
guaifenesin 300 mg
Uses: Bronchodilator, expectorant

Dilor-G Tablets:
dyphylline 200 mg
guaifenesin 200 mg
Uses: Bronchodilator, expectorant

Dimetane Decongestant:
brompheniramine 4 mg
phenylephrine 10 mg
Uses: Antihistamine, adrenergic

Dimetane-DC Cough Syrup:
Per 5 ml:
brompheniramine 2 mg

phenylpropanolamine 12.5 mg
codeine 10 mg
Uses: Antihistamine, analgesic

Dimetane-DX Cough Syrup:
Per 5 ml:
brompheniramine 2 mg
pseudoephedrine 30 mg
dextromethorphan 10 mg
Uses: Antihistamine, decongestant, antitussive

Dimetapp:
brompheniramine 4 mg
phenylpropanolamine 25 mg
Uses: Antihistamine

Dimetapp Cold & Allergy Chewable:
phenylpropanolamine 6.25 mg
brompheniramine 1 mg
Uses: Antihistamine

Dimetapp Cold & Flu:
phenylpropanolamine 12.5 mg
brompheniramine 2 mg
acetaminophen 500 mg
Uses: Antihistamine, analgesic

Dimetapp DM Elixir:
Per 5 ml:
phenylpropanolamine 12.5 mg
brompheniramine 2 mg
dextromethorphan 10 mg
Uses: Antihistamine, antitussive

Dimetapp Elixir:
Per 5 ml:
phenylpropanolamine 12.5 mg
brompheniramine 2 mg
Uses: Antihistamine

Dimetapp Extentabs:
phenylpropanolamine 75 mg
brompheniramine 12 mg
Uses: Antihistamine

Dimetapp Sinus:
pseudoephedrine 30 mg
ibuprofen 200 mg
Uses: Decongestant, analgesic

Diutensin-R:
methylclothiazide 2.5 mg

reserpine 0.1 mg
Uses: Antihypertensive
Doan's PM Extra Strength:
magnesium salicylate 500 mg
diphenhydramine 25 mg
Uses: Analgesic, antihistamine
Dolacet:
hydrocodone 5 mg
acetaminophen 500 mg
Uses: Analgesic
Donnatal:
phenobarbital 16.2 mg
hyoscyamine 0.1037 mg
atropine 0.0194 mg
scopolamine 0.0065 mg
Uses: Anticholinergic, barbiturate
Donnatal Elixir:
Per 5 ml:
phenobarbital 16.2 mg
hyoscyamine 0.1037 mg
atropine 0.0194 mg
scopolamine 0.0065 mg
23% alcohol
Uses: Anticholinergic, barbiturate
Donnatal Extentabs:
phenobarbital 48.6 mg
hyoscyamine 0.3111 mg
atropine 0.0582 mg
scopolamine 0.0195 mg
Uses: Anticholinergic, barbiturate
Donnazyme:
pancreatin 500 mg
lipase 1000 U
protease 12,500 U
amylase 12,500 U
Uses: Pancreatic enzymes
Dorcol Children's Cold Formula Liquid:
Per 5 ml:
pseudoephedrine 15 mg
chlorpheniramine 1 mg
Uses: Decongestant, antihistamine
Doxidan:
docusate calcium 60 mg
phenolphthalein 65 mg
Uses: Stool softener

Dristan Cold:
pseudoephedrine 30 mg
acetaminophen 500 mg
Uses: Decongestant, analgesic
Dristan Cold Maximum Strength Caplets:
pseudoephedrine 30 mg
brompheniramine 2 mg
acetaminophen 500 mg
Uses: Decongestant, antihistamine, analgesic
Dristan Cold Multi-Symptom Formula:
acetaminophen 325 mg
phenylephrine 5 mg
chlorpheniramine 2 mg
Uses: Analgesic, adrenergic, antihistamine
Dristan Sinus:
pseudoephedrine 30 mg
ibuprofen 200 mg
Uses: Decongestant, analgesic
Drixoral Allergy Sinus:
pseudoephedrine 60 mg
dexbrompheniramine 3 mg
acetaminophen 500 mg
Uses: Decongestant, antihistamine, analgesic
Drixoral Cold & Allergy:
pseudoephedrine 120 mg
dexbrompheniramine 6 mg
Uses: Decongestant, antihistamine
Drixoral Cold & Flu:
pseudoephedrine 60 mg
dexbrompheniramine 3 mg
acetaminophen 500 mg
Uses: Decongestant, antihistamine, analgesic
Drixoral Cough & Congestion Liquid Caps:
pseudoephedrine 60 mg
dextromethorphan 30 mg
Uses: Decongestant, antitussive
Drixoral Cough & Sore Throat Liquid Caps:
dextromethorphan 15 mg

acetaminophen 325 mg
Uses: Antitussive, analgesic
Drixoral Plus:
pseudoephedrine 60 mg
dexbrompheniramine 3 mg
acetaminophen 500 mg
Uses: Decongestant, antihistamine, analgesic
DT:
Per 5 ml dose:
diphtheria toxoid 2LfU
tetanus toxoid 5LfU
Uses: Vaccine
DTP:
Per 0.5 ml dose:
diphtheria toxoid 6.5LfU
tetanus toxoid 5LfU
pertussis 4LfU
Uses: Vaccine
Dura-Vent:
phenylpropanolamine 75 mg
guaifenesin 600 mg
Uses: Expectorant
Dura-Vent/A:
phenylpropanolamine 75 mg
chlorpheniramine 10 mg
Uses: Antihistamine
Dura-Vent/DA:
phenylephrine 20 mg
chlorpheniramine 8 mg
methscopolamine 2.5 mg
Uses: Adrenergic, antihistamine
Dyazide:
hydrochlorothiazide 25 mg
triamterene 37.5 mg
Uses: Diuretic
Dylline-GG Liquid:
dyphylline 300 mg
guaifenesin 300 mg
Uses: Bronchodilator, expectorant
Dynafed Asthma Relief:
ephedrine 25 mg
guaifenesin 200 mg
Uses: Adrenergic, expectorant
Dynafed Plus Maximum Strength:
pseudoephedrine 30 mg

acetaminophen 500 mg
Uses: Decongestant, analgesic
Dyphylline-GG Elixir:
Per 5 ml:
dyphylline 100 mg
guaifenesin 100 mg
Uses: Bronchodilator, expectorant
E-Pilo-1 Ophthalmic Solution:
1% epinephrine bitartrate
1% pilocarpine
Uses: Miotic
E-Pilo-2 Ophthalmic Solution:
1% epinephrine bitartrate
2% pilocarpine
Uses: Miotic
E-Pilo-4 Ophthalmic Solution:
1% epinephrine bitartrate
4% pilocarpine
Uses: Miotic
Elase-Chloromycetin Ointment:
Per gram:
fibrinolysin 1 U
desoxyribonuclease 666.6 U
chloramphenicol 10 mg
Uses: Enzyme, antiinfective
Elase Ointment:
Per gram:
fibrinolysin 1 U
desoxyribonuclease 666.6 U
Uses: Enzyme
Elixophyllin GG Liquid:
Per 5 ml:
theophylline 100 mg
guaifenesin 100 mg
Uses: Expectorant, bronchodilator
EMLA Cream:
lidocaine 2.5 mg
prilocaine 2.5 mg
Uses: Local anesthetic
Empirin w/Codeine #3:
aspirin 325 mg
codeine phosphate 30 mg
Uses: Analgesic
Empirin w/Codeine #4:
aspirin 325 mg

codeine phosphate 60 mg
Uses: Analgesic
Enduronyl:
methyclothiazide 5 mg
deserpidine 0.25 mg
Uses: Diuretic
Entex:
phenylephrine 5 mg
phenylpropanolamine 45 mg
guaifenesin 200 mg
Uses: Adrenergic, expectorant
Entex LA:
phenylpropanolamine 75 mg
guaifenesin 400 mg
Uses: Adrenergic, expectorant
Entex PSE:
pseudoephedrine 120 mg
guaifenesin 600 mg
Uses: Adrenergic, expectorant
Epifoam Aerosol Foam:
1% hydrocortisone
1% pramoxine
Uses: Topical corticosteroid
Esgic-Plus:
butalbital 50 mg
acetaminophen 500 mg
caffeine 40 mg
Uses: Barbiturate, analgesic
Esimil:
guanethidine 10 mg
hydrochlorothiazide 25 mg
Uses: Antihypertensive
Estratest:
esterified estrogens 1.25 mg
methyltestosterone 2.5 mg
Uses: Androgen, estrogen
Etrafon:
perphenazine 2 mg
amitriptyline 25 mg
Uses: Antipsychotic, antidepressant
Etrafon Forte:
perphenazine 4 mg
amitriptyline 25 mg
Uses: Antipsychotic, antidepressant
Excedrin Migraine:
aspirin 250 mg

acetaminophen 250 mg
caffeine 65 mg
Uses: Migraine agent
Excedrin P.M.:
acetaminophen 500 mg
diphenhydramine citrate 38 mg
Uses: Analgesic, antihistamine
Excedrin P.M. Liquid:
Per 30 ml:
acetaminophen 1000 mg
diphenhydramine 50 mg
Uses: Analgesic, antihistamine
Excedrin P.M. Liquigels:
acetaminophen 500 mg
diphenhydramine 25 mg
Uses: Analgesic, antihistamine
Excedrin Sinus Extra Strength:
pseudoephedrine 30 mg
acetaminophen 500 mg
Uses: Decongestant, analgesic
Fansidar:
sulfidoxine 500 mg
pyrimethamine 25 mg
Uses: Antimalarial
Fedahist:
pseudoephedrine 60 mg
chlorpheniramine 4 mg
Uses: Decongestant, antihistamine
Fedahist Expectorant Syrup:
Per 5 ml:
guaifenesin 200 mg
pseudoephedrine 20 mg
Uses: Expectorant, decongestant
Fedahist Gyrocaps:
pseudoephedrine 65 mg
chlorpheniramine 10 mg
Uses: Decongestant, antihistamine
Fedahist Timecaps:
pseudoephedrine 120 mg
chlorpheniramine 8 mg
Uses: Decongestant, antihistamine
Feen-A-Mint Pills:
docusate sodium 100 mg
phenolphthalein 65 mg
Uses: Laxative

◆ = Nursing alert   ⫸ = Herb-drug interaction   ⊘ = Do not crush

Fem-1:
acetaminophen 500 mg
pamabrom 25 mg
Uses: Nonnarcotic analgesic

Ferro-Sequels:
docusate sodium 100 mg
ferrous fumarate 150 mg
Uses: Laxative, hematinic

Fioricet:
acetaminophen 325 mg
caffeine 40 mg
butalbital 50 mg
Uses: Analgesic, barbiturate

Fioricet w/Codeine:
acetaminophen 325 mg
caffeine 40 mg
butalbital 50 mg
codeine 30 mg
Uses: Analgesic, barbiturate

Fiorinal:
aspirin 325 mg
caffeine 40 mg
butalbital 50 mg
Uses: Analgesic, barbiturate

Fiorinal with Codeine:
aspirin 325 mg
caffeine 40 mg
butalbital 50 mg
codeine 30 mg
Uses: Analgesic, barbiturate

FML-S Ophthalmic Suspension:
0.1% flurometholone
10% sulfacetamide
Uses: Ophth, antiinfective/antiinflammatory

Gas-Ban:
calcium carbonate 500 mg
simethicone 40 mg
Uses: Antiflatulent, antacid

Gas-Ban DS Liquid:
Per 5 ml:
aluminum hydroxide 400 mg
magnesium hydroxide 400 mg
simethicone 40 mg
Uses: Antiflatulent, antacid

Gaviscon:
magnesium trisilicate 20 mg
aluminum hydroxide 80 mg
Uses: Antacid, adsorbent, antiflatulent

Gaviscon Liquid:
Per 5 ml:
aluminum hydroxide 31.7 mg
magnesium carbonate 119.3 mg
Uses: Antacid, adsorbent, antiflatulent

Gelprin:
acetaminophen 125 mg
aspirin 240 mg
caffeine 32 mg
Uses: Analgesic

Gelusil:
aluminum hydroxide 200 mg
magnesium hydroxide 200 mg
simethicone 25 mg
Uses: Antacid, adsorbent, antiflatulent

Genatuss DM Syrup:
Per 5 ml:
guaifenesin 100 mg
dextromethorphan 10 mg
Uses: Expectorant, antitussive

Granulex Aerosol:
Per 0.82 ml:
trypsin 0.1 mg
balsam peru 72.5 mg
castor oil 650 mg
Uses: Top enzyme

Guaifenex PPA 75:
guaifenesin 600 mg
phenylpropanolamine 75 mg
Uses: Expectorant, decongestant

Guaifenex PSE 60:
pseudoephedrine 60 mg
guaifenesin 600 mg
Uses: Decongestant, expectorant

Guaifenex PSE 120:
pseudoephedrine 120 mg
guaifenesin 600 mg
Uses: Decongestant, expectorant

---

* = Canada only   Side effects: *italics* = common; **bold italics** = life-threatening

Haley's M-O Liquid:
Per 15 ml:
magnesium hydroxide 900 mg
mineral oil 3.75 ml
Uses: Laxative

Halotussin-DM Sugar Free Liquid:
Per 5 ml:
guaifenesin 100 mg
dextromethorphan 10 mg
Uses: Expectorant, antitussive

Helidac:
In a compliance package:
bismuth subsalicylate 262.4 mg tabs
metronidazole 250 mg tabs
tetracycline 500 mg caps
Uses: Antiinfective

Humibid DM Sprinkle Caps:
dextromethorphan 15 mg
guaifenesin 300 mg
Uses: Expectorant, antitussive

Humibid DM Tablets:
dextromethorphan 30 mg
guaifenesin 600 mg
Uses: Expectorant, antitussive

Hycodan:
hydrocodone 5 mg
homatropine 1.5 mg
Uses: Analgesic, mydriatic

Hycodan Syrup:
Per 5 ml:
hydrocodone 5 mg
homatropine 1.5 mg
Uses: Analgesic, mydriatic

Hycomine Compound:
chlorpheniramine 2 mg
acetaminophen 250 mg
phenylephrine 10 mg
hydrocodone 5 mg
caffeine 30 mg
Uses: Antihistamine, analgesic, adrenergic

Hycomine Syrup:
Per 5 ml:
hydrocodone 5 mg
phenylpropanolamine 25 mg
Uses: Analgesic, decongestant

Hycotuss Expectorant:
Per 5 ml:
guaifenesin 100 mg
hydrocodone 5 mg
10% alcohol
Uses: Expectorant

Hydro-Serp:
hydrochlorothiazide 50 mg
reserpine 0.125 mg
Uses: Antihypertensive

Hydrocet:
hydrocodone 5 mg
acetaminophen 500 mg
Uses: Narcotic, opioid analgesic

Hydrogesic:
hydrocodone 5 mg
acetaminophen 500 mg
Uses: Narcotic, opioid analgesic

Hydropres-50:
hydrochlorothiazide 50 mg
reserpine 0.125 mg
Uses: Antihypertensive

Hydroserpin #1:
hydrochlorothiazide 25 mg
reserpine 0.125 mg
Uses: Antihypertensive

Hyzaar:
losartan potassium 50 mg
hydrochlorothiazide 12.5 mg
potassium 4.24 mg
Uses: Antihypertensive

Iberet Filmtab:
ferrous sulfate 105 mg
ascorbic acid 150 mg
B-complex vitamins
Uses: Supplement

Iberet Liquid:
Per 5 ml:
ferrous sulfate 78.75 mg
ascorbic acid 112.5 mg
B-complex vitamins
Uses: Supplement

Imodium Advanced:
loperamide 2 mg
simethicone 125 mg
Uses: Antidiarrheal, antiflatulent

◆ = Nursing alert   ∥ = Herb-drug interaction   ⊘ = Do not crush

Inderide 40/25:
propranolol 40 mg
hydrochlorothiazide 25 mg
Uses: Antihypertensive

Innovar:
Per ml:
droperidol 2.5 mg
fentanyl 0.05 mg
Uses: Narcotic analgesic, general anesthetic

Iofed:
brompheniramine 12 mg
pseudoephedrine 120 mg
Uses: Antihistamine, adrenergic

Iofed PD:
brompheniramine 6 mg
pseudoephedrine 60 mg
Uses: Antihistamine, adrenergic

Iophen-C Liquid:
Per 5 ml:
iodinated glycerol 30 mg
codeine 10 mg
Uses: Expectorant, analgesic

Iophen-DM Liquid:
Per 5 ml:
iodinated glycerol 30 mg
dextromethorphan 10 mg
Uses: Expectorant, antitussive

Kondremul with Phenolphthalein:
Per 15 ml:
phenolphthalein 150 mg
55% mineral oil
Irish moss
Uses: Laxative

Lactinex:
Mixed culture of:
Lactobacillus acidophilus and
Lactobacillus bulgaricus
Uses: Supplement

Levsin PB Drops:
Per ml:
hyoscyamine 0.125 mg
phenobarbital 15 mg
5% alcohol
Uses: Anticholinergic, barbiturate

Levsin with Phenobarbital:
hyoscyamine 0.125 mg
phenobarbital 15 mg
Uses: Anticholinergic, barbiturate

Lexxel:
enalapril 5 mg
felodipine 5 mg
Uses: Antihypertensive

Librax:
chlordiazepoxide 5 mg
clidinium 2.5 mg
Uses: Antianxiety, anticholinergic

Lida-Mantel-HC-Cream:
0.5% hydrocortisone
3% lidocaine
Uses: Antiinflammatory, analgesic

Limbitrol DS 10-25:
chlordiazepoxide 10 mg
amitriptyline 25 mg
Uses: Antidepressant, antianxiety

Lobac:
salicylamide 200 mg
phenyltoloxamine 20 mg
acetaminophen 300 mg
Uses: Skeletal muscle relaxant, analgesic

Loestrin Fe 1.5/30:
norethindrone acetate 1.5 mg
ethinyl estradiol 30 µg
Uses: Oral contraceptive

Lomotil:
diphenoxylate 2.5 mg
atropine 0.025 mg
Uses: Antidiarrheal, anticholinergic

Lomotil Liquid:
Per 5 ml:
diphenoxylate 2.5 mg
atropine 0.025 mg
Uses: Antidiarrheal, anticholinergic

Lo Ovral:
ethinyl estradiol 30 µg
norgestrel 0.3 mg
Uses: Oral contraceptive

Lopressor HCT 50/25:
metoprolol 50 mg

hydrochlorothiazide 25 mg
Uses: Antihypertensive
Lopressor HCT 100/25:
metoprolol 100 mg
hydrochlorothiazide 25 mg
Uses: Antihypertensive
Lopressor HCT 100/50:
metoprolol 100 mg
hydrochlorothiazide 50 mg
Uses: Antihypertensive
Lorcet 10/650:
acetaminophen 650 mg
hydrocodone 10 mg
Uses: Analgesic
Lortab 2.5/500:
hydrocodone 2.5 mg
acetaminophen 500 mg
Uses: Analgesic
Lortab 5/500:
hydrocodone 5 mg
acetaminophen 500 mg
Uses: Analgesic
Lortab 7.5/500:
hydrocodone 7.5 mg
acetaminophen 500 mg
Uses: Analgesic
Lortab 10/500:
hydrocodone 10 mg
acetaminophen 500 mg
Uses: Analgesic
Lortab ASA:
aspirin 500 mg
hydrocodone 5 mg
Uses: Analgesic
Lortab Elixir:
Per 5 ml:
hydrocodone 2.5 mg
acetaminophen 167 mg
Uses: Analgesic
Lotensin HCT 5/6.25:
benazepril 5 mg
hydrochlorothiazide 6.25 mg
Uses: Antihypertensive
Lotensin HCT 10/12.5:
benazepril 10 mg
hydrochlorothiazide 12.5 mg

Uses: Antihypertensive
Lotensin HCT 20/12.5:
benazepril 20 mg
hydrochlorothiazide 12.5 mg
Uses: Antihypertensive
Lotensin HCT 20/25:
benazepril 20 mg
hydrochlorothiazide 25 mg
Uses: Antihypertensive
Lotrel 2.5/10:
amlopidine 2.5 mg
benazepril 10 mg
Uses: Antihypertensive
Lotrel 5/10:
amlodipine 5 mg
benazepril 10 mg
Uses: Antihypertensive
Lotrel 5/20:
amlodipine 5 mg
benazepril 20 mg
Uses: Antihypertensive
Lotrisone Topical:
0.05% betamethasone
1% clotrimazole
Uses: Local antiinfective, antiinflammatory
Lufyllin-EPG Elixir:
Per 5 ml:
dyphylline 150 mg
ephedrine 24 mg
guaifenesin 300 mg
phenobarbital 24 mg
Uses: Bronchodilator, expectorant
Lufyllin-EPG Tablets:
dyphylline 100 mg
ephedrine 16 mg
guaifenesin 200 mg
phenobarbital 16 mg
Uses: Bronchodilator, adrenergic, expectorant, barbiturate
Lufyllin-GG:
dyphylline 200 mg
guaifenesin 200 mg
Uses: Bronchodilator, expectorant
Lufyllin-GG Elixir:
dyphylline 100 mg

guaifenesin 100 mg
alcohol 17%
Uses: Bronchodilator, expectorant
M-M-R-II:
measles
mumps
rubella
Uses: Vaccine, toxoid
M-R Vax II:
measles
rubella
Uses: Vaccine, toxoid
Maalox:
aluminum hydroxide 200 mg
magnesium hydroxide 200 mg
Uses: Antacid, adsorbent, antiflatulent
Maalox Plus:
aluminum hydroxide 200 mg
magnesium hydroxide 200 mg
simethicone 25 mg
Uses; Antacid, adsorbent, antiflatulent
**Maalox Plus Extra Strength Sus-
pension:**
Per 5 ml:
aluminum hydroxide 500 mg
magnesium hydroxide 450 mg
simethicone 40 mg
Uses: Antacid, adsorbent, antiflatulent
Maalox Suspension:
Per 5 ml:
aluminum hydroxide 225 mg
magnesium hydroxide 200 mg
Uses: Antacid, adsorbent, antiflatu
lent
Mapap Cold Formula:
acetaminophen 325 mg
chlorpheniramine 2 mg
pseudoephedrine 30 mg
dextromethorphan 15 mg
Uses: Bronchodilator, expectorant
Marax:
ephedrine 25 mg
theophylline 130 mg

hydroxyzine 10 mg
Uses: Bronchodilator, sedative/
hypnotic
**Maxitrol Ophthalmic Suspension/
Ointment:**
Per ml:
0.35% neomycin
0.1% dexamethasone
polymyxin B 10,000 U
Uses: Ophthalmic antiinfective, antiinflammatory
Maxzide:
hydrochlorothiazide 50 mg
triamterene 75 mg
Uses: Antihypertensive, diuretic
Maxzide-25 MG:
hydrochlorothiazide 25 mg
triamterene 37.5 mg
Uses: Diuretic
Medi-Flu Liquid:
Per 5 ml:
pseudoephedrine 10 mg
chlorpheniramine 0.67 mg
dextromethorphan 5 mg
acetaminophen 167 mg
18.5% alcohol
Uses: Decongestant, antihistamine, antitussive, analgesic
Mepergan Fortis:
meperidine 50 mg
promethazine 25 mg
Uses: Analgesic, antihistamine
**Metimyd Ophthalmic Suspension/
Ointment:**
0.5% prednisolone
10% sodium sulfacetamide
Uses: Ophthalmic antiinfective, antiinflammatory
**Midol Maximum Strength Multi-
Symptom Menstrual Gelcaps:**
acetaminophen 500 mg
pyrilamine 15 mg
caffeine 60 mg
Uses: Analgesic
Midol PM:
acetaminophen 500 mg

diphenhydramine 25 mg
Uses: Analgesic, antihistamine

Midol PMS Maximum Strength Caplets:
acetaminophen 500 mg
pyrilamine 15 mg
pamabrom 25 mg
Uses: Analgesic

Midol, Teen:
acetaminophen 400 mg
pamabrom 25 mg
Uses: Analgesic

Midrin:
isometheptene 65 mg
acetaminophen 325 mg
dichloralphenazone 100 mg
Uses: Analgesic

Minizide 1:
prazosin 1 mg
polythiazide 0.5 mg
Uses: Antihypertensive

Minizide 2:
prazosin 2 mg
polythiazide 0.5 mg
Uses: Antihypertensive

Minizide 5:
prazosin 5 mg
polythiazide 0.5 mg
Uses: Antihypertensive

Modane Plus:
docusate sodium 100 mg
phenolphthalein 65 mg
Uses: Laxative

Moduretic:
hydrochlorothiazide 50 mg
amiloride 5 mg
Uses: Diuretic

Motrin IB Sinus:
pseudoephedrine 30 mg
ibuprofen 200 mg
Uses: Adrenergic, analgesic

Murocoll-2 Ophthalmic Drops:
0.3% scopolamine
10% phenylephrine
Uses: Ophth anticholinergic, mydriatic

Mycolog II Topical:
Per gram:
0.1% triamcinolone acetonide
nystatin 100,000 U
Uses: Local antiinfective, antiinflammatory

Mylanta:
aluminum hydroxide 200 mg
magnesium hydroxide 200 mg
simethicone 20 mg
Uses: Antacid, adsorbent, antiflatulent

Mylanta Double Strength Liquid:
Per 5 ml:
aluminum hydroxide 400 mg
magnesium hydroxide 400 mg
simethicone 40 mg
Uses: Antacid, adsorbent, antiflatulent

Mylanta Gelcaps:
calcium carbonate 311 mg
magnesium carbonate 232 mg
Uses: Antacid, adsorbent, antiflatulent

Naldecon Tablets:
phenylpropanolamine 40 mg
phenylephrine 10 mg
phenyltoloxamine 15 mg
chlorpheniramine 5 mg
Uses: Antihistamine, decongestant

Naldecon CX Adult Liquid:
Per 5 ml:
guaifenesin 200 mg
phenylpropanolamine 12.5 mg
codeine 10 mg
Uses: Antihistamine

Naldecon DX Adult Liquid:
Per 5 ml:
dextromethorphan 10 mg
guaifenesin 200 mg
phenylpropanolamine 12.5 mg
Uses: Expectorant, decongestant

Naldecon DX Children's Syrup:
Per 5 ml:
dextromethorphan 5 mg
guaifenesin 100 mg

◆ = Nursing alert   ✎ = Herb-drug interaction   🚫 = Do not crush

phenylpropanolamine 6.25 mg
Uses: Antihistamine, decongestant
Naldecon DX Pediatric Drops:
Per ml:
phenylpropanolamine 6.25 mg
dextromethorphan 5 mg
guaifenesin 50 mg
Uses: Antihistamine, decongestant
Naldecon EX Children's Syrup:
Per 5 ml:
guaifenesin 100 mg
phenylpropanolamine 6.25 mg
Uses: Antihistamine, decongestant
Naldecon EX Pediatric Drops:
Per ml:
phenylpropanolamine 6.25 mg
guaifenesin 50 mg
Uses: Antihistamine, decongestant
Naldecon Pediatric Drops:
Per ml:
phenylpropanolamine 5 mg
phenylephrine 1.25 mg
chlorpheniramine 0.5 mg
phenyltoloxamine 2 mg
Uses: Antihistamine, decongestant
Naldecon Pediatric Syrup:
Per 5 ml:
phenylpropanolamine 5 mg
phenylephrine 1.25 mg
chlorpheniramine 0.5 mg
phenyltoloxamine 2 mg
Uses: Antihistamine, decongestant
Naldecon Senior DX Liquid:
Per 5 ml:
dextromethorphan 10 mg
guaifenesin 200 mg
Uses: Expectorant, antitussive
Naldecon Syrup:
Per 5 ml:
chlorpheniramine 2.5 mg
phenylephrine 5 mg
phenylpropanolamine 20 mg
phenyltoloxamine 7.5 mg
Uses: Antihistamine, decongestant
Naphcon-A Ophthalmic Solution:
0.25% naphazoline

0.3% pheniramine
Uses: Ophth vasoconstrictor
Nasatab LA:
guaifenesin 500 mg
pseudoephedrine 120 mg
Uses: Expectorant, decongestant
NeoDecadron Ophthalmic Ointment:
0.35% neomycin
0.05% dexamethasone
Uses: Ophth antiinfective, antiinflammatory
NeoDecadron Ophthalmic Solution:
0.35% neomycin
0.1% dexamethasone
Uses: Ophth antiinfective, antiinflammatory
NeoDecadron Topical:
neomycin 0.5%
dexamethasone 0.1%
Uses: Top antiinfective, antiinflammatory
Neosporin Cream:
Per gram:
polymyxin B 10,000 U
neomycin 3.5 mg
Uses: Top antiinfective
Neosporin G.U. Irrigant:
Per ml:
neomycin 40 mg
polymyxin B 200,000 U
Uses: Antiinfective
Neosporin Ointment:
Per gram:
polymyxin B 5000 U
bacitracin zinc 400 U
neomycin 3.5 mg
Uses: Top antiinfective
Neosporin Ophthalmic Solution:
Per ml:
neomycin 1.75 mg
polymyxin B 10,000 U
gramicidin 0.025 mg
Uses: Ophthalmic antiinfective

Neosporin Ophthalmic Ointment:
Per gram:
neomycin 3.5 mg
polymyxin B 10,000 U
bacitracin zinc 400 U
Uses: Ophthalmic antiinfective

Neosporin Plus Cream:
polymyxin B 10,000 U
neomycin 3.5 mg
lidocaine 40 mg
Uses: Top antiinfective

Niferex-150 Forte:
ferrous sulfate 150 mg
vitamin B_{12} 25 μg
folic acid 1 mg
Uses: Supplement

Norgesic:
orphenadrine 25 mg
aspirin 385 mg
caffeine 30 mg
Uses: Skeletal muscle relaxant, analgesic

Norgesic Forte:
orphenadrine 50 mg
aspirin 770 mg
caffeine 60 mg
Uses: Skeletal muscle relaxant, analgesic

Novacet Lotion:
sodium sulfacetamine 10%
sulfur 5%
Uses: Acne agent

Novafed A:
pseudoephedrine 120 mg
chlorpheniramine 8 mg
Uses: Adrenergic, antihistamine

NuLytely:
PEG 3350/420 g
sodium bicarbonate 5.72 g
sodium chloride 11.2 g
potassium chloride 1.48 g
Uses: Laxative

NyQuil Hot Therapy:
Per packet:
acetaminophen 1000 mg
pseudoephedrine 60 mg

dextromethorphan 30 mg
doxylamine 12.5 mg
Uses: Analgesic, adrenergic, antitussive

NyQuil Nightime Cold/Flu Medicine Liquid:
Per 5 ml:
pseudoephedrine 10 mg
doxylamine 1.25 mg
dextromethorphan 5 mg
acetaminophen 167 mg
25% alcohol
Uses: Adrenergic, antitussive, analgesic

Octicair Otic Suspension:
hydrocortisone 1%
neomycin 5 mg/ml
polymyxin B 10,000 U/ml
Uses: Otic antiinflammatory, antiinfective

Opcon-A Ophthalmic Solution:
0.027% naphazoline
0.315% pheniramine
Uses: Ophth vasoconstrictor

Ornade:
phenylpropanolamine 75 mg
chlorpheniramine 12 mg
Uses: Antihistamine, decongestant

Ornex:
pseudoephedrine 30 mg
acetaminophen 500 mg
Uses: Adrenergic, analgesic

Ornex No Drowsiness Caplets:
acetaminophen 325 mg
pseudoephedrine 30 mg
Uses: Adrenergic, analgesic

Ortho-cept:
ethinyl estradiol 30 μg
desogestrel 0.15 mg
Uses: Oral contraceptive

Ortho-Novum 7/7/7:
Phase I:
0.5 mg norethindrone
35 μg ethinyl estradiol
Phase II:
0.75 mg norethindrone

Poly-Histine DM Syrup:
Per 5 ml:
brompheniramine 2 mg
phenylpropanolamine 12.5 mg
dextromethorphan 10 mg
Uses: Antihistamine, antitussive

Poly-Histine CS Syrup:
Per 5 ml:
phenylpropanolamine 12.5 mg
brompheniramine 2 mg
codeine 10 mg
Uses: Antihistamine, analgesic

Poly-Pred Ophthalmic Suspension:
Per ml:
0.5% prednisolone acetate
0.35% neomycin
polymyxin B 10,000 U
Uses: Ophth antiinflammatory, anti-
    infective

Polysporin Ointment:
Per gram:
polymyxin B 10,000 U
bacitracin zinc 500 U
Uses: Top antiinfective

Polysporin Ophthalmic Ointment:
Per gram:
polymyxin B 10,000 U
bacitracin zinc 500 U
Uses: Ophthalmic antiinfective

Polytrim Ophthalmic:
Per ml:
trimethoprim 1 mg
polymyxin B 10,000 U
Uses: Ophthalmic antiinfective

Premphase:
In a compliance package:
conjugated estrogens 0.625 mg
medroxyprogesterone 5 mg
Uses: Oral contraceptive

Prempro:
In a compliance package:
conjugated estrogens 0.625 mg
medroxyprogesterone 2.5 mg
Uses: Oral contraceptive

Premsyn PMS:
acetaminophen 500 mg

pamabrom 25 mg
pyrilamine 15 mg
Uses: Analgesic

Prevpac:
In a compliance package:
amoxicillin 500 mg caps
clarithromycin 500 mg tabs
lansoprazole 30 mg caps
Uses: Antiinfective

Primatene:
theophylline 130 mg
ephedrine 24 mg
phenobarbital 7.5 mg
Uses: Bronchodilator, barbiturate

Primatene Dual Action:
theophylline 60 mg
ephedrine 12.5 mg
guaifenesin 100 mg
Uses: Bronchodilator, expectorant, ad-
    renergic

Primaxin 250 mg
I.V. for Injection:
imipenem 250 mg
cilastatin sodium 250 mg
Uses: Antiinfective

Primaxin 500 mg
I.V. for Injection:
imipenem 500 mg
cilastatin sodium 500 mg
Uses: Antiinfective

Prinzide 10-12.5:
lisinopril 10 mg
hydrochlorothiazide 12.5 mg
Uses: Antihypertensive

Prinzide 20-12.5:
lisinopril 20 mg
hydrochlorothiazide 12.5 mg
Uses: Antihypertensive

Prinzide 20-25:
lisinopril 20 mg
hydrochlorothiazide 25 mg
Uses: Antihypertensive

Probampacin Oral Suspension:
Per single dose:
ampicillin 3.5 g

---

* = Canada only   Side effects: *italics* = common; ***bold italics*** = life-threatening

probenecid 1 g
Uses: Antiinfective
Proben-C:
colchicine 0.5 mg
probenecid 500 mg
Uses: Antigout agent
Proctofoam-HC Aerosol Foam:
1% hydrocortisone
1% pramoxine
Uses: Topical corticosteroid
Propacet 100:
propoxyphene-N 100 mg
acetaminophen 650 mg
Uses: Analgesic
Pseudo-Chlor:
pseudoephedrine 120 mg
chlorpheniramine 8 mg
Uses: Antihistamine
Pseudo-Gest Plus:
pseudoephedrine 60 mg
chlorpheniramine 4 mg
Uses: Antihistamine
P-V-Tussin:
phenindamine 25 mg
guaifenesin 200 mg
hydrocodone 5 mg
Uses: Antihistamine, analgesic
Quadrinal:
ephedrine 24 mg
theophylline 65 mg
potassium iodide 320 mg
phenobarbital 24 mg
Uses: Adrenergic, bronchodilator, barbiturate
Quelidrine Cough Syrup:
Per 5 ml:
dextromethorphan 10 mg
phenylephrine 5 mg
ephedrine 5 mg
chlorpheniramine 2 mg
ammonium chloride 40 mg
ipecac 0.005 ml
Uses: Expectorant, adrenergic, antihistamine
Quibron-300:
theophylline 300 mg

guaifenesin 180 mg
Uses: Bronchodilator, expectorant
Quibron:
theophylline, 150 mg
guaifenesin 90 mg
Uses: Bronchodilator, expectorant
R&C Shampoo:
0.3% pyrethrins
3% piperonyl butoxide
Uses: Scabicide, pediculicide
Rauzide:
bendroflumethiazide 4 mg
powdered rauwolfia serpentina 50 mg
Uses: Diuretic, antihypertensive
Regroton:
chlorthalidone 50 mg
reserpine 0.25 mg
Uses: Diuretic, antihypertensive
Regulace:
docusate sodium 100 mg
casanthranol 30 mg
Uses: Laxative
Renese-R:
polythiazide 2 mg
reserpine 0.25 mg
Uses: Diuretic, antihypertensive
Respahist:
pseudoephedrine 60 mg
brompheniramine 6 mg
Uses: Adrenergic, antihistamine
Respaire-60:
guaifenesin 200 mg
pseudoephedrine 60 mg
Uses: Expectorant, adrenergic
RID Shampoo:
0.3% pyrethrins
3% piperonyl butoxide
Uses: Scabicide, pediculicide
Rifamate:
isoniazid 150 mg
rifampin 300 mg
Uses: Antitubercular, antileprotic
Rifater:
rifampin 120 mg
isoniazid 50 mg

pyrazinamide 300 mg
Uses: Antitubercular
Riopan Plus Suspension:
Per 5 ml:
magaldrate 540 mg
simethicone 40 mg
Uses: Antacid, adsorbent, antiflatulent
Robaxisal:
methocarbamol 400 mg
aspirin 325 mg
Uses: Skeletal muscle relaxant, analgesic
Robitussin A-C Syrup:
Per 5 ml:
codeine 10 mg
guaifenesin 100 mg
3.5% alcohol
Uses: Analgesic, expectorant
Robitussin-CF Liquid:
Per 5 ml:
guaifenesin 100 mg
dextromethorphan 10 mg
phenylpropanolamine 12.5 mg
4.75% alcohol
Uses: Antitussive, expectorant
Robitussin Cold & Cough Liqui-Gels:
pseudoephedrine 30 mg
guaifenesin 200 mg
dextromethorphan 10 mg
Uses: Antitussive, expectorant
Robitussin-DAC Syrup:
Per 5 ml:
codeine 10 mg
guaifenesin 100 mg
pseudoephedrine 30 mg
1.4% alcohol
Uses: Analgesic, expectorant, adrenergic
Robitussin-DM Liquid:
Per 5 ml:
guaifenesin 100 mg
dextromethorphan 10 mg
Uses: Expectorant, antitussive

Robitussin Maximum Strength Cough and Cold Liquid:
dextromethorphan 15 mg
pseudoephedrine 30 mg
Uses: Antitussive, adrenergic
Robitussin Night Relief Liquid:
dextromethorphan 5 mg
pyrilamine 8.3 mg
pseudoephedrine 10 mg
acetaminophen 108.3 mg
Uses: Antitussive, adrenergic
Robitussin Pediatric Cough & Cold Liquid:
Per 5 ml:
pseudoephedrine 15 mg
dextromethorphan 7.5 mg
Uses: Antitussive, adrenergic
Robitussin-PE Syrup:
guaifenesin 100 mg
pseudoephedrine 30 mg
1.4% alcohol
Uses: Expectorant, adrenergic
Robitussin Severe Congestion Liqui-Gels:
guaifenesin 200 mg
pseudoephedrine 30 mg
Uses: Expectorant, adrenergic
Rolaids Calcium Rich:
magnesium hydroxide 80 mg
calcium carbonate 412 mg
Uses: Antacid, adsorbent, antiflatulent
Rondec:
pseudoephedrine 60 mg
carbinoxamine 4 mg
Uses: Adrenergic
Rondec DM Drops:
Per ml:
pseudoephedrine 25 mg
carbinoxamine 2 mg
dextromethorphan 4 mg
Uses: Adrenergic, antitussive
Rondec DM Syrup:
Per 5 ml:
pseudoephedrine 60 mg
carbinoxamine 4 mg

---

dextromethorphan 15 mg
Uses: Adrenergic, antitussive
Rondec Oral Drops:
Per 5 ml:
pseudoephedrine 25 mg
carbinoxamine 2 mg
Uses: Adrenergic
Roxicet:
Per 5 ml:
acetaminophen 325 mg
oxycodone 5 mg
Uses: Opioid analgesic
Roxicet 5/500:
oxycodone 5 mg
acetaminophen 500 mg
Uses: Opioid analgesic
Ru-Tuss:
phenylephrine 25 mg
phenylpropanolamine 50 mg
chlorpheniramine 8 mg
hyoscyamine 0.19 mg
atropine 0.04 mg
scopolamine 0.01 mg
Uses: Antihistamine, anticholinergic
Ru-Tuss DE:
pseudoephedrine 120 mg
guaifenesin 600 mg
Uses: Adrenergic, expectorant
Ru-Tuss Expectorant Liquid:
Per 5 ml:
guaifenesin 100 mg
pseudoephedrine 30 mg
dextromethorphan 10 mg
10% alcohol
Uses: Adrenergic, expectorant, antitussive
Ru-Tuss w/Hydrocodone Liquid:
Per 5 ml:
hydrocodone 1.7 mg
phenylephrine 5 mg
pyrilamine 3.3 mg
pheniramine 3.3 mg
phenylpropanolamine 3.3 mg
5% alcohol
Uses: Analgesic, adrenergic, decongestant

Ryna-C Liquid:
Per 5 ml:
pseudoephedrine 30 mg
chlorpheniramine 2 mg
codeine 10 mg
Uses: Adrenergic, antihistamine, analgesic
Ryna Liquid:
Per 5 ml:
pseudoephedrine 30 mg
chlorpheniramine 2 mg
Uses: Adrenergic, antihistamine
Rynatan:
phenylephrine 25 mg
chlorpheniramine 8 mg
pyrilamine 25 mg
Uses: Adrenergic, antihistamine
Rynatan Pediatric Suspension:
Per 5 ml:
phenylephrine 5 mg
chlorpheniramine 2 mg
pyrilamine 12.5 mg
Uses: Adrenergic, antihistamine
Rynatuss:
ephedrine 10 mg
carbetapentane 60 mg
chlorpheniramine 5 mg
phenylephrine 10 mg
Uses: Adrenergic, antihistamine
Salutensin:
hydroflumethiazide 50 mg
reserpine 0.125 mg
Uses: Antihypertensive
Salutensin Demi:
hydroflumethiazide 25 mg
reserpine 0.125 mg
Uses: Antihypertensive
Scot-Tussin DM Liquid:
Per 5 ml:
chlorpheniramine 2 mg
dextromethorphan 15 mg
Uses: Antihistamine, antitussive
Scot-Tussin Original 5-Action Liquid:
phenylephrine 4.2 mg

 = Nursing alert   = Herb-drug interaction   = Do not crush

pheniramine 13.3 mg
sodium citrate 83.3 mg
sodium salicylate 83.3 mg
caffeine citrate 25 mg
Uses: Adrenergic, analgesic
Scot-Tussin Senior Clear Liquid:
Per 5 ml:
guaifenesin 200 mg
dextromethorphan 15 mg
Uses: Antitussive, expectorant
Sedapap-10:
acetaminophen 650 mg
butalbital 50 mg
Uses: Analgesic, barbiturate
Semprex-D:
acrivastine 8 mg
pseudoephedrine 60 mg
Uses: Adrenergic, bronchodilator
Senokot-S:
docusate 50 mg
senna concentrate 187 mg
Uses: Laxative
Septra:
sulfamethoxazole 400 mg
trimethroprim 80 mg
Uses: Antiinfective
Septra DS:
sulfamethoxazole 800 mg
trimethroprim 160 mg
Uses: Antiinfective
Septra I.V. for Injection:
Per 5 ml:
trimethoprim 80 mg
sulfamethoxazole 400 mg
Uses: Antiinfective
Septra Suspension:
Per 5 ml:
trimethoprim 40 mg
sulfamethoxazole 200 mg
Uses: Antiinfective
Ser-Ap-Es:
hydrochlorothiazide 15 mg
reserpine 0.1 mg
hydralazine 25 mg
Uses: Diuretic, antihypertensive

Silafed Syrup:
Per 5 ml:
pseudoephedrine 30 mg
triprolidine 1.25 mg
Uses: Adrenergic, antihistamine
Silaminic Cold Syrup:
Per 5 ml:
phenylpropanolamine 12.5 mg
chlorpheniramine 2 mg
Uses: Antihistamine
Silaminic Expectorant Liquid:
Per 5 ml:
phenylpropanolamine 12.5 mg
guaifenesin 100 mg
Uses: Expectorant
Sinarest Extra Strength:
pseudoephedrine 30 mg
chlorpheniramine 2 mg
acetaminophen 500 mg
Uses: Adrenergic, antihistamine, analgesic
Sinarest No Drowsiness:
pseudoephedrine 30 mg
acetaminophen 500 mg
Uses: Adrenergic, analgesic
Sinarest Sinus:
pseudoephedrine 30 mg
chlorpheniramine 2 mg
acetaminophen 325 mg
Uses: Adrenergic, antihistamine, analgesic
Sine-Aid ID:
pseudoephedrine 30 mg
ibuprofen 200 mg
Uses: Adrenergic, analgesic
Sine-Aid Maximum Strength:
pseudoephedrine 30 mg
acetaminophen 500 mg
Uses: Adrenergic, analgesic
Sinemet 10/100:
carbidopa 10 mg
levodopa 100 mg
Uses: Antiparkinsonian
Sinemet 25/100:
carbidopa 25 mg

levodopa 100 mg
Uses: Antiparkinsonian
Sinemet 25/250:
carbidopa 25 mg
levodopa 250 mg
Uses: Antiparkinsonian
Sinemet CR 25-100:
carbidopa 25 mg
levodopa 100 mg
Uses: Antiparkinsonian
Sinemet CR 50-200:
carbidopa 50 mg
levodopa 200 mg
Uses: Antiparkinsonian
Sine-Off Maximum Strength No Drowsiness Formula Caplets:
pseudoephedrine 30 mg
acetaminophen 500 mg
Uses: Adrenergic, analgesic
Sine-Off Sinus Medicine:
pseudoephedrine 30 mg
chlorpheniramine 2 mg
acetaminophen 500 mg
Uses: Adrenergic, antihistamine, analgesic
Sinutab Maximum Strength Sinus Allergy:
acetaminophen 500 mg
pseudoephedrine 30 mg
chlorpheniramine 2 mg
Uses: Analgesic, adrenergic, antihistamine
Sinutab Maximum Strength Without Drowsiness:
acetaminophen 500 mg
pseudoephedrine 30 mg
Uses: Analgesic, adrenergic
Sinutab Non-Drying:
pseudoepedrine 30 mg
guaifenesin 200 mg
Uses: Adrenergic, expectorant
Slo-Phyllin GG Syrup:
theophylline 150 mg
guaifenesin 90 mg
Uses: Bronchodilator, expectorant

Synophylate-GG Syrup:
theophylline 150 mg
guaifenesin 100 mg
alcohol 15%
Uses: Bronchodilator, expectorant
Soma Compound:
carisoprodol 200 mg
aspirin 325 mg
Uses: Skeletal muscle relaxant, analgesic
Spec-T Lozenge:
dextromethorphan 10 mg
benzocaine 10 mg
Uses: Antitussive, topical anesthetic
St. Joseph Cold Tablets for Children:
phenylpropanolamine 3.125 mg
acetaminophen 80 mg
Uses: Decongestant, analgesic
Sudafed Cold & Cough Liquicaps:
pseudoephedrine 30 mg
dextromethorphan 10 mg
guaifenesin 100 mg
acetaminophen 250 mg
Uses: Adrenergic, antitussive, expectorant, analgesic
Sudafed Plus:
pseudoephedrine 60 mg
chlorpheniramine 4 mg
Uses: Adrenergic, antihistamine
Sudafed Severe Cold:
pseudoephedrine 30 mg
dextromethorphan 15 mg
Uses: Adrenergic, antitussive
Sudafed Sinus Maximum Strength:
pseudoephedrine 30 mg
acetaminophen 500 mg
Uses: Adrenergic, analgesic
Sudal 60/500:
pseudoephedrine 60 mg
guaifenesin 500 mg
Uses: Adrenergic, expectorant
Sudal 120/600:
pseudoephedrine 120 mg
guaifenesin 600 mg
Uses: Adrenergic, expectorant

Sultrin Triple Sulfa Vaginal Cream:
3.42% sulfathiazole
2.86% sulfacetamine
3.7% sulfabenzamide
Uses: Antiinfective

Sultrin Triple Sulfa Vaginal Tablets:
sulfathiazole 172.5 mg
sulfacetamide 143.75
sulfabenzamide 184 mg
Uses: Antiinfective

Synalgos-DC:
aspirin 356.4 mg
caffeine 30 mg
dihydrocodeine 16 mg
Uses: Analgesic

Talacen:
acetaminophen 650 mg
pentazocine 25 mg
Uses: Analgesic

Talwin Compound:
aspirin 325 mg
pentazocine 12.5 mg
Uses: Analgesic

Talwin NX:
pentazocine 50 mg
naloxone 0.5 mg
Uses: Analgesic, opioid antagonist

Tarka 182:
trandolapril 2 mg (immed rel)
verapamil 180 mg (sus rel)
Uses: Antihypertensive, calcium channel blocker

Tarka 241:
trandolapril 1 mg (immed rel)
verapamil 240 mg (sus rel)
Uses: Antihypertensive, calcium channel blocker

Tarka 242:
trandolapril 2 mg (immed rel)
verapamil 240 mg (sus rel)
Uses: Antihypertensive, calcium channel blocker

Tarka 244:
trandolapril 4 mg (immed rel)
verapamil 240 mg (sus rel)
Uses: Antihypertensive, calcium channel blocker

Tavist-D:
clemastine 1.34 mg
phenylpropanolamine 75 mg
Uses: Antihistamine, decongestant

Tavist Sinus:
acetaminophen 500 mg
pseudoephedrine 30 mg
Uses: Analgesic, adrenergic

Teczem:
enalapril 5 mg (extended release)
diltiazem 180 mg (extended release)
Uses: Antihypertensive, calcium channel blocker

Tedrigen:
ephedrine 22.5 mg
theophylline 120 mg
phenobarbital 7.5 mg
Uses: Adrenergic, bronchodilator, barbiturate

Tegrin-LT Shampoo:
0.33% pyrethrins
3.15% piperonyl butoxide
Uses: Scabicide, pediculicide

Tenoretic 50:
atenolol 50 mg
chlorthalidone 25 mg
Uses: Antihypertensive

Tenoretic 100:
atenolol 100 mg
chlorthalidone 25 mg
Uses: Antihypertensive

Terra-Cortril Ophthalmic Suspension:
1.5% hydrocortisone acetate
0.5% oxytetracycline
Uses: Ophth antiinflammatory, antiinfective

Terramycin with Polymycin B Sulfate Ophthalmic Ointment:
Per gram:
polymyxin B 10,000 units
oxytetracycline 5 mg
Uses: Ophth antiinfective

---

* = Canada only   Side effects: *italics* = common; **bold italics** = life-threatening

T-Gesic:
hydrocodone 5 mg
acetaminophen 500 mg
Uses: Analgesic

Theodrine:
ephedrine 22.5 mg
theophylline 120 mg
Uses: Adrenergic, bronchodilator

Theolate Liquid:
theophylline 150 mg
guaifenesin 90 mg
Uses: Bronchodilator, expectorant

Theophylline Kl Elixir:
theophylline 80 mg
potassium iodide 130 mg
Uses: Bronchodilator, expectorant

Thera-Flu, Flu & Cold Medicine Powder:
Per packet:
pseudoephedrine 60 mg
chlorpheniramine 4 mg
acetaminophen 650 mg
Uses: Adrenergic, antihistamine, analgesic

Thera-Flu, Flu, Cold & Cough Powder:
Per packet:
pseudoephedrine 60 mg
chlorpheniramine 4 mg
dextromethorphan 20 mg
acetaminophen 650 mg
Uses: Adrenergic, antihistamine, antitussive, analgesic

Thera-Flu NightTime Powder:
Per packet:
pseudoephedrine 60 mg
chlorpheniramine 4 mg
dextromethorphan 30 mg
acetaminophen 1000 mg
Uses: Adrenergic, antihistamine, antitussive, analgesic

Thera-Flu Non-Drowsy Flu, Cold & Cough Maximum Strength Powder
Per packet:
pseudoephedrine 60 mg
dextromethorphan 30 mg
acetaminophen 1000 mg
Uses: Adrenergic, antitussive, analgesic

Thera-Flu Non-Drowsy Formula Maximum Strength Caplets:
pseudoephedrine 30 mg
dextromethorphan 15 mg
acetaminophen 500 mg
Uses: Adrenergic, antitussive, analgesic

Timentin for Injection:
Per 3.1-g vial:
ticarcillin 3 g
clavulanic acid 0.1 g
Uses: Antiinfective

Timolide 10/25:
timolol 10 mg
hydrochlorothiazide 25 mg
Uses: Antihypertensive

Titralac Plus:
calcium carbonate 420 mg
simethicone 21 mg
Uses: Antacid, adsorbent, antiflatulent

Tobra Dex Ophthalmic Suspension/ Ointment:
tobramycin 0.3%
dexamethasone 0.1%
Uses: Ophth antiinfective, antiinflammatory

Triacin-C Cough Syrup:
Per 5 ml:
codeine 10 mg
pseudoephedrine 30 mg
triprolidine 1.25 mg
Uses: Analgesic, adrenergic, antihistamine

Tri-Hydroserpine:
hydralazine 25 mg
hydrochlorothiazide 15 mg
reserpine 0.1 mg
Uses: Antihypertensive

Tri-Levlen:
Phase I:
levonorgestrel 0.05 mg

◆ = Nursing alert   🍃 = Herb-drug interaction   🚫 = Do not crush

ethinyl estradiol 30 μg
Phase II:
levonorgestrel 0.075 mg
ethinyl estradiol 40 μg;
Phase III:
levonorgestrel 0.125 mg
ethinyl estradiol 30 μg
Uses: Oral contraceptive
Triaminic Allergy:
phenylpropanolamine 25 mg
chlorpheniramine 4 mg
Uses: Antihistamine
Triaminic AM Cough & Decongestant Formula Liquid:
Per 5 ml:
pseudoephedrine 15 mg
dextromethorphan 7.5 mg
Uses: Adrenergic, antitussive
Triaminic Cold:
phenylpropanolamine 12.5 mg
chlorpheniramine 2 mg
Uses: Decongestant, antihistamine
Triaminic-DM Syrup:
Per 5 ml:
dextromethorphan 5 mg
phenylpropanolamine 6.25 mg
Uses: Antitussive, decongestant
Triaminic Expectorant Liquid:
Per 5 ml:
guaifenesin 50 mg
phenylpropanolamine 6.25 mg
Uses: Expectorant, decongestant
Triaminic Expectorant DH Liquid:
Per 5 ml:
guaifenesin 100 mg
hydrocodone 1.67 mg
phenylpropanolamine 12.5 mg
pheniramine 6.25 mg
pyrilamine 6.25 mg
5% alcohol
Uses: Analgesic, expectorant, decongestant
Triaminic Expectorant w/Codeine Liquid:
Per 5 ml:
phenylpropanolamine 12.5 mg

codeine 10 mg
guaifenesin 100 mg
Uses: Expectorant, decongestant, analgesic
Triaminic Nite Light Liquid:
Per 5 ml:
pseudoephedrine 15 mg
chlorpheniramine 1 mg
dextromethorphan 7.5 mg
Uses: Adrenergic, antihistamine, antitussive
Triaminic Oral Infant Drops:
Per ml:
phenylpropanolamine 20 mg
pyrilamine 10 mg
pheniramine 10 mg
Uses: Decongestant, antihistamine
Triaminic Sore Throat Formula Liquid:
Per 5 ml:
pseudoephedrine 15 mg
dextromethorphan 7.5 mg
acetaminophen 160 mg
Uses: Adrenergic, antitussive
Triaminic Syrup:
Per 5 ml:
phenylpropanolamine 6.25 mg
chlorpheniramine 1 mg
Uses: Decongestant, antihistamine
Triaminicin Cold, Allergy, Sinus:
phenylpropanolamine 25 mg
chlorpheniramine 4 mg
acetaminophen 650 mg
Uses: Decongestant, antihistamine analgesic
Triaminicol Multi-Symptom Cough, Cold:
phenylpropanolamine 12.5 mg
chlorpheniramine 2 mg
dextromethorphan 10 mg
Uses: Decongestant, antihistamine, antitussive
Triaminicol Multi-Symptom Relief Liquid:
Per 5 ml:
phenylpropanolamine 12.5 mg

chlorpheniramine 2 mg
dextromethorphan 10 mg
Uses: Decongestant, antihistamine, antitussive

Triavil 2-10:
perphenazine 2 mg
amitriptyline 10 mg
Uses: Antidepressant, antipsychotic

Triavil 4-10:
perphenazine 4 mg
amitriptyline 10 mg
Uses: Antidepressant, antipsychotic

Triavil 2-25:
perphenazine 2 mg
amitriptyline 25 mg
Uses: Antidepressant, antipsychotic

Triminol Cough Syrup:
Per 5 ml:
dextromethorphan 10 mg
chlorpheniramine 2 mg
phenylpropanolamine 12.5 mg
Uses: Antitussive, antihistamine, decongestant

Trinalin Repetabs:
azatadine maleate 1 mg
pseudoephedrine 120 mg
Uses: Antihistamine

Triphasil:
Phase I:
levonorgestrel 0.05 mg
ethinyl estradiol 30 μg
Phase II:
levonorgestrel 0.075 mg
ethinyl estradiol 40 μg
Phase III:
levonorgestrel 0.125 mg
ethinyl estradiol 30 μg
Uses: Oral contraceptive

Triple Antibiotic Ophthalmic Ointment:
Per gram:
polymyxin B 10,000 U
neomycin 3.5 mg
bacitracin 400 U
Uses: Antiinfective

Tuinal 100 mg:
amobarbital 50 mg
secobarbital 50 mg
Uses: Sedative-hypnotic

Tuinal 200 mg:
amobarbital 100 mg
secobarbital 100 mg
Uses: Sedative-hypnotic

Tusibron-DM Syrup:
Per 5 ml:
guaifenesin 100 mg
dextromethorphan 15 mg
Uses: Expectorant, antitussive

Tussionex Pennkinetic Suspension:
Per 5 ml:
chlorpheniramine 8 mg
hydrocodone 10 mg
Uses: Antihistamine, analgesic

Tussi-Organidin NR Liquid:
Per 5 ml:
codeine 10 mg
guaifenesin 100 mg
Uses: Analgesic, expectorant

Tussi-Organidin DM NR Liquid:
Per 5 ml:
guaifenesin 100 mg
dextromethorphan 10 mg
Uses: Expectorant, antitussive

Tylenol Allergy Sinus, Maximum Strength Gelcaps:
acetaminophen 500 mg
chlorpheniramine 2 mg
pseudoephedrine 30 mg
Uses: Antihistamine, adrenergic, analgesic

Tylenol Children's Cold:
acetaminophen 80 mg
chlorpheniramine 0.5 mg
pseudoephedrine 7.5 mg
Uses: Antihistamine, adrenergic, analgesic

Tylenol Children's Cold Liquid:
Per 5 ml:
acetaminophen 160 mg
chlorpheniramine 1 mg
pseudoephedrine 15 mg

◆ = Nursing alert   ∥ = Herb-drug interaction   ⊘ = Do not crush

Uses: Antihistamine, adrenergic, analgesic

Tylenol Children's Cold Multi-Symptom Plus Cough Liquid:
Per 5 ml:
acetaminophen 160 mg
dextromethorphan 5 mg
chlorpheniramine 1 mg
pseudoephedrine 15 mg
Uses: Antihistamine, adrenergic, analgesic

Tylenol Children's Cold Plus Cough Chewable:
acetaminophen 80 mg
pseudoephedrine 7.5 mg
dextromethorphan 2.5 mg
chlorpheniramine 0.5 mg
Uses: Antihistamine, adrenergic, analgesic

Tylenol Cold Multi-Symptom:
acetaminophen 325 mg
chlorpheniramine 2 mg
pseudoephedrine 30 mg
dextromethorphan 15 mg
Uses: Antihistamine, adrenergic, analgesic

Tylenol Cold No Drowsiness:
acetaminophen 325 mg
pseudoephedrine 30 mg
dextromethorphan 15 mg
Uses: Analgesic, adrenergic, antitussive

Tylenol Flu Maximum Strength Gelcaps:
dextromethorphan 15 mg
pseudoephedrine 30 mg
acetaminophen 500 mg
Uses: Analgesic, adrenergic, antitussive

Tylenol Flu NightTime Maximum Strength Gelcaps:
pseudoephedrine 30 mg
chlorpheniramine 2 mg
acetaminophen 500 mg
Uses: Adrenergic, antihistamine, analgesic

Tylenol Flu NightTime Maximum Strength Powder:
pseudoephedrine 60 mg
diphenhydramine 50 mg
acetaminophen 1000 mg
Uses: Adrenergic, antihistamine, analgesic

Tylenol Headache Plus, Extra Strength:
acetaminophen 500 mg
calcium carbonate 250 mg
Uses: Analgesic, antacid

Tylenol Multi-Symptom Cough Liquid:
Per 5 ml:
dextromethorphan 10 mg
acetaminophen 216.7 mg
5% alcohol
Uses: Antitussive, analgesic

Tylenol Multi-Symptom Cough w/Decongestant Liquid:
Per 5 ml:
dextromethorphan 10 mg
acetaminophen 200 mg
pseudoephedrine 20 mg
Uses: Antitussive, analgesic, adrenergic

Tylenol Multi-Symptom Hot Medication:
Per packet:
acetaminophen 650 mg
chlorpheniramine 4 mg
pseudoephedrine 60 mg
dextromethorphan 30 mg
Uses: Analgesic, antihistamine, adrenergic, antitussive

Tylenol PM, Extra Strength:
acetaminophen 500 mg
diphenhydramine 25 mg
Uses: Analgesic, antihistamine

Tylenol Severe Allergy:
diphenhydramine 12.5 mg
acetaminophen 500 mg
Uses: Analgesic, antihistamine

Tylenol Sinus Maximum Strength:
pseudoephedrine 30 mg

acetaminophen 500 mg
Uses: Adrenergic, analgesic
Tylenol with Codeine Elixir:
Per 5 ml:
acetaminophen 120 mg
codeine 12 mg
Uses: Analgesic
Tylenol with Codeine No. 2:
acetaminophen 300 mg
codeine 15 mg
Uses: Analgesic
Tylenol with Codeine No. 3:
acetaminophen 300 mg
codeine 30 mg
Uses: Analgesic
Tylenol with Codeine No. 4:
acetaminophen 300 mg
codeine 60 mg
Uses: Analgesic
Tylox:
oxycodone 5 mg
acetaminophen 500 mg
Uses: Analgesic
Tyrodone Liquid:
Per 5 ml:
hydrocodone 5 mg
pseudoephedrine 60 mg
5% alcohol
Uses: Analgesic, adrenergic
Unasyn for Injection 1.5 g:
ampicillin 1 g
sulbactam 0.5 g
Uses: Antiinfective
Unasyn for Injection 3 g:
ampicillin 2 g
sulbactam 1 g
Uses: Antiinfective
Uniretic:
moexipril 7.5 mg
hydrochlorothiazide 12.5 mg
or moexipril 15 mg
hydrochlorothiazide 25 mg
Uses: Antihypertensive, diuretic
Unituss HC Syrup:
hydrocodone 2.5 mg

phenylephrine 5 mg
chlorpheniramine 2 mg
Uses: Analgesic, adrenergic, antihistamine
Urised:
methenamine 40.8 mg
phenylsalicylate 18.1 mg
atropine 0.03 mg
hyoscyamine 0.03 mg
benzoic acid 4.5 mg
methylene blue 5.4 mg
Uses: Antiinfective
Ursinus Inlay:
pseudoephedrine 30 mg
aspirin 325 mg
Uses: Adrenergic, analgesic
Vanquish:
aspirin 227 mg
acetaminophen 194 mg
caffeine 33 mg
Uses: Nonnarcotic analgesic
Vaseretic 10-25:
enalapril 10 mg
hydrochlorothiazide 25 mg
Uses: Antihypertensive, diuretic
Vasocidin Ophthalmic Ointment:
sulfacetamide 10%
prednisolone 0.5%
Uses: Ophthalmic antiinfective, antiinflammatory
Vasocidin Ophthalmic Solution:
sulfacetamide 10%
prednisolone 0.25%
Uses: Ophthalmic antiinfective, antiinflammatory
Vasocon-A Ophthalmic Solution:
naphazoline 0.05%
antazoline 0.5%
Uses: Ophthalmic vasoconstrictor
**Vicks 44D Cough & Head Conges-
tion Liquid:**
Per 5 ml:
dextromethorphan 10 mg
pseudoephedrine 20 mg
Uses: Antitussive, adrenergic

⬧ = Nursing alert   ✦ = Herb-drug interaction   ⊘ = Do not crush

Vicks 44E Liquid:
Per 5 ml:
dextromethorphan 6.7 mg
guaifenesin 66.7 mg
Uses: Antitussive, expectorant
Vicks 44M Cold, Flu, & Cough LiquiCaps:
dextromethorphan 10 mg
pseudoephedrine 30 mg
chlorpheniramine 2 mg
acetaminophen 250 mg
Uses: Antitussive, adrenergic, antihistamine, analgesic
Vicks 44 Non-Drowsy Cold & Cough LiquiCaps:
dextromethorphan 30 mg
pseudoephedrine 60 mg
Uses: Antitussive, adrenergic
Vicks Children's NyQuil Nighttime Cough/Cold Liquid:
Per 5 ml:
pseudoephedrine 10 mg
chlorpheniramine 0.67 mg
dextromethorphan 5 mg
Uses: Adrenergic, antihistamine, antitussive
Vicks Cough Silencers:
dextromethorphan 2.5 mg
benzocaine 1 mg
Uses: Antitussive, top anesthetic
Vicks DayQuil Allergy Relief 4 Hour:
phenylpropanolamine 25 mg
brompheniramine 4 mg
Uses: Decongestant, antihistamine
Vicks DayQuil Allergy Relief 12 Hour ER:
phenylpropanolamine 75 mg
brompheniramine 12 mg
Uses: Decongestant, antihistamine
Vicks DayQuil Liquid:
Per 5 ml:
dextromethorphan 3.3 mg
pseudoephedrine 10 mg
acetaminophen 108.3 mg
guaifenesin 33.3 mg

Uses: Antitussive, adrenergic, analgesic, expectorant
Vicks DayQuil Sinus Pressure & Pain Relief:
pseudoephedrine 30 mg
acetaminophen 500 mg
Uses: Adrenergic, analgesic
Vicks NyQuil Liquicaps:
pseudoephedrine 30 mg
doxylamine 6.25 mg
dextromethorphan 10 mg
acetaminophen 250 mg
Uses: Adrenergic, antihistamine, antitussive, analgesic
Vicks NyQuil Multi-Symptom Cold Flu Relief Liquid:
pseudoephedrine 10 mg
doxylamine 2.1 mg
dextromethorphan 5 mg
acetaminophen 167 mg
Uses: Adrenergic, antihistamine, antitussive, analgesic
Vicks Pediatric Formula 44e Liquid:
Per 5 ml:
dextromethorphan 3.3 mg
guaifenesin 33.3 mg
Uses: Expectorant, antitussive
Vicks Pediatric Formula 44 m Multi-Symptom Cough & Cold Liquid
pseudoephedrine 10 mg
chlorpheniramine 0.67 mg
dextromethorphan 5 mg
Uses: Adrenergic, antihistamine, antitussive
Vicodin:
acetaminophen 500 mg
hydrocodone 5 mg
Uses: Analgesic
Vicodin ES:
acetaminophen 750 mg
hydrocodone 7.5 mg
Uses: Analgesic
Vicodin HP:
hydrocodone 10 mg

---

acetaminophen 660 mg
Uses: Analgesic
VicodinTuss:
Per 5 ml:
hydrocodone 5 mg
guaifenesin 100 mg
Uses: Analgesic, expectorant
Vicoprofen:
hydrocodone 7.5 mg
ibuprofen 200 mg
Uses: Analgesic
Wigraine Suppositories:
ergotamine 2 mg
caffeine 100 mg
Uses: α-adrenergic blocker
Zestoretic 10/12.5:
lisinopril 10 mg
hydrochlorothiazide 12.5 mg
Uses: Antihypertensive
Zestoretic 20/12.5:
lisinopril 20 mg
hydrochlorothiazide 12.5 mg

Uses: Antihypertensive
Zestoretic 20/25:
lisinopril 20 mg
hydrochlorothiazide 25 mg
Uses: Antihypertensive
Ziac 2.5:
bisoprolol 2.5 mg
hydrochlorothiazide 6.25 mg
Uses: Antihypertensive
Ziac 5:
bisoprolol 5 mg
hydrochlorothiazide 6.25 mg
Uses: Antihypertensive
Ziac 10:
bisoprolol 10 mg
hydrochlorothiazide 6.25 mg
Uses: Antihypertensive
Zydone:
hydrocodone 5 mg
acetaminophen 500 mg
Uses: Analgesic

Appendix e

Rarely used drugs

aminocaproic acid (℞)

(a-mee-noe-ka-proe'ik)
Amicar, aminocaproic acid, EACA
Functional class.: Hemostatic

Dosage and routes: *Adult:* **PO/IV**
5 g loading dose, then 1-1.25 g q1h
if needed, not to exceed 30 g/day
Uses: Hemorrhage from hyperfibri-
nolysis, adjunctive therapy in hemophilia
Contraindications: Hypersensitivity, abnormal bleeding, postpartum
bleeding, DIC, upper urinary tract
bleeding, new burns

ammonium chloride
(ℙℴ-ℴ⊤ℭ, ⅳ-℞)

(ah-mohn'ee-um klor'ide)
ammonium chloride
Functional class.: Acidifier

Dosage and routes:
Alkalosis: Adult and child: **IV INF**
0.9-1.3 ml/min of a 2.14% sol, not
to exceed 5 ml/min
Acidifier: Adult: **PO** 4-12 g/day in
divided doses; *Child:* **PO** 75 mg/
kg/day in divided doses
Expectorant: Adult: **PO** 250-500 mg
q2-4h as needed
Uses: Alkalosis (metabolic), systemic and urinary acidifier, expectorant, diuretic
Contraindications: Hypersensitivity, severe hepatic disease, severe
renal disease

amyl nitrite (℞)

(am'il nye'trite)
amyl nitrite, Amyl Nitrite Aspirols,
Amyl Nitrite Vaporole
Functional class.: Coronary vasodilator

Dosage and routes:
Angina: Adult: **INH** 0.18-0.3 ml as
needed, 1-6 inhalations from 1 cap,
may repeat in 3-5 min
Cyanide poisoning: Adult: **INH** 0.3
ml ampule inhaled 15 sec until preparation of sodium nitrite infusion is
ready
Uses: Acute angina pectoris, cyanide poisoning
Investigational uses: Cardiac mur-
mur diagnosis
Contraindications: Hypersensitivity to nitrites, severe anemia, increased intracranial pressure, hypertension, pregnancy (X)

benzonatate (℞)

(ben-zoe'na-tate)
Tessalon Perles
Functional class.: Antitussive, non-
narcotic

Dosage and routes: *Adult and child:*
PO 100 mg tid, not to exceed 600
mg/day; *Child <10 yr:* **PO** 8 mg/kg
in 3-6 divided doses
Uses: Nonproductive cough
Contraindications: Hypersensitivity

benzoyl peroxide (OTC)
(ben'zoe-ill per-ox'ide)

Functional class.: Antiacne medication

Dosage and routes: *Adult and child:* **TOP** apply to affected area qd or bid
Uses: Mild to moderate acne
Contraindications: Hypersensitivity to benzoic acid derivatives

benzquinamide (℞)
(benz-kwin'a-mide)
Emete-Con

Functional class.: Antiemetic

Dosage and routes: *Adult:* **IM** 50 mg or 0.5-1 mg/kg, may be repeated in 1 hr, then q3-4h prn; **IV** 25 mg or 0.2-0.4 mg/kg as a one-time dose
Uses: To inhibit nausea, vomiting associated with anesthetic, surgery
Contraindications: Hypersensitivity, hypertension

beractant (℞)
(ber-ak'tant)
Survanta

Functional class.: Natural lung surfactant

Dosage and routes: INTRATRA-CHEAL INSTILL: 4 doses can be administered in the 1st 48 hrs of life; give doses no more frequently than q6h; each dose is 100 mg of phospholipids/kg birth weight (4 ml/kg)
Uses: Prevention and treatment (rescue) of respiratory distress syndrome in premature infants

chlorpropamide (℞)
(klor-proe'pa-mide)
Chloronase*, Chlorpropamide, Diabinese, Novopropamide*

Functional class.: Antidiabetic

Dosage and routes: *Adult:* **PO** 100-250 mg qd, initially, then 100-500 mg maintenance according to response; not to exceed 750 mg/day
Uses: Stable adult-onset diabetes mellitus (type II) NIDDM
Contraindications: Hypersensitivity to sulfonylureas, juvenile or brittle diabetes, pregnancy (D), lactation, renal failure

colfosceril (℞)
(kole-foss'er-ill)
Exosurf Neonatal

Functional class.: Synthetic lung surfactant

Dosage and routes:
Prophylactic treatment
• *Endotracheally:* 5 ml/kg as soon as possible after birth and repeat doses 12 and 24 hr later to infants remaining on mechanical ventilation
Rescue treatment
• *Endotracheally:* Administer in two 2.5 ml/kg doses; give initial dose after treatment of RDS, then second dose in 12 hr
Uses: Treatment of respiratory distress syndrome (RDS) in premature infants

cosyntropin (℞)
(koe-sin-troe'pin)
Cortrosyn, Synacthen*, Tetracosactrin

Functional class.: Pituitary hormone

Dosage and routes: *Adult and child >2 yr:* **IM/IV** 0.25-1 mg between blood sampling; *Child <2 yr:* **IM/IV** 0.125 mg

Uses: Testing adrenocortical function

Contraindications: Hypersensitivity

crotamiton (℞)

(kroe tam'i ton)

Functional class.: Scabicide

Dosage and routes:
Scabies: Adult and child: **CREAM** wash area with soap, water; remove visible crusts, apply cream, apply another coat in 24 hr, remove with soap, water in 48 hr
Pruritus: Massage into affected area, repeat as necessary

Uses: Scabies, pruritus

Contraindications: Hypersensitivity, skin inflammation, abrasions, breaks in skin, mucous membranes

delavirdine (℞)

(de-la-veer'din)

Rescriptor

Functional class.: Non-nucleoside reverse transcriptase inhibitor (NNRTI)

Dosage and routes: *Adult and child ≥16 yr:* 400 mg tid in combination with zidovudine or didanosine

Uses: HIV-1 in combination with zidovudine or didanosine

Contraindications: Hypersensitivity to this drug or atevirdine

desipramine (℞)

(dess-ip'ra-meen)

desipramine HCl, Norpramin, Pertofrane

Functional class.: Antidepressant tricyclic

Dosage and routes: *Adult:* **PO** 75-150 mg/day in divided doses; may increase to 300 mg/day or may give daily dose hs; *Adolescent and elderly:* **PO** 25-50 mg/day, may increase to 100 mg/day

Uses: Depression

Contraindications: Hypersensitivity to tricyclic antidepressants, recovery phase of myocardial infarction, narrow-angle glaucoma, convulsive disorders, prostatic hypertrophy, child <12 yr

dimercaprol (℞)

(dye-mer-cap'role)

BAL in Oil, British Anti-Lewisite*, dimercaptopropanol

Functional class.: Heavy metal antagonist

Dosage and routes:
Severe gold/arsenic poisoning
• *Adult:* **IM** 3 mg/kg q4h × 2 days then qid × 1 day, then bid × 10 days
Mild gold/arsenic poisoning
• *Adult:* **IM** 2.5 mg/kg qid × 2 days, then bid × 1 day, then qd × 10 days
Acute lead poisoning
• *Adult:* **IM** 4 mg/kg, then q4h with edetate calcium disodium 12.5 mg/kg **IM,** not to exceed 5 mg/kg/dose
Mercury poisoning
• *Adult:* **IM** 5 mg/kg, then 2.5 mg/kg/day or bid × 10 days

Uses: Arsenic, gold, mercury, lead poisoning

Contraindications: Hypersensitivity, anuria, hepatic insufficiency, poisoning of other metals, severe renal disease, child <3 yr, pregnancy (D)

Contraindications: Hypersensitivity, anuria, poisoning of other metals, severe renal disease, child <3 yr

disulfiram (R̸)

(dye-sul'fi-ram)
Antabuse, disulfiram
Functional class.: Alcohol deterrent

Dosage and routes: *Adult:* **PO** 250-500 mg qd × 1-2 wk, then 125-500 mg qd until fully socially recovered
Uses: Chronic alcoholism (as adjunct)
Contraindications: Hypersensitivity, alcohol intoxication, psychoses, CV disease, pregnancy (X), lactation

edetate calcium disodium (R̸)

(ee'de-tate)
calcium disodium versenate, calcium EDTA, edathamil calcium disodium, sodium calcium edetate
Functional class.: Heavy metal antagonist (antidote)

Dosage and routes:
Acute lead encephalopathy
• *Adult and child:* 1.5 g/m²/day × 3-5 days, with dimercaprol; may be given again after 4 days off drug
Lead poisoning
• *Adult:* **IV** 1 g/250-500 ml D₅W or 0.9% NaCl over 1-2 hr or q12h × 3-5 days; may repeat after 2 days; not to exceed 50 mg/kg/day; may be given as **CONT INF** over 8-24 hr
• *Adult:* **IM** 35 mg/kg bid
• *Child:* **IM** 35 mg/kg/day in divided doses q8-12h, not to exceed 50 mg/kg/day; may give for 3-5 days, off 4 days before next course
Uses: Lead poisoning, acute lead encephalopathy

estramustine (R̸)

(ess-tra-muss'teen)
Emcyt
Functional class.: Antineoplastic

Dosage and routes: *Adult:* **PO** 10-16 mg/kg in 3-4 divided doses/day; treatment may continue for ≥3 mo or 600 mg/m²/day in 3 divided doses
Uses: Metastatic prostate cancer
Contraindications: Hypersensitivity to estradiol, thromboembolic disorders, pregnancy (D)

floxuridine (R̸)

(flox-yoor'i-deen)
Floxuridine, FUDR
Functional class.: Antineoplastic, antimetabolite

Dosage and routes: *Adult:* **INTRAARTERIAL** by continuous inf 0.1-0.6 mg/kg/day × 1-6 wk; **HEPATIC ARTERY INJ** 0.4-0.6 mg/kg/day × 1-6 wk
Uses: GI adenocarcinoma metastatic to liver; cancer of breast, head, neck, liver, brain, gallbladder, bile duct
Contraindications: Hypersensitivity, myelosuppression, pregnancy (D), poor nutritional status, serious infections

fludarabine (R̸)

(floo-dar'a-been)
Fludara
Functional class.: Antineoplastic, antimetabolite

Dosage and routes: *Adult:* **IV** 25 mg/m² over 30 min qd × 5 days,

---

◆ = Nursing alert   ✒ = Herb-drug interaction   ⃠ = Do not crush

may repeat q28d; reconstitute with 2 ml of sterile water for inj; dissolution should occur in <15 sec
Uses: Chronic lymphocytic leukemia, non-Hodgkin's lymphoma
Contraindications: Hypersensitivity, pregnancy (D), lactation

---

glycerin, anhydrous (R)
(gli'ser-in, an-hye'drus)

Functional class.: Ophthalmic

Dosage and routes: *Adult:* **INSTILL** 1-2 gtt after local anesthetic
Uses: Reduce corneal edema
Contraindications: Hypersensitivity

---

halcinonide (R)
(hal-sin'oh-nide)

Functional class.: Corticosteroid, synthetic

Dosage and routes: *Adult:* **TOP** apply to affected area bid-tid
Uses: Inflammation of corticosteroid-responsive dermatoses
Contraindications: Hypersensitivity, viral infections, fungal infections

---

hydroquinone (R)
(hye-droh'quin-ohn)

Functional class.: Depigmenting agent

Dosage and routes: *Adult and child:* **TOP** apply to affected area qd-bid
Uses: Bleaching skin, including age spots, freckles, lentigo, chloasma
Contraindications: Hypersensitivity, inflamed skin, prickly heat, sunburn

hydroxyprogesterone (R)
(hye-drox-ee-pro-jess'te-rone)

Functional class.: Progestin, hormone

Dosage and routes:
Menstrual disorders: Adult: **IM** 125-375 mg q4wk; discontinue after 4 cycles
Uterine cancer: Adult: **IM** 1-5 g/wk
Uses: Uterine carcinoma, menstrual disorders (abnormal uterine bleeding, amenorrhea)
Contraindications: Breast cancer, hypersensitivity, thromboembolic disorders, genital bleeding (abnormal, undiagnosed), pregnancy (X)

---

indecainide (R)
(in-de-kane'ide)

Functional class.: Antidysrhythmic (Class IC)

Dosage and routes: *Adult:* **PO** 100-200 mg/day in divided dose q12h; 50 mg q12h initially, then increase dose by 25 mg increments q4d, max 400 mg/day
Uses: Life-threatening dysrhythmias, sustained ventricular tachycardia
Contraindications: 2nd- or 3rd-degree AV block, right bundle branch block, cardiogenic shock, hypersensitivity

---

iodoquinol (R)
(eye-oh-doh-kwin'ole)

Functional class.: Amebicide

Dosage and routes: *Adult:* **PO** 630-650 mg tid × 20 days, not to exceed 2 g/day; *Child:* **PO** 30-40 mg/kg/day in 2-3 divided doses × 20 days, not to exceed 1.95 g/24 hr × 20 days;

do not repeat treatment before 2-3 wk

Uses: Intestinal amebiasis

Contraindications: Hypersensitivity to this drug or iodine, renal disease, hepatic disease, severe thyroid disease, preexisting optic neuropathy

---

isotretinoin (℞)

(eye-soe-tret'i-noyn)

Functional class.: Antiacne agent

Dosage and routes: *Adult:* **PO** 0.5-2 mg/kg/day in 2 divided doses × 15-20 wk; if relapse occurs, repeat after 2 mo off drug

Uses: Severe recalcitrant cystic acne

Contraindications: Hypersensitivity, inflamed skin, pregnancy (X)

---

isoxsuprine (℞)

(eye-sox'syoo-preen)

Functional class.: Peripheral vasodilator

Dosage and routes: *Adult:* **PO** 10-20 mg tid or qid

Uses: Symptoms of cerebrovascular insufficiency, peripheral vascular disease including arteriosclerosis obliterans, thromboangitis obliterans, Raynaud's disease

Contraindications: Hypersensitivity, postpartum, arterial bleeding

---

ketamine (℞)

(keet'a-meen)
Ketalar

Functional class.: General anesthetic

Dosage and routes: *Adult and child:* **IV** 1-4.5 mg/kg over 1 min; **IM** 6.5-13 mg/kg; *Maintenance:* ½ to full induction dose may be repeated

Uses: Short anesthesia for diagnostic/surgical procedures

Contraindications: Hypersensitivity, CVA, increased intracranial pressure, severe hypertension, cardiac decompensation, child <2 yr

---

lincomycin (℞)

(lin-koe-mye'sin)

Functional class.: Antibacterial

Dosage and routes: *Adult:* **PO** 500 mg q6-8h, not to exceed 8 g/d; **IM** 600 mg/d or q12h; **IV** 600 mg-1 g q8-12h; dilute in 100 ml **IV sol;** infuse over 1 hr, not to exceed 8 g/day; *Child > 1 mo:* **PO** 30-60 mg/ kg/d in divided doses q6-8h; **IM** 10 mg/kg/d q12h; **IV** 10-20 mg/kg/d in divided doses q8-12h; dilute to 100 ml **IV sol;** infuse over 1 hr

Uses: Infections caused by group A β-hemolytic streptococci, pneumococci, staphylococci (respiratory tract, skin, soft tissue, urinary tract infections, osteomyelitis, septicemia)

Contraindications: Hypersensitivity, ulcerative colitis/enteritis, infants <1 mo

---

masoprocol (℞)

(mas-o-proe'cole)

Functional class.: Miscellaneous topical product

Dosage and routes: *Adult:* **TOP** apply to lesion bid × 2-4 wk

Uses: Actinic keratoses

Contraindications: Hypersensitivity, children

---

mazindol (R)
(may'zin-dole)
Functional class.: Anorexiant

Dosage and routes: *Adult:* **PO** 1 mg ac, or 2 mg 1 hr ac lunch
Uses: Exogenous obesity
Contraindications: Hypersensitivity to sympathomimetic amine, glaucoma, drug abuse, cardiovascular disease, children <12 yr, hypertension, severe arteriosclerosis, agitated states, hyperthyroidism

mefenamic acid (R)
(me-fe-nam'ik)
Functional class.: Nonsteroidal antiinflammatory

Dosage and routes: *Adult and child >14 yr:* **PO** 500 mg, then 250 mg q6h, use not to exceed 1 wk
Uses: Mild to moderate pain, dysmenorrhea, inflammatory disease
Contraindications: Hypersensitivity, asthma, severe renal disease, severe hepatic disease, ulcer disease

mefloquine (R)
(meh'floh-quin)
Functional class.: Antimalarial

Dosage and routes: *Adult:* **PO** 1250 mg as a single dose (treatment); 250 mg qwk × 4 wk, then 250 mg q2wk (prevention)
Uses: Treatment and prevention of *P. falciparum* malaria, *P. vivax*
Contraindications: Hypersensitivity

mepenzolate (R)
(me-pen'zoe-late)
Functional class.: GI anticholinergic

Dosage and routes: *Adult:* **PO** 25-50 mg qid with meals, hs; titrate to patient response
Uses: Treatment of peptic ulcer disease, irritable bowel syndrome in combination with other drugs; for other GI disorders
Contraindications: Hypersensitivity to anticholinergics, narrow-angle glaucoma, GI obstruction, myasthenia gravis, paralytic ileus, GI atony, toxic megacolon

methoxsalen (R)
(meth-ox'a-len)
Functional class.: Pigmenting agent

Dosage and routes:
Vitiligo: Adult and child >12 yr: **PO** 20 mg qd 2-4 hr before exposure to therapeutic ultraviolet rays; administer on alternate days; **TOP** apply 1-2 hr before exposure to UVA light; treatment intervals regulated by erythema response
Psoriasis: Adult: **PO** dosage individualized to weight; taken 2 hr before exposure to therapeutic ultraviolet rays
Uses: Vitiligo, psoriasis
Contraindications: Hypersensitivity, melanoma, LE, albinism, sunburn, cataracts, squamous cell cancer, child ≤12 yr, diseases associated with photosensitivity

methscopolamine (R)
(meth-skoe-pol'a-meen)
Functional class.: GI anticholinergic

Dosage and routes: *Adult:* **PO** 2.5-5 mg 1/2 hr ac, hs
Uses: Peptic ulcer disease
Contraindications: Hypersensitivity to anticholinergics, narrow-angle glaucoma, GI obstruction, myasthenia gravis, paralytic ileus, GI atony, toxic megacolon

methsuximide (R)
(meth-sux'i-mide)
Functional class.: Anticonvulsant

Dosage and routes: *Adult and child:* **PO** 300 mg/day; may increase by 300 mg/wk, not to exceed 1.2 g/day in divided doses
Uses: Refractory absence seizures (petit mal)
Contraindications: Hypersensitivity to succinimide derivatives

mitotane (R)
(mye'toe-tane)
Lysodren, p'-DDD
Functional class.: Antineoplastic

Dosage and routes: *Adult:* **PO** 9-10 g/day in divided doses tid or qid; may have to decrease dose for severe reaction
Uses: Adrenocortical carcinoma
Contraindications: Hypersensitivity

molindone (R)
(moe-lin'done)
Functional class.: Antipsychotic/neuroleptic

Dosage and routes: *Adult:* **PO** 50-75 mg/day increasing to 225 mg/day if needed
Uses: Psychotic disorders
Contraindications: Hypersensitivity, coma, child

papaverine (R)
(pa-pav'er-een)
Functional class.: Peripheral vasodilator

Dosage and routes: *Adult:* **PO** 100-300 mg 3-5×/day; **SUS REL** 150-300 mg q8-12h; **IM/IV** 30-120 mg q3h prn
Uses: Arterial spasm resulting in cerebral and peripheral ischemia; myocardial ischemia associated with vascular spasm or dysrhythmias; angina pectoris; peripheral pulmonary embolism; visceral spasm as in ureteral, biliary, GI colic, peripheral vascular disease
Contraindications: Hypersensitivity, complete AV heart block

paraldehyde (R)
(par-al'de-hyde)
Functional class.: Anticonvulsant

Dosage and routes:
Seizures: Adult: **IM** 5-10 ml; divide 10 ml into 2 inj; **IV** 0.2-0.4 ml/kg in **NS** inj; *Child:* **IM** 0.15 ml/kg; **RECT** 0.3 ml/kg q4-6h or 1 ml/yr of age, not to exceed 5 ml; may repeat in 1 hr prn; **IV** 5 ml/90 ml **NS** inj; begin infusion at 5 ml/hr; titrate to patient response

---

 = Nursing alert   = Herb-drug interaction   ◌ = Do not crush

Alcohol withdrawal: Adult: **PO/ RECT** 5-10 ml, not to exceed 60 ml; **IM** 5 ml q4-6h × 24 hr, then q6h on following days, not to exceed 30 ml

Sedation: Adult: **PO/REC** 4-10 ml; **IM** 5 ml; **IV** 3-5 ml in emergency only; *Child:* **PO/REC/IM** 0.15 ml/kg

Tetanus: Adult: **IV** 4-5 ml or 12 ml by gastric tube q4h diluted with water; **IM** 5-10 ml prn

Uses: Refractory seizures, status epilepticus, sedation, insomnia, alcohol withdrawal, tetanus, eclampsia

Contraindications: Hypersensitivity, gastroenteritis with ulceration

---

paramethadione (℞)

(par-a-meth-a-dye′one)

Functional class.: Anticonvulsant

Dosage and routes: *Adult:* **PO** 300 mg tid; may increase by 300 mg/ wk, not to exceed 600 mg qid; *Child >6 yr:* **PO** 0.9 g/day in divided doses tid or qid; *Child 2-6 yr:* **PO** 0.6 g/day in divided doses tid or qid; *Child <2 yr:* **PO** 0.3 g/day in divided doses tid or qid

Uses: Refractory absence (petit mal) seizures

Contraindications: Hypersensitivity, blood dyscrasias, pregnancy (D), lactation

---

paromomycin (℞)

(par-oh-moe-mye′sin)

Functional class.: Amebicide

Dosage and routes:
Intestinal amebiasis: Adult and child: **PO** 25-35 mg/kg/day in 3 divided doses × 5-10 day pc
Hepatic coma: Adult: 4 g qd in divided doses × 5-6 day

Uses: Intestinal amebiasis, adjunct in hepatic coma

Contraindications: Hypersensitivity, renal disease, GI obstruction

---

permethrin (OTC, ℞)

(per-meth′ren)

Functional class.: Pediculicide

Dosage and routes:
Lice (head): Adult and child: Wash hair, towel dry; apply liberally to hair, leave on 10 min, rinse with water
Scabies: Adult and child: **TOP** 5% cream applied and massaged into all skin surfaces; leave cream on 8-14 hr, then wash

Uses: Lice, nits, ticks, flea nits

Contraindications: Hypersensitivity

---

phenacemide (℞)

(fe-nass′e-mide)

Functional class.: Anticonvulsant

Dosage and routes: *Adult:* **PO** 500 mg tid, may increase by 500 mg/ wk, not to exceed 5 g/day; *Child 5-10 yr:* **PO** 250 mg tid, may increase by 250 mg/wk, not to exceed 1.5 g/day prn

Uses: Refractory, generalized tonic-clonic (grand mal), complex-partial (psychomotor), absence (petit mal), atypical seizures

Contraindications: Hypersensitivity, psychiatric condition, pregnancy (D), lactation

---

phendimetrazine (℞)

(fen-dye-me′tra-zeen)

Functional class.: Anorexiant

Dosage and routes: *Adult:* **PO** 35 mg bid-tid 1 hr ac, not to exceed 70

mg tid; **SUS REL** 105 mg qd ac AM
Uses: Exogenous obesity
Contraindications: Hypersensitivity, hyperthyroidism, hypertension, glaucoma, severe arteriosclerosis, severe cardiovascular disease, children <12 yr, agitated states, drug abuse

phenoxybenzamine (℞)
(fen-ox-ee-ben′za-meen)
Functional class.: Antihypertensive

Dosage and routes: *Adult:* **PO** 10 mg qd, increase by 10 mg qod, usual range: 20-40 mg bid-tid; *Child:* **PO** 0.2 mg/kg or 6 mg/m^2/day, max 10 mg; may increase q4d; maintenance dose 0.4-1.2 mg/kg/day or 12-36 mg/m^2/day divided doses tid or qid
Uses: Pheochromocytoma
Contraindications: Hypersensitivity, CHF, angina, cerebral vascular insufficiency, coronary arteriosclerosis

phentermine (℞)
(fen′ter-meen)
Functional class.: Cerebral stimulant

Dosage and routes: *Adult:* **PO** 8 mg tid 30 min before meals or 15-37.5 mg qd before breakfast
Uses: Exogenous obesity
Contraindications: Hypersensitivity, hyperthyroidism, hypertension, glaucoma, severe arteriosclerosis, angina pectoris, cardiovascular disease, pregnancy (C), child <12 yr

physostigmine (℞)
(fi-zoe-stig′meen)
Antilirium
Functional class.: Antidote, reversible anticholinesterase

Dosage and routes:
Overdose of anticholinergics:
Adult: **IM/IV** 2 mg; give no more than 1 mg/min; may repeat; *Child:* **IM/IV** inj 0.02 mg/kg, not more than 0.5 mg/min; may repeat at 5-10 min intervals until max dose of 2 mg
Postanesthesia: Adult: **IM/IV** 0.5-1 mg; give no more than 1 mg/min **(IV)**; can repeat at 10 to 30 min intervals
Uses: To reverse CNS effects of diazepam; anticholinergic, tricyclic antidepressant, Alzheimer's disease, hereditary ataxia
Contraindications: Hypotension, obstruction of intestine or renal system, asthma, gangrene, CV disease, choline esters, depolarizing neuromuscular blocking agents, diabetes

pinacidil (℞)
(pye-na′si-dill)
Functional class.: Antihypertensive

Dosage and routes: *Adult:* **PO** 12.5-25 mg bid
Uses: Severe hypertension not responsive to other therapy
Contraindications: Acute MI, dissecting aortic aneurysm, hypersensitivity, pheochromocytoma

◆ = Nursing alert   ⫯ = Herb-drug interaction   ⊘ = Do not crush

pralidoxime (R̶)

(pra-li-dox'eem)
Protopam Chloride
Functional class.: Cholinesterase re-activator

Dosage and routes:
Anticholinesterase overdose: Adult:
IV 1-2 g, then 250 mg q5min until desired response
Organophosphate poisoning: Adult:
IV INF 1-2 g/100 ml 0.9% NaCl over 15-30 min; may repeat in 1 hr;
PO 1-3 g q5h; *Child:* **IV INF** 20-40 mg/kg/dose diluted in 100 ml 0.9% NaCl over 15-30 min
Uses: Cholinergic crisis in myasthenia gravis, organophosphate poisoning antidote (early), relief of paralysis of respiratory muscles; used as an adjunct to systemic atropine administration
Contraindications: Hypersensitivity, carbamate insecticide poisoning

streptozocin (R̶)

(strep-toe-zoe'sin)
Zanosar
Functional class.: Antineoplastic alkylating agent

Dosage and routes: *Adult:* **IV** 500 mg/m² × 5 days q6wk until desired response; or 1 g/m² qwk × 2 wk, not to exceed 1.5 g/m² in 1 dose
Uses: Metastatic islet cell carcinoma of pancreas
Investigational uses: Prevention of spread of Hodgkin's disease, metastatic carcinoid tumor, pancreatic adenocarcinoma, colon malignancies
Contraindications: Hypersensitivity

teniposide (R̶)

(ten-i-poe'side)
Vumon, VM 26
Functional class.: Antineoplastic

Dosage and routes: *Child:* **IV INF** combo teniposide 165 mg/m² and cytarabine 300 mg/m² 2×/wk × 8-9 doses or combo teniposide 250 mg/m² and vincristine 1.5 mg/m² qwk × 4-8 wk and prednisone 40 mg/m² **PO** × 28 days
Uses: Childhood acute lymphoblastic leukemia (ALL), refractory childhood acute lymphocytic leukemia
Contraindications: Hypersensitivity, bone marrow depression, severe hepatic disease, severe renal disease, bacterial infection, pregnancy (D)

tolazamide (R̶)

(tole-az'a-mide)
Tolamide, tolazimide, Tolinase
Functional class.: Antidiabetic

Dosage and routes: *Adult:* **PO** 100 mg/day for FBS <200 mg/dl or 250 mg/day for FBS >200 mg/dl; dose should be titrated to response (1 g or less/day)
Uses: Type II (NIDDM) diabetes mellitus
Contraindications: Hypersensitivity to sulfonylureas, juvenile or brittle diabetes

tolbutamide (R̶)

(tole-byoo'ta-mide)
Mobenol*, Novobutamide*, Orinase, tolbutamide, Tolbutone*
Functional class.: Antidiabetic

Dosage and routes: *Adult:* **PO** 1-2 g/day in divided doses, titrated to patient response; **IV** 1 g (Fajans test)

Uses: Type II (NIDDM) diabetes mellitus

Contraindications: Hypersensitivity to sulfonylureas, juvenile or brittle diabetes

---

vasopressin (℞)

(vay-soe-press'in)
Pitressin Synthetic
Functional class.: Pituitary hormone

Dosage and routes:
Diabetes insipidus: Adult: **IM/SC** 5-10 units bid-qid as needed; **IM/SC** 2.5-5 units q2-3 days (Pitressin Tannate) for chronic therapy; *Child:* **IM/SC** 2.5-10 units bid-qid as needed; **IM/SC** 1.25-2.5 units q2-3 days (Pitressin Tannate) for chronic therapy

Abdominal distention: Adult: **IM** 5 units, then q3-4h, increasing to 10 units if needed (aqueous)

Uses: Diabetes insipidus (nonnephrogenic/nonpsychogenic), abdominal distention postoperatively, bleeding esophageal varices

Contraindications: Hypersensitivity, chronic nephritis

Appendix f

Local anesthetics

etidocaine (℞)
(eh-tie'doh-kane)
Duranest HCl
Func. class.: Local anesthetic
Chem. class.: Amide

Action: Competes with calcium for sites in nerve membrane that control sodium transport across cell membrane; decreases rise of depolarization phase of action potential

Uses: Peripheral nerve block, caudal anesthesia, central neural block, vaginal block

Dosage and routes:
• Varies with route of anesthesia
Available forms: Inj 1%, 1.5%

Side effects/adverse reactions:
CNS: Anxiety, restlessness, *convulsions, loss of consciousness,* drowsiness, disorientation, tremors, shivering

CV: Myocardial depression, cardiac arrest, dysrhythmias, bradycardia, hypotension, hypertension, *fetal bradycardia*

GI: Nausea, vomiting

EENT: Blurred vision, tinnitus, pupil constriction

INTEG: Rash, urticaria, allergic reactions, edema, burning, skin discoloration at injection site, tissue necrosis

RESP: Status asthmaticus, respiratory arrest, anaphylaxis

Contraindications: Hypersensitivity, child <12 yr, elderly, severe liver disease

Precautions: Severe drug allergies, pregnancy (B)

Pharmacokinetics: Onset 2-8 min, duration 3-6 hr; metabolized by liver, excreted in urine (metabolites)

Interactions:
• Dysrhythmias: epinephrine, halothane, enflurane
• Hypertension: MAOIs, tricyclic antidepressants, phenothiazines
• Decreased action of etidocaine: chloroprocaine

NURSING CONSIDERATIONS
Assess:
• B/P, pulse, respiration during treatment
• Fetal heart tones during labor
• Allergic reactions: rash, urticaria, itching
• Cardiac status: ECG for dysrhythmias, pulse, B/P during anesthesia

Administer:
• Only with crash cart, resuscitative equipment nearby
• Only drugs without preservatives for epidural or caudal anesthesia

Perform/provide:
• Use of new sol; discard unused portions

Evaluate:
• Therapeutic response: anesthesia necessary for procedure

Treatment of overdose: Airway, O_2, vasopressor, IV fluids, anticonvulsants for seizures

lidocaine (local) (℞)

(lye'doe-kane)

Dalcaine, Dilocaine, Duo-Trach Kit, L-Caine, lidocaine HCl, Lidoject-1, Lidoject-2, Nervocaine 1%, Nervocaine 2%, Octocaine HCl, Xylocaine HCl

Func. class.: Local anesthetic
Chem. class.: Amide

Action: Competes with calcium for sites in nerve membrane that control sodium transport across cell membrane; decreases rise of depolarization phase of action potential

Uses: Peripheral nerve block; caudal anesthesia; epidural, spinal, surgical anesthesia

Dosage and routes:
• Varies by route of anesthesia
Available forms: Inj 0.5%, 1%, 1.5%, 2%, 4%, 5%; inj with epinephrine 0.5%, 1%, 1.5%, 2%

Side effects/adverse reactions:
CNS: Anxiety, restlessness, *convulsions, loss of consciousness,* drowsiness, disorientation, tremors, shivering
CV: Myocardial depression, cardiac arrest, dysrhythmias, bradycardia, hypotension, hypertension, fetal bradycardia
GI: Nausea, vomiting
EENT: Blurred vision, tinnitus, pupil constriction
INTEG: Rash, urticaria, allergic reactions, edema, burning, skin discoloration at injection site, tissue necrosis
RESP: Status asthmaticus, respiratory arrest, anaphylaxis

Contraindications: Hypersensitivity, child <12 yr, elderly, severe liver disease

Precautions: Elderly, severe drug allergies, pregnancy (C)

Pharmacokinetics: Onset 4-17 min, duration 3-6 hr; metabolized by liver, excreted in urine (metabolites)

Interactions:
• Dysrhythmias: epinephrine, halothane, enflurane
• Hypertension: MAOIs, tricyclic antidepressants, phenothiazines
• Decreased action of lidocaine: chloroprocaine

NURSING CONSIDERATIONS

Assess:
• B/P, pulse, respiration during treatment
• Fetal heart tones if drug is used during labor
• For allergic reactions: rash, urticaria, itching
• Cardiac status: ECG for dysrhythmias, pulse, B/P during anesthesia

Administer:
• Only with crash cart, resuscitative equipment nearby
• Only drugs without preservatives for epidural or caudal anesthesia

Perform/provide:
• Use of new sol; discard unused portions

Evaluate:
• Therapeutic response: anesthesia necessary for procedure

Treatment of overdose: Airway, O_2, vasopressor, IV fluids, anticonvulsants for seizures

= Nursing alert   = Herb-drug interaction   = Do not crush

Appendix g

Look-alike/sound-alike drug names

Acetohexamide	Acetazolamide	Chlorpromazine	Chlorpropamide
Achromycin	Aureomycin	Chlorpromazine	Prochlorperazine
Adenosine	Adenosine	Clinoril	Clozaril
(Adenocard)	Phosphate	Clinoril	Oruvail
Adriamycin	Aredia	Clomipramine	Clomiphene
Adriamycin	Idamycin	Clomipramine	Norpramin
Albuterol	Atenolol		(Desipramine)
Allopurinol	Apresoline	Clonidine	Klonopin
Alprazolam	Lorazepam		(Clonazepam)
Altace	Alteplase	Cordarone	Inocor
Ambien	Amen	Corgard	Cognex
Amikin	Amicar	Coumadin	Compazine
Amiodarone	Amrinone	Cozaar	Zocor
Amitriptyline	Nortriptyline	Cyclobenzaprine	Cyproheptadine
Amoxapine	Amoxicillin	Cyclophosphamide	Cyclosporine
Amoxapine	Amoxil	Cyclosporine	Cycloserine
Amoxicillin	Amoxil	Cytovene	Cytosar
Artane	Altace	Cytoxan	Cytosar
Asacol	Ansaid		(Cytarabine)
Asacol	Os-Cal	Cytoxan	Cytotec
Atrovent	Alupent	Dantrium	Danazol
Bactocil	Pathocil	Daunorubicin	Doxorubicin
Bentyl	Aventyl	Decadron	Percodan
Betalin	Benylin	Depo Medrol	Solu-Medrol
Brethine	Banthine	Diabeta	Zebeta
Brevital	Brevibloc	Dialose Plus	Dialose Plus
Bumex	Buprenex	(Docusate	(Docusate
Cafergot	Carafate	Potassium/	Sodium/
Calcitriol	Calciferol	Casanthranol)	Phenolphthalein)
Carboplatin	Cisplatin	Diazepam	Ditropan
Cardene	Cardizem	Diflucan	Diprivan
Cardene SR	Cardizem SR	Dilaudid	Demerol
Cardizem CD	Cardizem SR	Diphenatol	Diphenidol
Cardura	Coumadin	Diphenhydramine	Dicyclomine
Cataflam	Catapres	Diupres	Daypro
Cefaclor	Cephalexin	Dobutrex	Diamox
Cefotan	Ceftin	Dopamine	Dobutamine
Cefprozil	Cafazolin	Doxorubicin	Idarubicin
Cefprozil	Cefuroxime	Edecrin	Eulexin
Ceftazidime	Ceftizoxime	Elavil	Mellaril
Cefuroxime	Cefotaxime	Eldepryl	Enalapril
Cefuroxime	Deferoxamine	Enalapril	Ramipril
Cefzil	Ceftin	Estratest	Estratab
Cefzil	Kefzol	Etidronate	Etretinate
Cephapirin	Cephradine	Etomidate	Etidronate

Eurax	Urex	Novolin 70/30	Novolin 70/30
Fioricet	Fiorinal	Penfill Prefilled	
Flumadine	Fludarabine	Nuprin	Lupron
Fluorouracil	Flucytosine	Ocufen	Ocuflox
FUDR	Fludara		(Ofloxacin)
Gamulin Rh	MICRhoGAM	Ocufen	Ocupress
Garamycin	Kanamycin	Oruvail	Elavil
Glucotrol	Glyburide	Paroxetine	Paclitaxel
Halotestin	Haloperidol	Paxil	Paclitaxel
Hycodan	Vicodin	Paxil	Taxol
Hydrocodone	Hydrocortisone	Pediaprofen	Prelone
Hydromorphone	Meperidine	Pentobarbital	Phenobarbital
Hydromorphone	Morphine	Phenergan	Theragran
Imferon	Roferon-A	Phenobarbital	Pentobarbital
Imipenem	Omnipen	Pindolol	Parlodel
Imipramine	Desipramine	Plendil	Pindolol
Imuran	Imferon	Plendil	Prinivil
Inderal LA	IMDUR	Pravachol	Prevacid
Klonopin	Clonidine	Prednisone	Methylprednisolone
Lamictal	Lomotil	Prednisone	Prednisolone
Lanoxin Lasix	Lomotil	Premarin	Primaxin
Leucovorin Leukine	Leukeran	Prepidil	Bepridil
Levsin	Levoxine	Prilosec	Prednisone
Librium	Librax	Prilosec	Prozac
Lithobid	Lithotabs	Prinivil	Prilosec
Lodine	Codeine	Prinivil	Proventil
Lortab	Lorabid	Prokine	Proleukin
Lotensin	Lioresal	Proloid	Prolixin
Lotensin	Loniten	Provera	Premarin
Lotrimin	Otrivin	Prozac Proscar	Prosom
Lupron	Lopurin	Psorion	Psorcon
Luvox	Lasix	Quinidine	Quinine
Mazicon	Mivacron	Ranitidine	Amantadine
Mepron	Mepron	Regian	Megace
(Atovaquone	(Meprobamate	Regroton	Hygroton
in U.S.)	in Australia)	Reserpine	Risperdal
Methyldopa	L-Dopa		(Risperidone)
	(Levodopa)	Ridaura	Cardura
Methylphenidate	Methadone	Rifampin	Rifabutin
Methylprednisolone	Medroxypro-	Rimantadine	Amantadine
	gesterone	Roxanol	Roxicet
Metolazone	Methotrexate	Sinequan	Serentil
Metolazone	Metoclopramide	Soma	Soma Compound
Metoprolol	Misoprostol	Stadol	Haldol
Monopril	Minoxidil	Sulfasalazine	Sulfisoxazole
Mylanta Gas	Mylicon	Symmetrel	Synthroid
Narcan	Norcuron	Taxol	Paxil
Nasalide	Nasalcrom	Tedral	Teldrin
Nicobid	Nitro-Bid	Tegretol	Toradol
Norflex	Noroxin	Temaril	Demerol
	(Norfloxacin)	Thiamine	Tenormin
Norpramin	Nortriptyline	Thyrar	Thyrolar
Norvasc	Navane	Timoptic	Viroptic
		Tobrex	Tobradex

Toradol	Inderal	Versed	Vepesid
Toradol	Torecan	Vincristine	Vinblastine
Toradol	Tramadol	Viroptic	Timoptic
Torsemide	Furosemide	Wymox	Tylox
Trifluoperazine	Trihexyphenidyl	Xanax	Lanoxin
Trimox	Diamox	Xanax	Tylox
Trimox	Tylox	Xanax	Zantac
Tronothane	Tronolane	Zantac	Xanax
Uridon	Vicodin	Zinacef	Zithromax
Urispas	Urised	Zocor	Zoloft
Vantin	Ventolin	Zofran	Zantac
Versed	Vistaril	Zosyn	Zofran

Appendix h

Herbal products

agrimony

Uses: Mild diarrhea, gastroenteritis, intestinal mucous secretion, inflammation of the mouth and throat, cuts and scrapes, amenorrhea

alfalfa

Uses: Poor appetite, hay fever and asthma, high cholesterol, nutrient source

aloe

Uses of aloe vera gel:
• *External:* Minor burns, skin irritations, minor wounds, frostbite, radiation-caused injuries
• *Internal:* To heal intestinal inflammation and ulcers, as a digestive aid to stimulate bile secretion

angelica

Uses: Heartburn, indigestion, gas, colic, poor blood flow to the extremities, bronchitis, poor appetite, psoriasis, vitiligo, as an antiseptic

arnica

Uses: Topical application for muscle and joint inflammation and swelling; in homeopathic preparations as a remedy for shock, injury, pain

astragalus

Uses: Immune stimulant, viral infections, HIV/AIDS, cancer, vascular disorders, improve circulation, lower blood pressure, possible efficacy in myasthenia gravis

bilberry

Uses: Diabetic retinopathy, macular degeneration, glaucoma, cataract, capillary fragility, varicose veins, hemorrhoids, mild diarrhea

black cohosh

Uses:
• *Menopause:* Hot flashes, nervous conditions associated with menopause
• *Dysmenorrhea:* Menstrual cramps, pain, inflammation

Adapted from: Debusk, Ruth, and Treadwell, Phillip. *Serious Drug/Herb Interactions.* Skidmore-Roth Publishing, Inc. 1999.

blessed thistle

Uses: Loss of appetite, indigestion, intestinal gas

blue cohosh

Uses: Menopausal symptoms, uterine and ovarian pain, improve flow of menstrual blood, antiinflammatory, antirheumatic, popular remedy in black ethnic medicine

borage

Uses: Antiinflammatory for premenstrual syndrome, rheumatoid arthritis, Raynaud's disease, other inflammatory conditions, atopic dermatitis, infant cradle cap, cystic fibrosis, high blood pressure, diabetes

calendula

Uses:
• *External:* Minor skin ailments
• *Internal:* Inflammation throughout the gastrointestinal tract, toxic liver and gallbladder, menstrual bleeding and pain, yeast infections

capsicum (cayenne)

Uses: Muscle spasms, pain of inflammation, neuromas, psoriasis, dry mouth, as an antioxidant food, as a food seasoning

cascara

Uses: Chronic constipation, hepatitis, gallstones

cat's claw

Uses: Cancer, herpes, HIV/AIDS, rheumatoid arthritis, gastritis, gout, wounds, gastric ulcers

chamomile

Uses:
• *External:* As an antiseptic and soothing agent for inflamed skin and minor wounds
• *Internal:* As an antispasmodic, gas-relieving, and antiinflammatory agent for the treatment of digestive problems; light sleep aid and sedative for adults and children; possible anticancer agent

chaparral

Uses: Not recommended— potentially toxic to the liver and kidneys

chicory

Uses: Coffee substitute, source of fructo-oligosaccharides, mild laxative for children, gout, rheumatism, loss of appetite, digestive distress

comfrey

Uses: Bruises, sprains, broken bones, acne, boils

cranberry

Uses: Urinary tract infections (UTIs); susceptibility to kidney stones

dong quai

Uses: To restore vitality to tired women; for a variety of gynecologic, menstrual, and menopausal symptoms; cirrhosis of the liver

echinacea

Uses: Low immune status, hard-to-heal superficial wounds, sun protection

elder (elderberry)

Uses: Susceptibility to colds, flu, yeast infections; nasal and chest congestion; earache associated with chronic congestion; hay fever

eleuthero (siberian ginseng)

Uses: Loss of concentration and mental alertness, fatigue, low productivity, stress, improve athletic performance, general tonic, immune stimulant, hyperglycemia

ephedra (ma huang)

Uses: Seasonal and chronic asthma, nasal congestion, cough

evening primrose

Uses: Premenstrual syndrome, arthritis and inflammatory disorders in general, dry skin, eczema, asthma, diabetes, migraines, chronic fatigue syndrome, heart disease and stroke, circulatory disorders, Raynaud's disease, NSAID use, multiple sclerosis

fenugreek

Uses: Loss of appetite, inflamed areas of the skin, water retention, cancer, constipation, diarrhea, high cholesterol, high blood sugar, calcium oxalate stones

feverfew

Uses: Migraines, cluster headaches, fever, psoriasis, inflammation

flaxseed

Uses: Constipation, as a source of omega-3 fatty acids

fo-ti

Uses: Tiredness, constipation, elevated cholesterol

garcinia cambogia

Uses: Appetite control, weight loss, high cholesterol

garlic

Uses: Vascular disease, elevated LDL, elevated triglycerides, low HDL, high blood pressure, poor circulation, risk of cancer, inflammatory disorders, childhood ear infection, yeast infection

ginger

Uses: Nausea, motion sickness, indigestion, inflammation

ginkgo

Uses: Poor circulation; age related decline in cognition, memory; diabetes; vascular disease; cancer; inflammatory disorders; impotence; degenerative nerve conditions

ginseng

Uses: Physical and mental exhaustion, stress, viral infections, diabetes, sluggishness, fatigue, weak immunity, convalescence

goldenseal

Uses: High blood pressure, poor appetite, infections, menstrual problems, minor sciatic pain, muscle spasms, eye washes

gotu kola

Uses: Chronic wounds, psoriasis

grape seed

Uses: Antioxidant, chronic disease prevention, inflammation

green tea

Uses: Cancer prevention, heart disease prevention, hypercholesterolemia, diarrhea

guggul

Uses: High LDL cholesterol, elevated triglycerides, weight loss

gymnema sylvestre

Uses: High blood sugar levels

hawthorn

Uses: Poor circulation, chest pain, irregular heartbeat, high blood fats, high blood pressure

horse chestnut

Uses: Fever, fluid retention, frostbite, hemorrhoids, inflammation, lower extremity swelling, phlebitis, varicose veins, wounds

kava kava

Uses: Nervous anxiety, restlessness, sleep disturbances, stress

kombucha

Uses: Numerous claims for a wide variety of ills; none has been substantiated to date

konjac

Uses: Blood sugar control, constipation, high blood fats, high blood pressure, excessive appetite

kudzu

Uses: Alcohol cravings, menopausal symptoms

lapacho (pau d'arco)

Uses: Cancer, inflammation, infection

lemon balm (melissa)

Uses: Abdominal gas and cramping, cold sores

licorice

Uses: Allergies, arthritis, asthma, constipation, esophagitis, gastritis, hepatitis, inflammatory conditions, peptic ulcers, poor adrenal function, poor appetite

maitake

Uses: Immunostimulant activity, diabetes, hypertension, high cholesterol, obesity

maté

Uses: Diuretic, depurative

melatonin

Uses: Jet lag, insomnia, cancer protection, oral contraceptive

milk thistle

Uses: Protection for alcoholic cirrhosis and hepatitis, antiinflammatory

monascus

Uses: Maintaining acceptable cholesterol levels

morinda

Uses: Headache, digestive, heart and liver conditions, arthritis

nettle

Uses: Diuretic, hay fever

octacosanol

Uses: Herpes, inflammation of the skin, physical endurance

passionflower

Uses: Antifungal, hypertension, sedative, group A hemolytic streptococcus

peppermint

Uses: GI disorders

pygeum

Uses: Benign prostate hypertrophy, antiinflammatory

st. john's wort

Uses: Depression, antiviral

sassafras

Uses: Banned in the United States

saw palmetto

Uses: Benign prostatic hypertrophy

schisandra

Uses: GI disorders, liver protection, tonic

scull cap

Uses: Antibacterial, sedative

senna

Uses: Laxative

tea tree oil

Uses: Topical use for infections; inhaled for respiratory disorders

uva ursi

Uses: Diuretic, urinary tract infections, contact dermatitis, arthritis

valerian

Uses: Sedative

yarrow

Uses: To decrease bleeding, Gi dis-orders, hypertension, thrombi, to improve circulation

yohimbine

Uses: Male organic impotence

Appendix i

FDA pregnancy categories

A   No risk demonstrated to the fetus in any trimester

B   No adverse effects in animals, no human studies available

C   Only given after risks to the fetus are considered; animal studies have shown adverse reactions, no human studies available

D   Definite fetal risks, may be given in spite of risks if needed in life-threatening conditions

X   Absolute fetal abnormalities; not to be used anytime during pregnancy

Note: **UK** = Unknown fetal risk (used in this text but not an official FDA pregnancy category).

Appendix j

Controlled substance chart

Drugs	United States	Canada
Heroin, LSD, peyote, marijuana, mescaline	Schedule I • High abuse potential • No currently accepted medical use	Schedule H
Opium (morphine), meperidine, amphetamines, cocaine, short-acting barbiturates (secobarbital)	Schedule II • High abuse potential; potentially severe psychologic or physical dependence • Currently accepted medical use but may be severely restricted • Telephone orders only in emergencies if written Rx follows promptly • No refills	Schedule G
Glutethimide, paregoric, phendimetrazine	Schedule III • Abuse potential less than the drugs/substances in Schedules I and II; potentially moderate or low physical dependence or high psychologic dependence • Currently accepted medical use • Telephone orders permitted • Prescriber may authorize limited refills	Schedule F

Drugs	United States	Canada
Chloral hydrate, chlordiazepoxide, diazepam, mazindol, meprobamate, phenobarbital (Canada—G)	Schedule IV • Low abuse potential relative to drugs/substances in Schedule III; potentially limited physical or psychological dependence • Currently accepted medical use • Telephone orders permitted • Prescriber may authorize limited refills	Schedule F
Antidiarrheals with opium (Canada—G), antitussives	Schedule V • Lowest abuse potential; potentially very limited physical or psychological dependence • Currently accepted medical use • Prescriber determines refills • Some products containing limited amounts of Schedule V substances (e.g., cough suppressants) available OTC to patients >18 yr	Schedule F

Appendix k

Abbreviations

AAS argininosuccinic acid synthetase

abd abdomen

ABG arterial blood gas

ac before meals

ACE angiotensin-converting enzyme

ADA American Diabetes Association

ADH antidiuretic hormone

ALT alanine aminotransferase

ANA antinuclear antibody

AP anteroposterior

APTT activated partial thromboplastin time

ASA acetylsalicylic acid, aspirin

ASHD arteriosclerotic heart disease

AST aspartate aminotransferase (SGOT)

AV atrioventricular

bid twice a day

BM bowel movement

BMR basal metabolic rate

B/P blood pressure

BPH benign prostatic hypertrophy

BPM beats per minute

BS blood sugar

BUN blood urea nitrogen

C Celsius (centigrade)

Ca cancer

CAD coronary artery disease

cap capsule

Cath catheterization or catheterize

CBC complete blood cell count

CC chief complaint

cc cubic centimeter

CHF congestive heart failure

cm centimeter

CNS central nervous system

CO$_2$ carbon dioxide

CONT continuous

COPD chronic obstructive pulmonary disease

CPAP continuous positive airway pressure

CPK creatine phosphokinase

CPR cardiopulmonary resuscitation

CPS carbamoyl phosphate synthetase

CrCl creatinine clearance

C&S culture and sensitivity

C sect cesarean section

CSF cerebrospinal fluid

CV cardiovascular

CVA cerebrovascular accident

CVP central venous pressure

D&C dilatation and curettage

DIR INF direct infusion

dr dram

D$_5$W 5% glucose in distilled water

ECG electrocardiogram (EKG)

EDTA ethylenediamine tetraacetic acid

EEG electroencephalogram

EENT ear, eye, nose, and throat

EPS extrapyramidal symptom

ESR erythrocyte sedimentation rate

EXT REL extended release

EXTRA STREN SUSP extra strength suspension

FBS fasting blood sugar

FHT fetal heart tones

FSH follicle-stimulating hormone

g gram

GABA γ-aminobutyric acid

GI gastrointestinal

gr grain

GT glucose tolerance test

gtt	drops
GU	genitourinary
H₂	histamine₂
HCG	human chorionic gonadotropin
Hct	hematocrit
HDCV	human diploid cell rabies vaccine
Hgb	hemoglobin
H & H	hematocrit and hemoglobin
5-HIAA	5-hydroxindoleacetic acid
HIV	human immunodeficiency virus (AIDS)
H₂O	water
HOB	head of bed
HR	heart rate
hr	hour
hs	at bedtime
IgG	immunolobulin G
IM	intramuscular
INF	infusion
INH	inhalation
Inj	injection
I&O	intake and output
INT	intermittent
IPPB	intermittent positive-pressure breathing
ITP	idiopathic thrombocytopenic purpura
IUD	intrauterine device
IV	intravenous
IVP	intravenous pyelogram
K	potassium
kg	kilogram
L	liter
lb	pound
LDH	lactic dehydrogenase
LE	lupus erythematosus
LFT	liver function test
LH	luteinizing hormone
LLQ	left lower quadrant
LMP	last menstrual period
LOC	level of consciousness
LR	lactated Ringer's solution
LT	leukotriene
LUQ	left upper quadrant
M	meter
m	minim
m²	square meter
MAC	monitored anesthesia care
MAOI	monoamine oxidase inhibitor

mEq	milliequivalent
mg	milligram
μg	microgram
μm	micron
MI	myocardial infarction
min	minute
ml	milliliter
mm	millimeter
mo	month
Na	sodium
neg	negative
ng	nanogram
NPO	nothing by mouth (Lat. *nulla per os*)
NS	normal saline
O₂	oxygen
OBS	organic brain syndrome
od	right eye
OR	operating room
os	left eye
OTC	over-the-counter
OU	each eye
oz	ounce
p̄	after
P56	plasma-lyte 56
PaCO₂	arterial carbon dioxide tension (pressure)
PaO₂	arterial oxygen tension (pressure)
PAT	paroxysmal atrial tachycardia
PBI	protein-bound iodine
pc	after meals
PCWP	pulmonary capillary wedge pressure
PEEP	positive end-expiratory pressure
PERRLA	pupils equal, round, react to light and accommodation
pH	hydrogen ion concentration
PO	by mouth
postop	postoperative
PP	postprandial
preop	preoperative
prn	as required
PT	prothrombin time
PTT	partial thromboplastin time
PVC	premature ventricular contraction
pwd	powder

q_{AM}	every morning

qAM every morning
qd every day
qh every hour
q2h every 2 hours
q3h every 3 hours
q4h every 4 hours
q6h every 6 hours
q12h every 12 hours
qid four times daily
qod every other day
qPM every night
qs sufficient quantity
qt quart
R right
RAIU radioactive iodine uptake
RBC red blood cell count or red blood cell
RECT rectal
RLQ right lower quadrant
ROM range of motion
RUQ right upper quadrant
SC subcutaneous
SIMV synchronous intermittent mandatory ventilation
SL sublingual
SLE systemic lupus erythematosus
SOB shortness of breath
sol solution
ss one half
suppos suppository
SUS REL sustained release
syr syrup

T&A tonsillectomy and adenoidectomy
tab tablet
tbsp tablespoon
temp temperature
tid three times daily
tinc tincture
TPN total parenteral nutrition
top topical
TRANS transdermal
TSH thyroid-stimulating hormone
tsp teaspoon
TT thrombin time
U unit
UA urinalysis
UTI urinary tract infection
UV ultraviolet
vag vaginal
VMA vanillylmandelic acid
vol volume
VS vital sign
WBC white blood cell count
wk week
wt weight
yr year
> greater than
< less than
= equal
° degree
% percent
γ gamma
β beta

Appendix I

Weights and equivalents

METRIC SYSTEM
Weight

kilogram	= kg	=	1000 grams
gram	= g	=	1 gram
milligram	= mg	=	0.001 gram
microgram	= μg	=	0.001 milligram

Volume

liter	= L	=	1 L
milliliter	= ml	=	0.001 L

AVOIRDUPOIS WEIGHT

1 ounce (oz)= 437.5 grains
1 pound (lb)= 16 ounces = 7000 grains

METRIC AND APOTHECARY EQUIVALENTS
Exact weight equivalents

Metric	Apothecary
1 mg	1/64.8 grain
64.8 mg	1 grain
324 mg	5 grains
1 g	15.432 grains
31.103 g	1 ounce = 480 grains

Exact volume equivalents

Metric	Apothecary		
1.00 ml	16.23 minims		
3.69 ml	1 fluidram	=	60 minims
29.57 ml	1 fluid ounce	=	480 minims
473.16 ml	1 pint	=	7680 minims
946.33 ml	1 quart	=	15,360 minims

Appendix m

Formulas for drug calculations

Surface area rule:

$$\text{Child dose} = \frac{\text{Surface area (m}^2)}{1.73\text{m}^2} \times \text{Adult dose}$$

Calculating strength of a solution:

Solution Strength: *Desired Solution:*

$$\frac{x}{100} = \frac{\text{Amount of drug desired}}{\text{Amount of finished solution}}$$

Calculating flow rate for IV:

$$\text{Rate of flow} = \frac{\text{Amount of fluid} \times \text{Administration set calibration}}{\text{Running time}}$$

$$\frac{x}{1} = \frac{\text{(ml) (gtt/min)}}{\text{min}}$$

Calculation of medication dosages:

Formula method:

$$\frac{\text{Amount ordered}}{\text{Amount on hand}} \times \text{Vehicle} = \text{Number of tablets, capsules, or amount of liquid}$$

Vehicle is the drug form or amount of liquid containing the dosage. Amounts used in calculation by formula must be in same system.

Ratio—proportion method:

1 tablet:tablet in mg on hand::x tablet order in mg

Know or have::Want to know or order

Multiply means and extremes, divide both sides by known amount to get X. Amounts used in equation must be in same system.

Dimensional analysis method:

$$\text{Order in mg} \times \frac{1 \text{ tablet or capsule}}{\text{What 1 tablet or capsule is in mg}}$$

$$= \text{Tablets or capsules to be given}$$

If amounts are in different systems:

$$\text{Order in mg} \times \frac{1 \text{ tablet or capsule}}{\text{What 1 tablet or capsule is in g}} \times \frac{1}{1000 \text{ mg}}$$

$$= \text{Tablets or capsules to be given}$$

Appendix n

Nomogram for calculation of body surface area

Place a straight edge from the patient's height in the left column to the patient's weight in the right column. The point of intersection on the body surface area column indicates the body surface area (BSA). (Reproduced from Behrman RE, and Vaughn VC (editors): *Nelson's textbook of pediatrics,* ed 12, Philadelphia, 1983, WB Saunders.)

Appendix o

Commonly used antibiotics in adults and children

amoxicillin
Adult: **PO** 750 mg-1.5 g qd in divided doses q8h
Child: **PO** 20-40 mg/kg/day in divided doses q8h

ampicillin
Adult: **PO** 1-2 g qd in divided doses q6h
IM/IV 2-8 g qd in divided doses q4-6h
Child: **PO** 50-100 mg/kg/day in divided doses q6h
IM/IV 100-200 mg/kg/day in divided doses q6h

cefaclor
Adult: **PO** 250-500 mg q8h
Child: **PO** 24-40 mg/kg/day in divided doses q8h

cephalexin
Adult: **PO** 250-500 mg q6h
Child: **PO** 25-50 mg/kg/day in 4 equal doses

chloramphenicol
Adult and child >3 mo: 50-100 mg/kg/day in divided doses q6h

clindamycin
Adult: **PO** 150-450 mg q6h
IM/IV 300 mg q6-12h
Child >1 mo: **PO** 8-25 mg/kg/day in divided doses q6-8h
IM/IV 15-40 mg/kg/day in divided doses q6-8h

erythromycin
Adult: 250-500 mg q6h
Child: 30-50 mg/kg/day in divided doses q6h

gentamicin
Adult: **IV INF** 3-5 mg/kg/day in divided doses q8h
Child: **IV/IM** 2-2.5 mg/kg q8h
Neonate and infant: **IV/IM** 2.5 mg/kg q8h

kanamycin
Adult and child: **IV INF/IM** 15 mg/kg/day in divided doses q8-12h

methicillin
Adult: **IM/IV** 4-12 g/day in divided doses q4-6h
Child: **IM/IV** 50-300 mg/kg/day in divided doses q4-12h
PO 25-50 mg/kg/day in divided doses q6h
Neonate: **IM** 10 mg/kg q12h

nafcillin
Adult: **PO/IM/IV** 2-6 g/day in divided doses q4-6h
Child: **IM** 25 mg/kg q12h
nitrofurantoin
Adult and child >12 yr: **PO** 50-100 mg qid pc
oxacillin
Adult: **PO** 2-6 g/day in divided doses q4-6h
IM/IV 2-12 g/day in divided doses q4-6h
Child: **PO/IM/IV** 50-100 mg/kg/day in divided doses q6h
penicillin G benzathine
Adult: **IM** 1.2 million U
penicillin G potassium
Adult: **PO** 400,000-500,000 U q6-8h
Child <12 yr: **PO** 25,000-90,000 U/kg/day in 3-6 divided doses
penicillin G procaine
Adult and child: **IM** 600,000-1.2 million U in 1-2 doses/day
Neonate: **IM** 50,000 U/kg qd
sulfisoxazole
Adult: **PO** 2-4 g loading dose, then 1-2 g qid
Child >2 mo: **PO** 75 mg/kg or 2 g/m^2 loading dose, then 150 mg/kg/day or 4 g/m^2/day in divided doses q6h
ticarcillin
Adult: **IV/IM** 12-24 g/day in divided doses q3-6h
Child: **IV/IM** 50-300 mg/kg/day in divided doses q4-8h
Neonate: **IV INF** 75-100 mg/kg q8-12h

Appendix p

Bibliography

Blumenthal M: *The complete German Commission E monographs: Therapeutic guide to herbal medicines,* Austin, 1998, American Botanical Council.

Clark JB, Queener SF, Karb VB: *Pharmacological basis of nursing practice,* ed 5, St Louis, 1998, Mosby.

Drug Information: Bethesda, American Hospital Formulary Service.

Facts and Comparisons: St Louis, updated monthly.

Gahart BL: *Intravenous medications,* ed 13, St Louis, 1999, Mosby.

Goodman A and others: *Goodman and Gilman's The pharmacological basis of therapeutics,* ed 10, New York, 1998, Pergamon Press.

McKenry LM, Salerno E: *Mosby's pharmacology in nursing,* ed 18, St Louis, 1996, Mosby.

Mediphor Editorial Group: *Drug interaction facts,* Philadelphia, updated quarterly, JB Lippincott.

Review of natural products: Philadelphia, updated monthly, *Facts and Comparisons.*

Index

Entries can be identified as follows: generic name, Trade Name, DRUG CATEGORY,
Combination Product, DISEASE/DISORDER.

Entries can be identified as follows: generic name, Trade Name, DRUG CATEGORY, *Combination Product, DISEASE/DISORDER.*

Entries can be identified as follows: generic name, Trade Name, DRUG CATEGORY, *Combination Product, DISEASE/DISORDER.*

Entries can be identified as follows: generic name, Trade Name, DRUG CATEGORY, *Combination Product, DISEASE/DISORDER.*

Entries can be identified as follows: generic name, Trade Name, DRUG CATEGORY, *Combination Product, DISEASE/DISORDER.*

Entries can be identified as follows: generic name, Trade Name, DRUG CATEGORY, *Combination Product, DISEASE/DISORDER.*

Entries can be identified as follows: generic name, Trade Name, DRUG CATEGORY, *Combination Product, DISEASE/DISORDER.*

Entries can be identified as follows: generic name, Trade Name, DRUG CATEGORY,
Combination Product, DISEASE/DISORDER.

Entries can be identified as follows: generic name, Trade Name, DRUG CATEGORY, *Combination Product, DISEASE/DISORDER.*

Entries can be identified as follows: generic name, Trade Name, DRUG CATEGORY, *Combination Product, DISEASE/DISORDER.*

Index

Entries can be identified as follows: generic name, Trade Name, DRUG CATEGORY,
Combination Product, DISEASE/DISORDER.

Entries can be identified as follows: generic name, Trade Name, DRUG CATEGORY, *Combination Product, DISEASE/DISORDER.*

Entries can be identified as follows: generic name, Trade Name, DRUG CATEGORY, *Combination Product, DISEASE/DISORDER.*

Entries can be identified as follows: generic name, Trade Name, DRUG CATEGORY,
Combination Product, DISEASE/DISORDER.

Entries can be identified as follows: generic name, Trade Name, DRUG CATEGORY, *Combination Product, DISEASE/DISORDER.*

Entries can be identified as follows: generic name, Trade Name, DRUG CATEGORY, *Combination Product, DISEASE/DISORDER.*

Entries can be identified as follows: generic name, Trade Name, DRUG CATEGORY,
Combination Product, DISEASE/DISORDER.

Entries can be identified as follows: generic name, Trade Name, DRUG CATEGORY,
Combination Product, DISEASE/DISORDER.

Entries can be identified as follows: generic name, Trade Name, DRUG CATEGORY, *Combination Product, DISEASE/DISORDER.*

Entries can be identified as follows: generic name, Trade Name, DRUG CATEGORY,
Combination Product, DISEASE/DISORDER.

Entries can be identified as follows: generic name, Trade Name, DRUG CATEGORY, *Combination Product, DISEASE/DISORDER.*

Entries can be identified as follows: generic name, Trade Name, DRUG CATEGORY, *Combination Product, DISEASE/DISORDER.*

Entries can be identified as follows: generic name, Trade Name, DRUG CATEGORY, *Combination Product, DISEASE/DISORDER.*

Entries can be identified as follows: generic name, Trade Name, DRUG CATEGORY,
Combination Product, DISEASE/DISORDER.